Comprehensive resources
for instructors and students
that engage, inform, and inspire on personal health topics.

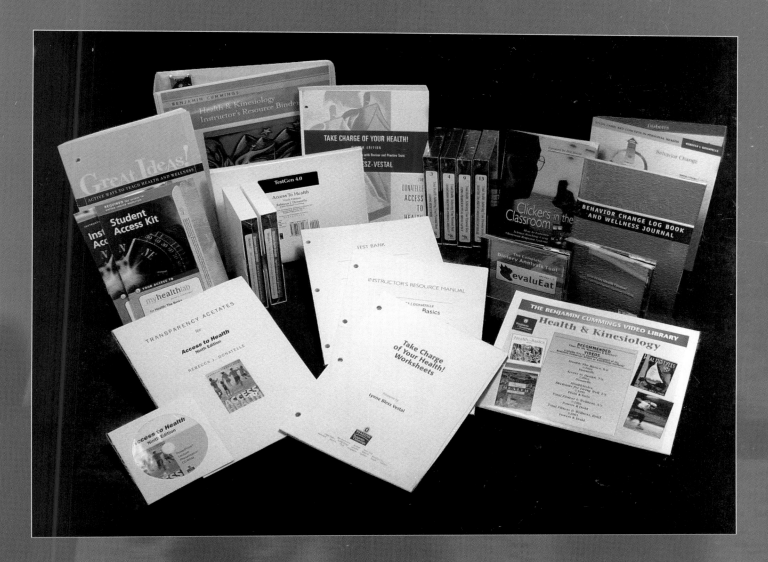

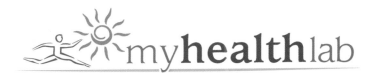

offers instructors and students access to a wealth of valuable class and study tools

MyHealthLab makes it easier than ever to organize your personal health class, personalize your students' educational experience, and push their learning to the next level. Powered by CourseCompass, the site provides a one-stop spot for accessing a wealth of preloaded content and tools, including:

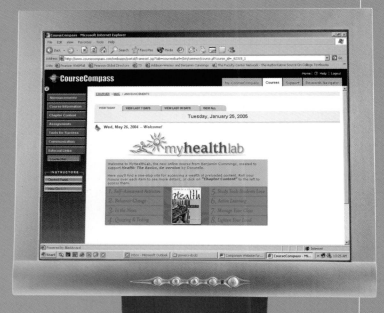

- **61 electronic self-assessments**
  including in-text self-assessments and chapter-specific "Take Charge of Your Health Worksheets"

- ***Discovery Health Channel* Health and Wellness video clips**

- **An interactive Ebook**

- **Behavior change tools**
  such as the "Behavior Change Log Book and Wellness Journal" with electronic journaling activities

- **Discussions of health issues in the news**
  from a variety of sources, including search-by-subject *New York Times* one year archive and Link Library on Research Navigator™

- **Course management tools,**
  including preloaded assignable quiz and test questions and a gradebook that automatically records student progress on assigned tests

- **Diagnostic testing and personalized study plan**
  that directs students to chapters in the book that they need to review

- Access to the Benjamin Cummings **Tutor Center**

- and more!

www.aw-bc.com/myhealthlab

Illustrate concepts and engage your students with interactive lecture tools

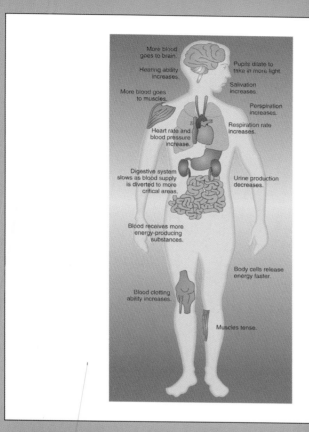

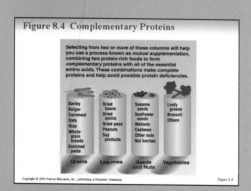

Transparency Acetates 0-8053-7851-0
Expand your classroom presentations by using bright, full-color transparency acetates of all the images in the textbook, such as this image of the body's response to stress. The transparency acetate package of 140 text-specific acetates includes all of the text's figures and tables, plus additional sexually transmitted infection photos.

NEW! Instructor Resource CD-ROM 0-8053-7853-7
This cross-platform CD-ROM includes all figures (in both PowerPoint® and jpeg formats) and tables from the book, selected photos, and PowerPoint® lecture outlines. These resources are provided in a format that may be easily customized for lecture presentation. Also includes ready-to-use questions for use with Classroom Response Systems, which let you ask students to respond electronically to in-class questions and see the results tabulated instantly.

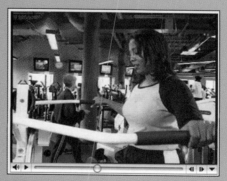

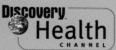

Discovery Health Channel **Health and Wellness Lecture Launcher Videos**
Volume 1 0-8053-5369-0; Volume 2 0-8053-6001-8; CD-ROM 0-8053-7830-8
Benjamin Cummings Lecture Launcher videos, created in partnership with the *Discovery Health Channel,* feature 24 video clips on health topics ranging from nutrition to stress management to substance abuse. Clips range from 5 to 12 minutes in length, and are available via a 2-volume VHS set or via CD-ROM.

More supplements to help teach your course with ease

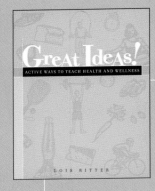

Great Ideas: Active Ways to Teach Health and Wellness
0-8053-2857-2
by Lois Ritter
This booklet contains active learning ideas for your classroom. It offers you access to innovative ideas in use among your peers, suitable for teaching to a large lecture hall or small group, in an urban or rural setting, and at a two-year or four-year institution.

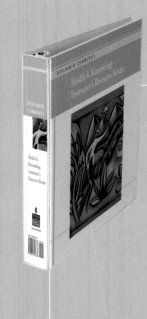

Instructor's Resource Binder
0-8053-5567-7
The Instructor's Resource Binder is handy for accommodating all print supplements that accompany *Access to Health*, Ninth Edition. (Note: All supplements are available separately.)

Instructor's Resource Manual and Media Guide 0-8053-7852-9
The Instructor's Resource Manual presents student and classroom activities, chapter objectives, lecture outlines, and Companion Website resources, all of which are designed to reinforce chapter concepts and encourage student learning. It also includes ideas for incorporating the *Discovery Health Channel* videos into your course and discussion questions for the text's "In the News" *New York Times* articles.

Printed Test Bank 0-8053-7855-3
Computerized Test Bank 0-8053-7854-5
The questions in the newly revised Printed Test Bank and Computerized Test Bank have been rigorously reviewed by a panel of instructors for relevance and accuracy. The Test Bank includes approximately 2,500 multiple-choice, short-answer, true/false, matching, and essay questions, all with answers and page references. The cross-platform TestGen CD-ROM, which includes the complete contents of the Printed Test Bank, enables you to create tests, edit questions, and add your own material to existing exams.

Electronic solutions to manage your course and interact with your students

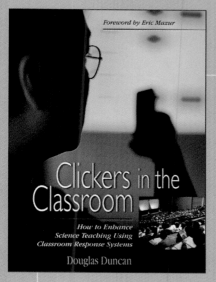

Clickers in the Classroom

0-8053-8728-5

Clickers (Classroom Response Systems) have quickly become one of the most popular and widely adopted new classroom teaching technologies in recent history. Whether you're a clicker novice or veteran, this is the book for learning how clickers can enhance your classroom lectures. In this handbook, experienced clicker educator Doug Duncan provides everything you need to know to successfully teach using clicker technology: What are the benefits of using clickers? What is the clicker experience like at other schools? What research has been published on clicker usage? How will clickers change the dynamic of your classroom? What types of clicker questions work best in lectures? How should I prepare my students before introducing clickers?

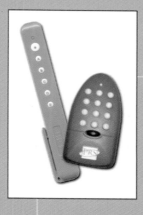

Classroom Response System

• Enhance interactivity
• Capture attention
• Get instant feedback
• Assess comprehension

Classroom Response Systems is a wireless polling system that enables you to pose questions, read results, and display those results instantly to your classroom. Whether you are considering a system for the first time or are interested in expanding a program department-wide, we can help you select the best system for your needs to accompany your Benjamin Cummings text.

Course Management Options

In addition to MyHealthLab, WebCT and BlackBoard are available to make it easy to integrate online course materials into your course. Password-protected courses feature a wealth of instructor and student resources, including a test bank specific to *Access to Health,* Ninth Edition.

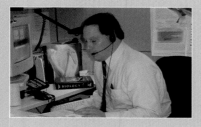

TECHNICAL SUPPORT
helps you make the most of your media

Benjamin Cummings is proud of its strong customer support. Whether you are looking for multimedia, textbook, or online assistance, our goal is to provide you with the best service possible. Visit us at www.aw-bc.com/technicalsupport for solutions to technical concerns, from physical media questions (CD-ROMs, installations, etc.) to website inquiries (registration, missing links, etc.).

Text features that keep students up-to-date on the most relevant content

IN THE NEWS

Worried Colleges Step Up Efforts Over Suicide

By Karen W. Arenson

Nicole Thompson had been at Columbia University for only a few weeks when she went out drinking with a group of friends downtown last year and became separated from them. She had skipped her medication for bipolar disorder. Now it was 3 A.M. and, crying and in a panic, she called friends; she told them, she said, that she "just wished the traffic would take me out."

Although she made it back to campus safely, her friends had already notified Columbia that they were worried about her. For Columbia officials, it was the first clue that Ms. Thompson faced any kind of mental health problems.

"I wasn't on Columbia's radar at all," said Ms. Thompson, who is back on campus now after being forced to take a medical leave.

Increasingly, college officials and mental health experts have come to realize that many of the most vulnerable students—the ones prone to self-injury and suicide—are like Ms. Thompson: they never go near the counseling centers or reveal anything about their experience before college. As a result, colleges are stepping up efforts to find them and to get them into treatment, sometimes forcing them to leave temporarily.

Read the complete article online in the eThemes section of this book's website: www.aw-bc.com/donatelle

Original article published December 3, 2004. Copyright © 2004 *The New York Times.* Reprinted with permission.

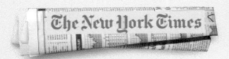

NEW! In the News
In the News chapter-opener articles, pulled from today's headlines, feature excerpts from *The New York Times*. These real-world news stories help demonstrate the relevance of health issues to students' everyday lives and draw students into the chapter's content.

NEW! Make it Happen
Make it Happen! sections help students assimilate the material from the Assess Yourself activities and put it into action. These end-of-chapter sections help students identify an area in which behavior change should be made, review the steps to follow in making a change, and give an example of a student's actual change.

TAKING CHARGE

MAKE IT HAPPEN!

Assessment The Assess Yourself box on page 42 gave you the chance to look at various aspects of your psychosocial health and compare your self-assessment with a friend's perceptions. Now that you have considered these results, you can take steps toward changing certain behaviors that may be detrimental to your psychosocial health.

Making a Change To change your behavior, you need to develop a plan. Follow these steps.

1. Evaluate your behavior, and identify patterns and specific things you are doing. What can you change now? What can you change in the near future?
2. Select one pattern of behavior that you'd like to change.
3. Fill out a Behavior Change Contract. It should include your long-term goal for change, your short-term goals, the rewards you'll give yourself for reaching these goals, potential obstacles along the way, and strategies for overcoming these obstacles. For each goal, list the small steps and specific actions that you can take.

4. Chart your progress in the journal. At the end of one week, consider how successful you were in following your plan.
5. Revise your plan as needed. Are the short-term goals attainable? Are the rewards satisfying?

One Student's Plan John assessed himself as a positive and upbeat person, but the assessment his friend gave him rated him as impatient and cynical. John resolved to slow down and become more appreciative of the good things around him. Among his short-term goals: listening to his sister without interrupting her, and expressing a sincere compliment to a family member or friend every other day. John found that paying compliments made him stop to think about the qualities he appreciated in friends and family. While he struggled to listen without interrupting, John found that he was learning a lot about his sister that he had never known before. After several weeks, John's friends commented on his calmer and happier demeanor.

Feature Boxes

highlight subjects of concern and interest to students and include cutting-edge research and topics.

HEALTH ETHICS: CONFLICT AND CONTROVERSY

The Science of Sex Selection

Parents have wanted the ability to choose the gender of their child since prehistoric times. Early drawings show sex selection efforts were being pursued by our earliest ancestors, while later history shows intense interest in sex selection in early Chinese, Egyptian, and Greek cultures. Even in these high tech times, people try a variety of avenues, most based on folklore, to conceive a particular sex. From diet, sex-

Currently, an FDA clinical trial of sophisticated sperm-sorting technology is more than halfway to completion. Approval of the technique by the FDA would add it to the arsenal of couples intent on having a baby of a particular sex. The *MicroSort method* is an experimental technique that separates X (female) chromosomes from Y (male) chromosomes. Sperm are stained with a fluorescent dye that binds to the chromosomes. X chromosomes are bigger than Y and soak up more dye. The sperm are then zapped with a laser that illuminates the dye. X chromosomes have

fluid. The heavy head of the sperm makes them swim downward. Sperm carrying the Y (male) chromosomes swim faster than those with X chromosomes, reaching the bottom of the tube faster. They can then be extracted and used for insemination. This technique claims to have a 78 to 85 percent chance of producing a boy, although critics says the odds are not better than 50:50.

Preimplantation genetic diagnosis, the third technique, was originally used for detecting genetic diseases. Doctors remove eggs from the woman and fertilize them with sperm in the lab, creating embryos. After three days, technicians extract a cell from each embryo. They can differentiate male and female embryos by examining their chromosomes. After determining the sex of the embryos, doctors implant the desired ones. While more invasive and costly than other methods, success is virtually guaranteed.

Source: Adapted from Karen Springen "Brave new babies." *Newsweek,* January 26, 2004, 45–53.

REALITY CHECK

Club Drugs on Campus

Every era seems to have its hot drug. At one point it was Valium, then LSD, and then crack. Currently the so-called club drugs are popular on college campuses. Three of note include Rohypnol (flunitrazepam), also called "ropies" or "roofies"; GHB (gamma hydroxybutyrate), or as it is known on the street, "grievous bodily harm"; and Special K (ketamine).

Rohypnol is a potent tranquilizer similar in nature to Valium, but many times stronger. The drug produces a sedative effect, amnesia, muscle relaxation, and slowed psychomotor responses. Commonly known as the "date rape drug," Rohypnol has gained notoriety as a growing problem on college campuses. The drug has been added to punch and other drinks at fraternity parties and college social gatherings, where it is reportedly given to female partiers in hopes of lowering their inhibitions and facilitating potential sexual conquests. The manufacturer changed the formula to give the drug a bright blue color that would make it easy to detect in most drinks, so would-be per-

petrators are turning to blue tropical drinks and punches to disguise the drug. While "ropie" fervor has subsided somewhat, it continues to be a concern. See the Reality Check box in Chapter 4 on strategies to protect yourself from being dosed with Rohypnol.

Rohypnol has been joined by a newer, liquid substance called GHB, or gamma-hydroxybutyrate. GHB is used as an aphrodisiac to increase one's sense of touch and sexual prowess, as a muscle builder, and as a tranquilizer. GHB is an odorless, tasteless fluid that can be made easily at home or in a chemistry lab. Like Rohypnol, GHB has been slipped into drinks without being detected, resulting in loss of memory, unconsciousness, amnesia, and even death. Other side effects of GHB include nausea, vomiting, seizures, memory loss, hallucinations, coma, and respiratory distress. During the 1980s, GHB was available in U.S. health food stores. Concerns about its use led the FDA to ban OTC sales in 1990, and GHB is now a Schedule I controlled substance.

The Special K we're referring to is not the breakfast cereal, but rather ketamine, used as an anesthetic in many hospital

and veterinary clinics. On the street, Special K is most often diverted in liquid form from veterinary offices or medical suppliers. Dealers dry the liquid (usually by cooking it) and grind the residue into powder. Special K causes hallucinations as it inhibits the relay of sensory input; the brain fills the resulting void with visions, dreams, memories, and sensory distortions. The effects of Special K are not as severe as those of Ecstasy, so it has grown in popularity among people who have to go to work or school after a night of partying.

Sources: U.S. Department of Health and Human Services, "Ketamine: A Fact Sheet," downloaded September 9, 2004, www.health.org/nongovpubs/ketamine; Office of National Drug Control Policy, "Rohypnol Fact Sheet," February 2003, www.whitehousedrugpolicy.gov/publications/factsht/rohypnol,; Office of National Drug Control Policy, "Gamma-Hydroxybutyrate (GHB) Fact Sheet," November 2002, www.whitehousedrugpolicy.gov.publications/factsht/gamma; T. Nordenberg, "The Death of the Party: All t... Go Unheeded," ... March–April 200... 200_toc.html

---

Other topics of current interest featured in the text include:

Low-carbohydrate diets
Prevalence of diabetes
Tanning beds and skin cancer
Unique stressors of non-traditional students
New contraceptive methods
Global increases in obesity rates
New forms of yoga
Glycemic index, *trans* fats, and other nutrition concerns
Debate over stem cell research

Help your students live healthier with behavior change resources

Print resources for students expand on the concepts presented within the text

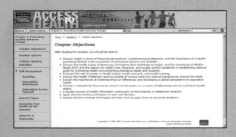

NAME: _____ DATE: _____

TAKE CHARGE WORKSHEET 1.1

Health Behavior Self-Assessment

DIRECTIONS: Answer the following questions about your health and behavior. After answering these questions, use the information to write a narrative description about yourself and your health risks.

Family Health History

Check any health problems that your parents or biological siblings have had.

____ Allergies	____ Alcoholism	____ Asthma	____ Angina
____ Breast cancer	____ Colon cancer	____ Lung cancer	____ Ovarian cancer
____ Prostate cancer	____ Skin cancer	____ Testicular cancer	____ Other cancer
____ Diabetes	____ Emphysema	____ Endometriosis	____ Fibromyalgia
____ Gout	____ High blood pressure	____ High cholesterol	____ HIV
____ Leukemia	____ Mononucleosis	____ Neurological disorder	____ Rheumatoid arthritis
____ Sickle cell anemia			

Other: _____

Personal Health History

1. List any chronic health problems you have.

2. List any surgeries you have had.

3. List any disabilities you have.

4. List any medications you take on a regular basis.

5. List any allergies you have.

Take Charge of Your Health! Self-Assessment Workbook with Review and Practice Tests 0-8053-7849-9
This student workbook includes assessment worksheets and review/practice tests. With a strong emphasis on evaluating one's current lifestyle and behaviors, this supplement is a useful tool for encouraging positive behavior change.

Take Charge of Your Health Worksheets 0-8053-6037-9
This sampling of 38 worksheets from the Take Charge! Self-Assessment Workbook is available in a convenient pad format.

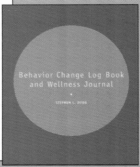

Behavior Change Log Book and Wellness Journal 0-8053-7844-8
by Stephen L. Dodd
This log book and journal encourages students to track daily exercise and nutritional intake in order to create a long-term nutrition and fitness prescription plan. It also suggests topics and gives space for journaling projects.

Electronic resources for students provide an interactive dimension to course material

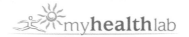

Companion website www.aw-bc.com/donatelle
This open access website is designed for easy navigation, offering a range of review activities including practice quizzes, open-ended critical thinking questions, hypothetical case studies, and weblinks. Students can practice and review key terms with the "Flashcard" program, featuring all key terms and definitions from the textbook. Also featured are eThemes of the Times–containing 30 *New York Times* articles reporting on the latest health news and research, including the complete articles found in the "In the News" textbook boxes. Students can easily test their knowledge with 61 electronic self-assessments including in-text self-assessments and chapter-specific "Take Charge of Your Health Worksheets".

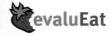

EvaluEat 0-8053-6779-9
EvaluEat diet analysis software helps students track their eating habits and evaluate the nutritional content of their diets. This software features a database of more than 6,200 food items and reports on dozens of different nutrients. Also allows users to input activity levels to create energy expenditure reports.

myhealthlab

MyHealthLab www.aw-bc.com/myhealthlab
MyHealthLab offers online access to a selection of print and media supplements geared toward personal health students. For details, see first page of this walk-through.

Access to Health

NINTH EDITION

REBECCA J. DONATELLE
Oregon State University

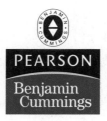

PEARSON

Benjamin Cummings

San Francisco Boston New York
Cape Town Hong Kong London Madrid Mexico City
Montreal Munich Paris Singapore Sydney Tokyo Toronto

Publisher: Daryl Fox
Senior Acquisitions Editor: Deirdre Espinoza
Development Manager: Claire Alexander
Senior Project Editor: Susan Malloy
Assistant Editor: Alison Rodal
Production Supervisor: Beth Masse
Senior Manufacturing Buyer: Stacey Weinberger
Cover Designer: Yvo Riezebos Design
Text Designer: Yvo Riezebos Design, Kathleen Cunningham Design
Production and Composition: The Left Coast Group
Photo Research: Kristin Piljay
Copy Editor: Carla Breidenbach
Proofreader: Martha Ghent
Cover Printer: Phoenix Color
Text Printer: Von Hoffman

Cover Photo: Charlie Edwards/Digital Vision/Getty Images

Credits can be found on page C-1.

ISBN 0-8053-7848-0
ISBN 0-8053-7897-9 (p-copy)

Library of Congress Cataloging-in-Publication Data
Donatelle, Rebecca J., 1950–
    Access to health / Rebecca J. Donatelle.—9th ed.
        p. cm.
    Includes bibliographical references and index.
    ISBN 0-8053-7848-0 (alk. paper)
    1. Health.   I. Title.
    RA776.D66 2006
    613—dc22

                                    2005001092

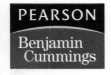

1 2 3 4 5—VHC—08 07 06 05

www.aw-bc.com

PREFACE

At no time in human history have so many people been concerned about health. Newspaper headlines proclaim that we are all too fat, that diabetes rates are soaring, and that if we fail to act, we will die prematurely while costing the health care system billions of dollars. Television news shows report dire warnings about the latest infectious diseases and employ doctors, health promotion specialists, nutrition experts, and other professionals to cover the latest health breakthroughs and threats. They exhort us to have better relationships, communicate more effectively, reduce stress, take care of our spiritual sides, and perform a host of other behaviors designed to improve our lives. We hear a constant litany of health do's and don'ts, facts and figures, and seemingly contradictory messages from the experts about what is good for us and what is bad for us. We worry about what illnesses we might catch from others; about environmental threats to health; about whether the foods we eat, the neighborhoods we live in, and the genes that we inherit pose health risks that require vigilance and constant monitoring.

The challenges to our health were unimaginable to our ancestors. Killer diseases that defy antibiotics, mysterious maladies that sap energy and restrict quality of life, harmful drugs that can lead to addiction, a health care system that excludes more and more people, and an increasingly degraded environment are all causes for great concern. Knowing how best to respond to these challenges, and which individual and societal resources should be enlisted in order to reduce health risks and promote health, is the responsibility of each individual.

Juxtaposed against the threats to health are positive developments: new insights into specific health problems, new strategies for reducing risks, and new policies and programs designed to help us be healthier. Protective measures to promote well-being include the banning of smoking in all public places in Corvallis, Oregon, and other cities; mandating the use of seat belts and bicycle helmets in many states; providing insurance coverage for mammograms; and improving labels so that they more accurately describe the contents of food products. Public health programs encourage safer sex through condom use, ensure that children get adequate nutrition, provide support for victims of domestic violence, protect our water and food supply, and require immunization of all children in the United States. Daily developments in the health field indicate that people are working hard to improve their own health and protect the health of others.

As a consumer, making the best choices to ensure health is challenging at best. Navigating the ever-changing sea of information about health may frustrate even the most knowledgeable among us. Not too long ago, disease and illness were shrouded in mystery, and the typical consumer had little power over health decision making. Few choices were available in foods, medicines, health care providers and services; and, consequently, health care decisions usually focused on cleanliness, avoiding people who were sick, and trusting the family doctor for advice.

In sharp contrast, today's health-conscious individuals have choices surrounding health that their grandparents could not have imagined: pharmacies loaded with prescription and over-the-counter drugs, health food stores with thousands of products that claim to cure illness, and telephone directories filled with doctors and alternative practitioners. Have a question about your health? Simply log on to the nearest computer and search an endless list of information, or go to your local library or bookstore. Making decisions even more difficult, unproven products are advertised alongside those that are scientifically validated. Many nutrition supplements are not regulated for consumer protection. Magazines often print information as fact when it is really only an advertisement. Overworked health professionals may be pressed for time to explain health issues and reassure patients. Some health organizations target worried consumers and play on their vulnerabilities and desires, promising quick fixes for those who want to lose weight, be sexy, or add years to life.

For health educators, preparing a new generation of students to be savvy consumers, armed with accurate information for making wise health decisions, is a formidable task. Writing an introductory health text for this population of students, in a field where information changes moment by moment, can be extremely challenging. Clearly, no single text can answer all of a student's questions, give solid advice about all possible topics, or even attempt to cover the vast spectrum of hotly debated health issues. After more than 30 years of teaching public health students and students from a wide array of health and nonhealth disciplines, we hope to provide the most accurate and up-to-date information about issues and topics that are most relevant to today's students. We strive to take students beyond what they were taught in high school and provide thought-provoking, scientifically valid information representing the culmination of years of research, rather than single-source and often spurious results of unsubstantiated research.

Helping students select the *best* sources for information and teaching them how to ask the right questions is one of our primary goals. We want to teach students how to evaluate information and process it in a systematic, reasoned way as they endeavor to make informed decisions about health. We believe that by challenging students to think about and discuss controversial health topics, they will become the citizens that future generations can rely on to develop sound policies, programs, and key health services. This opportunity to assist a new generation of students to become future agents for change in the area of health is something we take seriously. Although issues of individual decision making and lifestyle are key features of *Access to Health,* we believe that individual health is also strongly influenced by public health actions and policy. Thus, we also focus on policies, programs, and services that promote health and prevent premature disease and disability.

In addition, we are mindful of disparities in health and the underlying reasons for difference in risks based on race, ethnicity, age, gender, geographic region, and other factors. Recognizing that many of today's health problems know no national or international boundaries, we challenge students to think globally as they consider health risks and seek creative solutions to health problems. By reading, questioning, gaining greater understanding of the factors that contribute to individual and societal health, and contemplating possible actions that may reduce risk, *Access to Health* prepares students for their own development, as well as possible futures in the field.

As we prepared this text, we spent countless hours talking with students, interacting with them in classes, and testing what does and does not work in today's introductory health classes. Even more time was spent talking with course instructors, surveying selected features, and finding out how instructors assess whether such features benefit students. As always, we invited comments and suggestions on how to make this the *best* edition of *Access to Health* yet and the foremost personal health text on the market today.

We are pleased with the overwhelming success that *Access to Health* has enjoyed through its many revisions and changes, and we are gratified that many of you have continued to use this text. We hope that this edition once again meets the high standards we have previously established and that its rich foundation of scientifically valid and current citations, its wealth of technological tools and resources, and its thought-provoking exercises will continue to stimulate students to share our enthusiasm for health and to actively engage in health promotion and disease prevention.

New to this Edition

Each year as I face a new group of students, I reflect on the major changes that have occurred in health since I began teaching over 30 years ago. Each year is marked by remarkable discoveries, debunking of past "facts," and interesting additions to past knowledge. I am struck by the fact that I am very lucky to teach and do research in an area that is interesting and dynamic and that it is with great pleasure that I look forward to teaching students the things that I have learned in my own years of professional growth.

While there are many well-written textbooks on the market, very few are written by actual health professionals who are trained in health promotion and disease prevention and who actually teach students, talk with them daily about their interests and concerns, and see their reactions to health knowledge in the classrooms of major universities. I believe that this helps make this text a "stand-out" in the introductory health market. I am committed to making this book an excellent tool for learning—and, with the help of an outstanding publishing team, I feel that is the best edition to date.

As in our previous editions, we are committed to a tradition of excellence with the ninth edition of *Access to Health.* As such, this text maintains many features that it has become known for, while also focusing on exciting new health trends. The ninth edition has been updated, line by line, so that all facts and figures reflect cutting-edge research. Whether using classic references that helped set the stage for information, the latest research from professional journals, or reputable national data sources, we have tried to provide students with not only the most current information, but also references for further exploration. This careful attention to detail ensures that students will be getting the latest information about health topics as this text goes to press. The most noteworthy changes include the following:

- **New and expanded opportunities for self-assessment and behavior change.** The continued revision and replacement of many Assess Yourself boxes ensure that they ask the questions that are relevant to students' lives. For example, students have the opportunity to consider how tattoos and piercing, tanning beds, new forms of yoga and Pilates, and new diets affect their overall health. New assessments in several chapters help students take a quick measure of their own health status and plan strategies to change specific behaviors. These assessments can also be completed online.
- **New Make It Happen! sections.** Located at the end of each chapter, these sections reinforce the results of each chapter's self-assessment, give students the steps to follow for making a behavior change, and describe one student's behavior change in the area covered in the chapter. We hope to give students the tools that they need to make real and lasting behavior changes, and to see these

changes as something that can continue long after they have completed their health class.

- **New In the News selections.** Located at the beginning of each chapter, these sections give a preview of a *New York Times* article describing the latest research or developments in that chapter's subject. This encourages students to make connections between the content they are learning in school and "real world" issues. Students can access the complete, unabridged text of the article on this book's free website. These articles are part of an exciting new chapter design that is sure to capture student attention.

- **New Behavior Change Contracts.** Found at the front of the book and in the Health Resources section, contracts may be filled out as part of the students' Make It Happen! behavior change plans. An example of a completed contract is also included.

- **Updates on the leading causes of preventable death and the continued importance of tobacco, obesity, and other threats to overall health.** We cover the latest trends and threats to health and provide key information about risk reduction for major areas that are within individual control.

- **New information on reducing health disparities.** We are not created equal when it comes to health. Increasingly, health problems vary considerably by gender, race, education, ethnicity, age, socioeconomic status, sexual orientation, relationship status, culture, country of origin, and other factors. We provide current information about key disparities and their effects on health and about programs and policies to reduce disparities.

- **Increased coverage of global health issues.** In an era of constant travel and instant communication, we would be remiss in not addressing the interaction of individual, community, and global health. Textbooks that only focus on the individual concerns leave out an important factor: we all live and work in a broader community and are increasingly affected by factors that evolve in our external world. Knowing how to cope and how to reduce risks at all levels is crucial to overall health.

- **Expanded and updated coverage on violence, crime on campus, terrorism, and bioterrorism.** These topics are intended to increase student awareness of the tremendous toll that violence takes. New facts and figures include trends in crime, economic implications of crime, and the emotional and physical burden of violent crime among selected populations, particularly college students. Date rape, stranger rape, and marital rape are all discussed in terms of factors that contribute to these crimes, the impact on those affected by rape, and related societal issues.

- **Major revision of the fitness chapter reflecting ever-growing interest in this area.** Coverage has been increased on the role of strength training in weight control and increased metabolic activity, distinctions between physical activity and physical fitness, and information about newer forms of fitness activities and their benefits

and risks, including Pilates, newer forms of yoga, and tai chi. We also cover a unique, often ignored, area: exercise programs for overweight, obese, and very out-of-shape individuals. Information on factors to consider when buying exercise equipment and fitness club memberships should be of interest to students of all ages.

- **Major expansion of information on the global epidemic of obesity and the unique risks for people with weight problems.** Risk factors for obesity, new methods for assessing body composition, strategies for risk reduction, portion distortion, and the impact of advertising on the obesity epidemic are discussed.

- **Greatly expanded and updated sections on the new diets.** Coverage includes low-carb diets, low-fat diets, high-protein diets, and other weight management trends, as well as information about the glycemic index and eating to control blood glucose and energy balance.

- **Improved and updated nutrition chapter.** This includes the latest information about *trans* fats, the role of nutrition in disease prevention, and supplements such as vitamin E, antioxidants, flaxseed, and lycopene.

- **New coverage of metabolic syndrome** and its potential role in our increasing epidemic of diabetes.

- **New coverage of widely publicized drugs.** OxyContin, Ecstasy, ephedra, performance-enhancing drugs, and other drugs have been widely discussed in the media, but their risks are often misunderstood.

- **New information on the phenomenon of self-mutilation and cutting behavior.** We were the first in the personal health text field to provide material on self-inflicted cutting behaviors, and we have expanded and updated this section. This information is designed to prompt student thinking and discussion about an emerging problem among adolescents and young adults. Distinctions between self-inflicted violence and suicide, the lure of extreme sports, and related behaviors will help students better understand who is at risk, options for assistance, and ways to reduce risk.

- **Expanded coverage of environmental issues and concerns.** Included are discussions of our roles and responsibilities for environmental health, conservation, and protection of the environment. We added new information on potential risks from prolonged exposure to cell phones and dangers from molds and other environmental health risks at home and outdoors. Comparisons in consumption patterns between Americans and persons in other nations are designed to stimulate discussion and critical thinking.

- **New and expanded coverage of infectious and chronic diseases and conditions.** Topics include diabetes, West Nile virus, tickborne illnesses, antibiotic resistance, pathogens related to bioterrorism threats, hepatitis A, B, and C, tuberculosis, sleep apnea, and asthma. The December 2004 *World AIDS Report* and the growing global burden of disease from HIV/AIDS is presented. New statistics on cancer and heart disease and new guidelines for blood pressure and cholesterol monitoring are included.

- **New coverage of topics relevant to college-aged populations.** Whether the topic is information on new contraceptives such as NuvaRing, Ortho Evra, and Mirena; water and health; skin cancer and tanning booths; the connection between stress and health; or a vast array of other topics, we have tried to focus on areas of relevance to a new generation of healthy-savvy students. In many instances, we have updated facts and figures as we go to press and hope that you will find these data to be interesting and important. If you have topics that you would like to see included or expanded upon, please feel free to e-mail the author at Becky.Donatelle@orst.edu.

Maintaining a Standard of Excellence

With every edition, the challenge has been to make the book better than before and to provide information and material that surpass the competition at every level. As such, we have painstakingly considered our reviewer feedback from the previous edition and strengthened and improved pedagogical standards.

Chapter 1 establishes both the individual and social context of health and disease and the importance of health to society as a whole, a dual approach used throughout the text. In order to assist students in their efforts to achieve health, we provide a foundation for sound decision making based on well-established theories of health behavior.

Decision making through critical thinking and awareness continues to form the cornerstone of each chapter. Pedagogical aids such as the What Do You Think? questions throughout the chapter encourage students to apply information acquired from the chapter to their own lives.

The roles of the community, health policies, and health services in disease prevention and health promotion are integrated throughout the text. The public health approach is often ignored in health texts in favor of individual action only. We believe that optimum health changes will occur only in environments that are conducive to change, in which individuals can maximize resources to make long-term behavior changes.

Within a strong pedagogical framework, the importance of building health skills is emphasized and integrated consistently throughout the text. Readers will learn specific applications in every chapter through the Assess Yourself, Skills for Behavior Change, and Reality Check boxes throughout the text.

Special Features

Each chapter in *Access to Health* includes the following special feature boxes designed to help students think about healthy behavior skills, as well as how to apply the concepts in everyday life:

- **Assess Yourself** boxes help students evaluate their health behaviors and initiate positive changes.
- **Skills for Behavior Change** boxes focus on practical strategies that students can use to improve health or reduce their risks from negative health behaviors.
- **New Horizons in Health** boxes highlight new discoveries and research, as well as interesting trends in the health field.
- **Health Ethics: Conflict and Controversy** boxes highlight current controversial issues and allow students to explore their own opinions.
- **Reality Check** boxes offer current data about health trends, including potential risks and safety issues that affect students' lives.
- **Women's Health/Men's Health** boxes help students understand unique aspects of health for both genders.
- **Health in a Diverse World** boxes expand discussion of health topics to diverse groups within the United States and around the world.

Learning Aids

- Each chapter is introduced with **Chapter Objectives** to alert students to the key concepts to be covered in upcoming material.
- Designed to spark student interest and demonstrate the relevance of health to everyday life, **In the News sections** complete the introduction to each chapter.
- Groups of **What Do You Think? questions** that encourage students to think critically are highlighted and strategically placed throughout each chapter.
- To emphasize and support understanding of material, pertinent health terms are boldfaced in the text and defined in the **running glossary** appearing at the bottom of text pages. Key terms are also listed and defined in the Glossary at the end of the book.
- Appearing at the end of each chapter, **Accessing Your Health on the Internet** provides descriptions of relevant Internet websites, including organizations such as the World Health Organization (WHO), Centers for Disease Control and Prevention (CDC), WebMD, and the Mayo Clinic.
- At the end of each chapter, the **Taking Charge section** wraps up the chapter content with a focus on application by the student. The **Make It Happen! section** integrates the self-assessment results with the steps of behavior change and encourages student participation. In addition, the Summary, Questions for Discussion and Reflection, Accessing Your Health on the Internet, and Further Reading sections offer further opportunities to explore areas of interest.
- **Health Resources** provides practical information in a convenient format at the end of the book. The "Injury Prevention and Emergency Care" section describes procedures that may prevent injury and save lives. "Nutritive Value of

Selected Foods and Fast Foods" provides nutrient information for many common foods and can be used with the EvaluEat nutritional software described below. This section also includes a behavior change contract and a sample filled-in contract.

Student Supplements

Available with *Access to Health, Ninth Edition* is a comprehensive set of ancillary materials designed to enhance learning:

- **MyHealthLab (www.aw-bc.com/myhealthlab).** This online resource lets students access a wide range of print and media supplements that make studying convenient and fun. Contents include an interactive e-book, Discovery Health Channel Lecture Launcher video clips, over 60 electronic self-assessments, and an Individualized Study Plan directing students to the chapters they need to review. Also included are the Behavior Change Log Book and Wellness Journal, with an electronic behavior change contract and journal activities, and links to Research Navigator (three databases of credible and reliable source materials) and the text's Companion Website (described further below). The instructor resources on the site are described later in this preface.
- **Companion Website (www.aw-bc.com/donatelle).** This easy-to-navigate site offers the complete articles highlighted in the text's In the News feature and over 60 electronic self-assessments. The website also offers practice quizzes, open-ended critical-thinking questions, hypothetical case studies, and web links. The website includes the Flashcard program, with the entire list of terms and their definitions from the textbook available for study, and eThemes of the Times, containing 30 *New York Times* articles reporting on the latest health news and research.
- **Take Charge! Self-Assessment Workbook With Review and Practice Tests (0-8053-7849-9).** This workbook includes quizzes, self-assessment worksheets, behavior change projects, and review/practice tests for students.
- **Take Charge of Your Health! Worksheets (0-8053-6037-9).** This pad of 38 self-assessment activities (selected from the *Take Charge Workbook*) is available separately from the workbook.
- **Behavior Change Log Book and Wellness Journal (0-8053-7844-8).** This assessment tool helps students track daily exercise and nutritional intake and create a long-term nutrition and fitness prescription plan. It includes behavior change contracts and topics for journal-based activities.
- **EvaluEat Dietary Analysis Software (0-8053-7949-5).** This software can be used to do a single- or multiday diet analysis, create a variety of reports, and assess daily diets. Activity can also be tracked to provide a complete report.

Instructor Supplements

A full resource package accompanies *Access to Health* to assist the instructor with classroom preparation and presentation:

- **MyHealthLab (www.aw-bc.com/myhealthlab).** This online resource provides everything instructors need to teach health in one convenient location. MyHealthLab's course management system is loaded with valuable free teaching resources that make giving assignments and tracking student progress easy. Powered by CourseCompass™, the preloaded content in MyHealthLab includes Discovery Health Channel Lecture Launcher video clips, PowerPoint slides, Test Bank questions, Instructor's Manual material, and more.
- *Discovery Health Channel* **Health and Wellness Lecture Launcher Videos (CD-ROM, 0-8053-7830-8; VHS Volume I, 0-8053-5369-0; VHS Volume II, 0-8053-6001-8).** Created in partnership with *Discovery Health Channel,* these video materials offer lecture-launcher clips for digital presentation on topics from nutrition to stress management to substance abuse. There are 24 segments in all, ranging in length from 5 to 12 minutes. This supplement is available as a CD-ROM, a two-volume set of VHS tapes, and online at MyHealthLab.
- **Instructor Resource CD-ROM (0-8053-7853-7).** This cross-platform CD-ROM includes all of the text's figures (in PowerPoint and JPEG formats), plus tables from the book, selected photos, and PowerPoint lecture outlines, all easily customizable for lecture presentation. Also included are ready-to-use questions for use with Classroom Response Systems, which let you ask students to respond electronically to in-class questions and tabulate results immediately.
- **Transparency Acetates (0-8053-7851-0).** The figures and tables from the text are also available as 140 full-color transparencies.
- **Instructor's Resource Binder (0-8053-5567-7).** This three-ring binder accommodates all print supplements that accompany *Access to Health.*
- **Instructor's Resource Manual with Media Guide (0-8053-7852-9).** This teaching tool includes ideas for incorporating the Discovery Health Channel video clips into your course and discussion questions for the In the News *New York Times* articles. It also provides student and classroom activities, chapter objectives, lecture outlines, and additional Internet resources.
- **Printed Test Bank (0-8053-7855-3) and Computerized Test Bank (0-8053-7854-5).** The questions in the comprehensively revised test bank were reviewed by a panel of instructors for relevance and accuracy. The Test Bank includes approximately 2,500 multiple-choice, short-answer, true/false, matching, and essay questions, all with answers and page references. The cross-platform TestGen CD-ROM

enables you to create tests, edit questions, and add your own material to existing exams.

- **Great Ideas: Active Ways to Teach Health and Wellness (0-8053-2857-2).** This publication provides effective, proactive strategies for teaching health topics in a variety of classroom settings, contributed by health educators from around the country.
- **Clickers in the Classroom (0-8053-8728-5).** This handbook provides detailed guidance in enhancing lectures using clicker (Classroom Response Systems) technology.
- **Course Management.** In addition to MyHealthLab, WebCT and Blackboard are also available. Contact your Benjamin Cummings sales representative for details.

Acknowledgments

After writing nine editions of *Access to Health,* I can only marvel at the dedication and professionalism of the many fine publishing experts who have helped make such a text successful. With each subsequent edition of *Access,* their skills in dealing with the complexities and considerations of the publication process have become more apparent. Over the years, I have been extremely fortunate in having a steady stream of fine publishing teams to help me create the foundations of a text that was responsive to students, creative in approach, and reflective of the most important health trends of the times.

Senior Acquisitions Editor Deirdre Espinoza, Publisher Daryl Fox, and the outstanding group of editorial staff from Benjamin Cummings have helped make my experiences with Benjamin Cummings the best of my publishing years, and remarkably—it just keeps getting better! Particularly noteworthy has been the assistance of Susan Malloy, project editor for the last two editions of *Access to Health.* Although I have worked with many fine project editors over the years, I believe that Susan is "tops" in this category. She is extremely well organized, offers wonderful guidance, provides thoughtful suggestions, and "gets it" in terms of what college-aged students today really want in a personal health text. Importantly, she has been a strong, yet patient editor whose judgment I've come to trust over the last few years. Benjamin Cummings is very fortunate to have Susan on their editorial staff as she is truly one of the best out there! She is wonderful to work with, and I owe her a debt of gratitude for always going "above and beyond the call of duty" in her job.

In addition, I would like to acknowledge the wonderful editorial assistance provided by Developmental Editor Alice E. Fugate, who has been with this project for the last two editions. Her skill in helping merge text from *Health: The Basics* and *Access to Health* has been invaluable. In addition, she has made terrific suggestions on improving each edition of these texts based on reviewer comments and her own interests in the topics. I am very fortunate in having the Malloy/Fugate team assisting with the day-to-day details of publishing these texts.

Thank you to The Left Coast Group and Chris Schabow for invaluable assistance in final book development and refinement and to Alison Rodal, Assistant Editor, for overseeing the complete supplements package. I would also like to thank the Benjamin Cummings marketing and sales force, particularly Senior Marketing Manager Sandra Lindelof, who does a superb job of making sure that *Access to Health* gets into instructors' hands and that adopters receive the service they deserve. This is an important, often overlooked, part of selling texts, and without Sandy's direction and the superb work of a dedicated, professional sales force, *Access to Health* would not be as successful as it is. Part of the success of any book depends on those who work diligently to make sure that the strengths of the book are outlined and that instructors are able to make good decisions about what their students will be reading. In keeping with my overall experiences with Benjamin Cummings, the sales staff and editorial staff are among the best of the best. I am very lucky to have them working with me on this project and want to extend a special thanks to all of them!

Contributors to the Ninth Edition

Many colleagues, students, and staff members have provided the feedback, reviews, extra time and assistance, and encouragement that have helped me meet the demands of rigorous publishing deadlines over the years. With each edition of the book, your assistance has made the vision for *Access to Health* a reality. Rather than just creating an upscale version of a high school text, we have worked diligently to provide a text that is alive for readers. With each edition, we would not have developed a book like this one without the outstanding contributions of several key people. Whether acting as reviewers, generating new ideas, providing expert commentary, or writing chapters, each of these professionals has added his or her skills to our collective endeavor.

I would like to thank specific contributors to chapters in this edition: Dr. Patricia Ketcham (Oregon State University)—Chapter 7, Reproductive Choices; Chapter 11, Addictions and Addictive Behavior; Chapter 12, Drinking Responsibly; Chapter 13, Tobacco and Caffeine; and Chapter 14, Illicit Drugs; Dr. Donna Champeau (Oregon State University)—Chapter 6, Sexuality, and Chapter 20, Dying and Death; and Dr. Amy Eyler (St. Louis University)—Chapter 10, Personal Fitness.

I would also like to thank Ms. Karen Elliott, doctoral student and teaching assistant in the Department of Public Health, for her assistance in updating content in Chapter 17: Infectious Diseases and Sexually Transmitted Infections. Her thorough review and content updates helped make this chapter one of the most current and extensive available today.

Reviewers for the Ninth Edition

Clearly, *Access to Health* continues to be an evolving work in progress. With each new edition, we have built on the combined expertise of many colleagues throughout the country who are dedicated to the education and behavioral changes of students. We thank the many reviewers of the past eight editions of *Access to Health* who have made such valuable contributions. For the ninth edition, reviewers who have helped us continue this tradition of excellence include Avron Abraham, University of Delaware; Emmanuel Ahua, University of Southern Mississippi; Lois Beach, Plattsburgh State University; Randy Bergman, University of Tennessee; John Coldiron, American River College; Mariane Fahlman, Wayne State University; Michael Hall, University of Tennessee; Sarah Hansen, University of Iowa; Jay Johnson, University of Wisconsin Superior; Cathy Kennedy, Colorado State University; Lori Mallory, Johnson County Community College; Marcy Mauer, Austin Peay State University; Deborah Miller, College of Charleston; Mary Mock, University of South Dakota; Tanya Morgan, West Chester University; Diane Peterson, Mt. Hood Community College; David M. Pusey, University of the Ozarks; Michael Teague, University of Iowa; Kathleen Young, California State University Northridge.

We also had a panel of reviewers who scrutinized the Test Bank and made innumerable helpful comments and critiques: Emmanuel Ahua, University of Southern Mississippi; Lois Beach, State University of New York, Plattsburg; Randy Bergman, University of Tennessee, Knoxville; Michael Hall, University of Tennessee, Knoxville; Lynne Hamelton, West Chester University; and Tanya Morgan, West Chester University.

The colleagues who attended our Health Summits contributed invaluable feedback as well: Robert Alman, Indiana University of Pennsylvania; Fran Babich and her colleagues at Butte College; Steve Chandler, Florida A&M University; Jim Clarke, Modesto Junior College; Gail Grimm, Winona State University; Roger Imbrogno, Merced College; Bob Kostelnik, Indiana University of Pennsylvania; Miguel Perez, California State University–Fresno; Helda Pinzon-Perez, California State University–Fresno; Adele Smith, University of Louisiana–Lafayette; Michelle Stern, Bronx Community College; Debra Sutton, James Madison University. Many thanks to all.

Rebecca J. Donatelle
Health & Kinesiology
Benjamin Cummings
1301 Sansome Street
San Francisco, California 94111

BRIEF CONTENTS

CONTENTS

Part Three: Choosing a Healthy Lifestyle

FEATURE BOXES

Reality Check

Skills for Behavior Change

Women's Health/ Men's Health

Access to Health

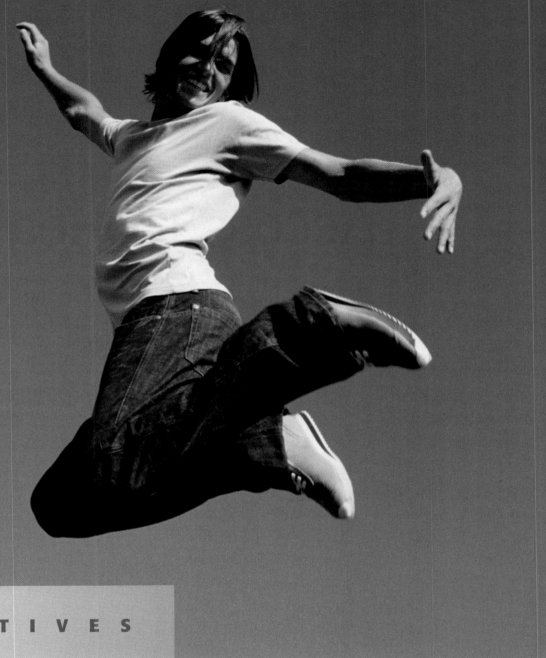

OBJECTIVES

- Discuss health in terms of historical perspectives and its multidimensional elements.

- Discuss the health status of Americans, the factors that contribute to health and illness, and the importance of *Healthy People 2010* and the *Agency for Health Care Research and Quality (AHRQ) Guidelines*.

- Evaluate the role of gender in health status, health research, and health training.

- Discuss the health challenges faced by people of various racial and cultural backgrounds.

- Explain the importance of developing a global perspective on health.

- Evaluate sources of health information, particularly the Internet, to determine reliability.

- Examine how predisposing factors, beliefs, attitudes, and significant others affect a person's behavior changes.

- Assess behavior change techniques, and learn how to apply them to personal situations.

PROMOTING HEALTHY BEHAVIOR CHANGE

IN THE NEWS

In Health Care, Gap Between Rich and Poor Persists, W.H.O. Says

By Elisabeth Malkin

Despite significant gains in medical science, disparities in public health persist between rich and poor countries, the World Health Organization said in a report released here on Wednesday.

The report, released in advance of a W.H.O. meeting here next week of health ministers from 30 countries, called for more research into how health care is delivered.

"Half of the world's deaths could be prevented with simple and cost-effective interventions," said the report. "But not enough is known about how to make these more widely available to the people who need them," it continued.

The study said that inadequate health systems in developing countries had been a constraint in global programs to fight AIDS, tuberculosis and malaria. "Countries with few resources struggle with creaking infrastructure, inadequate financing, migrating doctors and nurses and lack of basic information on health indicators," the study's authors concluded.

The study pointed to market reforms in the health sector, promoted by the World Bank in the 1980's, as one reason for steadily weakening public health systems in developing countries. The push toward privatization might have accentuated disparities in the health care available to rich and poor, the report said.

Read the complete article online in the eThemes section of this book's website: www.aw-bc.com/donatelle.

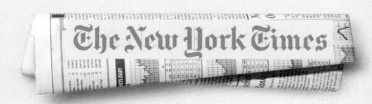

Concerned about your health? Worried about the air you breathe, the water you drink, or the food you eat? If so, you are not alone. At no time in our nation's history have so many individuals, government agencies, educational systems, community groups, businesses, and health organizations been so concerned about a growing list of health-related issues.

Today, it is nearly impossible to turn on the TV or read a newspaper and not see headlines that depict a nation in health trouble. Epidemic rates of obesity and diabetes, growing rates of HIV/AIDS, a food supply that seems threatened by mad cow disease, and other food-borne illnesses, increases in rates of certain cancers and heart disease, and other problems fuel our growing unease about health risks. Emerging health threats, such as West Nile virus, SARS, avian influenza, and other diseases, are subjects of frequent media warnings.

Juxtaposed against these futuristic images of impending threats to our health are the advertisements that offer pharmaceutical help for almost any problem. Drugs designed to increase sexual responsiveness, protect you from infectious diseases, reduce your levels of cholesterol, improve everything from cardiovascular functioning to memory, and treat stress and depression have exploded on the market. Books touting the newest "low carb" fix for obesity and fitness regimens promising to give you that "six-pack stomach" fly from bookstore shelves. We are told that there are solutions to our health problems, if we can only find them. Clearly, our health is a priority, and millions of us are working hard to try to change our lifestyles and improve our health. We are challenged to "Just do it, but don't overdo it"; "Be all you can be, but be yourself"; "Drink your milk, but maybe you should consider soy"; "Cut those bad carbs and reduce certain kinds of fat in the diet"; and "Eat more fruits and vegetables, but make sure they are organic"—and if you want to look and feel good, exercise, exercise, exercise!

Conflicting health claims abound, and research that would provide a clear message about the validity and safety of many so-called health behaviors is scarce or written in technical language that is hard for the typical person to interpret. Just when we start feeling pretty confident that what we are doing is right, a journal article or news release cautions us to be wary. Is it any wonder that so many people are confused about what they should and should not do? We often assume that the government, pharmaceutical industry, and medical profession will protect us or make everything better when we have a problem. Most of us are surprised when there isn't a drug to fix us or a treatment to make us better—or when we find out that the information we've received is, in fact, false.

As an example, for the past three decades doctors have advised women who've gone through menopause to take hormone replacement therapy as protection against heart disease and stroke. Research published in some of our most prestigious journals appeared to support this recommendation. However, beginning in 2002, and up to the current time, findings of more carefully controlled clinical trials dealt a considerable blow to the millions of American women in the United States and elsewhere who were taking these medications. Not only does hormone replacement therapy *not* protect against heart disease, stroke, and blood clots, but it actually seems to increase the risk for these diseases. Subsequent research has raised additional concerns over the use of estrogen-only therapy.[1] Health researchers, practitioners, and others on whom we rely for accurate information appear to have based long-standing prevention and treatment regimens on faulty premises.

In another example, practitioners treated stomach ulcers for decades with "milk-toast" bland diets, thinking that these diets would slow stomach secretions and aid in healing. Later, researchers found that the milk in these diets was often high in fat levels and actually caused stomach acid levels to increase, thereby irritating ulcers. More importantly, it was discovered that stomach acid was typically not the cause of ulcers; instead a bacterial pathogen caused the ulcer to develop in the stomach area, thus indicating that antibiotics are often a viable treatment.

Examples such as these cause us to question the validity of many current treatment and prevention strategies. How many of our existing health recommendations are false or misleading? Our best scientists often struggle to determine which research is valid and which provides only a preliminary indicator of hazards or benefits. How can the average person figure out what is accurate and what is not? How can we sort out the health information we are bombarded with daily and determine which warnings alert us to imminent danger and which should cause only minor concern?

Maneuvering through the "health-speak" of the twenty-first century is not simple. It is easy to see why individuals struggle so hard to get it right when it comes to making health decisions that affect them and those they care about. It should also come as no surprise that despite all of the emphasis on health in society today and all of our collective resources aimed at prevention, intervention, and treatment, the health status of Americans continues to be plagued by many old problems. To make healthy decisions, it is important to understand the behavior factors that contribute to the leading causes of death in the United States and the factors that increase our chances of living longer and more healthful lives (see the New Horizons in Health box).

Have you ever wondered how one of your friends managed to lose weight and is now out kayaking and running in triathlons when you can't seem to lose an ounce and the latest trip up the stairs leaves you panting for breath? Or why another friend seems to thrive under pressure, while it makes you break down into a screaming fit or tears? Why do so many good health intentions remain only intentions, without progressing to the action phase?

This text is not designed to provide a foolproof recipe for achieving health or to answer all of your questions. It is designed to provide fundamental knowledge about health topics, to help you utilize personal and community resources

What Americans Die From and What Really Causes Their Deaths

Although the leading causes of death in the United States are usually described as selected diseases and conditions, the actual causes of these diseases have often been presented only as a footnote. These actual causes, also referred to as modifiable behavioral risk factors, help us understand the effects of recent trends and the implications of missed prevention opportunities. As shown in the figure, recent data from the Centers for Disease Control and Prevention (CDC) reveal that smoking is the leading cause of mortality in the United States, with poor diet and physical inactivity likely to overtake tobacco use as leading culprits in sharply rising death rates.

Many of these underlying causes are preventable. Their prevalence, along with sky-rocketing health care costs and an aging population, graphically point to the fact that we must work aggressively on more prevention and intervention programs. Some actions that you can take as an individual to reduce your health risks include:

- Getting a good night's sleep (minimum of seven hours)
- Maintaining healthy eating habits
- Managing your weight

- Participating in regular physical exercise
- Avoiding tobacco use
- Limiting use of alcohol
- Practicing safer sex
- Wearing seat belts and driving cars with front and side airbags
- Scheduling regular self-exams and medical checkups
- Cultivating healthy relationships
- Finding creative outlets for fun and personal growth

- Avoiding unnecessary stressors and coping with unavoidable stress
- Recycling, reusing, and reducing excess waste to contribute to a healthy environment
- Enjoying nature and engaging in spiritual renewal
- Making time for yourself, while living unselfishly
- Being involved in activities designed to improve the health of the community

Leading Causes of Death and Actual Causes of Death in the United States, 2000

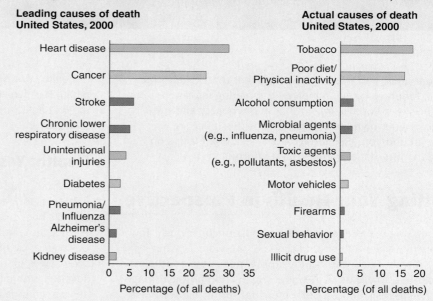

Sources: Leading causes data from A. M. Miniño, E. Arias, K. D. Kochanek, S. L. Murphy, and B. L. Smith, "Deaths: Final Data for 2000," *National Vital Statistics Reports* 50, no. 15 (Hyattsville, MD: National Center for Health Statistics, 2002), 1–120; actual causes data from A. Mokdad, J. Marks, D. Stroup, and J. Geberding, "Actual Causes of Death in the United States, 2000," *Journal of the American Medical Association* 291, no. 10 (2004): 1238–1245.

to create your own health profile, and to challenge you to think more carefully before making decisions that affect your health or the health of others. It shows how policies, programs, media, culture, ethnic background, gender, and socioeconomic status influence health, directly and indirectly, both in the United States and around the world.

It is our hope that you will gain appreciation for the many achievements that we've made in health and the many challenges that lie ahead. Additionally, it is our hope that you will begin to look at global health not in an ethnocentric way,

in which you are only able to appreciate those who look and talk like you and have habits and customs like yours, but rather in a more inclusive way.

Health decisions should be based on the best available research and should be consistent with who you are, your values and beliefs, and who you want to become. Although your health is not always totally within your control, certain behavior choices will affect you positively today and reduce future health risks. For those risk factors that are beyond your control, you must learn to react, adapt, respond

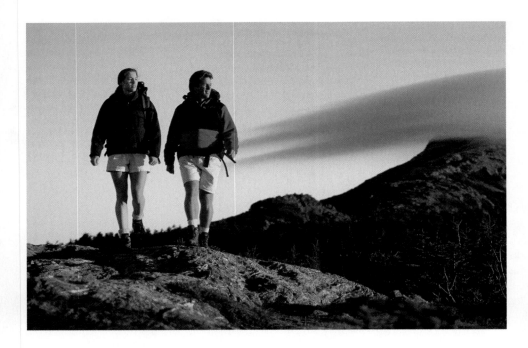

Today, health and wellness mean taking a positive, proactive attitude toward life, living it to its fullest.

appropriately, and use a reasoned, rather than purely emotional, rationale for your choices. By making informed, rational decisions, you will improve both the quality and the length of your own life and have a positive influence on those around you. (See the Reality Check box for tips on using the Internet to gather useful information.)

Putting Your Health in Perspective

Although we use the term **health** almost unconsciously, few people understand the broad scope of the word or what it really means. For some, *health* simply means the antithesis of sickness. To others, it means being in good physical shape and able to resist illness. Still others use terms like **wellness,** or *well-being,* to include a wide array of factors that seem to lead to positive health status. Why all of these variations? In part, the differences are due to an increasingly enlightened way of viewing health that has taken shape over time. In addition, as our collective understanding of illness has improved, so has our ability to understand the many nuances

of health. Our progress to current understandings about health has evolved over centuries, and we have a long way to go in achieving a truly comprehensive view of this complex subject.

Health: Yesterday and Today

Prior to the 1800s, if you weren't sick, you were not only regarded as lucky, but also healthy. When deadly epidemics such as bubonic plague, pneumonic plague, influenza, tuberculosis, and cholera killed millions of people, survivors were believed to be of hearty, healthy stock and congratulated themselves on their good fortune. Poor health was often associated with poor hygiene and unsanitary conditions, and certain stigmas were attached to households that harbored any of these illnesses. Not until the late 1800s and early 1900s did researchers slowly begin to discover that victims of these epidemics were not simply unhealthy or dirty. Rather, they were victims of environmental factors (microorganisms found in contaminated water, air, and human waste) that made them sick and over which they often had little control. Public health officials moved swiftly to address these problems, and as a result, the term *health* became synonymous with *good hygiene*. Colleges offered courses in health and hygiene, the predecessors of the course you are in today.

Throughout the years, perceptions of health were dominated by the **Medical Model,** in which health status focused primarily on the individual and a biological or diseased organ perspective. The surest way to bring about improved health was to cure or *treat* disease. Health and health status were primarily considered to be a result of something that happened to a person due to poor behavior, contact with a pathogen, or other negative influence on the body. Restoring health via medicines or therapy was the main goal of this

Health The ever-changing process of achieving individual potential in the physical, social, emotional, mental, spiritual, and environmental dimensions.

Wellness The achievement of the highest level of health possible in each of several dimensions.

Medical Model A model in which health status was focused primarily on the individual and a biological or diseased organ perspective.

Consumer Beware: Hoaxes, Rumors, and Other Perils of the Internet

Looking for reliable health information on the Internet? Wondering if that e-mail warning of a deadly pathogen in your hamburger is fact or fiction? Dazed by searching for a topic, only to be confronted with 300,000 websites in your search results? Each year more than 100 million people seek health information on the Internet. Many of them end up frazzled, confused, and—worst of all—misinformed.

Clearly, not all health websites are created equal. Where should you start? Here are some tips to point you in the right direction:

✔ Websites sponsored by an official government agency, a university or college, or a hospital/medical center typically offer accurate, up-to-date information about a wide range of health topics. Government sites are easily identified by their .gov extensions (for example, the National Institute of Mental Health is www.nimh.nih.gov); college and university sites typically have .edu extensions (Johns Hopkins University is www.jhu.edu). Hospitals often have an .org extension (Mayo Clinic is www.mayoclinic.org). Major philanthropic foundations, such as the Robert Wood Johnson Foundation, the Legacy Foundation, the Kellogg Foundation, and others, often provide information about selected health topics.

✔ Links associated with well-established, professionally peer-reviewed journals such as *The New England Journal of Medicine* (www.nejm.org) or *The Journal of the American Medical Association (JAMA)* (http://jama.amaassn.org) are good sources. While some of these sites require a fee for access to complete articles, often you can locate basic abstracts and information, such as a weekly table of contents, that can help you conduct a search. Other sites may require a basic fee for a certain number of hours of unlimited searching.

✔ For consumer news and updates on health-related hoaxes, consult the Centers for Disease Control and Prevention (CDC). The CDC provides consumer alerts on topics such as buying antibiotics online and e-mail health hoaxes. A sampler of recent e-mail scares: deliberate infections from concealed needles, poisonous perfume samples in the mail, and underarm deodorants causing breast cancer. If you receive an e-mail warning about a health topic, check the CDC hoax and rumor site (www.cdc.gov/hoax_ rumors.htm) before giving it credibility.

✔ Use discretion, and don't believe everything you read. Cross-check information against reliable sources to see if facts and figures are consistent. Quackery runs rampant on the Internet, particularly on sites that are trying to sell you a quick fix for a health problem. Just because a source claims to be a physician or an expert does not mean that this is true. When in doubt, check with your own medical doctor, health education professor, or state health division's website. There are many government and education-based sites that are independently sponsored and reliable. The following is just a sample; others are provided in each chapter as we cover specific topics.

Aetna Intelihealth: www.intelihealth.com

Dr. Koop.com: www.drkoop.com

Drug Infonet: www.druginfonet.com

Health AtoZ.com: www.healthatoz.com

WebMD: www.webmd.com

The American Accreditation Healthcare Commission (www.urac.org) has devised 50 criteria that health sites must meet to win its seal of approval, which makes it a little easier to determine a site's credibility. A rating scale and visible seal will tell you at a glance whether a site meets the commission's rigorous standards. In addition to policing the accuracy of health claims, this commission evaluates health information and provides a forum for reporting misinformation, privacy violations, and other complaints.

Source: From "Health Journal: Online Groups Step Up Attempts to Enforce Standards," *The Wall Street Journal, Eastern Edition,* July 20, 2001, by staff writer. © 2001 Dow Jones & Co. Reproduced by permission.

---

model, and government resources focused on initiatives that led to treatment of disease as a means of intervention. Even today, there are those who believe that it is cheaper to give someone a medicine to control a disease than it would be to prevent the disease from developing in the first place.

Around 1900, health professionals began to focus on an **Ecological or Public Health Model** of health. Under this model, diseases and other negative health events are viewed more as a result of an individual's interaction with his/her social and physical environment. Thus, polluted air and water, hazardous work conditions, negative influences in the home and social environment, abuse of drugs and alcohol, stress, unsafe behavior, diet, sedentary lifestyle, and cost,

quality, and access to health care all are viewed as potent forces affecting one's health status. If factors in the external environment and individual behaviors affect health risk, it seems logical that we must work to diminish these threats in order to prevent negative health outcomes. Under the Ecological or Public Health Model, prevention and intervention

> **Ecological or Public Health Model** A model in which diseases and other negative health events are viewed as a result of an individual's interaction with his/her social and physical environment.

America's Mixed Health Bag: Improvements, Disparities, and Continuing Problems

Our national preoccupation with health should make it easier to get healthy, stay healthy, and live a long and productive life. However, while we are doing better in some areas, we still have a long way to go in others. A national survey of trends in health behaviors from 1991–2000, known as the Behavioral Risk Factor Surveillance System (BRFSS), indicates that Americans are buckling up (seat belts) but chugging down (alcohol) more than ever, that they are fatter and less fit than at any time in our nation's history, and that they are getting their cancer screening tests but still smoking too much. Specific findings in this research are that:

- Binge drinking, particularly among college-aged adults, increased in one third of all states and declined in only three states. Increases concentrated in the South and Midwest, where Wisconsin had the highest amount of binge drinking in 1999 (19.6 percent, compared with 16.4 percent in 1991). Illinois had the greatest increase during the study, jumping from 7.3 to 13.9 percent.
- Most states reported increases in seat belt use, mammograms, adult vaccinations, and screening for cervical cancer.
- Levels of physical inactivity rose in 3 of 48 states and declined in 11 states.
- Cholesterol screening increased in 13 of 47 states and decreased in 5 states.

- Obesity rose in all states.
- Smoking increased in 14 of 47 states. It declined in only one state, Minnesota.

Another national report, summarizing trends in racial- and ethnic-specific health indicators in the United States as part of *Healthy People 2000,* indicates that although we are doing better as a population, there are still great disparities in our overall health status. According to Surgeon General David Satcher, "Americans of all ages and in every racial and ethnic group have better health today . . . but until all groups are equally protected, our work isn't done." Here are key points from this report:

- All racial and ethnic groups experienced improvements in rates for ten key health indicators: prenatal care, infant mortality, teen births, death rates for heart disease, homicide, motor vehicle crashes, work-related injuries, tuberculosis rates, syphilis rates, and air quality.
- Five more health indicators—total death rate and death rates for stroke, lung cancer, breast cancer, and suicide—improved in all groups except American Indians and Alaska Natives.
- The percent of children living in poverty improved for all groups except Asian or Pacific Islanders.
- Percent of low birthweight infants improved only among African American and non-Hispanic groups.

Still other findings from recent years highlight America's ongoing health concerns:

- Sales of red meat, butter, and other high-fat foods, once on the decline, are seeing an unprecedented rise.

- Salad bars, low-fat grilled items, and portion control are on the decline, as consumers opt for super-sized burgers and monster meals at popular restaurant chains.
- Cigarette smoking among our nation's young has declined, but certain groups—particularly young women—continue to smoke at high rates.
- Depression, mental health problems, certain infectious diseases, and other preventable ailments are on the rise.
- The diabetes rate among young adults is skyrocketing—up over 30 percent in the past decade.
- Increasing numbers of Americans lack access to basic health care.

As our population becomes more diverse—with growing numbers of Hispanics, Asians, and African Americans as well as other racial and ethnic minorities and persons who live in the United States illegally—poverty continues to be the single greatest barrier to health care, creating a burgeoning population of underserved or unserved individuals. One of the greatest lessons is that we need to tailor interventions and prevention activities to the unique needs of diverse groups.

Sources: National Center for Health Statistics, "*Healthy People 2000,* Trends in Racial and Ethnic-Specific Rates for Health Status Indicators: United States, 1990–1998," (PHS) Statistical Note No. 23, 2002, www.cdc .gov/nchs/releases/02news/ healthimpr .htm; Centers for Disease Control and Prevention, 2004, www.cdc.gov; National Institute for Mental Health, 2004, www.nimh .nih.gov; National Center for Health Statistics, 2004, www.cdc.gov/nchs/search/search .htm; Agency for Healthcare Research and Quality, 2004, www.ahcpr.gov

strategies become elevated to their proper place in improving the health of individuals and entire populations.

In the late 1940s, progressive thinkers in public health began to be more proactive in pushing for programs and policies that took an ecological approach to prevention. At an international conference in 1947 focusing on global health issues, the World Health Organization (WHO) took the landmark step of trying to clarify what *health* truly meant: "Health is the state of complete physical, mental, and social well-being, not just the absence of disease or infirmity."[2] For the first time, the concept of health came to be officially defined as more than the absence of disease.

Not until the 1960s and 1970s, however, did the definition of health began to more closely mirror the comprehensive ecological model that public health professionals had been advocating for decades. Scientists argued that health was much more than the absence of disease; in fact, their definition included the physical, social, and mental elements of life, as well as environmental, spiritual, emotional, and intellectual dimensions. To be truly healthy, a person must be capable of functioning at an optimal level in each of these areas, as well as interacting with others and the greater environment, in a productive and spiritually healthy manner. Public health leaders argued that it wasn't just length of life or the number of disease-free years that mattered, but rather living life to the fullest and reaching your potential for a happy, healthy, and productive life. Today, *quality of life* is recognized as being as important as years of life.

Investigation of environment as the primary cause of diseases has continued for decades, and the Medical Model still persists in some cultures, particularly those that are ravaged by outbreaks of disease and seemingly insurmountable poverty and poor social conditions. Today, however, more people understand that it is often a broken "system" that causes major diseases to spread unchecked. (See the "Achievements in Public Health" section for an indication of how public health has worked to improve health status.) As a classic example, consider life expectancy. In the early 1900s the average life expectancy in the United States was only 47 years, largely because of the vast numbers of individuals who died before age 5 from childhood diseases. Public health improvements in sanitation and the development of vaccines and antibiotics have added many years to the average life span since then.

Today, because most childhood diseases are preventable or curable and because massive public health efforts are aimed at reducing the spread of infectious diseases, average life expectancy in the United States is 76.9 years with many people living well into their eighties and nineties and more. According to **mortality** statistics, people are now living longer than at any previous time in our history. **Morbidity** rates also indicate that people less frequently contract the common infectious diseases that devastated previous generations. Longer life and less frequent disease are not proof that people are indeed *healthier,* however.

The Evolution toward Wellness

René Dubos, biologist and philosopher, aptly summarized the thinking of his contemporaries by defining *health* as "a quality of life, involving social, emotional, mental, spiritual, and biological fitness on the part of the individual, which results from adaptations to the environment."[3] The concept of *adaptability,* or the ability to successfully cope with life's ups and downs, became a key element of the overall health definition. Eventually the term *wellness* became popular and not only included the previously mentioned elements, but also implied that there were levels of health in each category. To achieve *high-level wellness,* a person would move

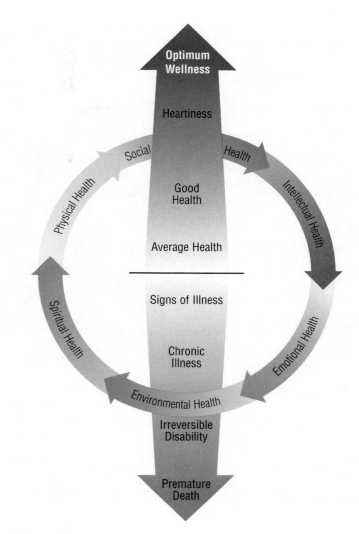

Figure 1.1
The Dimensions of Health and the Wellness Continuum

progressively higher on a continuum of positive health indicators. Those who fail to achieve these levels may move to the illness side of the continuum. Today, the terms *health* and *wellness* are often used interchangeably to mean the dynamic, ever-changing process of trying to achieve one's potential in each of several interrelated dimensions. These dimensions typically include those presented in Figure 1.1.

• *Physical health.* This dimension includes characteristics such as body size and shape, sensory acuity and responsiveness, susceptibility to disease and disorders, body functioning, physical fitness, and recuperative abilities. Newer definitions of physical health also include our ability

| **Mortality** | The proportion of deaths to population. |
| **Morbidity** | The relative incidence of disease. |

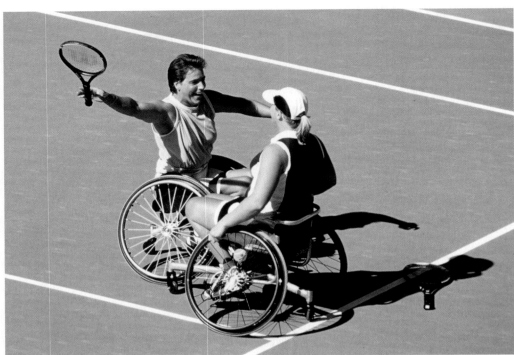

Self-love
Human
connection
Productivity
Spirituality

The motivation to improve quality of life within the framework of one's own unique capabilities is crucial to achieving health and wellness.

to perform normal **activities of daily living (ADLs),** or those tasks that are necessary to normal existence in today's society. Being able to get out of bed in the morning, being able to bend over to tie your shoes, or other daily tasks are examples of ADLs.

- *Intellectual health.* The ability to think clearly, reason objectively, analyze critically, and use "brainpower" effectively to meet life's challenges are all part of this dimension. Intellectual health means learning from successes and mistakes and making sound, responsible decisions that take into consideration all aspects of a situation.
- *Social health.* This dimension consists of the ability to have satisfying interpersonal relationships: interactions with others, adaptations to various social situations, and daily behaviors.
- *Emotional health.* This is the feeling component—being able to express emotions when appropriate, controlling them when not, and avoiding expressing them in an inappropriate manner. Feelings of self-esteem, self-confidence, self-efficacy, trust, love, and many other emotional reactions and responses are all part of emotional health.
- *Environmental health.* An appreciation of the external environment and the role individuals play in preserving, protecting, and improving environmental conditions are included.

- *Spiritual health.* This dimension may involve a belief in a supreme being or a specified way of living prescribed by a particular religion. Spiritual health also includes the feeling of unity with the environment—a feeling of oneness with others and with nature—and a guiding sense of meaning or value in life. It also may include the ability to understand and express one's purpose in life; to feel a part of a greater spectrum of existence; to experience love, joy, pain, sorrow, peace, contentment, and wonder over life's experiences; and to care about and respect all living things.

A *well* individual might display the following characteristics:

- A realistic sense of self, including personal capabilities and limitations.
- An appreciation of all living things, no matter how ugly or beautiful, how unique or different, or how great or small.
- A willingness to understand imperfection, to forgive others' mistakes, and to grow from personal mistakes or shortcomings.
- The ability to laugh, cry, and genuinely feel emotions without getting lost in emotional upsets.
- The ability to function at a reasonable level physiologically.
- The ability to maintain and support healthful relationships with family, friends, intimate partners, and strangers.
- An appreciation for one's role in preserving and protecting the environment.
- A sense of satisfaction with life and an appreciation for the stages of the life experience.

Activities of daily living (ADLs) Performance of tasks of everyday living, such as bathing and walking up the stairs.

- A zest for living, coupled with a curiosity about what each new encounter, each new day will bring.
- A respect for self, as well as a respect for others.
- A realistic perspective about life's challenges and the skills to cope with life's stresses and challenges.
- A balance in all things.

Many people believe that wellness can best be achieved by adopting a *holistic* approach, in which a person emphasizes the integration of and balance among mind, body, and spirit. Achieving wellness means attaining the optimal level of wellness for a given person's unique set of limitations and strengths. A physically disabled person may be functioning at his or her optimal level of performance; enjoy satisfying interpersonal relationships; work to maintain emotional, spiritual, and intellectual health; and have a strong interest in environmental concerns. In contrast, those who spend hours lifting weights to perfect the size and shape of each muscle but pay little attention to nutrition may *look* healthy but may not maintain a healthy balance in all areas of health. Although we often consider physical attractiveness and other external trappings in measuring the overall health of a person, appearance and physical performance indicators are actually only two signs of physical health, indicating little about the other dimensions. Complete the appraisal in the Assess Yourself box on page 12 to gain perspective on your own level of wellness in each dimension.

What do you think?

René Dubos, a renowned bacteriologist who developed many key philosophies about health, is credited with saying, "Measure your health by your sympathy with morning and spring." ■ *What do you think Dubos meant by this statement?* ■ *Discuss how well your own health measures up when weighed against this criterion.*

New Directions for Health

In response to the many indications that Americans were not as healthy as they should be, in 1990 the U.S. Surgeon General proposed a national plan for promoting health among individuals and groups. Known as *Healthy People 2000,* the plan outlined a series of long-term objectives.[4] Critics of this plan complained that it was just a large wish list, that it needed some unifying plan to help bring about the outlined changes, and that there was little financial support to ensure that the objectives could be achieved. Although many communities worked toward these goals and the plan helped solidify plans for many regions of the country, as a nation we still had a long way to go by the new millennium.

Healthy People 2010 and Other Initiatives

A new plan, *Healthy People 2010,* takes the *Healthy People 2000* initiative to the next level. *Healthy People 2010* is a nationwide program with two broad goals: (1) eliminate health disparities, and (2) increase the life span and quality of life. The plan includes 28 focus areas, each representing a public health priority such as nutrition, tobacco use, substance abuse, access to quality health services, and common health conditions (for example, heart disease and diabetes). Under these focus areas are a list of Leading Health Indicators (LHIs) that spell out specific health issues (Table 1.1 on page 18).

For each focus area, the plan presents specific objectives for the nation to achieve during the next decade. For instance, nutrition data show that only 42 percent of Americans aged 20 and older are at their healthy weight; the goal is to raise that number to 60 percent. In the focus area of physical activity and fitness, 40 percent of Americans aged 18 and older do not engage in any leisure-time physical activity. The objective is to reduce this number to 20 percent by 2010.[5]

Although the *Healthy People* documents provide a blueprint for health planning in the United States over the next decade, other programs and agencies also offer recommendations for improving overall health. In the public sector, the Agency for Health Care, Research, and Quality (AHRQ) offers additional direction for national health care efforts through its *AHRQ Guidelines,* a set of objectives for health care providers to meet in specific areas of practice. Other government agencies and research centers also address specific health concerns. Examples are the CDC's publication *Best Practices for Comprehensive Tobacco Control Programs,* which recommends budgets and treatment guidelines to curb smoking, and the Institute of Medicine's *The Future of Public Health in the 21st Century,* which recommends avenues of intervention for many critical public health issues.[6]

A New Focus on Health Promotion

The objectives of *Healthy People 2010* and other programs have prompted action to promote health and prevent premature disability through social, environmental, policy-related, and community-based programming. In addition, a new emphasis on assisting individuals in their pursuit of specific behavior changes is emerging. Changing behavior without help is not easy, however.

The term **health promotion** describes the educational, organizational, procedural, environmental, social, and financial supports that help individuals and groups reduce negative

---

Health promotion   Combined educational, organizational, policy, financial, and environmental supports to help people reduce negative health behaviors and promote positive change.

How Healthy Are You?

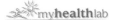

Fill out this assessment online at www.aw-bc.com/myhealthlab or www.aw-bc.com/donatelle

Although we all recognize the importance of being healthy, it can be a challenge to sort out which behaviors are most likely to cause problems or which ones pose the greatest risk. Even when we recognize our unique risks and know what to do, it isn't always easy to stay motivated enough to maintain a specific set of health behaviors. Before you decide where to start, it is important to take a careful look at your health status right now. Think carefully about where you believe that you are today in each of the dimensions of health. Circle the number in each category that you think best describes you. Rate your health status in each of the following dimensions by circling the number on the line that comes closest to describing the way you are most of the time.

	Poor Health		Average Health		Excellent Health
Physical health	1	2	3	4	5
Social health	1	2	3	4	5
Emotional health	1	2	3	4	5
Environmental health	1	2	3	4	5
Spiritual health	1	2	3	4	5
Intellectual health	1	2	3	4	5

After completing the above section, how would you rate your *overall* health?_____

Which area(s), if any, do you think you should work on improving? _____

If we were to ask your closest friends how healthy they think you are, which area(s) do you think they would say you need to work on and improve? _____

By completing the following assessment, you will have a clearer picture of health areas in which you excel and those that could use varying degrees of work. Taking this assessment will also help you to reflect on various components of health that you may not have thought much about.

Use the results from this assessment as a guide and as a way to begin analyzing potential areas for improvement and/or maintenance. Answer each question, then total your score for each section and fill it in on the Personal Checklist at the end of the assessment for a general sense of your health profile. Think about the behaviors that influenced your score in each category. Would you like to change any of them? Choose the area that you'd like to improve, then complete the Behavior Change Contract. Use the contract to think through and implement a behavior change over the course of this class.

Each of the categories in this questionnaire is an important aspect of the total dimensions of health, but this is not a substitute for the advice of a qualified health care provider. Consider scheduling a thorough physical examination by a licensed physician or setting up an appointment with a mental health counselor at your school if you think you need help making a behavior change.

For each of the following, indicate how often you think the statements describe you.

PHYSICAL HEALTH

	Never	Rarely	Some of the Time	Usually or Always
1. I am happy with my body size and weight.	1	2	3	4
2. I engage in vigorous exercises such as brisk walking, jogging, swimming, or running for at least 30 minutes per day, 3 to 4 times per week.	1	2	3	4
3. I do exercises designed to strengthen my muscles and increase endurance at least 2 times per week.	1	2	3	4
4. I do stretching, limbering up, and balance exercises such as yoga, Pilates, or tai chi to increase my body awareness and control and increase my overall physical health.	1	2	3	4

	Never	Rarely	Some of the Time	Usually or Always
5. I feel good about the condition of my body and would be able to respond to most demands placed upon it.	1	2	3	4
6. I get at least 7 to 8 hours of sleep each night.	1	2	3	4
7. I try to add moderate activity to each day, such as taking the stairs instead of the elevator and walking whenever I can instead of riding.	1	2	3	4
8. My immune system is strong, and my body heals itself quickly when I get sick or injured.	1	2	3	4
9. I have lots of energy and can get through the day without being overly tired.	1	2	3	4
10. I listen to my body; when there is something wrong, I try to make adjustments to heal it or seek professional advice.	1	2	3	4

Total score for section: _____

SOCIAL HEALTH

	Never	Rarely	Some of the Time	Usually or Always
1. When I meet people, I feel good about the impression I make on them.	1	2	3	4
2. I am open, honest, and get along well with other people.	1	2	3	4
3. I participate in a wide variety of social activities and enjoy being with people who are different from me.	1	2	3	4
4. I try to be a better person and work on behaviors that have caused problems in my interactions with others.	1	2	3	4
5. I get along well with the members of my family.	1	2	3	4
6. I am a good listener.	1	2	3	4
7. I am open and accessible to a loving and responsible relationship.	1	2	3	4
8. I have someone I can talk to about my private feelings.	1	2	3	4
9. I consider the feelings of others and do not act in hurtful or selfish ways.	1	2	3	4
10. I try to see the good in my friends and do whatever I can to support them and help them feel good about themselves.	1	2	3	4

Total score for section: _____

EMOTIONAL HEALTH

	Never	Rarely	Some of the Time	Usually or Always
1. I find it easy to laugh, cry, and show emotions like love, fear, and anger and try to express these in positive, constructive ways.	1	2	3	4
2. I avoid using alcohol or other drugs as a means of helping me forget my problems.	1	2	3	4
3. When viewing a particularly challenging situation, I tend to view the glass as half full rather than half empty and perceive problems as opportunities for growth.	1	2	3	4
4. When I am angry, I try to let others know in nonconfrontational and nonhurtful ways, trying to resolve issues rather than stewing about them.	1	2	3	4
5. I try not to worry unnecessarily and try to talk about my feelings, fears, and concerns rather than letting them become chronic issues.	1	2	3	4

(continues)

	Never	Rarely	Some of the Time	Usually or Always
6. I recognize when I am stressed and take steps to relax through exercise, quiet time, or other calming activities.	1	2	3	4
7. I feel good about myself and believe others like me for who I am.	1	2	3	4
8. I try not to be too critical and/or judgmental of others and to understand differences or quirks that I may note in others.	1	2	3	4
9. I am flexible and adapt or adjust to change in a positive way.	1	2	3	4
10. My friends regard me as a stable, emotionally well-adjusted person whom they trust and rely on for support.	1	2	3	4

Total score for section: _____

ENVIRONMENTAL HEALTH

	Never	Rarely	Some of the Time	Usually or Always
1. I am concerned about environmental pollution and actively try to preserve and protect natural resources.	1	2	3	4
2. I buy recycled paper and purchase biodegradable detergents and cleaning agents whenever possible.	1	2	3	4
3. I recycle my garbage, purchase refillable containers when possible, and try to minimize the amount of paper and plastics that I use.	1	2	3	4
4. I try to wear my clothes for longer periods between washing to reduce water consumption and the amount of detergents in our water sources.	1	2	3	4
5. I vote for pro-environment candidates in elections.	1	2	3	4
6. I write my elected leaders about environmental concerns.	1	2	3	4
7. I turn down the heat and wear warmer clothes at home in winter and use the air conditioner only when necessary or at higher temperatures in summer.	1	2	3	4
8. I am aware of lead pipes in my living area, chemicals in my carpet, and other potential hazards and try to reduce my exposure whenever possible.	1	2	3	4
9. I use both sides of the paper when taking class notes or doing assignments.	1	2	3	4
10. I try not to leave the faucet running too long when I brush my teeth, shave, or shower.	1	2	3	4

Total score for section: _____

SPIRITUAL HEALTH

	Never	Rarely	Some of the Time	Usually or Always
1. I believe life is a precious gift that should be nurtured.	1	2	3	4
2. I take time to enjoy nature and the beauty around me.	1	2	3	4
3. I take time alone to think about what's important in life— who I am, what I value, where I fit in, and where I'm going.	1	2	3	4
4. I have faith in a greater power, be it a God-like force, nature, or the connectedness of all living things.	1	2	3	4
5. I engage in acts of caring and goodwill without expecting something in return.	1	2	3	4
6. I feel sorrow for those who are suffering and try to help them through difficult times.	1	2	3	4
7. I look forward to each day as an opportunity for further growth and challenge.	1	2	3	4

	Never	Rarely	Some of the Time	Usually or Always
8. I work for peace in my interpersonal relationships, in my community, and in the world at large.	1	2	3	4
9. I have a great love and respect for all living things, and regard the natural world (animals, etc.), as containing important links in a vital living chain.	1	2	3	4
10. I go for the gusto and experience life to the fullest.	1	2	3	4

Total score for section: _____

INTELLECTUAL HEALTH

	Never	Rarely	Some of the Time	Usually or Always
1. I carefully consider my options and possible consequences as I make choices in life.	1	2	3	4
2. I learn from my mistakes and try to act differently the next time.	1	2	3	4
3. I follow directions or recommended guidelines, avoid risks, and act in ways likely to keep myself and others safe.	1	2	3	4
4. I consider myself to be a wise health consumer and check reliable information sources before making decisions.	1	2	3	4
5. I am alert and ready to respond to life's challenges in ways that reflect thought and sound judgment.	1	2	3	4
6. I have at least one hobby, learning activity, or personal growth activity that I make time for each week; something that improves me as a person.	1	2	3	4
7. I actively learn all I can about products and services before making decisions.	1	2	3	4
8. I manage my time well rather than let time manage me.	1	2	3	4
9. My friends and family trust my judgment.	1	2	3	4
10. I think about my self-talk (the things I tell myself) and then examine the evidence to see if my perceptions and feelings are sound.	1	2	3	4

Total score for section: _____

Although each of these six dimensions of health is important, there are some factors that don't readily fit one dimension. As college students, you face some unique risks that others may not have. For this reason, we have added an additional section to this self-assessment that focuses on personal health promotion and disease prevention. Answer these questions and add your results to the Personal Checklist in the following section.

PERSONAL HEALTH PROMOTION/DISEASE PREVENTION

	Never	Rarely	Some of the Time	Usually or Always
1. I know the warning signs of common sexually transmitted infections, such as genital warts (human papilloma virus, or HPV), chlamydia, and herpes, and read new information about these diseases as a way of protecting myself.	1	2	3	4
2. If I were to be sexually active, I would use protection such as latex condoms, dental dams, and other means of reducing my risk of sexually transmitted infections.	1	2	3	4
3. I find ways other than binge drinking when at parties or during happy hours to loosen up and have a good time.	1	2	3	4
4. When I have more than 1 or 2 drinks, I ask someone who is not drinking to drive me and my friends home.	1	2	3	4

(continues)

	Never	Rarely	Some of the Time	Usually or Always
5. I have eaten too much in the last month and have forced myself to vomit to avoid gaining weight.	4	3	2	1
6. I have several piercings and have found that I enjoy the rush that comes with each piercing event.	4	3	2	1
7. If I were to have a tattoo or piercing, I would go to a reputable person who follows strict standards of sterilization and precautions against blood-borne disease transmission.	1	2	3	4
8. I engage in extreme sports and find that I enjoy the highs that come with risking bodily harm through physical performance.	4	3	2	1
9. I am careful not to mix alcohol or other drugs with prescription and over-the-counter drugs.	1	2	3	4
10. I practice monthly breast/testicle self-examinations.	1	2	3	4

Total score for section: _____

PERSONAL CHECKLIST

Now, total your scores in each of the health dimensions and compare them to what would be considered optimal scores. Which areas do you need to work on? How does your score compare with how you rated yourself in the first part of the questionnaire?

	Ideal Score	Your Score
Physical health	40	_____
Social health	40	_____
Emotional health	40	_____
Environmental health	40	_____
Spiritual health	40	_____
Intellectual health	40	_____
Personal health promotion/disease prevention	40	_____

WHAT YOUR SCORES IN EACH CATEGORY MEAN

Scores of 35–40: Outstanding! Your answers show that you are aware of the importance of these behaviors in your overall health. More important, you are putting your knowledge to work for you by practicing good health habits that should reduce your overall risks. Although you received a very high score on this part of the test, you may want to consider areas where your scores could be improved.

Scores of 30–34: Your health practices in these areas are very good, but there is room for improvement. Look again at the items you answered that scored one or two points. What changes could you make to improve your score? Even a small change in behavior can help you achieve better health.

Scores of 20–29: Your health risks are showing! Find information about the risks you are facing and why it is important to change these behaviors. Perhaps you need help in deciding how to make the changes you desire. Assistance is available from this book, your professor, and student health services at your school.

Scores below 20: You may be taking unnecessary risks with your health. Perhaps you are not aware of the risks and what to do about them. Identify each risk area, and make a mental note as you read the associated chapter in the book. Whenever possible, seek additional resources, either on your campus or through your local community health resources, and make a serious commitment to behavior change. If any area is causing you to be less than functional in your class work or personal life, seek professional help. In this book you will find the information you need to help you improve your scores and your health. Remember that these scores are only indicators, not diagnostic tools.

MAKE IT HAPPEN!

Use the results of this self-assessment to begin your behavior change program. Follow the steps, use the examples on page 35 to complete your Behavior Change Contract , and use these resources to take action.

health behaviors and promote positive change. Health promotion programs identify healthy people who are engaging in **risk behaviors** (behaviors that increase susceptibility to negative health outcomes), motivate them to change their actions, and provide support that increases chances of success. Effective stop-smoking programs, for instance, don't simply say "Just do it." Instead, they provide information about risk behaviors and possible consequences to smokers and their sidestream smoke victims (educational supports); they encourage smokers to participate in smoking cessation classes and encourage employers to allow time off for worker attendance, or they set up buddy systems of social supports to help them (organizational supports); they establish rules governing smokers' behaviors and supporting their decisions to change, such as banning smoking in the workplace and removing cigarettes from vending machines (environmental supports); and they may provide monetary incentives to motivate people to participate (financial supports).[7]

Health promotion programs also encourage those with sound health habits to maintain them. By attempting to modify behaviors, increase skills, change attitudes, increase knowledge, influence values, and improve health-related decision making, health promotion goes well beyond the simple information campaign. By basing programs and services in communities, organizations, schools, and other places where many people spend their time, health promotion increases the likelihood of long-term success on the road to health and wellness.

Whether we use the term *health* or *wellness,* we are talking about a person's overall responses to the challenges of living. Occasional dips into the ice cream bucket and other dietary slips, failures to exercise every day, flare-ups of anger, and other deviations from optimal behavior should not be viewed as major failures. Actually, the ability to recognize that each of us is an imperfect being, attempting to adapt in an imperfect world, signals individual well-being.

We must also remember to be tolerant of others. Rather than be warriors against pleasure in our zeal to change the health behaviors of others, we need to be supportive, understanding, and nonjudgmental in recognizing our unique differences. Health bashing—intolerance or negative feelings, words, or actions aimed at people who fail to meet our own expectations of health—may indicate our own deficiencies in the psychological, social, and/or spiritual dimensions of health.

Disease Prevention

Most health promotion initiatives include the term *disease prevention.* What does it really mean? Historically, the health literature describes three types of prevention: primary, secondary, and tertiary.

In a general sense, *prevention* means taking positive actions *now* to avoid becoming sick *later.* Getting immunized against diseases such as polio, deciding not to smoke cigarettes, and practicing safer sex constitute **primary prevention**—actions designed to reduce risk and avoid health

problems before they start. **Secondary prevention** (also referred to as **intervention**) involves recognizing health risks or early problems and taking action (intervening) to stop the behavior before it leads to actual illness. Getting a young smoker to quit or reduce the number of cigarettes smoked is an example of secondary prevention. The third type of prevention, **tertiary prevention**, involves treatment and/or rehabilitation after the person is already sick. Typically, tertiary prevention is practiced by licensed health care professionals operating under the medical model of health.

In the United States, two of every three deaths and one of every three hospitalizations are linked to preventable lifestyle behaviors, such as tobacco use, sedentary lifestyle, alcohol consumption, and overeating. The chronic diseases these behaviors lead to impose an enormous financial and societal burden on the United States, accounting for 70 percent of the deaths of all Americans and 75 percent of the nation's annual health care costs.[8] This means that primary and secondary prevention offer our best hope for reducing the **incidence** (number of new cases) and **prevalence** (number of existing cases) of disease and disability.

It is clear that we need to move from a mind-set of tertiary prevention to focus on earlier intervention designed to remove barriers and help individuals succeed in their behavior change strategies. Health educators in U.S. schools and communities offer an affordable and effective delivery of prevention and intervention programs. **Certified Health Education Specialists (CHESs)** make up a trained cadre of public health workers with special credentials and competencies to plan, implement, and evaluate prevention programs that offer scientifically sound, behaviorally based methods to help individuals and communities increase the likelihood of success. As a nation that historically spends little on prevention

---

Risk behaviors Behaviors that increase susceptibility to negative health outcomes.

Disease prevention Actions or behaviors designed to keep people from getting sick.

Primary prevention Actions designed to stop problems before they start.

Secondary prevention (intervention) Intervention early in the development of a health problem.

Tertiary prevention Treatment and/or rehabilitation efforts.

Incidence The number of new cases.

Prevalence The number of existing cases.

Certified Health Education Specialists (CHESs) Academically trained health educators who have passed a national competency examination for prevention and intervention programming.

Table 1.1
What Is *Healthy People 2010*?

Overarching Goals
1. Increase quality and years of healthy life
2. Eliminate health disparities

Focus Areas
1. Access to quality health services
2. Arthritis, osteoporosis, and chronic back conditions
3. Cancer
4. Chronic kidney disease
5. Diabetes
6. Disability and secondary conditions
7. Educational and community-based programs
8. Environmental health
9. Family planning
10. Food safety
11. Health communication
12. Heart disease and stroke
13. Human immunodeficiency virus (HIV)
14. Immunization and infectious diseases
15. Injury and violence prevention
16. Maternal, infant, and child health
17. Medical product safety
18. Mental health and mental disorders
19. Nutrition and overweight
20. Occupational safety and health
21. Oral health
22. Physical activity and fitness
23. Public health infrastructure
24. Respiratory disease
25. Sexually transmitted disease
26. Substance abuse
27. Tobacco use
28. Vision and hearing

Leading Health Indicators
1. Physical activity
2. Overweight and obesity
3. Tobacco use
4. Substance abuse
5. Responsible sexual behavior
6. Mental health
7. Injury and violence
8. Environmental quality
9. Immunization
10. Access to health care

Source: Office of Disease Prevention and Health Promotion, U.S. Department of Health and Human Services, "Healthy People 2010," 2000, www.health.gov/healthypeople/About/hpfact.htm

(less than 5 percent of our total national funding for health goes to prevention), however, such a shift has been and will continue to be difficult.

Achievements in Public Health

To those of us in the field of public health, the saying "we've come a long way, baby" accurately reflects the health achievements of the past 100 years. According to the Centers for Disease Control and Prevention (CDC), here are the ten greatest public health achievements of the twentieth century:

1. *Vaccinations.* Vaccinations have eradicated smallpox, eliminated poliomyelitis, and significantly controlled a number of infectious diseases, including measles, rubella, tetanus, diphtheria, and *Haemophilus influenzae* type b, all of which claimed the lives of large numbers of people in the early 1900s.
2. *Motor vehicle safety.* Improvements in motor vehicle safety have resulted from engineering efforts to make both vehicles and highways safer and from successful efforts to change personal behavior, such as the use of seat belts, child safety seats, and motorcycle helmets and the avoidance of drinking and driving.
3. *Workplace safety.* Work-related health risks common at the beginning of the last century are now under better control or completely eliminated. Since 1980, the rate of fatal occupational injuries has fallen by 40 percent.
4. *Control of infectious diseases.* Clean water and improved sanitation have greatly reduced the development and transmission of infectious diseases since 1900. Antimicrobial therapy, such as the discovery of and treatment with antibiotics, has greatly reduced the risk of contracting diseases such as tuberculosis and sexually transmitted infections.
5. *Cardiovascular disease (CVD) and stroke deaths.* Efforts to educate the public on how to modify health risk factors, such as quitting smoking and controlling high blood pressure, coupled with improved access to early detection and better treatment, have reduced rates of CVD and stroke.
6. *Safe and healthy foods.* Since 1900, technology for eradicating microbial contaminants from foods has improved dramatically. Identification of essential micronutrients and establishment of food-fortification programs have almost eliminated major nutritional deficiency diseases such as rickets, goiter, and pellagra.
7. *Maternal and infant care.* Better hygiene and nutrition, improved availability of antibiotics, greater access to health care, and technological advances in medicine have greatly reduced the risks to infants and mothers. Since

1900, infant mortality has decreased by 90 percent, and maternal mortality has declined by 99 percent.

8. *Family planning.* Access to family planning and contraceptive services has altered social and economic roles of women. Family planning has provided health benefits that have reduced the number of infant, child, and maternal deaths; increased opportunities for preconception counseling and screening; and increased the use of barrier contraceptives to prevent unwanted pregnancies and sexually transmissible infections.

9. *Fluoridated drinking water.* Fluoridation of drinking water began in 1945 and by 1999 reached an estimated 144 million persons in the United States. Fluoridation safely and inexpensively prevents tooth decay, regardless of socioeconomic status or access to health care. It has played an important role in reducing tooth decay in children and tooth loss in adults.

10. *Recognition of tobacco as a health hazard.* Public antismoking campaigns have changed social norms to prevent initiation of tobacco use, promote cessation of use, and reduce exposure to environmental tobacco smoke. Since the 1964 Surgeon General's report on the health risks of smoking, millions of smoking-related health problems have been prevented and many lives have been saved.[9]

While past achievements are indeed remarkable, they also raise questions about where we're going in the new century. Will the future of our health rest solely in the hands of researchers, technological wizardry, and pharmaceutical houses? What roles will public health practitioners and the health care system play? What will our own roles be in health promotion and disease prevention in the twenty-first century? Interviews with leading experts in health-related fields offer some predictions.

- *New drugs.* By 2010, experts predict a new arsenal of medicines for diseases such as Alzheimer's and multiple sclerosis, which defy treatment today. Genetically targeted drugs will home in on certain conditions, and new, slow-release vaccinations will control diseases such as diabetes.

- *Cancer.* By the year 2015, cancer deaths are expected to drop by 21 percent, with 13 percent fewer people ever getting cancer. Although many of our cancer-producing behaviors (such as smoking) will persist, we will have better methods of genetic screening for risk, targeted vaccines that control certain cancers, and less invasive treatments. Cancer treatment will be less debilitating.

- *Bacteria and infectious diseases.* Infectious diseases are the number one cause of death worldwide, with emergent resurgent diseases on the increase. By 2010, new antibiotics will provide an improved prognosis for resistant diseases, but an as yet undiscovered virus could have the potential to wipe out over one-third of the world's population.

- *Spirituality.* Spirituality training will become a common element of traditional medical training. Insurers will reimburse it, and medical schools will teach alternative medicine.

- *Heart disease.* As baby boomers age, the prevalence of heart disease will increase, but better diagnostic tests will exist and better drug treatment will be developed, including proteins that create small arteries when main arteries are blocked.

- *Colds and flu.* Although there won't be a cure for the cold in 2010, new vaccines will cut the cost of inoculating a child in a developing country from $100 to 10 cents, and drugs will provide great relief for many. A pandemic flu also is projected, however.

- *Foods.* By 2010, we'll have more "medical" foods that combine supplements, micronutrient additives, and medicines to boost nutrient content, protect against disease, and bolster the immune system.

- *Aging.* By 2010, advances in medicine will include a "Methuselah" gene, which currently doubles or triples life span in roundworms; calorie-restricted meals that increase longevity; and proteins that might halt the brain declines found in Alzheimer's disease.[10]

While we've come a long way, the possibilities for health and well-being in the future defy the imagination. Living longer, living more disease-free years, and injecting more quality into the extra years of life will be major goals of the future. The more we learn about the remarkable resilience of the human body and spirit, and the more technology stretches our imagination and expands our possibilities, the more likely that the twenty-first century will rival the twentieth for major health-related achievements.

What do you think?

What do you consider the greatest achievements in public health in the twentieth century? ■ *What do you think will be the greatest health challenges of the twenty-first century?* ■ *What are five actions we could take today that would reduce the impact of these challenges in the future?*

Reducing Health Disparities: New Challenges

The dramatic improvements in the twentieth century in the health and life span of Americans are largely the result of changes in socioeconomic status, nutrition, and reproductive behavior, plus advances in public health, and, more recently, health care services.[11] However, it is important to note that these improvements have not been experienced uniformly by all of the diverse populations of the United States. Reasons for this have to do with who we are, where we live and work, the social and economic policies of our government, and many other factors that play a role in who gets sick and who remains healthy. When it comes to health, we are not all created equal.[12]

Recognizing the vast differences in health status, *Healthy People 2010* included strong language about the importance of reducing **health disparities,** the differences in the incidence, prevalence, mortality, and burden of diseases and other adverse health conditions that exist among specific population groups in the United States. Contributors to disparities include:

- Having no insurance or inadequate insurance
- Racism and other "-isms" that reduce opportunities or cause discrimination
- Inadequate transportation
- Lifestyle behaviors
- Cultural influences
- Diet
- Lack of exercise
- Obesity/overweight
- Sexual behaviors
- Stress
- Mental health issues
- Systemic barriers
- Access to health care
- Poverty
- Environmental factors

The effects of these disparities are seen in the vast differences in life expectancies and rates of chronic diseases (such as diabetes, certain cancers and CVD) by race, sex, and socioeconomic status. For example, people with lower socioeconomic status are most likely to die of tobacco-related problems. Knowing the factors that contribute to these differences and considering what actions might be taken to reduce these actions is a necessary part of any comprehensive efforts to improve the health of Americans.

As you consider each of the health issues raised throughout this text, think about the prevalence of the issue among people from different populations, in different regions of the country or world, and in people of differing races, cultures, gender, socioeconomic status, and other unique characteristics.

What do you think?

Go to the website for Health, United States, 2004 *at www.cdc.gov/nchs, and look up the leading causes of death. What are some noteworthy differences in these death rates based on race?* ■ *Gender?* ■ *Looking at the contributors to disparities listed above, what factors do you think have the greatest impact on these differences?* ■ *What policies, programs, and/or actions do you think would be most important in reducing these disparities?*

Health disparities   Differences in the incidence, prevalence, mortality, and burden of diseases and other health conditions among specific population groups.

Preparing for Better Health in the Twenty-First Century

Although we've made dramatic improvements in many health areas, there are clearly challenges ahead. To make additional strides, people must have a sense of both individual and social responsibility. Although it is important that each of us work to preserve and protect our own health, it is also important to become actively engaged in the health of our communities, our nation, and the global population. The mark of a truly healthy person is whether the individual focuses beyond the "me" aspects of human existence and becomes equally concerned with the "we" aspects of health, as well as having a sense of responsibility about the broader environment that we live in.

Focusing on Global Health Issues

Everyone's health is profoundly affected by economic, social, behavioral, scientific, and technological factors. The world economy has become increasingly interconnected and globalized; every day, 2 million people worldwide move across national borders. Global commerce and communication have benefited people in virtually every country while creating a remarkable degree of mutual interdependence.[13] In addition to their undoubted advantages, however, these changes also bring health risks that cannot be addressed by one country alone. Some obvious examples include infectious diseases, contaminated foodstuffs, terrorism, and illegal or banned toxic substances.[14]

Each of us must do our part to improve our own health, protect the health of others, and work for social justice in related health areas. This requires taking the time to understand the vast differences in health status across various social groups and actively promoting community actions that erase disparities.

What do you think?

What implications do developments in global health have for people living in the United States today? ■ *What international programs, policies, and/or services might help control the world's health problems in the next decade?* ■ *Are there actions that individuals can take to help?*

Focusing on Your Health

In this country, we tend to focus on the leading causes of death rather than those factors that threaten the lives or futures of young Americans. A 20-year-old typically does not view death from a heart attack, stroke, or cancer as an imminent threat; thus, the motivation for behavior change is not as great as it perhaps should be. It is important to consider how your current actions affect you right now and in the future. Also, think about how your actions may affect others and the global environment. For example, do you have days when you're tired all the time or disinterested in what is going on around you? Or perhaps you are a bit dissatisfied with yourself, your friends, your career choices, or other things in your life. In contrast, you probably also have days when you wake up full of energy, when you look forward to the next fun event, and when you later fall into bed exhausted, yet excited about the next day. Some of the time, you probably hear about the latest environmental threat or a catastrophe in another region of the world and "tune in" with great interest. Other times, you can hardly take time to worry about yourself, let alone others. What is the difference between the "blah" version of you and the "actively engaged" version? To a great extent, it probably depends on what you eat, the amount of exercise and sleep you get, the excitement you feel in meeting challenges and being rewarded, and whether you take time to refresh the spiritual side of your life. It also depends on how much time you've taken to inform yourself about community and global health problems. In short, your investment in healthy behaviors contributes to how well you live each day.

By focusing on health behaviors that energize and refresh you, you can become actively engaged in life. If you skip that early morning walk because you can't drag yourself out of bed, if you don't socialize because you are worried about how fat you might look or think you don't have anything to wear, if you find that your interactions with others cause stress, it may be time to reexamine your health status. What are your current health risks? Future health risks? What can you do to improve your current situation? While activities of daily living are performance-based measures typically used to assess functioning in the later years of life, perhaps we need to focus on them much earlier. In addition, rather than rating ourselves based on what everyone else is doing, we need to consider potential differences based on race, socioeconomic opportunity, gender, age, and other variables. It takes effort and sound decision making based on solid evidence to achieve our personal best.

> ### What do you think?
>
> *Based on the wellness dimensions discussed here, what are some of your strengths in each dimension?* ■ *What are some of your deficiencies?* ■ *What one or two things can you do to enhance your strong areas?* ■ *To improve on your weaknesses?*

Gender Differences and Health Status

You don't have to be a health expert to know that there are physiological differences between men and women. Although much of male and female anatomy is identical, major differences exist in susceptibility to disease and other health factors. Many disorders—osteoporosis, multiple sclerosis, and Alzheimer's disease, for example—are far more common in women than in men. Finally, although women live longer than men, they don't necessarily enjoy a better quality of life.[15]

Much of the current interest in exploring women's health came after 1990, when a highly publicized government study raised concern about the uneven numbers of women included in clinical trial research conducted by the National Institutes of Health (NIH). The NIH established the Office of Research on Women's Health (ORWH) in 1990 to oversee the representation of women in NIH studies. According to Vivian Pinn, ORWH's director, "For too long, medicine has viewed women as 'abnormal men' when considering health problems."[16]

Researchers have historically excluded women of childbearing age from clinical trials of many new drugs. One reason has been a concern about whether a medication might harm a fetus; another has been that women's menstrual cycles can influence the effects of a drug. Of course, men and women do vary physiologically, so the elimination of women from many studies means that the results from these studies cannot be applied to women directly. According to social psychologist Carol Tavris, "If you want to know the effects of Drug X and you throw women out of your study because the menstrual cycle affects their responses to medication, you cannot then extrapolate from your study of men to women, precisely because the menstrual cycle affects their responses to medication."[17] To address these concerns, the government has specified that equal amounts of money and time must be spent on men's and women's health research.[18] The National Heart, Blood, and Lung Institute is conducting the **Women's Health Initiative (WHI),** a 15-year, $625 million study focusing on the leading causes of death and disease in more than 160,000 postmenopausal women. WHI researchers hope to find out how a healthful lifestyle and increased medical attention can help prevent women's cancers, heart disease, and osteoporosis.[19] The breakthrough discoveries about hormone replacement therapy (page 4) are part of the WHI.

> ### What do you think?
>
> *Do you think there are true disparities between men's and women's health status?* ■ *What are some indicators or examples?* ■ *Can you think of programs, policies, or individual actions that would reduce such disparities?*

Women's Health Initiative (WHI) National study of postmenopausal women conducted in conjunction with the NIH mandate for equal research priorities for women's health issues.

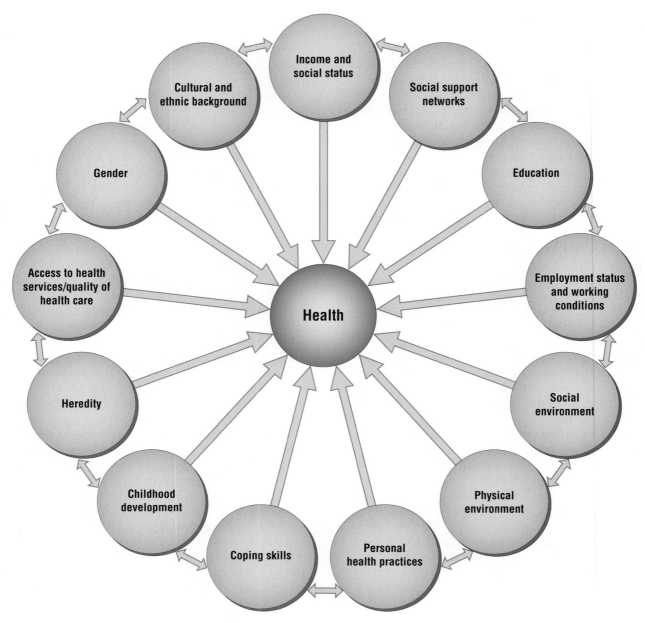

Figure 1.2
Key Determinants of Health
All of the factors shown influence your health. Can you think of others? How do these factors affect each other?

Improving Your Health

Table 1.2 summarizes the leading causes of death in the United States, by age. Note that Americans aged 15–24 are most likely to die from unintentional injuries, followed by homicide and suicide. Unintentional injuries are also the major killer in the next age group, ages 25–44, followed by malignant neoplasms and heart diseases.

Individual behavior is a major determinant of good health, but heredity, access to health care, and the environment can also influence health status (Figure 1.2). When these

factors are considered together and form the basis of a person's lifestyle choices, the net effect on health can be great.

Change is not always easy. All of us, no matter where we are on the wellness continuum, have to start somewhere. All people have faced personal and external challenges to their attempts to change health behaviors—some have not done so well, some have been extremely successful, and some have made only small changes that add up to significant improvements in how they feel and how they live. The key is to identify the behaviors most in need of change, determine goals and the actions necessary to achieve them,

Table 1.2
Leading Causes of Death in the United States by Age (Years), 2002

Rank	All Ages	Under 1 Year	1–4	5–14	15–24	25–44	45–64	65+
1.	Heart diseases 696,947	Congenital anomalies 5,623	Unintentional injuries 1,641	Unintentional injuries 2,718	Unintentional injuries 15,412	Unintentional injuries 29,279	Malignant neoplasms 143,028	Heart diseases 576,301
2.	Malignant neoplasms 557,271	Short gestation or low birth weight 4,410	Congenital anomalies 530	Malignant neoplasms 1,072	Homicide 5,219	Malignant neoplasms 19,957	Heart diseases 101,804	Malignant neoplasms 391,001
3.	Cerebrovascular diseases 162,672	Sudden infant death syndrome 2,234	Homicide 423	Congenital anomalies 417	Suicide 4,010	Heart diseases 16,853	Unintentional injuries 23,020	Cerebrovascular diseases 143,293
4.	Chronic lower respiratory diseases 124,816	Maternal complications 1,499	Malignant neoplasms 402	Homicide 356	Malignant neoplasms 1,730	Suicide 11,897	Cerebrovascular diseases 15,952	Chronic lower respiratory diseases 108,313
5.	Unintentional injuries 106,742	Complications of placenta, cord, membranes 1,018	Heart diseases 165	Suicide 264	Heart diseases 1,022	Homicide 7,728	Diabetes mellitus 15,518	Influenza and pneumonia 58,826
6.	Diabetes mellitus 73,249	Respiratory distress 1,011	Influenza and pneumonia 110	Heart diseases 255	Congenital anomalies 492	HIV 7,546	Chronic lower respiratory diseases 14,755	Alzheimer's disease 58,289
7.	Influenza and pneumonia 65,681	Unintentional injuries 976	Septicemia 79	Chronic lower respiratory diseases 136	Chronic lower respiratory diseases 192	Chronic liver disease and cirrhosis 3,528	Chronic liver disease and cirrhosis 13,313	Diabetes mellitus 54,715
8.	Alzheimer's disease 58,866	Bacterial sepsis 696	Conditions of perinatal period 72	Influenza and pneumonia 91	HIV 178	Cerebrovascular diseases 2,992	Suicide 9,926	Nephritis, nephritic syndrome, and nephrosis 34,316
9.	Nephritis, nephritic syndrome, and nephrosis 40,974	Diseases of circulatory system 622	In situ and benign neoplasms 60	Cerebrovascular diseases 91	Cerebrovascular diseases 171	Diabetes mellitus 2,806	HIV 5,821	Unintentional injuries 33,641
10.	Septicemia 33,865	Intrauterine hypoxia/birth asphyxia 534	Cerebrovascular diseases 53	In situ and benign neoplasms 89	Influenza and pneumonia 167	Influenza and pneumonia 1,316	Nephritis, nephritic syndrome, and nephrosis 5,348	Septicemia 26,670

Source: K. Kochanek, et al., "Deaths: Final Data for 2002," *National Vital Statistics Reports* 53, no. 5 (Hyattsville, MD: National Center for Health Statistics, 2004).

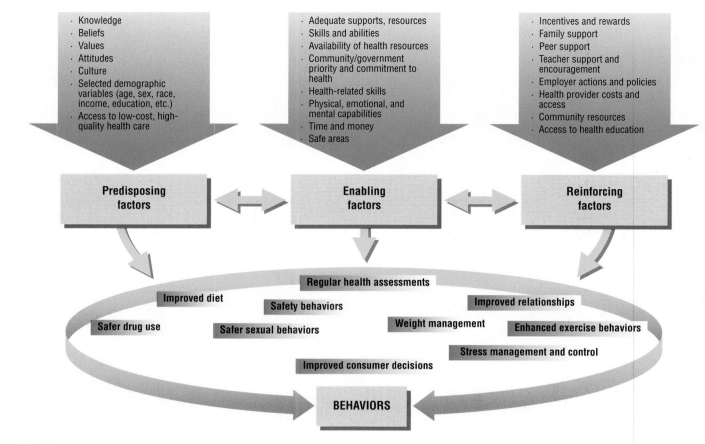

Figure 1.3
Factors That Influence Behavior-Change Decisions

set up a plan of action, and get started. But first, it is important to take a look at factors that contribute to current patterns of behavior.

Changing Your Health Behaviors

Mark Twain said that "habit is habit, and not to be flung out the window by anyone, but coaxed downstairs a step at a time." The chances of successfully changing negative habits improve when you identify a key behavior that you want to change and develop a plan for gradual change that allows you time to unlearn negative patterns and substitute positive ones. Many experts advocate dissecting a given health behavior into smaller parts and working on them one at a time in "baby steps" (see the Skills for Behavior Change box on page 26).

First, identify what is most important to you or what causes you the greatest immediate and long-term risks. For example, if you are concerned about your weight, assess your eating patterns and decide where you can make changes that you can live with. Too many of us decide on New Year's Day that we are going to lose weight, exercise more, find more friends, and essentially reinvent ourselves overnight! Is it any wonder that we don't keep most of these resolutions?

Factors That Influence Behavior Change

Figure 1.3 identifies major factors that influence behavior and behavior change decisions. They can be divided into three general categories: predisposing, enabling, and reinforcing.

Predisposing Factors   Our life experiences, knowledge, cultural and ethnic inheritance, and current beliefs and values are all *predisposing factors* influencing behavior and behavior change. Factors that may predispose us to certain conditions include age, sex, race, income, family background, educational background, and access to health care. For example, if your parents smoked, you are 90 percent more likely to start smoking than someone whose parents didn't. If your peers smoke, you are 80 percent more likely to smoke than someone whose friends don't.

Enabling Factors   Skills and abilities; physical, emotional, and mental capabilities; and resources and accessible facilities that make health decisions more convenient or difficult are *enabling factors*. Positive enablers encourage you to carry through on your intentions. Negative enablers work against your intentions to change. For example, if you would like to join a local fitness center but discover that the closest one is four miles away and the membership fee is $500, those negative enablers may convince you to stay home. On the other hand, if your school's fitness center is two blocks away, stays open until midnight, and offers a special student membership, those positive enablers will probably convince you to join. Identifying positive and negative enabling factors and devising alternative plans when the negative factors outweigh the positive are part of planning for behavior change.

Reinforcing Factors *Reinforcing factors* include the presence or absence of support, encouragement, or discouragement that significant people in your life bring to a situation. For example, if you decide to stop smoking and your family and friends continue smoking in your presence, you may be tempted to start smoking again. In other words, your smoking behavior was reinforced. If, however, you are overweight, you lose a few pounds, and all your friends tell you how terrific you look, then your positive behavior will be reinforced and you will be more likely to continue your weight-loss plan.

The manner in which you reward or punish yourself also plays a role. Accepting small failures and concentrating on your successes can foster further achievements. Berating yourself because you binged on ice cream or argued with a friend may create an internal environment in which failure becomes almost inevitable. Telling yourself that you're worth the extra time and effort and giving yourself a pat on the back for small accomplishments are often overlooked factors in positive behavior change.

Motivation

Wanting to change is a prerequisite of the change process, but there is much more to the process than motivation. Motivation must be combined with common sense, commitment, and a realistic understanding of how best to move from point A to point B.[20] *Readiness* is the state of being that precedes behavior change. People who are ready to change possess the knowledge, attitudes, skills, and internal and external resources that make change a likely reality. For someone to be ready for change, certain basic steps and adjustments in thinking must occur. The Skills for Behavior Change box on the following page describes the *Stages of Change* model of health behavior change.

Some of us need a little boost before we are able to change our behaviors. Rewards, or incentives for successfully reaching goals that we set, are effective ways to keep ourselves on track. Several studies have pointed out that those who set up a system of rewards for behavioral change are often successful. For example, allow yourself something that you really enjoy after losing 5 pounds, rather than depriving yourself until you lose all 30 of the pounds that you want to lose.[21]

Beliefs and Attitudes

We often assume that when rational people realize there is a risk in what they are doing, they will act to reduce that risk. But this is not necessarily true. Consider the number of health professionals who smoke, consume junk food, and act in other unhealthful ways. They surely know better, but their "knowing" is disconnected from their "doing." Why is this so? Two strong influences on behavior are beliefs and attitudes.

A **belief** is an appraisal of the relationship between some object, action, or idea (for example, smoking) and some attribute of that object, action, or idea (for example, smoking is expensive, dirty, and causes cancer—or it is relaxing). Beliefs may develop from direct experience (perhaps you have trouble breathing after smoking for several years) or from secondhand experience or knowledge conveyed by other people (maybe you watched your grandfather, a longtime smoker, die of lung cancer).[22] An **attitude** is a relatively stable set of beliefs, feelings, and behavioral tendencies in relation to something or someone.

Do Beliefs and Attitudes Influence Behavior? It seems logical to conclude that your beliefs will influence your behavior. If you believe (make the appraisal) that taking drugs (an action) is harmful (attribute of that action), you will not use drugs. If you believe that drinking and driving are incompatible, you will never drink and drive. Or will you?

Psychologists studying the relationship between beliefs and health behaviors have determined that although beliefs may subtly influence behavior, they may not actually cause people to change behavior. In 1966, psychologist I. Rosenstock developed a classic theory, the **Health Belief Model (HBM)**, to show when beliefs affect behavior change.[23]

Belief Appraisal of the relationship between some object, action, or idea and some attribute of that object, action, or idea.

Attitude Relatively stable set of beliefs, feelings, and behavioral tendencies in relation to something or someone.

Health Belief Model (HBM) Model for explaining how beliefs may influence behaviors.

Staging for Change

On any given morning, many of us get out of bed and resolve to change a given behavior that day. Whether it be losing weight, drinking less, exercising more, being nicer to others, managing time better, or some other change, we start out with enthusiasm and high expectations. Within a short time, however, a vast majority of people return to doing whatever it was they thought they shouldn't be doing.

Why do so many good intentions fail? According to Dr. James Prochaska, University of Rhode Island, and Dr. Carlos DiClemente, University of Maryland, it's because we are going about things in the wrong way. According to Prochaska and DiClemente, fewer than 20 percent of us are really prepared to take action. Yet, health professionals continue to exhort us to "Just Do It! And do it now!" After considerable research, Prochaska and DiClemente believe that behavior changes usually do not succeed if they start with the change itself. Instead, we must go through a series of stages to adequately prepare ourselves for that eventual change. Our chances of keeping those New Year's resolutions will be greatly enhanced if we have proper reinforcement and help during each of the following stages.

1. *Precontemplation.* People in the precontemplation stage have no current intention of changing. They may have tried to change a behavior before and given up, or they may be in denial and unaware of any problem.
Strategies for Change: Sometimes a few frank yet kind words from friends may be enough to make precontemplators take a closer look at themselves. This is not to say that you should become a warrior against pleasure or tell people what to do when they haven't asked for advice. Recommending readings or tactful suggestions, however, can be useful in helping precontemplators consider making a change.

2. *Contemplation.* In this phase, people recognize that they have a problem and begin to contemplate the need to change. Acknowledgment usually results from increased awareness, often due to feedback from family and friends or access to information. Despite this acknowledgment, people can languish in this stage for years, realizing that they have a problem but lacking the time or energy to make the change.
Strategies for Change: Often, contemplators need a little push to get them started. This may come in the form of helping them set up a change plan (for example, an exercise routine), buying a helpful gift (such as a low-fat cookbook), sharing articles about a particular problem, or inviting them to go with you to hear a speaker on a related topic. People often need time to think about a course of action or to build a skill. Your assistance can help them move off the point of indecision.

3. *Preparation.* Most people at this point are close to taking action. They've thought about what they might do and may even have come up with a plan. Rather than thinking about why they can't begin, they have started to focus on what they can do.
Strategies for Change: Follow a few standard guidelines: Set realistic goals (large and small), take small steps toward change, change only a couple of things at once, reward small milestones, and seek support from friends. Identify those factors that have enabled success or served as a barrier to success in the past, and modify them where possible. Fill out the Behavior Change Contract in this book to help you commit to making these changes.

4. *Action.* In this stage, people begin to follow their action plans. Those who have prepared for change, thought about alternatives, engaged social support, and made a plan of action are more ready for action than those who have given it little thought. Unfortunately, too many people start behavior change here rather than going through the first three stages. Without a plan, without enlisting the help of others, or without a realistic goal, failure is likely.
Strategies for Change: Publicly stating the desire to change helps ensure success. Encourage friends who are making a change to share their plans with you. Offer to help, and try to remove potential obstacles from the person's intended action plan. Social support and the buddy system can motivate even the most reluctant person.

5. *Maintenance.* Maintenance requires vigilance, attention to detail, and long-term commitment. Many people reach a goal, only to relax and slip back into the undesired behavior. In this stage, it is important to be aware of the potential for relapses and to develop strategies for dealing with such challenges. Common causes of relapse include overconfidence, daily temptations, stress or emotional distractions, and self-deprecation.
Strategies for Change: During maintenance, continue taking the same actions that led to success in the first place. Find fun and creative ways to maintain positive behaviors. This is where a willing and caring support group can be vital. Knowing where on your campus to turn for help when you don't have a close support network is also helpful.

6. *Termination.* By this point, the behavior is so ingrained that the current level of vigilance may be unnecessary. The new behavior has become an essential part of daily living. Can you think of someone you know who has made a major behavior change that has now become an essential part of that person's life?

Source: J. O. Prochaska, and C. C. DiClemente, "Stages and Processes of Self-change of Smoking: Toward an Integrative Model of Change," *Journal of Consulting and Clinical Psychology* 51 (1983), 390–395.

Although many other models attempt to explain the influence of beliefs on behaviors, the HBM remains one of the most widely accepted. It holds that several factors must support a belief before change is likely:

- *Perceived seriousness of the health problem.* How severe would the medical and social consequences be if the health problem was to develop or be left untreated? The more serious the perceived effects, the more likely that action will be taken.
- *Perceived susceptibility to the health problem.* Next, what is the likelihood of developing the health problem? People who perceive themselves at high risk are more likely to take preventive action.
- *Cues to action.* Those who are reminded or alerted about a potential health problem are more likely to take action.

Three other factors are linked to perceived risk for health problems: *demographic variables*, including age, gender, race, and ethnic background; *sociopsychological variables*, including personality traits, social class, and social pressure; and *structural variables*, including knowledge about or prior contact with the health problem.

The Health Belief Model is followed many times every day. Take, for example, smokers. Older smokers are likely to know other smokers who have developed serious heart or lung problems as a result of smoking. They are thus more likely to perceive tobacco as a threat to their health than does a teenager who has just begun smoking. The greater the perceived threat of health problems caused by smoking, the greater the chance a person will quit. However, many chronic smokers know the risks yet continue to smoke. Why do they fail to take actions to avoid further harm? According to Rosenstock, some people do not believe that they will be affected by a severe problem—they act as if they believe they have some kind of immunity—and are unlikely to change their behaviors. In some cases, they may think that even if they get cancer or have a heart attack, the health care system will cure them. They also may feel that the immediate pleasure outweighs the long-range cost.

Intentions to Change

Our attitudes tend to reflect our emotional responses to situations and also tend to follow from our beliefs. According to the **Theory of Reasoned Action,** our behaviors result from our intentions to perform actions. An intention is a product of our attitude toward an action and our beliefs about what others may want us to do.[24] A behavioral intention, then, is a written or stated commitment to perform an action.

In brief, the more consistent and powerful your attitudes about an action and the more you are influenced by others to take that action, the greater will be your stated intention to do so. The more you verbalize your commitment to change, the more likely you are to succeed.

Significant Others as Change Agents

Many of us are highly influenced by the approval or disapproval (real or imagined) of close friends, loved ones, and the social and cultural groups to which we belong. Such influences can support healthy behavior, or they can interfere with even the best intentions.

Your Family From the time of your birth, your parents have given you strong cues about which actions are socially acceptable and which are not. Brushing your teeth, bathing, wearing deodorant, and chewing food with your mouth closed are probably all behaviors that your family instilled in you long ago. Your family culture influenced your food choices, your religious beliefs, your political beliefs, and all your other values and actions. If you deviated from your family's norms, your mother or father probably let you know fairly quickly. Good family units share a dedication to the healthful development of all family members, unconditional trust, and a commitment to work out difficulties.

When the loving family unit does not exist, when it does not provide for basic human needs, or when dysfunctional, irresponsible individuals try to build a family under the influence of drugs or alcohol, it becomes difficult for a child to learn positive health behaviors. Healthy behaviors get their start in healthy homes; unhealthy homes breed unhealthy habits. Healthy families provide the foundation for a clear and necessary understanding of what is right and wrong, what is positive and negative. Without this fundamental grounding, many young people have great difficulties.[25]

Your Social Bonds Like family, personal environments also mold behaviors. If you deviated from the actions expected in your hometown, you probably suffered strange looks, ostracism by some high school cliques, and other negative social reactions. The more you value the opinions of other people, the more likely you are to change a behavior that offends them. If you couldn't care less what they think, you probably brush off their negative reactions or suggested changes. How often have you told yourself, "I don't care what so-and-so thinks. I'll do what I darn well please"? Although most of us have thought or said these words, often we care too much about what even the insignificant people in our lives think. In general, the lower your level of self-esteem and self-efficacy, the higher the chances that others will influence your actions.

Sometimes, the influence of others can be a powerful social support for positive behavior changes.[26] At other times, we are influenced to drink too much, party too hard,

> **Theory of Reasoned Action** Model for explaining the importance of our intentions in determining behaviors.

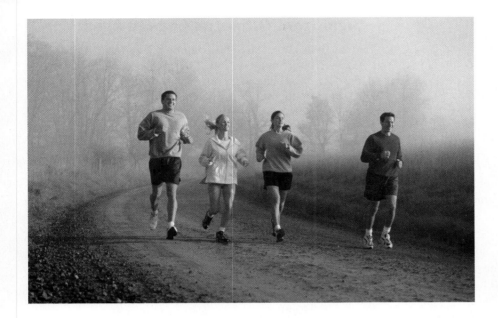

The support and encouragement of friends who have similar goals and interests will strengthen your commitment to develop and maintain positive health behaviors.

eat too much, or engage in some other negative action because we don't want to be left out or criticized. Understanding the subtle and not-so-subtle ways in which other people influence our actions is an important step toward changing our behaviors.

Choosing a Behavior-Change Strategy

Once you have analyzed all the factors that influence what you do, you must decide which behavior-change technique will work best for you. Options include shaping, visualization, modeling, controlling the situation, reinforcement, and changing self-talk.

Shaping

Regardless of how motivated you are, some behaviors are almost impossible to change immediately. To reach your goal, you may need to take a number of individual steps, each designed to change one small piece of the larger behavior. This process is known as **shaping.**

For example, suppose that you have not exercised for a while. You decide that you want to get into shape, and your goal is to be able to jog three to four miles every other day.

> **Shaping**   Using a series of small steps to gradually achieve a particular goal.
>
> **Imagined rehearsal**   Practicing, through mental imagery, to become better able to perform an event in actuality.

You realize that you'd face a near-death experience if you tried to run even just a few blocks in your current condition. So you decide to start slowly and build up to your desired fitness level gradually. During week 1, you will walk for one hour every other day at a slow, relaxed pace. During week 2, you will walk for the same amount of time but will speed up your pace and cover slightly more ground. During week 3, you will speed up even more and will try to go even farther. You will continue taking such steps until you reach your goal.

Whatever the desired behavior change, all shaping involves the following items:

- Starting slowly and trying not to cause undue stress during the early stages of the program.
- Keeping the steps small and achievable.
- Being flexible and ready to change if the original plan proves uncomfortable.
- Refusing to skip steps or to move to the next step until the previous step has been mastered.

Behaviors don't develop overnight, so they won't change overnight.

Visualization

Mental practice and rehearsal can help change unhealthy behaviors into healthy ones. Athletes and others use a technique known as **imagined rehearsal** to reach their goals. By visualizing their planned action ahead of time, they will be prepared when they put themselves to the test.

For example, suppose you want to ask someone out on a date. Imagine the setting for the action (walking together to class). Then practice in your mind and out loud exactly what you're going to say ("Mary, there's a great concert this Sunday, and I was wondering if . . ."). Mentally anticipate different responses ("Oh, I'd love to, but I'm busy that evening") and what you will say in reaction ("How about if I call you sometime this week?"). Careful mental and verbal rehearsal (you could even try out your scenario on a good friend) will greatly improve the likelihood of success.

Modeling

Modeling, or learning behaviors through careful observation of other people, is one of the most effective strategies for changing behavior. For example, suppose that you have trouble talking to people you don't know very well. One of the easiest ways to improve your communication skills is to select friends whose "gift of gab" you envy. Observe their social skills. Do they talk more or listen more? How do people respond to them? Why are they such good communicators? If you carefully observe behaviors you admire and isolate their components, you can model the steps of your behavior-change strategy on a proven success.

Controlling the Situation

Sometimes, the right setting or the right group of people will positively influence your behaviors. Many situations and occasions trigger certain actions. For example, in libraries, houses of worship, and museums, most people talk softly. Few people laugh at funerals. The term **situational inducement** refers to an attempt to influence a behavior by using situations and occasions to control it.

For example, you may be more apt to stop smoking if you work in a smoke-free office, a positive situational inducement. But a smoke-filled bar, a negative situational inducement, may tempt you to resume. Careful consideration of which settings will help and which will hurt your effort to change, and your decision to seek the first and avoid the second, will improve your chances for change.

Reinforcement

A **positive reinforcement** seeks to increase the likelihood that a behavior will occur by presenting something positive as a reward for it. Each of us is motivated by different reinforcers. Although a special T-shirt may be a positive reinforcer for young adults entering a race, it would not be for a 40-year-old runner who dislikes message-bearing T-shirts.

Most positive reinforcers can be classified under five headings: consumable, activity, manipulative, possessional, and social.

- *Consumable reinforcers* are delicious edibles such as candy, cookies, or gourmet meals.
- *Activity reinforcers* are opportunities to watch TV, go on a vacation, go swimming, or do something else enjoyable.
- *Manipulative reinforcers* are incentives such as lower rent in exchange for mowing the lawn or the promise of a better grade for doing an extra-credit project.
- *Possessional reinforcers* are tangible rewards such as a new TV or sports car.

- *Social reinforcers* are signs of appreciation, approval, or love, such as loving looks, affectionate hugs, and praise.

When choosing reinforcers, determine what would motivate you to act in a particular way. Research has shown that people can be motivated to change their behaviors, such as not smoking during pregnancy or abstaining from cocaine, if they set themselves up on a *token economy* system, whereby they earn tokens or points that can be exchanged for meaningful rewards such as financial incentives.[27] The difficulty often lies in determining *which* incentive will be most effective. Your reinforcers may initially come from others (extrinsic rewards); but as you see positive changes in yourself, you will begin to reward and reinforce yourself (intrinsic rewards). Keep in mind that reinforcers should immediately follow a behavior, but beware of overkill. If you reward yourself with a movie every time you go jogging, this reinforcer will soon lose its power. It would be better to give yourself this reward after, say, a full week of adherence to your jogging program.

What do you think?

What consumable reinforcers (food or drink) would be a healthy reward for your new behavior? ■ *If you could choose one activity reinforcer to reward yourself after one day of success in your new behavior, what would it be?* ■ *If you could obtain something (possessional reinforcer) after you reach your goal, what would it be?* ■ *If you maintain your behavior for one week, what type of social reinforcer would you like to receive from your friends?*

Changing Self-Talk

Self-talk, or the way you think and talk to yourself, can also play a role in modifying health-related behaviors. Here are some cognitive procedures for changing self-talk.

Rational-Emotive Therapy   This form of cognitive therapy, or self-directed behavior change, is based on the premise that there is a close connection between what people say to themselves and how they feel. According to psychologist Albert Ellis, most everyday emotional problems and related

---

Modeling   Learning specific behaviors by watching others perform them.

Situational inducement   Attempt to influence a behavior through situations and occasions that are structured to exert control over that behavior.

Positive reinforcement   Presenting something positive following a behavior that is being reinforced.

Evaluating Personal Risk

A simple glance at newspaper headlines or a session watching the evening news can easily make your hair stand on end. Anthrax, West Nile virus, polluted water, diabetes, HIV, and a host of other health risks seem to be stalking us. Making sense of these potential threats is often challenging and requires an understanding of the concept of *risk*. Essentially, risk implies that there is some chance that something bad may happen to you. The question is when it is likely to happen. Is it inevitable? Is it something you can prevent through changes in your own behavior?

Clearly, each of us is born with a genetic propensity toward certain risks. Diseases like diabetes, sickle-cell anemia, and hypercholesterolemia are among a long list of diseases that appear to have distinct genetic links. If your grandparents and parents had one of these conditions, chances are increased that you will also have that disease.

Another factor that increases your risk is age, or relative longevity. If you live long enough, you will be likely to develop certain conditions, such as arthritis, certain memory-sapping dementias, several of the cardiovascular diseases, and various forms of cancer. For example, although you may hear that a woman has a 1 in 8 chance of contracting breast cancer, in truth, that is a woman's risk in the later years of her life. The risk is much lower for women in their twenties and thirties. A quick look at the leading causes of death by age (see Table 1.2 on page 23) indicates which risks are greatest for each age group.

Other factors that increase your risk include the environment that you live in, your exposure to toxic chemicals, your socioeconomic status, your ethnic background, and lifestyle behaviors. These and a host of other factors, either individually or collectively, can spell health or disease risk for each of us.

QUESTIONS TO ASK

When we can read information that tells us that we are at risk, many of us are left wondering what we can do to reduce our risk or whether we should believe all of the hype to begin with. Although there are many reputable sources of information available, the best place to start is by checking information from government agencies, institutions of higher education resources, or top-ranked peer-reviewed journals. (Such journals require a panel of professional experts review the scientific merits of a study and resultant health claims and determine whether the claims are valid and/or reliable.) There are several additional things that you can do to ensure that you are getting the most accurate information available.

1. *Cross-check the information from two or three of the above sources.* Are they basically saying the same thing? Is conflicting information being given? If there is conflicting information, you'll need to continue your search and confirm information with additional sources.

2. *Is the source reliable?* Just because a magazine is published and in your library doesn't mean that it uses good science in making health claims. Even in your doctor's office, you may find trade magazines that publish articles written by people who may be good writers but lack sufficient expertise to make the claims that they are making or by people who are paying for space to advertise and have a vested interest in making a claim, even though it may be false.

3. *What are the credentials of the authors?* Just because someone has a PhD, MD, or other set of initials behind his or her name doesn't mean that he or she is an expert. For example, someone with a PhD in counseling may decide to write about a particular exercise program, or a medical doctor with little background in the area may decide to write an article about teen pregnancy. Look for information on the specific background of the authors. What are their degrees in? Where are they working now? Have they published related research in peer-reviewed journals? Those working, teaching, or doing research in the area that they are writing about have more credibility than those who are not in the field.

4. *Where does the research come from?* Who paid for the research? Was it a drug company, business, or service provider who may have a vested interest in a particular outcome?

5. *What research methods were used?* Was it part of a randomized, controlled trial that is representative of the people being studied and about whom the claims are being made? Taking a course in research methods and basic statistics while in college will help you assess the merits of a particular study. In general, studies that include randomized, controlled samples that are applicable to populations are the

behaviors stem from irrational statements that people make to themselves when events in their lives are different from what they would like them to be.[28]

For example, suppose that after doing poorly on an exam, you say to yourself, "I can't believe I flunked that easy exam. I'm so stupid." By changing this irrational, "catastrophic" self-talk into rational, positive statements about

what is really going on, you can increase the likelihood that positive behaviors will occur. Positive self-talk might be phrased as follows: "I really didn't study enough for that exam, and I'm not surprised I didn't do very well. I'm certainly not stupid. I just need to prepare better for the next test." Such self-talk will help you to recover quickly from disappointment and take positive steps to correct the situation.

most reliable. However, be careful not to make decisions about risk based on the results of only one study that hits the nightly news. Compare the characteristics of more and less reliable research studies:

Less reliable

Small number of subjects (small sample size)

Unpublished (and therefore not likely to have been peer-reviewed)

Not repeated (so results may have been a fluke)

Tests performed on nonhuman subjects but results are extrapolated to humans

Results not related to group in question (for example, men vs. women)

No limitations mentioned

Not compared to other research

Author credentials unclear

More reliable

Larger number of subjects (larger sample size)

Published in peer-reviewed journal

Results verified in multiple studies

Tests performed on human subjects and results are interpreted for humans

Results related to group in question (for example, men vs. women)

Limitations discussed

Compared to other research

Author credentials clear

6. *How does this risk compare to others?* While you may very well be afraid of being killed in an airplane crash, statistically your risk is much smaller than that of being killed while driving your car to campus each day. Keeping your risk in perspective is an important factor in being able to rationally cope with life's challenges.

7. *Is the risk real?* Sometimes health risks are sensationalized or played up in the media because of their shock value rather than because they are real risks for you. For example, you may hear a lot about a murder in your area (although chances are low that you would be a victim) and not hear much at all about the fact that a sexually transmitted infection is raging through the campus community. You might be led to worry about a small risk that appears to be big and to ignore big risks that appear to be small.

8. *What do the numbers really mean?* If rates are listed as 1 in 100, remember that this is the same as 1 percent, or 10 in 1,000, or 10,000 out of 1 million. Normally health risks are listed per 100,000 people.

Remember that when you consider risks you should look at your risk at a particular point in time, whether you are looking at it today or in 30 years. Then, consider what science tells you is the best course of action for reducing risk. Also, consider these questions:

✔ What actions are best for me? Which are most compatible with my current situation? How much time/effort am I really willing to invest? What sacrifices will I have to make for a given result?

✔ Where can I find information that will help me make a better decision?

KNOW YOUR "RISK" TERMINOLOGY

Once you've evaluated whether there is a real risk for you, you should also familiarize yourself with the risk terminology that is typically used in reporting epidemiological data.

Risk-specific attack rate is the number of persons who became ill who reported the risk behavior divided by the total number of people who reported the risk behavior. For example, if 150 students went to a dormitory picnic, all ate warm potato salad, and 30 got sick, there would be 30 cases and 120 noncases for an attack rate of 25 percent.

Relative risk is the attack rate among those exposed to the risk factor divided by the attack rate in those who were not exposed. If those who ate potato salad were no more likely to become ill than those who did not, the attack rates would be equal and the relative risk would be 1. If those who ate potato salad were more likely to become ill than those who did not, this ratio would be greater than 1, and potato salad would be a risk factor for illness.

Overall, knowing what the terms mean, assessing the reliability and validity of the source, and keeping abreast of new studies will help you have a better understanding of what the threats to your health are and what you can do to reduce risk. Careful study of the information found in the following chapters should provide the necessary foundation for risk reduction.

Sources: Health Insight, "A Consumer's Guide to Taking Charge of Health Information," August 2002, www.healthinsight .harvard.edu/guide.html; and K. E. Nelson, C. Williams, and N. Graham, *Infectious Disease Epidemiology: Theory and Practice* (Aspen Publishers, 2001), 140–142.

Meichenbaum's Self-Instructional Methods   In Meichenbaum's behavioral therapies, clients are encouraged to give themselves self-instructions ("Slow down, don't rush") and positive affirmations ("My speech is going fine—I'm almost done!") instead of self-defeating thoughts ("I'm talking too fast—my speech is terrible") whenever a situation seems to be getting out of control. Behavioral psychologist Donald Meichenbaum is perhaps best known for a process known as stress inoculation, which subjects clients to extreme stressors in a laboratory environment. Before a stressful event (for example, going to the doctor), clients practice individual coping skills (such as deep-breathing exercises) and self-instructions ("I'll feel better once I know what's causing my pain"). Meichenbaum demonstrated that clients who practiced coping techniques and self-instruction were less likely to resort to negative behaviors in stressful situations.

OBSTACLE	STRATEGY
Stress (intrinsic and extrinsic)	Identify potential sources of stress. Find constructive ways to lower stress level.
Social pressures to repeat old habits	Enlist the support of friends. Identify specifics of these pressures.
Not accepting mistakes, being a perfectionist, hypercritical	Accept that slips are inevitable, but maintain control. Acknowledge that humans are imperfect beings.
Self-blame for poor coping or a weak personality	Blame pressures from the environment or lack of skills, rather than innate weakness.
Lack of effort, lack of motivation	Assess effort and make sure it is adequate. Provide rewards for successes.
Faulty beliefs, low self-efficacy	Develop new skills, focus on successes, and plan ahead for difficult situations. Change self-talk.

Figure 1.4

Overcoming Obstacles to Behavior Change

There are several types of obstacles that can make it difficult to succeed in making a behavior change. Each strategy can help overcome these obstacles.

Source: From *Self-Directed Behavior: Self-Modification for Personal Adjustment,* 7th ed. by D. L. Watson and R. G. Tharp. © 1997 Reprinted with permission of Wadsworth Publishing, a division of Thomson Learning. www.thomsonrights.com. Fax 800-730-2215.

Blocking/Thought Stopping By purposefully blocking or stopping negative thoughts, a person can concentrate on taking positive steps toward behavior change. For example, suppose you are preoccupied with your ex-partner, who has recently deserted you for someone else. You consciously stop thinking about the situation and force yourself to think about something more pleasant (perhaps dinner tomorrow with your best friend). By refusing to dwell on negative images and forcing yourself to focus elsewhere, you can avoid wasting energy, time, and emotional resources and move on to positive change.

Changing Your Behavior

Many strategies have proved effective in making behavior changes. Before you begin this process, take stock of what has contributed to maintaining the behavior.

Self-Assessment: Antecedents and Consequences

Behaviors, thoughts, and feelings always occur in a context—the situation. Situations can be divided into two components: the events that come before and after. Antecedents are the setting events for a behavior; they cue or stimulate a person to act in certain ways. Antecedents can be physical events, thoughts, emotions, or the actions of other people. Consequences—the results of behavior—affect whether a person will repeat a behavior.[29] Consequences can also consist of physical events, thoughts, emotions, or the actions of other people.

Suppose you are shy and must give a speech in front of a large class. The antecedents include walking into the class, feeling frightened, wondering if you are capable of doing a good job, and being unable to remember a word of your speech. If the consequences are negative—if your classmates make fun of you or you get a low grade—your terror about speaking in public will be reinforced, and you will continue to dread this kind of event. In contrast, if you receive positive feedback from the class and instructor, you may actually learn to like speaking in public.

Learning to recognize the antecedents of a behavior and acting to modify them is one method of changing behavior. A diary noting your undesirable behaviors and identifying the settings in which they occur can be a useful tool. Figure 1.4 identifies several factors that can make behavior change more difficult.

Analyzing Personal Behavior

Successful behavior change requires determining what you want to change. All too often we berate ourselves by using generalities: "I'm lousy to my friends; I need to be a better person." Determining the specific behavior you would like to change—in contrast to the general problem—will allow you to set clear goals. What are you doing that makes you a lousy friend? Are you gossiping or lying about your friends? Have you been a taker rather than a giver? Or are you really a good friend most of the time? Let's say the problem is gossiping. You can now analyze this behavior by examining the following components:

- *Frequency.* How often are you gossiping—all the time or only once in a while?
- *Duration.* How long have you been doing this?
- *Seriousness.* Is your gossiping just idle chatter, or are you really trying to injure the other person? What are the consequences for you? For your friend? For your friendship?
- *Basis for problem behavior.* Is your gossip based on facts, perceptions of facts, or deliberate embellishment of the truth?
- *Antecedents.* What kinds of situations trigger your gossiping? Do some settings or people bring out the gossip in you more than others? What triggers your feelings of dislike for or irritation toward your friends? Why are you talking behind their backs?

Decision Making: Choices for Change

Choosing among alternatives isn't easy, particularly when friends, family, media influences, and pleasurable options tempt you. "Just saying no" is usually easier said than done. However, if you are trying to fit in, be liked, or satisfy other emotional needs, decision making will become even more difficult. That's why anticipating what might occur in a given setting and thinking through all possible safe alternatives is important as you implement behavior changes.

For example, knowing that you are likely to be offered a drink when you go to a party, what kind of response could you make that would be okay in your social group? If someone is flirting with you and the situation takes on a distinct sexual overtone, what might you do to prevent the situation from turning bad? Advance preparation will help you stick to your behavior plan.

Fill out a Behavior Change Contract (Figure 1.5) to help you set a goal, anticipate obstacles, and create strategies to overcome those obstacles. Remember that things typically don't "just happen." Making a commitment by completing a contract helps you stay alert to potential problems, be aware of your alternatives, maintain a good sense of your own values, and stick to your beliefs under pressure.

Setting Realistic Goals

Changing behavior is not easy, but sometimes we make it even harder by setting unrealistic and unattainable goals. To start making positive changes, ask yourself these questions.

- *What do I want?* What is your ultimate goal—to lose weight? Exercise more? Reduce stress? Have a lasting relationship? Whatever it is, you need a clear picture of the eventual target outcome.
- *Which change is the greatest priority at this time?* Often people decide to change several things all at once. Suppose that you are gaining unwanted weight. Rather than saying, "I need to eat less, start jogging, and really get in shape," you need to be specific about your current behavior. Are you eating too many sweets? Too many foods high in fat? Perhaps a realistic goal, therefore, would be, "I am going to try to eat less fat during dinner every day." Choose the behavior that constitutes your greatest problem, and tackle that first. You can always work on something else later. Take small steps, experiment with alternatives, and find the best way to meet your unique goals.
- *Why is this important to me?* Think through why you want to change. Are you doing it because of your health? To look better? To win someone else's approval? Usually, doing things because it's right for you rather than to win others' approval is a sound strategy. If you are doing it for someone else, what happens when that other person isn't around?
- *What are the potential positive outcomes?* What do you hope to accomplish with this change?
- *What health-promoting programs and services can help me get started?* Nearly all campuses and communities have programs and services designed to support positive behavior change. It may mean buying a self-help book, speaking to a counselor, or enrolling in an aerobics class at the local fitness center.
- *Are there family or friends whose help I can enlist?* Social support is one of your most powerful allies. Getting a friend to walk with you on a regular basis, asking your partner to help you stop smoking by quitting at the same time, and making a commitment with a friend to never let each other drive if you've had something to drink—these are all examples of how people can help each other make positive changes.

What do you think?

Why is it sometimes hard to make decisions?
- *What factors influence your decision making?*
- *Select one behavior that you want to change and refer to the Behavior Change Contract.* ■ *Using the goal-setting strategies discussed here, outline a plan for change.*

Behavior Change Contract

Complete the Assess Yourself questionnaire, and read the Skills for Behavior Change box describing the stages of change. After reviewing your results and considering the various factors that influence your decisions, choose a health behavior that you would like to change, starting this quarter or semester. Sign the contract at the bottom to affirm your commitment to making a healthy change, and ask a friend to witness it.

My behavior change will be:

_____

My long-term goal for this behavior change is:

_____

These are three obstacles to change (things that I am currently doing or situations that contribute to this behavior or make it harder to change):

1. _____

2. _____

3. _____

The strategies I will use to overcome these obstacles are:

1. _____

2. _____

3. _____

Resources I will use to help me change this behavior include:

a friend/partner/relative: _____

a school-based resource: _____

a community-based resource: _____

a book or reputable website: _____

In order to make my goal more attainable, I have devised these short-term goals:

_____	_____	_____
short-term goal	target date	reward
_____	_____	_____
short-term goal	target date	reward
_____	_____	_____
short-term goal	target date	reward

When I make the long-term behavior change described above, my reward will be:

_____ target date: _____

I intend to make the behavior change described above. I will use the strategies and rewards to achieve the goals that will contribute to a healthy behavior change.

Signed: _____   Witness: _____

Date: _____   Date: _____

Figure 1.5
Behavior Change Contract

Use this contract to set short-term and long-term goals for behavior change. Anticipate obstacles and develop strategies to overcome these obstacles, and investigate resources to help you along the way. Be sure to include rewards for reaching your goals. There are additional contracts for your use at the front of this book and in the Health Resources section.

MAKE IT HAPPEN!

Assessment: The Assess Yourself box earlier in this chapter (page 12) gave you the chance to look at the status of your health in several dimensions. Now that you have considered these results, you can begin to take steps toward changing certain behaviors that may be detrimental to your health.

Making a Change: In order to change your behavior, you need to develop a plan. Follow these steps:

1. Evaluate your behavior and identify patterns and specific things you are doing. What can you change now? What can you change in the near future?
2. Select one pattern of behavior that you want to change.
3. Fill out the Behavior Change Contract (see Figure 1.5). It should include your long-term goal for change, your short-term goals, the rewards you'll give yourself for reaching these goals, potential obstacles along the way, and strategies for overcoming these obstacles. For each goal, list the small steps and specific actions that you will take.
4. Chart your progress in a journal. At the end of a week, consider how successful you were in following your plan. What helped you be successful? What made change more difficult? What will you do differently next week?
5. Revise your plan as needed: Are the short-term goals attainable? Are the rewards satisfying?

One Student's Plan: Felipe assessed his health and discovered that his score in the Personal Health promotion section was low—25 points—because of some risky behaviors in which he was engaging. In particular, he realized that he had driven several times after drinking and that he was not performing monthly testicle self-examinations. Felipe decided to tackle one of these issues at a time. He completed a Behavior Change Contract to drive only when he had had fewer than two drinks. Steps in his contract included finding out about designated driver programs, moderating his drinking so that he was sober and competent to drive at the end of a night out with friends, and finding concerts and other events to attend that did not involve drinking. The rewards he chose for these steps included tickets to a concert and a new computer game. After a few months Felipe realized that he had been in several situations in which he might previously have driven under the influence. Instead, he had given himself alternatives such as designated drivers, budgeting for a taxi, and moderating his drinking, and thus had avoided unsafe situations.

Next month, Felipe will get a pamphlet from the health center on testicular self-exams and choose a day of the month to be his self-examination day. Every month that he does the exam, he'll sleep in an extra hour that weekend as a reward.

Summary

- Health encompasses the whole dynamic process of fulfilling one's individual potential in the physical, social, emotional, spiritual, intellectual, and environmental dimensions of life. Wellness means achieving the highest level of health possible along several dimensions.
- Although the average American life span has increased over the past century, we need to increase the span of quality life. The programs *Healthy People 2000* and *Healthy People 2010* and documents such as the *AHRQ Guidelines* have established a set of national objectives for achieving longer life and quality of life for all Americans through health promotion and disease prevention.
- Health disparities have become increasingly recognized as contributors to increased disease risks. Factors such as gender, race, and socioeconomic status continue to play a major role in health status and care. Women live longer but have more medical problems than do men. The recent inclusion of women in medical research and training and greater emphasis on minority populations are attempts to close the gap in health care.
- For the U.S. population as a whole, the leading causes of death are heart disease, cancer, and stroke. But in the 15- to 24-year-old age group, the leading causes are unintentional injuries, homicide/legal intervention, and suicide. Many of the risks associated with heart disease, cancer, and stroke can be reduced through lifestyle changes. Many of the risks associated with accidents, homicide, and suicide can be reduced through preventive measures.
- Worldwide commerce and travel are bringing dramatic changes in global health. In nonindustrialized countries, noncommunicable diseases such as depression and heart disease are replacing infectious disease and malnutrition as leading causes of disability and death.

- Several factors contribute to a person's health status, and a number of them are within our control. Beliefs and attitudes, intentions to change, support from significant others, and readiness to change are factors over which individuals have some degree of control. Access to health care, genetic predisposition, health policies that support positive choices, and other factors are all potential reinforcing, predisposing, and enabling factors that may influence health decisions.

- Applying behavior-change techniques, such as shaping, visualizing, modeling, controlling the situation, reinforcing, and changing self-talk help people succeed in making behavior changes.
- Decision making has several key components. Each person must explore his or her own problems, the reasons for making change, and the expected outcomes. The next step is to plan a course of action best suited to individual needs and fill out a Behavior Change Contract.

Questions for Discussion and Reflection

1. How are the terms *health* and *wellness* similar? What, if any, are important distinctions between these terms? What is health promotion? Disease prevention? What does it really mean to be healthy? Considering the various dimensions of health, describe someone that you believe has many of these characteristics.

2. How healthy is the U.S. population today? Are we doing better or worse in terms of health status in this country? Who is not doing better in an era when health is the "buzz" and everyone seems to be interested in improving health? What factors influence today's disparities in health?

3. What are some of the major global health problems today? Why is it increasingly important that we consider individual, community, U.S., and global health when we consider the health of populations?

4. What are some of the major differences in the way males and females are treated in the health care system? Why do you think these differences exist? Why are people treated differently based on race, sexual orientation, religion, marital status, and age?

5. What are the leading causes of death across different ages and races? What are the leading causes of death for people ages 15 to 24? Why are these statistics so different? Explain why it is important to look at these statistics by age rather than just in total. What lifestyle changes can you make to lower your risks for contracting major diseases?

6. What major differences exist between the leading causes of death for Americans and for people in other regions of the world?

7. What is the Health Belief Model? What is the Theory of Reasoned Action? How may each of these models be working when a young woman decides to smoke her first cigarette? Her last cigarette?

8. Explain the predisposing, reinforcing, and enabling factors that might influence a young mother who is dependent on welfare as she decides whether to sell drugs to support her children.

9. Using the Stages of Change model, discuss what you might do (in stages) to help a friend stop smoking. Why is it important that a person be ready to change before trying to change?

Accessing Your Health on the Internet

Visit the following Internet sites to explore further topics and issues related to personal health. To visit an organization's website, go to the Companion Website for *Access to Health, Ninth Edition* at www.aw-bc.com/donatelle, click on the book image, and select "Accessing Your Health on the Internet" from the navigation menu.

1. *CDC Wonder.* Clearinghouse for comprehensive information from the Centers for Disease Control and Prevention (CDC), including special reports, guidelines, and access to national health data.

2. *Mayo Clinic.* Reputable resource for specific information about health topics, diseases, and treatment options. Easy to navigate and consumer friendly.

3. *National Center for Health Statistics.* Outstanding place to start for information about health status in the United States. Links to key documents such as *Health United States* (published annually), national survey information, and information on mortality by age, race, gender, geographic location, and other important data. Includes comprehensive information provided by the CDC, as well as easy links to at least ten of the major health resources currently being utilized for policy and decision making about health in the United States.

4. *National Health Information Center.* An excellent resource for consumer information about health.

5. *WebMD.* Reputable and comprehensive overview of various diseases and conditions. Written for the public in an easy-to-understand format with links to more in-depth information.

Further Reading

Centers for Disease Control and Prevention, *Health United States: 2004.* (Washington, DC: Government Printing Office, 2004).

Provides an up-to-date overview of U.S. health statistics, risk factors, and trends.

Institute of Medicine, *Who Will Keep the Public Healthy: Educating Public Health Professionals for the 21st Century* (Washington, DC: National Academies Press, 2003).

An edited text featuring experts from throughout the country discussing the role of health professionals in health change. It outlines an ecological approach to improving the nation's health and has served as a catalyst for initiatives focused on current health issues and future plans to improve health and prevent premature death and disability.

Institute of Medicine, *The Future of Public Health in the 21st Century* (Washington, DC: National Academies Press, 2003).

The summary of a national effort to examine the nation's health status describes how key individuals and organizations can work as a public health system to create conditions in which people can be healthy. This text also recommends the evidence-based actions necessary to make the U.S. health system work effectively.

Lee, Philip and Carroll Estes, *The Nation's Health,* 7th ed. (Sudbury, MA: Jones and Bartlett, 2003).

An overview of key writings on public health and issues affecting individuals and populations. Special emphasis is placed on health determinants, emerging threats to health, the health of diverse populations, and issues of health care quality, costs, and access.

U.S. Department of Health and Human Services, *Healthy People 2010: National Health Promotion and Disease Prevention Objectives for the Year 2010* (Washington, DC: Government Printing Office, 1998).

A plan containing the Surgeon General's long-range goals for improving the life span for all Americans by three years and improving access to health for all Americans, regardless of sex, race, socioeconomic status, and other variables.

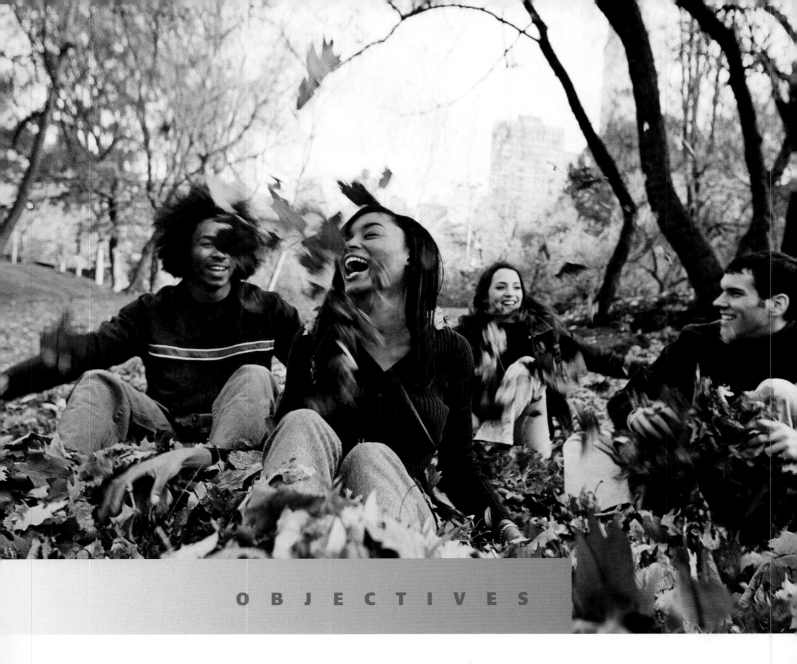

OBJECTIVES

- Define psychosocial health in terms of its mental, emotional, and social components, and identify the basic traits shared by psychosocially healthy people.

- Consider how each of the internal and external factors that influence psychosocial health may affect you.

- Discuss the positive steps you can take to enhance psychosocial health.

- Discuss the dimension of spirituality and the role that it plays in health and wellness.

- Discuss the mind–body connection and show how emotions (including optimism and happiness) influence health status.

- Identify and describe common psychosocial problems of adulthood, and explain their causes, methods of prevention, and available treatments.

- Describe different types of anxiety disorders and their key risk factors.

- Discuss warning signs of suicide and actions that can be taken to help a suicidal individual.

- Explain the goals and methods of different types of health professionals and therapies. Build a strategy for selecting a good therapist.

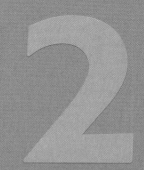

PSYCHOSOCIAL HEALTH

BEING MENTALLY, EMOTIONALLY, SOCIALLY, AND SPIRITUALLY WELL

IN THE NEWS

Worried Colleges Step Up Efforts Over Suicide

By Karen W. Arenson

Nicole Thompson had been at Columbia University for only a few weeks when she went out drinking with a group of friends downtown last year and became separated from them. She had skipped her medication for bipolar disorder. Now it was 3 A.M. and, crying and in a panic, she called friends; she told them, she said, that she "just wished the traffic would take me out."

Although she made it back to campus safely, her friends had already notified Columbia that they were worried about her. For Columbia officials, it was the first clue that Ms. Thompson faced any kind of mental health problems.

"I wasn't on Columbia's radar at all," said Ms. Thompson, who is back on campus now after being forced to take a medical leave.

Increasingly, college officials and mental health experts have come to realize that many of the most vulnerable students—the ones prone to self-injury and suicide—are like Ms. Thompson: they never go near the counseling centers or reveal anything about their experience before college. As a result, colleges are stepping up efforts to find them and to get them into treatment, sometimes forcing them to leave temporarily.

Read the complete article online in the eThemes section of this book's website: www.aw-bc.com/donatelle.

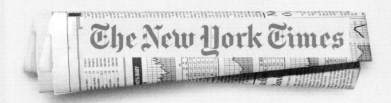

Have there been days when you felt mentally and physically exhausted? Were you so tired that you found it hard to stay awake long enough to study or go out with friends? In contrast, have there been other days when you felt energized from the moment you woke up in the morning? Although you were busy all day, you may have felt too awake to even think about going to bed.

Your experience illustrates the close link between psychosocial and physical health. Although often overlooked during the pursuit of a fit body, a fit mind is equally important to your well-being.

All of us go through difficult times. A study of nearly 14,000 students who sought help from a Midwestern university counseling center over a 13-year period revealed that students frequently have more complex problems today than they did a decade ago. Issues included both the expected difficulties—relationships and developmental issues—and more severe problems such as depression, effects of sexual assault, and thoughts of suicide. Some of these increases were dramatic. The number of students seen each year with depression doubled, the number of suicidal students tripled, and the number of students counseled after a sexual assault quadrupled.[1]

However, human beings possess a resiliency that enables us to cope, adapt, and thrive, regardless of life's challenges. How we feel and think about ourselves, those around us, and our environment can tell us a lot about our psychosocial health and whether we are healthy emotionally, spiritually, and mentally. Increasingly, health professionals recognize that having a solid social network, being emotionally and mentally healthy, and developing spiritual capacity don't just add years to life—they put life into years.

Defining Psychosocial Health

Psychosocial health encompasses the mental, emotional, social, and spiritual dimensions of health (Figure 2.1). It is the result of a complex interaction between a person's history and conscious and unconscious thoughts and interpretations of the past. Psychosocially healthy people are emotionally, mentally, socially, intellectually, and spiritually resilient. They respond to challenges and frustrations in appropriate ways most of the time, despite occasional slips. Most authorities identify several basic elements shared by psychosocially healthy people:[2]

- *They feel good about themselves.* Healthy people are not typically overwhelmed by fear, love, anger, jealousy, guilt, or worry. They know who they are, have a realistic sense of their capabilities, and respect themselves even though they realize they aren't perfect.

Psychosocial health The mental, emotional, social, and spiritual dimensions of health.

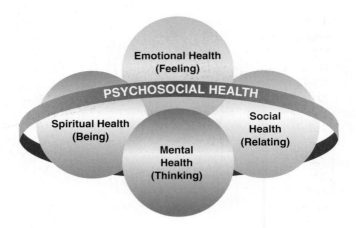

Figure 2.1
Psychosocial Health
Psychosocial health is a complex interaction of the mental, emotional, social and spiritual dimensions of health.

- *They feel comfortable with other people.* Healthy people enjoy satisfying and lasting personal relationships and do not take advantage of others, nor do they allow others to take advantage of them. They can give love, consider others' interests, respect personal differences, and feel responsible for their fellow human beings.
- *They control tension and anxiety.* They recognize the underlying causes and symptoms of stress and anxiety in their lives and consciously work to avoid irrational thoughts, hostility, excessive excuse making, and blaming others for their problems.
- *They meet the demands of life.* They try to solve problems as they arise, accept responsibility, and plan ahead. Acknowledging that change is inevitable, they welcome new experiences.
- *They curb hate and guilt* by acknowledging and combating their tendencies to respond with anger, thoughtlessness, selfishness, vengeful acts, or feelings of inadequacy. Rather than knocking others aside to get ahead, they reach out to help others—even those they don't particularly care for.
- *They maintain a positive outlook.* Psychosocially healthy people approach each day with a presumption that things will go well. They block out most negative and cynical thoughts and give star billing to the good things in life. They look to the future with enthusiasm rather than dread.
- *They enrich the lives of others* because they recognize that there are people whose needs are greater than their own.
- *They cherish the things that make them smile.* Reminders of good experiences brighten their day. Fun is an integral part of their lives. So is making time for themselves.
- *They value diversity.* Healthy people do not feel threatened by those of a different race, gender, religion, sexual orientation, ethnicity, or political party. They appreciate creativity in others as well as in themselves.
- *They respect nature.* They take time to enjoy their surroundings and are conscious of their place in the universe.

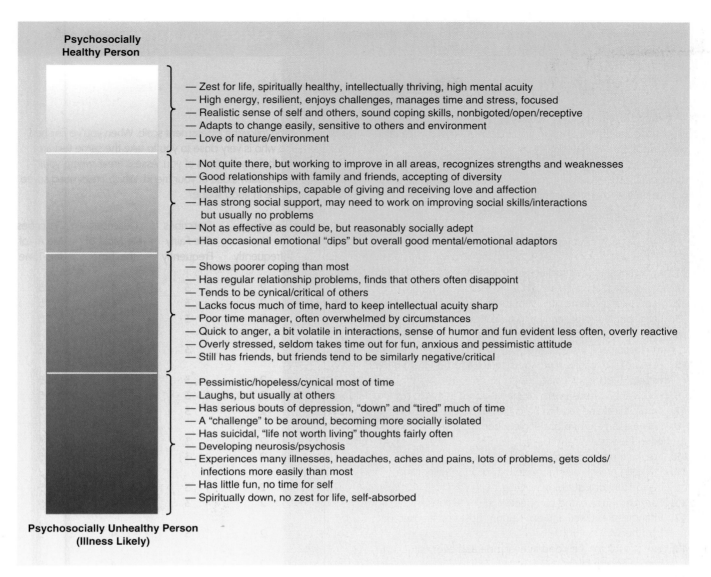

Psychosocially Healthy Person

— Zest for life, spiritually healthy, intellectually thriving, high mental acuity
— High energy, resilient, enjoys challenges, manages time and stress, focused
— Realistic sense of self and others, sound coping skills, nonbigoted/open/receptive
— Adapts to change easily, sensitive to others and environment
— Love of nature/environment

— Not quite there, but working to improve in all areas, recognizes strengths and weaknesses
— Good relationships with family and friends, accepting of diversity
— Healthy relationships, capable of giving and receiving love and affection
— Has strong social support, may need to work on improving social skills/interactions but usually no problems
— Not as effective as could be, but reasonably socially adept
— Has occasional emotional "dips" but overall good mental/emotional adaptors

— Shows poorer coping than most
— Has regular relationship problems, finds that others often disappoint
— Tends to be cynical/critical of others
— Lacks focus much of time, hard to keep intellectual acuity sharp
— Poor time manager, often overwhelmed by circumstances
— Quick to anger, a bit volatile in interactions, sense of humor and fun evident less often, overly reactive
— Overly stressed, seldom takes time out for fun, anxious and pessimistic attitude
— Still has friends, but friends tend to be similarly negative/critical

— Pessimistic/hopeless/cynical most of time
— Laughs, but usually at others
— Has serious bouts of depression, "down" and "tired" much of time
— A "challenge" to be around, becoming more socially isolated
— Has suicidal, "life not worth living" thoughts fairly often
— Developing neurosis/psychosis
— Experiences many illnesses, headaches, aches and pains, lots of problems, gets colds/infections more easily than most
— Has little fun, no time for self
— Spiritually down, no zest for life, self-absorbed

Psychosocially Unhealthy Person
(Illness Likely)

Figure 2.2
Characteristics of Psychosocially Healthy and Unhealthy People
Where do you fall on this continuum?

Of course, no one ever achieves perfection. Attaining psychosocial health and wellness involves many complex processes (Figure 2.2). This chapter will help you understand not only what it means to be psychosocially well, but also why we may run into problems. Learning how to assess your own health and to help yourself or seek help from others are important parts of psychosocial health (see the Assess Yourself box on page 42).

What do you think?

Which psychosocial qualities do you value the most in your friends? ■ *Do you think that you are strong in these areas?* ■ *Explain your answer.*

Mental Health: The Thinking You

The term **mental health** is often used to describe the "thinking" part of psychosocial health. As a thinking being, you have the ability to reason, interpret, and remember events from a unique perspective; to sense, perceive, and evaluate what is happening; and to solve problems. In short, you are intellectually able to sort through the clutter of events, contradictory messages, and uncertainties of a situation and attach meaning (either positive or negative) to it. (People often refer to this subset of mental health as *intellectual health*).

Mental health The thinking part of psychosocial health; includes your values, attitudes, and beliefs.

Assessing Your Psychosocial Health

Fill out this assessment online at www.aw-bc.com/myhealthlab or www.aw-bc.com/donatelle

Being psychosocially healthy requires both introspection and the willingness to work on areas that need improvement. Begin by

completing t[...]d,
ask someon[...]d
respond with[...]
responses di[...]me
work? Which[...]

	Never Describes Me	In[...]	[...]ibes ll of ime
1. My actions and interactions indicate that I am confident in my abilities.	1		
2. I am quick to blame others for things that go wrong in my life.	1		
3. I am spontaneous and like to have fun with others.	1		
4. I am able to give love and affection to others and show my feelings.	1		
5. I am able to receive love and signs of affection from others without feeling uneasy.	1		
6. I am generally positive and upbeat about things in my life.	1		
7. I am cynical and tend to be critical of others.	1		
8. I have a large group of people whom I consider to be good friends.	1		
9. I make time for others in my life.	1		
10. I take time each day for myself for quiet introspection, having fun, or just doing nothing.	1		
11. I am compulsive and competitive in my actions.	1		
12. I handle stress well and am seldom upset or stressed out by others.	1		
13. I try to look for the good in everyone and every situation before finding fault.	1		
14. I am comfortable meeting new people and interact well in social settings.	1		
15. I would rather stay in and watch TV or read than go out with friends or interact with others.	1		
16. I am flexible and can adapt to most situations, even if I don't like them.	1		
17. Nature, the environment, and other living things are important aspects of my life.	1		

Your values, attitudes, and beliefs about your body, your family, your relationships, and life in general are usually—at least in part—a reflection of your mental health.

A mentally healthy person is likely to respond in a positive way even when things do not go as expected. For example, a mentally healthy student who receives a D on an exam may be disappointed but will try to assess why she did poorly. Did she study enough? Did she attend class and ask questions when she didn't understand? Even though the test result may be important to her, she will find constructive

ways to d[...]
velop mo[...]
more tim[...]
unhealth[...]
rationally[...]
her or tha[...]
allow her[...]
could spe[...]
school, tr[...]
roommat[...]

[...], de-
[...]ote
[...]entally
[...]nd ir-
[...]get
[...]nay
[...]e. She
[...]to quit
[...]her

	Never Describes Me	Describes Me Infrequently	Describes Me Fairly Frequently	Describes Me Most of the Time	Describes Me All of the Time
18. I think before responding to my emotions.	1	2	3	4	5
19. I am selfish and tend to think of my own needs before those of others.	1	2	3	4	5
20. I am consciously trying to be a better person.	1	2	3	4	5
21. I like to plan ahead and set realistic goals for myself and others.	1	2	3	4	5
22. I accept others for who they are.	1	2	3	4	5
23. I value diversity and respect others' rights, regardless of culture, race, sexual orientation, religion, or other differences.	1	2	3	4	5
24. I try to live each day as if it might be my last.	1	2	3	4	5
25. I have a great deal of energy and appreciate the little things in life.	1	2	3	4	5
26. I cope with stress in appropriate ways.	1	2	3	4	5
27. I get enough sleep each day and seldom feel tired.	1	2	3	4	5
28. I have healthy relationships with my family.	1	2	3	4	5
29. I am confident that I can do most things if I put my mind to them.	1	2	3	4	5
30. I respect others' opinions and believe that others should be free to express their opinions, even when they differ from my own.	1	2	3	4	5

INTERPRETING YOUR SCORES

Look at items 2, 7, 11, 15, and 19. Add up your score for these five items and divide by 5. Is your average for these items above or below 3? Did you score a 5 on any of these items? Do you need to work on any of these areas? Now look at your scores for the remaining items. (There should be 25 items.) Total these scores and divide by 25. Is your average above or below 3? On which items did you score a 5? Obviously you're doing well in these areas. Now remove the items having from this grouping of 25, and add up your scores for the remaining items. Then divide your total by the number of items included. Now what is your average?

Do the same for the scores completed by your friend or family member. How do your scores compare? Which ones, if any, are different, and how do they differ? Which areas do you need to work on? What actions can you take now to improve your ratings in these areas?

MAKE IT HAPPEN!

Use the results of this self-assessment to begin your behavior change program. Follow the steps and use the examples on page 66 to complete your Behavior Change Contract and use these resources to take action.

If a person's mental health begins to deteriorate, he or she may experience sharp declines in rational thinking ability and increasingly distorted perceptions. The person may become cynical and distrustful, experience volatile mood swings, or choose to be isolated from others. Extremely negative reactions may even threaten the life and health of others. People who show such extreme behavior are classified as having mental illnesses, discussed later in this chapter.

Emotional Health: The Feeling You

The term **emotional health** is often used interchangeably with *mental health*. Although the two are closely intertwined, emotional health more accurately refers to the "feeling," or

> **Emotional health**   The feeling part of psychosocial health, includes your emotional reactions to life.

subjective, side of psychosocial health. **Emotions** are intensified feelings or complex patterns of feelings that we experience on a minute-by-minute, day-to-day basis. Love, hate, frustration, anxiety, and joy are only a few of the many emotions we feel. Typically, emotions are described as the interplay of four components: physiological arousal, feelings, cognitive (thought) processes, and behavioral reactions. Each time you are placed in a stressful situation, you react physiologically while your mind tries to sort things out. You consciously or unconsciously react based on how rationally you interpret the situation.

Psychologist Richard Lazarus has indicated that there are four basic types of emotions: (1) emotions resulting from harm, loss, or threats; (2) emotions resulting from benefits; (3) borderline emotions, such as hope and compassion; and (4) more complex emotions, such as grief, disappointment, bewilderment, and curiosity.[3] Each of us may experience any of these feelings in any combination at any time. As rational beings, it is our responsibility to evaluate our individual emotional responses, the environment that is causing them, and the appropriateness of our actions.

Emotionally healthy people are usually able to respond in an appropriate manner to upsetting events. When they feel threatened, they are not likely to overreact, behave inconsistently, or adopt an offensive attack mode. Even when their feelings are trampled upon or they suffer agonizing pain because of a lost love, they keep their emotions in perspective. Emotionally unhealthy people are much more likely to let their feelings overpower them. They may be highly volatile and prone to unpredictable emotional outbursts and inappropriate, sometimes frightening responses. An ex-boyfriend who is so jealous of your new relationship that he hits you is showing an extremely unhealthy and dangerous emotional reaction. Such violent responses have become a problem of epidemic proportions in the United States (see Chapter 4).

Emotional health also affects social health. Someone feeling hostile, withdrawn, or moody may become socially isolated. People in the midst of emotional turmoil may be grumpy, irritable, or overly quiet; they may cry easily or demonstrate other disturbing emotional responses. Since they are not much fun to be around, their friends may avoid them at the very time they are most in need of emotional support. Social isolation is just one of the many potential negative consequences of unstable emotional behavior.

Emotions Intensified feelings or complex patterns of feelings we constantly experience.

Social health Aspect of psychosocial health that includes interactions with others, ability to use social supports, and ability to adapt to various situations.

Social bonds Degree and nature of interpersonal contacts.

Social support Network of people and services with whom you share ties and get support.

Social health also reflects the way we react to others. In its most extreme forms, a lack of social health may be represented by aggressive acts of prejudice toward other individuals or groups. In its most obvious manifestations, **prejudice** is reflected in acts of discrimination, hate, and bias, and in purposeful intent to harm individuals or groups.

Just as supportive ties promote health and longevity, the loss of such relationships threatens health. For example, on average, widows and widowers are at increased risk of mental and physical illness for up to two years after their spouse dies.

Spiritual Health: An Inner Quest for Well-Being

Although mental and emotional health are key factors in overall psychosocial functioning, it is possible to be mentally and emotionally healthy and still not achieve optimal well-being. What is missing? For many people, the difficult-to-describe element that gives zest to life is the spiritual dimension.

Most experts agree that **spirituality** refers to a belief in some unifying force that gives meaning to life, a sense of belonging to a scheme of being that is greater than the purely physical or personal dimensions of existence. For some, this unifying force is nature; for others, it is a feeling of connection to other people; for still others, the unifying force is a god or other spiritual symbol. Dr. N. Lee Smith, internist and associate professor of medicine at the University of Utah, defines spiritual health in the following ways:[5]

- The quality of existence in which one is at peace with oneself and in good standing with the environment
- A sense of empowerment and personal control that includes feeling valued and in control over one's responses (but not necessarily in control of one's environment)
- A sense of connectedness to one's deepest self, to other people, and to all that is generally regarded as good
- A sense of meaning and purpose, which provides a sense of mission by finding meaning and wisdom in the here and now
- Enjoying the process of growth and having a vision of one's potential
- Having hope, which translates into positive expectations

On a day-to-day basis, many of us focus on acquiring material possessions and satisfying basic needs. But there comes a point when we discover that material possessions do not automatically bring happiness or a sense of self-worth. This realization may be triggered by a crisis. A failed relationship, a terrible accident, the death of a close friend or family member, or other loss often prompts a search for meaning, for the answer to the proverbial question, Is that all there is? Whatever the reason, this search brings new opportunities for understanding ourselves. As we develop into spiritually healthy beings, we recognize our identity as unique individuals. We gain a better appreciation of our strengths and shortcomings and our place in the universe. Perhaps most important, we gain an appreciation for the here-and-now, rather than living for aspirations that we may never achieve.

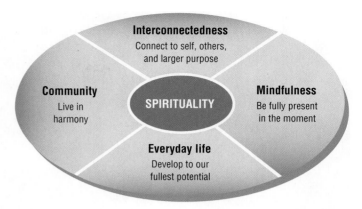

Figure 2.3
Four Major Themes of Spirituality

In its purest sense, spirituality addresses four main themes: interconnectedness, the practice of mindfulness, spirituality as a part of everyday life, and living in harmony with the community (Figure 2.3).

- *Interconnectedness.* The term **interconnectedness** expresses a sense of harmony with oneself, with others, and with a larger meaning or purpose. Connecting with oneself involves exploring feelings, taking time to consider how you feel in a given situation, assessing your reactions to people and experiences, and taking mental notes when things or people cause you to lose equilibrium. It also involves considering your values and achieving congruence between your goals and what you can do to achieve them without compromising your values.
- *Practice of mindfulness.* **Mindfulness** refers to the ability to be fully present in the moment. Mindfulness has been described as a way of nurturing greater awareness, clarity, and acceptance of present-moment reality or a form of inner flow—a holistic sensation you feel when you are totally involved in the moment.[6] According to mindfulness experts, you can achieve this inner flow through an almost infinite range of opportunities for enjoyment and pleasure, either through the use of physical and sensory skills ranging from athletics to music to yoga or through

Prejudice A negative evaluation of an entire group of people that is typically based on unfavorable and often wrong ideas about the group.

Spirituality A belief in a unifying force that gives meaning to life and transcends the purely physical or personal dimensions of existence.

Interconnectedness A web of connections, including our relationship to ourselves, to others, and to a larger meaning or purpose in life.

Mindfulness Awareness and acceptance of the reality of the present moment.

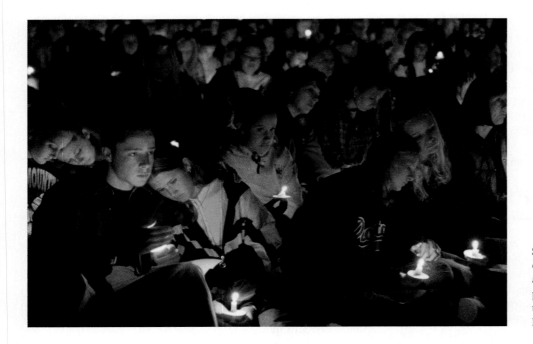

Spirituality does not have to involve organized religion. These students at a memorial service are participating in a community ritual that strengthens their spiritual health.

the development of symbolic skills in areas such as poetry, philosophy, or mathematics.[7] The psychologist Abraham Maslow referred to these moments as peak experiences, during which a person feels integrated, synergistic, and at one with the world.

- *Spirituality as a part of daily life.* Spirituality is embodied in the ability to discover and articulate our own basic purpose in life; to learn how to experience love, joy, peace, and fulfillment; and to help ourselves and others achieve their full potential.[8] This ongoing process of growth fosters three convictions: faith, hope, and love. **Faith** is the belief that helps us realize our purpose in life; **hope** is the belief that allows us to look confidently and courageously to the future; and **love** involves accepting, affirming, and respecting self and others, regardless of who they are.[9]

- *Living in harmony with our community.* Our values are an extension of our beliefs about the world and attitude toward life. They are formed over time through a series of life experiences, and they are reflected in our hopes, dreams, desires, goals, and ambitions.[10] Though most people have some idea of what is important to them, many spend life largely unaware of how their values impact themselves or those around them until a life-altering event shakes up their perspective on life.

Faith   Belief that helps each person realize a unique purpose in life.

Hope   Belief that allows us to look confidently and courageously to the future.

Love   Acceptance, affirmation, and respect for the self and others.

Spirituality: A Key to Health and Wellness   Although many experts affirm the importance of spirituality in achieving health and wellness, the specific impact of this dimension remains elusive. Some researchers describe the spiritual dimension as a factor of well-being, which is achieved when four basic kinds of needs are satisfied:[11]

1. The need for having
2. The need for relating
3. The need for being
4. The need for *transcendence,* or that sense of well-being that is experienced when a person finds purpose and meaning in life. Nonphysical in nature, transcendence can best be described as spiritual.

A Spiritual Resurgence   Over recent decades, studies have shown that most Americans believe in God and consider spirituality to be important in their lives, although not necessarily in the form of religion.[12] Many find spiritual fulfillment in music, poetry, literature, art, nature, and intimate relationships.[13] Many religious groups have spawned new philosophies that are more inclusive and often influenced by "New Age" ideas, such as using positive thought to achieve your goals and striving to find your rightful place in the world. An estimated 32 million baby boomers have turned to Eastern practices, New Age philosophies, 12-step programs, Greek mythology, shamanistic practices, massage, yoga, and a host of other traditions and practices.[14]

For some, spirituality means a "quest for self and self-lessness"—a form of therapy and respite from a sometimes challenging personal environment. This quest for a "life force," which helps people deeply experience the moments of their lives rather than just living through them, has received much scholarly and popular attention. Self-help

Spirituality and Health: Separating Fact from Fiction

It wasn't too long ago that doctors and researchers avoided the study of spirituality and shook their heads in quiet disbelief over claims that spirituality was responsible for improvements in health. However, research in the last decade has given preliminary support for the importance of the mind–body connection in maintaining physical and psychological health. Scientists are increasingly investigating this connection, as shown by the fact that the National Institutes of Health has more than doubled research funding for studies examining this phenomenon.

Critics of research supporting a relationship between spirituality and health point to the fact that the populations of these studies are often skewed in favor of the elderly, and thus results may not be generalizable. They indicate that flaws in design, sample size, and methods make conclusive statements about effect questionable. A new generation of researchers hope to have sufficient funding to reduce research problems and sufficiently test hypotheses that seem promising.

Studies have examined the role of spirituality in bolstering immune response; others have pointed to the role of spirituality in improving social connections and thereby indirectly improving health and healing. Studies have looked into the correlations between spirituality and the following:

- *Depression.* A study at Duke University Medical Center revealed that patients who sought a connection with a benevolent God as well as support from clergy and church members were less depressed and rated their quality of life as higher.
- *Blood pressure.* Researchers at Duke University studied nearly 4,000 people aged 65 and older, and discovered that people who both attended religious services at least once a week and prayed or studied the Bible at least daily had consistently lower blood pressure than those who did so less frequently or not at all.
- *Stress.* The Alameda County Study, which has tracked over 7,000 Californians from 1965 to the present, showed that West Coast worshippers who participate in church-sponsored activities are markedly less stressed over finances, health, and other daily concerns than their nonreligious counterparts.
- *HIV/AIDS.* A study of HIV/AIDS patients showed that the long-term survivors scored significantly higher on such measures of spirituality and religiousness as sense of peace, faith in God, and compassionate views of others than did individuals in a comparison group. Long-term survivors were also more likely to be less judgmental and to pray more than the control group.
- *Breast cancer.* A study of women with breast cancer found that both receiving help from fellow patients and giving help to fellow patients led to self-transcendence, which directly affect emotional well-being.
- *Immune system responsiveness.* People who are altruistic and strive to work for the common good have been shown to have lower levels of the stress hormone cortisol. By lowering cortisol levels, risks to the immune system are thought to also be lowered.

Although the exact mechanisms are not known, it appears that people who are more spiritual tend to have more social interactions, manage stress levels more effectively, and have more hope for the future than do their nonspiritual counterparts. People who value their interactions with nature also tend to take more time relaxing in nature and, therefore, control their stress levels more effectively.

Sources: D. Ko, "Religious Coping Plays a Role in Recovery from Depression," *MHToday,* www.mental-health-today.com/articles/spirituality.htm; H. G. Koenig et al., "The Relationship Between Religious Activities and Blood Pressure in Older Adults," *International Journal of Psychology in Medicine* 28, no. 2 (1998), 189–213; C. Westlake and K. Dracup, "Role of Spirituality in Adjustment of Patients with Advanced Heart Failure," *Progress in Cardiovascular Nursing* 16 no. 3 (2001), 119–125; G. Ironson, G. F. Solomon et al., "The Ironson-Woods Spirituality/Religiousness Index Is Associated with Long Survival, Health Behaviors, Less Distress, and Low Cortisol in People with HIV/AIDS," *Annals of Behavioral Medicine* 24, no. 1 (2002), 34–38; R. J. Davidson and J. Kabat-Zinn et al., "Alterations in Brain and Immune Function Produced by Mindfulness Meditation," *Psychosomatic Medicine Journal* 65, no. 4 (2003), 564–570.

books that focus on spirituality consistently top the bestseller lists. Television programs promote the virtues of a spiritual or natural existence. Writers and psychologists such as William James, Carl Jung, Gordon Allport, Erich Fromm, Viktor Frankl, Abraham Maslow, and Rollo May have made spirituality a major focus of their work.

Spiritual health courses have emerged in public health and medical school training. For example, the Harvard Medical School of Continuing Education offers a course called "Spirituality and Healing in Medicine," which brings together scholars and medical professionals from around the world to discuss the role of spirituality in treating illness and chronic pain. Self-help workshops focusing on spiritual elements of health are popular throughout the world. The New Horizons in Health box above describes several studies that examine the link between spirituality and health.

What do you think?

What do social and emotional health mean to you?
■ *What are your strengths and weaknesses in these areas?* ■ *What can you do to enhance your strengths?* ■ *How can you improve areas that are not as strong?*

Factors That Influence Psychosocial Health

Most of our mental, emotional, and social reactions to life are a direct outcome of our experiences and social and cultural expectations. Our psychosocial health is based, in part, on how we perceive life experiences.

External Factors

While some life experiences are under our control, others are not. External influences are those factors in life that we do not control, such as who raised us and where we lived in our youth.

The Family   Families have a significant influence on psychosocial development. Children raised in healthy, nurturing, happy families are more likely to become well-adjusted, productive adults. Children raised in **dysfunctional families**—which show characteristics such as violence, distrust, anger, dietary deprivation, drug abuse, parental discord, sexual, physical, or emotional abuse—may have a harder time adapting to life. In dysfunctional families, love, security, and unconditional trust are so lacking that children often become confused and psychologically bruised. Yet not all people raised in dysfunctional families become psychosocially unhealthy, and not all people from healthy environments are well adjusted. Obviously, more factors are involved in our "process of becoming" than just our family.

The Wider Environment   Although isolated negative events may do little damage to psychosocial health, persistent stressors, uncertainties, and threats can cause significant

---

Dysfunctional families   Families in which there is violence; physical, emotional, or sexual abuse; parental discord; or other negative family interactions.

Self-efficacy   Belief in one's own ability to perform a task successfully.

Personal control   Belief that one's own internal resources can control a situation.

Self-esteem   Sense of self-respect or self-confidence.

---

problems. Children raised in environments where crime is rampant and daily safety is in question, for example, run an increased risk of psychosocial problems. Drugs, crime, violent acts, school failure, unemployment, and a host of other bad things can happen to good people. But it is believed that certain protective factors, such as having a positive role model in the midst of chaos, may help children from even the worst environments remain healthy and well adjusted.

Another important influence is access to health services and programs designed to enhance psychosocial health. Going to a support group or a trained therapist can be a crucial first step in prevention and intervention efforts. Individuals from poor socioeconomic environments who cannot afford such services often find it difficult to secure help in improving their psychosocial health.

Social Bonds   Although often overlooked, a stable, loving support network of family and friends is key to psychosocial health. The social support of close relationships helps us get through even the most difficult times. Having those with whom we can talk, share thoughts, and practice good and bad behaviors without fear of losing their love is an essential part of growth.

Internal Factors

Many internal factors also shape a person's development. These factors include hereditary traits, hormonal functioning, physical health status (including neurological functioning), physical fitness, and certain elements of mental and emotional health.

Self-Efficacy and Self-Esteem   During our formative years, successes and failures in school, athletics, friendships, intimate relationships, our jobs, and every other aspect of life subtly shape our beliefs about our own personal worth and abilities. These beliefs in turn become internal influences on our psychosocial health.

Psychologist Albert Bandura used the term **self-efficacy** to describe a person's belief about whether he or she can successfully engage in and execute a specific behavior. Prior success in academics, athletics, or social interactions will lead to expectations of success in the future. In general, the more self-efficacious a person is and the more positive past experiences have been, the more likely this person will keep trying to execute a specific behavior successfully. Self-efficacious people are more likely to feel a sense of **personal control** over situations, that their own internal resources allow them to control events. On the other hand, someone with low self-efficacy may give up easily or never even try to change a behavior. Always being the last chosen to play basketball or having long-term difficulty with making friends may make failure seem inevitable.

Self-esteem refers to one's sense of self-respect or self-worth. It can be defined as one's evaluation of oneself and one's own personal worth as an individual. People with high self-esteem tend to feel good about themselves and express a positive outlook on life. People with low self-esteem often do not like themselves, constantly demean themselves, and doubt their ability to succeed.

Our self-esteem is a result of the relationships we have with our parents and family during our formative years, with our friends as we grow older, with our significant others as we form intimate relationships, and with our teachers, coworkers, and others throughout our lives. If we felt loved and valued as children, our self-esteem allows us to believe that we are inherently lovable individuals.

Learned Helplessness versus Learned Optimism   Psychologist Martin Seligman has proposed that people who continually experience failure may develop a pattern of responding known as **learned helplessness** in which they give up and fail to take any action to help themselves. Seligman ascribes this in part to society's tendency toward "victimology," blaming one's problems on other people and circumstances. While viewing ourselves as victims may make us feel better temporarily, it does not address the underlying causes of a problem. Ultimately, it erodes self-efficacy and fosters learned helplessness by making us feel that we cannot do anything to improve the situation.[15]

Countering this is Seligman's principle of **learned optimism:** Just as we learn to be helpless, so can we teach ourselves to be optimistic. His research provides growing evidence for the central place of mental health in overall positive development.[16]

In one study, university freshmen who had been identified as pessimistic on the basis of a questionnaire were randomly assigned to an experimental group or a control group. The experimental group attended a 16-hour workshop in which they practiced social and study skills and learned to dispute chronic negative thoughts. The control group did not participate. Eighteen months later, 15 percent of the control group members were experiencing severe anxiety and 32 percent were suffering from moderate to severe depression. In contrast, only 7 percent of workshop participants suffered from anxiety and 22 percent from depression. Seligman concluded that even relatively brief interventions, such as this workshop, can produce measurable improvements in coping skills.[17]

Personality   Your personality is the unique mix of characteristics that distinguish you from others. Hereditary, environmental, cultural, and experiential factors influence how each person develops. Personality determines how we react to the challenges of life, interpret our feelings, and resolve conflicts.

Most of the recent schools of psychosocial theory promote the idea that we have the power not only to understand our behavior, but also to actively change it and thus mold our own personalities. Yet although much has been written about the importance of a healthy personality, there is little consensus on what that concept really means. In general, people who possess the following traits often appear to be psychosocially healthy.[18]

- *Extroversion,* the ability to adapt to a social situation and demonstrate assertiveness, power, and/or interpersonal involvement.
- *Agreeableness,* the ability to conform, be likable, and demonstrate friendly compliance as well as love.
- *Openness to experience,* the willingness to demonstrate curiosity and independence (also referred to as *inquiring intellect*).
- *Emotional stability,* the ability to maintain social control.
- *Conscientiousness,* the qualities of being dependable and demonstrating self-control, discipline, and a need to achieve.[19]

Life Span and Maturity   Our personalities are not static. Rather, they change as we move through the stages of our lives. Our temperaments also change as we grow, as is illustrated by the extreme emotions experienced by many people in early adolescence. Most of us learn to control our emotions as we advance toward adulthood.

The college years mark a critical transition period for young adults as they move away from families and establish themselves as independent adults. For most, this step toward maturity entails changing the nature of the relationship to parents. Managing personal finances, career strategies, and interpersonal communication are among the developmental tasks college students must accomplish. Older students often have to balance the responsibilities of family, career, and school.

The transition to independence will be easier for those who have successfully accomplished earlier developmental tasks such as learning how to solve problems, make and evaluate decisions, define and adhere to personal values, and establish both casual and intimate relationships. People who have not fulfilled these earlier tasks may find their lives interrupted by recurrent crises left over from earlier stages. For example, if they did not learn to trust others in childhood, they may have difficulty establishing intimate relationships as adults.

What do you think?

Over which external factors does an individual have the most control? ■ *Which factors had the greatest impact on making you who you are today?*

Learned helplessness   Pattern of responding to situations by giving up because of repeated failure in the past.
Learned optimism   Teaching oneself to think optimistically.

Tips for Building Self-Esteem

How can you build self-esteem? Many things you can do daily can have a significant impact on the way you feel about yourself. Practice these tips regularly to bolster your self-esteem.

- *Pay attention to your own needs and wants.* Listen to what your body, your mind, and your heart are telling you.
- *Take very good care of yourself.* Eat healthful foods, avoid junk foods, exercise, and plan fun activities for yourself.
- *Take time to do things you enjoy.* Make a list of things you enjoy doing. Then do something from that list every day.
- *Do something that you have been putting off.* Cleaning out your closet, going on a diet, or paying a bill that you've been putting off will make you feel like you've accomplished something.
- *Give yourself rewards.* Acknowledge that you are a great person by rewarding yourself occasionally.
- *Spend time with people.* People who make you feel better about yourself are great self-esteem boosters. Avoid people who treat you badly or make you feel bad about yourself.
- *Display items that you like.* You may have items that remind you of your achievements, your friends, or of special times. Keep those special items close by.
- *Make your meals a special time.* Get rid of distractions like the television and really concentrate on enjoying your meal, whether by yourself or with others.
- *Learn something new every day.* Take advantage of any opportunity to learn something new every day—you'll feel better about yourself and be more productive.
- *Do something nice for another person.* There is no greater way to feel better about yourself than to help someone in greater need. Check out local volunteer opportunities or make a special effort to be nice to those around you such as your parents or siblings.

Sources: A. L. Story, "Self-Esteem and Self-Certainty: A Mediational Analysis," *European Journal of Personality* 18, no. 2 (March 2004), 115; and M. E. Copeland, "Building Self-Esteem: A Self-Help Guide," Center for Mental Health Services [online booklet] www.mentalhealth.org/publications/allpubs /SMA-3715/default.asp

Enhancing Psychosocial Health

Attaining self-fulfillment is a lifelong, conscious process that involves building self-esteem, understanding and controlling emotions, and learning to solve problems and make decisions. The Skills for Behavior Change box will provide ideas for improving your psychosocial health. In addition to the advice in this chapter, see Chapter 3 for tips on effective stress reduction, relaxation techniques, and other tools for enhancing psychosocial health.

Developing and Maintaining Self-Esteem and Self-Efficacy

There are several ways to build self-esteem and self-efficacy. These include finding a support group, completing required tasks, forming realistic expectations, making time for yourself, maintaining your physical health, and examining your problems and seeking help.

Find a Support Group   The best way to build self-esteem is through a support group—peers who share your values. The prime prerequisite for a support group is that it makes you feel good about yourself and forces you to take an honest look at your actions and choices. Although the idea of finding a support group seems to imply establishing a wholly new group, remember that old ties are often the strongest.

Keeping in contact with old friends and important family members can provide a foundation of unconditional love that will help you through the many life transitions ahead. Try to be a support for others, too. Join a discussion, political action, or recreational group. Write more postcards and "thinking of you" notes to people who matter. This will build both your own self-esteem and that of your friends.

Complete Required Tasks   Develop a history of success by completing required tasks well. You are less likely to succeed in your studies if you leave term papers until the last minute or fail to ask about points that are confusing to you. Most college campuses provide study groups and learning centers that offer tips for managing time, understanding assignments, dealing with professors, and preparing for tests. Poor grades, or grades that do not meet expectations, are major contributors to emotional distress among college students.

Form Realistic Expectations   Set realistic expectations for yourself. If you expect perfect grades, a steady stream of Saturday-night dates and soap-opera romances, and the perfect job, you may be setting yourself up for failure. Assess your current resources and the direction in which you are heading. Set small, incremental goals that are possible to meet.

Make Time for You   Taking time to enjoy yourself is another way to boost self-esteem and psychosocial health. Trying to view each new activity as something to look forward to and an opportunity to have fun is an important part of keeping the excitement in your life. Wake up focusing on the fun things you have to look forward to each day, and try to make this anticipation a natural part of your day.

Maintain Physical Health   Regular exercise fosters a sense of well-being. Nourishing meals can help you avoid the weight gain experienced by many college students. (See Chapter 9 for information on nutrition and Chapter 10 for more on the importance of exercise).

Examine Problems and Seek Help when Necessary
Sometimes you can handle life's problems alone; at other times you may need assistance. Recognize your strengths, act appropriately, and know when to seek help from friends, support groups, family, or professionals.

Sleep: The Great Restorer

Sleep serves at least two biological purposes: (1) conservation of energy so that we are rested and ready to perform during high-performance daylight hours and (2) restoration so that neurotransmitters that have been depleted during waking hours can be replenished. This process clears the brain of daily minutiae to prepare for a new day. Getting enough sleep to feel ready to meet daily challenges is a key factor in physical and psychosocial health.

All of us can identify with that tired, listless feeling caused by sleep deprivation during periods of high stress. Either we can't find enough hours in the day for sleep, or once we get into bed, we can't fall asleep or stay asleep. **Insomnia**—difficulty in falling asleep quickly, frequent arousals during sleep, or early morning awakening—is a common complaint among 20 to 40 percent of Americans. Insomnia is more common among women than among men, and its prevalence is correlated with age and low socioeconomic status.

Some people have difficulty getting a good night's rest due to other sleep disorders. An increasingly common condition is **sleep apnea,** which is characterized by periodic episodes when the sleeper stops breathing completely for 10 seconds or longer at a time or when the sleeper is breathing but not getting enough oxygen.[20] Typically caused by upper respiratory tract problems in which weak muscle tone allows part of the airway to collapse, sleep apnea results in poor air exchange. This in turn raises blood pressure and lowers blood oxygen levels. Sleep apnea can pose a serious health risk.

How much sleep do we need? This depends on many factors. There is a genetically based need for sleep, and it differs for each species. Sleep duration is also controlled by *circadian rhythms*, which are linked to the hormone *melatonin*. People may also alter sleep patterns by staying up late, drinking coffee, getting lots of physical exercise, eating a heavy meal, or using alarm clocks.

Most of us follow characteristic stages of sleep, ranging from *wakefulness* to *drowsiness* to *light sleep,* and then

moving to *deeper sleep*. The most important period of sleep, known as the time of *rapid eye movement (REM)* sleep, is essential to feeling rested and refreshed. In REM sleep, heart rate increases, respiration speeds up, and dreaming tends to occur. If we miss REM sleep, we are left feeling groggy and sleep deprived.

Though many people turn to over-the-counter sleeping pills, barbiturates, or tranquilizers, the following methods for conquering sleeplessness are more effective and less risky:[21]

- Establish a consistent sleep schedule. Go to bed and get up at about the same time every day.
- Evaluate your sleep environment, and change anything that could be keeping you awake. If it's noise, wear earplugs or use a white-noise item such as running a fan. If it's light, try room-darkening shades.
- Exercise regularly; it's hard to feel drowsy if you have been sedentary all day. Don't exercise right before bedtime, however, because activity speeds up your metabolism and makes it harder to go to sleep.
- Limit caffeine and alcohol. Caffeine can linger in your body for up to 12 hours and cause insomnia. While alcohol may make you drowsy at first, it interferes with the normal sleep–wake cycle and can make you wake up early.
- Avoid eating a heavy meal, particularly at bedtime. Don't drink large amounts of liquid before bed.
- If you're unable to get to sleep in 30 minutes, get up and do something else for awhile. Read, play solitaire, or try other relaxing activities, and return to bed when you feel drowsy.
- If you nap, do so only during the afternoon when circadian rhythms make you especially sleepy. Don't let naps interfere with your normal sleep schedule.
- Establish a relaxing nighttime ritual that puts you in the mood to sleep. Take a warm shower, relax in a comfortable chair, don your favorite robe. Doing this consistently will cue your mind and body that it's time to wind down.[22]

The Mind–Body Connection

Can negative emotions make us physically sick? Can positive feelings help us stay well? Researchers are exploring the interaction between emotions and health, especially in conditions of uncontrolled, persistent stress. According to one theory, the brain of an emotionally overwrought person sends signals to the adrenal glands, which respond by secreting cortisol and epinephrine (adrenaline), the hormones that

---

Insomnia   Difficulty in falling asleep or staying asleep.

Sleep apnea   Disorder in which a person has numerous episodes of breathing stoppage during a normal night's sleep.

activate the body's stress response. These chemicals are also known to suppress immune functioning, possibly causing subtle immune changes. What remains to be shown is whether these changes affect overall health.

Happiness: A Key to Well-Being

Although we can list the actions that we should perform to become physically healthy, such as eating the right foods, getting enough rest, exercising, and so on, it is less clear how to achieve that "feeling-good state" that researchers call **subjective well-being (SWB)**. This refers to that uplifting feeling of inner peace and wonder that we call happiness. Psychologists David Myers and Ed Deiner completed a major study of happiness and noted that people experience it in many different ways, based on age, culture, gender, and so on.[23] However, in spite of these differences, SWB is defined by three central components:[24]

1. *Satisfaction with present life.* People who are high in SWB tend to like their work and are satisfied with their current personal relationships. They are sociable, outgoing, and willing to open up to others. They also like themselves and enjoy good health and self-esteem.
2. *Relative presence of positive emotions.* People high in SWB more frequently feel pleasant emotions, mainly because they evaluate the world around them in a generally positive way. They have an optimistic outlook, and they expect success in what they undertake.
3. *Relative absence of negative emotions.* Individuals with a strong sense of subjective well-being experience fewer and less severe episodes of such negative emotions as anxiety, depression, and anger.

What do you think?

How do you rate on each of the components of subjective well-being? ▪ *What factors influence your SWB?* ▪ *How has it changed over the course of your life?*

Myths and Misperceptions about Happiness

Do you have to be happy all the time to achieve subjective well-being? Of course not. Everyone experiences disappointment, unhappiness, and times when life seems unfair. However, people with SWB are typically resilient, able to look on the positive side and get themselves back on track fairly quickly, and less likely to fall into deep despair over setbacks.

Subjective well-being (SWB)   That uplifting feeling of inner peace and wonder that we call happiness.

There are several myths about happiness: that it depends on age, gender, race, and socioeconomic status. Research and empirical evidence, however, have debunked a variety of myths and instead support the following conclusions.[25]

- *There is no "happiest age."* Age is not a predictor of SWB. Most age groups exhibit similar levels of life satisfaction, although the things that bring joy often change with age.
- *Happiness has no gender gap.* Women are more likely than men to suffer from anxiety and depression, and men are more at risk for alcoholism and personality disorders. However, equal numbers of men and women report being fairly satisfied with life.
- *There are minimal racial differences in happiness.* For example, African Americans and European Americans report nearly the same levels of happiness, and African Americans are slightly less vulnerable to depression. Despite racism and discrimination, members of disadvantaged minority groups generally seem to think optimistically by making realistic self-comparisons and attributing problems less to themselves than to unfair circumstances.
- *Money does not buy happiness.* Wealthier societies report greater well-being. However, once the basic necessities of food, shelter, and safety are provided, there is a very weak correlation between income and happiness. Having no money is a cause of misery, but wealth itself does not guarantee happiness.

Fortunately, humans are remarkably resourceful creatures. We respond to great loss or a traumatic event, such as the death of a loved one, with an initial period of grief, mourning, and sometimes rage. Yet, with time and the support of loving family and friends, we pick ourselves up, brush off the bad times, and manage to find satisfaction and peace. Typically, humans learn from suffering and emerge even stronger and more ready to deal with the next crisis. Most find some measure of happiness after the initial shock and pain of loss. Those who are otherwise healthy, in good physical condition, and part of a strong social support network can adapt and cope effectively.

Does Laughter Enhance Health?

Remember the last time you laughed so hard that you cried? Remember how relaxed you felt afterward? Scientists are just beginning to understand the role of humor in our lives and health:

- Stressed-out people with a strong sense of humor become less depressed and anxious than those whose sense of humor is less well developed.
- Students who use humor as a coping mechanism report that it predisposes them to a positive mood.
- In a study of depressed and suicidal senior citizens, patients who recovered were the ones who demonstrated a sense of humor.
- Telling a joke, particularly one that involves a shared experience, increases our sense of belonging and social cohesion.

Strategies for Resolving Conflict

Stereotyped gender roles have often taught men and women different ways to communicate. These differences frequently translate into conflict both at home and in the workplace. Women tend to be more indirect, less comfortable with conflict, less willing to force an issue, and more interested in collaborating. Men tend to thrive on direct conflict, express their opinions loudly, be more data driven and opinionated, and avoid anything too emotional.

Depending on the situation, both approaches have value. Assertiveness and conviction are effective for conveying information and making rapid decisions, especially in formal hierarchies, while a collaborative style is valuable for promoting cooperation and building consensus. When these communication styles clash, they can lead to misunderstanding and conflict.

You can't avoid conflict so it's best to learn how to handle tensions construc-tively as they arise. Leslie A. Perlow, author of *When You Say Yes But Mean No: How Silencing Conflict Wrecks Relationships and Companies . . . and What You Can Do About It*, writes, "The goal in effectively expressing difference is to replace vicious silent spirals with virtuous spirals of speaking up." Some tips for resolving conflict include the following.

1. *Seek mutual understanding by putting others first.* Be sure to start with facts, not feelings. Facts enable us to start with what we know rather than what we feel, which can make a big difference in resolving conflict.

2. *Turn the situation around by being honest and upfront.* Take some time to calm down and think about what to do. Acknowledge the differences you are experiencing. Make sure that you have expressed yourself clearly. Then seek to turn the situation around by finding alternative ways to express yourself or by gathering more information to support your viewpoint.

3. *Speak up, but don't forget to listen.* Bring up and talk about the real issues, even ones that may be difficult to discuss with the other person. Speaking up and expressing your thoughts, feelings, and goals can help you achieve mutual understanding while acknowledging each other's positions. At the same time, keep listening because that is where resolution begins.

Confronting someone, whether male or female, is never easy, but it can lead to better understanding and a more productive use of time. The basic principles of conflict resolution should always transcend gender.

Sources: K. Ludeman and E. Erlandson, "Coaching the Alpha Male," *Harvard Business Review* 82, no. 5 (May 2004), 61; R. Levine, "Male Speak, Female Speak: Bridging the Gap," *Medical Meetings* 30, no. 5 (July/August 2003), 41; L. A. Perlow, *When You Say Yes But Mean No: How Silencing Conflict Wrecks Relationships and Companies . . . and What You Can Do About It* (New York: Crown Business/Random House, 2003); C. L. Gillan, "Putting Out the Fires of Conflict," *Child Care Information Exchange* 151 (May–June 2003), 71–74.

Laughter helps us in many ways. People like to be around others who are fun-loving and laugh easily. Learning to laugh puts more joy into everyday experiences and increases the likelihood that fun-loving people will keep company with us.

Psychologist Barbara Fredrickson argues that positive emotions such as joy, interest, and contentment serve valuable life functions. Joy is associated with playfulness and creativity. Interest encourages us to explore our world, enhancing knowledge and cognitive ability. Contentment allows us to savor and integrate experiences, an important step to achieving mindfulness and insight. By building our physical, social, and mental resources, these positive feelings empower us to cope effectively with life's challenges. While the actual emotions may be transient, their effects can be permanent and provide lifelong enrichment.[26]

Laughter also seems to have positive physiological effects. A number of researchers, such as Lee Berk, MD, and Stanley Tan, MD, have noted that laughter sharpens our immune systems by activating T cells and natural killer cells and increasing production of immunity-boosting interferon.[27] It also reduces levels of the stress hormone cortisol.

In one experiment, Fredrickson monitored the cardiovascular responses of human subjects who suffered fear and anxiety induced by an unsettling film clip. Some of them then viewed a humorous film clip, while others did not. Those who watched the humorous film returned more quickly to their baseline cardiovascular state, indicating that laughter may counteract some of the physical effects of negative emotions.[28]

In another study, 50 women with advanced breast cancer who were randomly assigned to a weekly support group lived an average of 18 months longer than 36 cancer patients not in the support group. The implication of this finding is that the women in the support group cheered each other on, and this encouraged them to sleep and eat better, which promoted their survival. Other researchers have found that a fighting spirit and the determination to survive are vital adjuncts to standard cancer therapy.[29]

Relaxation therapies such as meditation and yoga offer the chance to practice self-initiated contentment, thus providing practical skills for dealing with day-to-day stress. These therapies have proved to be effective treatments for physical ailments such as headaches, chronic pain, and high blood pressure.[30]

While positive emotions appear to benefit physical health, evidence is accumulating that negative emotions can impair it. Studies of widowed and divorced people reveal below-normal immune system functioning and higher rates of illness and death than among married people. Other studies have shown unusually high rates of cancer among depressed people.[31]

Some researchers believe that certain psychosocial behaviors actually make people vulnerable to illness. Psychologist Lydia Temoshok studied people with malignant melanoma (a potentially deadly skin cancer) and found that 75 percent shared common traits. They tended to be unfailingly pleasant, repress their negative feelings and emotions, and make extraordinary attempts to accommodate others. She hypothesized that this "Type C" personality signals emotional repression, which may suppress the immune system.[32]

Do these studies provide conclusive evidence of a mind–body connection? Not necessarily, because they do not account for other factors known to be relevant to health. For example, some researchers suggest that people who are divorced, widowed, or depressed are more likely to drink and smoke, use drugs, eat and sleep poorly, and be sedentary—all of which may affect the immune system. In fact, the immune system changes measured in studies of the mind–body connection are relatively small. The health consequences of such minute changes are difficult to gauge because the body can tolerate a certain amount of reduced immune function without contracting illness. The exact amount it is able to tolerate and under what circumstances are still in question.[33]

A large body of evidence points to an association between the emotions and physical health. Does an emotional state trigger negative behaviors that impair immune function? Or do emotions directly affect health by stimulating the production of hormones that tax the immune system? We still have much to learn about this relationship. In the meantime, however, it appears that happiness and an optimistic mind-set don't just feel good—they are also good for you.

When Psychosocial Health Deteriorates

Sometimes circumstances overwhelm us to such a degree that we need outside assistance to help us get back on track toward healthful living. Abusive relationships, stress, anxiety, loneliness, financial upheavals, and other traumatic events

---

can sap our spirits, causing us to turn inward or to act in ways that are outside of what might be considered normal. Chemical imbalances, drug interactions, trauma, neurological disruptions, and other physical problems also may contribute to these behaviors. **Mental illnesses** are disorders that disrupt thinking, feeling, moods, and behaviors, and cause a varying degree of impaired functioning in daily life. They are believed to be caused by life events in some cases and by actual biochemical and/or brain dysfunction in other instances.[34]

As with physical disease, mental illnesses can range from mild to severe and exact a heavy toll on the quality of life, both for those with the illnesses and those who come in contact with them. Although mental illness often is not discussed as openly as physical ailments, mental illness is universal. Recent reports by the World Health Organization, the World Bank, and Harvard University indicate that mental illness is the second leading cause of disability and premature death in developed countries—right behind cardiovascular disease and just ahead of cancer.[35] Or consider this from the Mayo Clinic:

> Imagine attending a 25th reunion at your local high school. Studies tell us that, on average, out of every 100 people on the dance floor, 28 have coped with a mental or substance abuse disorder in the past year. Of these, a dozen or so have had symptoms of an anxiety disorder, such as panic disorder or social phobia. Ten have struggled with an addiction, most likely to be alcohol, and about 10 have lived with a mood disorder, perhaps depression or bipolar disorder. These numbers add up to more than 28 because some people experience more than one illness at the same time, just as high blood pressure, diabetes, and asthma may occur together. Although these conditions are common, fear of seeming weak or defective makes many people reluctant to acknowledge mental or emotional distress.[36]

Although there are many types of mental illnesses, we will focus here on those most likely to be experienced by large numbers of college students. For information about other disorders, consult the websites at the end of this chapter or ask your instructor for local resources.

Depression: The Full-Scale Tumble

In a recent meeting of the American Psychological Association, the organization's president remarked, "Depression has been called the common cold of psychological disturbances, which underscores its prevalence, but trivializes its impact."[37] In any one-year period, nearly 10 percent, or 20 million, American adults suffer from a depressive illness.[38] Many of them are misdiagnosed, underdiagnosed, and not receiving treatment, despite its availability.[39]

Major Depressive Disorder It is normal to feel blue or depressed in response to certain experiences, such as the death of a loved one, divorce, loss of a job, or an unhappy ending

---

Mental illnesses Disorders that disrupt thinking, feeling, moods, and behaviors, and impair daily functioning.

to a long-term relationship. However, people with **major depressive disorder** experience a form of **chronic mood disorder** that involves, on a day-to-day basis, extreme and persistent sadness, despair, and hopelessness. People with this disorder typically feel discouraged by life and circumstances and experience feelings of intense guilt and worthlessness. They may be hypercritical of others and feel disappointed by others most of the time. Usually they show some impairment of social and occupational functioning, although their behavior is not necessarily bizarre. Approximately 15 percent of them eventually attempt suicide or succeed in committing suicide.[40] Untold numbers of others victimize their families, cause disruptions, or display outwardly violent acts.

Depression can strike at any age, but the first episode usually occurs before age 40. (Table 2.1 lists common symptoms.) Some people experience one bout of depression and never have problems again, but others suffer recurrences throughout their lives. Stressful life events are often catalysts for these recurrences.

Risks for Depression

Major depressive disorder is caused by the interaction between biology, learned behavioral responses, and cognitive factors. Chemical and genetic processes may predispose people to depression, and irrational ideas and beliefs can guide them to negative coping behaviors.[41] Some people, because of genetic history, environment, situational triggers and stressors, poor behavioral skills, and brain–body chemistry, may be particularly vulnerable.

Facts and Fallacies about Depression

Although it is one of the fastest-growing problems in U.S. culture, depression remains one of the most misunderstood mental disorders. Myths and misperceptions about the disease abound; and research results now support the following.[42]

- *True depression is not a natural reaction to crisis and loss.* It is a pervasive and systemic biological problem. Symptoms may come and go, and their severity will fluctuate, but they do not simply go away. Crisis and loss can lead an already depressed person over the edge to suicide or other problems, but crisis and loss do not inevitably result in depression.
- *People will not snap out of depression by using a little willpower.* Telling a depressed person to "snap out of it" is like telling a diabetic to produce more insulin. Medical intervention in the form of antidepressant drugs and therapy is often necessary for recovery. Understanding the seriousness of the disease and supporting people in their attempts to recover are key elements.
- *Frequent crying is not a hallmark of depression.* Some depressed people bear their burdens in silence or may even be the life of the party. Some don't cry at all. In fact, biochemists theorize that crying may actually ward off depression by releasing chemicals that the body produces as a positive response to stress.

Table 2.1
Are You Depressed?

Sadness and despair are the main symptoms of depression. Other common signs include:

- Loss of motivation or interest in pleasurable activities
- Preoccupation with failures and inadequacies; concern over what others are thinking
- Difficulty concentrating; indecisiveness; memory lapses
- Loss of sex drive or interest in close interactions with others
- Fatigue and loss of energy; slow reactions
- Sleeping too much or too little; insomnia
- Feeling agitated, worthless, or hopeless
- Withdrawal from friends and family
- Diminished or increased appetite
- Recurring thoughts that life isn't worth living, thoughts of death or suicide
- Significant weight loss or weight gain

Some depressed people mask their symptoms with a forced, upbeat sense of humor or high energy levels. Communication may cease or seem frantic.

- *True depression is not "all in the mind."* Depression isn't a disease of weak-willed, powerless people. In fact, research suggests that depressive illnesses originate with an inherited chemical imbalance in the brain. In addition, some physiological conditions, such as thyroid disorders, multiple sclerosis, chronic fatigue syndrome, and certain cancers have depressive side effects. Certain medications also are known to prompt depression-like symptoms.
- *In-depth psychotherapy is not the only cure for long-term clinical depression.* No single psychotherapy method works for all cases of depression.

Depression and Gender

According to the National Institute of Mental Health (NIMH), women experience depression at nearly two times the rate of men: 8 to 11 percent of men compared to 19 to 23 percent of women. About 6 percent of women and 3 percent of men have experienced episodes severe enough to require hospitalization.[43]

Many hormonal factors may contribute to the increased rates in women, particularly such events as menstrual cycle changes, pregnancy, miscarriage, postpartum period, premenopause, and menopause. In fact, an NIMH study indicated that in the case of severe premenstrual

---

Major depressive disorder Severe depression that entails chronic mood disorder, physical effects such as sleep disturbance and exhaustion, and mental effects such as the inability to concentrate.

Chronic mood disorder Experience of persistent sadness, despair, and hopelessness.

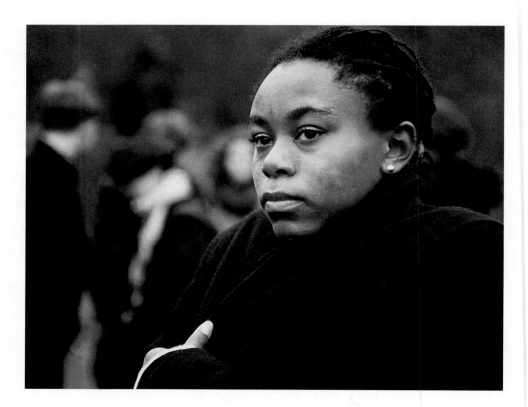

When experiencing problems such as depression, it is unwise to try to "go it alone." A qualified, caring therapist can help.

syndrome (PMS), women with a pre-existing vulnerability to PMS experienced relief from mood swings and physical symptoms when their sex hormones were suppressed. Shortly after the hormones were reintroduced, they again developed symptoms of PMS. Women with no history of PMS reported no effects of hormonal manipulation.[44]

Although adolescent and adult females have been found to experience depression at twice the rate of males, the college population seems to represent a notable exception, with equal rates experienced by males and females. Why? Several theories have been suggested:[45]

- The social institutions of the college campus provide more egalitarian roles for men and women.
- College women experience fewer negative events than do high school females. Men in college report more negative events than they experienced in high school.
- College women report smaller and more supportive social networks.

Depression is often preceded by a stressful event. Some psychologists therefore theorize that women are under more stress than men and thus more prone to become depressed. However, women do not report more stressful events than men do.

Finally, researchers have observed gender differences in coping strategies (responses to certain events or stimuli) and have proposed that some women's strategies make them more vulnerable to depression. Presented with a list of things people do when depressed, college students were asked to indicate how likely they were to engage in each behavior. Men were more likely to assert that "I avoid thinking of reasons why I am depressed," "I do something physical," or "I play sports." Women were more likely to answer "I try to determine why I am depressed," "I talk to other people about my feelings," and "I cry to relieve the tension." In other words, the men tried to distract themselves from a depressed mood whereas the women focused on it. If focusing obsessively on negative feelings intensifies these feelings, women who do this may predispose themselves to depression. This hypothesis has not been directly tested, but some supporting evidence suggests its validity.[46]

Overall, the rate of depression among men may be increasing. Certain factors, such as family history, undue stress, loss of a loved one, or serious illness, seem to increase the risk.[47] Men are less likely than women to admit to depression, and doctors are less likely to suspect it. Men's depression is also more likely to be hidden by alcohol or drug abuse or by the socially acceptable habit of working excessively long hours. Depression typically shows up in men not as feeling hopeless and helpless, but as being irritable, angry, and discouraged. One marker of the problem is that, although more women attempt suicide, the rate of suicide in men is actually four times that of women. In fact, after age 70, the rate of men's suicide rises, reaching a peak after age 85.[48]

Interestingly, depression seems also to be more lethal for men than women in terms of physical health. Although depression is associated with an increased risk of coronary heart disease in both genders, only men suffer a high death rate.[49] Because even men who realize they may be depressed are less likely to seek help than women, encouragement and support from concerned friends and family members are crucial.

Table 2.2
Drug Treatments for Depression

	SSRIs (Selective Serotonin Reuptake Inhibitors)	TCAs (Tricyclic Antidepressants)	MAOIs (Monoamine Oxidase Inhibitors)
How They Work	An SSRI works by stabilizing levels of serotonin, an important neurotransmitter. Low levels of serotonin have been linked to depression and other mood disorders.	An earlier family of anti-depressant drugs, TCAs increase the brain's levels of norepinephrine, a neurotransmitter.	MAOIs increase the levels of epinephrine, norepinephrine, and serotonin in the brain.
Commonly Prescribed Antidepressant Drugs	Zoloft, Prozac, Luvox, Paxil, Paxil CR, Celexa, Lexapro	Adapin, Endep, Norpramin, Pamelorf, Sinequan, Effexor	Nardil, Pamate, Remeron, Wellbutrin
Advantages	Relatively few side effects and no withdrawal symptoms. An SSRI is generally the first choice of most physicians.	Some patients respond better to TCA medication than they do to SSRIs.	May be used if other depression medications fail to treat the condition.
Disadvantages	Possible increase in suicidal tendencies under investigation. Can be transferred in breast milk; may cause weight gain, reduced sexual desire.	More side effects than SSRIs. May cause sensitivity to heat, which makes it harder for the body to adapt to temperature changes. Must be discontinued slowly or withdrawal symptoms may occur.	A strict dietary regime must be followed. Failure to do so can result in hypertensive crisis, which can be fatal. Many other medications react badly with MAOIs.

Source: "Selective Serotonin Reuptake Inhibitors" from Treatment-for-Depression.com. Copyright © NCER, LLC, Oceanside, CA. Reprinted by permission.

Depression in Selected Populations There are a few exceptions to the findings on depression and gender. Among Jews, males are equally as likely as females to experience major depressive episodes.[50] In recent years, there has also been a noteworthy increase in depression among children, the elderly, and adolescents, particularly adolescent girls, and perhaps in Native American and homosexual young people as well.[51] Writers, composers, and entertainers also seem to have higher than expected rates of major depression, and people experiencing chronic, unrelenting pain have the highest rates of any group.[52]

Depression in older adults is often undiagnosed. Sufferers may be even less likely to report hopelessness, sadness, loss of interest in normally pleasurable activities, or prolonged grief than their younger counterparts. Sometimes their depression is attributed to drug reactions or the aging process, rather than to an underlying problem. As the elderly person becomes more isolated and has fewer social contacts, it becomes more difficult for anyone to recognize that depressed behaviors are unusual, and the symptoms may become progressively worse without treatment.

Treating Depression The best treatment involves determining the person's type and degree of depression and its possible causes. Both psychotherapeutic and pharmacological modes of treatment are recommended for clinical (severe and prolonged) depression. Drugs often relieve the symptoms of depression, such as loss of sleep or appetite, while psychotherapy can be equally helpful by improving the ability to function (Table 2.2).[53]

In some cases, psychotherapy alone may be the most successful treatment. The two most common psychotherapeutic treatments for depression are cognitive therapy and interpersonal therapy. *Cognitive therapy* aims to help a patient look at life rationally and correct habitually pessimistic thought patterns. It focuses on the here and now rather than analyzing a patient's past. To pull a person out of depression, cognitive therapists usually need 6 to 18 months of weekly sessions comprising reasoning and behavioral exercises. *Interpersonal therapy*, sometimes combined with cognitive therapy, also addresses the present but focuses on correcting chronic relationship problems. Interpersonal therapists focus on patients' relationships with their families and other people.

Antidepressant drugs relieve symptoms in nearly 80 percent of people with chronic depression. Several types of the medications known as *tricyclic* antidepressants (TCAs) are available and work by preventing excessive absorption of mood-altering neurotransmitters. Tricyclics can take six weeks to three months to become effective. Newer antidepressant drugs, called *tetracyclics*, work in one or two weeks.

In recent years, Zoloft and Prozac have become such a common part of our vocabulary that it doesn't seem at all unusual to know someone who is taking an antidepressant. This could lead one to think that antidepressants can be taken like aspirin. However, countless emergency room visits occur when people misuse antidepressants, try to quit by going "cold turkey," or suffer reactions to the drugs.

The potency and dosage of each vary greatly. Antidepressants should be prescribed only after a thorough psychological and physiological examination. Recently, the U.S. Food and Drug Administration has asked the makers of antidepressant drugs to add a warning to the labels advising that patients taking these drugs should be monitored for "worsening depression or the emergence of suicidality." This warning applies to commonly prescribed drugs such as Prozac, Zoloft, Paxil, Luvox, Celexa, Lexapro, Wellbutrin, Effexor, Serzone, and Remeron.[54]

If your doctor suggests an antidepressant, ask these questions first:

- What biological indicators are you using to determine whether I really need this drug? (Beware of the health professional who gives you a five-minute exam, asks you if you are feeling down or blue, and prescribes an antidepressant to fix your problems.)
- What is the action of this drug? What will it do, and when will I start to feel the benefits?
- What is your rationale for selecting this antidepressant over others?
- What are the side effects of using this drug?
- How long can I be on this medication without significant risk to my health?
- What happens if I stop taking it?
- How will you follow up or monitor the levels of this drug in my body? How often will I need to be checked?

Electroconvulsive therapy (ECT) is another treatment for depression. A patient given ECT is sedated under light general anesthesia, and electric current is applied to the patient's temples for five seconds at a time for 15 or 20 minutes. Ten to 20 percent of people with depression who do not respond to drug therapy are responsive to ECT. However, because it carries a risk of permanent memory loss, some therapists do not recommend ECT under any circumstances.

Clinics have been established in large metropolitan areas to offer group support for depressed people. Some clinics treat all types of depressed people; others restrict themselves to specific groups, such as widows, adolescents, or families and friends of people with depression.

Bipolar disorder   Form of depression characterized by alternating mania and depression.

Anxiety disorders   Disorders characterized by persistent feelings of threat and anxiousness in coping with everyday problems.

Bipolar Disorder   Also known as manic-depressive illness, **bipolar disorder** is considered another form of depression. It is characterized by alternating emotional highs (mania) and lows (depression). Symptoms can vary from mild to disabling and severe. Bipolar disorder affects more than 2 million adult Americans, about 1 percent of the population age 18 and older. It often begins in adolescence and can last for weeks or months at a time—sometimes it may persist for life. In the depression phase, symptoms follow the same pattern as in a major depressive syndrome. In the manic phase, symptoms may include feelings of euphoria, extreme optimism and inflated self-esteem; rapid speech, racing thoughts, agitation, and increased physical activity; poor judgment and recklessness; difficulty sleeping; tendency to be easily distracted; inability to concentrate; and extreme irritability.[55]

Although the exact cause of bipolar disorder is unknown, biological, genetic, and environmental factors seem to be involved in causing episodes of the illness. Evidence indicates that neurotransmitters in people with the disorder differ from those in people without the disorder. Bipolar disorder tends to run in families, with about 60 percent of cases showing a family history. Thus, a genetic predisposition to have abnormal genes regulating neurotransmitter action may be a risk factor.[56] Factors that are believed to trigger episodes include drug abuse and stressful or psychologically traumatic events. Once diagnosed, persons with bipolar disorder have a number of counseling and pharmaceutical options, and most will be able to live a healthy, functional life while being treated.

Anxiety Disorders: Facing Your Fears

Anxiety disorders, which are characterized by persistent feelings of threat and worry, are a little-understood yet common psychological problem. Consider John Madden, former head coach of the Oakland Raiders and a true "man's man," who has outfitted his own bus and drives every weekend across the country to serve as commentator on NFL football games. What's the reason behind this exhausting driving schedule? Madden is terrified of getting on a plane.

Anxiety disorders are the number-one mental health problem in the United States, affecting over 19 million people aged 18 to 54 each year, or about 13 percent of all adults.[57] Some sources place the number as high as 25 percent. Anxiety is also a leading mental health problem among adolescents, affecting 13 million youngsters aged 9 to 17. Costs associated with an overly anxious populace are growing rapidly; conservative estimates cite nearly $50 billion a year spent in doctors' bills and workplace losses in America. According to a study by the World Health Organization (WHO), the odds of developing an anxiety disorder have doubled in the past four decades.[58] These numbers don't begin to address the human costs incurred when a person is too fearful to leave the house or to talk to anyone outside the immediate family. Anxiety-related ailments include generalized anxiety disorders, panic disorder, specific phobias, and social phobias.

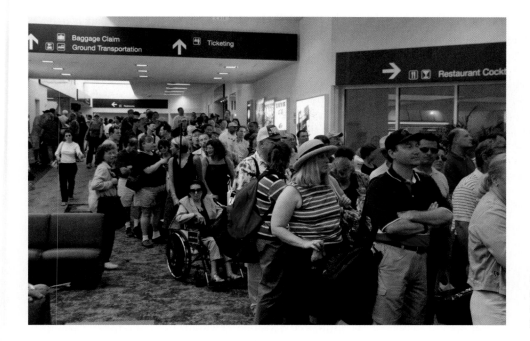

Overcrowded airports and increased security make travel even more difficult for people susceptible to panic attacks brought on by flying.

Generalized Anxiety Disorder One common form of anxiety disorder, **generalized anxiety disorder (GAD),** is severe enough to significantly interfere with daily life. Generally, the person with this disorder is a consummate worrier who develops a debilitating level of anxiety. Often multiple sources of worry exist, and it is hard to pinpoint the root cause of the anxiety. A diagnosis of GAD depends on showing at least three of the following symptoms for more days than not during a period of six months.[59]

1. Restlessness or feeling keyed up or on edge
2. Being easily fatigued
3. Difficulty concentrating or mind going blank
4. Irritability
5. Muscle tension
6. Sleep disturbances (difficulty falling or staying asleep or restless sleep)

Often GAD runs in families and is readily treatable with benzodiazepines such as Librium, Valium, and Xanax, which calm the person for short periods. Individual therapy can be a more effective long-term treatment.

Panic Disorders On a recent trip to a professional conference, Marilyn Erickson (not her real name) boarded a connecting flight at O'Hare International Airport, only to find that her husband John, a professor at a major university, was missing. Marilyn got off the plane and searched frantically throughout the airport for him. Finally, long after the plane had departed, she found John sitting on a bench outside the terminal; he was vomiting, dizzy, and distraught over the mere thought of boarding the plane. When Marilyn suggested catching another flight, he trembled violently and refused to move from the bench. They returned to their home on the West Coast on a bus and missed their scheduled conference appearance.

Professor Erickson suffered a **panic attack,** a form of acute anxiety reaction that brings on an intense physical reaction. This reaction may be so severe that you fear you will have a heart attack and die—or you may dismiss it as the jitters from too much stress. Between 10 and 20 percent of Americans experience panic attacks at some time in their lives. Although highly treatable, it is also growing in incidence, particularly among young women. Panic attacks may become debilitating and destructive, particularly if they happen often and lead the person to avoid going out in public or interacting with others.

A panic attack typically starts abruptly, peaks within 10 minutes, lasts about 30 minutes, and leaves the person tired and drained.[60] In addition to those just described, symptoms can include increased respiration rate, chills, hot flashes, shortness of breath, stomach cramps, chest pain, difficulty swallowing, and a sense of doom or impending death.

Although researchers aren't sure of causation, heredity, stress, and certain biochemical factors may play a role. Your chances of having a panic attack increase if you have a close family member who has them. Some researchers believe that people who suffer panic attacks are experiencing an over-reactive fight-or-flight physical response (see Chapter 3).

As with other anxiety-based disorders, medication and cognitive behavioral therapy are often the keys to treatment. Some individuals are given antidepressants, which often

Generalized anxiety disorder (GAD) A constant sense of worry that may cause restlessness, difficulty in concentrating, tension, and other symptoms.

Panic attack Severe anxiety reaction in which a particular situation, often for unknown reasons, causes terror.

prevent future attacks. In some cases, a medication to relieve anxiety is effective given alone or with other drugs.[61] Cognitive therapy can help sufferers recognize and avoid triggers or deal with triggers through meditation, deep breathing, and other relaxation techniques. Patients usually show improvement within eight to ten sessions.

Specific Phobias   In contrast to panic disorders, **phobias,** or phobic disorders, involve a persistent and irrational fear of a specific object, activity, or situation, often out of proportion to the circumstances. About 13 percent of Americans suffer from phobias, such as fear of spiders, snakes, public speaking, and so on. Social phobias are perhaps the most common phobic response.[62]

Social Phobias   A **social phobia** is an anxiety disorder characterized by the persistent fear and avoidance of social situations. Essentially, the person dreads these situations for fear of being humiliated, embarrassed, or even looked at.[63] These disorders vary in scope. Some cause difficulty only in specific situations, such as getting up in front of the class to give a report. In more extreme cases, a person avoids all contact with others.

Sources of Anxiety Disorders   Because anxiety disorders vary in complexity and degree, scientists have yet to find clear reasons why one person develops them and another doesn't. The following factors are often cited as possible causes.

- *Biology.* Some scientists trace the origin of anxiety to the brain and brain functioning. Using sophisticated positron emission tomography scans (PET scans), scientists can analyze areas of the brain that react during anxiety-producing events. Families appear to display similar brain and physiological reactivity, so we may inherit our tendencies toward anxiety disorders.
- *Environment.* Anxiety may also be a learned response. Though genetic tendencies may exist, experiencing a repeated pattern of reaction to certain situations programs the brain to respond in a certain way. For example, mon-

keys separated from their mothers at an early age are more fearful and their stress hormones fire more readily than those that stayed with their mothers. If your mother (or father) screamed whenever a large spider crept into view or if other anxiety-raising events occurred frequently, you might be predisposed to react with anxiety to similar events later in your life. Animals also experience such anxieties—perhaps from being around their edgy owners.

- *Social and cultural roles.* Because men and women are taught to assume different roles in society (such as man as protector, woman as victim), women may find it more acceptable to scream, shake, pass out, and otherwise express extreme anxiety. Men, on the other hand, have learned to repress such anxieties rather than act upon them. See the Reality Check box information on another psychological disorder of growing concern— self-mutilation.

Seasonal Affective Disorder (SAD)

An estimated 6 percent of Americans suffer from **seasonal affective disorder (SAD),** a type of depression, and an additional 14 percent experience a milder form of the disorder known as the winter blues. SAD strikes during the winter months and is associated with reduced exposure to sunlight. People with SAD suffer from irritability, apathy, carbohydrate craving, and weight gain, increases in sleep time, and general sadness. Researchers believe that SAD is caused by a malfunction in the hypothalamus, the gland responsible for regulating responses to external stimuli. Stress may also play a role.

Certain factors seem to put people at risk for SAD. Women are four times more likely to suffer from it than men. Although SAD can occur at any age, people aged 20 to 40 appear to be most vulnerable. Certain families appear to be at risk. Residents of northern states, where there are fewer hours of sunlight during the winter, are more at risk than those living in the South. An estimated 10 percent of the population in Maine, Minnesota, and Wisconsin experience SAD, compared to fewer than 2 percent of those in Florida and New Mexico.

Therapies for SAD are simple but effective. The most beneficial is light therapy, which exposes patients to lamps that simulate sunlight. Eighty percent of patients experience relief from their symptoms within four days of treatment. Other treatments for SAD include diet change (eating more complex carbohydrates), increased exercise, stress management techniques, sleep restriction (limiting the number of hours slept in a 24-hour period), psychotherapy, and antidepressants.

Schizophrenia

Perhaps the most frightening of all mental disorders is **schizophrenia,** which affects about 1 percent of the U.S. population. Schizophrenia is characterized by alterations of the senses (including auditory and visual hallucinations); the

---

Phobia   A deep and persistent fear of a specific object, activity, or situation that results in a compelling desire to avoid the source of the fear.

Social phobia   A phobia characterized by fear and avoidance of social situations.

Seasonal affective disorder (SAD)   A type of depression that occurs in the winter months, when sunlight levels are low.

Schizophrenia   A mental illness with biological origins that is characterized by irrational behavior, severe alterations of the senses (hallucinations), and often an inability to function in society.

Cutting through the Pain

Self-injury is an alarming phenomenon on the rise that especially affects bright, middle-class teens and young adults. Also called self-mutilation, self-hurt, self-abuse, or self-harm, self-injury is deliberate harm inflicted on one's own body in an attempt to alter a mood state. Cutting (with razors, glass, knives, etc.) is the most common way that people choose to hurt themselves, followed by burning, bruising, excessive nail biting, breaking bones, and pulling out hair. Those who self-injure don't feel the pain because they are in a state of dissociation, or mentally removed from reality.

Self-injury is a coping mechanism used to deal with stress and sadness. Some studies suggest that when people who self-injure feel emotionally overwhelmed, inflicting physical pain reduces tension and stress almost immediately and calms them down.

The typical self-injurer is female, single, has average to high intelligence, low self-esteem, and comes from middle- to upper-middle-class families. Self-injury usually starts during puberty (most of the self-injurers range in age from 11 to 17, although some are adults). About half say they were physically or sexually abused in their childhoods, although some experts estimate up to 90 percent have been abused. New York psychotherapist Steven Levenkron has written six books on the subject, and his research shows that 85 percent of those who self-injure are girls; boys tend to direct their emotions toward others, while girls turn their feelings inward.

Experts estimate anywhere from 1 to 4 percent of the population in the United States purposely hurt themselves in some way. Dr. Armando Favazza, a psychiatry professor at the University of Missouri-Columbia Medical School, says about 1,500 per 100,000 Americans self-mutilate today.

Signs of self-injury include scars or current cuts or abrasions and flimsy excuses for these wounds. A self-injurer may wear long sleeves and pants in warm weather to hide the wounds. Difficulty handling anger, social withdrawal, sensitivity to rejection, or body alienation may also be symptoms of self-injury.

Treatments currently being explored range from psychotherapy to medications such as antidepressants and mood stabilizers. What all of the treatments have in common is the goal to end the feelings that prompt the behavior, not just to stop the behavior itself.

Self-cutters who are currently in treatment offer the following tips for dealing with the desire to cut:

✔ *Do something creative with your hands.* Keep your hands busy with painting, making a collage, or even cleaning.
✔ *Play with your pets.* Taking care of and playing with animals diverts your attention and your hands.
✔ *Communicate your feelings.* Tell someone you trust how you are feeling. You don't need to explain yourself, just let them know what you are going through.
✔ *Start a journal.* This is a place to write your thoughts and feelings down. Write in the journal as often as you need to.
✔ *Share your secrets.* Confide in someone whom you trust, but only when you feel that it's safe.

For more information, try these books and websites.

Fiction: P. McCormick, *Cut* (New York: Scholastic, 2002); S. Levenkron, *The Luckiest Girl in the World* (New York: Penguin USA, 1998).

Nonfiction: K. Conterio and W. Lader, *Bodily Harm: The Breakthrough Healing Program for Self-Injurers* (New York: Hyperion, 1998); S. Levenkron, *Cutting: Understanding and Overcoming Self-Mutilation* (New York: W.W. Norton, 1998); M. Strong, *A Bright Red Scream: Self-Mutilation and the Language of Pain* (New York: Viking Press, 1998); A. R. Favazza, *Bodies Under Siege: Self-Mutilation and the Body Modification in Culture and Society,* 2nd ed. (Baltimore, MD: John Hopkins University Press, 1996).

Websites: Discovery Health Channel "Cutters: Self-Abuse" http://health .discovery.com/premiers/cutters/cutters /html; National Self-Harm Network, www.nshn.co.uk; SAFE Alternatives, www.selfinjury.com; Secret Shame: Self-Injury Information and Support, www .crystal.palace.net/~llama/selfinjury

Sources: S. Dobie, Oregon State University; "Cutting (Self-mutilation)," MayoClinic .com, www.mayoclinic.com/invoke.cfm? objectid=74946FF7-B41B-456F -AF3E97F9BA898021; A. Derovin and T. Bravender, "Living on the Edge: The Current Phenomenon of Self-mutilation in Adolescents," *MCN The American Journal of Maternal Child* Nursing 29, no. 1 (2004): 12–18; "Student Self-Harm: Silent School Crisis," *Education Week* 23 no. 14 (2003): 1; K. Goetz, "Cutting through the Pain," *The Cincinnati Enquirer*, July 28, 2002, www .enquirer.com/editions/2002/07/28/loc _cutting_through_pain.html; D. Martinson, "Self-Injury: A Quick Guide to the Basics," 1998, www.palace.net/~llama/psych /guide.html

inability to sort out incoming stimuli and to make appropriate responses; an altered sense of self; and radical changes in emotions, movements, and behaviors. Victims of this disease often cannot function in society. Contrary to popular belief, schizophrenia is not the same as split personality or multiple personality disorder.

For decades, scientists believed that schizophrenia was an environmentally provoked form of madness. They blamed abnormal family interactions or early childhood traumas. Since the mid-1980s, however, magnetic resonance imaging (MRI) and PET scans have allowed closer study of brain function, and scientists have recognized that schizophrenia is a biological disease of the brain. The brain damage occurs very early in life, possibly as early as the second trimester of fetal development. However, symptoms most commonly appear in late adolescence.

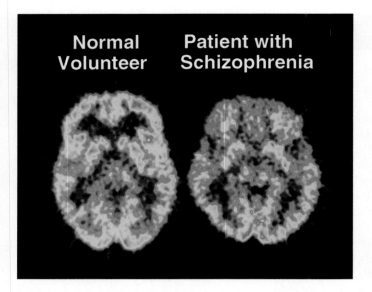

These brain images reveal significant differences between normal brain activity and that of a person with schizophrenia.

At present, schizophrenia is treatable but not curable. Treatments usually include some combination of hospitalization, medication, and supportive psychotherapy. Supportive psychotherapy, as opposed to psychoanalysis, can help the patient acquire skills for living in society.

Even though environmental theories of the causes of schizophrenia have been discarded in favor of biological theories, a stigma remains attached to the disease. Families of people with schizophrenia often experience anger and guilt associated with misunderstandings about the causes of the disease. They often need information, family counseling, and advice on how to meet the schizophrenic person's needs for shelter, medical care, vocational training, and social interaction.

Gender Issues in Psychosocial Health

Unfortunately, gender bias can hinder the correct diagnosis of psychosocial disorders. In one study, for instance, 175 mental health professionals of both genders were asked to diagnose a patient based upon a summarized case history. Some of the professionals were told that the patient was male, others that the patient was female. The gender of the patient made a substantial difference in the diagnosis (though the gender of the clinician did not). When subjects thought the patient was female, they were more likely to diagnose hysterical personality, which is often thought of as a women's disorder. When they believed the patient to be male, the more likely diagnosis was antisocial personality, frequently perceived as a male disorder.

PMS: Physical or Mental Disorder? A major controversy is the inclusion of a provisional diagnosis for premenstrual syndrome (PMS) in the American Psychiatric Association's *Diagnostic and Statistical Manual of Mental Disorders* (fourth

edition; known as *DSM-IV*). The provisional inclusion, in an appendix to *DSM-IV*, signals that PMS merits further study and may be included as an approved diagnosis in future editions of the *DSM*. In other words, PMS could be considered a mental disorder in the future.

PMS is characterized by depression, irritability, and other symptoms of increased stress typically occurring just prior to menstruation and lasting for a day or two. A more severe case of PMS is known as *premenstrual dysphoric disorder*, or *PMDD*. Whereas PMS is somewhat disruptive and uncomfortable, it does not interfere with daily functions; PMDD does. To be diagnosed with PMDD, a woman must have at least five symptoms of PMS for a week to 10 days, with at least one symptom being serious enough to interfere with her ability to function at work or at home. In these more severe cases, antidepressants may be prescribed. The point of contention lies in whether administering this treatment indicates that PMDD is viewed as a mental disorder rather than a physical problem.[64] Is it legitimate to attach a label indicating dysfunction and disorder to symptoms experienced only once or twice a month? Further controversy stems from the possible use (or misuse) of the diagnostic label to justify excluding women from certain desirable jobs.

Suicide: Giving Up on Life

Each year there are over 35,000 reported suicides in the United States. Experts estimate that there may actually be closer to 100,000 cases, due to the difficulty in determining the causes of many suspicious deaths. More lives are lost to suicide than to any other single cause except cardiovascular disease and cancer. Suicide often results from poor coping skills, lack of social support, lack of self-esteem, and the inability to see one's way out of a bad situation. Factors contributing to suicide are common risks in many regions of the world. The Health in a Diverse World box provides key indicators of this.

College students are more likely than the general population to attempt suicide; suicide is the third leading cause of death in people between the ages of 15 and 24. In fact, this age group now accounts for nearly 20 percent of all suicides.[65] The pressures, joys, disappointments, challenges, and changes of the college environment are believed to be partially responsible. However, young adults who choose not to go to college but who are searching for direction in careers, relationships, and other life goals are also at risk.

Risk factors for suicide include a family history of suicide, previous suicide attempts, excessive drug and alcohol use, prolonged depression, financial difficulties, serious illness in the suicide contemplator or in his or her loved ones, and loss of a loved one through death or rejection. Societal pressures often serve as a catalyst.

In most cases, suicide does not occur unpredictably. In fact, 75 to 80 percent of people who commit suicide give a warning of their intentions.

Suicide: A Neglected Problem among Diverse Populations

One of the most underrated public health problems facing Americans today, suicide accounts for more than 35,000 preventable deaths each year, nearly 10,000 more than deaths from homicide. It touches all ages, races, and social groups and is on the rise in many segments of the population.

- Suicide rates for youths and young adults aged 15 to 24 has tripled since 1950, and suicide is now the third leading cause of death in this age group.

- Over 30 percent of Hispanic female high school students reported seriously considering suicide, the highest rate of any racial or ethnic group in the country.
- American Indian/Alaska Native adolescents are more than twice as likely to commit suicide as any other racial/ethnic group.
- Rates of suicide are generally higher in western states and lower in the Eastern and Midwestern states.
- Suicide rates among the elderly are highest for those who are divorced or widowed.
- Men had a higher frequency of suicide and a greater overall mortality than women.

Sources: Centers for Disease Control and Prevention, National Center for Injury Prevention and Control, "Suicide in the United States," 2004, www.cdc.gov/ncipc/factsheets/suifacts.htm; R. H. Asletine Jr. and R. DeMartino, "An Outcome Evaluation of the SOS Suicide Prevention Program," *American Journal of Public Health* 94 no. 3, 446; Congressional testimony of Cheryl A. King, PhD, Professor of Psychology, University of Michigan, before the Subcommittee on Substance Abuse and Mental Health Services, U.S. Senate Committee on Health, Education, Labor and Pensions Hearing, "Suicide Preven-tion and Youth: Saving Lives," March 2, 2004, www.apa.org/ppo/issues/youthsuictest304.html

Warning Signs of Suicide

Common signs of possible suicide include:[66]

- Recent loss and a seeming inability to let go of grief
- Change in personality—sadness, withdrawal, irritability, anxiety, tiredness, indecisiveness, apathy
- Change in behavior—inability to concentrate, loss of interest in classes
- Diminished sexual interest—impotence, menstrual abnormalities
- Expressions of self-hatred
- Change in sleep patterns
- Change in eating habits
- A direct statement about committing suicide, such as "I might as well end it all."
- An indirect statement, such as "You won't have to worry about me anymore."
- Final preparations such as writing a will, repairing poor relationships with family or friends, giving away prized possessions, or writing revealing letters

- A preoccupation with themes of death
- A sudden and unexplained demonstration of happiness following a period of depression
- Marked changes in personal appearance
- Excessive risk taking and an "I don't care what happens to me" attitude

Taking Action to Prevent Suicide

Most people who attempt suicide really want to live but see death as the only way out of an intolerable situation. Crisis counselors and suicide hotlines may help temporarily, but the best way to prevent suicide is to get rid of conditions that may precipitate attempts, including alcoholism, drug abuse, loneliness, isolation, and access to guns.

If someone you know threatens suicide or displays any warning signs, take the following actions:

- Monitor the warning signals. Keep an eye on the person, or see that there is someone around the person as much as possible.
- Take any threats seriously. Don't brush them off.
- Let the person know how much you care about him or her. State that you are there to help.
- Listen. Empathize, sympathize, and keep the person talking. Try not to discredit or be shocked. Talk about stressors and listen to the responses.
- Ask directly, "Are you thinking of hurting or killing yourself?"
- Do not belittle the person's feelings. Don't say that he or she doesn't really mean it or couldn't succeed at suicide. To some people, these comments offer the challenge of proving you wrong.

What do you think?

If your roommate showed some of the warning signs of suicide, what action would you take? ■ *Who would you contact first?* ■ *Where on campus might your friend get help?* ■ *What if someone in class whom you hardly know gave some of the warning signs? What would you then do?*

- Help the person think about alternatives. Be ready to offer choices. Offer to go for help together. Call your local suicide hotline, and use all available community and campus resources. Recommend a counselor or other person to talk to.
- Remember that your relationships with others involve responsibilities. If you need to stay with the person, take the person to a health care facility, provide support, and give of yourself and your time.
- Tell your friend's spouse, partner, parents, siblings, or counselor. Do not keep your suspicions to yourself. Don't let a suicidal friend talk you into keeping your discussions confidential. If your friend succeeds in a suicide attempt, you may find that others will question your decision and you may blame yourself.

Seeking Professional Help

A physical ailment will readily send most of us to the nearest health professional, but many people view seeking professional help for psychosocial problems as an admission of personal failure. However, increasing numbers of Americans are turning to mental health professionals, and nearly one in five seeks such help. Researchers cite dysfunctional families, breakdowns in support systems, and high societal expectations of the individual as three major reasons why more people are asking for assistance than ever before.

Consider seeking help if any of the following apply to you.

- You think you need help.
- You experience wild mood swings.
- A problem is interfering with your daily life.
- Your fears or feelings of guilt frequently distract your attention.
- You begin to withdraw from others.
- You have hallucinations.
- You feel that life is not worth living.
- You feel inadequate or worthless.
- Your emotional responses are inappropriate to various situations.
- Your daily life seems to be nothing but repeated crises.
- You feel you can't "get your act together."
- You are considering suicide.
- You turn to drugs or alcohol to escape from your problems.
- You feel out of control.

Getting Evaluated for Treatment

If you are considering treatment for a psychosocial problem, schedule a complete evaluation first. Start with your campus health center. Consult a credentialed health professional for a thorough examination, which should include three parts:

- A physical checkup, which will rule out thyroid disorders, viral infections, and anemia—all of which can result in

---

Table 2.3
Questions to Ask When Choosing a Therapist

A qualified mental health professional should be willing to answer all your questions during an initial consultation. Questions to ask include the following.

- Can you interview the therapist before starting treatment? An initial meeting will help you determine whether this person will be a good fit for you.
- Do you like the therapist as a person? Can you talk to him or her comfortably?
- Is the therapist watching the clock or easily distracted? *You* should be the main focus of the session.
- Does the therapist demonstrate professionalism? Be concerned if your therapist is frequently late or breaks appointments, suggests social interactions outside your therapy sessions, talks inappropriately about himself or herself, has questionable billing practices, or resists releasing you from therapy.
- Will the therapist help you set your own goals? A good professional should evaluate your general situation and help you set small goals to work on between sessions. The therapist should not tell you how to help yourself but help you discover the steps.

Remember, in most states, the use of the title *therapist* or *counselor* is unregulated. Make your choice carefully.

---

depression-like symptoms—and a neurological check of coordination, reflexes, and balance, to rule out brain disorders.
- A psychiatric history, which will attempt to trace the course of the apparent disorder, genetic or family factors, and any past treatments.
- A mental status examination, which will assess thoughts, speaking processes, and memory, as well as an in-depth interview with tests for other psychiatric symptoms.[67]

Once physical factors have been ruled out, you may decide to consult a professional who specializes in psychosocial health.

Mental Health Professionals

Several types of mental health professionals are available to help you. The most important criterion is not how many degrees this person has, but whether you feel you can work together. Table 2.3 presents fundamental criteria to help you choose the best therapist for your needs.

Psychiatrist A **psychiatrist** is a medical doctor. After obtaining an MD degree, a psychiatrist spends up to 12 years studying psychosocial health and disease. As a licensed physician, a psychiatrist can prescribe medications for various mental or emotional problems and may have admitting privileges at a local hospital. Some psychiatrists are affiliated with hospitals, while others are in private practice.

Table 2.4
Traditional Forms of Psychotherapy: Assumptions, Goals, and Methods

Type of Therapy	Basic Assumptions	Goals and Methods
Psychoanalysis	Behavior is motivated by intrapsychic conflict and biological urges.	Discover the sources of conflict and resolve them through insight.
Psychodynamic therapy	Behavior is motivated by both unconscious forces and interpersonal experiences.	Understand and improve interpersonal skills by modifying the client's inappropriate schemas about interpersonal relationships.
Humanistic and gestalt therapy	People are good and have innate worth.	Use techniques to enhance personal awareness and feelings of self-worth to promote personal growth and self-actualization and to enhance clients' awareness of bodily sensations and feelings.
Behavior and cognitive-behavior therapy	Behavior is largely controlled by environmental contingencies, people's perception of them, or a combination.	Change maladaptive behavior and thinking patterns by manipulating environmental variables, restructuring thinking patterns, and correcting faulty thinking or irrational beliefs.
Family/couples therapy	Problems in relationships require treatment of everybody involved in them.	Analyze relationship patterns and others' roles in order to discover how interactions influence problems in individual functioning.

Source: From Neil R. Carson and William Buskist, *Psychology: The Science of Behavior,* 5th ed. (Boston: Allyn & Bacon, 1994), 629. Copyright © 1994 Pearson Education. Reprinted by permission of the publisher.

Psychologist A **psychologist** usually has a doctor of philosophy (PhD) degree in counseling or clinical psychology. In addition, many states require licensure. Psychologists are trained in various types of therapy, including behavior and insight therapy. Most can conduct both individual and group counseling sessions. Psychologists may also be trained in certain specialties, such as family counseling or sexual counseling.

Psychoanalyst A **psychoanalyst** is a psychiatrist or psychologist with special training in psychoanalysis. Psychoanalysis is a type of therapy that helps patients remember early traumas that have blocked personal growth. Facing these traumas helps them resolve conflicts and begin to lead more productive lives.

Clinical/Psychiatric Social Worker A **social worker** has at least a master's degree in social work (MSW) and two years of experience in a clinical setting. Many states require an examination for accreditation. Some social workers work in clinical settings, whereas others have private practices.

Counselor A **counselor** often has a master's degree in counseling, psychology, educational psychology, or related human service. Professional societies recommend at least two years of graduate coursework or supervised practice as a minimal requirement. Many counselors are trained to do individual and group therapy. They often specialize in one type of counseling, such as family, marital, relationship, children, drug, divorce, behavioral, or personal counseling.

Psychiatric Nurse Specialist Although all registered nurses can work in psychiatric settings, some continue their education and specialize in psychiatric practice. The **psychiatric nurse specialist** can be certified by the American Nursing Association in adult, child, or adolescent psychiatric nursing.

What to Expect in Therapy

Many different types of counseling exist, ranging from individual therapy, which involves one-on-one work between therapist and client, to group therapy, in which two or more clients meet with a therapist to discuss problems. Table 2.4 identifies traditional forms of psychotherapy.

The first trip to a therapist can be extremely difficult. Most of us have misconceptions about what therapy is and

---

Psychiatrist A licensed physician who specializes in treating mental and emotional disorders.

Psychologist A person with a PhD degree and training in psychology.

Psychoanalyst A psychiatrist or psychologist with special training in psychoanalysis.

Social worker A person with an MSW degree and clinical training.

Counselor A person with a variety of academic and experiential training who deals with the treatment of emotional problems.

Psychiatric nurse specialist A registered nurse specializing in psychiatric practice.

about what it can do. That first visit is a verbal and mental sizing up between you and the therapist. You may not accomplish much in that first hour. If you decide that this professional is not for you, you will at least have learned how to present your problem and what qualities you need in a therapist.

Before meeting, briefly explain your needs. Ask what the fee is. Arrive on time, wear comfortable clothing, and expect to spend about an hour during your first visit. The therapist will want to take down your history and details about the problems that have brought you to therapy. Answer as honestly as possible. Many will ask how you feel about aspects of your life. Do not be embarrassed to acknowledge your feelings. It is critical to the success of your treatment that you trust this person enough to be open and honest.

Do not expect the therapist to tell you what to do or how to behave. The responsibility for improved behavior lies with you. Ask if you can set your own therapeutic goals and timetables.

If after your first visit (or even after several visits), you feel you cannot work with this person, say so. You have the right to find a therapist with whom you feel comfortable.

What do you think?

Have you ever thought about seeing a therapist?
■ *What made you decide to go or not go?* ■ *If you were to consult a therapist, what factors would you take into consideration in choosing one who is right for you?*

TAKING CHARGE

MAKE IT HAPPEN!

Assessment: The Assess Yourself box on page 42 gave you the chance to look at various aspects of your psychosocial health and compare your self-assessment with a friend's perceptions. Now that you have considered these results, you can take steps toward changing certain behaviors that may be detrimental to your psychosocial health.

Making a Change: To change your behavior, you need to develop a plan. Follow these steps.

1. Evaluate your behavior, and identify patterns and specific things you are doing. What can you change now? What can you change in the near future?
2. Select one pattern of behavior that you'd like to change.
3. Fill out a Behavior Change Contract. It should include your long-term goal for change, your short-term goals, the rewards you'll give yourself for reaching these goals, potential obstacles along the way, and strategies for overcoming these obstacles. For each goal, list the small steps and specific actions that you can take.

4. Chart your progress in a journal. At the end of one week, consider how successful you were in following your plan.
5. Revise your plan as needed. Are the short-term goals attainable? Are the rewards satisfying?

One Student's Plan: John assessed himself as a positive and upbeat person, but the assessment his friend gave him rated him as impatient and cynical. John resolved to slow down and become more appreciative of the good things around him. Among his short-term goals: listening to his sister without interrupting her and expressing a sincere compliment to a family member or friend every other day. John found that paying compliments made him stop to think about the qualities he appreciated in friends and family. While he struggled to listen without interrupting, John found that he was learning a lot about his sister that he had never known before. After several weeks, John's friends commented on his calmer and happier demeanor.

Summary

- Psychosocial health is a complex phenomenon involving mental, emotional, social, and spiritual health.
- Many factors influence psychosocial health, including life experiences, family, the environment, other people, self-esteem, self-efficacy, and personality. Some of these are modifiable; others are not.

- Developing self-esteem and self-efficacy and getting enough sleep are key to enhancing psychosocial health.
- Many people believe spirituality is important to wellness. Though the exact reasons have not been established, many studies show a connection between the two.

- Happiness is a key factor in determining overall reaction to life's challenges. The mind–body connection is an important link in overall health and well-being.
- Indicators of deteriorating psychosocial health include depression. Identifying depression is the first step in treating this disorder.
- Other common psychosocial problems include bipolar disorder, anxiety disorders, panic disorders, phobias, seasonal affective disorder, and schizophrenia.

- Suicide is a result of negative psychosocial reactions to life. People intending to commit suicide often give warning signs of their intentions. They can often be helped.
- Mental health professionals include psychiatrists, psychoanalysts, psychologists, clinical/psychiatric social workers, counselors, and psychiatric nurse specialists. A great variety of therapy methods exist, including group and individual therapy. It is wise to carefully interview a therapist before beginning treatment.

Questions for Discussion and Reflection

1. What is psychosocial health? What indicates that you are or aren't psychosocially healthy? Why might the college environment provide a real challenge to psychosocial health?
2. Discuss the factors that influence your overall level of psychosocial health. Which factors can you change? Which ones may be more difficult to change?
3. What steps could you take today to improve your psychosocial health? Which steps require long-term effort?
4. What are four main themes of spirituality, and how are they expressed in daily life?
5. Why is laughter therapeutic? How can humor help you better achieve wellness?
6. What factors appear to contribute to psychosocial difficulties and illnesses? Which of the common psychosocial illnesses is likely to affect people in your age group?

7. What are the warning signs of suicide? Of depression? Why is depression so pervasive among young Americans today? Why are some groups more vulnerable to suicide and depression than others? What would you do if you heard a friend in the cafeteria say to no one in particular that he was going to "do the world a favor and end it all"?
8. Discuss the different types of health professionals and therapies. If you felt depressed about breaking off a long-term relationship, which professional and which therapy do you think would be most beneficial to you? Explain your answer. What services are provided by your student health center? What fees are charged to students?
9. What psychosocial areas do you need to work on? Which are most important to you, and why? What actions can you take today?

Accessing Your Health on the Internet

Visit the following Internet sites to explore further topics and issues related to personal health. To visit an organization's website, go to the Companion Website for *Access to Health, Ninth Edition* at www.aw-bc.com/donatelle, click on the book image, and select "Accessing Your Health on the Internet" from the navigation menu.

1. *American Foundation for Suicide Prevention.* Resources for suicide prevention and support for family and friends of those who have committed suicide.
2. *American Psychological Association Help Center.* Includes information on psychology at work, the mind–body connection, psychological responses to war, and other topics.

3. *Anxiety Disorders Association of America.* Offers links to treatment resources, self-help tools, information on clinical trials, and other information.
4. *National Alliance for the Mentally Ill.* A support and advocacy organization of families and friends of people with severe mental illnesses. Over 1,200 state and local affiliates; local branches can often help with finding treatment.
5. *National Institute of Mental Health (NIMH).* Overview of mental health information and new research relating to mental health.
6. *National Mental Health Association.* Works to promote mental health through advocacy, education, research, and services.

Further Reading

Dalai Lama and H. C. Cutler. *The Art of Happiness: A Handbook for Living.* New York: Riverhead, 1998.

Through a series of interviews, the authors explore questions of meaning, motives, and the interconnectedness of life, including the reasons why so many people are unhappy, and offer strategies for becoming happy.

Julie Norem. *The Positive Power of Negative Thinking.* New York: Basic Books, 2002.

Explores reasons for negative thinking and mechanisms for changing the way you think. Includes self-tests and analysis for helping you retrain your thinking processes.

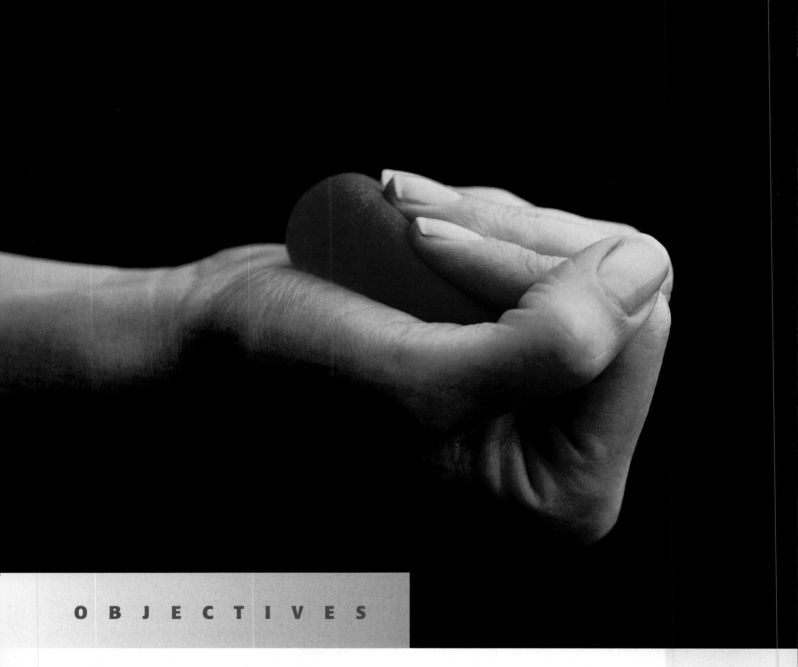

OBJECTIVES

- Define stress, and examine the potential impact of stress on health, relationships, and success in college.

- Explain the three phases of the general adaptation syndrome, and describe what happens physiologically when we experience a real or perceived threat.

- Examine the health risks that may occur with chronic stress.

- Discuss psychosocial, environmental, and self-imposed sources of stress. Examine ways in which you might reduce risks from these stressors or inoculate yourself against stressful situations.

- Examine the special stressors that affect college students and strategies for reducing risk.

- Explore techniques for coping with unavoidable stress, reducing exposure to stress, and making optimum use of positive stressors to promote growth and enrich life experiences.

- Examine the role of spirituality in enhancing the ability to deal with stress.

3

MANAGING STRESS

COPING WITH LIFE'S CHALLENGES

IN THE NEWS

Too Much Stress May Give Your Genes Gray Hair

By Benedict Carey

Some stressful events seem to turn a person's hair gray overnight.

Now a team of researchers has found that severe emotional distress—like that caused by divorce, the loss of a job, or caring for an ill child or parent—may speed up the aging of the body's cells at the genetic level.

The findings, being reported today, are the first to link psychological stress so directly to biological age.

The researchers found that blood cells from women who had spent many years caring for a disabled child were, genetically, about a decade older than those from peers who had much less caretaking experience. The study, which appears in *Proceedings of the National Academy of Sciences,* also suggests that the perception of being stressed can add years to a person's biological age.

Though doctors have linked chronic psychological stress to weakened immune function and an increased risk of catching colds, among other things, they are still trying to understand how tension damages or weakens tissue.

Read the complete article online in the eThemes section of this book's website: www.aw-bc.com/donatelle.

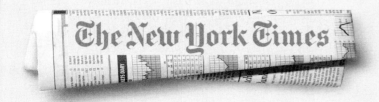

Rising tuition, crowded dorms, roommates who bug you, social-life drama, pyramids of empty beer cans on the windowsills and coffee tables, too much noise, no privacy, long lines at the bookstore, pressure to get good grades, never enough money, worries over war and terrorism. STRESS! You can't run from it, you can't hide from it, and it invades your waking and sleeping hours. Even when you are out socializing with friends, you feel guilty about not enough time and so much left to do.

The normal stresses of college life and a full course load are enough to put circles under the eyes of any college student. Add to that the fact that more than half of the students on some campuses are also working one, two, or even three jobs to keep themselves afloat, and the result is increasing health problems caused by stress.

Often, stress is insidious, and we don't even notice the things that affect us. As we sleep, it encroaches on our psyche through noise or incessant worries over things that need to be done. While we work at the computer, stress may interfere in the form of noise from next door, strain on our eyes, and tension in our backs. The exact toll stress exacts from us during a lifetime of stress overload is unknown, but it is much more than an annoyance. Rather, it is a significant health hazard that can rob the body of needed nutrients, damage the cardiovascular system, raise blood pressure, and dampen the immune system's defenses, leaving us vulnerable to infections and a host of diseases. In addition, it can drain our emotional reserves, contribute to depression, anxiety, and irritability, and punctuate social interactions with hostility and anger. Stress is a major concern in the United States, and it appears to be getting worse: one-third of U.S. workers report an increase in job-related stress over the past year.[1] Although much has been written about stress, we are only beginning to understand the multifaceted nature of the stress response and its tremendous potential for harm or benefit.

Stress   Mental and physical responses to change.

Stressor   A physical, social, or psychological event or condition that requires our bodies to make an adjustment.

Adjustment   The attempt to cope with a given situation or event.

Strain   The wear and tear sustained by the body and mind in adjusting to or resisting a stressor.

Eustress   Stress that presents opportunities for personal growth.

Distress   Stress that can have a negative effect on health.

Fight-or-flight response   Physiological arousal response in which the body prepares to combat a real or perceived threat.

What Is Stress?

Often, we think of stress as an externally imposed factor. But for most of us, stress results from an internal state of emotional tension that occurs in response to the various demands of living. Most current definitions state that **stress** is the mental and physical response of our bodies to the changes and challenges in our lives. Inherent in these definitions is the idea that we sometimes take ourselves too seriously: that we should loosen up, worry less, and gain greater control over our minds as well as our bodies. A **stressor** is any physical, social, or psychological event or condition that causes our bodies to adjust to a specific situation. Stressors may be tangible, such as an angry parent or a disgruntled roommate, or intangible, such as the mixed emotions associated with meeting your significant other's parents for the first time. **Adjustment** is the attempt to cope with a given situation. **Strain** is the wear and tear the body and mind sustain during the adjustment process.

Stress and strain are associated with most daily activities. Generally, positive stress, or stress that presents the opportunity for personal growth and satisfaction, is called **eustress.** Getting married, starting school, beginning a career, developing new friendships, and learning a new physical skill all give rise to eustress. **Distress,** or negative stress, is caused by events that result in debilitative stress and strain (such as financial problems, the death of a loved one, academic difficulties, and the breakup of a relationship).

We cannot get rid of distress entirely: like eustress, it is a part of life. However, we can train ourselves to recognize the events that cause distress and to anticipate our reactions to them. We can learn coping skills and strategies that will help us manage stress more effectively (see the Assess Yourself box on page 74).

The Body's Response to Stress

Whenever we're surprised by a sudden stressor, such as someone swerving into our lane of traffic, the adrenal glands jump into action. Emotional reactions to a perceived threat trigger these two almond-sized glands sitting atop the kidneys to secrete adrenaline and other hormones into the bloodstream. As a result, the heart speeds up, breathing rate increases, blood pressure rises, and the flow of blood to the muscles increases with a rapid release of blood sugars into the bloodstream. This sudden burst of energy and strength is believed to provide the extra edge that has helped generations of humans survive during adversity. Known as the **fight-or-flight response,** this physiological reaction is believed to be one of our most basic, innate survival instincts. It is a point at which our bodies go on the alert either to fight or to escape.

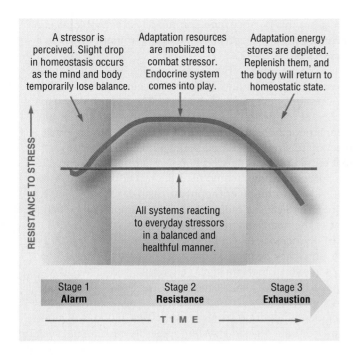

Figure 3.1
The General Adaptation Syndrome

The General Adaptation Syndrome (GAS)

What we have just described in very general terms is a complicated physiological response to stress in which our bodies move from **homeostasis,** a level of functioning in which systems operate smoothly and maintain equilibrium, to one of crisis, in which the body attempts to return to homeostasis. This adjustment is referred to as an **adaptive response.** First characterized by Hans Selye in 1936, this internal fight to restore balance is known as the **general adaptation syndrome (GAS)** (Figure 3.1), which has three distinct phases: alarm, resistance, and exhaustion.[2]

Alarm Phase   When the body is exposed to a stressor, whether real or perceived, the fight-or-flight response kicks into gear. Stress hormones flow into the body, and it prepares to do battle. The subconscious perceptions and appraisal of the stressor stimulate the areas in the brain responsible for emotions. Emotional stimulation, in turn, starts the physical reactions that we associate with stress (Figure 3.2 on page 72). This entire process takes only a few seconds.

Suppose that you are walking to your car on a dimly lit campus after a late-night class. As you pass a particularly dark area, you hear someone cough behind you and sense that this person is fairly close. You walk faster, only to hear the quickened footsteps of the other person. Your senses become increasingly alert, your breathing quickens, your heart races, and you begin to perspire. The stranger is getting closer and closer. In desperation you stop, clutching your

book bag in your hands, determined to use force if necessary to protect yourself. You turn around quickly and let out a blood-curdling yell. To your surprise, the only person you see is Mrs. Fletcher, a woman in your class, who has been trying to stay close to you out of her own anxiety about walking alone in the dark. She screams and jumps back off the curb, only to trip and fall. You look at her in startled embarrassment, help her to her feet, and nervously laugh about your reaction. You have just experienced the *alarm phase* of GAS.

When the mind perceives a stressor (either real or imaginary), such as a potential attacker, the **cerebral cortex,** the region of the brain that interprets the nature of an event, is called to attention. If the cerebral cortex perceives a threat, it triggers an **autonomic nervous system (ANS)** response that prepares the body for action. The ANS is the portion of the central nervous system that regulates bodily functions that we do not normally consciously control, such as heart function, breathing, and glandular function. When we are stressed, the activity rate of all these bodily functions increases dramatically to give us the physical strength to protect ourselves or to mobilize internal forces.

The ANS has two branches: sympathetic and parasympathetic. The **sympathetic nervous system** energizes the body for either fight or flight by signaling the release of several stress hormones that speed the heart rate, increase the breathing rate, and trigger many other stress responses. The **parasympathetic nervous system** functions to slow all the systems stimulated by the stress response. Thus, the parasympathetic branch of the ANS serves as a system of checks and balances on the sympathetic branch. In a healthy person, these two branches work together in a balance that controls the negative effects of stress. However, long-term stress

Homeostasis   A balanced physical state in which all the body's systems function smoothly.

Adaptive response   Form of adjustment in which the body attempts to restore homeostasis.

General adaptation syndrome (GAS)   The pattern followed in the physiological response to stress, consisting of the alarm, resistance, and exhaustion phases.

Cerebral cortex   The region of the brain that interprets the nature of an event.

Autonomic nervous system (ANS)   The portion of the central nervous system that regulates bodily functions that a person does not normally consciously control.

Sympathetic nervous system   Branch of the autonomic nervous system responsible for stress arousal.

Parasympathetic nervous system   Branch of the autonomic nervous system responsible for slowing systems stimulated by the stress response.

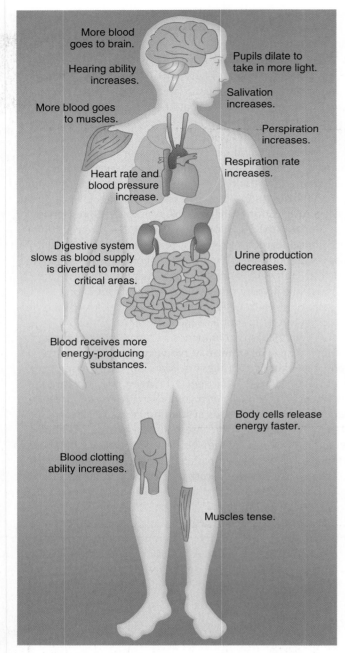

Figure 3.2
The General Adaptation Syndrome: The Alarm Phase

Labels in figure:
More blood goes to brain.

Hearing ability increases.

More blood goes to muscles.

Pupils dilate to take in more light.

Salivation increases.

Perspiration increases.

Heart rate and blood pressure increase.

Respiration rate increases.

Digestive system slows as blood supply is diverted to more critical areas.

Urine production decreases.

Blood receives more energy-producing substances.

Body cells release energy faster.

Blood clotting ability increases.

Muscles tense.

Hypothalamus   A section of the brain that controls the sympathetic nervous system and directs the stress response.

Epinephrine   Also called adrenaline, a hormone that stimulates body systems in response to stress.

Adrenocorticotropic hormone (ACTH)   A pituitary hormone that stimulates the adrenal glands to secrete cortisol.

Cortisol   Hormone released by the adrenal glands that makes stored nutrients more readily available to meet energy demands.

can strain this balance, and chronic physical problems can occur as stress reactions become the dominant forces in a person's body.

The responses of the sympathetic nervous system to stress involve a complex series of biochemical exchanges between different parts of the body. The **hypothalamus,** a section of the brain, functions as the control center of the sympathetic nervous system and determines the overall reaction to stressors. When the hypothalamus perceives that extra energy is needed to fight a stressor, it stimulates the adrenal glands, located near the top of the kidneys, to release the hormone **epinephrine,** also called adrenaline. Epinephrine causes more blood to be pumped with each beat of the heart, dilates the bronchioles (air sacs in the lungs) to increase oxygen intake, increases the breathing rate, enhances hearing, stimulates the liver to release more glucose (which fuels muscular exertion), and dilates the pupils to improve visual sensitivity. The body is then poised to act immediately.

As epinephrine secretion increases, blood is diverted away from the digestive system, possibly causing nausea and cramping if the distress occurs shortly after a meal, and drying of nasal and salivary tissues, producing dry mouth. The alarm phase also provides for longer-term reaction to stress. The hypothalamus triggers the pituitary gland, which in turn releases another powerful hormone, **adrenocorticotropic hormone (ACTH).** ACTH signals the adrenal glands to release **cortisol,** a hormone that makes stored nutrients more readily available to meet energy demands. Finally, other parts of the brain and body release endorphins, the body's naturally occurring opiates, which relieve pain that may be caused by a stressor.

Resistance Phase   The resistance phase of the GAS begins almost immediately after the alarm phase starts. In this stage, the body has reacted to the stressor and adjusted in a way that allows the system to return to homeostasis. As the sympathetic nervous system energizes the body via the actions of epinephrine, norepinephrine, cortisol, and other hormones, the parasympathetic nervous system helps control these energy levels and return the body to normal functioning.

Exhaustion Phase   In the exhaustion phase of the GAS, the physical and emotional energy used to fight a stressor have been depleted. The toll it takes on the body depends on the type of stress or the period of time spent under stress. Short-term stress probably would not deplete all of a person's energy reserves, but chronic stress experienced over a period of time can create continuous states of alarm and resistance, resulting in total depletion of energy and susceptibility to illness. The key to warding off the effects of stress lies in what many researchers refer to as *adaptation energy stores*, the physical and mental foundations of our ability to cope with stress.

Two levels of adaptation energy stores exist: deep and superficial. We apparently have little control over deep stores, as their size appears to be preset by heredity.

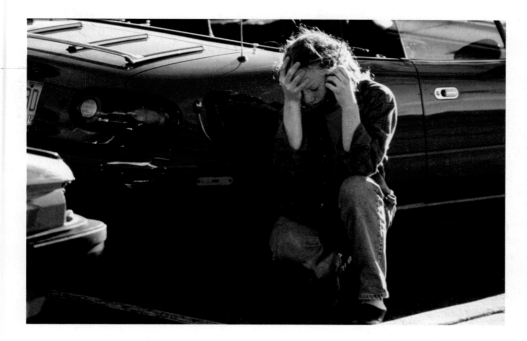

The fight-or-flight response was once responsible for our survival, but the response and its aftereffects now can lead to serious health issues.

Superficial adaptation energy stores, however, are renewable and present the first line of defense against stress, as they are tapped into initially when the body fights stress. Only when superficial stores are exhausted does the body tap into the deep energy stores. As our adaptation energy stores are depleted, we tire more quickly and require more rest. Without this replenishing sleep, the alarm and resistance phases eventually will limit our ability to rebound properly.

As the body adjusts to chronic unresolved stress, the adrenal glands continue to release cortisol, which remains in the bloodstream for longer periods of time due to slower metabolic responsiveness. Over time, without relief, cortisol can reduce **immunocompetence,** or the ability of the immune system to respond to various onslaughts. Blood pressure can remain dangerously elevated, and our body systems become unable to respond with the same vigor they once did. The net effect? Greater chance of minor illnesses at one end of the continuum; greater risk of life-threatening disease at the other end.

Stress management, therefore, depends on the ability to replenish superficial stores and conserve deep stores. Besides getting adequate rest, adaptation energy stores can be replenished by aerobic exercise, finding a balance between work and relaxation, practicing good nutritional habits, setting realistic goals, and maintaining supportive relationships.

What do you think?

What are your greatest sources of stress right now? ■ *On a scale of 1 to 10, with 10 being the highest level, how stressed are you?* ■ *Have you noticed any symptoms of stress?* ■ *How can you reduce your stress?*

Stress and Your Health

Although much has been written about the negative effects of stress, researchers have only recently begun to untangle the complex web of physical and emotional interactions that can break down the body over time. Stress is often described as a "disease of prolonged arousal" that leads to other negative health effects. Nearly all body systems are potential targets, and the long-term effects may be devastating. Much of the initial impetus for studying the health effects of stress came from indirect observations. Cardiologists in the Framingham Heart Study and other research projects noted that highly stressed individuals seemed to experience significantly greater risks for cardiovascular disease (CVD) and hypertension.[3] Monkeys exposed to high levels of unpredictable stressors in studies showed significantly increased levels of disease and mortality.[4] In a landmark study, M. D. Jeremko observed that chronic stress activation can result in headaches, asthma, hypertension, ulcers, lower back pain, and other medical conditions, a finding substantiated by a meta-analysis of over one hundred similar studies.[5] A Harvard study concluded that mental health was the most important predictor of physical health.[6] While the battle over the legitimacy of these observations continues to be waged in research labs around the world, the theory that chronic stress increases susceptibility to certain ailments has gained credibility.

Immunocompetence   The ability of the immune system to respond to assaults.

How Stressed Are You?

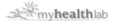

Fill out this assessment online at www.aw-bc.com/myhealthlab or www.aw-bc.com/donatelle

Each of us reacts differently to life's little challenges. Faced with a long line at the bookstore, most of us will get anxious for a few seconds before we start grumbling or shrug and move on. But for others—the one in five of us whom researchers call *hot reactors*— such incidents are part of a daily health assault. These individuals may get very angry outwardly, or they may appear calm and

collected. It is what is going on under the surface that affects health. Surges in heart rate and blood pressure, nausea, sweating, and a host of other hot reactor indicators may occur. Completing the following assessment will help you think about the nature and extent of stress in your life and how you respond to daily stressors. Although this survey is just an indicator of what stress levels might be, it will help you focus on areas that you may need to work on.

PART ONE: WHAT IS STRESSING YOU OUT?

For each statement, indicate how often the following stressful situations or feelings are part of your daily life.

	Never	Rarely	Sometimes	Often	All the time
1. I find that there are not enough hours in the day to finish everything I have to do.	1	2	3	4	5
2. I am nervous/anxious about how I am performing in my classes.	1	2	3	4	5
3. People don't seem to notice whether I do a good job or not.	1	2	3	4	5
4. I am tired and feel like I don't have the energy to do everything that I need to get done.	1	2	3	4	5
5. I am irritable and seem to be easily bothered by things that people do.	1	2	3	4	5
6. I worry about what is happening in my family (health of a loved one, financial problems, relationship problems).	1	2	3	4	5
7. I'm worried about my finances and having enough money to pay my bills.	1	2	3	4	5
8. I don't have enough time for fun.	1	2	3	4	5
9. I am unhappy with my body (weight, fitness level, etc.).	1	2	3	4	5
10. My family and friends count on me to help them with their problems.	1	2	3	4	5
11. I am concerned about my current relationship or lack of a relationship.	1	2	3	4	5
12. I am impatient/intolerant of the weaknesses of others.	1	2	3	4	5
13. My house/apartment is a mess, and I'm embarrassed to have others see it.	1	2	3	4	5
14. I worry about whether I'll get a job and be able to support myself after graduation.	1	2	3	4	5
15. I worry that people don't like me or think that I'm not someone that they'd like to be friends with.	1	2	3	4	5

Your Total Score: _____

INTERPRETING YOUR SCORES

Scores of 61–75: Your stress level is probably quite high. Prioritize the areas where you scored 5's, and list two or three things for each area that you could do to reduce your stress level. Note any increase in headaches, backaches, or insomnia; that's your

body telling you to lighten your load. Plan at least one fun thing to do for yourself each day. Make yourself more of a daily priority.

Scores of 46–60: Your stress level is moderate. Look at those areas that are 5's and pick out two or three that you would like to change now. Make a list of things you can do to help yourself reduce stress levels today. Practice at least one stress manage-ment technique each day. Make more time for yourself. Use the Behavior Change Contract to plan how you will reduce stress.

Scores of 30–45: You seem to have a lower level of stress—this is good. However, there are still areas that you could work on. Think about what these are, and list things you could do now to reduce stress.

Scores Below 30: You seem to be doing a great job. Even when stressful events do occur—and they will—your health probably won't suffer. Remember, each of us has "stress slips" along the way. Think about your reactions to situations like those above. Whenever possible, make conscious choices to reduce stress.

PART TWO: HOW DO YOU RESPOND TO STRESS?

Respond to each of the following stressful events with a rating of how likely you are to react to it.

SCENARIO 1

You've been waiting 20 minutes for a table in a crowded restaurant, and the hostess seats a group that arrived after you.

	Never	Rarely	Sometimes	Often	All the time
1. You feel your anger rise as your face gets hot and your heart beats faster.	1	2	3	4	5
2. You yell, "Hey! I was here first!" in an irritated voice to the hostess.	1	2	3	4	5
3. You angrily confront the people who are being seated before you and tell them you were there first.	1	2	3	4	5
4. You say, "Excuse me" in a polite voice and inform the other group and/or the hostess that you were there first.	1	2	3	4	5
5. You note it, but don't react. It's no big deal, and the hostess obviously didn't notice the order of arrival.	1	2	3	4	5

SCENARIO 2

You get to a movie theater early so that you and a friend can get great seats. You strategically pick a seat that will give you a good view. Then, although the theater is nearly empty, a very large, very tall man plops himself in the seat directly in front of you. Try as you might, you cannot see the screen.

1. You say in a very loud voice: "Dang it, there's a whole theater, and he has to sit right in front of us!"	1	2	3	4	5
2. You yell directly at the man, saying, "Can't you go sit somewhere else? I can't see!"	1	2	3	4	5
3. You tap the man on the shoulder and say, "Excuse me. I wonder if you could slide down a seat. I can't see."	1	2	3	4	5
4. You calmly nudge your friend and decide to get up and move.	1	2	3	4	5
5. You aren't bothered by the person in front of you; this is just part of going to the movies and no big deal.	1	2	3	4	5

MULTIPLE SCENARIOS

1. Your sister calls out of the blue and starts to tell you how much you mean to her. Uncomfortable, you change the subject without expressing what you feel.	1	2	3	4	5

(continues)

	Never	Rarely	Sometimes	Often	All the time
2. You come home to find the kitchen looking like a disaster area and your spouse/roommate lounging in front of the TV. You tense up and can't seem to shake your anger, but you decide not to bring it up.	1	2	3	4	5
3. Faced with a public speaking event, you get keyed up and lose sleep for a day or more, worrying about how you'll do.	1	2	3	4	5
4. Your boyfriend/girlfriend/partner is seen out with another person and appears to be acting quite close to the person. You are a trusting individual and decide not to worry about it. If your significant other has anything to tell you, you know that he/she will talk to you.	1	2	3	4	5
5. You aren't able to study as much as you'd like for an exam, yet you think that you really "nailed" the exam after you have taken it. When you get it back, you find that you actually did horribly. You make an appointment to talk with the professor and determine what you can do to improve on the next exam. You acknowledge that you are responsible for the low grade this time but vow to do better next time. You are disappointed, but don't dwell on it.	1	2	3	4	5

INTERPRETING YOUR SCORES

Look carefully at each of these scenarios. Obviously, none of us is perfect, and we sometimes react in ways that we later regret. The key here is to assess how you react most of the time.

If stressful events occur and you are able to remain calm, not experience increases in heart rate or blood pressure, and avoid outward displays or inner signs of anxiety, anger, or frustration, you are probably a cool reactor, someone who tends to roll with the punches when a situation is out of your control. This is usually indicative of a good level of coping and overall, this type of person will suffer fewer health consequences when stressed. The key here is that you really feel calm and unworried about the situation.

If you fret and stew about a stressor, can't sleep, or tend to react by hostile confrontation, anger, or other negative physiological overreactions, you probably are a hot reactor, someone who responds to mildly stressful situations with a fight-or-flight adrenaline rush that drives up blood pressure and can lead to heart rhythm disturbances, accelerated clotting, and damaged blood

vessel linings. Some hot reactors can seem cool as a cucumber on the outside, but inside their bodies are silently killing them. They may be on edge or jumpy or unable to sleep, even though most people would never suspect that they are in trouble. Before you honk or make obscene gestures at the guy who cuts you off in rush hour traffic, remember that getting angry can destroy thousands of heart muscle cells within minutes. Robert S. Eliot, author of *From Stress to Strength,* says hot reactors have no choice but to calm themselves down with rational thought. Look at ways to change your perceptions and cope more effectively. Ponder the fact that the only thing you'll hurt by reacting is your own health. "You have to stop trying to change the world," Eliot advises, "and learn to change your response to it."

MAKE IT HAPPEN!

Use the results of this self-assessment to begin your behavior change program. Follow the steps and use the examples on page 96 to complete your Behavior Change Contract and use these resources to take action.

Stress and CVD

Since Friedman and Rosenman's classic study of Type A and Type B personalities and heart disease in the late 1960s and (discussed later in this chapter), researchers have tried to definitively link personality, emotions, and a host of other variables to heart disease.[7] Results of numerous meta-analyses, summarizing many studies, have consistently pointed to a

correlation between chronic, unresolved stress and prolonged elevations in heart rate and blood pressure. This increased pressure can cause turbulence in blood flow and is believed to damage the inner lining of blood vessels. Once this damage occurs, fatty substances seem to stick to this site more readily, leading to the buildup of atherosclerotic plaque. Recent studies point to increased risk of sudden heart attack (myocardial infarction) due to prolonged stress in the environment.[8] A large number of epidemiological studies have related the incidence of heart disease deaths to type of employment, particularly jobs in which a person is subject to many demands but has little control in decision-making and daily tasks.[9]

Historically, the increased risk of CVD from chronic stress has been linked to increased plaque buildup due to elevated cholesterol, hardening of the arteries, alterations in heart rhythm, increased and fluctuating blood pressures, and difficulties in cardiovascular responsiveness due to all of the above. While these continue to be considered major risks, recent research also points to inflammation in blood vessels, perhaps due to lingering viral effects, as a major contributor to heart disease. (For more information about CVD, see Chapter 15.)

Stress and Impaired Immunity

A new area of scientific investigation known as **psycho-neuroimmunology (PNI)** analyzes the intricate relationship between the mind's response to stress and the ability of the immune system to function effectively. An article in the *Journal of the American Medical Association* reviews the research linking stress to adverse health consequences.[10] Among the findings: too much stress over a long period of time can negatively regulate various aspects of the cellular immune response. In particular, stress disrupts bidirectional communication networks between the nervous, endocrine, and immune systems. When these networks fail, messenger systems that regulate hormones, blood cell formation, and a host of other health-regulating systems begin to falter or send faulty information.[11]

During prolonged stress, elevated levels of adrenal hormones destroy or reduce the ability of certain white blood cells, known as natural killer T cells, to aid the immune response. When killer T cells are suppressed and other regulating systems aren't working correctly, illness may occur.

A study of older adults under chronic stress uncovered higher-than-normal levels of *interleukin-6 (IL-6),* an immune-system protein in the blood that promotes inflammation.[12] IL-6 has been linked with various age-related conditions such as heart disease, diabetes, osteoporosis, frailty, and certain cancers. The researchers compared the health of 117 caregivers for patients suffering from dementia with a control group of 106 adults with no caregiving role. Caregivers experienced consistently higher stress levels, worked longer hours, slept less, and reported more isolation and loneliness. Over the course of the six-year study, IL-6 levels increased an average of four times faster among caregivers. In cases where spouses died, IL-6 levels rose and, for many, remained elevated for several years. (These caregivers' immune systems did not rebound as quickly as expected, perhaps because of the dual effects of stress and depression.)

Earlier findings by this research team showed that stress levels had a detrimental effect on the effectiveness of certain vaccines, the speed of wound healing, and the impact of even short-term stress events, such as arguments and test-taking, on the immune response.

Other studies that link stress with infectious diseases include:

- Mice that are forced to live in crowded cages prior to and after infection with tuberculosis have much poorer outcomes than mice in less crowded situations. Social disruption in mice also seems to trigger outbreaks of herpes viruses.[13]
- Caregivers of Alzheimer's patients who were vaccinated against the flu still had a much greater chance of getting the flu or becoming ill than noncaregivers who received the same vaccine.[14]
- People with self-reported high stress levels were much more likely to develop upper respiratory infections than those who reported lower levels of stress.[15]
- People with high stress levels who skip breakfast and consume a high level of fats catch many more colds than those who eat healthily and have low stress levels.[16]
- Certain changes in lifestyle may increase resistance to infectious diseases. These changes include broadening one's social involvement (for example, joining social or spiritual groups, having a confidant, spending time with supportive friends) and maintaining healthful practices, such as proper diet, exercise, and sleep.[17]
- Students' disease-fighting mechanisms are weaker during high-stress times, such as exam weeks and on days when they are upset. In one experiment, a stressful event increased the severity of symptoms in a group of volunteers who were knowingly infected with a cold virus. In another, 47 percent of subjects living high-stress lives developed colds after a virus was dropped into their noses, but only 27 percent of those living relatively stress-free lives caught these colds.[18]

Although strong indicators support the hypothesis of a relationship between high stress and increased risk for disease, we are only beginning to understand this link. Some research indicates that other factors, such as genetics and environmental stimuli, may be involved. However, in spite of questions, studies supporting this relationship outnumber those that don't.[19]

Stress and Diabetes

The effect of stress on blood sugar levels makes its impact on diabetes management crucial. First, people under lots of stress often don't get enough sleep, don't eat well, and may drink or take other drugs to help them get through a stressful

---

Psychoneuroimmunology (PNI) Science of the interaction between the mind and the immune system.

Nontraditional Students: Uniquely Different With Unique Stressors

Unprecedented numbers of adults who do not match the traditional student profile—18 years old, right out of high school—are enrolling in America's colleges and universities. In fact, nontraditional is becoming the norm, with as many as 47 percent of college students now over the age of 25. Students not only are older, but more diverse, with more life and work experiences, and often the added responsibilities of family, home, and job on top of the demands of college. Are schools ready to accommodate the unique needs of this population and to be supportive of their diverse responsibilities and schedules?

The stressors facing all college students include academic, financial, time, health-related, and self-imposed ones. Add to these for older students issues such as children, family, dependent care, job schedules, commutes to/from other areas, family expectations for career and income improvements, and the pressure to succeed among a younger, more technologically savvy group of students, and it is easy to see why older students might be prone to be unusually stressed.

Even the way assignments are given in classes might be unusually stressful for these students. For example, instructors often assume when they give group projects that class members are readily available to meet with others on campus and that all are equally motivated. Now consider these excerpts from a survey of nontraditional students and their views about working in groups with their younger classmates:

I have a family that is depending on me to get a job and support them with the degree I will earn. I find it difficult to be a member of a group based on factors such as family life, commitments to my children, and travel issues. (I live 45 miles from campus.) When the younger students are always confiding their problems to me, it begins to wear me down . . . I am NOT their mom.

I am a single mother, and I find it very difficult to meet in groups. I work and attend school and feel like evenings are my time at home with my son. I also feel that it would be impossible for me to afford to pay someone to watch my child in the evenings or during the extra meeting times required of cooperative learning. Although there are tons of non-trad students, classes and organizations are still geared toward 18-year-olds who don't have the same outside responsibilities as we do.

You or some of your classmates may share some of these frustrations. If you are feeling the effects of being a nontraditional student, try the following strategies to help reduce stress:

- *Plan your time wisely.* Use your commuting time and nonclass time on campus. Tape lectures and use driving time to listen to lectures again. Many colleges have special areas for quiet study between classes.
- *Analyze your tendencies to overachieve.* Many nontraditional students spend inordinate amounts of time on projects, often much more than an assignment requires. Try to prioritize and resist the tendency to prove that you are older, wiser, and can do the best job in class. Do your best, but don't obsess about perfection.
- *Find a support group.* One of the difficulties faced by many nontraditional students is that they feel "out of it" on campus. If you don't engage in the traditional college social life you may only get to know others from class, and with larger class sizes, it is especially difficult to meet and interact with people with common interests. Seek out nontraditional student groups on campus. Check with your college health center personnel or counselors about ways in which your campus brings together nontraditional students for fun activities. Don't isolate yourself from younger students. Often, these relationships become important avenues for information, support in time of need, and general self-validation.
- *Work hard to reduce tensions between student groups.* Differences in psychological and life stages may cause tensions between traditional and nontraditional students. To older students, traditional-age students may appear less serious about their studies, while younger students may see older students as monopolizing class and instructor time or as being preoccupied with work, families, and other issues. Keep the lines of communication open, be sure that individuals respect other's right to opinions, and given limited class times, be sure all have a chance to participate.
- *Speak up.* Although many nontraditional students are reluctant to speak up about the difficulties of group projects, you should be respectful but firm about your role. Take charge if necessary, but delegate specific responsibilities and let the group participate in evaluations of everyone's efforts. Many younger students are equally frustrated by the lack of motivation that some students display.
- *Find time for yourself.* Often you may find yourself flying around all day at school and then going home to family or to work and facing another set of stressors. Find time to be alone, to refresh and rejuvenate.

Sources: K. Droege, "One Size Does NOT fit All" (unpublished paper, University of Wisconsin, Stout, March, 2004); R. Misra, and M. McKean, "College Students' Academic Stress and its Relation to Their Anxiety, Time Management, and Leisure Satisfaction," *American Journal of Health Studies* 16 (2000): 41–51.

time. All of these behaviors can alter blood sugar levels. Second, when a person is stressed, his or her body releases stress hormones (the fight-or-flight hormones discussed previously), and the body begins to increase blood sugars to ensure the extra fuel is available to fight or flee. In a person with diabetes, if his pancreas is not functioning properly and insulin isn't produced in sufficient levels or if it isn't as effective, blood sugar levels may stay high and begin to damage body organs (such as the kidneys) or blood vessels in the extremities and eyes. Particularly for people with type 2 diabetes, mental stress causes blood sugar levels to soar. Physical stress, such as from illness or injury, also causes blood sugar levels to rise precipitously in both type 1 and type 2 diabetics.[20] While an occasional stress reaction might not harm you, high stress jobs, situations that remain unresolved and cause stress, and chronic stress may make a diabetic's struggle in controlling blood sugar extremely difficult.

Controlling stress levels is critical for successful short- and long-term diabetes management. Exercise and relaxation techniques are particularly important. Even a short 15-minute walk can cause glucose levels to drop dramatically, as well as having other stress-reducing effects. Losing weight is also important. Being at a healthy weight contributes to overall glucose control and prevents the stress that people feel when they are overweight.

Stress and the Mind

Stress may be one of the single greatest contributors to mental disability and emotional dysfunction in industrialized nations. Whether it be from lost work productivity, difficulties in relationships, abuse of drugs and other substances, displaced anger and aggressive behavior, or a host of other problems, stress overload does much more than cause the heart rate to soar. Evidence suggests a strong relationship between stress and the potential for negative mental health reactions. Consider the following:[21]

- Numerous researchers have demonstrated that when stressors are combined with low self-esteem and/or maladaptive coping styles, depression and anxiety increase.
- Depression and drug abuse are highly correlated with excessive exposure to stress.
- Among college students, low self-esteem or depression and concerns about stress and health were identified as unresolved problems for 35 percent and 20 percent of the respondents, respectively.
- Mature coping styles predict happiness, occupational and social success, enjoyment, and absence of addictions.
- People with high nervous tension have increased risk for mental illness, suicide, and coronary heart disease.
- A recent national study of Americans aged 15 to 54 found that almost half will suffer a mental and addictive disorder during their lifetime. Many of these disorders are believed to be stress related.
- Mental illness is on the increase in almost all segments of U.S. society.

Sources of Stress

Both eustress and distress have many sources. They include psychosocial factors, environmental stressors, and self-imposed stress.

Psychosocial Sources of Stress

Psychosocial stress refers to the factors in our daily lives that cause stress. Interactions with others, the subtle and not-so-subtle expectations we and others have of ourselves, and the social conditions we live in force us to readjust continually. Psychosocial stressors include change, hassles, pressure, inconsistent goals and behaviors, conflict, overload, burnout, and discrimination.

Change Any time change occurs in your normal routine, whether good or bad, you will experience stress. The more changes you experience and the more adjustments you must make, the greater the stress effects may be. In 1967, Drs. Thomas Holmes and Richard Rahe analyzed the social readjustments experienced by over 5,000 patients, noting which events seemed to occur just prior to disease onset.[22] They determined that certain events (both positive and negative) were predictive of increased risk for illness. They called their scale for predicting stress overload and the likelihood of illness the Social Readjustment Rating Scale (SRRS).[23] The SRRS has since served as the model for scales for certain groups, including college-age students, as shown in Table 3.1. Although many other factors must be considered, in general, the more of these stressors you experience, the more you need to change your behaviors or situation before problems occur.

Hassles While Holmes and Rahe focused on major stressors, psychologists such as Richard Lazarus have focused on petty annoyances and frustrations, collectively referred to as *hassles*.[24] Minor hassles—losing your keys, slipping and falling in front of everyone as you walk to your seat in a new class, finding that you went through a whole afternoon with a big chunk of spinach stuck in your front teeth—seem unimportant, but their cumulative effects may be harmful in the long run.

Pressure Pressure occurs when we feel forced to speed up, intensify, or shift the direction of our behavior to meet a higher standard of performance.[25] Pressures can be based on our personal goals and expectations, concern about what others think, or outside influences. Among the most significant outside influences are society's demands that we compete and be all that we can be. The forces that push us to compete for the best grades, nicest cars, most attractive significant others, and highest-paying jobs create significant pressure to be the personification of success.

Table 3.1
Chronic Stressors for College Students

Here are some chronic stressors often experienced by college students. Each has the potential to cause serious health problems, particularly if experienced on a fairly regular basis (i.e., at least two or three times per week for the past month).

1. Roommate conflict	13. Uncertainty over the right major	25. Conflict with parents
2. Homesickness	14. Missing distant friends	26. Academic performance
3. Friend conflict	15. Family illness	27. Overweight
4. Writing major papers	16. Loneliness	28. Don't fit in; no friends
5. Dieting	17. Job pressures	29. Living/housing situations
6. Money/financial problems	18. Lack of privacy	30. Tuition bills/book costs
7. Long-distance relationship	19. Friends with problems	31. Health problems/not feeling well
8. Juggling school and job	20. Parental problems/family problems	32. Difficult class or instructor
9. Time management	21. Not enough sex/intimacy	33. Unsure of job future
10. Noisy dorm or apartment	22. Behind in schoolwork	34. Not enough sleep
11. No car or car not working	23. Problem with lover	35. Problem with drugs/alcohol
12. Underweight	24. Not enough exercise	

Source: Adapted from Kluwer Academic Publishers *Journal of Youth and Adolescence* 25, no. 2 (1996) 199–217, "Chronic Stress in the Lives of College Students: Scale Development and Prospective Predictions of Distress," by L. Towbes and L. Cohen. With the kind permission of Springer Science and Business Media.

Inconsistent Goals and Behaviors For many of us, negative stress effects are magnified when there is a disparity between our goals (what we value or hope to obtain in life) and our behaviors (actions that may or may not lead to these goals). For instance, you may want good grades, and your family may expect them. But if you party and procrastinate throughout the term, your behaviors are inconsistent with your goals, and significant stress in the form of guilt, last-minute frenzy before exams, and disappointing grades may result. On the other hand, if you dig in and work and remain committed to getting good grades, this may eliminate much of your negative stress. Thwarted goals can lead to frustration, and frustration has been shown to be a significant disrupter of homeostasis.

Determining whether behaviors are consistent with goals is an essential component of maintaining balance in life. If we consciously strive to attain our goals in a direct manner, we greatly improve our chances of success.

Conflict Conflict occurs when we are forced to make difficult decisions between competing motives, behaviors, or impulses, or when we are forced to face incompatible demands, opportunities, needs, or goals.[26] What if your best friends all choose to smoke marijuana and you don't want to smoke but fear rejection? Conflict often occurs as our values are

tested. College students who are away from home for the first time often face conflict between parental values and their own set of developing beliefs.

Overload Excessive time pressure, too much responsibility, high expectations of yourself and those around you, and lack of support can lead to **overload,** a state of being overburdened. Have you ever felt you had so many responsibilities that you couldn't possibly begin to fulfill them all? Have you longed for a weekend when you could just take time out with friends and not feel guilty? These feelings are symptoms of overload. Students suffering from overload may experience anxiety about tests, poor self-concept, a desire to drop classes or drop out of school, and other problems. In severe cases, in which they are unable to see any solutions to their problems, students may suffer from depression or turn to substance abuse.

Burnout People who regularly suffer from overload, frustration, and disappointment may eventually experience **burnout,** a state of physical and mental exhaustion caused by excessive stress. People involved in the "helping professions," such as teaching, social work, drug counseling, nursing, and psychology, experience high levels of burnout, as do people such as police officers and air-traffic controllers who work in high-pressure, dangerous jobs.

Other Forms of Psychosocial Stress Other forms of psychosocial stress include problems with overcrowding, discrimination, and socioeconomic difficulties such as unemployment and poverty. People of different ages or ethnic backgrounds may face a disproportionately heavy impact from these sources of stress. In addition to all of these we face increasing threats from technological stressors. For more information see the New Horizons in Health box.

Overload A condition in which a person feels overly pressured by demands.

Burnout Physical and mental exhaustion caused by excessive stress.

Taming Technostress

Cell phones that ring constantly or cut out in the middle of a conversation; e-mail lists that grow on your desktop like an out-of-control fungus; laptop computers that somehow end up in your luggage when you go on vacation; electronic organizers that beep at the movies; voice message systems that don't let you talk to a live person; and slow, slow, slow downloading of information. Can you feel your heart rate speeding up just reading this?

If you are like millions of other people today, you find that technology is often a daily terrorizer that raises your blood pressure, frustrates you, and prevents you from ever really "getting away from it all." In short, you may unknowingly be a victim of stressors that previous generations only dreamed (or had nightmares) about. Known as *technostress*, this problem is defined as "personal stress generated by reliance on technological devices, . . . a panicky feeling when they fail, and a state of near-constant stimulation, or being perpetually 'plugged in.'" When technostress grabs you, it may interact with other forms of stress to create a synergistic, never-ending form of stimulation that keeps your stress response reverberating all day.

Part of the problem, ironically, is that technology enables us to be so productive. Because it encourages polyphasic activity, or multitasking, people are forced to juggle multiple thoughts and actions at the same time, such as driving and talking on cell phones or checking handheld devices for appointments. There is clear evidence that such multitasking contributes to auto accidents and other harmful consequences. What is less clear is what happens to someone who is always plugged in.

What are the symptoms of technology overload? It evokes typical stress responses by increasing heart rate and blood pressure and by causing irritability and memory disturbances. Over time, many stressed-out people lose the ability to relax and find that they feel nervous and anxious when they are supposed to be having fun. Headaches, stomach and digestive problems, skin irritations, colds, slow wound healing, lack of sleep, ulcers, and a host of other problems may result. A study conducted by Yale University indicates that chronic stress may even thicken the waistline; increased secretions of cortisol caused even slender women to store more fat in the abdomen.

Authors Michelle Weil and Larry Rosen describe *technosis*, a syndrome in which people get so immersed in technology that they risk losing their own identity. If you answer "yes" to questions such as "Do you rely on preprogrammed systems to contact others?" or "Do you feel stressed if you haven't checked your e-mail within the last 12 hours?" you may be too dependent on technology.

TIPS FOR FIGHTING TECHNOSTRESS

- *Exercise.* Get away from any form of technology. Quiet walks or runs away from the blare of music and the sound of machines (typical in fitness centers) are best. Try to find a place that has few people and little noise—that usually means outdoors.
- *Become aware of what you are doing.* Track the time you spend on e-mail, voice mail, and so on. Set up a schedule to limit your use of technology. For example, limit all e-mail responses to two to three lines. Spend no more than a half hour per day writing and answering e-mails.
- *Set up strict rules for when you can go online,* and don't log on at other times.
- *Give yourself more time for everything you do.* If you are surfing the web for resources for a term paper, start early rather than the night before the paper is due.
- *Manage the telephone—don't let it manage you.* Rather than interrupting what you're doing to answer, screen calls with an answering machine. Get rid of call waiting, which forces you to juggle multiple calls, and subscribe to a voice mail service that takes messages when you're on the phone.
- *Set "time out" periods.* During these times, don't answer the phone, listen to the stereo, turn on the computer or TV. Switch off e-mail notification systems so you aren't beeped during these periods.
- *Take regular breaks.* Every hour or so, get up, walk around, stretch, do deep breathing, or get a glass of water,
- *If you are working on the computer, look away from the screen and focus on something far away* every 30 minutes or so. Stretch your shoulders and neck periodically as you work. Playing soft background music can help you relax.
- *Resist the urge to buy the newest and fastest technology.* Such purchases not only cause financial stress, but also add to stress levels with the typical glitches that occur when installing and adjusting to new software.
- *Do not take laptops, hand-held devices, or other technological gadgets on vacation.* If you must take a cell phone for emergencies, turn it and your voice messaging system off, and use the phone only in true emergencies.
- *Back up materials on your computer at regular intervals.* Writing a term paper only to lose it during a power outage will send you into hyperstress very quickly.
- *If you have a technical problem, resist the urge to start trial-and-error button pushing,* which often makes the situation worse. Read the manual or contact technical support.
- *Accept that a certain amount of technology-driven aggravation is inevitable.*

Sources: "Taming Technostress" from *Technostress: Coping with Technology@Work@Home @Play* by Dr. Michelle M. Weil and Dr. Larry D. Rosen. © 1997. Used by permission of the author; M. Weil, and L. Rosen, "Technostress: Are you a Victim of Technosis?," 2004, www.technostress.com/tstechnosis.htm; D. Zielinksi, "Techno-stressed?," *Presentations* 18, no. 2 (2004): 28–34; Yale University, "Stress May Cause Excess Abdominal Fat In Otherwise Slender Women, Study Conducted At Yale Shows," *ScienceDaily*, November 23, 2000; MayoClinic.com, "Are You a Slave to the Telephone?," November 1, 2000, www.mayoclinic.com

What do you think?

Think about the changes that you have made during the past couple of years. Which of them would you regard as positive? As negative? ■ How did you react to these changes initially? ■ Did your reactions change later? ■ What are the biggest and most important changes that students must make as they enter colleges and universities, and what can they do to cope with unexpected changes?

Stress and "-isms"

Today's racially and ethnically diverse group of students, faculty members, and staff enriches everyone's educational experience yet also challenges everyone to deal with differences. Students come to the campus from vastly different contexts and life experiences. Often, those who act, speak, dress, or appear different face additional pressures that do not affect students considered more typical. Students perceived as different may become victims of subtle and not-so-subtle forms of bigotry, insensitivity, harassment, or hostility. Race, ethnicity, religious affiliation, age, sexual orientation, or other *"-isms"*—different viewpoints and backgrounds—may hang like a dark cloud over these students.[27]

Evidence of the health effects of excessive stress abound in the general population. Black Americans suffer higher rates of hypertension, CVD, and most forms of cancer than their white counterparts do. Gay men and lesbians have higher rates of suicide and are more likely to become victims of violent acts. Although poverty and socioeconomic status have been blamed for much of the spike in hypertension rates for African Americans and other marginalized groups, this chronic, physically debilitating stress may reflect real and perceived status in society more than actual poverty. Feeling that they occupy a position of low status, either due to living conditions, financial security, or job status, can be a source of stress. The problem is exacerbated for those who are socially disadvantaged early in life and grow up without a nurturing environment. Many believe that stressors for ethnic minority students may contribute to a wide range of difficulties on college campuses.[28]

Imagine what it would be like to come to campus and find yourself isolated, lacking friends, and ridiculed on the

Background distressors Environmental stressors of which people are often unaware.

Cognitive stress system The psychological system that recognizes stressors and processes emotional responses to stress.

basis of who you are or how you look. Even worse, consider the fate of Matthew Shepard, a young student in Wyoming who was brutally murdered for being gay, or of countless other students who have been victimized because of race, nationality, or religious affiliation. In addition to "making the grade" in classes, they must deal with hidden fears, suffering, and difficulties caused by intolerant factions on campus. (Chapter 4 focuses on the incidence and prevalence of violence on campus.)

Environmental Stress

Environmental stress results from events occurring in the physical environment as opposed to social surroundings. Environmental stressors include natural disasters, such as floods and hurricanes, and industrial disasters, such as chemical spills and explosions. Often as damaging as one-time disasters are **background distressors,** such as noise, air, and water pollution, although we may be unaware of them, and their effects may not become apparent for decades. As with other distressors, our bodies respond to environmental distressors with the general adaptation syndrome. People who cannot escape background distressors may exist in a constant resistance phase, which can contribute to the development of stress-related disorders.

Self-Imposed Stress

Self-Concept and Stress The **cognitive stress system** is the psychological system that helps us recognize stressors; evaluate them on the basis of self-concept, past experiences, and emotions; and decide how to cope with them.[29]

Sensory organs serve as input channels for information reaching the brain. From that point on, attention to the problem, memory, reasoning processes, and problem solving are organized in various parts of the brain. This occurs before we act on the stressor. Because learning and memory involve the changing of various proteins in brain neurons, the emotions experienced during the stress response also "tickle" the memory storage neurons and contribute to responses. Behaviorally, we will respond to the stressor in ways consistent with our memories of similar situations.

Self-esteem is closely related to the emotions engendered by past experiences. Low self-esteem can lead to helpless anger. People suffering helpless anger have usually learned that they are wrong to feel anger, so instead of expressing it in healthy ways they turn it inward. They may "swallow" their rage in food, alcohol, or other drugs, or act in other self-destructive ways. Donna Shalala, former U.S. Secretary of Health and Human Services, has instituted a program called Girl Power, designed to improve the self-esteem of young women between the ages of 9 and 14, a time when low self-esteem is thought to trigger a host of negative health behaviors.

Research indicates that self-esteem significantly affects various disease processes. People with low self-esteem create

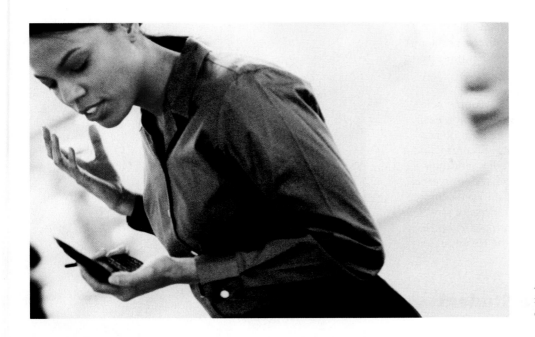

As technology becomes more important in everyday life, it can cause stress in new ways.

a self-imposed distressor that can depress the immune system and increase the symptoms of diseases such as acquired immunodeficiency syndrome (AIDS), herpes, multiple sclerosis, and Epstein-Barr syndrome.

Personality Types and Hardiness   Personality may contribute to the kind and degree of self-imposed stress we experience. In 1974, physicians Meyer Friedman and Ray Rosenman identified two stress-related personality types: Type A and Type B.[30] Type A personalities are hard-driving, competitive, anxious, time-driven, impatient, angry, and perfectionistic. Type B personalities are relaxed and noncompetitive. According to Rosenman and Friedman, people with Type A characteristics are more prone to heart attacks than their Type B counterparts.

Researchers today believe that more needs to be discovered about personality types before we can say that all Type A's have greater risks for heart disease. First of all, most people are not one personality type all the time. Second, many other unexplained variables must also be explored, such as why some Type A people seem to thrive in stress-filled environments. Sometimes labeled Type C personalities (not to be confused with the cancer-prone Type C discussed in Chapter 2), these individuals appear to succeed more often than Type B personalities. They enjoy good overall health even while displaying Type A patterns of behavior.

Critics argue that these attempts to base ill health on personal behavioral patterns are crude. For example, researchers at Duke University contend that the Type A personality may be more complex than previously described. They have identified a "toxic core" in some Type A personalities. People who have this toxic core are angry, distrustful of others, and have above-average levels of cynicism. People who are angry and hostile often have below-average levels of social support and other increased risks for ill health. It may be this toxic core rather than the hard-driving nature of the Type A personality that makes people more vulnerable to self-imposed stress.[31]

According to psychologist Susanne Kobasa, **psychological hardiness** may negate self-imposed stress associated with Type A behavior. Psychologically hardy people are characterized by *control, commitment,* and *challenge.*[32] People with a sense of control are able to accept responsibility for their behaviors and change behaviors that they discover to be debilitating. People with a sense of commitment have good self-esteem and understand their purpose in life. People with a sense of challenge see changes in life as stimulating opportunities for personal growth.

Because some Type A behavior is learned, it can be modified. Some Type A's are able to slow down and become more tolerant, patient, and better humored. Unfortunately, many people do not decide to modify their Type A habits until after they become ill or suffer a heart attack. Prevention of heart and circulatory disorders resulting from stress entails recognizing and changing dangerous behaviors before damage is done. See the section on managing emotional responses to stress (page 88) for more on how to change these behaviors.

Self-Efficacy   Whether people cope successfully with stressful situations often depends on their level of self-efficacy, or their belief in their skills and performance abilities.[33] If they have succeeded in mastering similar problems in the past, they will be more likely to believe in their own effectiveness.

Psychological hardiness   A personality trait characterized by control, commitment, and challenge.

Similarly, people who have repeatedly tried and failed may lack confidence in their abilities to deal with life's problems. In some cases, this insecurity may prevent them from trying to cope.

External Versus Internal Locus of Control   People who believe they lack control in a situation may become easily frustrated and give up. Those who feel they have no personal control tend to have an *external locus of control* and a low level of self-efficacy. People who are confident their behavior will influence the outcome tend to have an *internal locus of control*. Individuals who feel that they have limited control over their lives often show higher levels of stress. In extreme cases, this feeling of little control can contribute to post-traumatic stress, as discussed in the Health in a Diverse World box.

Stress and the College Student

For many young adults, their college years are the best times of their lives. For the first time, they are on their own, free to make their own choices, interact, and spend their time focusing on a future career. However, for some students, these "best of times" lead to the "worst of times," as they buckle under overwhelming pressures and responsibilities. These students experience numerous distressors, including changes related to being away from home for the first time, pressure to make friends in a new and sometimes intimidating setting, the feeling of anonymity imposed by large classes, and academic pressures and test-taking anxiety (see the Skills for Behavior Change box on page 86).

We thrive under a certain amount of stress, but excessive levels can leave students overwhelmed and underenthused about classes and social interactions. Some 29 percent of students surveyed for the National College Health Assessments reported that stress was the number-one factor affecting their individual academic performance, followed closely by stress-related problems such as sleep difficulties (21.3 percent) and cold/flu/sore throats (21.2 percent).[34]

A recent study by the Higher Education Research Institute at University of California (Los Angeles) reported that current college freshmen are more stressed than any class of freshmen before them. These researchers define **psychological stress** as the relationship between a person and the environment that the person judges to be beyond his or her resources and jeopardizes his or her well-being.[35] Freshmen

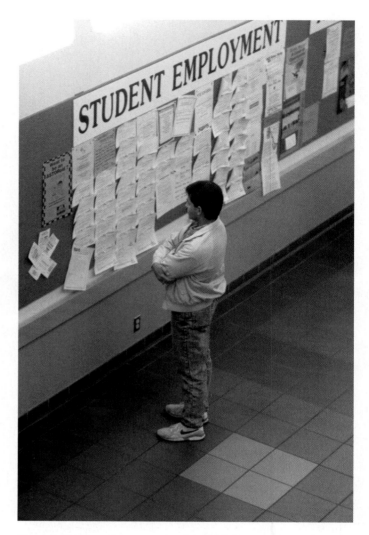

Many college students are dealing with financial responsibilities for the first time. Finding and keeping a job while attending school, pursuing financial aid, and keeping to a budget all can contribute to stress.

seem to be the most vulnerable to the negative effects of psychological stress, with relationships, race relations, school events, physical assault (or being stalked), and feeling deviance from school norms being noted as particularly distressful. Not only did freshmen report more problems with these issues, they also reported more emotional reactivity in the form of anger/hostility/frustration and a greater sense of being out of control. Sophomores and juniors reported fewer problems with these issues, and seniors reported the fewest problems, which perhaps indicates progressive emotional growth through experience, maturity, increased awareness of support services, and more social connections.[36]

In a large study of chronic stressors, male and female college students differed significantly in the things they perceived to be significant stressors.[37] Women indicated that among their most frequent stressors were trying to diet, being overweight, having an overload of school work, and gaining weight. Men, in contrast, tended to list the following

Psychological stress   Stress caused by being in an environment perceived to be beyond one's control and endangering one's well-being.

Post-traumatic stress disorder   An acute stress disorder caused by experiencing an extremely traumatic event, such as rape or combat.

Post-Traumatic Stress: Dealing With the Aftermath

For many of us, the vivid images of the planes hitting the World Trade Center towers on September 11, 2001, will be etched in our memory forever. Anger, horror, frustration, and a host of other emotions brought tears, stomach upset, and other bodily ills to those of us who sat helplessly watching the events following the attack. As horrible as this experience was for those who sat watching, the real trauma for those who lost loved ones, coworkers, and friends may have only begun.

According to the National Institutes of Health, 5 to 8 percent of the American public suffer from chronic stress as a result of a traumatic experience. Historically, rape victims and survivors of torture and concentration camps have been among those most likely to experience such problems, with women experiencing it at almost twice the prevalence of men.

In severe cases, an individual's response may be considered **post-traumatic stress disorder (PTSD).** This acute stress disorder with extreme anxiety and behavioral disturbances develops within the first hours or days after a traumatic event. Many persons suffering from PTSD have been soldiers returning from war, particularly those who saw friends killed or mangled or who experienced terrible suffering and pain themselves. Many of these soldiers continue to suffer from these experiences for decades afterward. Other extreme traumatic events include terrorist attacks, rape or other severe physical attacks, near-death experiences in accidents, witnessing a murder or death, street crime or assault, abuse, or being caught in a natural disaster.

Typical symptoms of PTSD include:

- *Dissociation,* or perceived detachment of the mind from the emotional state or even the body. In dissociation, people may have a sense of the world as a dreamlike or unreal place and have poor memory of the events—a form of *dissociative amnesia.*
- *Acute anxiety* or nervousness, in which people are hyperaroused, may cry easily or experience mood swings, and experience flashbacks, nightmares, and recurrent thoughts or visual images. They may sense vague uneasiness or feel like the event is happening again and again. Some may experience intense physiological reactions, such as shaking or nausea when something reminds them of the events. In some cases, they may have difficulty returning to areas that remind them of the trauma.
- *Persistent stress symptoms.* Sufferers may have two or more of these symptoms: difficulty falling or staying asleep; irritability or outbursts of anger or other emotions; difficulty concentrating; hypervigilance; exaggerated startle response.

If these symptoms last more than one month, post-traumatic stress disorder may be diagnosed, either as an *acute form* (less than 3 months' duration) or as a *chronic form* (longer than 3 months). A *delayed onset* form of PTSD may appear months after the event. In most people, symptoms disappear within 6 months.

TIPS FOR COPING

It is important to acknowledge the trauma and address its effects. Ways to recover include:

- *Talking about it* and encouraging others to share their perspectives.
- *Taking care of yourself.* Get plenty of rest and exercise. Do things you find relaxing and soothing. As soon as possible, get back to normal routines.

- *Staying connected to friends and family.* Make plans to visit family or others who can offer reassurance and stability. If you can't travel or are nervous about it, use phone or e-mail contact.
- *Doing something positive* that will help you gain a sense of control, such as giving blood, taking a first aid class, or donating food or clothing. Get involved with campus activities planned in response to a disaster, such as candlelight vigils, benefits, or discussion groups and speakers.
- *Asking for help* if you are feeling overwhelmed or out of control. It's not a sign of weakness. Talk with a trusted friend or faith leader. Consult on-campus resources such as the counseling center or student health center. If you don't know where to go, talk with your health professor about options. If your feelings of sadness, depression, or excessive anxiety persist, seek professional help.

WHEN THE TRAUMA IS TOO GREAT

Therapies designed to help trauma victims recover are increasingly effective as our knowledge about this disorder grows. Schools, communities, and workplaces now routinely bring in crisis experts immediately after an event to help survivors talk through their feelings and gain support from others. A supportive family, employer, and friends and access to professional counseling are important in the recovery process. New generations of antianxiety drugs can help individuals who have difficulties. Sleep aids and other options are available to ease short-term symptoms.

Sources: National Mental Health Association, "Coping with Disaster," 2001, www.nmha.org /reassurance/collegetips.cfm; Posttraumatic Stress Disorder Society, "Posttraumatic Stress Disorder," 2003, www.mentalhealth.com /dis/p20-an06.html; *Mental Health: A Report to the Surgeon General,* 1999, www .surgeongeneral.gov/library/mentalhealth /chapter4/sec2.html; National Center for Post Traumatic Stress, 2004, www.ncptsd.org

Overcoming Test-Taking Anxiety

Doing well on a test is an ability needed far beyond college. Tests are a fact of life in government, insurance, medicine, and other fields—and stress is a fact of tests!

There are things you can do to get the upper hand on your anxiety. Here are some helpful hints to try on your next exam.

BEFORE THE EXAM

1. *Manage your time.* Plan to start studying a week before your test (longer if it's a professional exam required for your career). The more in advance the studying is done, the less anxiety you will feel. The final night should be limited to review, and you should try to get a good night's sleep. Arrive at the test a half hour early for a final run-through. You will find that this will ease your anxiety and increase your confidence.
2. *Build your test-taking self-esteem.* First, take a 3 x 5 inch card, and write down the three reasons you will pass the exam. Carry the card with you and look at it whenever you study. Second, when you get the test, write your three reasons on the test or on a piece of scrap paper. Positive affirmations such as this will help you succeed.
3. *Get adequate sleep.* You need to be alert, so get a little extra sleep for a few nights before your exam.
4. *Eat a balanced meal before the exam.* Sugar doesn't give you energy—in fact, it tires you. Avoid rich or heavy foods (they'll make you sleepy) as well as foods that might upset your stomach. You want to feel your best.
5. *Take a moderate amount of caffeine an hour before the test.* Research shows that caffeine promotes alertness, motor performance, and the capacity for work, as well as decreases fatigue. A cup of coffee, tea, or a cola drink is sufficient. Be aware, though, that some people shouldn't use caffeine. Avoid it if it makes you feel shaky or if you do not regularly consume it. Test day is not the day to find our how your body reacts to caffeine.

DURING THE TEST

1. *Manage your time during the test.* If you have 60 minutes to answer 30 multiple-choice questions, you might decide to spend the first 45 minutes taking the test (1 ½ minutes per question) and 15 minutes reviewing your answers (30 seconds per question). Hold to this schedule. After 15 minutes, you should have completed the first ten questions. If you don't know an answer or the question is taking too long, skip it and move on. Since you allotted yourself time at the end to review, you will be able to go back and work on these questions. Test makers usually allow sufficient time to complete and review a test. However, if you feel that you are a slow reader and need more time, talk to your teacher or test administrator before the exam.
2. *Slow down.* When you open your test book, always write RTFQ (Read the Full Question) at the top. Make sure you understand the question before answering.
3. *Stay on track.* If you begin to get anxious, reread your three reasons for success.

---

items as major stressors: being underweight, problems relating to commuting to school, not having someone to date, not having enough sex, being behind in schoolwork, not having enough friends, and concerns about drug or alcohol use.[38]

College students may be especially vulnerable because they are in a period of transition, often being away from home for the first time, striking out on their own, and forging new relationships. From the moment they start packing, these transitions cause them to face key developmental tasks as their lives begin to make dramatic changes, such as achieving emotional independence from family; choosing and preparing for a career; preparing for a major relationship, commitment, and/or family life; facing economic independence; and developing their own values and ethical system. These tasks require that the college student develop new social roles and modify old ones. Such changes can result in role strain as they attempt to form a new identity and can lead to chronic stress responses.

If you experience any of the stressors listed in Table 3.1 (page 80), act promptly to reduce their impact. Most colleges offer stress management workshops through health centers or student counseling departments. Do not ignore the symptoms of stress overload, which include a vague sense of anxiety or nervousness; changes in sleep, diet, or exercise patterns; headaches; dizziness; short temper; increased negativism, cynicism, anger, or frustration; recurring colds and minor illnesses; persistent time pressures; increased difficulty in completing tasks; inability to concentrate; wanting to get away from others; and less tolerance of petty annoyances.

If stress is not dealt with, it can lead to long-lasting problems. According to researchers, many mental health problems may be traced to stress-related trauma that occurs at key periods of life, particularly during the college years. Some of the threats to college students' mental well-being are outlined below:[39]

- Depression affects over 19 million American adults annually, including college students. According to a recent national college health survey, 10 to 13 percent of college students have been diagnosed with depression.

- Anxiety levels among college students have been rising since the 1950s. In 2000, almost seven percent of college students reported experiencing anxiety disorders within the previous year. Women are five times as likely to experience anxiety disorders as men.
- Eating disorders affect 5 to 10 million women and 1 million men, with the highest rates occurring in college-aged women.
- Suicide was the third biggest killer for those aged 15 to 24 and the second leading killer in the college population in 1998.
- According to the Centers for Disease Control and Prevention, 7.8 percent of men and 12.3 percent of women aged 18 to 24 report frequent mental distress.
- More than 30 percent of college freshmen report feeling overwhelmed a great deal of the time; about 38 percent of college women report feeling frequently overwhelmed.

Managing Your Stress

Recognizing stress is the first step toward making positive changes. Being on your own in college poses many challenges; however, it also lets you evaluate your unique situation and take steps that fit your own schedule and lifestyle in order to reduce negative stressors in your life. One of the most effective ways to combat stressors is to build skills and coping strategies that will help inoculate you against them. Such efforts are known collectively as *stress management techniques* and may range from doing something as simple as taking 20 minutes each day to be alone to developing an elaborate time management plan for eating, socializing, and exercising.

Any stress management technique that you select should be developed in a series of steps. Be careful not to change too many things at once, or your new stress management program could stress you out! It is also important to recognize the factors that exacerbate your negative reactions to stress. Physical and mental fatigue from sleeplessness, excessive use of alcohol and drugs, unhealthy relationships, or the presence of chronic disease may make it difficult for you to cope. Recognizing these threats, and trying to prevent those you can, is one of your best coping strategies.

Building Skills to Reduce Stress

Dealing with stress involves assessing all aspects of a stressor, examining your response and how you can change it, and learning to cope. Often we cannot change the requirements at our college, assignments in class, or unexpected distressors. Inevitably, we will be stuck in classes that bore us and for which we find no application in real life. We feel powerless when a loved one dies. However, although we cannot alter the facts, we can change our reactions to them.

Assessing Your Stressors After recognizing a stressor, evaluate it. Can you alter the circumstances to reduce the amount of distress you are experiencing, or must you change

your behavior and reactions to reduce stress levels? For example, if five term papers for five different courses are due during the semester, your professors are unlikely to drop such requirements. You can, however, change your behavior by beginning the papers early and spacing them over time to avoid last-minute stress.

Changing Your Responses Changing your responses requires practice and emotional control. If your roommate is habitually messy and this causes you stress, you can choose among several responses. You can express your anger by yelling, you can pick up the mess and leave a nasty note, or you can defuse the situation with humor. The first reaction that comes to mind is not always the best. Stop before reacting to gain the time you need to find an appropriate response. Ask yourself, "What is to be gained from my response?"

Many people change their responses to potentially stressful events through *cognitive coping strategies*. These strategies help them prepare for stressors through gradual exposure to increasingly higher stress levels.

Learning to Cope Everyone copes with stress in different ways. Some people drink or take drugs, others seek help from counselors, and still others try to forget about it or engage in positive activities such as exercise. **Stress inoculation,** one of the newer coping techniques, helps people prepare for stressful events ahead of time. For example, suppose you are petrified over speaking in front of a class. Practicing in front of friends or in front of a video camera are strategies that may inoculate and prevent your freezing up on the day of the presentation. Some health experts compare stress inoculation to a vaccine given to protect against a disease. Regardless of how you cope with a situation, your conscious effort to deal with it is an important step in stress management.

Downshifting More and more people recognize that today's lifestyle is hectic and pressure-packed, and stress often comes from trying to keep up. Many people are questioning whether "having it all" is worth it, and they are taking a step back and simplifying their lives. This trend is known as **downshifting.** Moving from a large urban area to a smaller town, exchanging the expensive SUV for a modest four-door sedan, and a host of other changes in lifestyle typify this move. Some dedicated downshifters have given up television, microwaves, phones, and even computers.

Downshifting involves a fundamental shift in values and honest introspection about what is important in life.

Stress inoculation Newer stress management technique in which a person consciously tries to prepare ahead of time for potential stressors.

Downshifting Conscious attempt to simplify life in an effort to reduce the stresses and strains of modern living.

When considering any form of downshifting or perhaps even starting your career this way, it's important to move slowly and consider the following:

- *Determine your ultimate goal.* What is most important to you, and what will you need to reach that goal? What can you do without? Where do you want to live?
- *Make a short-term and long-term plan for simplifying your life.* Set up your plan in doable steps, and work slowly toward each step. Begin saying no to requests for your time, and determine those people with whom it is important for you to spend time.
- *Complete a financial inventory.* How much money will you need to do the things you want to do? Will you live alone or share costs with roommates? Do you need a car, or can you rely on public transportation? Pay off credit cards and eliminate current debt or consider debt consolidation. Get used to paying with cash. If you don't have the cash, don't buy. Remember your lifestyle may be different as a student than when you were working or living at home.
- *Plan for health care costs.* Make sure that you budget for health insurance and basic preventive health services if you're not covered under your parents' plan. This should be a top priority. Be sure you understand your coverage so you're not caught off guard.
- *Select the right career.* Look for work that you enjoy and that isn't necessarily driven by salary. Can you be happy taking a lower-paying job that is less stressful and allows you the opportunity to have a life?
- *Consider options for saving money.* Downshifting doesn't mean you renounce money; it means you choose not to let money dictate your life. It's still important to save. If you're just getting started, you need to prepare for emergencies and for future plans.
- *Clear out/clean out.* A cluttered life can be distressing. Take an inventory of material items, and get rid of things you haven't worn or used in the last year. Donate items to charity.

Managing Social Interactions

As you plan your stress management program, don't underestimate the importance of social networks and social bonds. Consider the nature and extent of your friendships. Do you have someone with whom you can share intimate thoughts and feelings? Is there someone you could call if you needed help in an emergency? Do you trust your friends to keep your confidences? Be supportive? Be honest with you if you are doing something risky or inappropriate? Having someone to "vent" with when you are frustrated and who can give helpful advice is an invaluable stress reducer. It isn't necessary to have a large number of friends; however, different friends often serve different needs so having more than one is usually beneficial. Particularly for those who lack close ties with family, friends often serve as family away from home. As you work to develop and cultivate friendships, look for individuals who:

- Have values that are similar to your own
- Share common interests (but remain open to people with different interests who encourage you to stretch, grow, and explore new possibilities)
- Are good listeners, tolerant, give and share freely, and do not rush to judgment
- Are trustworthy and have your best interests at heart
- Are not unusually critical, negative, selfish, or only bring you down. Avoid people who enjoy stirring things up and always seem to be in some crisis themselves. Such friends often precipitate, rather than reduce, stress responses.
- Are responsible, value doing well in school, but also know when and how to have fun
- Enjoy balance in their lives
- Are willing to be exercise and diet buddies or study partners and share with a mutual interest in a healthy lifestyle
- Know how to laugh, cry, engage in meaningful conversation, and listen to the silence

Just as it is important to find some or all of these characteristics in your friends, it is also important for you to bring these qualities to your friendships. Sometimes focusing on others may help you get your own problems into better focus and control.

Managing Emotional Responses

Have you ever gotten all worked up about something only to find that your perceptions were totally wrong? We often get upset not by reality, but by our faulty perceptions. For example, suppose you found out that everyone except you is invited to a party. You might easily begin to wonder why you were excluded. Does someone dislike you? Have you offended someone? Such thoughts are typical. However, the reality of the situation may have absolutely nothing to do with your being liked or disliked. Perhaps you were sent an invitation and it didn't get to you.

Stress management requires that you examine your *self-talk* and your emotional responses to interactions with others. With any emotional response to a distressor, you are responsible for the emotion and the behaviors elicited by the emotion. Learning to tell the difference between normal emotions and those based on irrational beliefs can help you either stop the emotion or express it in a healthy and appropriate way.

Learning to Laugh and Cry Have you noticed that you feel better after a good laugh or cry? It isn't your imagination. Laughter and crying stimulate the heart and temporarily rev up many body systems. Heart rate and blood pressure then decrease significantly, allowing the body to relax.

Hostility: The Lethal Reaction Personality type as a source of self-imposed stress was discussed earlier in this chapter. One characteristic in particular can have severe effects on cardiovascular health: the tendency toward **hostility.** Hostility has three components: (1) *cognitive*—negative beliefs about and attitudes toward others, including cynicism and mistrust; (2) *affective*—anger, which can range from irritation to rage and be assessed with regard to frequency, intensity, and target; and (3) *behavioral*—an action intending to harm others, either verbally or physically, usually in an aggressive way. A wide range of studies have identified hostility as an independent risk factor for coronary heart disease (CHD), hypertension, and premature mortality. Hostility is thought to harm individuals by influencing health behaviors that themselves confer risk, such as smoking or fast driving, by being associated with sociodemographic characteristics that are in turn associated with risk for CHD, or by being associated with aberrations in physiological states that increase risk for atherosclerosis.[40] White males and people with low socioeconomic status appear to be at highest risk for hostility, along with people who are overweight or obese, smokers, and people with excessive alcohol consumption, sedentary lifestyle, hypertension, or high total cholesterol.

Fighting the Anger Urge   We all know what it means to be angry, whether it is the feeling we get when someone puts a ding on our car or the response when someone hurts someone we love. It may vary in intensity from mild irritation to rage and may be acted out as cynicism, sarcasm, intimidation, frustration, impatience, quick flaring of temper, distrust, or anxiety. It is important to remember that not all anger is inherently bad. Sometimes, it can give us the energy we need to fight back if attacked or the resolve to work even harder to accomplish a goal. It is unresolved anger—the kind that festers and clouds our reasoning and our reactions—that we need to worry about and take action to control.

Anger varies according to its source and can be an internal feeling of anger at ourselves for doing something foolish or anger at classmates, teachers, politicians, cancelled airline flights, or a host of other life events. Anger usually results when we feel we have lost control of a situation and/or are frustrated by a situation that we can do little about. The five main sources of anger are related to threats to (1) safety and well-being; (2) power; (3) perfectionism and pride; (4) self-sufficiency and autonomy; and (5) self-esteem and status.[41]

Each of us has learned by this point in our lives that we have three main approaches to dealing with anger: expressing it, suppressing it, or calming it. You may be surprised to find out that *expressing* your anger is probably the healthiest thing to do in the long run, particularly if you express anger in an assertive, rather than aggressive way. However, it's a natural reaction to want to respond aggressively, and that is what we must learn to keep at bay. To be able to do this, there are several things that you can do:[42]

- Understand what anger is and how you tend to express it.
- Develop an awareness and acceptance of your own tendency to anger.
- Recognize your anger patterns: When do you get angry and how often? Who makes you angry and under what circumstances?
- Learn and practice good communication.
- Respect others and yourself.

If all of the above sounds too good to be true, remember that this is no easy task. In truth, controlling and deescalating anger is one of the more difficult stress management techniques that you can try to do. To enhance your likelihood of success, the following strategies may be useful:

1. *Calm yourself.* There are many relaxation techniques. Find one that works for you, and bring yourself back to a level feeling.
2. *Change your thoughts about the situation.* When angry, many people act out in verbally abusive or other dramatic ways. Instead of screeching and yelling, tell yourself that you are justified in being angry and that you have a right to be upset, but don't act overtly. Remember that "get it all out of your system with cathartic soul cleansing" impulse is really not productive. It only makes you feel good for a bit and then you realize that you have hurt others and said much more than you should have, and in the end, nothing is changed. Avoid thoughts or statements such as "never" or "always." Stay in the present.
3. *Improve your communication with the person who has made you angry or frustrated.* Talk with them when you are calm. Be direct and assertive. Let them know how you feel without being aggressive or attacking them. Direct your anger at the person who deserves it, not at anyone who happens to be around. Social psychologist Carol Tavris, in her book *Anger: The Misunderstood Emotion,* says that anger should be expressed directly at the person or object that is perceived to have violated personal space, values, or identity, not randomly.[43] If you can't express it immediately, try writing down your feelings and thoughts in a journal, and describe what you'd like to see changed. Be clear when you talk with the person and try to keep your comments to "I" rather than "you" statements (e.g., "I feel like I have been insulted in some way," rather than "You insulted me.")
4. *Don't fight back.* It is natural to get upset if you feel attacked or criticized. Instead of reacting with anger, listen to what the person is saying, ask clarifying questions, and keep your cool. When the person has finished talking, acknowledge that you have heard, and then express your own feelings.
5. *Use humor if possible.* Sometimes, the sheer volatility of a situation requires a bit of defusing, sort of like the comic relief that accompanies a long dramatic passage in a movie or play. Try to defuse the situation if possible, and don't allow it to escalate. However, this doesn't mean sitting there with a smirk on your face or laughing at the other person or being sarcastic. Try to get the other person to laugh with you.
6. *Recognize that certain situations may cause little things to blow out of proportion.* Drinking alcoholic beverages, not getting enough sleep, responding to loss, and other

---

Hostility   The cognitive, affective, and behavioral tendencies toward anger and cynicism.

Relaxation Techniques for Stress Management

Relaxation techniques for stress reduction have been practiced for centuries, and you have a wide selection from which to choose. Finding the one that works best for you may take some time—the activities that calm and renew your friends could make you tense and nervous. Four to consider are yoga, qigong, deep breathing, and progressive muscle relaxation.

YOGA

An estimated 20 million adults in America actively engage in yoga, an ancient tradition that combines meditation, stretching, and breathing exercises designed to relax, refresh, and rejuvenate. There are several popular versions.

Hot yoga, also known as bikram yoga, differs from traditional yoga in that classes are held in rooms where the temperatures are up to 105 degrees. After going through up to 26 poses, students emerge from these classes drained of energy, drenched in sweat, and feeling cleansed. Although bikram centers have sprung up across the country, there have been reports of heat exhaustion, dehydration, and other problems. This style of yoga is risky for those with hypertension, certain respiratory conditions, and other cardiovascular risks. If you feel weak, dizzy, nauseated, or have other ill effects, use caution. Before attending a class, speak with your doctor if you have questions or concerns, and make sure you go to a reputable facility with qualified staff.

Popularized by Madonna, *ashtanga yoga* is designed to improve sport performance with deep breathing and a progressive series of postures. Less well known than other forms, this type of yoga is growing in popularity.

Kripalu is a gentle, introspective practice in which much emphasis is placed on breathing techniques and releasing emotional blockages. Initially practitioners concentrate mainly on poses and deep breathing followed by emotional exercises.

In the later stages, practitioners focus primarily on poses. This form of yoga is particularly suited for those who want to go slowly and gently or who have underlying injuries or problems.

Classical yoga is the ancestor of nearly all of the above forms; many of them have components of the classical yoga techniques. Breathing, poses, and verbal mantras are often a part of classical yoga.

QIGONG

Qigong (pronounced chee-kong) is one of the fastest growing and most widely accepted forms of mind–body health exercises. Even some of the country's largest health care organizations, such as Kaiser Permanente, have incorporated this relaxation technique into their system, particularly for chronic pain sufferers and those who are chronically stressed. Like acupuncture, qigong taps into a complex system of internal pathways called meridians, which are thought to run along the length of the body. According to Chinese medicine, meridians carry chi, or vital energy, throughout your body. If your chi becomes stagnant or blocked, you'll feel sluggish or

---

situations may make people short fused. Avoid conflict when you are tired or too drained to respond appropriately, and respect these needs in others.

7. *Seek help.* If you feel about yourself or have others telling you that you are a chronically hostile or angry person, seek help. Your school has counselors who are able to help you. Talk with them or someone else you trust.

Taking Mental Action

Stress management calls for mental action in two areas. First, positive self-esteem, which can help you cope with stressful situations, comes from learned habits and responses to people and events. Successful stress management involves mentally developing and practicing self-esteem skills, thinking positively about yourself, and examining self-talk to reduce irrational responses. Focus on the here and now rather than on past problems.

Second, because you can't always anticipate what the next stressor will be, develop the mental skills necessary to manage your reactions after it occurs. The ability to react productively and appropriately comes with time, practice, patience, and experience with a variety of stressful situations.

Changing the Way You Think   Once you realize that some of your thoughts may be irrational or overreactive, make a conscious effort to adjust your thinking, reframe or change the way you've been thinking, and focus on more positive patterns. Here are specific actions you can take to develop these mental skills:

- *Worry constructively.* Don't waste time and energy worrying about things you can't change or events that may never happen.
- *Look at life as being fluid.* If you accept that change is a natural part of living and growing, the jolt of change may become less stressful.
- *Consider alternatives.* Remember, there is seldom only one appropriate action. Anticipating options will help you plan for change and adjust more rapidly.
- *Moderate expectations.* Aim high, but be realistic about your circumstances and motivation.
- *Weed out trivia.* Cardiologist Robert Eliot offers two rules for coping with life's challenges: (1) "Don't sweat the small stuff," and (2) Remember that "it's all small stuff."
- *Don't rush into action.* Think before you act.

powerless. Thus, a series of flowing movements, mental visualization exercises, and vocalizations of healing sounds such as "shhhhuuuu" are designed to invigorate and refresh through easy-to-perform techniques.

DIAPHRAGMATIC OR DEEP BREATHING

Typically, we breathe using only the upper chest and thoracic region rather than the abdominal region. Diaphragmatic breathing is deep breathing that involves the movement of the lower abdomen to maximally expand the chest. This technique is commonly used in yoga exercises in various forms. Diaphragmatic breathing process occurs in stages:

1. *Assume a comfortable position.* Whether sitting or lying down on your back, find the most natural position to be in. Close your eyes, unbutton shirts or binding clothes, remove belts or unbutton pants. Often it works best to fold your hands over your abdomen and get used to feeling the rise and fall of your stomach.

2. *Concentrate on the act of breathing.* Shut out external noise. Focus on inhaling, exhaling, and the route the air is following. Try saying to yourself, "Feel the warm air coming into your nose, warming your windpipe, and flowing into your lungs. Feel your stomach rise and fall as you inhale slowly and exhale slowly, noting the air flowing out of your nose or mouth." Repeat this action several times.

3. *Visualize.* The above stages seem to work best when combined with visualization. A common example is to visualize clean, fresh, invigorating air slowly entering the nose, and being exhaled as gray, stale air that has accumulated in the body. Such processes, particularly when they involve the whole body, seem to help deep breathers become more refreshed from their experience.

PROGRESSIVE MUSCLE RELAXATION

Progressive muscle relaxation (PMR) is another common form of relaxation technique. This involves systematically contracting and relaxing each of several

muscle groups; proper breathing and concentration are part of this process. Again, find a comfortable position, similar to that discussed above, and begin a deep breathing cycle. The difference is that, as you concentrate on inhaling, you also contract a particular muscle group (for example, the hand and fingers). Hold that position for a short period, and then, as you exhale, slowly release the muscles that you have been tightening. Repeat and add more and more muscle groups. You might start with a hand, then move to the forearm, to the entire arm, to the neck, to the shoulders, back, buttocks, foot, and thigh. You can add components of other relaxation techniques to this experience by saying, "My hands are getting warmer, my arm is getting warmer," and so on as you work to gain maximum control of blood flow and muscle tension in a region.

Source: Paragraph on Qigong from C. Dold, "The New Yoga," *Health,* May, 2004, 73–77.

- *Tolerate mistakes by yourself and others.* Rather than getting angry or frustrated by mishaps, evaluate what happened and learn from them.
- *Live simply.* Eliminate unnecessary objects and obligations. Prioritize. Commitments should be to things you have to and want to do.

Once you have improved your mental outlook and gained a more positive perspective on life, you will find it easier to cope with stressors.

Taking Physical Action

Physical activities can complement the emotional and mental strategies of stress management.

Exercise Exercise reduces stress by raising levels of endorphins—mood-elevating, pain killing hormones—in the bloodstream. As a result, it boosts energy, reduces hostility, and improves mental alertness. It can also be a source of social interaction, which further reduces stressor effects.

Most of us have relieved stress by engaging in aggressive physical activity: chopping wood when we are angry is one example. Exercise performed as an immediate response

can help alleviate stress symptoms. However, a regular exercise program yields even more substantial benefits. Try to engage in at least 25 minutes of aerobic exercise three or four times a week. Even simply walking up stairs, parking farther away from your destination, or standing rather than sitting helps to conserve and replenish your adaptive energy stores. Although it may not improve your aerobic capacity, a quiet walk alone or with friends can refresh your mind and calm your stress response. Plan walking breaks with friends. Stretch after prolonged periods of study at your desk. A short period of physical exercise may provide the break you really need. For more information on the beneficial effects of exercise, see Chapter 10.

Relaxation Like exercise, relaxation can help you cope with stressful feelings, preserve adaptation energy stores, dissipate excess hormones associated with GAS, and refocus your energies. (The role of yoga and relaxation techniques as stress management strategies is discussed in the Skills for Behavior Change box. See Chapter 10 for information on doing yoga to increase your flexibility and fitness.) Practice relaxation daily until it becomes a habit. You will probably find that you enjoy it.

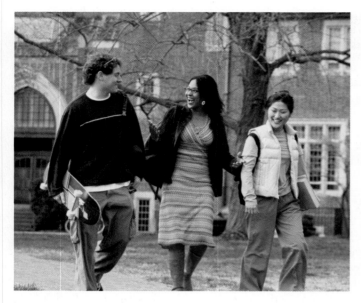

Spending time with friends is an important part of stress reduction.

Once you have learned simple relaxation techniques, you can use them at any time—during a difficult exam or stressful confrontation, for example. If you're facing a tough exam, for example, choose to relax before it or at intervals during it. As your body relaxes, your heart rate slows, your blood pressure and metabolic rate decrease, and many other body-calming effects occur, allowing you to channel energy appropriately.

Eating Right   Is food really a destressor? Whether foods can calm us and nourish our psyches is a controversial question. Much of what has been published about hyperactivity and its relation to the consumption of candy and other sweets has been shown to be scientifically invalid. While vitamins are part of a healthy diet, megadoses are of questionable value. However, it is clear that eating a balanced, healthful diet will help provide the stamina you need to get through problems and will stress-proof you in ways that are not fully understood. It is also known that undereating, overeating, and eating the wrong kinds of foods can create distress in the body. For more information about the benefits of sound nutrition, see Chapter 8.

Managing Your Time

Time. Everybody needs more of it, especially students trying to balance the demands of classes, social life, earning money for school, and family obligations. Include the following time management tips in your stress management program.

- *Take on only one thing at a time.* Don't try to pay bills, clean the bathroom, wash clothes, and write your term paper all at once. Stay focused.
- *Clean off your desk.* According to Jeffrey Mayer, author of *Winning the Fight Between You and Your Desk,* most of us spend many stressful minutes each day looking for things that are lost on our desks or in our homes. Go through the items on your desk, toss what's unnecessary, and file the papers relating to tasks that you must do.
- *Find a clean, comfortable place to work.* Go somewhere where you won't be distracted.
- *Never handle papers more than once.* When bills and other papers come in, take care of them immediately. Write a check and hold it for mailing. Get rid of the envelopes. Read your mail and file it or toss it. For most papers, if you haven't looked at something in over a year, toss it.
- *Prioritize your tasks.* Make a daily "to do" list and try to stick to it. Categorize the things you must do today, the things that you have to do but not immediately, and the things that it would be nice to do. Prioritize the *Must Do Now* and *Have to Do Later* items, and put deadlines next to each. Only consider the *Nice to Do* items if you finish the others or if the *Nice to Do* list includes something fun for you. Give yourself a reward as you finish each task.
- *Don't be afraid to say no.* All too often we do things out of fear of what someone may think. Set your school and personal priorities. Please yourself as often as you can.
- *Avoid interruptions.* When you've got a project that requires your total concentration, schedule uninterrupted time. Unplug the phone or let your answering machine get it. Close your door and post a *Do Not Disturb* sign. Go to a quiet room in the library or student union where no one will find you.
- *Reward yourself for being efficient.* You've planned to take a certain amount of time to finish a task and you finish early? Take some time for yourself. Have a cup of coffee or hot chocolate. Go for a walk. Start reading something you've wanted to read but haven't had time for. Differentiate between rest breaks and work breaks. Work breaks simply mean switching tasks for awhile. Rest breaks give you time to yourself. Make sure that your rest breaks help you recharge and refresh your energy levels.
- *Become aware of your own time patterns.* We all have 168 hours in a week; how do you spend yours? Keep a time journal for one week (Figure 3.3). Note the time that was wasted and the time spent in productive work or restorative pleasure. Assess how you could be more productive and make more time for yourself.
- *Use time to your advantage.* If you're a morning person, schedule activities to coincide with when you're at your best. Study and write papers in the morning, and take breaks when you start to slow down. Take a short nap when you need it.
- *Break overwhelming tasks into small pieces, and allocate a certain amount of time to each.* If you are floundering in a task, move on and come back to it when you're refreshed.
- *Remember that time is precious.* Many people learn to value their time only when they face a terminal illness. Try to value each day. Time spent not enjoying life is a tremendous waste of potential.

More Stress Management Techniques

Popular stress fighters include hypnosis, massage therapy, meditation, and biofeedback.

Activity	Monday	Tuesday	Wednesday	Thursday	Friday	Saturday	Sunday	Total Hours
Getting ready								
On the road								
In class								
Working for pay								
Exercising								
Eating (meals & snacks)								
Studying								
Watching TV, videos								
Using computer (school-related)								
Using computer (recreational)								
Spending time with friends								
Leisure activities								
Other (specify)								
Total Hours								

Figure 3.3

How Do You Spend Your Time?

Fill in your daily activities for a week and assess how you spend your time. Are there any activities you can cut back or that you would like to increase?

Hypnosis Hypnosis is a process that requires a person to focus on one thought, object, or voice, thereby freeing the right hemisphere of the brain to become more active. The person then becomes unusually responsive to suggestions. Whether self-induced or induced by someone else, hypnosis can reduce certain types of stress.

Massage Therapy If you have ever had someone massage your stiff neck or aching feet, you know that massage is an excellent way to relax. Massage techniques vary from vigorous Swedish massage to the gentler acupressure and Esalen massage. Before selecting a massage therapist, check his or her credentials carefully. The therapist should have training from a reputable program that teaches scientific principles for anatomic manipulation and be certified through the American Massage Therapy Association (AMTA).

Meditation There are many different forms of **meditation.** Most involve sitting quietly for 15 to 20 minutes, focusing on a particular word or symbol, controlling breathing, and getting in touch with the inner self. Practiced by Eastern

religions for centuries, meditation is believed to be an important form of introspection and personal renewal. As a stress management tool, it can calm the body and quiet the mind, creating a sense of peace.

Biofeedback Biofeedback involves using a machine to self-monitor physical responses to stress and attempts to control them. The machine records perspiration, heart rate, respiration, blood pressure, surface body temperature, muscle tension, and other stress responses. Then, by trial and error, the person using biofeedback techniques learns to

Hypnosis A process that allows people to become unusually responsive to suggestion.

Meditation A relaxation technique that involves deep breathing and concentration.

Biofeedback A technique involving using a machine to self-monitor physical responses to stress.

Social Connections and Social Support as a Stress Buffer

Although a number of buffers may inoculate us from the negative health effects of stress, social support may be more important than all others. Consider the following points, derived from several studies assessing the role of social support and social connections in dealing with stress.

✔ Social environment can have a buffering effect on stress. An example: when a stressor is given to an animal that is alone, its plasma cortisol levels increase by 50 percent; however, when the same stressor is given to an animal surrounded by familiar companions, its plasma cortisol levels do not increase at all.

✔ Being well integrated socially reduces all age-adjusted mortality by a factor of 2, about as much as having low versus high serum cholesterol levels or being a smoker versus a non-smoker. Furthermore, the nature of one's position in the social hierarchy, including relatively higher status within the same social class, has health consequences.

✔ Although women enjoy as much or more social support as men, they may not derive as many physical health benefits from it. Social support provided in relationships characterized by emotionality or ambivalence may have an adverse effect on health.

✔ People are statistically more likely to die right after, rather than before, birthdays and important holidays, events that include social interactions.

✔ Randomized trials have provided evidence that psychosocial support is associated with longer survival for patients with breast cancer, malignant melanoma, and lymphoma.

✔ Studies looking at the relationship between widowhood (regarded as a high stressor) and depression have found repeatedly that the death of a spouse is more strongly associated with depression among men than women.

How can we explain the final item on the list? Though some argue that men depend more on women for activities of daily living, studies show that widowed men tend to cut off or reduce ties with surviving parents and adult children after such an event, presumably as they begin to search for a new partner. Women, on the other hand, maintain and, in fact, increase their social connections during this time, which may serve as a stress buffer.

Sources: L. Powell. and L. Matthews, "New Directions in Understanding the Link between Stress and Health in Women," *International Journal of Behavioral Medicine* 9, no. 3 (2002): 173–176; B. Uchino et al., "Nuances of Interpersonal Relationships Influence Blood Pressure," *Heart Disease Weekly,* August 17, 2003; R. Lee and K. Keough, "Social Connectedness, Social Appraisal, and Perceived Stress in College Men and Women," *Journal of Counseling and Development* 80, no. 3 (2002): 355; S. Levine, D. M. Lyons, and A. F. Schatzberg, "Psychobiological Consequences of Social Relationships," *The Annals of the New York Academy of Science* 89 no. 7, (1997): 210–218; M. G. Marmot et al., "Contributions of Psychosocial Factors to Socio-economic Difference in Health," *Milbank Quarterly* 76 (1998): 403–448; D. P. Phillips, T. E. Ruth, and L. M. Wagner, "Psychology and Survival," *Lancet* 342 (1993): 1142–1145; D. Ornish et al., "Intensive Lifestyle Changes for Reversal of Coronary Heart Disease," *Journal of the American Medical Association* 280 (1998): 2001–2007; and D. Spiegel, "Healing Words: Emotional Expression and Disease Outcome," *Journal of the American Medical Association* (1999).

lower his or her stress responses through conscious effort. Eventually, the person develops the ability to lower stress responses at will, without using the machine.

Making the Most of Support Groups

Support groups are an important part of stress management. Friends, family members, and coworkers can provide emotional and physical support. See the Reality Check box for additional information about the beneficial effects of social support. Although the ideal support group differs for each of us, you should have one or two close friends in whom you are able to confide and neighbors with whom you can trade favors. Try to participate in community activities at least once a week. A healthy committed relationship can also provide vital support.

If you do not have a close support group, find out where to turn when the pressures of life seem overwhelming. Family members are often a steady base of support on which you can rely. But if friends or family are unavailable or unsupportive, most colleges and universities offer counseling services at no cost for short-term crises. Clergy, instructors, and dorm supervisors may also be excellent resources. If university services are unavailable or if you are concerned about confidentiality, most communities offer low-cost counseling through mental health clinics.

Developing Your Spiritual Side: Mindfulness

A final piece of the stress puzzle is the role of spirituality in managing stress. In discussions of spirituality, the concept of mindfulness often emerges. As a meditative technique, mindfulness—the ability to be fully present in the moment—can aid relaxation, reduce emotional and physical pain, and help us connect more effectively with ourselves, with others, and with nature. Practicing mindfulness includes strategies and activities that contribute to overall health and wellness. In fact, mindfulness and wellness are interconnected and can be developed concurrently, reinforcing each other.

We can think of spirituality as encompassing four dimensions: physical, emotional, social, and intellectual.

The Physical Dimension: Moving in Nature

A delightful way to strengthen the body, build endurance, and bring peace of mind is to interact with the natural environment. Activities such as walking, jogging, biking, and swimming foster this interaction, providing sensory experience (feeling, smelling, touching, listening, and hearing) while strengthening muscles and the cardiovascular system. By focusing on the sounds of birdsong or the crunch of your shoes on freshly fallen snow, you can free yourself of worry or anxious thoughts. Appreciating and absorbing the beauty of nature allow us to unwind emotionally even as our bodies are at work.

The Emotional Dimension: Dealing with Negative Emotions

Each of us has positive and negative emotions that govern moods and behaviors throughout the day. We often take joy, happiness, and contentment for granted since we tend not to notice the *absence* of stress and distress. However, we typically are aware of negative emotions, such as jealousy, hatred, and anger because they deplete our energy reserves and cause us problems in interacting with others.

To improve our emotional health and access our spiritual side, we must take notice of the situations that trigger negative emotions, such as anger. (See "Fighting the Anger Urge" page 89). By stopping in the midst of anger and concentrating on physical reactions, we begin to realize the full extent of the damage we inflict upon ourselves when we allow negativity to get the best of us. We might ask ourselves, "Is it worth it?"—and probably we will conclude: "I don't like allowing this kind of hit on my body. I've got to get a handle on this before I hurt myself or someone else." By practicing thought-stopping, blocking negative thoughts, and focusing on positive emotions via self-talk and other methods of diversion, we can help ourselves through a negative experience.

Just as important as control of negative emotions is the development of spiritual wholeness characterized by faith, hope, and love, the beliefs mentioned in Chapter 2. These beliefs contribute to spiritual growth and lessen the negative effects of stress.

The Social Dimension: Interacting, Listening, and Communicating

Developing the spiritual side is not an individual internal process. It is also a social process that enhances relationships with others. The abilities to give and take, speak and listen, and forgive and move on are all integral to spiritual development.

Today, life is busier than ever. While constantly juggling responsibilities, it is easy to get so caught up in the stresses of our own lives that we find it difficult to give to others. Here again, we need to stop and think about how being too self-enmeshed can affect relationships and the ability to communicate with others. Communication is a two-way process in which listening is every bit as important as speaking. The ability to *listen actively* is a potent asset. Active listeners take note of content, intent, and feelings being expressed. They listen to all levels of the communication. Sensitivity and honesty are also essential to the give and take of communication. Ask specific questions, rephrase the speaker's ideas, and focus genuine attention on the speaker. Through such active participation, we gain a greater insight into the other person, who in turn will be encouraged to share more. Sharing becomes more intimate and relationships more connected when people feel that others care for them and are genuinely interested in their well-being. Both parties benefit from such an interchange.

Similar behaviors enhance interactions in a group or work setting, too. How many times in the past week have you sat in class and "zoned out" on what was happening? These are lost moments of potential learning and experience. What made you withdraw from discussing a particularly hot political topic—fear of rejection? Insecurity? Before you pull away from group activities or connections with others, ask yourself the following questions:

- What prevents me from listening and contributing here? What do I fear? What effect does this situation have on me?
- What thoughts and feelings are getting in the way? Can I put these aside for a moment? What's the worst thing that could happen if I engage in this interaction?
- Are there things that I would feel comfortable sharing with this group? How could I let others know that I have something to say?

The Intellectual Dimension: Sharpening Intuition

Take the time to carefully assess events in life, their causes, and your own involvement in them. This often involves putting aside our emotional dimension for a moment to reflect, read, and ponder. Sometimes this process leads to startling new insights—"Ah-ha! Now I get it; this all makes sense!" Such moments mean so much, but few people include this mental activity in daily rituals. Examining the past, how we've gotten to where we are in the present, and what actions might have changed the course of events is a critical element of spiritual growth. By using our minds for objective reasoning, we develop the intellectual dimension of spiritual health.

MAKE IT HAPPEN!

Assessment: The Assess Yourself box earlier in this chapter (page 74) gave you the chance to look at your stress levels and identify situations in your life that particularly cause stress. Now that you are aware of these patterns, you can change a behavior that leads to increased stress.

Making a Change: In order to change your behavior, you need to develop a plan. Follow these steps:

1. Evaluate your behavior and identify patterns.
2. Select one pattern of behavior that you want to change.
3. Fill out a Behavior Change Contract. It should include your long-term goal for change, your short-term goals, the rewards for reaching these goals, potential obstacles along the way, and strategies for overcoming these obstacles.
4. Chart your progress in a journal.
5. Revise your plan as needed: Are the short-term goals attainable? Are the rewards satisfying?

One Student's Plan: Kim discovered that much of her stress was caused by school deadlines. She wanted to learn how to manage her time more efficiently. Kim filled out a Behavior Change Contract, with a goal of finishing her history term paper five days before its due date in order to give herself enough time to study for her biology final. She broke the paper-writing process into manageable steps of research, writing, revising, and proofreading. Each time she finished a stage she rewarded herself with a movie or a trip to the local coffeehouse. She fell behind when her sister unexpectedly visited her for two days, but she got back on schedule when she worked on her paper instead of watching her afternoon soap opera. Kim completed her paper in plenty of time, was able to study efficiently for her biology exam, and didn't come down with her usual finals-period cold.

Summary

- Stress is an inevitable part of our lives. Eustress refers to stress associated with positive events, distress to negative events.
- The alarm, resistance, and exhaustion phases of the general adaptation syndrome (GAS) involve physiological responses to both real and imagined stressors and cause a complex cascade of hormones to rush through the body. Prolonged arousal may be detrimental to health.
- Undue stress for extended periods of time can compromise the immune system and result in serious health consequences. Psychoneuroimmunology is the science that analyzes the relationship between the mind's reaction to stress and the function of the immune system. While increasing evidence links disease susceptibility to stress, much of this research remains controversial. However, stress has been linked to numerous health problems including CVD, cancer, and increased susceptibility to infectious diseases.
- Multiple factors contribute to stress and the stress response. Psychosocial factors include change, hassles, pressure, inconsistent goals and behaviors, conflict, overload, and burnout. Other factors are environmental stres-

sors and self-imposed stress. Persons subjected to discrimination or bias due to *"-isms"* may face unusually high levels of stress.
- College can be especially stressful. Recognition of the signs of stress is the first step toward better health. Learning to reduce test anxiety and cope with multiple stressors is also important.
- Managing stress begins with learning simple coping mechanisms: assessing stressors, changing responses, and learning to cope. Finding out what works best for you—probably some combination of managing emotional responses, taking mental or physical action, downshifting, learning time management, and using alternative stress management techniques—will help you cope with stress in the long run.
- Developing the spiritual side involves practicing mindfulness and its many dimensions. These include the physical dimension—moving in nature; the emotional dimension—identifying and controlling negative emotions and feelings; the social dimension—interacting, listening, and communicating; and the intellectual dimension—sharpening intuition.

Questions for Discussion and Reflection

1. Compare and contrast distress and eustress. Are both types of stress potentially harmful?
2. Describe the alarm, resistance, and exhaustion phases of the general adaptation syndrome and the body's physiological response to stress. Does stress lead to more emotionality, or does emotionality lead to stress? Provide examples.
3. What are some of the health risks that result from chronic stress? How does the study of psychoneuroimmunology link stress and illness?
4. What major factors seem to influence the nature and extent of a person's susceptibility to stress? Explain how social support, self-esteem, and personality can make a person more or less susceptible to stress.
5. Why are some students more susceptible to stress than others? What services are available on your campus to help you deal with excessive stress?
6. What can college students do to inoculate themselves against negative stress effects? What actions can you take to manage your stressors? How can you help others to manage their stressors more effectively?
7. How does anger affect the body? Discuss the steps you can take to fight your own anger urge and to help your friends control theirs.
8. What can you do to develop the dimensions of spirituality in your life? How can you apply the social dimension of spirituality to your current relationships?

Accessing Your Health on the Internet

Visit the following Internet sites to explore further topics and issues related to personal health. To visit an organization's website, go to the Companion Website for *Access to Health, Ninth Edition* at www.aw-bc.com/donatelle, click on the book image, and select "Accessing Your Health on the Internet" from the navigation menu.

1. *American College Counseling Association.* The website of the professional organization for college counselors offers useful links and articles.
2. *American College Health Association.* Information and data from the National College Health Assessment survey is available here.
3. *Center for Anxiety and Stress Treatment.* Provides resources and services regarding a broad range of stress-related topics.
4. *Hampden-Sydney College.* Links to useful tips for dealing with stressful issues college students commonly experience.
5. *Mind Tools.* Focuses on all aspects of stress and stress management.
6. *National Institute of Mental Health.* A resource for information on all aspects of mental health, including the effects of stress.

Further Reading

Lovallo, W. R. *Stress and Health: Biological and Psychological Interactions,* 2d ed. Thousand Oaks, CA: Sage, 2004.

Latest scientific findings from psychology, neuroscience, and medicine on the relationship between stress and health.

Health and Stress: Newsletter of the American Institute of Stress. www.stress.org/news.htm.

Excellent monthly resource on stress. Reports on latest developments in all areas of stress research. Each issue contains a listing of meetings of interest and a book review.

Romas, J. A. and M. Sharma. *Practical Stress Management,* 3rd ed. San Francisco: Benjamin Cummings, 2004.

An accessible text that combines theory and principles with hands-on exercises to manage stress. Includes an audio CD with guided relaxation techniques such as progressive muscle relaxation, deep breathing, and visual imaging.

Schindler, W. *Adults in College: A Survival Guide for Nontraditional Students.* Mt. Pleasant, TX: Dallas Publishing, 2002.

Focus on how older students cope with the stress of being an adult surrounded by recent high school graduates.

Seaward, B. *Managing Stress: Principles and Strategies for Health and Well-Being,* 4th ed. Sudbury, MA: Jones & Bartlett, 2004.

Spirituality and stress expert provides complete overview of stress and health effects, as well as strategies for reducing risk.

Stepanek, M. *Heartsongs.* New York: Hyperion, 2002.

Verse focused on peace and the human spirit, showing how this young poet, who died in 2004, used spirituality to cope with the stress of terminal illness.

Weil, A. *Ask Dr. Weil.* New York: Random House, 2003.

Weil, a holistic doctor, has written this and other books giving overviews of mind–body health and alternative strategies for coping with life's challenges.

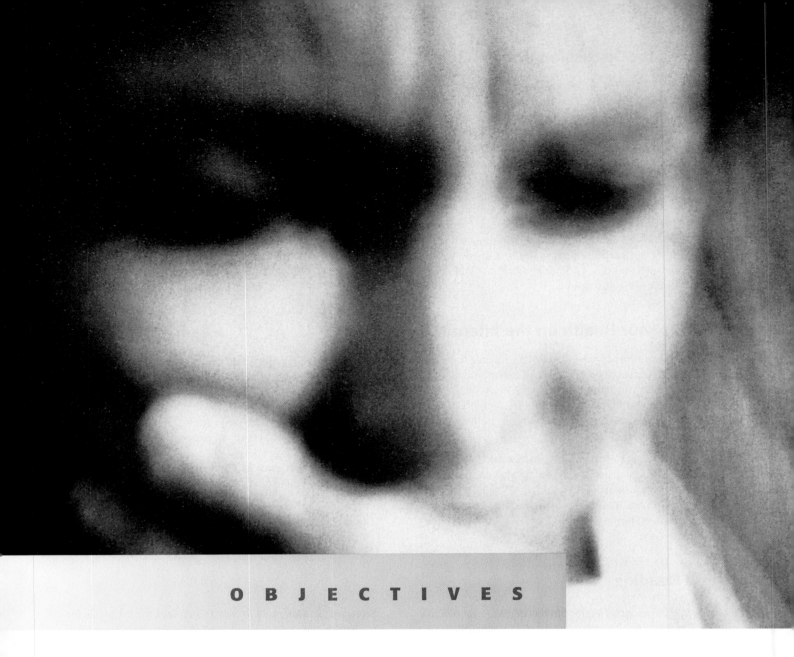

OBJECTIVES

- Differentiate between intentional and unintentional injuries, and discuss societal and personal factors that contribute to violence in American society.

- Discuss factors that contribute to homicide, domestic violence, sexual victimization, and other intentional acts of violence.

- Explain how terrorism can affect individuals and populations, and summarize practical steps to lower your risk from terrorist attacks.

- Discuss strategies to prevent intentional injuries and reduce their risk of occurrence.

- Explain how the campus community, law enforcement officials, and individuals can prevent crimes that are common on campuses.

- Discuss the impact of unintentional injuries on American society, and explain actions that might contribute to personal risk of injuries of all types.

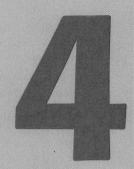

VIOLENCE AND ABUSE

CREATING HEALTHY ENVIRONMENTS

IN THE NEWS

As Anxiety Grows, So Does Field of Terror Study

By Claire Hoffman

On a summer evening in a TriBeCa classroom at Metropolitan College of New York, graduate students pored over spreadsheets, calculating how prepared the elderly residents of Harlem would be for a dirty-bomb attack. In a course titled "The Impact of Disaster on Communities," the students analyzed the catastrophic possibilities for New York City and its residents.

Motivated by the terror attacks of 9/11, colleges have rushed to create counterterrorism and homeland security courses, and thousands of students in New York and elsewhere are pursuing degrees in that area, making disaster one of the fastest-growing fields in academia.

Drawn together under the unofficial banner of homeland security studies, these programs, which include undergraduate degrees as well as master's and doctoral programs, use an interdisciplinary approach, teaching students how to psychoanalyze terrorists, conduct crowd control and remain calm in front of reporters.

"You are dealing with the dark side of humanity," said Olymar Alsina, 27, who will graduate next spring from Metropolitan College with a master's degree in emergency and disaster management. "But the fact that you are addressing it or minimizing the damage reflects some sort of hope that what you do will have an outcome."

Read the complete article online in the eThemes section of this book's website: www.aw-bc.com/donatelle.

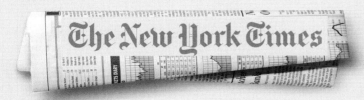

The New York Times

Across the land, waves of violence seem to crest and break, terrorizing Americans in cities and suburbs, in prairie towns and mountain hollows.

To millions of Americans few things are more pervasive, more frightening, more real today than violent crime. . . . The fear of being victimized by criminal attack has touched us all in some way.

Among urban children ages 10–14, homicides are up 150 percent, robberies are up 192 percent, assaults are up 290 percent.

Y ou might think these are statements from today's newspapers or television news. But they're not. The first quotation comes from President Herbert Hoover's 1929 inauguration speech, the second from the 1860 Senate report on crime, and the third from a 1967 report on children's violence.[1] Clearly, violence and our concern over its rising rates are not new concepts.

The term **violence** is used to indicate a set of behaviors that produce injuries, regardless of whether they are **intentional injuries** (committed with intent to harm) or **unintentional injuries** (committed without intent to harm, often accidentally), as well as the outcome of these behaviors. Any definition of *violence* implicitly includes the use of force, regardless of the intent, but as you'll see, some forms of violence are also extremely subtle.

In this chapter, we focus on the various types of intentional and unintentional violence, the underlying causes of or contributors to these problems, strategies to reduce risk of encountering violence, and possible methods for preventing violence. Although certain indicators of violence, such as murders and deadly assaults, seem to be on the decline, other forms of violence, such as rape, hate crimes, and suicides are on the increase.

Even more important is that for all we know about violence incidence and prevalence, a great deal remains unknown. Just how many people suffer in silence, failing to report violent acts due to fear of repercussions or accepting violence as "the way it is," remains unknown.

Violence in the United States

Even though violence has long been a major concern in American society, it was not until 1985 that the U.S. Public Health Service formally identified violence as a leading pub-

Violence   A set of behaviors that produce injuries, as well as the outcomes of these behaviors (the injuries themselves).

Intentional injuries   Injuries committed on purpose with intent to harm.

Unintentional injuries   Injuries committed without intent to harm.

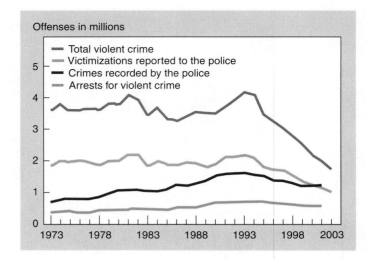

Figure 4.1
Changes in Crime Rates, 1973–2002
Note: Total violent crime is the number of homicides recorded by police plus the number of rapes, robberies, and aggravated assaults reported in the National Crime Victimization Survey. *Victimization* is the number of homicides recorded by the police plus other serious crimes that respondents to the survey said were reported to the police. *Crimes recorded by police* and *arrests* are based on law enforcement reports to the FBI.

Source: Bureau of Justice Statistics, "Key Crime and Justice Facts at a Glance," August, 2003, www.ojp.usdoj.gov/bjs/glance.htm

lic health problem that contributed significantly to death and disability. The Centers for Disease Control and Prevention (CDC) created the Division of Violence Prevention and considers violence a form of chronic disease that is pervasive at all levels of American society. Vulnerable populations, such as children, women, black males, and the elderly, were listed as being at high risk.

Recent numbers indicate that we have made dramatic improvements in certain areas. Since 1973, statistics from the Federal Bureau of Investigation (FBI) show that overall crime and certain types of violent crime have actually decreased each year (Figure 4.1). In 2003, overall rates of crime continued to decline, down as much as 3.2 percent over 2002. Out of all violent crime categories, murder was the only one to increase slightly, rising 1.1 percent.[2] In addition, a recent Department of Justice report on crime and safety on college campuses suggests that colleges and universities are relatively safe.[3] However, many question the accuracy of such reports, since petty theft, date rape, fighting, and other common campus incidents are not always reported to police. There have also been criticisms that campuses have been reluctant to report such incidents over concerns about reputation and potential financial impact. Although a person's chances of being murdered or violently assaulted may have declined, the odds of being a victim of crimes such as burglary, theft, and minor assault in general are on the increase.[4] It is important to note that 70.8 percent of all deaths among persons aged 10 to 24 have violent elements and stem from just four causes: motor vehicle crashes (particularly where alcohol is involved), other unintentional injuries, homicide, and suicide.[5]

Why should we be concerned about a violence-prone society? Violence affects everyone, directly or indirectly. Although the direct victims of violence and those close to them obviously suffer the most, others suffer in various ways because of the climate of fear that violence generates. Women are afraid to walk alone at night. The elderly are often afraid to go out even in the daytime. After terrorist episodes such as the 2001 World Trade Center attack, some people are afraid to fly, work in tall buildings, or live in heavily populated areas. The cost of homeland security is staggering. You might be surprised to learn that international travelers often fear coming to the United States in much the same way that some Americans fear traveling to other regions of the world where attacks on U.S. citizens have taken place. Tourists are afraid of being brutalized in many of our nation's cities, hearing of children dodging bullets while playing in city neighborhoods or of drivers being carjacked. Many of these reports are carried in the international news media, depicting the United States as a violent nation. Even people who live in supposedly safe areas can become victims of violence within their own homes or at the hands of family members.

Costs of Violence

Although the greatest costs of violence, those of human suffering and loss, are impossible to calculate, the direct and indirect economic toll is staggering. According to a recent World Health Organization report, many nations spend more than 4 percent of their total Gross Domestic Product dealing with violence-related injuries.[6] Estimates for the costs of violence in the United States total more than $300 billion per year. Specific costs include $55.4 billion related to adult criminality related to child abuse. Intimate partner violence against women costs $6 billion annually.[7] The remainder of the costs are attributed to gun violence, homicides and legal intervention by adults, and other adult criminal activity. Societies face a monumental task in paying for violence-related problems, funding prisons, and providing assistance to victims (Figure 4.2). At the very least, we all pay higher tax bills for law enforcement and prisons and higher insurance premiums for damage done to others' or our own property. In the United States, the Department of Homeland Security must also be funded for protection from and prevention of terrorist activities.

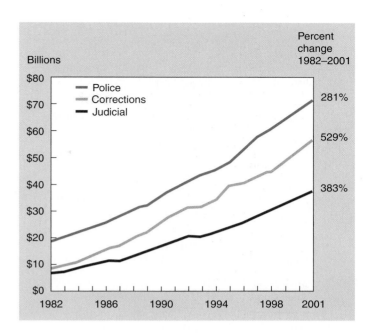

Figure 4.2
Increasing Costs of Crime Control in the United States, 1982–2001

Source: Bureau of Justice Statistics, "Key Crime and Justice Facts at a Glance," 2004, www.ojp.usdoj.gov/bjs/glance/exptyp.htm

Societal Causes of Violence

Several social, cultural, and individual factors increase the likelihood of violent acts (Figure 4.3 on page 102), including:

- *Poverty.* Low socioeconomic status and poor living conditions can create an environment of hopelessness, leaving people feeling trapped and seeing violence as the only way to obtain what they want.
- *Unemployment.* It is a well-documented fact that when the economy goes sour, violent crime, suicide, assault, and other crimes increase.
- *Parental influence.* Violence is cyclical. Children raised in environments in which shouting, slapping, hitting, and other forms of violence are commonplace are more apt to act out these behaviors as adults. Horrifying reports in recent years have made this pattern impossible to ignore.
- *Cultural beliefs.* Cultures that objectify women and empower men to be tough and aggressive show increased rates of violence in the home.
- *The media.* A daily dose of murder and mayhem can take a toll on even resistant minds.
- *Discrimination/oppression.* Whenever one group is oppressed by another, seeds of discontent are sown and hate crimes arise.
- *Religious differences.* Religious persecution has been a part of the human experience throughout history.

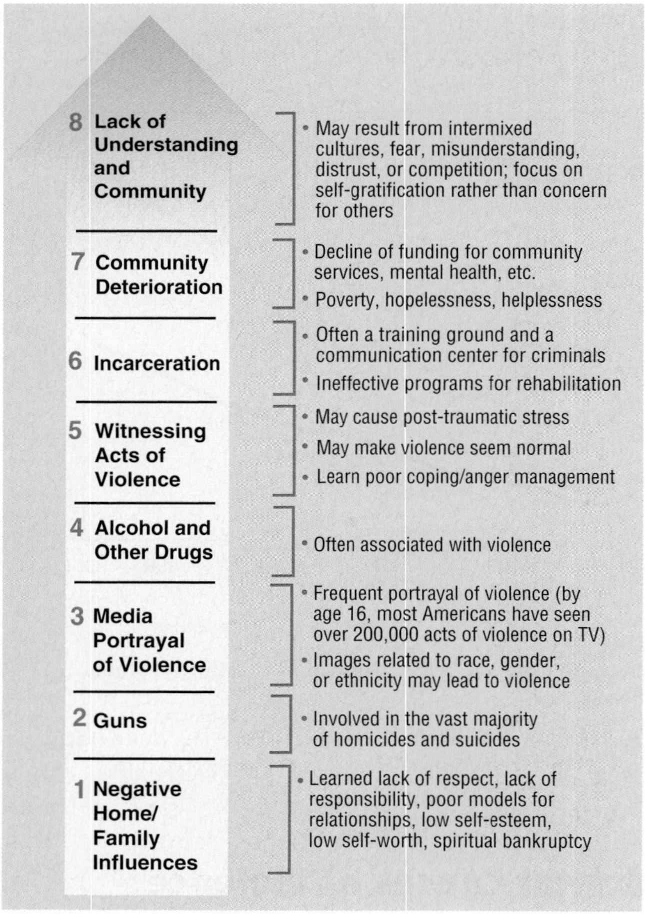

The figure shows a large upward-pointing arrow labeled 1 through 8 from bottom to top:

8 Lack of Understanding and Community
- May result from intermixed cultures, fear, misunderstanding, distrust, or competition; focus on self-gratification rather than concern for others

7 Community Deterioration
- Decline of funding for community services, mental health, etc.
- Poverty, hopelessness, helplessness

6 Incarceration
- Often a training ground and a communication center for criminals
- Ineffective programs for rehabilitation

5 Witnessing Acts of Violence
- May cause post-traumatic stress
- May make violence seem normal
- Learn poor coping/anger management

4 Alcohol and Other Drugs
- Often associated with violence

3 Media Portrayal of Violence
- Frequent portrayal of violence (by age 16, most Americans have seen over 200,000 acts of violence on TV)
- Images related to race, gender, or ethnicity may lead to violence

2 Guns
- Involved in the vast majority of homicides and suicides

1 Negative Home/Family Influences
- Learned lack of respect, lack of responsibility, poor models for relationships, low self-esteem, low self-worth, spiritual bankruptcy

Figure 4.3
Correlates to Violence

- *Breakdowns in the criminal justice system.* Overcrowded prisons, lenient sentences, early releases from prison, and trial errors subtly encourage violence in a number of ways.
- *Stress.* People who are in crisis or under stress are more apt to be highly reactive, striking out at others or acting irrationally.
- *Heavy use of alcohol and other substances.* Alcohol and drug abuse are often catalysts for violence, and risk factors for domestic violence, rape, child abuse, homicide, and other crimes.[8] (Chapter 14 discusses the abuse of drugs. Chapter 12 goes into further detail about social and health problems related to alcohol abuse).

Primary aggression Goal-directed, hostile self-assertion that is destructive in character.

Reactive aggression Emotional reaction brought about by frustrating life experiences.

Some say that the prevalence of guns in our society also contributes to the high death rate caused by violent acts (see the Health Ethics: Conflict and Controversy box on the next page). In addition to these broad, societally based factors, many personal factors also can lead to violence.

What do you think?

Why do you think there is so much violent behavior in the United States? ■ *What actions can you take personally to prevent violence from occurring?* ■ *What could be done to reduce risk on your campus?* ■ *In your community?*

Personal Precipitators of Violence

If you are like most people, you probably acted out your anger more readily as a child than you do today. However, even the worst behaved children usually grow up. As we mature, we learn to control outbursts of anger and approach conflict rationally.

Yet others go through life acting out their aggressive tendencies in much the same ways they did as children or their families did. Why do two children from the same neighborhood, or even from the same family, go in different directions when it comes to violence? There are several predictors of future aggressive behavior, including anger and substance abuse.

Anger *Anger* is a spontaneous, usually temporary, biological feeling or emotional state of displeasure that occurs most frequently during times of personal frustration. Since life is stressful, anger becomes a part of daily experience. Anger can range from slight irritation to *rage,* a violent and extreme form of anger.[9] When it is acted out at home or on the road, the consequences can be deadly. (See the Skills for Behavior Change box on page 104.)

What makes some people flare up at the slightest provocation? Often, people who anger quickly have a low tolerance for frustration, believing that they should not have to put up with inconvenience or petty annoyances. The cause may be genetic or physiological; there is evidence that some people are born unstable, touchy, or easily angered. Another cause of anger is sociocultural. People who are taught not to express anger in public do not know how to handle it when it reaches a level that can no longer be hidden. Family background may be the most important factor. Typically, anger-prone people come from families that are disruptive, chaotic, and not skilled in emotional expression.[10] In fact, the single largest predictor of future violence is past violence.[11]

Aggressive behavior is often a key aspect of violent interactions. **Primary aggression** is goal-directed, hostile

Gun Control: Issues and Choices

Almost 40 years ago, *Time* magazine ran a feature entitled "The Gun in America," which summarized the feelings of a nation reeling from the murders of John F. Kennedy, Robert Kennedy, and Martin Luther King, Jr. The national disgust that followed led to the Gun Control Act of 1968, a milestone law that banned most interstate gun sales, licensed most gun dealers, and barred felons, minors, and the mentally ill from owning firearms.

Today, gun violence has spread to our nation's playgrounds and schools. There are nearly as many firearms in the United States as people, more than 235 million by some estimates. At a time when crime rates are dropping, gun crime is dropping, too—gun murders in the United States are still far more common than they were 30 years ago and much more common than they are in other Western industrialized nations.

Since the 1968 gun control legislation, the only major gun laws to date were the Brady Bill, which requires background checks of purchasers, and the assault-gun ban. The ban on assault weapons expired in September 2004 and has not been renewed. Although there is talk about a gun safety-lock law and special "owner-use only" imprinting on guns, Congress is unlikely to pass any major gun control measures in the near future. In fact, the trend is toward more deregulation of guns and state laws that permit concealed weapons. Since 1985, the number of states that permit citizens who pass a background check to carry concealed weapons has risen from 8 to 30. A recent book, *More Guns, Less Crime: Understanding Crime and Gun Laws*, analyzed crime rates in the 10 states that passed right-to-carry laws between 1977 and 1992. The author contends that after these laws were enacted, murders fell an average of 8 percent, rapes 5 percent, and aggravated assaults by 7 percent at a time when murders, rapes, and assaults were increasing in states without such laws. Criminologists, researchers, and gun control lobbyists say that the book's research has been poorly conducted, its statistics are suspect, and its conclusions dangerous. Who are we to believe?

Millions of Americans believe that their right to bear arms, their personal safety, and their hunting rights should not be curtailed. They believe that outgunned police forces and the typical citizen on the street face undue risks from criminals who have access to illegal weapons. Some argue that school shootings might be prevented if teachers had the right to carry guns for protection. As violence seems to escalate, many of us have wondered about buying guns to protect ourselves. Concealed weapons appeal to those who fear for their own safety and want a means to fight back. But what's to say that people won't overreact to perceived threats?

Recent lawsuits against gun manufacturers raise yet another controversial issue. Are gun manufacturers liable for violent homicides, in much the same way that the tobacco industry is being held liable for deaths from cigarette smoking? The attorneys general of several states feel they are and are taking these suits to court as of this writing. They argue that many deaths are preventable through better monitoring of sales and curtailing production of armor-piercing bullets and automatic assault weapons (which can fire bullets in very rapid succession). They believe that it is possible to manufacture guns that fire only if the original owner is operating them but that gun manufacturers refuse to produce them.

In the future, we will all be called upon to make choices that may affect the lives of our families, coworkers, and friends. What can you do?

- Investigate the facts about gun-related violence. Your best data sources are federal and state crime statistics, rather than information from special interest groups on either side.
- Consider the pros and cons of antigun legislation. Would these laws discourage recreational hunters from buying rifles or homeowners from purchasing handguns for their own protection? Would user IDs on guns, which would not allow anyone but the original purchaser to operate the weapon, be an acceptable solution? Why or why not?
- Analyze the voting records of your state and national political representatives regarding gun control. Are they voting in ways that support your own beliefs?

Do you feel there should be additional restrictions on use or ownership of guns? Explain your answer. Do the risks of gun ownership outweigh the benefits? Do the benefits outweigh the risks?

Source: From R. Lacayo, "Still Under the Gun," *Time,* July 6, 1998, 32–56.

---

self-assertion that is destructive in nature. **Reactive aggression** is more often part of an emotional reaction brought about by frustrating life experiences. Whether aggression is reactive or primary in nature, it is most likely to flare up in times of acute stress, during relationship difficulties or loss, or when a person is so frustrated that he or she feels the only recourse is to strike out at others.

What do you think?

What are some examples of primary aggression? ■ *Reactive aggression?* ■ *Can both result in the same degree of harm?* ■ *Do you think our laws are more lenient when violent acts result from reactive aggression? Why or why not?*

Road Rage!

We pulled out into traffic and immediately were serenaded by a blaring horn from a car speeding by in the next lane. Apparently we had pulled out in front of the car, causing the driver to swerve quickly to avoid hitting us. We felt bad and were thankful that nothing serious had happened, but the other driver wasn't so quick to forgive. For several miles she maneuvered to make us pull over or slowed down in the neighboring lane to pull alongside our car. I wanted nothing to do with this and slowed down as well to avoid facing her. Finally, she pulled over as she approached a right-hand turn, and as we went by, she stuck her head out the window and screamed venomous slurs our way. I'll never forget the expression on the woman's face as we passed. It was filled with such hatred, such rage.

—From the author's files

If you drive at all, you have probably encountered road rage. While drunk driving remains a critical problem, the facts about aggressive driving are surely as ominous. According to the National Highway Transportation Safety Association, 43,220 people died on the highways last year. An estimated two-thirds of these fatalities were caused at least in part by aggressive driving behavior.

Why is road rage becoming more common? One reason is sheer overcrowding. In the last decade, the number of cars on the roads has increased by more than 11 percent, and the number of miles driven has increased by 35 percent; however, the number of new road miles has only increased by 1 percent. That means more cars in essentially the same amount of space; and the problem is magnified in urban areas. Also, people have less time and more things to do. When people try to fit more activities into the day, stress levels rise. Stress creates anxiety, which leads to short tempers and road rage.

ARE YOU IMMUNE TO ROAD RAGE?

You may think you are the last person who would drive aggressively, but you might be surprised. Have you ever tailgated a slow driver, honked long and hard at another car, or sped up to keep another driver from passing? If you recognize yourself in any of these situations, watch out!

AVOID THE "RAGE" (YOURS AND OTHER DRIVERS')

Whether you are getting angry at other drivers, or another driver is visibly upset with you, there are things you can do to avoid major confrontations. The key is to discharge your emotion in a healthy way. If you are the target of another driver's rage, do everything possible to get away safely:

- Avoid eye contact!
- If you need to use your horn, do it sparingly.
- Get out of the way. Even if the other guy is speeding, it's safest to not make a point by staying in your lane.
- If someone is following you after an on-the-road encounter, drive to a public place or the nearest police station.
- Report any aggressive driving incidents to the police department immediately. You may be able to prevent further occurrences by the same driver.
- Above all, always buckle your seat belt! Seat belts save 9,500 lives each year.

Source: Reprinted with permission of Allstate Insurance Co., "Don't Be Blinded by Road Rage," Allstate Insurance website, www.allstate.com/safety/auto/rage.html

Substance Abuse   Although much has been written about a link between substance abuse and violence, we have yet to show that substance abuse actually causes violence. In fact, many violent episodes are carefully planned actions that involve no alcohol or drug abuse. In some situations, however, psychoactive substances appear to be a form of "ignition" for violence:

- Consumption of alcohol—by perpetrators of the crime, the victim, or both—immediately preceded over half of all violent crimes, including murder.[12]
- Chronic drinkers are more likely than others to have histories of violent behavior.[13]
- Criminals using illegal drugs commit robberies and assaults more frequently than nonusing criminals and do so especially during periods of heavy drug use.[14]
- In domestic assault cases, more than 86 percent of the assailants and 42 percent of victims reported using alcohol at the time of the attack. Nearly 15 percent of victims and assailants reported using cocaine at the time of the attack.[15]
- Ninety-two percent of assailants and 42 percent of victims reported using alcohol or other drugs on the day of the assault.[16]
- Mentally ill patients who fail to adhere to prescription drug regimens and abuse alcohol and/or other drugs are significantly more likely to be involved in a serious violent act.[17]
- Substance abuse markedly increases the risk of both homicide and suicide. Problems at work due to drinking, hospitalization for a drinking problem, use of illicit drugs, and arrest for use of illicit drugs all place subjects at risk for violent death by homicide. The combination of depression and alcohol or other drugs increases homicide and suicide rates threefold.[18]

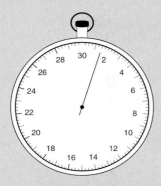

Every 2.7 seconds: One crime index offense

Every 3.0 seconds: One property crime
Every 4.5 seconds: One larceny-theft
Every 14.7 seconds: One burglary
Every 25.3 seconds: One motor vehicle theft

Every 22.1 seconds: One violent crime
Every 35.3 seconds: One aggravated assault
Every 1.2 minutes: One robbery
Every 5.5 minutes: One forcible rape
Every 32.4 minutes: One murder

Figure 4.4
Crime Clock: How Often Is a Crime Committed?

Source: Federal Bureau of Investigation, "Crime in the United States, 2002," www.fbi.gov

Intentional Injuries

Anytime someone sets out to harm other people or their property, the incident may be referred to as intentional violence. Such acts often result in intentional injuries, which come in many forms. Whether the situation entails a simple outburst of anger or a fatal attack with a weapon, the resulting intentional injuries cause pain and suffering at the very least and disability or death at the worst. Although nonviolent criminal acts are much more common, violent crimes occur all too frequently (Figure 4.4).

Gratuitous Violence

Violence can manifest itself in many ways. Often the most shocking or gratuitous crimes gain the greatest attention, such as stories of innocent victims of drive-by shootings or young students who turn their internal rage outward on family, classmates, and teachers.

Assault/Homicide Homicide, death that results from intent to injure or kill, accounts for over 19,000 premature deaths in the United States.[19] These numbers are down significantly

from recent years but still represent a signifi⟨cant⟩ to life lost in certain segments of the popula⟨tion⟩ homicide was the nineteenth leading caus⟨e of death in the⟩ United States among all age groups in 20⟨0_. It is the sec⟩ond leading cause of death for persons aged 1⟨5_.⟩ Homicide is the leading cause of death for black male⟨s aged⟩ 15 to 24 and the second leading cause of death for young Hispanic males. Homicide is an area in which disparities among races are particularly clear. Asian/Pacific Islanders, Hispanic or Latino, and African American groups all list homicide among the top ten causes of death, while homicide is not among the top ten killers of white or American Indians.

As measured by years of potential life lost, homicide exacts a heavy toll (Table 4.1 on page 106). For every violent death, at least one hundred nonfatal injuries are caused by violence. In 1999, an estimated 28,874 firearm-related deaths occurred, including large numbers of homicides and suicides.[21] For every person shot and killed by a firearm, almost three others were treated annually for nonfatal shootings, many of them children under age 10.[22]

For an American, the average lifetime probability of being murdered is 1 in 153—but the average masks large differences for specific segments of the population. For white women, the risk of murder is 1 in 450; for black men, it is 1 in 28. For a black man in the 20- to 22-year-old age group, the risk is 1 in 3. Combined across races, males represent 77 percent of all murder and nonnegligent manslaughter victims. Black males are 1.14 times more likely than white males to be murder victims; white females are 1.5 times more likely than black females to be victims.[23] Over half of all homicides occur among people who know one another. In two-thirds of these cases, the perpetrator and the victim are friends or acquaintances; in one-third, they belong to the same family.[24] Living in certain regions of the country also seems to increase one's risk for homicide.

What do you think?

Why do you think there are such disparities in homicide rates among various groups? ■ *What can be done to reduce these disparities?*

Bias and Hate Crimes

In spite of national efforts in workplaces, schools, and communities to promote understanding and diversity-related appreciation, intolerance of differences continues to smolder in many parts of U.S. society. The killings of James Byrd and Matthew Shepard, the murder of two gay men in California,

---

Homicide Death that results from intent to injure or kill.

Table 4.1
Years of Potential Life Lost (per 100,000)

Years of Potential Life Lost (YPLL) is a rough measure of the impact of a specific disease or societal event/condition on a given population. It is calculated by subtracting the age at death of a person from the expected life expectancy for this person. In this table, the total years are those lost before age 75 per 100,000 population under the age of 75. It provides a glimpse of the overall impact of a problem on the lives of particular populations.

Some questions to consider: Where are the greatest disparities in YPLL among males? Among females? What factors do you think contribute to the low rates of suicide in some groups? High rates of assault?

	Unintentional Injury	Suicide	Assault (Homicide)
Male			
White	1,475.9	624.7	253.9
African American	1,888.7	388.1	1,753.5
American Indian/Alaska Native	2,771.7	850.8	568.3
Asian/Pacific Islander	637.1	308.8	210.2
Hispanic	1,536.8	346.6	676.8
White, non-Hispanic	1,440.8	657.6	167.1
Female			
White	586.8	154.4	95.0
African American	676.9	67.0	370.2
American Indian/Alaska Native	1,276.8	219.7	205.8
Asian/Pacific Islander	309.6	102.5	80.2
Hispanic	461.8	306.3	121.9
White, non-Hispanic	599.1	164.4	88.2

Note: The groups of white, African American, Asian/Pacific Islander, and American Indian/Alaska Native include persons of Hispanic and non-Hispanic origin. Conversely, persons of Hispanic origin may be of any race.

Source: Department of Health and Human Services, National Institutes of Health, Centers for Disease Control and Prevention, "Health United States," 2001, www.cdc.gov

and the arson attacks on several U.S. synagogues remind Americans that violence based on race and other "-isms" still occurs. International terrorist acts often reflect the hatred of one religious or political group for another that is considered to be of less value due to differences in religion, language, or other characteristics. Recent acts of violence against different racial groups by police, beatings in public schools and on the streets that are racially motivated gang events, and other hate crimes are common events on the nightly news.

According to the FBI's most recent Hate Crime Statistics Report, 8,825 bias-motivated crimes were reported in 2002. Of the total reported incidents, 49 percent were motivated by racial bias, 19 percent by religious bias, 17 percent by sexual orientation bias, and 15 percent were related to ethnicity/national-origin bias.[25]

Since the 2001 terrorist attack in the United States and the conflicts in Iraq and Afghanistan, reports of hate-related incidents, beatings, and other physical and verbal assaults have escalated, even as other rates of violent crime decreased. In particular, persons of Muslim or Middle-Eastern descent reported civil rights violations at work, in mass transit, and in communities throughout the United States. Many

believe that the reported incidents are but the tip of the iceberg and actual numbers of bias/hate-related crimes are much higher, but people do not report them out of fear of possible retaliation.

Hate crimes vary along two dimensions: (1) the way they are carried out and (2) their effects on victims. Vicious gossip, nasty comments, and devilish pranks may not make headlines, but they can hurt nonetheless. Generally, about 30 percent of all hate crimes are against property, with the other 70 percent being against the person. Recent studies have identified three additional characteristics of hate crimes:[26]

- Excessively brutal
- Perpetrated at random on total strangers
- Perpetrated by multiple offenders

In addition, the perpetrators tend to be motivated by thrill, defensive feelings, or a hate-mongering mission.

Academic settings are not immune to hatred and bias. According to a report in the *Chronicle of Higher Education,* nearly one-third of our nation's campuses have reported incidents of hate crimes. Another study of four campuses found that victimization rates varied widely, from 12 percent of

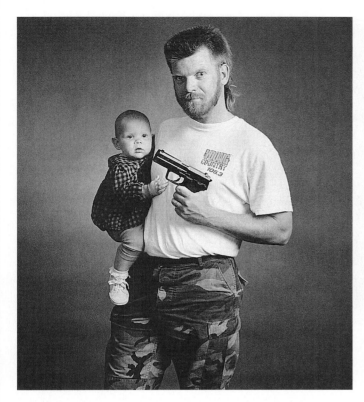

Guns are a common part of life in many households in this country. What effect might this have on the children in these homes?

Often intolerance stems from a fear of change and a desire to blame others when forces such as the economy and crime seem to be out of control. What can you do to be part of the solution rather than the problem?

- Support educational programs that foster understanding and appreciation for differences in people. Many colleges now require diversity classes as part of their academic curriculum.
- Examine your own attitudes and behaviors. Are you intolerant of others? Do you engage in racist, sexist, or similar behaviors meant to demean a group of individuals? If you have problems with a particular group, why?
- Do you discourage hurtful jokes and other forms of social or ethnic bigotry? Do not participate in such behaviors, and express your dissatisfaction with those who do.
- Educate yourself. Read, interact with, and attempt to understand people who appear to be different from you. Remember that you do not have to like everything about them. They may not like everything about you, either. However, respecting people's right to be different is a part of being a healthy, integrated individual.
- Examine your own values in determining the relative worth of your friends and others in your life. Are you judgmental? Do you judge people on appearances, or do you take time to know them as individuals?
- Encourage your legislators to support antihate and antibias legislation. Vote for those who support antidiscrimination policies and programs.

Jewish students to as high as 60 percent of Hispanic students. White students were victimized at rates ranging from 5 to 15 percent.[27] The sad truth is, however, that many minor assaults go unreported, so this may be only part of the picture.

The tendency toward violent acts on campus might best be defined as campus **ethnoviolence,** a term that reflects relationships among groups in the larger society and is based on prejudice and discrimination. Although ethnoviolence often is directed randomly at persons affiliated with a particular group, the group itself is specifically targeted apart from other people, and that differentiation is usually ethnic in nature. Typically, the perpetrators agree that the group is an acceptable target. For example, in a largely Christian community, Jews and Muslims may be considered acceptable targets.[28] Students bring with them attitudes and beliefs from past family and life experiences.

Prejudice and discrimination are always at the base of ethnoviolence. **Prejudice** is a set of negative attitudes toward a group of people. To say that a person is prejudiced against some group is to say that the person holds a set of beliefs about the group, has an emotional reaction to the group, and is motivated to behave in a certain way toward the group. **Discrimination** constitutes actions that deny equal treatment or opportunities to a group of people, often based on prejudice.

What do you think?

Think about the bias or hate crimes that you have heard about in the past six months. Who were the victims? ■ *Did you know any of them?* ■ *Why do you think people are motivated to initiate such crimes against people they don't know?* ■ *What can you do to reduce such crimes in your area?* ■ *What should be done nationally?*

Gang Violence   The growing influence of street gangs has had a harmful impact on our country. Drug abuse, gang shootings, beatings, thefts, carjackings, and the possibility of being caught in the middle between gangs at war have led to

Ethnoviolence   Violence directed randomly at persons affiliated with a particular, usually ethnic, group.

Prejudice   A negative evaluation of an entire group of people that is typically based on unfavorable and often wrong ideas about the group.

Discrimination   Actions that deny equal treatment or opportunities to a group, often based on prejudice.

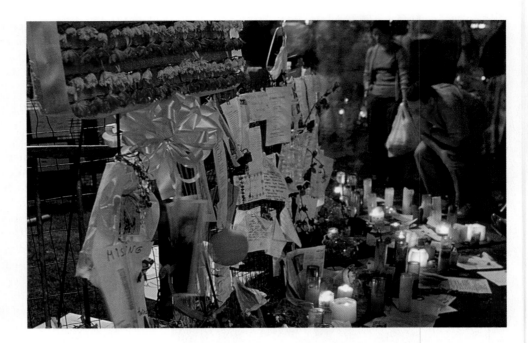

The events of September 11, 2001, were a grim reminder of the power and senselessness of hatred. This memorial was one of hundreds of tributes to those who lost their lives that day.

whole neighborhoods being held hostage by gang members. Once thought to occur only in inner-city areas, gang violence now also appears in rural and suburban communities, particularly in the southeast, southwest, and western regions of the country.

Why do young people join gangs? Although the reasons are complex, gangs seem to meet many of their needs. Gangs provide a sense of belonging to a "family" that gives them self-worth, companionship, security, and excitement. In other cases, gangs provide economic security through criminal activity, drug sales, or prostitution. Once young people become involved in the gang subculture, it is difficult to leave. Threats of violence or fear of not making it on their own discourage even those who are most seriously trying to get out.

Who is at risk for gang membership? Membership varies considerably from region to region. The age range of gang members is typically 12 to 22 years. Risk factors include low self-esteem, academic problems, low socioeconomic status, alienation from family and society, a history of family violence, and living in gang-controlled neighborhoods.

The best way to prevent someone from joining a gang is to keep that person connected to positive influences and programs. From a child's early years, the focus should be on establishing bonds among friends, family, and school. Any student who has learning disabilities or other problems that make it hard to keep up should be involved in alternative activities that foster success and prevent a sense of alienation. Community-based programs that coordinate involvement of families, social service organizations, and law enforcement, school, and city officials have proved effective in keeping students out of gangs. Also, community members must begin to think of gang members not merely as trouble-making

delinquents, but as people whose circumstances make them susceptible to the gang lifestyle.

In part because the number of gangs and gang-related crimes grows daily, the U.S. Congress passed a crime bill in the early 1990s that included the hiring of 100,000 additional police officers, a ban on assault weapons, reform of the welfare system, the creation of a national network of neighborhood banks to boost communities' economic development, and the establishment of "boot camps" for young nonviolent offenders. (Similar additions to our national policing and surveillance capabilities have been initiated post–September 11.) These boot camps were designed to keep offenders out of prison and instill discipline, self-esteem, and respect for the law. Preliminary results indicate that such "tough love" programs are not as effective as many had hoped. Public health professionals have long advocated prevention rather than the current efforts spent on intervention. Examining the underlying causes of violence should provide evidence for supporting systemwide changes in the social environment.

Terrorism: Increased Risks from Multiple Sources

Not so long ago, Americans thought acts of terrorism occurred only in distant cities, seldom amounting to more than a blip on the evening news. The bombing of an Oklahoma City federal building in 1995 focused national attention on terrorism briefly. Most of us, however, went about our daily business after the event, acknowledging that it was the act of a madman and sympathizing with the victims. On September 11, 2001, Americans received a huge wake-up call. Terrorist attacks on the World Trade Center and Pentagon revealed the vulnerability of our nation to domestic and international threats. The terms *terrorist attack, bioterrorism,* and *biological weapons* catapulted us into the new millennium with an emotional reaction unlike any ever seen. America had lost its innocence and its illusion of invulnerability. An undercurrent of fear and anxiety about potential threats from faceless strangers shook many of us in ways that we had never even considered. Today, the specter of a terrorist attack looms ever present. Any time there is a national holiday or occasion where many Americans gather, we worry about a terrorist event.

What Is Terrorism?   According to the FBI, **terrorism** is the use of unlawful force or violence against persons or property to intimidate or coerce a government, the civilian population, or any segment thereof, in furtherance of political or social objectives. Typically, terrorism is of two major types:

1. *domestic terrorism,* which involves groups or individuals whose terrorist activities are directed at elements of our government or population without foreign direction, and
2. *international terrorism,* which involves groups or individuals whose terrorist activities are foreign-based, transcend national boundaries, and are directed by countries or groups outside the United States.

Clearly, terrorist activities may have immediate impact in loss of lives and resources. However, the 2001 attacks also had far-reaching effects on the U.S. economy, airlines, and transportation systems. Perhaps most damaging in the aftermath of the attacks was the fear, anxiety, and altered behavior of countless Americans. How many people will fear working in skyscrapers for years to come? How many will fear climbing on a plane, crossing a bridge, or getting on the subway? Will worry about biological weapons and future terrorist attacks disrupt our lives and our interactions with others? (See the New Horizons in Health box on page 110.)

As the media spur our anxieties about germ, chemical, and nuclear warfare and the multitude of ways that terrorists can breach our defenses, is it any wonder that an already stressed American public is demonstrating increasing concern? What can we do to reduce our risk of terrorist attack?

The CDC has a wide range of ongoing programs and services to help Americans respond to terrorist threats and prepare for possible attacks. Information is available on the CDC website and is updated regularly. A new government entity, the Department of Homeland Security, has been established to prevent future attacks, and the FBI and other government agencies have also prepared a sweeping set of procedures and guidelines for ensuring citizen safety. Here are some things you can do to help reduce the risk of terrorist attacks.

- *Be aware of your own reactions to stress, anxiety, and fear.* Try to assess how much of your fear is justifiable in a given situation and how much is a product of media sensationalism. Practice stress reduction techniques, determine the source of your stressors, and react as prudently

as possible. (See Chapter 3 for more information on post-traumatic stress disorder, which can be caused by exposure to events such as terrorist attacks.)
- *Be conscious of your surroundings.* If you notice suspicious activities or irregularities, report them to a person in authority. Being a passive observer and not speaking up when warranted may put you and others at risk.
- *Stay informed.* Try to stay on top of the news and understand the underlying roots of violent activity. Persistent poverty, pervasive religious or political fanaticism, and political situations in which there is an imbalance of power can provide fodder for violent acts. Consider when a self-righteous contempt for others may lead to persecution and violation of human rights. Be skeptical of acts perpetrated in the name of some cause, and intervene if possible to defuse violence.
- *Seek understanding.* Whenever two opposing groups stop engaging with each other mentally or communication breaks down, hatred, bigotry, and anger may result. Knowing about each other's customs, cultures, and beliefs and keeping the lines of communication open are good steps to avoid separation.
- *Seek information.* When political parties fight for power in election years, know your candidates. What are their underlying beliefs regarding national defense, spending for consumer protection, policies on immigration, human rights violations, diversity issues, hate crimes, gun control, and so forth? Are they more aligned with one ideology than another? What is their stance on government interference and control, punishment of offenders, and other key issues?
- *Know what to do in an emergency.* Who would you call? How would you access local and regional assistance? Do you have the necessary provisions—food, water, prescription medications, first aid? What happens when your electricity is off, your phone and communication systems are down, and your access to health care is limited?

Domestic Violence

In the 1980s a popular country-western song crooned, "No one knows what goes on behind closed doors." Domestic violence shows us just how true that refrain can be. **Domestic violence** refers to the use of force to control and maintain

---

Terrorism   The use of unlawful force or violence against persons or property to intimidate or coerce a government, the civilian population, or any segment thereof, in furtherance of political or social objectives.

Domestic violence   The use of force to control and maintain power over another person in the home environment, including both actual harm and the threat of harm.

Bioterrorism: Pandora's Box

For many, the threat of a viable attack on the United States was incomprehensible until the World Trade Center and Pentagon attacks in 2001. As shocking as those events were, they may pale in comparison to the unleashing of a Pandora's box of biological killers, which could threaten the global population. Before the 2001 terrorist attacks, many people had never heard of diseases such as anthrax, but within a few days Americans watched as endless newscasts discussed the potential horrors of biological warfare.

As chilling as these threats might be, the actual potential for bioterrorism is more far-reaching than any of us might imagine. Included are a wide range of threats from both biological diseases and chemical agents, as indicated below. A complete listing of potential agents and diseases, plus information on preparing for and dealing with emergencies is on the CDC website, www.bt.cdc.gov.

BIOLOGICAL AGENTS/DISEASES

Category A diseases are pathogens rarely seen in the United States and pose a risk to national security because they (1) can be easily disseminated or transmitted person-to-person; (2) cause high mortality, with potential for major public health impact; (3) might cause widespread panic and social disruption; and (4) require special action for public health preparedness. The category A threats of greatest concern are highlighted below.

- *Bacillus anthracis* **(anthrax):** An acute infectious disease caused by a bacterium, anthrax typically occurs in host animals but can also infect humans. Three major forms of anthrax may occur: inhalation, cutaneous (skin), and intestinal anthrax, all with symptoms that usually appear within seven days after infection. Early symptoms of inhalation anthrax resemble a common cold, followed by respiratory symptoms and shock, which is often fatal. The intestinal form appears initially as nausea, vomiting, loss of appetite, and fever, followed by abdominal pain, bloody vomit, and severe diarrhea. It is believed that direct person-to-person spread of anthrax is very rare; thus, immunization and treatment of contacts are not recommended. Antibiotics are effective treatments in the early stages. Vaccination is also effective.

- *Clostridium botulinum* toxin **(botulism):** Botulism is an acute muscle-paralyzing disease caused by a toxin produced by a bacterium. There are three major forms of botulism. Food-borne, the most common strain, leads to illness within hours. Infant botulism affects babies who harbor the organism in their intestines. Wound botulism occurs when cuts are infected. Fortunately, botulism is not spread from person to person. Symptoms include double vision, blurred vision, slurred speech, difficulty swallowing, and muscle weakness that descends through the body. It can eventually paralyze the ability to breathe and kill the person.

- *Yersinia pestis* **(plague):** An infectious disease of animals and humans that is found in many parts of the world, plague is caused by a bacterium carried by rodents and their fleas. The plague organism infects the lungs. Fever, headache, weakness, and a watery, blood-laden cough are frequent symptoms. Pneumonia follows quickly, and over 2 to 4 days may cause septic shock. Without treatment, plague can be fatal. Per-

power over another person in the home environment. It can involve emotional abuse, verbal abuse, threats of physical harm, and actual physical violence ranging from slapping and shoving to beatings, rape, and homicide. Today, domestic violence is at epidemic levels in America. An estimate of nearly 700,000 incidents against a current or former spouse or romantic partner are projected for 2004; 85 percent of the attacks will be against women.[29]

Women as Victims While young men are more apt to become victims of violence from strangers, women are much more likely to become victims of violent acts perpetrated by spouses, lovers, ex-spouses, and ex-lovers. Forty percent of offenders were described as friends, 20 percent as intimates, and 7 percent as relatives, leaving only 31 percent of the men who attack women in the "stranger" category.[30] In 2002, more than 5 million women were victims of assault.

In fact, six of every ten women in the United States will be assaulted at some time in their lives by someone they know.[31] Every year, according to a national survey, approximately 12 percent of married women are the victims of physical aggression perpetrated by their husbands.[32] This aggression often includes pushing, slapping, and shoving, but it can take more severe forms.

Each year about 4 percent of married women are beaten, threatened, or actually injured by knives or guns.[33] In fact, acts of aggression by a husband or boyfriend are one of the most common causes of death for young women, and roughly 2,200 women in the United States are killed each year by their partners or ex-partners.[34] Over a recent ten-year period, according to the National Crime Victimization Survey, on average, more than 2 million assaults on women occurred each year. More than two-thirds of these assaults were committed by someone the woman knew.[35]

son-to-person contact with transfer of respiratory droplets spreads the disease. A vaccine has not been developed, but several antibiotics are effective if given early.

• Variola major (smallpox): Although smallpox was eliminated from the world in 1977, stockpiling of the virus that causes this disease has occurred in many regions of the world. Smallpox spreads from person to person by infected saliva droplets and is most contagious during the first week of illness. Initial symptoms include high fever, fatigue, and head- and back-aches. In two to three days a characteristic rash develops, with flat red lesions that evolve into pustules that are most prominent on the face, arms, and legs. Lesions crust early in the second week. Scabs develop, separate, and fall off after about three to four weeks. Most people who get smallpox recover, but death occurs in up to 30 percent of cases. Although most Americans were vaccinated prior to 1972, it is uncertain whether these shots conferred lasting immunity. Although vaccines are effective, the current supply is limited. Treatment for smallpox focuses on relieving symptoms, but new antiviral agents are being tested.

Category B diseases are of concern but are less easily transmitted or have a lower mortality rate than those in category A. Examples include *Coxiella burnetii* (Q fever), *Brucella* species (brucellosis), *Burkholderia mallei* (glanders), ricin toxin from *Ricinus communis* (castor beans), epsilon toxin of *Clostridium perfringens*, and staphylococcal enterotoxin B.

Category C diseases are emerging pathogens that could be engineered for bioterrorism in the future, because they have the potential for high morbidity and mortality rates and could be easily produced and disseminated. Examples include Nipah virus, hantavirus, tick-borne hemorrhagic fever, tickborne encephalitis viruses, yellow fever, and multidrug-resistant tuberculosis.

CHEMICAL AGENTS

These agents are classified by the body system they damage or the effects they produce.

Blister/Vesicants
Distilled mustard (HD)
Lewisite
Various forms of nitrogen mustard and
  Lewisite combinations

Blood
Arsine
Cyanogen chloride
Hydrogen chloride
Hydrogen cyanide

Choking/Lung/Pulmonary Damage
Chlorine
Diphosgene
Nitrogen oxide
Zinc oxide

Incapacitating
Agent 15
BZ
Canniboids
Fentanyls
Lysergic acid diethylamide (LSD)
Phenothiazines

Nervous system
Cyclohexyl sarin
Sarin

Riot control/tearing
Bromobenzyl cyanide (CA)
Chloroacetophenone (CN)

Vomiting
Adamsite

Source: Centers for Disease Control and Prevention, "Emergency Preparedness and Response," 2004, www.bt.cdc.gov

---

The following U.S. statistics indicate the seriousness of this long-hidden problem.[36]

• The most vulnerable women are African American and Hispanic, live in large cities far from their families, and are young and unmarried.
• Every 15 seconds, someone batters a woman.
• Only 1 in every 250 such assaults is reported to the police.
• More than a third of female victims of domestic violence are severely abused on a regular basis.
• About five women are killed every day in domestic violence incidents.
• Three of every four women murdered are killed by their husbands.
• Domestic violence is the single greatest cause of injury to women, surpassing rape, mugging, and auto accidents combined.

• About 25 to 45 percent of all women who are battered sustain such attacks during pregnancy.
• One-quarter of suicide attempts by women occur as a result of domestic violence.
• In 2002, 71 percent of all violent crime victims did not face an armed perpetrator.[37]

Although the ultimate result of these assaults can be murder, there are other devastating effects as well. Depression, panic attacks, disordered eating, chronic neck or back pain, migraine and other headaches, sexually transmitted infections, ulcers, and social isolation can all be results of domestic violence.

How many times have you heard of a woman who is repeatedly beaten by her partner and wondered, "Why doesn't she just leave him?" There are many reasons why some women find it difficult to break their ties with their

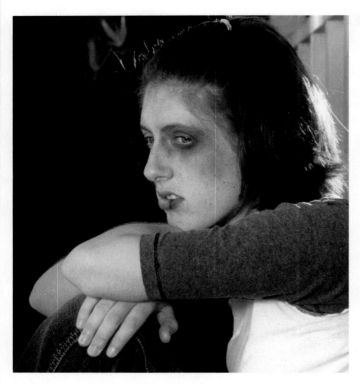

Despite obvious physical and psychological injury, it can be difficult for a person to leave an abusive partner.

abusers. Many women, particularly those with small children, are financially dependent on their partners. Others fear retaliation against themselves or their children. Some hope the situation will change with time (it rarely does), and others stay because cultural or religious beliefs forbid divorce. Finally, some women still love the abusive partner and are concerned about what will happen to him if they leave.[38]

Psychologist Lenore Walker developed a theory known as the "cycle of violence" to explain how women can get caught in a downward spiral without realizing it.[39] The cycle has three phases:

1. *Tension building.* In this phase, minor battering occurs, and the woman may become more nurturant, more pleasing, and more intent on anticipating the spouse's needs to forestall further violence. She assumes guilt for doing something to provoke him and tries hard to avoid doing it again.
2. *Acute battering.* At this stage, pleasing her man doesn't help, and she can no longer control or predict the abuse. Usually, the spouse is trying to "teach her a lesson," and when he feels he has inflicted enough pain, he'll stop. When the acute attack is over, he may respond with shock and denial about his own behavior. Both batterer and victim may soft-pedal the seriousness of the attacks.
3. *Remorse/reconciliation.* During this "honeymoon" period, the batterer may be kind, loving, and apologetic, swearing he will never act violently again. He may "behave" for sev-

eral weeks or months, and the woman may come to question whether she overreacted. However, when the tension that precipitated past abuse resurfaces, the man beats her again. Unless some form of intervention breaks this downward cycle of abuse, contrition, further abuse, denial, and contrition, it will repeat itself again and again—perhaps ending only in the woman's (or, rarely, the man's) death.

For most women who get caught in this cycle (which may include forced sexual relations and psychological and economic abuse as well as beatings), it is very hard to summon the resolution to extricate themselves. Most need effective outside intervention.

Men as Victims   Are men also victims of domestic violence? Some women do abuse and even kill their partners. Approximately 12 percent of men reported that their wives had engaged in physically aggressive behaviors against them in the past year—nearly the same percentage of reported claims as for women.

The difference between male and female batterers is twofold. First, although the frequency of physical aggression may be similar, the impact is drastically different: women are injured in domestic incidents two to three times more often than men.[40] These injuries tend to be more severe and have resulted in significantly more deaths. Women do engage in moderate aggression, such as pushing and shoving, at rates almost equal to those of men, but severe aggression that is likely to land the victim in the hospital is almost always male-against-female.

Second, a woman who is physically abused by a man is generally intimidated: she fears that he will use his power and control over her in some fashion. Men, however, generally report that they do not live in fear of their wives.

Causes of Domestic Violence   There is no single explanation for why people tend to be abusive in relationships. Although alcohol abuse is often associated with such violence, marital dissatisfaction is also a predictor.[41] Numerous studies also point to differences in the communication patterns between abusive and nonabusive relationships.[42] While some argue that the hormone testosterone causes male aggression, studies have failed to show a strong association between physical abuse in relationships and this hormone.[43] Many experts believe that men who engage in severe violence are more likely than other men to suffer from personality disorders.[4] Clearly, more research is needed to understand abusive relationships.[4]

Regardless of the cause, it is the dynamics that *both* people bring to a relationship that result in violence and allow it to continue. Community support and counseling services can help determine underlying problems and allow the victim and batterer to break the cycle. The Assess Yourself box on page 114 may help you determine if you are involved in an abusive relationship.

Child Abuse and Neglect   Children raised in families in which domestic violence and/or sexual abuse occur are at great risk for damage to personal health and well-being. The effects of such violent acts are powerful and long-lasting. **Child abuse** refers to the systematic harm of a child by a caregiver, generally a parent.[45] The abuse may be sexual, psychological, physical, or any combination of these. Although exact figures are lacking, many experts believe that over 2.5 million cases of child abuse and neglect occur every year in the United States, involving severe injury, permanent disability, or death. Of these, 35 percent involve physical abuse, 15 percent involve sexual abuse, and 50 percent involve neglect.[46]

Child abusers exist in all gender, social, ethnic, religious, and racial groups, but they tend to share certain characteristics: a history of abuse as a child, a poor self-image, feelings of isolation, extreme frustration with life, higher stress or anxiety levels than normal, a tendency to abuse drugs and/or alcohol, and unrealistic expectations of the child. It is estimated that one-half to three-quarters of men who batter their female partners also batter children. In fact, spousal abuse is the single most identifiable risk factor for predicting child abuse. Children with disabilities or other "differences" are more likely to be abused.

Child Sexual Abuse   **Sexual abuse of children** by adults or older children includes sexually suggestive conversations; inappropriate kissing; touching; petting; oral, anal, or vaginal intercourse; and other kinds of sexual interaction. The most frequent abusers are a child's parents or the companions or spouses of the child's parents. Next most frequent are grandfathers and siblings. Girls are more commonly abused than boys, although young boys are also frequent victims, usually of male family members. Between 20 and 30 percent of all adult women report having had an unwanted childhood sexual encounter with an adult male, usually a father, uncle, brother, or grandfather. It is a myth that mental illness accounts for most of these incidents: "Stories of retrospective incest patients typically involved perpetrators who are 'Everyman'—attorneys, businessmen, farmers, teachers, doctors, and clergy."[47]

Most sexual abuse occurs in the child's home. The following situations raise the risk:[48]

1. The child lives without one of his or her biological parents.
2. The mother is unavailable because she is disabled, ill, or working outside the home.
3. The parents' marriage is unhappy.
4. The child has a poor relationship with his or her parents or is subjected to extremely punitive discipline.
5. The child lives with a stepfather.

To appreciate the impact of child abuse on later life, consider these points: 99 percent of the inmates in the maximum security prison at San Quentin were either abused or raised in abusive households; and 300,000 children between the ages of 8 and 15 are living on the nation's streets, willing to prostitute themselves to survive rather than return to the abusive households they ran away from.[49]

Although most people who were abused as children do not end up as convicts or prostitutes, many do bear spiritual, psychological, and/or physical scars. Clinical psychologist Marjorie Whittaker has found that "of all forms of violence, incest and childhood sexual abuse are considered among the most 'toxic' because of their violations of trust, the confusion of affection and coercion, the splitting of family alignments, and serious psychological and physical consequences."[50]

Parents and caretakers of children should be aware of behavioral changes that may signal sexual abuse:[51]

- Noticeable fear of a certain person or place
- Unusual or unexpected response when the child is asked if he or she has been touched by someone
- Unreasonable fear of a physical exam
- Drawings that show sexual acts
- Abrupt changes in behavior such as bed-wetting
- Sudden or unusual awareness of genitals or sexual acts
- Attempts to get other children to perform sexual acts

Not all child violence is physical. Health can be severely affected by psychological violence—assaults on personality, character, competence, independence, or general dignity as a human being. The negative consequences of this kind of victimization can be harder to discern and therefore harder to combat. They include depression, low self-esteem, and a pervasive fear of offending the abuser.

What do you think?

What factors in society lead to child abuse and neglect? ■ *What are common characteristics of children's abusers?* ■ *Why are family members often the perpetrators of child abuse and child sexual abuse?* ■ *What actions can be taken to prevent such behaviors?*

Sexual Victimization

As with all forms of violence, men and women alike are susceptible to sexual victimization. However, sexual violence against women is of epidemic proportions, so we will focus

---

Child abuse   The systematic harming of a child by a caregiver, typically a parent.

Sexual abuse of children   Sexual interaction between a child and an adult or older child; includes, but is not limited to, sexually suggestive conversations, inappropriate kissing, touching, petting, and oral, anal, or vaginal intercourse.

Relationship Violence: Are You at Risk?

myhealthlab

Fill out this assessment online at www.aw-bc.com/myhealthlab or www.aw-bc.com/donatelle

Although we all want to have healthy relationships, sometimes we get caught in patterns of behavior that are a direct result of past experiences. Sometimes we don't even recognize that we are acting inappropriately. Other times we know we should act in a particular way, but we get caught up in our own emotions and act out in ways that are physically or emotionally abusive to

others. If you have been a victim of emotional or physical violence, you may have become so used to certain behaviors that you might not even realize they're inappropriate. To prevent violence, we have to be able to recognize it, deal with it in appropriate ways, and take action to avoid it. We can start by examining our intimate relationships. Answer the following questions about your current or past relationships.

How Often Does Your Partner

	Never	Sometimes	Often
1. Criticize you for your appearance (weight, clothing, hair, etc.)?	❑	❑	❑
2. Embarrass you in front of others by putting you down?	❑	❑	❑
3. Blame you or others for his or her mistakes?	❑	❑	❑
4. Curse at you, say mean things, or mock you?	❑	❑	❑
5. Demonstrate uncontrollable anger?	❑	❑	❑
6. Criticize your friends, family, or others who are close to you?	❑	❑	❑
7. Threaten to leave you if you don't behave in a certain way?	❑	❑	❑
8. Manipulate you to prevent you from spending time with friends or family?	❑	❑	❑
9. Express jealousy, distrust, and anger when you spend time with other people?	❑	❑	❑
10. Tell you that you are crazy, irrational, or paranoid?	❑	❑	❑
11. Call you names to make you lose confidence in yourself?	❑	❑	❑
12. Make all the significant decisions in your relationship?	❑	❑	❑
13. Intimidate or threaten you, making you fearful or anxious?	❑	❑	❑
14. Make threats to harm others you care about?	❑	❑	❑

on women. In fact, sexual battering is the single greatest cause of injury to women in the United States, occurring more frequently than car accidents, muggings, and rapes combined.[52] Physical battering and emotional abuse often leave psychological as well as physical scars. One-quarter to one-third of high school and college students report involvement in dating violence, as perpetrators, victims, or both.[53]

Sexual Assault and Rape **Sexual assault** is any act in which one person is sexually intimate with another person without that person's consent. This may range from simple

touching to forceful penetration and may include such things as ignoring indications that intimacy is not wanted, threatening force or other negative consequences, and actually using force. Nearly six out of ten rapes and sexual assaults are reported by victims as occurring in their own or a friend's home.[54]

Rape, the most extreme form of sexual assault, is defined as "penetration without the victim's consent."[55] Whether committed by an acquaintance, a date, or a stranger, rape is a criminal activity that usually has serious emotional, psychological, social, and physical consequences for the victim. Typically, victims are young females, with 29 percent under 11 years of age, 32 percent between the ages of 11 and 17, and 22 percent between ages of 18 and 24.[56] Women age 16 to 19 are four times as likely as the general population to be rape victims.[57]

One of the most startling aspects of sex crimes is how many go unreported, usually out of a belief that this is a private matter, fear of reprisal by the assailant, or unwarranted

Sexual assault Any act in which one person is sexually intimate with another person without that person's consent.

Rape Sexual penetration without the victim's consent.

	Never	Sometimes	Often
15. Prevent you from going out by taking your car keys?	❏	❏	❏
16. Control your telephone calls, listen in on your messages, or read your e-mail?	❏	❏	❏
17. Punch, hit, slap, or kick you?	❏	❏	❏
18. Gossip about you to turn others against you or make them think bad things about you?	❏	❏	❏
19. Make you feel guilty about something?	❏	❏	❏
20. Use money or possessions to control you?	❏	❏	❏
21. Force you to have sex or perform sexual acts that make you uncomfortable?	❏	❏	❏
22. Threaten to kill himself or herself if you leave?	❏	❏	❏
23. Control your money and make you ask for what you need?	❏	❏	❏
24. Set rules that you must abide by?	❏	❏	❏
25. Follow you, call to check on you, or demonstrate a constant obsession with what you are doing?	❏	❏	❏

If you answered "sometimes" to one or more of these questions, you may be at risk for emotional or physical abuse. If you answered "often" to any question, you may need to talk with someone about immediate threats to your emotional or physical health. Typically, such potentially abusive patterns only get worse over time as a person gains control and power in a relationship. If you are nervous or anxious about talking to your partner, seek counseling through your campus counseling center, student health center, or community services. If you don't know where to go, ask your instructor for possible options.

After you have completed the test about your partner's behavior, ask the same questions about your own behavior. If any of the questions describe your actions in a relationship, you should seek help to change these behavioral patterns. These actions are not conducive to healthy relationships and may result in harm to you or your loved ones. Seek help now to ensure healthier relationships in the future.

MAKE IT HAPPEN!

Use the results of this self-assessment to begin your behavior change program. Follow the steps and use the examples on page 125 to complete your Behavior Change Contract and use these resources to take action.

---

feelings of guilt and responsibility. It is thought that one out of every three women is the victim of an attempted or completed rape in her lifetime. Although as many as two-thirds of all rapes are never reported, there were over 683,000 reported cases of rape, attempted rape, or sexual assault in 2003.[58]

Incidents of rape generally fall into one of two types—aggravated or simple. An **aggravated rape** involves multiple attackers, strangers, weapons, or physical beatings. A **simple rape** is perpetrated by one person, whom the victim knows, and does not involve a physical beating or use of a weapon. Most incidents are classified as simple rapes, with one report suggesting that 82 percent of female rape victims have been victimized by acquaintances (53 percent), current or former boyfriends (16 percent), current or former spouses (10 percent), or other relatives (3 percent). With almost half of all rape charges dismissed before the cases reach trial and a perceived lack of male understanding of how rape affects women, it's easy to understand why experts feel that so-called "simple" rape is seriously underreported and ignored.

Acquaintance or Date Rape Although the terms *date rape*, *friendship rape*, and *acquaintance rape* have become standard terminology, they are typically misused. Not all rapes occur on dates, not all the relationships are friendships, and sometimes the term *acquaintance* is used all too loosely. Many acquaintance rapes occur as the result of incidental contact at a party or when groups of people congregate at one person's

Aggravated rape Rape that involves multiple attackers, strangers, weapons, or a physical beating.

Simple rape Rape by one person known to the victim that does not involve a physical beating or use of a weapon.

house. These are crimes of opportunity, not necessarily a prearranged date. This is an important distinction because the term *date* suggests some type of reciprocal interaction arranged in advance. While most date or acquaintance rapes happen to women age 15 to 21 years, the 18-year-old new college student is the most likely victim.[59]

In a study of 6,000 college students from 32 different universities, researchers uncovered the following data.[60]

- More than 50 percent of the college women surveyed had experienced some form of sexual abuse.
- More than 25 percent had been the victims of rape or attempted rape.
- Eighty-four percent of the assault victims knew their assailants.
- Fifty-seven percent of the assaults occurred on dates.
- Forty-one percent of the women raped were virgins at the time of the assault.
- Seventy-three percent of the assailants and 55 percent of the victims had used alcohol or drugs prior to the assault.
- Forty-two percent of the victims indicated that they had sex with the offender again (it is unknown whether the subsequent sex was voluntary).
- Twenty-five percent of the men admitted to some degree of aggressive sexual behavior.
- Men were most likely to commit sexual assaults during their senior year in high school or first year in college.

Date rape is not simply miscommunication; it is an act of violence. Well-known expert on interpersonal relationships Susan Jacoby puts it this way:

> Some women (especially the young) initially resist sex not out of real conviction, but as part of the elaborate persuasion and seduction rituals accompanying what was once called courtship. And it is true that many men (again, especially the young) take pride in their ability to coax a woman further than she intended to go. But these mating rituals do not justify or even explain date rape. Even the most callow youth is capable of understanding the difference between resistance and genuine fear; between a halfhearted "no, we shouldn't" and tears or screams.[61]

Marital Rape   While the legal definition of marital rape varies within the United States, marital rape can be defined as any unwanted intercourse or penetration (vaginal, anal, or oral) obtained by force, threat of force, or when the wife is unable to consent.[62] Some researchers estimate that marital rape may account for 25 percent of all rapes; rape in marriage may be an extremely prevalent form of sexual violence.

Although this problem has undoubtedly existed since the origin of marriage as a social institution, it is noteworthy

that marital rape did not become a crime in all 50 states until 1993. Even more noteworthy is the fact that in 33 states, there are still exemptions from rape prosecution, meaning that the judicial system may treat it as a lesser form of crime.

Who is most vulnerable to marital rape? In general, women under the age of 25 and those from lower socioeconomic groups are at highest risk. Women from homes where other forms of domestic violence are common and where there is a high rate of alcoholism and/or substance abuse also tend to be victimized at greater rates. Women who are subjected to marital rape often report multiple offenses over a period of time and that these events are more likely to be forced anal and oral experiences.[63]

Again, abuse of power and a need to control and dominate seem to be key factors in the husband-rapist profile. Marital rape can have devastating short- and long-term consequences for women, including injuries to the vaginal and anal areas, lacerations, soreness, bruising, torn muscles, fatigue, panic attacks, sexually transmitted diseases, broken bones, wounds, and other emotional and physical scars.

Sexual Harassment   If we think of violence as including verbal abuse and the threat of coercion, then sexual harassment is a form of violence. Under Title VII of the Civil Rights Act, **sexual harassment** is defined as "unwelcomed sexual advances, requests for sexual favors, and other verbal or physical contact of a sexual nature." Despite what might appear to be a clear definition, sexual harassment is often difficult to identify. While many people would say that sexual harassment is anything the offended person *believes* is harassment, others say that this explanation is too nebulous.

The issue of sexual harassment was brought to the collective consciousness of society in the early 1990s when Anita Hill charged Supreme Court Justice nominee Clarence Thomas with sexual harassment in a previous employment environment. The alleged harassment was partly in the form of sexually offensive humor, not all directed at Hill. What had long been dismissed as harmless behavior became a cause for concern in business, academia, and government. More recently, the Paula Jones and Monica Lewinsky scandals have kept sexual harassment issues in the news and have focused attention on additional aspects such as improper touching, improper suggestions, and inappropriate uses of power. Most universities now offer courses on identifying and preventing sexual harassment, and most schools and companies have established policies and procedures for dealing with it.

It's always important to watch what you say and how you say it. Learning now what constitutes sexual harassment may save you embarrassment or worse in the future. A simple compliment on someone's appearance can be offensive if stated without sensitivity, regardless of the intent. "You look very nice today" can become offensive if stated as, "That dress looks great on your body." Even if the person enjoys your comment, remember that others may overhear.

Most schools and companies have sexual harassment policies in place, as well as procedures for dealing with it.

Sexual harassment   Any form of unwanted sexual attention.

Gender Violence: A Global Phenomenon

Over the last decade, the issue of gender violence, or violence against women, has increasingly captured the world's attention. Sexual, physical, and psychological violence are believed to cause as much ill health and death among women aged 15 to 44 as cancer and more than malaria and traffic accidents combined. Although men and women are both affected by violence, women bear a disproportionate burden, reflecting significant gender disparity. Consider the following facts:

- Globally, the World Health Organization believes that at least one woman in five has been physically or sexually abused by a man at some time in her life, usually by a husband, father, or neighbor rather than a stranger.

- Forty-eight surveys on intimate partner violence around the world asked whether a partner had ever hit you with his fist or other object that could hurt you; between 10 and 69 percent of women answered "yes."
- Studies in Mexico and the United States indicate that 40 to 52 percent of women who have been physically abused have also been sexually assaulted.
- Many large studies of women indicated that they had never told anyone about the violence they experienced. In Canada, 22 percent of women had remained silent before being asked for the study; in Chile, 30 percent; in Nicaragua, 37 percent; in the United Kingdom, 38 percent; in Egypt, 47 percent; and in Bangladesh, 68 percent.
- In many countries of the world, women whose husbands beat them feel it is justified; in Egypt, as many as 81 percent felt this way.
- Recent research in the United Kingdom found that 50 percent of boys and 33 percent of girls thought it was OK to hit a woman or force her to have sex in certain circumstances, and 36 percent of boys thought they might personally hit a woman or force her to have sex.
- According to several researchers, physical and sexual abuse lie behind some of the most intractable reproductive health issues of our times: unwanted pregnancies, HIV and other sexually transmitted infections, and complications from pregnancy.

What are your thoughts about each of these statistics? What factors contribute to them? How do societal values and beliefs contribute to global violence against women? Who are the most likely victims? What actions can be taken to reduce the rate of violence?

Source: World Health Organization, "The WHO Multi-Country Study on Women's Health and Domestic Violence Against Women," 2004, www.who.int/gender /violence/multicountry/en

---

If you feel you are being harassed, the most important thing you can do is be assertive. Immediately after the incident occurs, follow these guidelines:

- *Tell the harasser to stop.* Be clear and direct about what is bothering you and why you are upset: "I don't like this joke/touch/remark/look. It makes me feel uncomfortable and it makes it hard for me to come to class/participate/be your friend," and so on. This may be the first indication the person has ever had that such behavior is inappropriate. This will usually stop the harassment.
- *Document the harassment.* Make a record of the incident. If the harassment becomes intolerable, having a record of exactly what occurred (and when and where) will be helpful in making your case.
- *Complain to a higher authority.* Talk to your instructor, adviser, or counseling center about what happened. If they don't take you seriously, find out what the grievance procedures are for your school.
- *Remember that you have not done anything wrong.* You will likely feel awful after being harassed (especially if you report it). However, feel proud that you are not keeping silent. The person who is harassing you is wrong, not you. If the situation becomes so uncomfortable that it interferes with your studies, why put up with it?

What do you think?

Why do you think people are often reluctant to report sexual harassment? ■ *Why do you think so many people report that they were unaware of their own sexually harassing behaviors?* ■ *What can be done to increase awareness in this area?*

Social Contributors to Sexual Assault   According to many experts, certain common assumptions in our society prevent recognition by both the perpetrator and the wider public of the true nature of sexual assault.[64] These assumptions include the following:[65]

- *Minimization.* It is often assumed that sexual assault of women is rare because official crime statistics, including the Uniform Crime Reports of the FBI, show very few rapes per thousand population. However, rape is the most underreported of all serious crimes. Researchers have found that nearly 25 percent of women in the United States have been raped.

- *Trivialization.* Incredibly enough, sexual assault of women is still often viewed as a jocular matter. During a gubernatorial election in Texas a few years back, one of the candidates reportedly compared a bad patch of weather to rape: "If there's nothing you can do about it, just lie back and enjoy it." (He lost the election—to a woman.)
- *Blaming the victim.* Many discussions of sexual violence against women display a sometimes unconscious assumption that the woman did something to provoke the attack—that she flirted or dressed revealingly, for example.
- *"Boys will be boys."* According to this assumption, men just can't control themselves once they become aroused.

Over the years, psychologists and others have proposed several theories to explain why many males sexually victimize women. In one of the first major studies to explore this issue, almost two-thirds of the male respondents had engaged in intercourse unwanted by the woman, primarily because of male peer pressure.[66] By all indicators, these trends continue today. Peer pressure is certainly a strong factor, but a growing body of research suggests that sexual assault is encouraged by the socialization processes that males experience daily.[67]

- *Male socialization.* Throughout our lives, we are exposed to social norms that objectify women—make them appear as objects that can be used. Media portrayals of half-dressed and undressed women in seductive poses promoting products, for instance, contribute to sex-role stereotyping. These portrayals often show males as aggressors and females as targets. In addition, men are exposed from an early age to antifemale jokes and vulgar and obscene terms for women. These reinforce the idea that females are lesser beings who may be pushed around with impunity.[68] Males are also discouraged from acting in ways that society views as feminine. They are told to act tough and unemotional; strive for power, status, and control; be aggressive and take risks.
- *Male attitudes.* Several studies have confirmed a greater tolerance of rape among men who accept the myth that rape is something women secretly desire, who believe in adversarial relationships between men and women, who condone violence against women, or who hold traditional attitudes toward sex roles. Such men are apt to blame the victim and more likely to commit rape themselves if they think they can get away with it.[69]
- *Male sexual history and hostility.* Most rapists do not appear abnormal or psychologically disturbed. They typically are employed, often married with families, and have a history of multiple sexual experiences (both forced and voluntary) during childhood. Many feel hostility toward women.[70]

- *Male misperceptions.* Men who are convinced that women really want sex even if they say they don't are more likely to perpetrate sexual assaults. They more readily misinterpret a woman's words and behavior and act on their misperceptions—only to be surprised later when the woman says that she has been assaulted.[71]
- *Situational factors.* Several factors increase the likelihood of sexual assault. Dates in which the male makes all the decisions, pays, drives, and in general controls what happens are more likely to end in aggression. Alcohol and drug use increase the risk and severity of assault. Length of relationship is another important situational factor: the more long-standing the relationship, the greater the chance of aggression. Finally, males who belong to a close-knit social group involving intense interaction are more prone to engage in a peer-pleasing assault.

What do you think?

What factors make men likely to commit sexual assault or rape? ■ *What measures might be effective in preventing such behaviors?*

Crime on Campus: A Safe Haven?

Although the majority of crimes on campuses today consist of vandalism, theft, and setting off fire alarms illegally, the rates of certain violent crimes continues to increase. Recent Department of Justice statistics indicate that in a population of approximately 7.7 million U.S. college students aged 18 to 24, an average of 526,000 students per year experience a violent crime (rape, robbery, aggravated, or simple assault).[72] Important facts include:

- Most of the violent crimes occurred off campus.
- Female college students were about half as likely as male college students to be victims of violent crime. There were an annual average of 47 violent crimes per 1,000 female students versus 91 violent crimes per 1,000 male students.
- Student victims reported that the offender was believed to be under the influence of alcohol or other drugs in 41 percent of incidents.
- About six in ten victims did not know the offender.
- Overall, college students were less likely to be victims of violent crime than their same-aged population in the general population. Only Hispanic students experienced rates of violent victimization equivalent to those of the same age in the general population.

Traditionally, most campus crimes were handled internally. This has changed as more states have passed legislation requiring that colleges and universities warn their students about crime and danger both on campus and in off-campus housing that they recommend.[73] In 1992, Congress passed the Campus Sexual Assault Victim's Bill of Rights, known as the Ramstad Act. The act gives victims the right to call in off-campus authorities to investigate serious campus crimes. In addition, universities must set up educational programs and notify students of available counseling. More recent provisions of the act specify received notification procedures and options for victims, rights of victims and the accused perpetrators, and consequences if schools do not comply. It also requires the Department of Education to publish campus crime statistics annually.

Sexual Assault on Campus Most studies of sexual assault among college students indicate that 25 percent to 60 percent of college men have engaged in some form of sexually coercive behavior.[74] This is consistent with the 27 percent of college women who have reported experiencing rape or attempted rape since they were 14 years old, and the 54 percent who claim to have been sexually victimized (forced to endure unwanted petting, kisses, and other advances).[75] In one survey, only 39 percent of the men sampled denied coercive involvement, 28 percent admitted to having used a coercive method at least once, and 15 percent admitted that they had forced a woman to have intercourse at least once.[76] According to a large, nationally representative sample of college and university students, 25 percent of the male respondents had been involved in some form of sexual assault since age 14.[77] Since this early national study, many smaller studies have reported similar statistics.

As with the general public, the incidence of sexual assault on campuses is believed to be seriously underreported. In a recent report, one major university familiar to the author claimed there were no rapes on campus. However, based on national averages, it seems highly unlikely that no forcible sexual encounters would occur in a setting where nearly 16,000 students date, drink, and socialize every week. The fact is that coercive sex and date rape are seldom reported to campus police, and when a rape victim seeks help at the campus health center, the center is not required to report the crime. In one study, 20 percent of female respondents at a midwestern university said they had been raped by someone they knew, but only 8 percent of them had reported it to the police. At another midwestern university, 20 percent of 247 women interviewed said they had experienced date rape, but few had reported it.[78] Needless to say, other sexual violations, such as obscene phone calls, stalking, sexual molestation that does not result in penetration, exhibitionism, voyeurism, and attempted rape, go equally unreported.[79]

Sexual Harassment on Campus How pervasive is sexual harassment at U.S. schools? According to a national study by the American Association of University Women, four out of five students attending public schools have been sexually harassed by other students. Over one-third of these incidents occurred before the seventh grade. Another study indicates that 90 percent of undergraduate women and 52 percent of graduate women report at least one negative experience from male students and that the students most likely to harass these women are members of fraternities, athletic teams, and all-male groups and cliques; men who are defiant or angry at women; and those who have been abused themselves.[80]

While peers pose a threat of harassment, a study by the Institute of Social and Economic Research at Cornell University found that 61 percent of juniors, seniors, and graduate students experienced "unwanted sexual attention from someone of authority within the university."[81] Typically, these attentions come from male professors and may include affairs of male faculty with married and unmarried female students; demands for sex, with threats of lower grades for noncompliance; and sexually offensive and hostile environments in the classroom.[82] Many universities have strict codes of conduct relating to faculty–student consensual as well as nonconsensual relationships. Many of these policies stem from reported difficulties with power and control between faculty and students and the potential for negative consequences.

What do you think?

What policies does your school have regarding consensual relationships between faculty members and students? ■ *Do you think that consenting adults should have the right to interact, regardless of their positions within a system or workplace?* ■ *What are the potential dangers of such interactions?*

Reducing Your Risk

After a violent act is committed against someone we know, we acknowledge the horror of the event, express sympathy, and go on with our lives—but the person who has been brutalized may take months or years to recover. It is far better to prevent a violent act than to recover from it.

Self-Defense against Rape

Rape can occur no matter what preventive actions you take, but commonsense tactics can lower the risk. Self-defense is a process that includes learning increased awareness, self-defense techniques, reasonable precautions, and the self-confidence and judgment needed to determine appropriate responses to different situations.[83] Figure 4.5 identifies practical tips for preventing personal assaults.

In Your Car

- Always keep your doors and windows locked.
- Purchase cars with an alarm system and remote entry.
- Don't stop for vehicles in distress; call for help.
- If your car breaks down, lock the doors and wait for help from the police.
- If you think someone is following you, do not drive to your home; drive to a busy place and attract attention.
- Stick to well-traveled routes.
- Keep your car in good running order and always filled with gas.
- On long trips, don't make it obvious you're traveling alone.
- Do not sleep in your car along interstate highways.
- Carry a cell phone with programmed emergency numbers.

On the Street

- Walk or jog at a steady pace.
- Walk or jog with others.
- At night, avoid dark parking lots, wooded areas, and any place that offers an assailant good cover.
- Listen for footsteps and voices.
- Be aware of cars that keep driving around in your area.
- Vary your running or walking routes.
- Carry pepper spray or other deterrents, or walk or jog with a dog... the bigger, the better!
- Carry a cell phone or change to make a phone call.
- Tell others where you are going, your route, and when you'll return.

Figure 4.5
Preventing Personal Assaults

Taking Control Most rapes by unknown assailants are planned in advance. They are frequently preceded by a casual, friendly conversation. Although many women have said that they started to feel uneasy during this conversation, they denied the possibility of an attack to themselves until it was too late. Listen to your feelings and trust your intuition. Be assertive and direct to someone who is getting out of line or threatening—this may convince the would-be rapist to back off. Stifle your tendency to be "nice," and don't fear making a scene. Let him know that you mean what you say and are prepared to defend yourself.

- *Speak in a strong voice.* Use statements such as "Leave me alone" rather than questions like "Will you please leave

me alone?" Sound like you mean it. Avoid apologies and excuses.
- *Maintain eye contact with the would-be attacker.*
- *Stand up straight, act confident, and remain alert.* Walk as if you own the sidewalk.

Many rapists use certain ploys to initiate their attacks. Among the most common are:

- *Request for help*. This allows him to get close—to enter your house to use the phone, for instance.
- *Offer of help.* This can also help him gain entrance to your home: "Let me help you carry that package."
- *Guilt trip.* "Gee, no one is friendly nowadays. I can't believe you won't talk with me for just a little while."
- *Deliberate accident.* He may bump into the back of your car, and then assault you when you get out to see the damage. Don't stop unless you have to in these situations, and if you do stop, stay in your car with the doors locked.
- *Authority.* Many women fall for the old "policeman at the door" ruse. If anyone comes to your door or vehicle dressed in uniform, ask him or her to show an ID before you unlock the door. You can also call the police department to confirm the ID.

If you are attacked, act immediately. Don't worry about causing a scene. You *want* to draw attention to yourself and your assailant. Scream "Fire" loudly. Research has shown that passersby are much more likely to help if they hear the word *fire* rather than just a scream or calls using the word *help*. Your attacker may also be caught off balance by the action.

To prevent an attack, remember the following points:

- *Always be vigilant.* Rapes occur in even the safest cities and towns. Don't be fooled by a sleepy-little-town atmosphere.
- *Use campus escort services whenever possible.*
- *Be assertive in demanding a well-lit campus.*
- *Don't use the same routes all the time.* Vary your movement patterns.
- *Don't leave a bar alone with a friendly stranger.* Stay with your friends, and let the stranger come along. Don't give your address to anyone you don't know.
- *Let friends and family know where you are going, what route you'll take, and when to expect your return.*
- *Stay close to others.* Avoid shortcuts through dark or unlit paths. Don't be the last one to leave the lab or library late at night.
- *Keep your windows and doors locked.* Don't open the door to strangers.

What to Do if a Rape Occurs

If you are a rape victim, report the attack. This gives you a sense of control. Follow these steps:

- Call 911 (if available).
- Do not bathe, shower, douche, clean up, or touch anything the attacker may have touched.

Drug-Facilitated Rapes: Rohypnol and Other Dangers

Of the over 600,000 sexual assaults and rapes that occur each year in the United States, many involve drugs or alcohol. In the late 1990s, rape crisis centers became alarmed over reports of drugs being used to immobilize victims and make them unable to defend themselves from sexual attacks. Known as "roofies" or "liquid ecstasy," these "date rape" drugs are typically slipped into the drinks of unsuspecting women, who wake up after being raped and can remember few details of the assault. Two of the most common drugs used are Rohypnol and GHB. Although these drugs are often called date rape drugs, their use is often unrelated to a date. Many times, these drugs are slipped into the drinks of women whose only meeting with the male perpetrator is to be bought a drink at a bar or handed a drink at a party. There is no date involved—just an opportunity to gain control of a woman, any woman, and remove any chance of resistance.

Although not approved for sale in the United States, Rohypnol (flunitrazepam) is widely available in other countries as a sleep aid. Street names for it include Roaches, LaRocha, rope, Rib Roche, Roches, roofies, Ruffies, Mexican Valium, and roach-2. When put in a drink, Rohypnol produces a sedative-hypnotic effect that includes muscle relaxation and amnesia. Generally, sedative effects occur within 20 to 30 minutes and incapacitation within 1 to 2 hours, often lasting for hours. People who take it may appear drunk or sleepy, be dizzy, or seem confused. Tablets are white and contain the name "Roche" and an encircled "1" or "2" on one side, indicating dosage. The manufacturer has now released a new, lower dose blue tablet designed to be impossible to slip into a drink without detection. Tests are available at rape crisis centers, emergency rooms, and through law enforcement agencies to see if Rohypnol has been administered.

GHB (gamma-hydroxybutyrate) is known as Liquid E, Liquid Ecstasy, Liquid X, Grievous Bodily Harm, and Easy First. Illicitly used for its euphoric, sedative, and anabolic (body-building) effects, today GHB is more commonly used than Rohypnol in sexual assaults. GHB is usually a colorless, odorless liquid that may taste salty. Used as a surgical anesthetic in Europe, it is not legal in the United States and can induce short-term coma, slowed heart rate, decreased breathing, seizures, and death.

A drug that has recently appeared and that causes similar reactions is Burundanga, a light yellow powder that has no taste and an immediate effect. This drug affects the central nervous system and can be highly dangerous.

Each year, there are several deaths from these rape-facilitating drugs. Victims must cope with the fact that they have been violated without a chance to defend themselves. To reduce your risk, follow these guidelines:

✔ *Do not accept drinks from strangers.* In fact, do not take any beverages from someone you do not know well and trust.
✔ *Never leave a drink unattended.* If you get up to dance, have someone watch your drink, or take it with you.
✔ *At a bar or club, accept drinks only from the bartender or wait staff.* Watch the bartender pour the drink, and keep the drink in sight until it's in your hand.
✔ *At parties, do not accept open-container drinks from anyone.*
✔ *Be alert to the behavior of friends.* If they seem disproportionately "out of it" in relation to what they've had to drink, stay with them and watch them carefully.
✔ *Go out with friends and leave with friends.* Make a rule never to leave a bar or party with someone you don't know well.
✔ *If you think you may have been slipped something in a drink, tell a friend and have him or her get you to an emergency room.* Call 911 if anyone appears to be unusually "out of it" or experiences seizures, difficulty breathing, or other complications.

Source: National Institute of Drug Abuse, "NIDA Info Facts: Rohypnol and GHB," March 30, 2004, www.nida.nih.gov/infofax/RohypnolGHB.html

---

- Do not throw away or launder the clothes you were wearing. They will be needed as evidence.
- Bring a clean change of clothes to the clinic or hospital.
- Contact the rape assistance hotline in your area, and ask for advice on therapists or counseling if you need additional help or advice.

    If a friend is raped, here's how you can help:

- Believe her. Don't ask questions that may appear to implicate her in the assault.

- Recognize that rape is a violent act and the victim was not looking for this to happen.
- Encourage her to see a doctor immediately. She may have medical needs but feel too embarrassed to seek help on her own. Offer to go with her.
- Encourage her to report the crime.
- Be understanding, and let her know you will be there for her.
- Recognize that this is an emotional recovery, and it may take six months to a year for her to bounce back.
- Encourage her to seek counseling.

A Campuswide Response to Violence

Increasingly, college campuses have become microcosms of the greater society, complete with the risks, hazards, and dangers people face in the world. Many college administrators have been proactive in establishing violence prevention policies, programs, and services.[84]

Changing Roles To increase student protection, campus law enforcement has changed over the years in both numbers and authority to prosecute student offenders. Campus police are responsible for emergency responses to situations that threaten overall safety, human resources, the general campus environment, traffic and bicycle safety, and other dangers. They have the power to enforce laws with students in the same way they are handled in the general community. In fact, many campuses now hire state troopers or local law enforcement officers to deal with campus issues rather than maintain a separate police staff.

Many of these law enforcement groups follow a *community policing* model in which officers have specific responsibilities for certain areas of campus, departments, or events. By narrowing the scope of each officer's territory, officers get to know people in the area and are better able to anticipate and prevent risks. This differs from earlier policies, in which campus security typically swooped down only in times of trouble.

Prevention Efforts Many universities now hire crime prevention and safety specialists. They commonly recommend the following activities:

- A rape awareness and education program for members of the campus community.
- A crime prevention orientation program for new faculty and staff, as well as students.
- Specialized safety workshops for particular groups, such as commuters, international students, athletes, and students with disabilities.
- Printed and electronic educational messages about personal safety.
- A notification process to distribute information about special hazards.
- Alcohol and drug programs dealing with policy, awareness, education, and enforcement.
- A "grounds safety" program, including measures such as installing good lighting and removing shrubs from dark areas.
- Emergency call boxes or telephones across campus.
- Escort services for students who must be out after dark.
- Motorist assistance programs for people with car trouble.
- Antitheft programs, including regular patrols of parking lots and other areas.
- Victim advocacy programs, such as rape and abuse counseling.

How many of these are available on your campus?

The Role of Student Affairs Although there may be some overlap with law enforcement activities, student affairs offices need to play a vital role in all on-campus programs, both to prevent trouble and to resolve problems that do occur. Student groups should monitor progress, identify potential threats, and advocate for improvements in any areas found to be deficient. A student affairs office can play a key role in making sure that mental health services, student assistance programs, and other services are high quality, easily accessible, and meet student needs. A human services or student affairs office should seek to involve the entire student body and ensure that all are aware of its services. Any programs that are not visible or proactive in ensuring campus safety should be evaluated carefully. Student leaders can play a major role in shaping such services and advocating for the campus population.

Community Strategies for Preventing Violence

Since the causes of homicide and assaultive violence are complex, community strategies for prevention must be multidimensional. Successful strategies include the following.[85]

- Developing and implementing educational programs to teach people communication, conflict resolution, and coping skills.
- Working with individuals to help them develop self-esteem and respect for others.
- Rewarding youngsters for good behavior, and never spanking a child when angry. (Children need to know that anger is sometimes acceptable, but violence never is. Use family meetings to resolve conflicts.)
- Establishing and enforcing policies that forbid discrimination on the basis of gender, religious affiliation, race, sexual orientation, marital status, and age.
- Increasing and enriching educational programs for family planning.
- Increasing efforts by health care and social service programs to identify victims of violence.
- Improving treatment and support for victims.
- Treating the psychological as well as the physical consequences of violence.

Unintentional Injuries

As stated at the beginning of the chapter, unintentional injuries occur without planning or intention to harm. Examples of unintentional injuries include car accidents, falls, water accidents, accidental gunshots, recreational accidents, and workplace accidents. None of these injuries happen on purpose, yet they may result in pain, suffering, and possibly even death. Most efforts to prevent unintentional injuries focus on changing something about the *person,* the *environment,* or the *circumstances* (policies, procedures) that put people in harm's way.

Residential Safety

Injuries within the home typically take the form of falls, burns, or intrusions by others. Some populations, such as the elderly, are particularly vulnerable. However, the elderly are not the only victims; each year, hundreds of children suffer severe burns or die from accidental fires, falls, and other home-based injuries. To reduce the risk of accidents, consider the following.

Fall-Proof Your Home

- Eliminate clutter, particularly objects you may stumble over in the dark. Leave nothing lying around on the floor or stairs.
- Fasten all rugs securely to the floor so they don't wrinkle or slide when stepped on. Inexpensive rubberized mats or strips will hold rugs in place.
- Train your pets to stay away from your feet. Many an unsuspecting person has ended up on the floor while trying to avoid a pet.
- Make sure handrails are secure and within easy reach. All stairs should have slip-proof treads.
- Install slip-proof mats or decals in showers and tubs. Add handrails and places to grab for stability in bathtubs and showers.

Avoid Burns

- Extinguish all cigarettes in ashtrays before you go to bed.
- Don't smoke and drink before bed. In fact, don't smoke in bed at any time! Sparks can smolder in mattresses or upholstered furniture, and then flare into flames.
- Don't throw spent matches in the trash with combustibles. Soak matches in water before discarding.
- Set lamps away from drapes, linens, and paper, particularly halogen lights or specialty lamps that can get extremely hot.
- Keep hotpads and kitchen cloths away from stove burners. When not using a cloth, set it on a counter far from the stove.
- Keep candles under control and away from combustibles. Although it may seem romantic to go to sleep by candlelight, it is highly risky. Don't do it.
- Use caution when lighting barbecue grills and other home-based fires. Never spray combustible fluids such as lighter fluid directly onto the fire.
- Check chimneys and fireplaces regularly for buildup of flammable soot.
- Service furnaces annually, and be sure to change the filters.

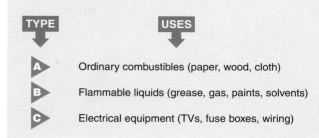

Fire extinguishers are labeled A, B, and C, depending on the kind of fire they are designed to extinguish. They also are numbered according to the size of the fire they can put out. The higher the number, the greater the capacity.

TYPE	USES
A	Ordinary combustibles (paper, wood, cloth)
B	Flammable liquids (grease, gas, paints, solvents)
C	Electrical equipment (TVs, fuse boxes, wiring)

Figure 4.6
Do You Have the Right Fire Extinguisher?

- Avoid overloading electrical circuits with appliances and cords. Older buildings are at particular risk for fire from such overloads.
- Program phones with emergency numbers for speed dialing, and keep these numbers in clear sight near phones as well.
- Replace batteries in smoke alarms periodically, and test them regularly to make sure the batteries are working.
- Have the proper fire extinguishers ready in case of fire (Figure 4.6).

Prevent Intruders

- Close blinds and drapes whenever you are away and in the evening when you are home. Remove large bushes and obstructions from around your windows and doors so that anyone lurking outside will be visible.
- Install dead-bolt locks on all doors and locks on windows. Put a peephole in the main entryway to your home, and do not let anyone in without checking.
- If you have a screen door, lock it. If an unfamiliar visitor comes to the door, this door can serve as a barrier.
- Install a home alarm system.
- Rent apartments that require a security code or clearance to gain entry, and do not distribute that code to friends or delivery people.
- Avoid apartments that are easily accessible, such as first-floor units with large patio doors.
- Don't give information about your home or schedule to telephone solicitors. Try to vary the times of day that you come home for lunch or run errands.
- Don't let repairmen in without identification. Preferably, landlords should inform you about such visits well in advance. Have someone else with you when repairmen are there working. Just because a person is licensed to fix refrigerators does not mean he can be trusted.

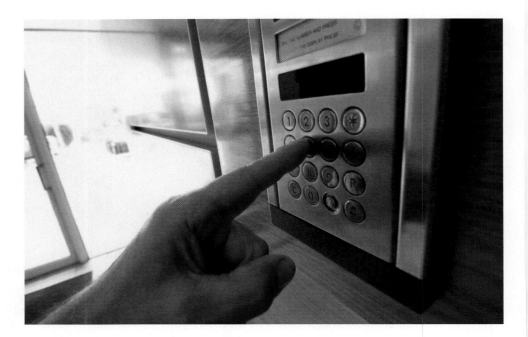

Security systems that control access can make dormitories and apartment buildings safer, but are not a substitute for other precautions.

- Avoid dark parking structures, laundry rooms, and the like. Try to use these areas only when others are around.
- Use initials for first names on mailboxes and in phone listings. Keep your address out of phone books.
- Keep a cell phone near your bed, and program it to 911. Unlike what you see on TV, many intruders do not cut phone lines. More often, they simply pick up the receiver in another room as they walk through, thereby disabling a bedroom phone.
- Get to know your neighbors. Organize a neighborhood watch.
- Be careful of "doggy doors." Some thieves let their smallest associate crawl through and unlock the door.
- Be careful of skylights and other areas that open from the outside. Keep them locked and bolted.
- When away, put the lights in different rooms on timers set to come on and go off at different times. Stop your mail and newspaper deliveries.

Although no amount of security will prevent all threats of intrusion, following these precautions, as well as actively searching for well-maintained housing in low-crime areas, are good steps toward preventing break-ins. Usually intruders are searching for items to sell and enter with theft in mind. If you encounter an intruder, it is far better to give up your money than to fight.

Workplace Safety

American adults spend most of their waking hours on the job. While most job situations are pleasant and productive, others pose physical and emotional hazards. Stress, burnout, hostile or abusive interactions with others, discrimination,

What do you think?

Do a "spot check" of your home. What areas might pose a risk for home accidents or forced entry? ■ *Do you know the numbers of your local fire and police departments?* ■ *Do you have a fire extinguisher in your house? Do you know how to use it?* ■ *What would you do if the house caught on fire and you needed to escape immediately?*

power struggles, sexual harassment, and a host of other threats are possible whenever people are cloistered together for prolonged periods of time. The nature of the job itself, the corporate culture, and the policies and procedures that characterize certain professions can add to workplace stress.

Fatal Injuries Certain industries are inherently more hazardous than others; outdoor occupations show the highest fatality and injury rates. Although workplaces have instituted programs and services to reduce risks, the following statistics indicate a continuing problem:[86]

- In 1999, job-related fatalities reached their highest levels since recordkeeping began. Rates have decreased slightly since then but continue to surpass most previous fatality reports. In 2002, 5,524 people lost their lives at work.
- Highway crashes were the leading cause of on-the-job fatalities and accounted for over 25 percent of fatal work injury totals in 2002. Most involved truck drivers.
- Sixteen percent of worker fatalities resulted from other types of transportation-related incidents, such as tractors

and forklifts overturning in fields or warehouses, workers being struck by vehicles, aircraft and railway crashes, and water vehicles crashing or capsizing.

- Workplace homicides have declined in recent years but continue to be a major cause of workplace danger; over 600 people were murdered at work in 2002. Cashiers and managers of food and lodging establishments accounted for the majority of victims. Disputes with coworkers or former coworkers and shootings during the course of robbery were the most common situations leading to deaths. Homicides also occur at workplaces as a carryover of domestic violence, when a violent spouse or partner comes to seek revenge.
- Falls, being struck by objects, and electrocutions are also significant causes of worker fatality, accounting for 13 percent of work-related deaths in 2002.
- On average, about 17 workers were fatally injured each day in 2002. Hundreds more were permanently or temporarily disabled. Overall, there were 1.4 million injuries that required time off work.
- Men between the ages of 35 and 54 are the most likely victims of fatal occupational injuries.

Nonfatal Work Injuries   Although deaths capture media attention, other workers may be seriously injured or disabled. Chronic, debilitating pain and other injuries can cause great economic strain on organizations due to workers' compensation claims and days lost from work. Injuries that cause the greatest number of lost-work days include carpal tunnel syndrome, hernia, amputation of a limb, fractures, sprains and strains (often of the back), cuts or lacerations, and chemical burns.[87] For example, nearly half of all workers with carpal tunnel syndrome miss 30 days or more of work each year. Because so many work injuries are due to repetitive motion, overexertion, or inappropriate motion, they are largely preventable through training and techniques designed to reduce employees' risks.

What do you think?

What can be done to prevent injuries? ▪ *Are students on your campus at risk from any of the problems discussed?* ▪ *Does your school have programs in place to prevent injuries?* ▪ *Do you think more can be done, and if so, what?*

TAKING CHARGE

MAKE IT HAPPEN!

Assessment: The Assess Yourself box on page 114 gave you a chance to think about symptoms of abuse. If any of the symptoms describe a relationship you or someone you know is experiencing, you should consider taking action.

Making a Change: To change your behavior, you need to develop a plan. Follow these steps.

1. Evaluate your behavior and identify patterns. What can you change now? What can you change in the near future?
2. Select one pattern of behavior that you want to change.
3. Fill out a Behavior Change Contract. It should include your long-term goal for change, your short-term goals, the rewards for reaching these goals, potential obstacles along the way, and strategies for overcoming these obstacles. For each goal, list the small steps and specific actions that you will take.

4. Chart your progress in a journal. At the end of a week, consider how successful you were in following your plan. What helped you be successful? What will you do differently next week?
5. Revise your plan as needed. Are the short-term goals attainable? Are the rewards satisfying?

One Student's Plan: Sondra thought that her roommate Jessie was experiencing several symptoms of abuse. Jessie's boyfriend Carl sometimes belittled her in front of her friends. He broke Jessie's cell phone by throwing it against a wall next to her and seemed resentful when she spent time with anyone but him. Sondra talked to Jessie about her perceptions, and Jessie agreed that she sometimes was afraid of Carl's actions. As a first step, Sondra helped Jessie make immediate appointments at the school counseling center, one for herself and one for her and Carl together.

Summary

- Intentional injuries result from actions committed with intent to harm. Unintentional injuries are the result of actions involving no intent to harm. Violence is at epidemic levels in the United States. Many factors lead people to be violent. Among them are anger, substance abuse, and root causes of oppression, poor mental health, and economics.

- Acts of terrorism are becoming more common in the United States. In addition to their immediate impact, terrorist activities can exert damaging long-term effects by fostering an atmosphere of fear and anxiety.

- Violence affects everyone in society—from the direct victims, to those who live in fear, to those who pay higher taxes and insurance premiums. Over half of homicides are committed by people who know their victims. Bias and hate crimes divide people, but teaching tolerance can reduce risks. Gang violence continues to grow but can be

combated by programs that reduce the problems that lead to gang membership. Violence on campus may be increasing, but victims' rights have also increased as a result of major legislation.

- Prevention of violent acts begins with avoiding potentially dangerous situations. There are several avenues available for reducing risks, including community, school, workplace, and individual strategies. Many crimes of general society are now commonplace at universities and colleges, including personal assaults, harassment, hate crimes, and even murder.

- Unintentional injuries frequently occur in homes and worksites and can produce serious consequences, including death. By following commonsense guidelines, you can significantly reduce your risk of falls, burns, and other injuries.

Questions for Discussion and Reflection

1. What major types of crimes are committed in the United States? What is the difference between primary and reactive aggression?
2. What major factors lead to violent acts?
3. Who tends to be susceptible to the appeal of gang membership? What actions can be taken to keep kids out of gangs?
4. What is terrorism, and why does it occur? What can you do to protect yourself against terrorist attacks?
5. Compare domestic violence against men and against women: What are the differences and similarities? What causes domestic violence?
6. What conditions put a child at risk for abuse? What can be done to prevent or decrease child abuse?
7. What is sexual harassment, and what factors contribute to it in the workplace? On campus?
8. What factors increase risk for sexual assault?
9. What are the most effective violence prevention strategies on your campus?
10. What steps can you take to lower your risk of accidental injuries?

Accessing Your Health on the Internet

Visit the following Internet sites to explore further topics and issues related to personal health. To visit an organization's website, go to the Companion Website for *Access to Health, Ninth Edition* at www.aw-bc.com/donatelle, click on the book image, and select "Accessing Your Health on the Internet" from the navigation menu.

1. ***American College Counseling Association.*** Provides useful information on a variety of violence issues facing college students.
2. ***Communities Against Violence Network.*** An extensive, searchable database for information about violence against women, with articles about everything from domestic violence to legal information and statistics.
3. ***Crimes on College Campuses.*** Comprehensive source of information and statistics on colleges and universities across America.
4. ***National Center for Injury Prevention and Control.*** The WISQARS database of this CDC section provides sta-

tistics and information on fatal and nonfatal injuries, both intentional and unintentional.

5. ***National Center for Victims of Crime.*** Provides information and resources for victims of crimes ranging from hate crimes to sexual assault. Its "Get Help" series provides information on a wide range of crime victim topics, from bullying and harassment to identity theft.
6. ***National Institute for Occupational Safety and Health (NIOSH).*** Excellent reference for national statistics on injury and violence, in both the community and the workplace.
7. ***Washington Votes.*** This nonpartisan organization allows you to research your senator and congressional representative's votes on 50 issues, including criminal law and firearms.
8. ***Workplace Solutions.*** Provides information that helps promote well-being by helping people understand the nature of interpersonal conflict, stress, and violence at work.

Further Reading

Hoffman, A., J. Schuh, and R. Fenske. *Violence on Campus.* Gaithersburg, MD: Aspen, 1998.

Overview of violence on campus, unique factors that lead to violence and abuse on college campuses, and current programs and policies designed to reduce risk.

Ottens, A. and K. Hotelling (eds.). *Sexual Violence on Campus: Policies, Programs, and Perspectives.* New York: Springer Publishing, 2001.

Overview of trends, causes, and contributors to violence on campus, as well as policies and programs designed to prevent violence.

U.S. Department of Health and Human Services. "Inventory of Federal Data Systems for Injury, Surveillance, Research and Prevention Activities." Washington, DC: Government Printing Office, 2001.

Excellent reference for data, reporting mechanisms, and instruments used in assessing U.S. violence statistics.

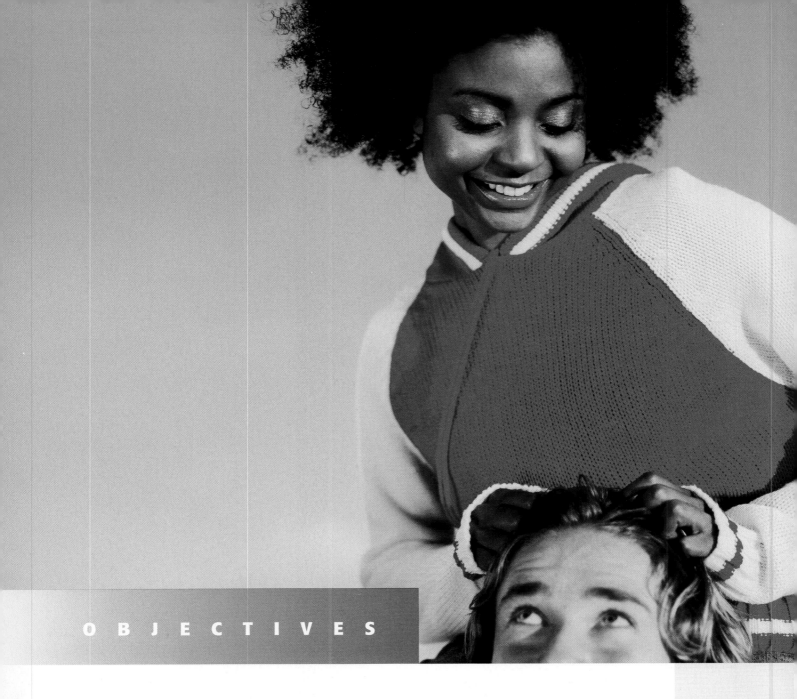

OBJECTIVES

- Discuss ways to improve communication skills and interpersonal interactions.

- Explain the characteristics of intimate relationships and how to maintain them effectively.

- Discuss similarities and differences between men and women in communication styles and in how they make decisions.

- Discuss the barriers to intimate relationships and factors that inhibit successful communication. Explain how these barriers can be overcome.

- Discuss the importance of commitment, honesty, and mutual respect in relationships.

- Examine factors that are important in determining the success of an intimate relationship.

- Discuss factors that affect life decisions, such as whether to remain single and whether to have children.

- Describe signs of relationship decline and where to get help with relationship problems.

- Discuss actions that can improve interpersonal interactions.

HEALTHY RELATIONSHIPS

COMMUNICATING EFFECTIVELY WITH FRIENDS, FAMILY, AND SIGNIFICANT OTHERS

IN THE NEWS

For Younger Latinas, a Shift to Smaller Families

By Mireya Navarro

Rocío Yñiguez grew up in a family of seven children in Jalisco, Mexico. She remembers how friends of her parents proudly displayed a clock in their living room with a picture of each of their 12 children, a son or daughter for every hour.

Ms. Yñiguez, 35, a department store cashier who now lives in Redwood City in the San Francisco Bay Area, said she could not imagine having more than the three children she has, not if she wants to educate them and ferry them to soccer games, dance lessons and play dates. And she does not want to diverge from the goal that brought her to this country.

"You need to work to get ahead, and with children it's too hard," she said.

Her decision to stop at three has made her part of a trend that is catching some demographers by surprise.

Latina women are choosing to have smaller families, in some cases resisting the social pressures that shaped the Hispanic tradition of big families.

Read the complete article online in the eThemes section of this book's website: www.aw-bc.com/donatelle.

Original article published December 5, 2004. Copyright © 2004 The *New York Times*. Reprinted with permission.

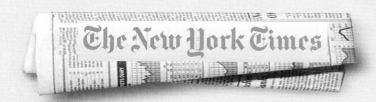

Humans are social animals—we have a basic need to fit in to a human "pack," to feel loved and appreciated by others. We thrive in environments where we feel secure, needed, and respected; particularly if we are cared about by people who really matter to us. Although we can exist without these close interactions, our lives are enhanced and our days are more fulfilling when we can share our successes and failures with others. In fact, a study done by researchers at the Harvard School of Public Health shows that the ability to relate well with people throughout your life can have almost as much impact on your health as exercise and good nutrition.[1]

All relationships involve a degree of risk. Only by taking these risks, however, can we grow and truly experience all that life has to offer. In this chapter, we examine healthy relationships and the communication skills necessary to create and maintain them. Why is communication so important? For one thing, the way we communicate influences whether or not we are accepted by others. For another, most of us sincerely want to express ourselves clearly and honestly in our relationships. Clear communication can help us bridge our differences, and it can also affect health. Several studies point to links between the inability to identify and communicate feelings and increased health risks. For example, an ongoing study of 2,500 Finnish men, aged 42 to 60, has found that the "stoic personality" may in fact promote dramatic increases in mortality. Many other studies have linked suppressed emotions with health problems such as hypertension and inflammatory bowel disease.[2] (See the New Horizons in Health box for more research into this connection.)

Expressing ourselves well and knowing how to understand what others are saying are both vitally important to communication. These abilities lay the groundwork for healthy relationships, and satisfying relationships are significant factors in overall health.

The Communication Process: Getting Started

Many of us find it difficult to tell people what we really think or to express how we feel. We constantly worry about making people angry, hurting their feelings, being misinterpreted, saying too much, or not saying enough. You may have communication problems with friends, family, lovers, coworkers, professors, or others, and this is nothing new. Humans have found communication to be difficult ever since people began living together and forming common bonds. Some of this difficulty stems from our individual communication styles. Some of it comes from technology that allows us to whip

---

Communication The transmission of information and meaning from one individual to another.

---

expletives over the Internet whenever we feel the need—and some of it stems from the fact that learning to communicate effectively is something that never comes easily, even to those who consciously work at it.

Much of our communication difficulty is inherent in the complexity of language itself. As our nation becomes more diverse, numerous languages, dialects, and vocal inflections make understanding each other more difficult. If you were raised in northern Wisconsin, you may not only have a different accent than individuals from Texas or Massachusetts; you may find that you express yourself in a different manner overall, have different gestures and facial expressions, have a different speed and manner of speaking, and that certain words may sound downright odd. Even a simple word or gesture can cause confusion, send mixed messages, and create misunderstanding. When there are no eyes to look into or no body language to interpret, as with e-mail communication, it is no wonder that we can quickly take offense, get frustrated, or misinterpret what others are saying.

Problems arise when we assume that others mean the same thing that we mean when we say certain words. Your friend's definition of *love* may be very different than what it means to you, and if the two of you are saying it and meaning two different things, the result may be disastrous. To someone raised in a home where yelling and angry outbursts are common occurrences that are quickly forgotten, a small raising of the voice or cursing on the phone may mean very little. To someone raised in an environment where peace and even-tempered discussions prevail, loud outbursts may be difficult to comprehend or downright offensive. Awareness of the subtleties of language and the ways in which we react to various life situations, both verbally or nonverbally, is an important aspect of the communication process.

Different cultures, too, not only have different languages and dialects, but also different ways of expressing themselves and using body language.[3] Some cultures gesture wildly; others maintain a closed and rigid manner of speaking. Some cultures are offended by apparent "fixed and dilated" staring; others welcome a steady look in the eyes.

This doesn't mean that one sex, culture, or group is better at communicating or should be a model for the others. It does mean that we have to be willing to accept differences and work to keep communication lines open and fluid. Remaining interested, actively engaged in the interaction, and open and willing to exchange ideas is something that we typically learn with practice and hard work.

Symbolism in Communication

How often have you heard someone say "We just can't communicate" or "You're sending me mixed messages"? These exchanges occur regularly as people struggle to solve a problem, learn a new skill, start a relationship, or work through difficulties in an existing relationship.[4] Whereas people typically use the word **communication** to mean "talking and listening, sending messages with words or your body,"

Can Positive Relationships Improve Physical Health?

Although it has been well documented that positive relationships and a strong social support network can enhance emotional and social health, research supporting the role of these positive interactions in enhancing physical health has emerged much more slowly. In the late 1990s some of the first studies appeared that supported the theory that certain relationship characteristics served as protective functions against illnesses. Characteristics that have been shown to increase the risk of disease and illness include a lack of social support, hostility, criticism, and blame within the family, family perfectionism and rigidity, and the presence of psychopathology. Some

examples of the research supporting this connection include:

- An unhappy marriage can increase the likelihood that you will become ill by 35 percent and shorten your life an average of four years.
- Children growing up in distressed marriages tend to have higher levels of chronic stress, resulting in increased physical illnesses.
- Stressful marital interactions lead to an increase in cardiovascular reactivity, which increases the risk of chronic heart disease and premature mortality.
- People who experience undefined organic seizure are more likely to have grown up in a family that had difficulty defining family roles and that had dysfunctional communication patterns.
- Lack of strong social support and interpersonal relationships increases risk for conditions such as heart disease.

- Women who are not close to their extended families and have little sense of family heritage are more likely to take sexual risks that lead to contracting sexually transmitted infections (STIs) and HIV.

In Jennifer Holmes' summary of this research, such findings provide "a very strong argument for supporting individuals, families, and communities through preventative psychosocial education programs (teaching people relationship skills, how to take care of themselves, and how to take care of their loved ones) to improve their relationships and in turn increase their chances for remaining physically healthy."

Source: J. Holmes, "Healthy Relationships: Their Influence on Physical Health," BC Council for Families, July 2004, www.bccf.bc.ca/learn/health_relations.html

communication experts tend to describe this act as "the symbolic process of shared meanings."[5] Symbols transmit messages and represent people, events, places, or objects. Words or verbal expressions, facial expressions, vocal tone, eye contact, gestures, movement, body posture, appearance, context, and spatial distance all reflect various communication symbols. Gifts, food, cards, e-mails, and other objects are also forms of symbolic communication. The multiplicity of symbolic gestures and ways of interpreting them can make communication a challenge. Sometimes we think we are saying something quite clearly, but even an attentive listener may misunderstand the symbols we use and thus our meaning.

Because communication is a process, our every action, word, and other symbols become part of our history with others—part of the evolving impression we make. If we are nasty and hostile with someone, even for a short period of time, those messages form a permanent part of our shared history. Each time we interact and communicate, this history evolves, for better or for worse. This is complicated by the fact that each person brings emotional "baggage" (both good and bad) from the past into an interaction. For example, a person who has become cynical and distrustful may be critical and guarded during interactions with others. Our interpretations of communication also become part of shared

history, and interpretation can be tricky. If someone says, "I love you," it may mean friendship, the love shared by family members, or the passion reserved for a deep and intimate relationship. Knowing how to seek clarification, ask for what you want, and interpret words in the context of the situation are critical skills.

How Perception Affects Communication

Perception is the process by which people filter and interpret information from the senses in order to create a meaningful picture of the world.[6] It is the lens through which we view the world. Gender, culture, educational level, family behaviors, and a host of other factors influence this view. Important factors that affect your perceptions, and therefore your communication effectiveness, include the way you define yourself (*self-concept*) and the way you evaluate yourself (*self-esteem*). Your self-concept is like a mental mirror that reflects how you view your physical features, emotional states, talents, likes and dislikes, values, and roles.[7] Are you a student, a mother, an honors student, a Democrat, a pianist? How you define

Perception The process of filtering and interpreting information gathered through the senses.

yourself is your self-concept. How you feel about yourself or evaluate yourself constitutes your self-esteem. You might consider yourself an excellent student, a horrible singer, a great lover, or a "10" in terms of appearance—such judgments indicate your level of self-esteem or self-evaluation.

Self-perceptions influence communication choices. If you feel unattractive, uncomfortable, or inferior to others, you may choose not to interact with them or to avoid social events. If you feel self-conscious and ill at ease around people who seem different, you might avoid or feel suspicious of them. Conversely, if you feel secure about your unique characteristics and talents, that positive self-concept will make it easier to interact with a variety of people in a healthy, balanced way.

What do you think?

Take a few minutes to identify who you are, using characteristics that describe the following:

- *Your moods or feelings*
- *Your appearance and physical condition*
- *Your social traits*
- *The talents you possess or lack*
- *Your intellectual capacity*
- *Your strong beliefs or philosophies*
- *Your social roles*
- *Your economic status*
- *Your "fit" in society and with friends*
- *Your capacity for giving and receiving love*

Write your responses, then ask someone you know well and trust to write their evaluation of you using the same questions. ■ *Do your observations match?*

Improving Your Communication Skills

All of us can learn to be better communicators. This lifelong process involves several challenges. We can start by learning how to share information through self-disclosure. This form of sharing will allow others to better understand us. Likewise, we can work at becoming better listeners—a critical skill for starting or maintaining any relationship. A third skill involves understanding nonverbal communication—both how we convey nonverbal messages and how others use their bodies and facial expressions to convey information. Through understanding how to deliver and interpret information, we can enhance the relationships in our lives. In order to have

Self-disclosure The process of revealing one's inner thoughts, feelings, and beliefs to another person.

healthy interactions with others and keep stress levels under control, it is important to deal with problems as early as possible. Learning communication skills that quickly resolve fights and misunderstandings can reduce unnecessary stress and lead to happier, more productive relationships.

Learning Appropriate Self-Disclosure

Self-disclosure is the sharing of personal information with others. If you are willing to share personal information with others, they will likely share personal information with you. In other words, if you want to learn more about someone, you have to be willing to share parts of your personal self with that person. Self-disclosure is not storytelling or sharing secrets; rather, it is revealing how you are reacting to the present situation and giving any information about the past that is relevant to the other person's understanding of your current reactions.[8]

Self-disclosure can be a double-edged sword, for there is risk in divulging personal insights and feelings. If you sense that sharing feelings and personal thoughts will result in a closer relationship, you will likely take such a risk. On the other hand, if you believe that the disclosure may result in rejection or alienation, you may not open up so easily. If the confidentiality of previously shared information has been violated, you may hesitate to disclose yourself in the future.

However, the risk in not disclosing yourself to others is that you will lack close relationships. Psychologist Carl Rogers stressed the importance of understanding yourself and others through self-disclosure. Rogers believed that weak relationships were characterized by inhibited self-disclosure.[9]

If self-disclosure is a key element in creating healthy communication, but fear is a barrier to that process, what can we do? The following suggestions can help:

- *Get to know yourself.* Remember that your self includes your feelings, beliefs, thoughts, and concerns. The more you know about yourself, the more likely it is that you will be able to communicate with others about yourself. Think about who you are, what you are passionate about, and your strengths and limitations. Which of these do you feel good about? Which cause you concern?
- *Become more accepting of yourself.* No one is perfect or has to be. Even the people you look up to have their flaws. Only by accepting your imperfections can you expect others to accept them, too.
- *Be willing to discuss your sexual history.* In a culture that puts many taboos on discussions of sex in everyday conversation, it's no wonder we find it hard to disclose our sexual feelings to those with whom we are intimate. However, with the soaring rate of sexually transmitted infections and the ever-looming threat of AIDS, there has never been a more important time to disclose sexual feelings and history. The life-altering effects of an unwanted pregnancy or contracting the HIV virus underscore the need to communicate about sex *before* you become intimate.

- *Choose a safe context for self-disclosure.* Context refers to the setting in which the self-disclosure occurs. When and where you make such disclosures and to whom may greatly influence the response. Choose a setting in which you feel safe to let yourself be known.

Being a Better Listener

Listening is a vital part of interpersonal communication; it allows us to share feelings, express concerns, communicate wants and needs, and let our thoughts and opinions be known. We must do the necessary work to improve both our speaking and listening skills, which will enhance our relationships, improve our grasp of information, and allow us to interpret more effectively what others say. We listen best when (1) we believe that the message is somehow important and relevant to us, (2) the speaker holds our attention through humor, dramatic effect, use of the media, or other techniques, and (3) we are in the mood to listen (free of distractions and worries).

When we really listen effectively, we try to understand what people are thinking and feeling from their perspective. We not only hear the words, but we try to understand what is really being said. How many times have you been caught pretending to be listening when you were not? After several moments of nodding and saying "uh-huh" your friend finally asks you a question, and you haven't a clue about what she has been saying. Sometimes this tuned-out behavior is due to a lack of sleep, stress overload, being preoccupied, having too much to drink, or being under the influence of drugs. Other times it's because speakers are motor-mouths who talk for the sake of talking or because you find them or what they are talking about is boring. Some of the most common listening difficulties are things that we can work to improve:[10]

- Being so interested in what you are going to say that you listen mainly to find an opening to get the floor
- Nodding your head vigorously or gesturing with every word that is said, displaying an obvious anxiousness to get "in" the conversation
- Mentally formulating a rebuttal to what is being said rather than really listening

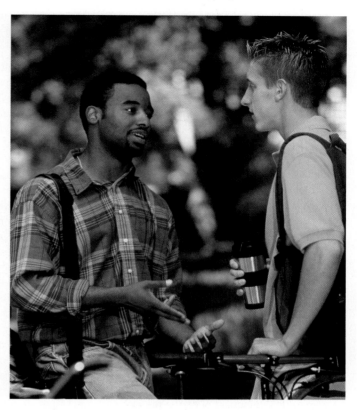

"The better part of one's life consists of his friendships."
—Abraham Lincoln

- Evaluating or making judgments about the speaker or the message
- Not asking for clarification when there are things that you are unclear about
- Being frustrated because the other person is speaking in limited English or in another language
- Being so biased or emotional about your opinion that you are thinking of a counterargument the entire time the other person is speaking
- Engaging in side conversations with others while someone is speaking

Other external factors or things about the speaker that may make listening difficult and that could be improved include:

- Speaker speaks too fast or jumps from point to point
- Speaker speaks too loudly or too quietly
- External noise, commotion around you, or distractions
- Bad phone connections
- Lack of familiarity with a language or dialect

See the Skills for Behavior Change box on page 134 for suggestions for improving your listening.

The Three Basic Listening Modes There are three main ways in which we listen. Knowing when to use each of these

Learning to Really Listen

Most of us have lamented the fact that someone "never listens" and seems to monopolize the entire conversation. Although we are quick to recognize such flaws in others, we are often less likely to spot listening problems of our own. On a daily basis, we all have times when we just tune out. When a professor drones on about a subject we don't relate to, we begin doodling or put on a fake interested facial expression, even though we are thinking about dinner or what to wear to the movies that night. When that boring friend tells the same story over and over again, we say "uh-huh," "yes," and worry that we'll be caught when he asks a question and we don't have a clue what he is talking about. We grimace at the thought of certain people calling but dash for the phone when the caller ID indicates that it is someone we love to talk with. What is the difference? Why do we tune out when some people speak and tune in for others?

We gravitate toward those who seem to understand us and with whom we have fun and interesting interactions. If the truth be told, most of us are only mediocre listeners. What does it take to be an excellent listener? Practicing the following skills and consciously using them on a daily basis is an important part of improved communication.

- *Be present in the moment.* Contrary to what is often believed, good listeners don't just sit back with their mouths shut. They participate and acknowledge what the other person is saying. (Nodding, smiling, saying "yes" or "uh-huh," and asking questions at appropriate times are all part of this. Take care, however, not to numbly say "uh-huh" to every word, which is distracting and conveys insincerity.)

- *Use positive body language and voice tone.* Show that you are "with" the speaker by turning toward him or her and staying focused (wandering eyeballs are a sure sign that your mind is elsewhere). Avoid barrier gestures such as shaking your head "no," making negative faces, or folding your arms across your chest or stomach; smile at appropriate times and maintain appropriate eye contact (deadpan stares can also be distracting). Voice tone, posture, and an attitude that conveys interest are all key.

- *Show empathy and sympathy.* Watching for verbal and nonverbal clues to the other person's feelings and trying to relate can be very useful. For example, saying, "That must have been really hard for you" can encourage the speaker to talk and feel more comfortable with you as an understanding listener.

- *Ask for clarification.* If you aren't sure what the speaker means, indicate that you're not sure you understand, or paraphrase what you think you heard. This kind of feedback is invaluable in avoiding misinterpretation and lapses in overall communication. As a speaker, you may ask, "What did you think I was just saying?," but be sure to say this in a nonthreatening manner.

- *Control that deadly desire to interrupt.* Some people start nodding and gesturing before you ever get a word out of your mouth. If you are like that, squelch it, even if you have to put an inconspicuous hand over your mouth. Try taking a deep breath for two seconds, then hold your breath for another second and really listen to what is being said as you slowly exhale. Don't be so enthusiastically empathetic that you finish speakers' sentences or put words in people's mouths.

- *Avoid snap judgments based on what other people look like or are saying.* If you notice some strange mannerism, try to focus on what is being said, not how it is being said. Avoid stereotyping or labeling.

- *Resist the temptation to "set the other person straight."* Control your urge to correct errors or react defensively. Listen and hear without reacting or trying to rationalize what the speaker is trying to say.

- *Try to focus on the speaker.* Sometimes it is very tough to listen to someone who is trying to talk about a painful situation, especially if we are experiencing or have recently experienced the same thing. Hold back the temptation to "tell all" and fly off into your own rendition of a similar situation. Give the speaker the moment and later, after he or she is done talking, you may want to discuss your own experience as a way of validating the feelings expressed. Don't tell him how he is feeling or how he should feel.

- *Be tenacious.* Stick with the speaker and try to stay on the topic. If they seem to wander, gently nudge them back by saying, "You were just saying . . ." Offer your thoughts and suggestions, but remember that you should only advise up to a certain point. Clarify statements with "this is my opinion" as a reminder that it is only opinion, rather than fact.

will enhance the way in which you listen and improve the outcome.

1. *Competitive,* or *combative, listening* happens when we are more interested in promoting our own point of view than in understanding or exploring someone else's view. We listen either for openings to take the floor or for flaws and weak points that we can attack. Looking at your watch, sighing, nodding vigorously, staring into space, or other actions are meant to put speakers in their place or cause them to relinquish the floor.

2. *Passive,* or *attentive, listening* occurs when we are genuinely interested in hearing and understanding the other person's point of view. By being attentive and passively listening, we encourage further discussion. We assume that we heard and understand correctly, but we stay passive and don't verify it.

3. *Active,* or *reflective, listening* is the single most useful and important listening skill. In active listening, we are also genuinely interested in understanding what the other person is thinking, feeling, and wanting in addition to what the message means, and we are active in checking out our understanding before we respond with our own new message. We restate or paraphrase our understanding of the other person's meaning and reflect it back to the sender for verification. This verification or feedback process is what distinguishes active listening and makes it effective.[11]

Benefits of Active Listening The most obvious benefit of active listening is that it reduces the risk of misunderstanding or, if a misunderstanding does occur, makes it immediately apparent. Other benefits include:[12]

- Sometimes people just need to be heard and acknowledged before they are willing to consider an alternative or soften their position.
- It is often easier for people to listen to and consider the other's position when they know the other person is listening to and considering theirs.
- It helps people spot the flaws in their reasoning when they hear it played back without criticism.
- Active listening helps identify areas of agreement so that the areas of disagreement are put into perspective and diminished rather than magnified.
- Reflecting back what we hear each other say makes each of us aware of the different levels of communication that are going on below the surface. This helps to bring issues into the open, where they can be resolved more readily.
- If we listen and try to understand other people's point of view, we can more effectively help them see the flaws in their position or discover the flaws in our own reasoning.

What do you think?

Think about a topic that you and a friend have been disagreeing about. Ask him or her to take some time to discuss it. Discuss your feelings about what has happened in past conversations and what each of you would need to have happen to come to an agreement. Also talk about your hopes and expectations. Try having another discussion about this topic and use active listening and the strategies listed above and in the Skills for Behavior Change box.

Using Nonverbal Communication

Understanding what someone is saying often involves much more than listening and speaking. Often, what is *not* actually said may speak louder than any words. Rolling the eyes, looking at the floor or ceiling rather than maintaining eye contact, body movements, hand gestures—all these nonverbal clues influence the way we interpret messages.[13] Researchers have found that an astounding 93 percent of the meaning of a message comes from nonverbal cues![14]

Nonverbal communication includes all unwritten and unspoken messages, both intentional and unintentional. Because expressions and actions can mean so many different things and be interpreted in so many ways, it is easy to be confused by nonverbal messages. This confusion increases when what a person says seems to contradict what he or she does. How would you interpret the following?

- Edie assures Becky that she loves her spaghetti sauce, yet only picks at it and leaves most of it on her plate.
- Brent tells Nicole that he loves her deeply, but whenever they go out, he constantly watches other women and acts detached and uninterested in Nicole.
- Heather tells Joselyn that she has forgiven her for gossiping about her, yet she avoids Joselyn on campus and does not look at her when Joselyn speaks to her.

In most cases, when differences exist between what is being said and what is being done, people tend to agree with the old saying "Actions speak louder than words." Effective communicators learn to observe nonverbal cues and carefully differentiate between what someone is saying and what is really being said.

Expressing Difficult Feelings

How many times have you struggled to find just the right words in an emotionally charged situation? Imagine that Sarah has been dating Charles and, while she feels he is a great person, he is not the one she wants to date exclusively. She wants to tell him that she likes him a lot, but she is not in love with him. Like most people, Sarah finds it difficult to express her feelings in a way that is not hurtful to another person. Professionals offer the following guidelines for expressing feelings:[15]

- *Try to be specific rather than general about how you feel.* Consistently using only one or two words to say how you are feeling, such as *unhappy* or *upset,* is too vague. Explain what you mean by *upset:* irritated, agitated, mad, anxious, uncomfortable, angry, frightened, bothered?

Nonverbal communication All unwritten and unspoken messages, both intentional and unintentional.

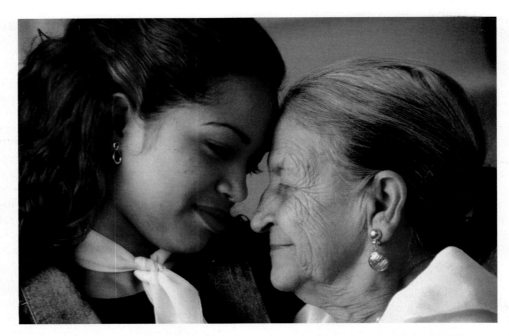

The emotional bonds that characterize intimate relationships often span the generations and help individuals gain insight and understanding into each other's worlds.

- *Specify the degree of feelings, and you will reduce the chances of being misunderstood.* When you say *angry*, someone may think you are enraged when you are just a bit irritated.
- *When expressing anger or irritation, first describe the specific behavior you don't like, then your feelings.* The other person may become immediately defensive or intimidated when he or she first hears "I am angry with you" and could miss the message.
- *If you have mixed feelings, say so; express each feeling, and explain what each feeling is about.* For example: "I really like your sense of humor and your values, but I don't feel comfortable around you 24–7." "I am thankful that I met you and we can be friends, but I don't have the depth of feeling that I think needs to be there for a relationship. We just are too different."

In general, the most tried and true techniques for expressing your feelings involve using **"I" messages** that include feelings like those stated above, rather than "you" statements that imply blame or something that the other person did wrong. "I" messages ("I like being with you"; "I'm sorry that I missed practice") are a direct, clear, and effective way to send information to others. When using "I" messages, the speaker takes responsibility for communicating his or her

own feelings, thoughts, and beliefs. People who practice using "I" messages tend to have more positive interactions and generate less defensiveness from listeners.

The opposite of an "I" message is a "you" message. "You" messages are easy to distinguish because they begin with the communicator saying "you" ("You made me so mad"; "You never say you're sorry about anything"). "You" messages put the receiver of the information on the defensive and ready to attack. Consider this of "I" and "you" messages: Terry and Jim have been working together on a class project for most of the term. Although they are both supposed to contribute 50 percent to the final product, Jim has done very little work thus far. Terry is very angry, but rather than saying, "Jim, you're really lazy, and you are not holding up your part of this assignment," she says, "Jim, I really am feeling overburdened by all of the work I've been putting into this project. I don't want to feel 'used' in this process, and I want both of us to get as much out of the effort as we can." Because Terry is putting this discussion in terms of how she is feeling (using "I" messages) rather than attacking Jim with "you" statements that make him want to defend himself, they are more likely to communicate constructively. Jim is apt to get the message and start contributing to the project.

To practice using "I" messages, follow these steps:

1. *"When you . . ."* Start by thinking about a problem behavior or situation that you want to discuss. Choose something specific—not a vague, sweeping complaint such as "My roommate is such a slob, and he needs to change." Concentrate on a particular ("When you leave your clothes all over the floor . . .").

"I" messages Messages in which a person takes responsibility for communicating his or her own feelings, thoughts, and beliefs by using statements that begin with "I," not "you."

2. *"I feel . . ."* Identify how the behavior or incident makes you feel, and state those feelings by starting your sentence with "I." Adding a feeling statement allows you to share your reaction honestly without placing blame or exerting power ("I feel frustrated and angry").

3. *"Because . . ."* Add a statement to explain, from your perspective, why the feeling occurred (". . . because I spend so much time trying to keep the place looking good").

Now put these steps together into one simple sentence: "When you leave your clothes on the floor, I feel frustrated and angry because I spend so much time trying to keep the place looking good."

Communicating Assertively

Communicating assertively means using direct, honest communication that maintains and defends your rights in a positive manner. **Assertive communicators** are people who get their points across while at the same time respecting the rights of others. Assertiveness demands both verbal and nonverbal skills. Verbally, assertive communicators speak calmly, directly, and clearly to those around them. Nonverbally, they maintain direct eye contact, sit or stand facing the person they are speaking to, and sit or stand with an erect posture that indicates confidence and control.

Assertiveness is often distinguished from two other styles of communication that produce poor results: *nonassertiveness* and *aggressiveness*. **Nonassertive communicators** tend to be shy and inhibited. Verbally, nonassertive communicators may speak too rapidly, use a tone that is too low to be heard easily, or not say directly what's on their minds. Nonverbally, their body language frequently reveals timidity: their shoulders slump, they don't face the person they are talking to, or they avoid direct eye contact. Nonassertive people fear that if they really express how they feel, it will upset others. This fear leaves them without positive ways of communicating their needs and concerns. (See the Assess Yourself box on page 138.)

Aggressive communicators tend to employ an angry, confrontational, hostile manner in their interactions with others. Their communications are typically loud and verbally abusive, and they often blame others when things don't go their way. Someone who constantly uses "you" messages, causing the receiver of the information to feel on the defensive immediately, is usually an aggressive communicator.

What do you think?

How would you describe your communication style—nonassertive, assertive, or aggressive? ■ *Do you tend to use more "I" or "you" messages?* ■ *Should you alter your communication style in any way? If so, why?*

Establishing a Proper Climate

An open climate for communication does not simply happen. Although selecting a safe place and a trustworthy confidant are important, carefully consider your own role in establishing a supportive climate for conversation. If you follow these steps when you speak, the other person is more likely to engage in an open, honest conversation.[16]

- *Watch judgmental statements.* Words such as *stupid, ridiculous, great, crummy,* or *fantastic* show that an evaluation has already been made. Many of these judgmental statements leave no room for another opinion. Instead, use descriptive statements that reveal your feelings without labeling them as good, bad, right, or wrong. Say, "Your borrowing my car makes me very nervous," rather than, "You stupid jerk, you'll wreck my car and hurt yourself!"

- *Keep an open mind.* Since absolute statements tend to close off other opinions, thereby restricting communication, use qualifying statements to invite others to state their opinions. Say, "This may not always be true, depending on the circumstances," or, "I could be wrong, but it's what I think."

- *Avoid lecturing or projecting superiority.* If you really want someone's opinion, then respect it as having some value. As you learn to show respect for others' opinions, your own viewpoint will become more respected. Monitor your facial expressions, voice pitch and intonation, word choice, and actions to see whether they express true interest and respect.

- *Don't ask for feedback unless you want an honest answer.* How many times have you asked people what they thought, only to be hurt or angry when they told you? If you become visibly upset by honest feedback, people won't give it to you. Look at such feedback as an attempt to help. No one enjoys criticism, but you can't correct a negative action unless you are aware of it.

- *Avoid people who tend to give negative feedback.* Some people have such low self-esteem that they delight in criticizing others. Try to determine the underlying motives of such people, and then avoid them if possible.

Assertive communicators People who use direct, honest communication that maintains and defends their rights in a positive manner.

Nonassertive communicators Individuals who tend to be shy and inhibited in their communication with others.

Aggressive communicators People who use hostile, loud, and blaming communication styles.

Standing Up for Yourself

myhealthlab

Fill out this assessment online at www.aw-bc.com/myhealthlab or www.aw-bc.com/donatelle

You know that sinking feeling. Someone asks you to do something, and your stomach lurches. You don't want to go along, but you can't come up with a good excuse. It's hard to say no. How often are you caught in the "I can't say no" trap? Read the following situations and assess your responses according to the following 5-point scale:

	Never 1	Very seldom 2	Sometimes 3	Frequently 4	Always 5
1. Friends ask you to ride home with them after they've all been drinking. You know you shouldn't go, but you think one of them is cute, and you don't want to seem like a prude. You take the ride.	1	2	3	4	5
2. Your decisions can be easily swayed by a strong argument from someone else pushing you in the opposite direction.	1	2	3	4	5
3. You feel strongly about a political issue, but it is the opposite of the opinion your parents hold. You remain silent rather than getting into an argument.	1	2	3	4	5
4. You start out by saying no to something but get talked into doing it after a short time.	1	2	3	4	5
5. You're stressed out, with too much to do and too little time, but you can't seem to say no when someone asks for a favor.	1	2	3	4	5
6. Someone says something really nasty about someone you like. You jump to the defense of the person being criticized, even though you are in the minority opinion.	1	2	3	4	5
7. You would describe yourself as assertive and tend to quickly let others know your thoughts about certain issues.	1	2	3	4	5
8. Someone is critical of something you do. You quickly defend your actions by explaining why you did what you did.	1	2	3	4	5

INTERPRETING YOUR SCORE

Think about your responses to each statement. Do your responses indicate an assertive communication style in which you stand up for your feelings or beliefs? What factors cause you to hold back when you should probably speak up? How can you work to improve your communication behaviors in this area? For statements 1 to 5, do you have several "5" responses? If yes, you should consider what skills you could develop to help you communicate more assertively.

MAKE IT HAPPEN!

Use the results of this self-assessment to begin your behavior change program. Follow the steps and use the examples on page 157 to complete your Behavior Change Contract and use these resources to take action.

Conflict An emotional state that arises when the behavior of one person interferes with the behavior of another.

Managing Conflict

A **conflict** is an emotional state that arises when the behavior of one person interferes with the behavior of another. Conflict is inevitable whenever people live or work together. Not all conflict is bad; in fact, airing feelings and coming to some form of resolution over differences can sometimes strengthen strained relationships. **Conflict resolution** and successful conflict management are a systematic approach to resolving differences fairly and constructively, rather than allowing them to fester. The goal of conflict resolution is to solve differences peacefully and creatively.

Most conflicts revolve around two message components: content and relationship. *Content* is usually easy to discern, as it is the subject of the sentences used by the participants. It deals with the issues on the surface. *Relationship* is more difficult to discern because it embodies the interactions between the people involved and usually involves issues that are much more deeply rooted. Because of the double-pronged nature of messages, many arguments arise out of seemingly innocuous situations. For instance, a housemate comes home from the library, walks into the kitchen, and asks, "What's for dinner?" The other responds, "Whatever you make! When are you going to take care of yourself for once?" On the surface, the conflict may be about dinner, the content. From a relationship standpoint, however, one roommate feels used and underappreciated.

Prolonged conflict can destroy relationships unless the parties agree to resolve points of contention in a constructive manner. As two people learn to negotiate and compromise on their differences, the number and intensity of conflicts should diminish. Conflict resolution can therefore be a growth process as people learn to recognize problems and solutions based on past experience.

During a heated conflict, try to pause for a moment before responding, consider the possible impact of your comments or actions, and speak slowly and state your point positively and constructively. You can also dismiss yourself from the situation and walk away by saying something like "I can see we aren't going to resolve this right now. Let's save it for a time when we've both cooled off and can discuss this more calmly."

Rude or inconsiderate behavior usually develops in situations in which a person fails to recognize the feelings or rights of another. To avoid this type of behavior, try to see the other person's point of view, listen actively, avoid interrupting, and avoid making gestures, such as head-shaking or finger-pointing, that indicate disagreement. A key element of managing conflict successfully is to validate others' opinions and treat them as you would like to be treated. Maintain respect and concern for others' welfare at all times.

Here are some strategies for conflict resolution.[17]

1. *Focus on one topic at a time, and make other preoccupations clear,* such as in, "I may seem angry, but I had a bad day at school today and I'm really worried about my grades." This takes the heat off the other person.
2. *Stop the action and cool down before things get out of control.* One sign of major distress in a couple is escalating hostility, often in the form of nagging that provokes angry responses. The escalation seems unstoppable once it gets started. Never send an e-mail to someone when you are upset. E-mails make it very easy to misinterpret what

someone feels or intends. Talk in person: eye contact, gestures, and body language all speak louder than written words. (See the Reality Check box on page 140 for more on constructive e-mail use.)

3. *Be specific in your criticisms or praises.* Prevent small complaints that you may stew over. You could say, "When I see your clothes on the floor, I feel that you are not doing your share of the work in the house and I feel taken advantage of," instead of, "You're a slob."
4. *Learn to "edit" what you say before you say it* to avoid remarks that would be needlessly hurtful. For example, don't dredge up past events and old grudges during a fight. Don't bring up additional issues before you've resolved the one at hand.
5. *Think about possible solutions that involve compromises for both parties.* Do some brainstorming to discover options that work for both of you. Consider all the options first, then eliminate those that aren't acceptable to both of you. Be committed to change.
6. *Never think in terms of winning an argument.* Think instead of ways to prevent an argument from starting. By doing so, both parties win. Avoid becoming too invested in getting your way. Remember, your reality is not the only reality!

What do you think?

When you have conflicts, does the content of your language accurately represent what you want to convey? ■ *How could you improve your conflict resolution skills?*

Characterizing and Forming Intimate Relationships

Most people think of intimacy as two people having a loving, intense, often sexual, relationship in which there is a mutual desire for closeness, touching, and physical expression. However, in her book *The Dance of Intimacy*, Dr. Harriet Goldhor Lerner defines intimacy as "being who we are in a relationship and allowing the other person to be the same. An intimate relationship is one in which neither party silences or betrays the self and each party expresses strength and vulnerability, weakness and competence in a balanced way."[18] Thus, intimacy is less a physical state and has more to do with the mind, heart, and essence of those who share it. It may culminate in a physical way, but it is much more complex than the act of sexual intercourse or sexual expression.

Conflict resolution A concerted effort by all parties to resolve points in contention in a constructive manner.

Cybercommunication: Improving E-mail Communication and Making Safe Online Connections

Ten years ago, the thought of sharing intimate details with a faceless stranger in cyberspace would have been unthinkable. Today, such meetings may lead to excitement, intrigue, or "happy-ever-after" encounters. They may also lead to disappointment as the computer persona turns out to be a rather ordinary person in real life. Occasionally, they can even lead to victimization and death. In one case, a woman had been communicating daily with an online friend for several months. When her friend began to use increasingly vivid and kinky sexual references and seemed to know more about her than she wished, she became uncomfortable and tried to back off. She was relentlessly "stalked" on her home and work computers, and it became evident that her online stalker knew her address and much about her personal life. Eventually, she was found dead, the result of a vicious attack by the person she knew only via computer.

Though this incident is an extreme example of computer interactions gone wrong, it is important to remember that there are inherent risks in communicating with people you don't know in any traditional sense. Less seriously, but more commonly, misunderstandings caused by the nature of e-mail communication can lead to arguments, disagreements, or worse. Conversations held in real time over instant messaging (IM) or on e-mail lack the clues of eye contact, body language, and other helpful ways of conveying meaning, and can be land mines for both users and senders. Even worse, that nasty little retort that you typed and sent lasts forever, clearly visible for anyone as evidence of your emotional reactivity and/or irrational responses.

Remembering these key points of computerized communication may save you many hours of worry and frustration.

✔ Never give your real name or vital information (for example, credit card numbers or Social Security number) to a computer chat partner. Use a screen name only, and avoid giving information that could help chat partners home in on you personally.

✔ If conversations become suggestive, threatening, or make you uncomfortable in any way, terminate the session. Report such violations to your Internet service provider.

✔ Never arrange to meet strangers at your home or their homes. Pick a safe public meeting place, and bring a friend. Do not give specific identifying information until you know much more about the person. Keep information such as where you work out of initial conversations, except in generic terms.

✔ Think before you write. If you are tempted to write a flame (an expression of extreme emotion or opinion), use the 24-hour rule: write the e-mail and hold it for at least 24 hours. Getting your emotions out on paper is a cathartic exercise. When you reread the note when some time has passed, you are likely to think twice about sending it. It is almost al-ways better to talk face to face about emotional issues than over e-mail.

✔ When you receive an upsetting message, try to assume the good intentions of the other person. As with active listening, try to think about what the sender must have been feeling, what their motivation for writing was, and what they may want from you in your response.

✔ Don't overuse emoticons or audibles. It is usually better to talk about things in person rather than to send angry faces or insulting audibles. Emoticons only really work with people who know what they are and who also recognize their limitations.

✔ When it appears that the e-mail is getting tense or if you are unclear about meaning, don't just plunge in with a response using your own assumptions. Consider other alternatives such as a phone call or, better yet, a meeting to discuss any difficult areas or problems.

✔ When you are wrong or have made a mistake, promptly admit it. If you responded tersely or in anger, tell the recipient that you were really upset and apologize. Ask for a face-to-face meeting to discuss.

✔ Don't forward personal or confidential e-mails without asking for permission from the original sender.

✔ Don't invade your roommate's or partner's e-mail space. Treat this information as private and not for your eyes without permission.

✔ When you write an e-mail, keep it concise. Save lengthy personal missives for face-to-face conversation. Remember that once an e-mail is sent, it can't be taken back.

In fact, intimacy is sometimes described as an attitude; one that defines the quality of how two people relate to one another and their level of emotional and spiritual connectedness to each other in the times between lovemaking, as well as during lovemaking.

Experts in the field of interpersonal relationships define **intimate relationships** in terms of four characteristics: *behavioral interdependence, need fulfillment, emotional attachment,* and *emotional availability.* Each of these characteristics may be related to interactions with family, close friends, and romantic partners.[19]

Intimate relationships Relationships with family members, friends, and romantic partners, characterized by closeness and understanding.

Behavioral interdependence refers to the mutual impact that people have on each other as their lives and daily activities intertwine. What one person does influences what the other person wants to do and can do. Behavioral interdependence may become stronger over time to the point that each person would feel a great void if the other were gone.

Intimate relationships also fulfill psychological needs and so are a means of *need fulfillment*. Through relationships with others, we fulfill our needs for:

- *Intimacy,* someone with whom we can share our feelings freely
- *Social integration,* someone with whom we can share worries and concerns
- *Nurturance,* someone whom we can take care of and who will take care of us
- *Assistance,* someone to help us in times of need
- *Affirmation,* someone who will reassure us of our own worth and tell us that we matter

In rewarding, intimate relationships, partners and friends meet each other's needs. They disclose feelings, share confidences, and provide support and reassurance. Each person comes away feeling better for the interaction and validated by the other person.

In addition to behavioral interdependence and need fulfillment, intimate relationships involve strong bonds of *emotional attachment,* or feelings of love and attachment. *Emotional availability,* the ability to give to and receive from others emotionally without fear of being hurt or rejected, is the fourth characteristic of intimate relationships. At times, all of us may limit our emotional availability—for example, after a painful breakup we may decide not to jump into another relationship immediately. Holding back can offer time for introspection and healing as well as considering the "lessons learned." However, because of intense trauma, some people find it difficult ever to be fully available emotionally. This limits their ability to experience and enjoy intimate relationships.

In the early years of life, families provide the most significant relationships. Gradually, the circle widens to include friends, coworkers, and acquaintances. Ultimately, most of us develop romantic relationships with a significant other. Each of these relationships plays a significant role in psychological, social, spiritual, and physical health.

Families: The Ties That Bind

The United Nations defines seven basic types of families, including single-parent families, communal families (unrelated people living together for ideological, economic, or other reasons), extended families, and others. But most Americans think of family in terms of either the family of origin or the nuclear family.

The **family of origin** includes the people present in the household during a child's first years of life—usually parents and siblings. The family of origin may also include stepparents, grandparents, aunts or uncles, partners, and friends. The family of origin has a tremendous impact on the child's psychological and social development. The **nuclear family** consists of parents (usually married, but not necessarily) and their offspring.

The modern American family looks quite different from those of previous generations. The *Leave It to Beaver* model encouraged during the 1950s—composed of Mom with her apron, staying at home and content with her role as mother and spouse; Dad with his briefcase, trying to move up the corporate ladder; and two or three happy, well-adjusted children—is not the norm. Over half of today's moms work outside the home, and large numbers of children are cared for by single parents, grandparents, relatives, stepparents, friends, nannies, day care centers, and other caregivers. No particular family structure is inherently good or bad. Families that promote the most positive health outcomes for all members are those that offer a sense of security, safety, love, and the opportunity for members to grow through positive interactions.

If parents are willing to share feelings, affection, and love with each other and their offspring, their children are likely to become emotionally connected adults. If the home environment provides stability and seems safe, it is likely that the children will learn to express feelings and develop intimacy skills. Sibling interactions provide a way to learn and practice interpersonal skills. When the family itself is healthy, people can practice positive behaviors and learn the rights and wrongs of negative behaviors in a safe, nonjudgmental environment. However, if the family is psychologically or physically unhealthy, it may pose significant barriers to later relationships, as we will discuss later in this chapter.

Establishing Friendships

A Friend is one who knows you as you are, understands where you've been, accepts who you've become, and still gently invites you to grow. —Author Unknown

Good friends—they can make a boring day fun, a cold day warm, or a gut-wrenching worry disappear. They can make us feel that we matter and that we have the strength to get through just about anything. They can also make us angry, disappoint us, or seriously jolt our comfortable ideas about right and wrong. No friendship is perfect, and most need careful attention if they are to remain stable over time. Psychologists believe that people are attracted to and form

---

Family of origin   People present in the household during a child's first years of life—usually parents and siblings.

Nuclear family   Parents (usually married, but not necessarily) and their offspring.

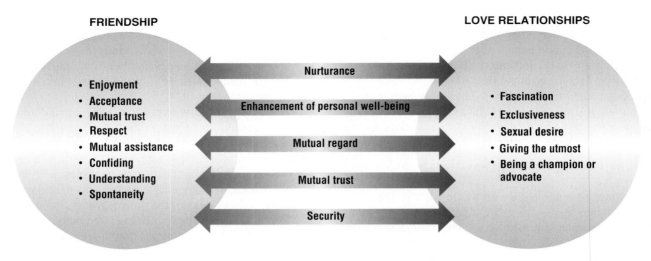

Figure 5.1
Common Bonds of Friends and Lovers

relationships with people who give them positive reinforcement and that they dislike those who punish or overcriticize them. The basic idea is simple: you like people who like you. Another factor that affects the development of a friendship is a real or perceived similarity in attitudes, opinions, and background.[20] In addition, true friends have a sense of *equity* in which they share confidences, contribute fairly and equally to maintaining the friendship, and consistently try to give as much as they get back from the interactions.[21]

Though we all know that friends enrich our lives, most people don't realize that real health benefits result from strong social bonds. Social support has been shown to boost the immune system, improve the quality and possibly the length of life, and even reduce the risks of heart disease.[22]

Although most of us have a fairly clear idea of the distinction between a friend and a lover, this difference is not always easy to verbalize. Some people believe that the major difference is that no intimate physical involvement exists between friends. Others have suggested that intimacy levels are much lower between friends than between lovers. However, as we have stated, people can be intimate with each other without being sexually involved. Also, many people have sex with others more as friends than as true lovers and partners. Confused? You are not alone. Surprisingly, little research has been done to clarify these terms. Psychologists Jeffrey Turner and Laurna Rubinson summarized the consensus among experts on characteristics that make a good friendship:[23]

- *Enjoyment.* Although temporary states of anger, disappointment, or mutual annoyance may occur, friends enjoy each other's company most of the time.
- *Acceptance.* Friends accept each other as they are, without trying to change or make the other into a different person.

- *Mutual trust.* Each assumes that the other will act in his or her friend's best interest.
- *Respect.* Friends respect each other; each assumes that the other exercises good judgment in making life choices.
- *Mutual assistance.* Friends are inclined to assist and support one another. Specifically, they can count on each other in times of need, trouble, or personal distress.
- *Confiding.* Friends share experiences and feelings with each other that they don't share with other people.
- *Understanding.* Friends have a sense of what each person values. They are not puzzled or mystified by each other's actions.
- *Spontaneity.* They feel free to be themselves in the relationship, without being required to play a role or inhibit revelation of personal traits.

According to psychologist Dan McAdams, most of us are fortunate to develop one or two lasting friendships in a lifetime.[24]

Significant Others, Partners, Couples

Most people choose at some point to enter into an intimate sexual relationship with another person. Numerous studies have analyzed the ways in which couples form significant partnering relationships. Most partners fit into one of four categories: married heterosexual couples, cohabiting heterosexual couples, lesbian couples, and gay male couples. These groups are discussed in greater detail later in this chapter.

Love relationships in each of these four groups typically include all the characteristics of friendship as well as other characteristics related to passion and caring:[25]

- *Fascination.* Lovers tend to pay attention to the other person even when they should be involved in other activities.

Is it love? Look for these signs:

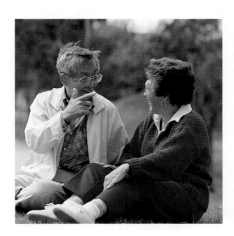

— **Verbally expressing affection,** such as saying "I love you"

— **Offering self-disclosure,** such as revealing intimate facts about oneself

— **Giving nonmaterial evidence,** such as emotional and moral support in times of need, and respecting the other's opinion

— **Expressing nonverbal feelings,** such as feeling happy, more content, more secure when the person is present

— **Giving material evidence** (such as gifts, flowers, or small favors) or doing more than one's own share of a task

— **Physically expressing love,** such as hugging, kissing, making love

— **Tolerating the other,** such as accepting his or her idiosyncrasies, peculiar routines, or forgetfulness

— **Wanting to promote** the partner's welfare

— **Feeling happiness** with the partner

— **Holding the partner** in high regard

— **Being able to count on the partner** in time of need

— **Being able to understand** each other

— **Sharing oneself and one's possessions** with the partner

— **Giving emotional support** to the partner

— **Being able to communicate** about intimate things

— **Valuing the partner's presence** in one's own life

Figure 5.2
Common Experiences of Love

Source: B. Strong, C. DeVault, and B. Sayad, *Human Sexuality* (Mountain View, CA: Mayfield, 1999). Reprinted by permission of The McGraw-Hill Companies.

They are preoccupied with the other and want to think about, look at, talk to, or merely be with that person.

- *Exclusiveness.* Lovers have a special relationship that usually precludes having the same bond with a third party. The love relationship takes priority over all others.
- *Sexual desire.* Lovers want physical intimacy with the partner, desiring to touch, hold, and engage in sexual activities with each other.
- *Giving the utmost.* Lovers care enough to give the utmost when the other is in need, sometimes to the point of extreme sacrifice.
- *Being a champion or advocate.* Lovers actively champion each other's interests and attempt to ensure that the other succeeds.

For obvious reasons, the best love relationships share friendships, and the best friendships include several love components. Both relationships share common bonds of nurturance, enhancement of personal well-being, and a genuine sense of mutual regard, trust, and security. Healthy friendships and love relationships greatly enhance overall health and lead to sustained personal growth throughout life (see Figure 5.1).

This Thing Called Love

What is love? Defining it may be more difficult than listing the characteristics of a loving relationship. The term *love* has more entries in *Bartlett's Familiar Quotations* than any other word except *man.*[26] This four-letter word has been written about and engraved on walls; it has been the theme of countless novels, movies, and plays. There is no one definition of *love,* and the word may mean different things to people depending on cultural values, age, gender, and situation. Yet, we all know what it is when it strikes (Figure 5.2).

Many social scientists maintain that love may be of two kinds: *companionate* and *passionate.* Companionate love is a secure, trusting attachment, similar to what we may feel for family members or close friends. In companionate love, two people are attracted, have much in common, care about each other's well-being, and express reciprocal liking and respect. Passionate love, in contrast, is defined as a state of high arousal, filled with the ecstasy of being loved and the agony of being rejected.[27] The person experiencing passionate love tends to be preoccupied with his or her partner and to perceive the love object as perfect.[28]

According to Elaine Hatfield and G. William Walster, passionate love will not occur unless three conditions are met.[29] First, the person must live in a culture in which the concept of "falling in love" is idealized. Second, a "suitable" love object must be present. If someone has been taught by parents, movies, books, and peers to seek partners of a certain appearance, socioeconomic status, or racial background, and if no such partner is available, the person may find it difficult to become involved. Finally, for passionate love to occur, there must be some type of physiological arousal that occurs when a person is in the presence of the beloved. Often this arousal takes the form of sexual excitement.

In his article "The Triangular Theory of Love," researcher Robert Sternberg attempts to clarify love by isolating three key ingredients:

- *Intimacy,* the emotional component, which involves feelings of closeness
- *Passion,* the motivational component, which reflects romantic, sexual attraction
- *Decision/commitment,* the cognitive component, which includes the decisions you make about being in love and the degree of commitment to your partner

According to Sternberg's model, the higher the levels of intimacy, passion, and commitment, the more likely a person is to be involved in a healthy, positive love relationship.

According to anthropologist Helen Fisher (and others), attraction and falling in love follow a fairly predictable pattern based on (1) *imprinting,* in which our evolutionary patterns, genetic predispositions, and past experiences trigger a romantic reaction; (2) *attraction,* in which neurochemicals produce feelings of euphoria and elation; (3) *attachment,* in which endorphins—natural opiates—cause lovers to feel peaceful, secure, and calm; and (4) *production of a "cuddle chemical,"* in which the brain secretes the chemical *oxytocin,* thereby stimulating sensations during lovemaking and eliciting feelings of satisfaction and attachment.[30]

Lovers who claim that they are swept away by passion may not, therefore, be far from the truth.

> A meeting of the eyes, a touch of the hands, or a whiff of scent may set off a flood that starts in the brain and races along the nerves and through the blood. The familiar results—flushed skin, sweaty palms, heavy breathing—are identical to those experienced when under stress. Why? Because the love-smitten person is secreting chemical substances such as dopamine, norepinephrine, and phenylethylamine (PEA) that are chemical cousins of amphetamines.[31]

Although attraction may in fact be a "natural high," with PEA levels soaring, this hit of passion loses effectiveness over time as the body builds up a tolerance. Needing a continual fix of passion, many people may become attraction junkies, seeking the intoxication of love much as the drug user seeks a chemical high.[32]

Fisher speculates that PEA levels drop significantly over a three to four year period, leading to the "four-year itch" that shows up in the peaking fourth-year divorce rates present in over 60 cultures. Romances that last beyond the four-year decline of PEA are influenced by another set of chemicals, the endorphins.[33]

Other researchers describe the first stage as the *lust phase,* in which our biological and genetic histories converge to pique our interest and intensity of response. In the lust

---

Genderlect The "dialect," or individual speech pattern and conversational style, of each gender.

---

phase, if someone comes into our range of awareness, a chemical surge can trigger our enthusiastic response. Known as *pheromones,* these triggers, said to be as unique as our fingerprints, are scent-infused chemicals found in perspiration under the armpits. They trigger a unique sensory reaction in the nose and result in attraction if their producer is a match for you.[34]

Following these pheromone triggers comes the *attraction phase*, often labeled the falling in love phase, and then the *attachment phase*. The two hormones which are most important in this last phase are oxytocin and vasopressin. Oxytocin not only increases the bond between lovers, but is also one of the chemicals responsible for contractions during childbirth and milk expression when breastfeeding and is released by both sexes during orgasm. The theory goes, therefore, that the more sex a couple have, the greater the bond between them.[35]

Vasopressin has been described as the "monogamy chemical." Much of what we know about oxytocin and vasopressin's roles in the chemistry of love comes from observations of voles, tiny mouse-size mammals that mate over a 24-hour period and bond for life. They prefer to spend their days together, nest together, and show affection toward one another and their offspring. In laboratory settings, if these two chemicals are blocked, voles' relationships become more like one-night stands, and they actively seek out other mates. If the chemicals are injected into voles, their monogamous ways continue. Although there are many other factors involved and the science is relatively new and specific to one species, there are interesting implications for humans.[36]

In addition to such possible chemical influences, past experiences significantly affect our attractions for others. Our parents' modeling of traits we believe are desirable or undesirable may play a role in drawing us to people with similar traits.

Gender Issues in Relationships

When it comes to relationships, are men really from Mars and women from Venus? If they are not planets apart, how far apart are they, and what are the implications of the disparities? In her landmark book *You Just Don't Understand: Women and Men in Conversation,* psychologist Deborah Tannen coined the term **genderlect** to characterize differences in word choices, interruption patterns, questioning patterns, language interpretations and misinterpretations, and vocal influences based on gender.[37] Tannen is not alone in her research. In fact, communication patterns between women and men have been studied for generations, with similar results. Recent research validates much of Tannen's work and indicates that women tend to be more expressive, relationship oriented, and concerned with creating and maintaining intimacy; men tend to be more instrumental, task oriented, and concerned with gathering information or establishing and maintaining social status or power.[38] Unlike women,

men tend to believe that they are not supposed to show emotions and are brought up to believe that "being strong" is often more important than having close friendships. As a result, men are generally less likely to share their innermost thoughts. Figure 5.3 summarizes some of these characteristics found in each gender.

What do you think?

Who are the people with whom you feel most comfortable talking about personal issues?
■ *Do you talk with both males and females about these issues, or do you tend to gravitate toward just one sex?* ■ *Why do you think you do this?*

Styles in Decision Making

According to classic research conducted by Harvard professor Carol Gilligan, men and women may make very different decisions when facing ethical dilemmas.[39] Gilligan believes that women tend to think and speak differently from men because of the two genders' contrasting images of self. Because of these self-image differences, Gilligan believes that there is a feminine ethic of *care* and a masculine ethic of *justice*.[40] Following this line of thinking, she suggests that women view sensitivity to others, loyalty, responsibility, self-sacrifice, and peacemaking as key factors to consider in making ethical decisions. In contrast, men are more interested in individual rights, equality before law, and fair play—factors that are much more impersonal. Because such gender differences would affect both the encoding and decoding of messages, difficulties in communication might result.[41] Today, as gender differences have become less pronounced, decisions are influenced more by past experiences and behaviors. Men are more likely than ever to express caring ethics and women to express justice ethics.

What do you think?

What changes in society have blurred the gender differences in decision making proposed by Gilligan? ■ *Can you think of examples that support or refute her thinking?*

Picking Partners

For both males and females, the choice of partners is influenced by more than just chemical and psychological processes. One important factor is *proximity,* or being in the same place at the same time. The more you see a person in your hometown, at social gatherings, or at work, the more likely that interaction will occur. Thus, if you live in

Men
- Talk is primarily a means of preserving independence and negotiating and maintaining status.
- Men are more likely to give advice, tell a joke, change the subject, or remain silent when trouble arises.
- When women offer sympathy to men, men may feel that they are being placed in a lower-status position and find it condescending.
- Men are more likely to be avoidant.

Women
- Talk is primarily a means of rapport, a way of establishing connections and negotiating relationships. Emphasis is on displaying similarities and matching experiences.
- Women are more likely to share a similar problem or openly express sympathy, and to expect sympathy in return.
- When men give advice, women feel that their feelings are being invalidated, their problems are being minimized, or that the simple "fix" provided is condescending.
- Women are likely to be supportive.

Figure 5.3
Troubles Talk: How Men and Women Respond

Source: From S. L. Michaud and R. Warner, "Gender Differences in Self-Reported Responses in Troubles Talk," *Sex Roles: A Journal of Research* 37, no. 7-8 (1997): 527.

New York, you'll probably end up with another New Yorker. If you live in Texas, you'll probably end up with another Texan. (With the advent of the Internet, geographic proximity is less important, as discussed in the Reality Check box on computer dating and e-mail communication, page 140.)

You also choose a partner based on *similarities* (in attitudes, values, intellect, and interests); the old adage that "opposites attract" usually isn't true. If your potential partner expresses interest or liking, you may react with mutual regard known as *reciprocity.* The more you express interest, the safer it is for someone else to return the regard, and the cycle spirals onward.

A final factor that apparently plays a significant role in selecting a partner is *physical attraction.* Whether such attraction is caused by chemical reactions or socially learned behavior, males and females appear to have different attraction criteria. Men tend to select their mates primarily on the basis of youth and physical attractiveness. While women also value physical attractiveness, they tend to place higher emphasis on partners who are somewhat older, have good financial prospects, and are dependable and industrious.

What do you think?

What factors do you consider most important in a potential partner? ■ *Which are absolute musts?* ■ *Are there any differences between what you believe to be important in a relationship and the things your parents feel are important?*

Sharing Feelings

Although men tend to talk about intimate issues with women more frequently than with men, women still complain that men do not communicate enough about what is really on their minds. This may reflect the powerfully different socialization processes experienced by women and men, which influence their communication styles. Throughout their lives, females are offered opportunities to practice sharing their thoughts and feelings with others. In contrast, males receive strong societal messages to withhold their feelings. The classic example of this training in very young males is the familiar saying "Big boys don't cry." Men learn very early that certain emotions are not to be shared, with the result that they are more information-focused and businesslike in their conversations. Understandably, such differences in communication styles contribute to misunderstandings and conflict. (See the Women's Health/Men's Health box.)

Although men are often perceived as being less emotional than women, do they really feel less or do they just have more difficulty expressing their emotions? In one study, when men and women were shown scenes of people in distress, the men exhibited little outward emotion, whereas the

---

Leveling   The communication of a clear, simple, and honest message.

Editing   The process of censoring comments that would be intentionally hurtful or irrelevant to the conversation.

Documenting   Giving specific examples of issues being discussed.

Validating   Letting your partner know that although you may not agree with his or her point of view, you still respect the fact that he or she thinks or feels that way.

---

women communicated feelings of concern and distress. However, physiological measures of emotional arousal (such as heart rate and blood pressure) indicated that the male subjects were actually as affected emotionally as the female subjects but inhibited the expression of their emotions, whereas the women openly expressed them. In other studies, men and women responded very differently to the same test.[42]

When men are angered, they tend to interpret the cause of their anger as something or someone in their environment and are likely to turn their anger outward in an aggressive manner. Women, on the other hand, tend to see themselves as the source of the problem and turn their anger inward, suppressing direct expression of it.[43]

Communication between Couples

The following techniques can promote good communication between couples:[44]

1. **Leveling** refers to sending your partner a clear, simple, and honest message. The purposes of leveling are to: (1) make communication clear; (2) clarify the expectations you and your partner have of each other; (3) clear up pleasant and unpleasant feelings and thoughts from past incidents; (4) make clear what is relevant and what is irrelevant; and (5) become aware of the things that draw you together or push you apart.
2. **Editing** means censoring remarks that may be hurtful or are irrelevant. Often, when people are upset, they let everything fly, bringing up old issues and incidents that cause pain and put a partner on the defensive. Editing means taking the time and making the effort not to say inflammatory things. Leveling and editing help establish genuine communication characterized by caring and sensitivity.
3. **Documenting** refers to giving specific examples of issues under discussion. Documenting helps you avoid gross generalizations that tend to be accusatory, such as "You always" and "You never." If you provide specific examples of when and how an incident occurred, your partner will gain a concrete understanding of the issue. In documenting, you can also include specific suggestions for changing or improving the situation.
4. **Validating** means letting a partner know that although you may not agree with his or her point of view, you still respect the person's thoughts and feelings ("I don't agree with you, but I can see how you might view things that way"). This does not mean that you are giving in to your partner; you are simply recognizing that your opinions differ.

We All Want to Be Understood

The bottom line is simple: both men and women want to be heard and understood. Understanding gender differences in communication patterns, rather than casting blame at each

---

How Different Are Men and Women? Recognizing and Acknowledging Uniqueness

Although men and women may make decisions differently, act differently in terms of their sexual and partnering behaviors, and act in ways that are somewhat distinctive to their genders, these lines have begun to blur over time. Books such as *Men Are from Mars, Women Are from Venus* that focus on these differences capture media attention, but they also have their critics. According to Dr. Cynthia Burggraf Torppa at Ohio State University, differences in communication between men and women are really quite minor. What she says is most important is the way in which men and women interpret or process the same message. She indicates that studies support the idea that women, to a greater extent then men, are sensitive to the interpersonal meanings that lie between the lines in the messages they exchange with their mates. This is because societal expectations often make women responsible for regulating intimacy. Men, on the other hand, are more sensitive than women to subtle messages about status. For them, societal expectations dictate that they negotiate hierarchy, or who's the captain and who's the crew.

There are some gender-specific communication patterns and behaviors that are obvious to the casual observer, however. Recognizing these differences and how they make us unique is a good first step in avoiding unnecessary frustrations and irritations.

Men	Women
Body Language	
Occupy more space; gesture away from the body; lean back when listening; less feedback through body language; more forceful gestures (backslapping, stronger handshakes); overt fidgeting	Take up less space; movement is light and easy; gesture toward the body; lean forward when listening; provide feedback via body language; less likely to invade another's space; more gentle when touching others
Facial Expressions	
Often avoid eye contact; show less warmth in facial expression; frown more often	Maintain better eye contact; smile and nod more often
Speech Patterns	
More likely to interrupt, mumble, and use fewer speech tones (approximately three); voices are lower-pitched and usually louder; sound more abrupt; talk less personally about selves; make more direct statements than feeling statements; use fewer adjectives and descriptive statements; use fewer terms of endearment; tendency to lecture	Interrupt less often; articulate more clearly; use more speech tones (approximately five); may sound more emotional; voices are higher pitched and softer; more likely to discuss feelings and disclose more personal information; make more tentative statements ("kind of," "isn't it?")
Behavioral Differences	
More inclined to be analytical; give fewer compliments; use more sarcasm and teasing to show affection; cry less often; more argumentative; difficulty in expressing intimate feelings; hold fewer grudges; gossip less; less likely to ask for help; tend to take rejection less personally; apologize less often	More emotional approach to issues; give more compliments; show more expression; express feelings more readily; greater tendency to hold grudges; inclined to gossip more; more likely to ask for help; take rejection more personally; apologize more frequently

Sources: C. Burggraf Torppa, "Gender Issues: Communication Differences in Interpersonal Relationships," Family Life Packet, 2002, http://ohioline.osu.edu/flm02/FS04.html; J. Wood, *Gendered Lives: Communication, Gender, and Culture,* 4th ed (Belmont, CA: Wadsworth, 2001); Kings Communications, "Men and Women Are Different!," 2002, www.KingsCommunications.com. Reprinted by permission; and M. L. Knapp and A. L. Vangelisti, *Interpersonal Communication and Human Relationships* (Boston: Allyn & Bacon, 2000).

other, is the first step toward promoting effective communication. Tannen suggests that expecting persons of the other sex to change their style of communication is not an effective way to deal with the gender gap. Instead, learn to interpret messages while explaining your own unique way of communicating. Working to understand the different ways in which males and females use language will help us all achieve the goal of clear and honest communication.

What do you think?

Do you believe that men and women really communicate in different styles? ▪ *What can you do to improve your communication with members of the other sex?*

Overcoming Barriers to Intimacy

Obstacles to intimacy include lack of personal identity, emotional immaturity, and a poorly developed sense of responsibility. The fear of being hurt, low self-esteem, mishandled hostility, chronic "busyness" (and its attendant lack of emotional presence), a tendency to "parentify" loved ones, and a conflict of role expectations may be equally detrimental. In addition, individual insecurities and difficulties in recognizing and expressing emotional needs can lead to an intimacy barrier. These barriers to intimacy may have many causes, including miscommunication, a dysfunctional family background, and jealousy.

Barriers to Communication

In today's world of instant messages, cell phones, pagers, and technologically advanced information systems, communication problems have grown exponentially. Our current means of communication differ greatly from those of our ancestors. In addition to physical changes in communication, people around the world must increasingly interact with others of vastly different backgrounds and values. Finding a means of communicating that accommodates everyone can be difficult. Barriers to communication take many forms.

Differences in Background Age, education, social status, gender, culture, political beliefs, and many other variables can lead to differences between communicators. Your closest friends from high school, with whom you grew up, shared many similar experiences with you. Shared experiences contribute to shared meaning and understanding. At college, however, you may suddenly find yourself among people having few shared experiences. Remember that the goal of good communication is not necessarily to have everyone agree with you; rather, it is to have others understand you.

Dysfunctional family A family in which the interaction between family members inhibits rather than enhances psychological growth.

Jealousy An aversive reaction evoked by a real or imagined relationship involving a person's partner and a third person.

Alcohol and Drugs Perhaps nothing stands in the way of effective communication more than alcohol and drugs. With an inhibited ability to encode messages, you may not be understood correctly. With an inhibited ability to decode messages, you may misinterpret someone else's message. Is it any wonder that 90 percent of campus rapes take place under the influence of alcohol? Avoiding date rape depends on a woman's ability to be clear in her own mind about what she wants and then to make herself clearly understood. It also depends on a man's ability to listen and hear what is being said, rather than what he thinks is being said. In most college campus sexual encounters that lead to date rape complaints, alcohol and drugs have played a role.

Dysfunctional Families

As noted earlier, the ability to sustain genuine intimacy is largely developed in the family of origin. If you were to examine even the most pristine family under a microscope, you would likely find some problems. No group of people can interact perfectly all the time, but this does not necessarily make them dysfunctional. In a truly **dysfunctional family**, interaction between family members inhibits psychological growth, self-love, emotional expression, and individual development. Negative interactions are the norm rather than the exception.

Children raised in dysfunctional settings tend to face tremendous obstacles to growing up healthy. Coming to terms with past hurts may take years. However, with introspection, support from loved ones, and counseling when needed, children from even the worst homes have proved to be remarkably resilient. Many are able to forget the past and focus on the future, developing into healthy, well-adjusted adults. Some will have problems throughout their lives.[45]

For example, many adult children of alcoholics (ACOAs) claim that they become involved in unhealthy relationships and have difficulty trusting others, communicating with partners, and defining a healthy relationship.[46] Research supporting this theory is conflicting, and many questions remain concerning how past experiences affect relationships for ACOAs.

Another tragically large group of people struggling with intimacy problems originating in the family of origin are survivors of childhood emotional, physical, and sexual abuse (see Chapter 4). It is important to note that dysfunctional families are found in every social, ethnic, religious, economic, and racial group.

Jealousy in Relationships

"Jealousy is like a San Andreas fault running beneath the smooth surface of an intimate relationship. Most of the time, its eruptive potential lies hidden. But when it begins to rumble, the destruction can be enormous."[47] **Jealousy** has been described as an aversive reaction evoked by a real or imagined relationship involving one's partner and a third person. Contrary to what many of us believe, jealousy is not a sign of intense devotion. Instead, jealousy often indicates underlying problems that may prove to be a significant barrier to a healthy intimate relationship. Causes of jealousy typically include:

- *Overdependence on the relationship.* People who have few social ties and who rely exclusively on their significant others tend to be fearful of losing them.
- *High value on sexual exclusivity.* People who believe that sexual exclusiveness is a crucial indicator of love are more likely to become jealous.
- *Low self-esteem.* People who feel good about themselves are less likely to feel unworthy and fear that someone is going to snatch their partners away. The underlying question that torments people with low self-esteem is "Why would anyone want me?"
- *Fear of losing control.* Some people need to feel in control of any situation. Feeling that they may be losing the attachment of or control over a partner can cause jealousy.

In both sexes, jealousy is related to the expectation that it would be difficult to find another relationship if the current one should end. For men, jealousy is positively correlated with the degree to which the man's self-esteem is affected by his partner's judgments. Though a certain amount of jealousy can be expected in any loving relationship, it doesn't have to threaten a relationship as long as partners communicate openly about it.[48]

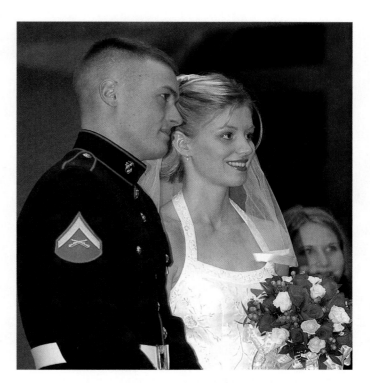

For many people, marriage or partnership ceremonies serve as the ultimate symbol of commitment between two people and validate their love for each other.

What do you think?

"Jealousy is not a barometer by which the depth of love can be read. It merely records the depth of the lover's insecurity" (anthropologist Margaret Mead, 1901–1978). Do you agree or disagree with this statement? ■ *What other factors may play a role in jealousy?*

Committed Relationships

Commitment in a relationship means that there is an intent to act over time in a way that perpetuates the well-being of the other person, oneself, and the relationship. Polls show that the majority of Americans—as many as 96 percent—strive to develop a committed relationship. These relationships can take several forms, including marriage, cohabitation, and gay and lesbian partnerships.

Marriage

In many societies around the world, traditional committed relationships take the form of marriage. In the United States, marriage means entering into a legal agreement that includes shared financial plans, property, and responsibility for raising children. Many Americans also view marriage as a religious sacrament that emphasizes certain rights and obligations for each spouse.

Close to 90 percent of all Americans marry at least once. U.S. Census Bureau data shows that we are marrying later than ever before. In 1970 the median age for first marriage was 22.5 years for men and 20.6 years for women; by 2000, this had risen to 27 years for men and 25 years for women.[49] This trend appears to be continuing.

Many Americans believe that marriage involves **monogamy,** or exclusive sexual involvement with one partner. In fact, the lifetime pattern for many Americans appears to be **serial monogamy,** which means that a person has a monogamous sexual relationship with one partner before moving on to another monogamous relationship. However, some people prefer an **open relationship,** or open marriage, in which both partners agree that there may be sexual involvement for each person outside their relationship.

Monogamy   Exclusive sexual involvement with one partner.

Serial monogamy   A series of monogamous sexual relationships.

Open relationship   A relationship in which partners agree that sexual involvement can occur outside the relationship.

Humans are not naturally monogamous; most of us are capable of being sexually and/or emotionally involved with more than one person at a time. Sexual infidelity is an extremely common factor in divorces and breakups. So why do we continue to get married?

Certainly marriage is socially sanctioned and highly celebrated in our culture, so there are numerous incentives for couples to formalize their relationship with a wedding ceremony. A healthy marriage provides emotional support by combining the benefits of friendship and a loving committed relationship. A happy marriage also provides stability for both the couple and for those involved in the couple's life. Considerable research indicates that married people live longer, feel happier, remain mentally alert longer, and suffer fewer physical and mental health problems.[50] Even people who divorce seem to miss being married: nearly 80 percent of them remarry.

While a successful marriage can bring much satisfaction, traditional marriage does not work for everyone. Some research suggests that today's women who choose marriage may not be as happy as their mothers were.[51] This may reflect increasing pressure on women to perform multiple roles such as taking care of a family while working outside the home. Other studies suggest that the happiness of never-married men has increased. However, traditional marriage is not the only path to a successful committed relationship.

Cohabitation

Cohabitation is defined as two people with an intimate connection who live together in the same household. For a variety of reasons, increasing numbers of Americans are choosing cohabitation. These relationships can be very stable and happy, with a high level of commitment between the partners. In some states, cohabitation that lasts a designated number of years (usually seven) legally constitutes a **common-law marriage** for purposes of real estate and other financial obligations.

Cohabitation can offer many of the same benefits that marriage does: love, sex, companionship, and the ongoing opportunity to know a partner better over time. In addition to enjoying emotional and physical benefits, some people may cohabit for practical reasons such as the opportunity to share bills and housing costs. While many cohabitors are young, some older adults choose this lifestyle because they would lose income, such as Social Security or a late spouse's pension, if they were to marry.

Successful cohabitations can also offer benefits not found in marriage. Partners may feel greater autonomy and independence than they might find in a traditional arrangement. Furthermore, if they decide to separate, they do not experience the legal problems and expense of a divorce.

Although cohabitation has its advantages, it also has some drawbacks. Perhaps the greatest disadvantage is the lack of societal validation for the relationship, especially if the couple then have children. Many cohabitors must deal with pressures from parents and friends, difficulties in obtaining insurance and tax benefits, and legal issues over property. In 1996, the U.S. Congress reaffirmed tax advantages for married couples and effectively blocked cohabiting heterosexual and homosexual couples from these benefits through the Defense of Marriage Bill. Today, controversy continues over whether traditional marriage should remain the only means of eligibility for tax deductions, health insurance, and other benefits. In general, there appears to be a trend toward recognizing the validity of unmarried relationships. The state of Vermont, for example, was among the first states to allow partners to form "civil unions."[52] Some companies now offer insurance benefits to employees' unmarried partners.

Gay and Lesbian Partnerships

Most adults want intimate, committed relationships, whether they are gay or straight, men or women. Lesbians and gay men seek the same things in primary relationships that heterosexual partners do: friendship, communication, validation, companionship, and a sense of stability.

The 2000 U.S. Census revealed a significant increase in the number of same-sex partner households across the country—more than three times the total reported in the 1990 Census. The states with the most reported same-sex households are California, New York, Florida, Illinois, and Georgia. According to Lee Badgett, research director of the Institute for Gay and Lesbian Strategic Studies, the actual number of households is probably much higher. Many gay and lesbian partners hesitate to report their relationship due to concerns about discrimination.[53]

Studies of lesbian couples indicate high levels of attachment and satisfaction and a tendency toward monogamous long-term relationships. Gay men, too, tend to form committed, long-term relationships, especially as they age, much like their heterosexual counterparts.

Challenges to successful lesbian and gay male relationships often stem from discrimination and difficulties dealing with social, legal, and religious doctrines. For lesbian and gay couples, obtaining the same level of "marriage benefits," such as tax deductions, power-of-attorney, child custody, and other rights, continues to be a challenge. However, commitment ceremonies and marriage ceremonies are becoming more frequent in some U.S. cities and in several countries. In 2004, courts in Massachusetts legalized marriages between same-sex partners. The city of San Francisco also challenged the state by performing same-sex marriages until halted by court order. Controversy and legal challenges continue in both cases. In Canada, several provinces have legalized same-sex marriages, and hundreds have been performed without incident.

Cohabitation   Living together without being married.

Common-law marriage   Cohabitation lasting a designated period of time (usually seven years) that is considered legally binding in some states.

Staying Single

Increasing numbers of adults of all ages are electing to marry later or to remain single altogether. The percentage of women aged 20 to 24 who had never been married doubled between 1970 and 2000, from 36 percent to a whopping 73 percent. Likewise, men in this age group postponed marriage in increasing numbers, with over 84 percent remaining unmarried in 2000. The number of women aged 30 to 34 who had never married tripled during that time, from 6 percent in 1970 to 22 percent in 2000, while the number of men this age who had never married grew from 9 percent in 1970 to over 30 percent in 2000. According to the most recent figures from the U.S. Census Bureau and National Center for Health Statistics, the number of unmarried women aged 15 and older will soon surpass the number of married women.[54] The number of unmarried men is also increasing. Other changes are reflected in the following facts.

- Over 10 percent of all people say they would never marry.
- People marrying today have more than a 50 percent chance of divorcing.
- As more women enjoy financial independence, they are less likely to remarry after divorce.
- Increasing numbers of widows and widowers are opting not to remarry.
- The percentage of children living with one parent has increased from 9 percent in 1960 to 28 percent in 2002.

Today, large numbers of people prefer to remain single or to delay marriage. Singles clubs, social outings arranged by communities and religious groups, extended family environments, and a large number of social services support the single lifestyle. Many singles live rich, rewarding lives and maintain a large network of close friends and families. Although sexual intimacy may or may not be present, the intimacy achieved through other interactions with loved ones is a key aspect of the single lifestyle.

Some research indicates that single people live shorter lives, are more unhappy, and are more likely to experience financial and health problems than their married peers. However, other studies refute these conclusions. Few studies to date have controlled for other confounding variables, such as environmental conditions, past histories, and other factors that may carry more weight than the married or single state.

What do you think?

Although there are advantages and disadvantages in marriage, many people feel that it is a desirable option. Are there any advantages in remaining single? ■ What are potential disadvantages? ■ Are there any societal or organizational supports for the single lifestyle?

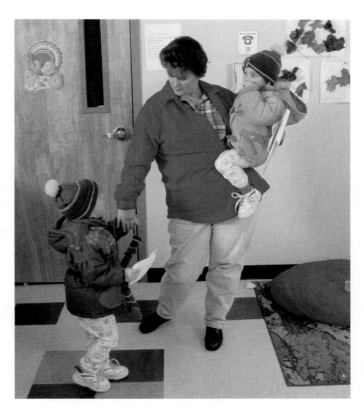

Single parents face additional challenges in juggling their work and family responsibilities. Many use community resources such as after-school day care centers.

Success in Relationships

Our definition of success in a relationship tends to be based on whether a couple stays together over the years. Learning to communicate, respecting each other, and sharing a genuine fondness are crucial to relationship success. Many social scientists agree that the happiest committed relationships are flexible enough to allow the partners to grow throughout their lives.

Partnering Scripts

Parents often believe that their children will achieve happiness by living much as they have. Accordingly, most children are reared with a very strong script for what is expected of them as adults. Each group in society has its own partnering script that includes similarities of sex, age, social class, race, religion, physical attributes, and personality types. By adolescence, people generally know exactly what type of person they are expected to befriend or date. By which partnering script were you raised? Just picture whom you could or couldn't bring home to meet your family.

Society provides constant reinforcement for traditional couples, but it may withhold this reinforcement from couples of the same sex, mixed race, mixed religion, or mixed age.

People who have not chosen an "appropriate" partner are subject to a great deal of external stress. In addition to denying recognition to such couples, friends and family often blame the "inappropriateness" of the couple if the relationship fails. Recognizing that this stress is external to the relationship can help alleviate criticism and distancing between the partners.

Nonetheless, many nontraditional relationships survive and flourish. For example, the number of interracial marriages has quadrupled since the late 1960s, and the number of same-sex partner households has grown from 145,130 to almost half a million over the past ten years.[55]

What do you think?

What characteristics are most important to you in a potential partner? ■ *Which of these would be important to your parents or friends?* ■ *If your parents or friends didn't like a potential partner, how important would their opinion be to you?* ■ *What would you do in this situation?*

Being Self-Nurturant

It is often stated that you must love yourself before you can love someone else. What does this mean? Learning how you function emotionally and how to nurture yourself through all life's situations is a lifelong task. You should certainly not postpone intimate connections with others until you have achieved this state. However, a certain level of individual maturity helps in maintaining a committed relationship. For example, divorce rates are much higher for couples under age 30 than for older couples.

Two concepts that are especially important to a good relationship are accountability and self-nurturance. **Accountability** means that both partners in a relationship see themselves as responsible for their own decisions and actions. They don't hold the other person responsible for positive or negative experiences.

Self-nurturance goes hand in hand with accountability. In order to make good choices in life, a person needs to maintain a balance of sleeping, eating, exercising, working,

---

Accountability Accepting responsibility for personal decisions, choices, and actions.

Self-nurturance Developing individual potential through a balanced and realistic appreciation of self-worth and ability.

Power The ability to make and implement decisions.

---

relaxing, and socializing. When the balance is disrupted, as it will inevitably be, self-nurturing people are patient with themselves and try to put things back on course. It is a lifelong process to learn to live in a balanced and healthy way. Two people who are on a path of accountability and self-nurturance together have a much better chance of maintaining a satisfying relationship.

Confronting Couple Issues

Couples seeking a long-term relationship have to confront a number of issues that can enhance or ruin their chances of success. Some of these issues involve gender roles and power sharing.

Changing Gender Roles   Throughout history, women and men have taken on various roles in their relationships. In agricultural America, gender roles were determined by tradition, and each task within a family unit held equal importance. Our modern society has very few gender-specific roles. Women and men alike drive cars, care for children, operate computers, manage finances, and perform equally well in the tasks of daily living. Rather than taking on the traditional female and male roles, many couples find it makes more sense to divide tasks on the basis of schedule, convenience, and preference. However, while it may make sense to divide household chores, it rarely works out that the division is equal. Today's working woman, living in a dual-career family and coping with the responsibilities of being a partner, a mother, and a professional, is often stressed and frustrated. Men, who may have expected a more traditional role for their partners, may experience difficulties. Even when women work full time, they tend to bear heavy family and household responsibilities. Over time, if couples are unable to communicate about how they feel about performing certain tasks, the relationship may suffer.

Sharing Power   **Power** can be defined as the ability to make and implement decisions. There are many ways to exercise power, but powerful people are those who know what they want and have the ability to attain it. In traditional relationships, men were the wage earners and consequently had decision-making power. Women exerted much influence, but in the final analysis they needed a man's income for survival. As women became wage earners in increasing numbers, the power dynamics between women and men changed. Within individual households, however, the dynamics have shifted considerably, with greater numbers of women working and enjoying their own financial resources. Part of the increase in the divorce rate undoubtedly reflects the recognition by working women that they can leave bad relationships in which they previously felt trapped. In general, successful couples have power relationships that reflect their unique needs rather than popular stereotypes.

Having Children . . . or Not?

When a couple decides to raise children, their relationship changes. Resources of time, energy, and money are split many ways, and the partners no longer have each other's undivided attention. Babies and young children do not time their requests for food, sleep, and care to the convenience of adults. Therefore, individuals or couples whose own basic needs for security, love, and purpose are already met make better parents. Any stresses that already exist in a relationship will be further accentuated when parenting is added to the responsibilities. Having a child does not save a bad relationship—in fact, it only seems to compound the problems that already exist. A child cannot and should not be expected to provide the parents with self-esteem and security.

Changing patterns in family life affect the way children are raised. In modern society, it is not always clear which partner will adjust his or her work schedule to provide the primary care of children. Nearly half a million children each year become part of a blended family when their parents remarry; remarriage creates a new family of stepparents and stepsiblings. In addition, an increasing number of individuals are choosing to have children in a family structure other than a heterosexual marriage. Single women or lesbian couples can choose adoption or alternative (formerly called "artificial") insemination as a way to create a family. Single men can choose to adopt or can obtain the services of a surrogate mother. According to the 2000 Census, over 9 percent of all U.S. households were headed by a man or woman raising a child alone, reflecting a growing trend in America and in the international community (Figure 5.4).[56] Regardless of the structure of the family, certain factors remain important to the well-being of the unit: consistency, communication, affection, and mutual respect

Some people become parents without a lot of forethought. Some children are born into a relationship that was supposed to last and didn't. This does not mean it is too late to do a good job of parenting. Children are amazingly resilient and forgiving if parents show respect and communicate about household activities that affect their lives. Even children who grew up in a household of conflict can feel loved and respected if the parents treat them fairly. This means that parents must take responsibility for their own emotions and make it clear to children that they are not the reason for the conflict.

Today, many families find that two incomes are needed just to make ends meet. Consider the financial implications of deciding to have a child: it is estimated that a family that had a child in 2004 will spend close to $250,000 to raise the child over the next 17 years, and this does not take into account the costs of college.[57] Indeed, more than 80 percent of all mothers with children under the age of 5 work outside the home. Day care, extended family and friends, grandparents, neighbors, and nannies "mind the kids." Some employers offer family leave arrangements that allow parents more latitude in taking time from work.

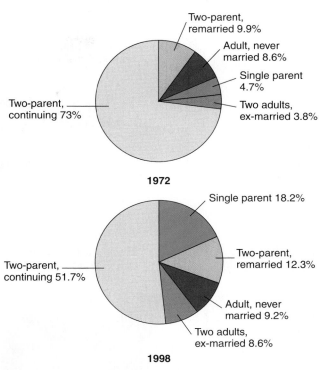

Percentage of children in various types of families

1972

1998

Figure 5.4
Changes in Family Types, 1972–1998

Note: Single parent = one adult in household; two-parent, continuing = married couple, never divorced; two-parent, remarried = married couple, at least one remarried (unknown if children came before or after remarriage); two adults, ex-married = two or more adults, previously but not currently married; adult, never married = two or more adults, never married (also includes some other family structures)

Source: General Social Survey News Number 13, August 1999. From National Opinion Research Center. Reprinted by permission of NORC.

What do you think?

What characteristics of a healthy family environment are important to you? ■ *Do you think that day care centers, extended families, and full-time babysitters can provide a positive environment for children? Why or why not?*

When Relationships Falter

Breakdowns in relationships usually begin with a change in communication, however subtle. Either partner may stop listening, ceasing to be emotionally present for the other. In turn, the other feels ignored, unappreciated, or unwanted. Unresolved conflicts increase, and unresolved anger can

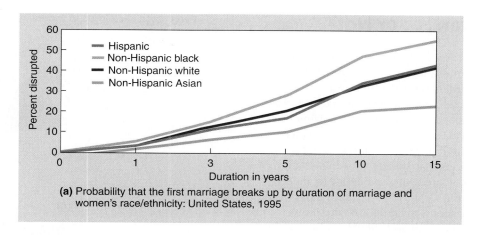

(a) Probability that the first marriage breaks up by duration of marriage and women's race/ethnicity: United States, 1995

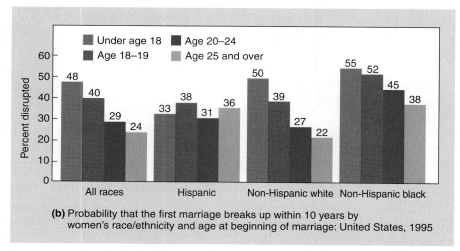

(b) Probability that the first marriage breaks up within 10 years by women's race/ethnicity and age at beginning of marriage: United States, 1995

Figure 5.5

Effects of Women's Age and Ethnicity on Marriage Success

(a) Probability that first marriage breaks up, by duration of marriage and women's race/ethnicity; (b) Probability that first marriage breaks up within 10 years, by women's race/ethnicity and age at beginning of marriage

Source: National Center for Health Statistics, "Cohabitation, Divorce, and Remarriage in the United States," *National Vital Statistics Report* 23, no. 22 (July 2002): 1–103.

cause problems in sexual relations, sometimes leading to infidelity. Over time, relationships with such difficulties may end in divorce. Age at first marriage, race, and socioeconomic status also affect the success of relationships (Figure 5.5).

When a couple who previously enjoyed spending time together find themselves continually in the company of others, spending time apart, or preferring to stay home alone, it may be a sign that the relationship is in trouble. Of course, the need for individual privacy and **autonomy** (the ability to care for oneself emotionally, socially, and physically) is not a

cause for worry—it's essential to health. If, however, a partner decides to change the amount and quality of time spent together without the input or understanding of the other, it may be a sign of hidden problems.

College students, particularly those who are socially isolated and far from family and hometown friends, may be particularly vulnerable to staying in unhealthy relationships. They may become emotionally dependent on a partner for everything from eating meals to recreational and study time, and mutual obligations such as shared rental arrangements, transportation, and child care can make it tough to leave.

It's also easy to mistake sexual advances for physical attraction or love. Without a network of friends and supporters to talk with, to obtain validation for feelings, or to share concerns, a student may feel stuck in a relationship that is headed nowhere.

Autonomy The ability to care for oneself emotionally, socially, and physically.

Honesty and verbal affection are usually positive aspects of a relationship. In a troubled relationship, however, they can be used to cover up irresponsible or hurtful behavior. "At least I was honest" is not an acceptable substitute for acting in a trustworthy way. The words "But I really do love you" should not be used as a license to be inconsiderate or rude.

Getting Help

The first place most people look for help for relationship problems is a trusted friend. However, although friends can offer support during trying times, few have the training and detachment necessary to resolve serious relationship problems.

Most communities have trained therapists who specialize in relationship difficulties. These practitioners may be psychiatrists, licensed psychologists, social workers, or counselors with advanced degrees. Most student health centers or on-campus counseling centers offer these services at low cost. If you don't know how to find such services, ask your instructor for suggestions.

If a couple's commitment to the relationship is strong, their chances of solving problems increase. The counselor typically interviews the partners separately and together, gradually helping them recognize and change the behaviors and attitudes that are detrimental to the relationship. Counseling may take a few weeks, several months, or even years as couples examine their values and reestablish their commitment.

Beware of the counselor who tells you during the first visit to drop the relationship or who tries to give advice without hearing the full story. Most good counselors will spend a good deal of time letting you tell them what you want and helping you work through your feelings rather than adopting theirs.

Trial Separations

Sometimes a relationship becomes so dysfunctional that even counseling cannot bring about significant change. Moving apart for a period of time may allow some preliminary healing and give both parties an opportunity to reassess themselves and their commitment. Trial separations do not guarantee that the situation will improve, nor do they mean the relationship is ending. If both people are involved in counseling or have other support systems and mutually agree on the need for a trial separation, it may be a way to regroup and save a failing relationship.

When and Why Relationships End

Based on recent statistics, it has been predicted that 20 percent of those who marry today will divorce within 5 years; one-third may divorce within 10 years; and 40 percent will divorce before their fifteenth anniversary. Ultimately, half of

Table 5.1
World Divorce Rates: United States Ranked Number Two

Countries with the highest rates of divorce are in bold; the lowest-ranking nations are in italics. Divorce is legal in the countries shown in this list; the divorce rates are per 100 marriages.

Austria	**43.4**	Moldova	28.1
Belarus	**52.9**	Netherlands	38.3
Belgium	**44.0**	Norway	40.4
Bulgaria	21.1	*Poland*	*17.3*
Canada	37.0	Portugal	26.2
Czech Republic	**43.3**	Romania	19.1
Denmark	**44.5**	**Russia**	**43.3**
Finland	**51.2**	*Spain*	*15.2*
France	38.3	**Sweden**	**54.9**
Germany	39.4	Switzerland	25.5
Greece	*15.7*	*Turkey*	*6.0*
Hungary	37.5	Ukraine	40.0
Italy	*10.0*	**United Kingdom**	**42.6**
Luxembourg	**47.4**	**United States**	**54.8**

Sources: Americans for Divorce Reform, "World Divorce Rates," 2002, www.divorcereform.org; *Recent Demographic Developments in Europe, 2001* (Strasbourg, France: Council of Europe Publishing, 2001); Jean-Paul Sardon, "Recent Demographic Trends in the Developed Countries," *Population: English Edition* 57 (January–February 2002): 111–156.

all marriages will end in divorce.[58] Rates of divorce have declined slightly in the last two years, however. This may be due to people getting married later in life, when they are more mature and financially stable. Table 5.1 compares the American divorce rate with that of other countries.

While the divorce rate may seem alarming, the actual number of failed relationships is probably much higher. Many people never go through a legal divorce process and, as a result, are not counted in these statistics. Cohabitors and unmarried partners, who raise children, own homes together, and exhibit all the outward appearances of marriage without the license, are also not included.

Why do relationships end? There are many reasons, including illness, financial concerns, and career problems. Other breakups arise from unmet expectations. Many people enter a relationship with certain expectations about how they and their partner will behave. Failure to communicate these beliefs can lead to resentment and disappointment. Differences in sexual needs may also contribute to the demise of a relationship. Table 5.2 on page 156 summarizes important factors in relationship failure.

Under stress, communication and cooperation between partners can break down. Conflict and negative interactions as well as a general lack of respect between partners can erode even the most loving relationship. One of the greatest predictors of divorce appears to be husband dissatisfaction in the first five years of marriage.

Table 5.2
Key Factors Predicting Success and Failure in Marriages and Relationships

Traits that Predict Success	Traits that Predict Failure	Common Reasons for Marriage and Relationship Failure
Individual • High self-esteem • Flexibility • Assertiveness • Sociability	**Individual** • Neurotic characteristics • Anxiety, depression, impulsiveness, anger/hostility • Self-consciousness • Vulnerability to stress • Dysfunctional beliefs	• Poor communication • Financial problems • Lack of commitment to the marriage • Dramatic change in priorities • Infidelity • Failed expectations or unmet needs • Addictions and substance abuse • Physical, sexual, or emotional abuse • Lack of conflict-resolution skills
Couple • Similarity • Long acquaintanceship • Good communication skills • Good conflict-resolution skills	**Couple** • Dissimilarity • Short acquaintanceship • Premarital sex with many partners • Premarital pregnancy • Cohabitation • Poor communication and conflict-resolution skills	
Context • Older age • Healthy family-of-origin experiences • Happy parental marriage • Parents' and friends' approval • Significant education or career preparation	**Context** • Younger age • Unhealthy family-of-origin experiences • Parental divorce or chronic conflict • Parents' and friends' disapproval • Pressure to marry • Little education or career preparation	

Source: American Academy of Matrimonial Lawyers, "Making Marriage Last," 2000, www.aaml.org/Marriage_Last/MarriageMain.htm

---

What do you think?

What factors do you think contribute to the high U.S. divorce rate? ■ *How would you explain Americans' attitudes about marriage and divorce to a friend from another country?*

Coping with Loneliness

When a relationship ends, it is normal to experience painful emotions of anger, guilt, rejection, and unworthiness. No matter how miserable the relationship was, feelings of failure are common. Counselors estimate that it can take at least a year and often longer to recover from the loss of a major relationship, whether by death or separation.

Although it may be painful, reflecting on the past relationship can help prevent similar mistakes in the future. Con-

Psychoeducation The teaching of crucial psychological skills, giving people knowledge so they can help themselves.

centrating on the negative aspects of an ex-partner is a natural tendency, but it is equally important to remember what you loved in the other person and what is lovable about you. When we accept the risk and challenge of close relationships, we accept one of the greatest gifts life has to offer. With time, support from others, and community or professional help, most people do recover and establish rewarding new relationships.

Building Better Relationships

Most relationships start with great optimism and true love. So why do so many run into trouble? "We just don't know how to handle the negative feelings that are the unavoidable by-product of the differences between two people, the very differences that attract them to each other in the first place. Think of it as the friction any two bodies would generate rubbing against each other countless times each day," says Howard Markman, PhD, professor of psychology at the University of Denver.[59] According to Markman, most unhappy couples don't need therapy; they need education in how relationships work and the special skills that make them work well. Markman and others promote **psychoeducation,** the teaching of crucial psychological skills—giving people knowledge so they can help themselves. Psychoeducation courses aren't therapy per se, but they typically have a therapeutic effect on couples.

Elements of Healthy Relationships

Stable, satisfying relationships are characterized by good communication, intimacy, friendship, and other factors discussed in this chapter. In addition, they share certain identifiable traits. A key ingredient is **trust**, the degree of confidence felt in a relationship. Without trust, intimacy will not develop and the relationship could fail. Trust includes three fundamental elements:

- *Predictability* means that you can predict your partner's behavior, based on the knowledge that your partner acts in consistently positive ways.
- *Dependability* means that you can rely on your partner to give support in all situations, particularly those in which you feel threatened with hurt or rejection.
- *Faith* means that you feel absolutely certain about your partner's intentions and behavior.

Trust can develop even when it is initially lacking. This requires opening yourself to others, which carries the risk of hurt or rejection.

Other characteristics of happy relationships include the following items.

- Partners interpret each other's behavior in the context of their own relationship, without overreacting to behaviors that remind them of past relationships. For example, if a previous partner continually flirted with other people and cheated on you, the sight of your current partner dancing with someone else at a party could trigger unpleasant memories. However, don't assume that your current partner will behave the same way.

- Partners who like each other and find each other interesting are happier than those who don't. Many people describe their partners as their best friends. Although most relationships have their share of ups and downs, members of successful couples are able to talk, listen, and touch each other in an atmosphere of caring. They value a good sense of humor and exhibit clear communication, cooperation, and the ability to resolve conflicts constructively.
- Sexual intimacy is a major component of healthy relationships, but sex is not a major reason for the existence of the relationship. Some couples admit to sexual dissatisfaction but find the relationship itself more important than sexual pleasure. Many couples report that as communication and trust increase, the sexual relationship also improves.
- Another important quality is a shared and cherished history, including private jokes, special places where key events have occurred, nicknames, rituals, emotions, and significant shared time and activities.

After reading this chapter, it should be apparent that relationships—whether with partners, parents, friends, or others—involve complex interactions that don't always work the way you'd like them to. Occasionally, they'll lead to frustration and disappointment. However, they also will be a source of great joy and fulfillment. Developing skills that will protect you in a relationship and also help your relationship grow and flourish is an important step in achieving good relationship health. In addition, learning not to take yourself quite so seriously, to forgive others' slips, and to overcome your own fears and overreactions will help keep relationships on course.

Trust The degree of confidence felt in a relationship.

TAKING CHARGE

MAKE IT HAPPEN!

Assessment: The Assess Yourself box earlier in this chapter (page 138) gave you the chance to look at how you communicate in certain situations. It is important to be able to communicate assertively and to feel that you can stand up for yourself. Now that you have considered your responses to the statements, you may want to take steps toward becoming a more assertive communicator.

Making a Change: In order to change your behavior, you need to develop a plan. Follow these steps:

1. Evaluate your behavior, and identify patterns. What can you change now? What can you change in the near future?
2. Select one pattern of behavior that you want to change.
3. Fill out a Behavior Change Contract. It should include your long-term goal for change, your short-term goals, the

rewards for reaching these goals, potential obstacles along the way, and strategies for overcoming these obstacles. For each goal, list the small steps and specific actions that you will take.

4. Chart your progress in a journal. At the end of a week, consider how successful you were in following your plan. What helped you be successful? What made change more difficult? What will you do differently next week?

5. Revise your plan as needed: Are the short-term goals attainable? Are the rewards satisfying?

One Student's Plan: When Stacey assessed her responses to the statements about assertiveness she realized that she tended to say "yes" when someone asked her for a favor, no matter how busy or stressed out she was. Stacey decided she

wanted to learn to say no when she needed to. She set a goal of imagining certain situations that she had faced recently and how she would handle them more assertively. The first week, she imagined her older sister asking her to babysit her son at the last minute and her roommates asking her for car rides while she was in the middle of studying. She planned what she would say and how she would explain her reasons for saying no.

The second week, when her roommates asked for a ride to the movies, Stacey calmly stated that she was busy and needed two hours more for studying before she could take a break. Her roommates decided to walk to the video store instead, where they rented a movie they could all watch together when Stacey was ready for a break.

Summary

- Communication is a complex process that dictates how we interact with others. Understanding each other's words and symbols is an important part of communication. Our perceptions of these words and symbols, or our way of interpreting incoming information, is equally consequential as we forge relationships throughout our lives.

- To improve our ability to communicate with others, we need to address a number of factors. These include learning how to use self-disclosure, listen effectively, convey and interpret nonverbal communication, establish a proper climate for communicating, and manage and resolve conflicts.

- Intimate relationships have certain important characteristics, including behavioral interdependence, need fulfillment, emotional attachment, and emotional availability. These characteristics influence how we interact with others and the types of intimate relationships we form. Family, friends, and partners or lovers provide the most common opportunities for intimacy. Each relationship may include healthy and unhealthy characteristics that may affect daily functioning.

- Gender differences in communication can include different conversation styles as well as differences in sharing feelings and disclosing personal facts and fears. These differences explain why men and women may relate differently in intimate relationships. Understanding these differences and learning how to deal with them are important aspects of healthy relationships.

- Barriers to intimacy often involve barriers in communication, which could result from a difference in background or the effects of alcohol and drugs. Other barriers may

include the different emotional needs of both partners, jealousy, and emotional wounds that could result from being raised in a dysfunctional family.

- Commitment is an important ingredient in successful relationships for most people. The major types of committed relationships include marriage, cohabitation, and gay and lesbian partnerships.

- Success in committed relationships requires understanding the roles of partnering scripts, the importance of self-nurturance, the elements of a good relationship, and the ability to confront couple issues.

- Life decisions such as whether to marry or whether to have children require serious consideration. Remaining single is more common than ever before. Most single people lead healthy, happy, and well-adjusted lives. Those who decide to have or not to have children can also lead rewarding, productive lives as long as they have given this decision the utmost thought, weighing the pros and cons of each alternative in the context of their lifestyles. Today's family structure may look different from that of previous generations, but love, trust, and commitment to a child's welfare continue to be the cornerstones of successful childrearing.

- Before relationships fail, often many warning signs appear. By recognizing these signs and taking action to change behaviors, partners may save and enhance their relationship.

- There are many strategies for building better relationships. Examining one's own behaviors to determine what to change and how to change it is an important ingredient of success.

Questions for Discussion and Reflection

1. Why are symbolism and individual perception so critical to the communication process?
2. How are self-esteem and stress directly related to physical well-being? How does communication improve self-esteem and reduce stress?
3. Why is self-disclosure so important to mental well-being? At what times is it better not to disclose personal information?
4. What is nonverbal communication, and why is it important to develop skills in this area? Give examples of some things that you do to communicate without words.
5. What are the characteristics of intimate relationships? What are behavioral interdependence, need fulfillment, emotional attachment, and emotional availability, and why is each important in relationship development?
6. Why are relationships with family important? Explain how your family unit was similar to or different from the traditional family unit in early America. Who made up your family of origin? your nuclear family?
7. How can you tell the difference between a love relationship and one that is based primarily on attraction? What characteristics do love relationships share?
8. What problems can form barriers to intimacy? What actions can you take to reduce or remove these barriers?
9. What are common elements of good relationships? Warning signs of trouble? What actions can you take to improve your own interpersonal relationships?
10. Name some common misconceptions about people who choose to remain single and about couples who choose not to have children. Do you want to have children? Why or why not? What characteristics show that a couple is ready to have children?
11. How have gender roles changed over the past twenty years? Do you view the changes as positive for women? For men?

Accessing Your Health on the Internet

Visit the following Internet sites to explore further topics and issues related to personal health. To visit an organization's website, go to the Companion Website for *Access to Health, Ninth Edition* at www.aw-bc.com/donatelle, click on the book image, and select "Accessing Your Health on the Internet" from the navigation menu.

1. *Couples National Network.* Link into a network for same-sex couples and singles, with resources about gay and lesbian issues.
2. *Mental Health Notes.* User-friendly information about dysfunctional families from a licensed clinical psychologist. Includes links to related mental health articles.
3. *National Center for Health Statistics.* This division of the Centers for Disease Control and Prevention has up-to-date statistics on trends in marriage, divorce, and cohabitation.
4. *Relationship Growth Online.* Provides information, quizzes, games, advice, and links to more information on how to build better relationships.
5. *University of Missouri Counseling Center Self-Help Area.* Provides a bibliography of books and other resources dealing with intimacy issues.

Further Reading

Bailey, J. *Slowing Down to the Speed of Love.* New York: McGraw-Hill, 2005.

A faculty member at the Center for Spirituality and Healing at the University of Minnesota School of Medicine gives his advice on love and relationships.

Busby, D. and V. Loyer-Carlson. *Pathways to Marriage with RELATE Online Relationship Inventory: Premarital and Early Marital Relationships.* Boston: Allyn & Bacon/Longman, 2003.

Step-by-step approach to building better relationships.

Erber, R. and M. Wang-Erber. *Intimate Relationships: Issues, Theories, and Research.* Boston: Allyn & Bacon, 2001.

Overview of common issues in relationships, theories about why relationships succeed and fail, and discussions of relevant research.

Fisher, H. *Why We Love: The Nature and Chemistry of Romantic Love.* New York: Henry Holt, 2004.

Overview of biological and chemical physiological reactions that stimulate love, lust, and romantic attachment.

Galvin, K. and P. Cooper. *Making Connections.* Los Angeles: Roxbury Publishing, 2000.

Outstanding overview of the importance of interpersonal communication in everyday lives. Provides practical strategies to assist us at all stages of life.

Sichel, M. *Healing from Family Rifts.* New York: McGraw-Hill, 2004.

The author, a therapist and clinical social worker, provides advice on dealing with family issues and problems that may seem insurmountable.

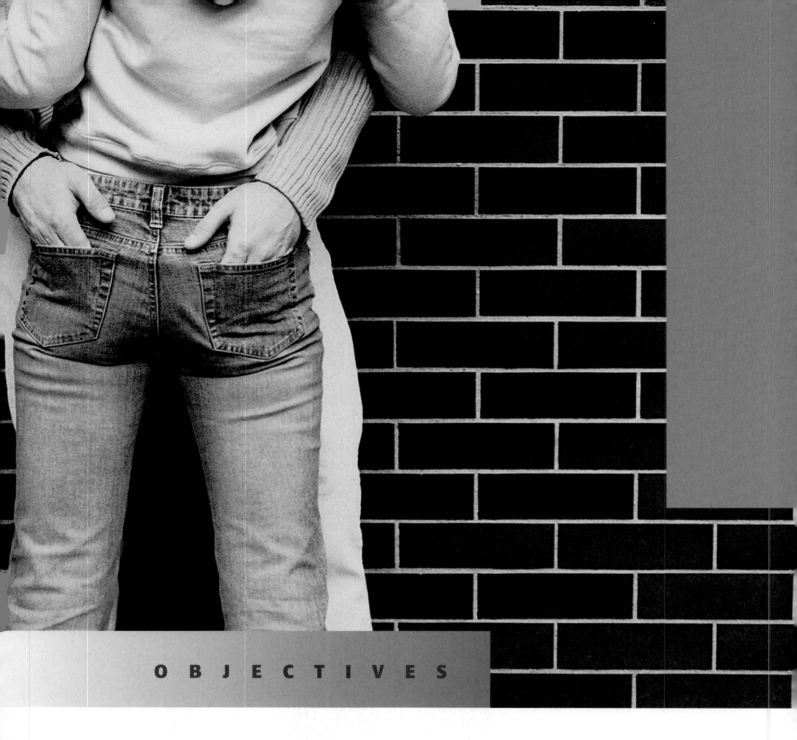

- Define *sexual identity,* and discuss the major components of sexual identity, including biology, gender identity, gender roles, and sexual orientation.

- Identify major features and functions of sexual anatomy and physiology.

- Discuss the options available for the expression of one's sexuality.

- Classify sexual dysfunctions, and describe major disorders.

6

SEXUALITY

CHOICES IN SEXUAL BEHAVIOR

IN THE NEWS

More Data Sought on Drug for Sex Drive

By Andrew Pollack

A federal advisory panel voted unanimously yesterday that the first drug to enhance the sex drive of women should not be approved because of a lack of information about its long-term safety.

Members of the committee said that the possible risks of the drug—a patch containing the hormone testosterone developed by Procter & Gamble—outweighed what some saw as only a modest benefit in increasing desire and the frequency of sex.

"I am not devaluing the importance of this symptom and its treatment," said Dr. Steven Nissen, a cardiologist at the Cleveland Clinic and a panel member. "But I also don't want to expose several million American women to the risk of heart attack and stroke, with their devastating consequences, in order to have one more sexual experience per month."

The Food and Drug Administration, which convened the meeting, will have the final say on the hormone patch, which is called Intrinsa. But the agency usually follows the advice of its advisory panels, which are made up of outside experts.

Read the complete article online in the eThemes section of this book's website: www.aw-bc.com/donatelle.

Original article published December 3, 2004. Copyright © 2004 *The New York Times*. Reprinted with permission.

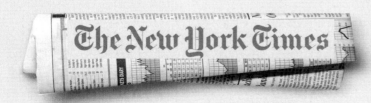

Human sexuality can be fascinating, complex, contradictory, and sometimes frustrating. In reality, sexuality is interwoven into every aspect of being human. No single theory or perspective can explain all its subtleties. It presents challenges in the areas of personal values, interpersonal relationships, cultural traditions, social norms, new technologies, current research findings, and changing political agendas.

Most college students are or have been sexually active. The 2000 National College Health Assessment reports that about 72 percent of respondents said they were sexually active.[1] Other studies have found that four out of five college students have had sexual intercourse at some point during their life; one in four reported that they have had six or more sexual partners in their lifetime. About 80 percent of sexually active college students reported using some form of contraception the last time they had intercourse, although only about 38 percent said they used a condom during their last experience of intercourse. Thirty-five percent of college students said they have either been pregnant or gotten someone else pregnant.

In this chapter, we provide information and insights into the major components of sexual identity, including biology, gender identity, gender roles, and sexual orientation. Understanding your sexual identity will prepare you to make healthful, responsible, and satisfying decisions about your sexuality and will help you have fulfilling and rewarding relationships.

Your Sexual Identity

Sexual identity, the recognition and acknowledgment of oneself as a sexual being, is determined by a complex interaction of genetic, physiological, environmental, and social

factors. The beginning of sexual identity occurs at conception with the combining of chromosomes that determine sex. It is the biological father who determines whether a baby will be a boy or a girl. All eggs (ova) carry an X chromosome; sperm may carry either an X or a Y chromosome. If a sperm carrying an X chromosome fertilizes an egg, the resulting combination of sex chromosomes (XX) provides the blueprint to produce a female. If a sperm carrying a Y chromosome fertilizes an egg, the XY combination produces a male.

Not all people, however, have XX or XY chromosomes, nor do they all necessarily exhibit exclusively female or male primary and secondary sex characteristics. **Intersexuality** may occur as often as one in 100 live births (see the Health in a Diverse World box).

The genetic instructions included in the sex chromosomes lead to the differential development of male and female **gonads** (reproductive organs) at about the eighth week of fetal life. Once the male gonads (testes) and the female gonads (ovaries) are developed, they play a key role in all future sexual development because the gonads are responsible for the production of sex hormones. The primary sex hormones produced by females are estrogen and progesterone. In males, the sex hormone of primary importance is testosterone, which is converted from androgens, hormones secreted by the adrenal glands. The release of testosterone in a maturing fetus signals the development of a penis and other male genitals. If no testosterone is produced, female genitals form.

At the time of **puberty,** sex hormones again play major roles in development. Hormones released by the pituitary gland, called gonadotropins, stimulate the testes and ovaries to make appropriate sex hormones. The increase of estrogen production in females and testosterone production in males leads to the development of **secondary sex characteristics.** Male secondary sex characteristics include deepening of the voice, development of facial and body hair, and growth of the skeleton and musculature. Female secondary sex characteristics include growth of the breasts, widening of the hips, and the development of pubic and underarm hair.

Thus far, we have described sexual identity only in terms of a person's biology. While biology is an important facet of sexual identity, the relationship between biology and culture is much more complicated than the popular notion of sex as biology and gender as social. Biological facts are themselves always understood and interpreted within the cultural framework that gives meaning to those facts. Sex simply refers to the biological condition of being male or female based on physiological and hormonal differences.

Gender is the practice of behaving in masculine or feminine ways as defined by the society in which one lives and as a component of our identity, while sex is more related to physical form and function. In this sense, gender is a performance, something we do rather than something we have, and we learn gender through the process of **socialization.** Through interactions with family, peers, teachers, media, and other social organizations, we learn to act in ways that

---

Sexual identity Recognition of oneself as a sexual being; a composite of biological sex characteristics, gender identity, gender roles, and sexual orientation.

Intersexuality Not exhibiting exclusively female or male primary and secondary sex characteristics.

Gonads The reproductive organs in a male (testes) or female (ovaries).

Puberty The period of sexual maturation.

Secondary sex characteristics Characteristics associated with gender but not directly related to reproduction, such as vocal pitch, degree of body hair, and location of fat deposits.

Gender The psychological condition of being feminine or masculine as defined by the society in which one lives.

Socialization Process by which a society communicates behavioral expectations to its individual members.

Intersexuality

Intersexual people are born with various levels of male and female biological characteristics, ranging from different chromosomal arrangements to a variety of primary and secondary sex characteristics. While most people are born with either XX or XY chromosomes, some are born with XXY or XO chromosomes (where O signifies a missing or damaged chromosome). In some people, gonads do not develop fully into ovaries or testicles, and in others external genitalia may be ambiguous. For example, a person may possess a phallus that could be a large clitoris or a small penis and a structure that resembles partially fused labia or a split scrotum.

Common forms of intersexuality include:

- *Androgen insensitivity syndrome (AIS).* Two forms of AIS exist: complete and partial. In complete AIS, people with XY chromosomes develop testes and produce androgens (hormones that produce male characteristics), but their bodies cannot respond to androgen and, therefore, their external genitalia are female. In adolescence, they experience breast development and sparse pubic hair growth but do not menstruate. In partial AIS, external genitalia are ambiguous.
- *Gonadal dysgenesis.* Like AIS, gonadal dysgenesis has two forms: complete and partial. In complete gonadal dysgenesis, people with XY chromosomes do not develop testes capable of producing androgen, and they have female external genitalia. People with partial gonadal dysgenesis develop ambiguous external genitalia.
- *Congenital adrenal hyperplasia (CAH).* In CAH, excess adrenal androgens lead to the development of ambiguous genitalia in people with XX chromosomes. People with CAH have masculine features, such as facial hair, grow quickly but stop growing before they should, have difficulty fighting off infections, and may have difficulty retaining enough salt. People with mild CAH usually have irregular periods and may have trouble becoming pregnant.
- *Turner's syndrome.* People with Turner's syndrome have a single X chromosome and a missing or damaged X chromosome. Turner's occurs in about 1 out of 3,000 live births. Symptoms include short stature, webbed neck, absent or retarded development of secondary sex characteristics, absence of menstruation, and drooping eyelids.
- *Klinefelter's syndrome.* People with Klinefelter's syndrome have an extra sex chromosome—XXY instead of XY. This chromosome arrangement occurs in 1 in 500 to 1,000 male births. Not all XXY males will develop Klinefelter's syndrome, and many will never know

they have an extra chromosome. Those who do develop the syndrome will have male external genitalia, although the penis may be smaller than in most males. They may develop breasts, lack facial and body hair, develop rounder bodies, and be overweight. They may also have some degree of language impairment.

Intersexuality has often been treated as a birth defect. Very often parents and physicians make determinations about the sex of a child born with ambiguous genitalia and have surgery performed to make the child's genitalia conform to expectations for the assigned sex. Many members of the intersex community have begun to protest this practice as a form of genital mutilation. They argue that conditions that are not life-threatening should not be surgically altered and society should become more accepting of the wide range of sexual differences.

Sources: Intersex Society of North America, "Intersexuality Basics," 2004, www.itpeople.org /frameset.html; S. Shaw and J. Lee, "Learning Gender in a Diverse Society," *Women's Voices, Feminist Visions: Classic and Contemporary Readings* (Mountain View, CA: Mayfield Publishing, 2001); The Johns Hopkins Children's Center, "Syndromes of Abnormal Sex Differentiation," 2004, www.hopkinsmedicine.org /pediatricendocrinology/intersex/index.html; and National Institute of Child Health and Human Development, "A Guide for XXY Males and Their Families," 2004, http://156.40.88.3 /publications/pubs/klinefelter.htm

---

society deems appropriate. Think about the television shows you watch. Do the characters play out traditional gender roles?

Each of us expresses our maleness or femaleness to others on a daily basis by the **gender roles** we play. **Gender identity** refers to the personal sense or awareness of being masculine or feminine, a male or a female. It may sometimes be difficult to express one's true sexual identity because of the bounds established by **gender-role stereotypes**, or generalizations about how males and females should express themselves and the characteristics each possesses. Our traditional sex roles are an example of gender-role stereotyping. Men are expected to be independent, aggressive, better in math and science, logical, and always

in control of their emotions. Women, on the other hand, are traditionally expected to be passive, nurturing, intuitive, sensitive, and emotional.

Gender roles   Expression of maleness or femaleness in everyday life.

Gender identity   Personal sense or awareness of being masculine or feminine, a male or a female.

Gender-role stereotypes   Generalizations concerning how males and females should express themselves and the characteristics each possesses.

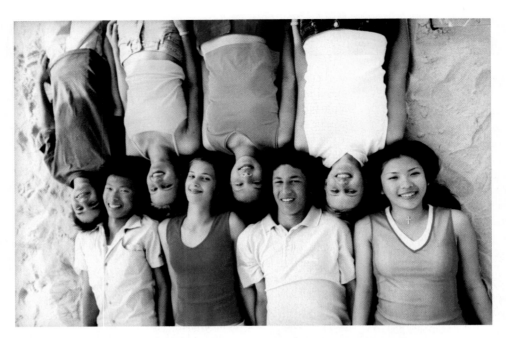

Signs of physical maturity are not always indicators of emotional adulthood.

Androgyny is the combination of traditional masculine and feminine traits in a single person. Androgynous people do not always follow traditional sex roles but instead choose behaviors based on the given situation.

Other people consider themselves to be **transgendered.** These people refuse to follow the sexual and gender scripts prescribed to them based on their biology and resist the division of gender into two distinct categories.[2]

Androgyny   Combination of traditional masculine and feminine traits in a single person.

Transgendered   Refusing to follow the sexual and gender scripts prescribed based on biology and resisting the division of gender into two distinct categories.

Transsexuality   Condition in which a person is psychologically of one sex but physically of the other.

Sexual orientation   A person's enduring emotional, romantic, sexual, or affectionate attraction to other persons.

Heterosexual   Experiencing primary attraction to and preference for sexual activity with people of the other sex.

Homosexual   Experiencing primary attraction to and preference for sexual activity with people of the same sex.

Bisexual   Experiencing attraction to and preference for sexual activity with people of both sexes.

Transsexuality, also known as gender dysphoria, refers to a condition in which a person is in a state of conflict between gender identity and physical sex. Simply stated, a transsexual is a mind physically trapped in the body of the opposite sex. The condition is not related to sexual orientation, nor should it be confused with transvestism, or cross-dressing.

By now you can see that defining sexual identity is not a simple matter. It is a lifelong process of growing and learning. Your sexual identity is made up of the unique combination of your biology, gender identity, chosen gender roles, sexual orientation, and personal experiences. It is up to you to take every opportunity to get to know and like yourself so that you may enjoy your life to the fullest.

What do you think?

How often do you challenge existing gender-role stereotypes? ■ *What is the outcome?* ■ *Do you think men and women have the same degree of freedom in gender-role expression?*

Sexual Orientation

Sexual orientation refers to a person's enduring emotional, romantic, sexual, or affectionate attraction to other persons. You may be primarily attracted to members of the other sex (**heterosexual**), your same sex (**homosexual**), or both sexes (**bisexual**).

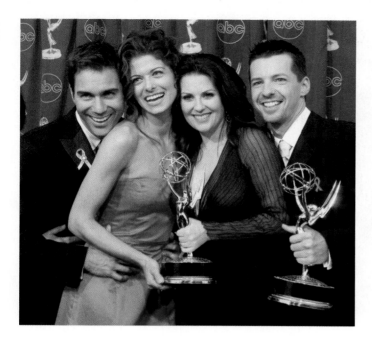

The presence of gay and lesbian characters and their friends, such as those portrayed by these actors on TV's *Will and Grace,* contributes to the increasing acceptance of gay relationships in everyday life.

Many homosexuals prefer the terms **gay** and **lesbian** to describe their sexual orientations, as these terms go beyond the exclusively sexual connotation of the term *homosexual.* The term *gay* can apply to both men and women, but *lesbian* refers specifically to women.

Throughout history, scientists and laypersons alike have debated the mental health status of gay men and lesbians. In 1973 the American Psychiatric Association's board of trustees unanimously voted that homosexuality was not a mental illness or psychiatric disorder. This position was affirmed by the American Psychological Association and the Sexuality Information and Education Council of the United States (SIECUS). Recently, the issue of homosexuality as a treatable "disease" has been resurrected. Therapies labeled as conversion or reparative therapies are being promoted in national newspapers and television ads. Mental health professionals have found these ads so troubling that the American Psychological Association passed a resolution reaffirming that homosexuality is not a disease in need of a "cure."[3]

Most researchers today agree that sexual orientation is best understood using a multifactorial model, which incorporates biological, psychological, and socioenvironmental factors. Biological explanations focus on research into genetics, hormones (perinatal and postpubertal), and differences in brain anatomy, while psychological and socioenvironmental explanations examine parent–child interactions, sex roles, and early sexual and interpersonal interactions. Collectively, this growing body of research suggests that the origins of homosexuality, like heterosexuality, are complex. To diminish the complexity of sexual orientation to "a choice" is a clear misrepresentation of current research. Homosexuals do not "choose" their sexual orientation any more than heterosexuals do.

Irrational fear or hatred of homosexuality creates anti-gay prejudice and is expressed as **homophobia.** Homophobic behaviors range from avoiding hugging same-sex friends to name-calling and physical attacks. Herek and colleagues surveyed 2,259 gay and lesbian people and found that one in five women and one in four men had been victimized in the preceding five years because of their sexual orientation.[4]

> **What do you think?**
>
> *Why is sexual orientation so controversial in our society?* ■ *Do you think homophobic behavior is on the decline?* ■ *What can you do to help prevent hate crimes?*

Sexual Anatomy and Physiology

An understanding of the functions of the male and female sexual systems will help you make responsible choices regarding your own sexual health, derive pleasure and satisfaction from your sexual relationships, and be sensitive to your partner's wants and needs.

Female Sexual Anatomy and Physiology

The female sexual system includes two major groups of structures, the external genitals (Figure 6.1 on page 166) and the internal genitals (Figure 6.2 on page 167). The **external female genitals** include all structures that are outwardly visible and are enclosed in a region known as the **vulva.** Specifically, the external genitalia include the mons pubis, the labia minora and majora, the clitoris, the urethral and vaginal openings,

Gay Sexual orientation involving primary attraction to people of the same sex; usually but not always applies to men attracted to men.

Lesbian Sexual orientation involving primary attraction of women to other women.

Homophobia Irrational hatred or fear of homosexuals or homosexuality.

External female genitals The mons pubis, labia majora and minora, clitoris, urethral and vaginal openings, and the vestibule of the vagina and its glands.

Vulva The female's external genitalia.

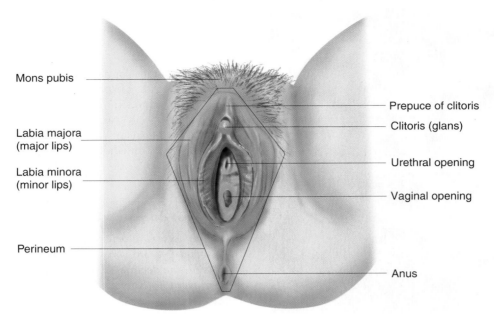

Figure 6.1
External Female Genital Structures

Source: From Richard McAnulty and Michele Burnette. *Exploring Human Sexuality: Making Healthy Decisions.* Published by Allyn & Bacon, Boston, MA. Copyright © 1999 by Pearson Education. Reprinted by permission of the publisher.

Mons pubis Fatty tissue covering the pubic bone in females; in physically mature women, the mons is covered with coarse hair.

Labia minora "Inner lips," or folds of tissue just inside the labia majora.

Labia majora "Outer lips," or folds of tissue covering the female sexual organs.

Clitoris A pea-sized nodule of tissue located at the top of the labia minora.

Urethral opening The opening through which urine is expelled.

Hymen Thin tissue covering the vaginal opening in some women.

Perineum Tissue that forms the "floor" of the pelvic region; it covers a kite-shaped region including the external genitalia and anus.

Internal female genitals The vagina, uterus, uterine (fallopian) tubes, and ovaries.

Vagina The passage in females leading from the vulva into the uterus.

Uterus (womb) Hollow, pear-shaped muscular organ whose function is to contain the developing fetus.

and the vestibule of the vagina. The **mons pubis** is a pad of fatty tissue covering the anterior part of the pubic bone. The mons serves to protect the bone, and after puberty it becomes covered with coarse hair. The **labia minora** are folds of thin skin, and the **labia majora** are folds of skin and tissue that enclose the urethral and vaginal openings. The labia minora are found just inside the labia majora.

The **clitoris** is the female sexual organ whose only known function is sexual pleasure. It is located at the upper end of the labia minora and beneath the mons pubis. Directly below the clitoris is the **urethral opening** through which urine leaves the body. Below the urethral opening is the vaginal opening. In some women, the vaginal opening is covered by a thin membrane called the **hymen.** It is a myth that an intact hymen is proof of virginity. The **perineum** is the "floor" that supports the endmost regions of the urogenital and gastorintestinal tracts (see Figure 6.1). Although not technically part of the external genitalia, the tissue in this area has many nerve endings and is sensitive to touch; it can play a part in sexual excitement.

The **internal female genitals** of the reproductive system include the vagina, uterus, fallopian tubes, and ovaries. The **vagina** is a tubular organ that serves as a passageway from the uterus to the outside of a female's body. This passageway allows menstrual flow to exit from the uterus during a female's monthly cycle and serves as the birth canal during childbirth. The vagina also receives the penis during intercourse. The **uterus,** also known as the womb, is a hollow,

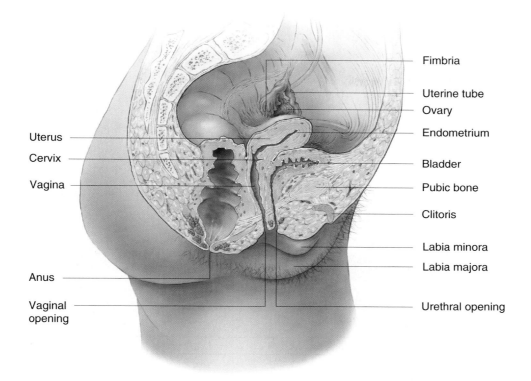

Figure 6.2
Side View of Female Reproductive Organs

muscular, pear-shaped organ. Hormones acting on the inner lining of the uterus, called the **endometrium,** either prepare the uterus for implantation and development of a fertilized egg or signal that no fertilization has taken place, in which case the endometrium deteriorates and its tissue and blood become menstrual flow.

The lower end of the uterus, the **cervix,** extends down into the vagina. The **ovaries** are almond-size structures suspended on either side of the uterus. The ovaries produce the hormones estrogen and progesterone and are also the reservoir for immature eggs. All the eggs a female will ever have are present in the ovaries at birth. Eggs mature and are released from the ovaries in response to hormone levels. Extending from the upper end of the uterus are two thin, flexible tubes called the **uterine (fallopian) tubes.** The uterine tubes, which do not actually touch the ovaries, capture eggs as they are released from the ovaries during ovulation, and they are where sperm and egg meet and fertilization takes place. Following fertilization, the uterine tubes serve as the passageway to the uterus, where the fertilized egg is implanted in the wall and development continues.

The Onset of Puberty and the Menstrual Cycle With the onset of **puberty,** the female reproductive system matures, and the development of secondary sex characteristics transforms young girls into young women. The first sign of

puberty is the beginning of breast development, which occurs around age 11. Under the direction of the endocrine system, the **pituitary gland,** the **hypothalamus,** and the ovaries all secrete hormones that act as chemical messengers among

Endometrium   Soft, spongy matter that makes up the uterine lining.

Cervix   Lower end of the uterus that opens into the vagina.

Ovaries   Almond-size organs that house developing eggs and produce hormones.

Uterine (fallopian) tubes   Tubes that extend from near the ovaries to the uterus.

Puberty   The maturation of the female or male reproduction system.

Pituitary gland   The endocrine gland located deep within the brain; controls reproductive functions.

Hypothalamus   An area of the brain located near the pituitary gland. The hypothalamus works in conjunction with the pituitary gland to control reproductive functions.

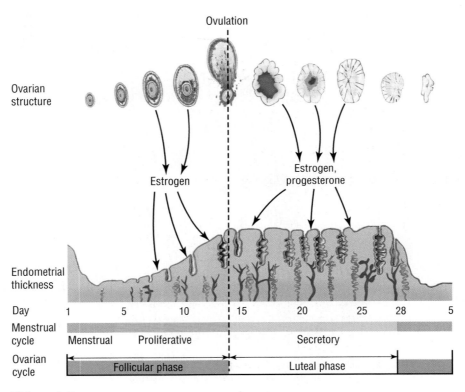

Ovulation

Ovarian
structure

Estrogen

Estrogen,
progesterone

Endometrial
thickness

| Day | 1 | 5 | 10 | 15 | 20 | 25 | 28 | 5 |

Menstrual
cycle   Menstrual   Proliferative   Secretory

Ovarian
cycle   Follicular phase   Luteal phase

Figure 6.3
Phases of the Menstrual (Uterine) and Ovarian Cycle

Source: From Richard McAnulty and Michele Burnette. *Exploring Human Sexuality: Making Healthy Decisions.* Published by Allyn & Bacon, Boston, MA. Copyright © 1999 by Pearson Education. Reprinted by permission of the publisher.

them. Working in a feedback system, hormonal levels in the bloodstream act as the trigger mechanism for release of more or different hormones.

Gonadotropin-releasing hormone (GnRH)   Hormone that signals the pituitary gland to release gonadotropins.

Follicle-stimulating hormone (FSH)   Hormone that signals the ovaries to prepare to release eggs and to begin producing estrogens.

Luteinizing hormone (LH)   Hormone that signals the ovaries to release an egg and to begin producing progesterone.

Estrogens   Hormones secreted by ovaries; control the menstrual cycle.

Progesterone   Hormone secreted by the ovaries; helps keep the endometrium developing in order to nourish a fertilized egg; also helps maintain pregnancy.

Menarche   The first menstrual period.

Ovarian follicles (egg sacs)   Areas within the ovary in which individual eggs develop.

At around age $9\frac{1}{2}$ to $11\frac{1}{2}$ in females, the hypothalamus receives the message to begin secreting **gonadotropin-releasing hormone (GnRH).** The release of GnRH in turn signals the pituitary gland to release hormones called gonadotropins. Two gonadotropins, **follicle-stimulating hormone (FSH)** and **luteinizing hormone (LH),** signal the ovaries to start producing **estrogens** and **progesterone.** Increased estrogen levels assist in the development of female secondary sex characteristics. In addition, estrogens regulate the reproductive cycle. The normal age range for the onset of the first menstrual period, termed **menarche,** is 9 to 17 years, with the average age being $11\frac{1}{2}$ to $13\frac{1}{2}$ years. Body fat heavily influences the onset of puberty, and increasing rates of obesity in children may account for the fact that girls here and in other countries seem to be reaching puberty much earlier than they used to.[5] Very thin girls, such as young athletes, tend to start menstruating later.

The average menstrual cycle is 28 days long and consists of three phases: the menstrual phase, the proliferative phase, and the secretory phase (Figure 6.3). During the proliferative phase, the pituitary gland releases FSH and LH. The FSH acts on the ovaries to stimulate the maturation process of several **ovarian follicles (egg sacs).** These follicles secrete estrogens and, in response to this estrogen stimulation, the lining of the uterus, the endometrium, begins to grow and develop. The inner walls of the uterus become coated with a thick, spongy lining composed of blood and mucus. In the event of fertilization, this endometrial tissue will become a nesting place for the developing embryo. The increased estrogen level also signals the pituitary to slow down FSH production but increase LH secretion. Of the several follicles developing in the ovaries, only one each month normally reaches complete maturity. Under the influence of LH, this one ovarian follicle rapidly matures; and, about the fourteenth day of the proliferative phase, it releases an ovum into the uterine tube—a process referred to as **ovulation.** This is the follicular phase of the ovarian cycle. Just prior to ovulation, the mature egg's follicle begins to increase secretion of progesterone, the first function of which is to spur the addition of further nutrients to the developing endometrium.

After ovulation, the secretory phase begins. The ovarian follicle is converted into the corpus luteum, or yellow body, which secretes an increased level of estrogen and progesterone. In addition, FSH also falls back to preproliferative levels. Essentially, the woman's body is "waiting" to see whether fertilization will occur. During this time, LH declines and progesterone levels rise, causing additional tissue growth in the endometrium.

If fertilization takes place, cells surrounding the developing embryo release a hormone called **human chorionic gonadotropin (HCG).** HCG increases estrogen and progesterone secretion, which maintains the endometrium while signaling the pituitary gland not to start a new menstrual cycle. This is roughly the luteal phase of the ovarian cycle.

When fertilization does not occur, the egg gradually disintegrates within approximately 72 hours. The corpus luteum gradually becomes nonfunctional, causing levels of progesterone and estrogen to decline. As hormonal levels decline, the endometrial lining of the uterus loses its nourishment, dies, and is sloughed off as menstrual flow.

Menstrual Problems   Premenstrual syndrome (PMS) comprises the mood changes and physical symptoms that occur in some women during one or two weeks prior to menstruation. Symptoms may include any or all of the following: breast swelling and tenderness, fatigue, trouble sleeping, upset stomach, bloating, constipation or diarrhea, headache, changes in appetite or food cravings, joint or muscle pain, weight gain, swelling of hands and feet, poor concentration, and feeling blue or irritable.

As many as 80 percent of women have some negative symptoms associated with the menstrual cycle. Of these, about 3 to 5 percent have symptoms that are similar to but more severe than PMS. Collectively these symptoms are labeled **premenstrual dysphoric disorder, or PMDD.** Unlike PMS, PMDD symptoms are severe and difficult to manage. In addition to the physical symptoms described for PMS, PMDD is marked by severe mood disturbances including depressed mood, anxiety, irritability, angry outbursts, and/or periods of sudden tearfulness or sadness. Many PMDD sufferers also experience insomnia and difficulty in concentrating. Women with PMDD experience significantly impaired lives for one to

two weeks every month, and the quality of their social relationships is often affected. Only about 25 percent of women who seek medical attention for this disorder are actually diagnosed with this rare condition. Women usually do not develop PMDD until their late twenties or early thirties, and PMDD worsens until menopause.[6]

Many natural approaches to managing PMS can also help PMDD. These strategies include: (1) eating more carbohydrates (grains, fruits, and vegetables); (2) reducing caffeine and salt intake; (3) exercising regularly; and (4) taking measures to reduce stress. Recent investigation into methods of controlling the severe emotional swings has led to the use of antidepressant medications for treating PMDD. A particular type of antidepressant, selective serotonin reuptake inhibitors (SSRIs such as Prozac and Zoloft), has been shown to be beneficial in reducing the mood disturbances associated with PMDD. Overall, more than 60 percent of women with PMDD respond to SSRIs, even in low doses and when taking them only while premenstrual. Side effects are generally minimal.

Toxic shock syndrome (TSS), although rare today, is still something of which you should be aware. It is caused by a bacterial infection facilitated by tampon or diaphragm use (see Chapters 7 and 17). Since the early 1980s, the U.S. Food and Drug Administration (FDA) has mandated that manufacturers of tampons conduct a battery of tests for safety clearance, but regardless of the safeguards, all women who use tampons should be aware of the potential for TSS. Symptoms are sometimes hard to recognize because they mimic the flu and include sudden high fever, vomiting, diarrhea, dizziness, fainting, or a rash that looks like sunburn during one's period or a few days after. Proper treatment usually assures recovery in two to three weeks.

Ovulation   The point of the menstrual cycle at which a mature egg ruptures through the ovarian wall.

Human chorionic gonadotropin (HCG)   Hormone that calls for increased levels of estrogen and progesterone secretion if fertilization has taken place.

Premenstrual syndrome (PMS)   Comprises the mood changes and physical symptoms that occur in some women during one or two weeks prior to menstruation.

Premenstrual dysphoric disorder (PMDD)   Collective name for a group of negative symptoms similar to but more severe than PMS, including severe mood disturbances.

Toxic shock syndrome (TSS)   A potentially life-threatening disease that occurs when specific bacterial toxins are allowed to multiply unchecked in wounds or through improper use of tampons or diaphragms.

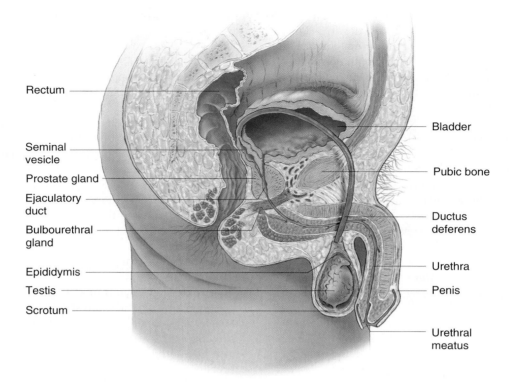

Rectum

Seminal vesicle

Prostate gland

Ejaculatory duct

Bulbourethral gland

Epididymis

Testis

Scrotum

Bladder

Pubic bone

Ductus deferens

Urethra

Penis

Urethral meatus

Figure 6.4
Side View of the Male Reproductive Organs

Dysmenorrhea is a condition that causes pain or discomfort in the lower abdomen just before or after menstruation. Primary dysmenorrhea usually begins one to two years after a woman's first period, while secondary dysmenorrhea is caused by a specific disease or disorder and may appear years after regular menstruation begins.

Many women find relief for painful menstrual periods through over-the-counter nonsteroidal anti-inflammatory drugs (NSAIDs) such as ibuprofen and aspirin. Applying a heating pad to the abdomen, taking a hot bath or shower, and massaging the abdomen may also provide relief.

Dysmenorrhea   Condition that causes pain or discomfort in the lower abdomen just before or after menstruation.

Menopause   The permanent cessation of menstruation, generally between the ages of 40 and 60.

Hormone replacement therapy (HRT)   or **menopausal hormone therapy**   Use of synthetic or animal estrogens and progesterone to compensate for decreases in estrogens in a woman's body.

Menopause   Just as menarche signals the beginning of a female's potential reproductive years, **menopause**—the permanent cessation of menstruation—signals the end. Generally occurring between the ages of 40 and 60, and at age 51 on average, menopause results in decreased estrogen levels, which may produce troublesome symptoms in some women. Decreased vaginal lubrication, hot flashes, headaches, dizziness, and joint pain have all been associated with the onset of menopause.

Hormones, such as estrogen and progesterone through **hormone replacement therapy (HRT),** have long been prescribed to relieve menopausal symptoms and reduce the risk of heart disease and osteoporosis. (The National Institutes of Health prefers the term **menopausal hormone therapy,** since hormone treatment is not a replacement and does not restore the physiology of youth.) However, recent studies, including results from the Women's Health Initiative (WHI), suggest that hormone therapy may actually do more harm than good. In fact, the WHI terminated this research ahead of schedule due to concerns about participants' increased risk of breast cancer, heart attack, stroke, blood clots, and other health problems.[7] All women need to discuss the risks and benefits of HRT with their health care provider and come to an informed decision. It is crucial to find a doctor who specializes in women's health and keeps up to date with the

Circumcision: Risk versus Benefit

New parents must decide whether their infant son will be circumcised. Circumcision involves the surgical removal of the foreskin (prepuce), a fold of skin covering the end (glans) of the penis. Most circumcisions in the United States are performed for religious or cultural reasons or because of concerns about hygiene. (The foreskin is fully attached to the glans at birth and naturally separates from it anywhere from weeks to several years after birth.)

Some studies suggest that uncircumcised males have a slightly greater risk of penile cancer and some sexually transmitted infections (STIs), including syphilis, gonorrhea, and HIV. The reason is suspected to be poor hygiene—not cleaning between the foreskin and glans as recommended. (Uncircumcised males should regularly wash the area under the foreskin with soap and water.) However, other apparently stronger data suggest that uncircumcised men are no more likely to contract STIs than circumcised men. Furthermore, the rate of penile cancer is so low that an equal number of deaths occur from circumcision-related complications as from penile cancer.

The American Academy of Pediatrics does not consider circumcision to be medically necessary. Parents who choose to circumcise do so for religious, aesthetic, or other personal reasons. If it is performed, pain relief should be given to the infant.

What decision do you think you would make for your son? Give your reasons. If you are male, does your circumcised or uncircumcised status affect your opinion?

Sources: American Academy of Pediatrics, "Just the Facts: Circumcision," 2003, www.aap .org/mrt/factscir.html; American Academy of Pediatrics, "Care of the Uncircumcised Penis," 2001, www.aap.org/family/uncirc.html; American Academy of Pediatrics Task Force on Circumcision, "Circumcision Policy Statement," *Pediatrics* 103 (1999): 686–693; E. O. Laumann, C. M. Masi, and E. W. Zuckerman, "Circumcision in the United States: Prevalence, Prophylactic Effects, and Sexual Practices," *Journal of the American Medical Association* 277 (1997), 1052–1057; and H. Shingleton and C. W. Heath, "Letter to Dr. Peter Rappo, American Academy of Pediatrics, from the American Cancer Society," 1996, www.nocirc.org/position/acs.html

---

latest research findings. Certainly a healthy lifestyle, such as regular exercise, a balanced diet, and adequate calcium intake, can also help protect postmenopausal women from heart disease and osteoporosis.

Male Sexual Anatomy and Physiology

The structures of the male sexual system may be divided into external and internal genitals (Figure 6.4). The penis and the scrotum make up the **external male genitals.** (See the Health Ethics box on circumcision for a discussion of the controversy surrounding removal of the foreskin of the penis.) The **internal male genitals** include the testes, epididymides, ductus deferentia, and urethra and three other structures—the seminal vesicles, the prostate gland, and the bulbourethral (Cowper's) glands—that secrete components that, with sperm, make up semen. These three structures are sometimes referred to as the **accessory glands.**

The **penis** serves as the organ that deposits sperm in the vagina during intercourse. The urethra, which passes through the center of the penis, acts as the passageway for both semen and urine to exit the body. During sexual arousal, the spongy tissue in the penis becomes filled with blood, making the organ stiff, or erect. Further sexual excitement leads to **ejaculation,** a series of rapid, spasmodic contractions that propel semen out of the penis.

Situated behind the penis and also outside the body is a sac called the **scrotum.** The scrotum protects the testes and also helps control the temperature within the testes, which is vital to proper sperm production. The **testes** (singular: *testis*) are egg-shaped structures in which sperm are manufactured. The testes also contain cells that manufacture **testosterone,** the hormone responsible for the development of male secondary sex characteristics.

The development of sperm is referred to as **spermatogenesis.** Like the maturation of eggs in the female, this

---

External male genitals   The penis and scrotum.

Internal male genitals   The testes, epididymides, vasa deferentia, ejaculatory ducts, urethra, and accessory glands.

Accessory glands   The seminal vesicles, prostate gland, and bulbourethral (Cowper's) glands.

Penis   Male sexual organ that releases sperm into the vagina.

Ejaculation   The propulsion of semen from the penis.

Scrotum   Sac of tissue that encloses the testes.

Testes   Two organs, located in the scrotum, that manufacture sperm and produce hormones.

Testosterone   The male sex hormone manufactured in the testes.

Spermatogenesis   The development of sperm.

process is governed by the pituitary gland. FSH is secreted into the bloodstream to stimulate the testes to manufacture sperm. Immature sperm are released into a comma-shaped structure on the back of the testis called the **epididymis** (plural: *epididymides*), where they ripen and reach full maturity.

The epididymis contains coiled tubules that gradually "unwind" and straighten out to become the **ductus (vas) deferens.** The two ductus (vasa) deferentia, as they are called in the plural, make up the tubular transportation system whose sole function is to store and move sperm. Along the way, the **seminal vesicles** provide sperm with nutrients and other fluids that compose **semen.**

The ductus deferentia eventually connect the epididymides to the ejaculatory ducts, which pass through the prostate gland and empty into the urethra. The **prostate gland** contributes more fluids to the semen, including chemicals that aid the sperm in fertilizing an ovum and neutralize the acidic environment of the vagina to make it more conducive to sperm motility (ability to move) and potency (potential for fertilizing an ovum).

Just below the prostate gland are two pea-shaped nodules called the **bulbourethral (Cowper's) glands.** The bulbourethral glands secrete a fluid that lubricates the urethra and neutralizes any acid that may remain in the urethra after urination. Urine and semen do not come into contact with each other. During ejaculation of semen, a small valve closes off the tube to the urinary bladder.

Human Sexual Response

Psychological traits greatly influence sexual response and sexual desire. Thus, we may find relationships with one partner vastly different from those we might experience with others.

Epididymis   A comma-shaped structure atop the testis where sperm mature.

Ductus (vas) deferens   A tube that transports sperm toward the penis.

Seminal vesicles   Storage areas for sperm where nutrient fluids are added to them.

Semen   Fluid containing sperm and nutrient fluids that increase sperm viability and neutralize vaginal acid.

Prostate gland   Gland that secretes nutrients and neutralizing fluids into the semen.

Bulbourethral (Cowper's) glands   Glands that secrete a fluid that lubricates the urethra and neutralizes any acid remaining in the urethra after urination.

Vasocongestion   The engorgement of the genital organs with blood.

Sexual response is a physiological process that generally follows a pattern. Both males' and females' sexual responses are somewhat arbitrarily divided into four stages: excitement/arousal, plateau, orgasm, and resolution (Figure 6.5). Researchers agree that each individual has a personal response pattern that may or may not conform to these phases. Regardless of the type of sexual activity (stimulation by a partner or self-stimulation), the response stages are the same.

During the first stage, excitement/arousal, **vasocongestion,** or increased blood flow in the genital region, stimulates male and female genital responses. Increased blood flow to these organs causes them to swell. The vagina begins to lubricate in preparation for penile penetration, and the penis becomes partially erect. Both sexes may exhibit a "sex flush," or light blush all over their bodies. Excitement/arousal can be generated by touching other parts of the body, by kissing, through fantasy, by viewing films or videos, or by reading erotic literature.

During the plateau phase, the initial responses intensify. Voluntary and involuntary muscle tensions increase. The female's nipples and the male's penis become erect. The penis secretes a few drops of preejaculatory fluid, which may contain sperm. During the orgasmic phase, vasocongestion and muscle tensions reach their peak, and rhythmic contractions occur through the genital regions. In females, these contractions are centered in the uterus, outer vagina, and anal sphincter. In males, the contractions occur in two stages. First, contractions within the prostate gland begin propelling semen through the urethra. In the second stage, the muscles of the pelvic floor, urethra, and anal sphincter contract. Semen usually, but not always, is ejaculated from the penis. In both sexes, spasms in other major muscle groups also occur, particularly in the buttocks and abdomen. Feet and hands may also contract, and facial features often contort.

Muscle tension and congested blood subside in the resolution phase, as the genital organs return to their prearousal states. Both sexes usually experience deep feelings of wellbeing and profound relaxation. Following orgasm and resolution, many females can become aroused again and experience additional orgasms. However, some men experience a refractory period, during which their systems are incapable of subsequent arousal. This refractory period may last from a few minutes to several hours, and tends to lengthen with age.

Men and women experience the same stages in the sexual response cycle; however, the length of time spent in any one stage varies. Thus, one partner may be in the plateau phase while the other is in the excitement/arousal or orgasmic phase. Such variations in response rates are entirely normal. Some couples believe that simultaneous orgasm is desirable for sexual satisfaction. Although simultaneous orgasm is pleasant, so are orgasms achieved at different times.

Sexual pleasure and satisfaction are also possible without orgasm or intercourse. Expressing sexual feelings for

1. Excitement/Arousal Phase

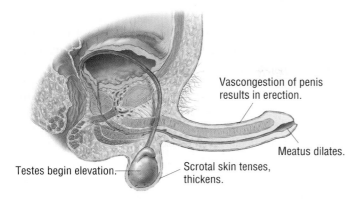

Vascongestion of penis results in erection.

Meatus dilates.

Testes begin elevation.

Scrotal skin tenses, thickens.

1. Excitement/Arousal Phase

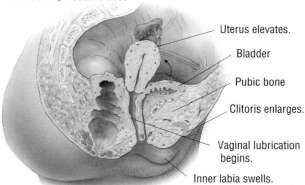

Uterus elevates.

Bladder

Pubic bone

Clitoris enlarges.

Vaginal lubrication begins.

Inner labia swells.

2. Plateau Phase

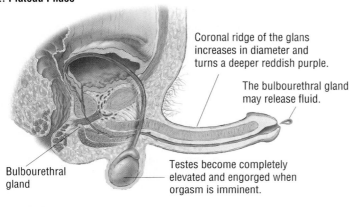

Coronal ridge of the glans increases in diameter and turns a deeper reddish purple.

The bulbourethral gland may release fluid.

Bulbourethral gland

Testes become completely elevated and engorged when orgasm is imminent.

2. Plateau Phase

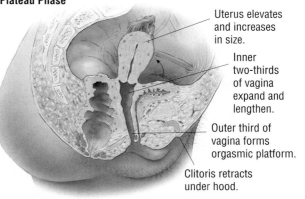

Uterus elevates and increases in size.

Inner two-thirds of vagina expand and lengthen.

Outer third of vagina forms orgasmic platform.

Clitoris retracts under hood.

3. Orgasmic Phase

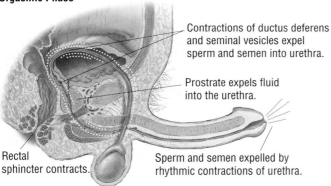

Contractions of ductus deferens and seminal vesicles expel sperm and semen into urethra.

Prostrate expels fluid into the urethra.

Rectal sphincter contracts.

Sperm and semen expelled by rhythmic contractions of urethra.

3. Orgasmic Phase

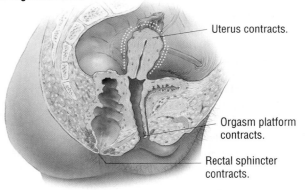

Uterus contracts.

Orgasm platform contracts.

Rectal sphincter contracts.

4. Resolution Phase

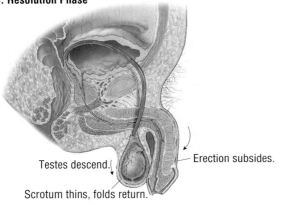

Testes descend.

Erection subsides.

Scrotum thins, folds return.

4. Resolution Phase

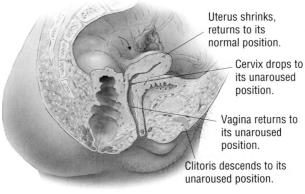

Uterus shrinks, returns to its normal position.

Cervix drops to its unaroused position.

Vagina returns to its unaroused position.

Clitoris descends to its unaroused position.

Figure 6.5
Comparison of Male and Female Sexual Responses

another person involves many pleasurable activities, of which intercourse and orgasm may only be a part.

What do you think?

Why do we place so much importance on orgasm? ■ *Can sexual pleasure and satisfaction be achieved without orgasm?* ■ *What is the role of desire in sexual response?*

Sexual Responses among Older Adults

Older adults are commonly stereotyped as being incapable of or uninterested in sexual relations. The truth is, though we do experience some physical changes as we age, these changes generally do not cause us to stop enjoying sex.

In women, the most significant physical changes follow menopause. Skin becomes less elastic; most internal sexual organs, including the uterus and cervix, shrink somewhat; the vaginal walls become thinner; and vaginal lubrication during sexual arousal may decrease. The resulting increased friction during penetration can be painful. The typical physical change during orgasm is that the duration tends to be shorter. In fact, as W. H. Masters and V. Johnson's research showed, postmenopausal women experience sexual relations much the same as they did prior to menopause, only less intensely and for shorter periods of time.[8] Women who remain sexually active report fewer problems with age-related changes in sexual functioning. The use of artificial lubricants usually resolves the problem of insufficient lubrication.

Although men do not experience menopause, their bodies also change as a result of the aging process. They require more direct and prolonged stimulation to achieve an erection, and erections become less firm. They are slower to obtain a full erection and to reach orgasm, and their refractory periods are longer. Older men also experience a decrease in the intensity of ejaculation. Semen seeps out during ejaculation rather than being forcefully expelled as is typical in younger men. However, the majority of healthy older men, like healthy older women, enjoy a regular and satisfying sex life.

Expressing Your Sexuality

Finding healthy ways to express your sexuality is an important part of developing sexual maturity. Many avenues of sexual expression are available.

Celibacy State of not being involved in a sexual relationship.

Sexual Behavior: What Is "Normal"?

Most of us want to fit in and be identified as normal, but how do we know which sexual behaviors are considered normal? What or whose criteria should we use? These are not easy questions.

Every society sets standards and attempts to regulate sexual behavior. Boundaries arise that distinguish good from bad, acceptable from unacceptable, and result in criteria used to establish what is viewed as normal or abnormal. Common sociocultural standards for sexual behavior in Western culture today include:[9]

- *The heterosexual standard.* Sexual attraction should be limited to members of the other sex.
- *The coital standard.* Penile–vaginal intercourse (coitus) is viewed as the ultimate sex act.
- *The orgasmic standard.* All sexual interaction should lead to orgasm.
- *The two-person standard.* Sex is an activity to be experienced by two.
- *The romantic standard.* Sex should be related to love.
- *The safer sex standard.* If we choose to be sexually active, we should act to prevent unintended pregnancy or disease transmission.

These are not laws or rules, but rather social scripts that have been adopted over time. Sexual standards often shift through the years, and many people choose not to follow them. We are a pluralistic nation, and that pluralism extends to our sexual practices. Rather than making blanket judgments about normal versus abnormal, we might ask the following questions:[10]

- Is a sexual behavior healthy and fulfilling for a particular person?
- Is it safe?
- Does it lead to the exploitation of others?
- Does it take place between responsible, consenting adults?

In this way, we can view behavior along a continuum that takes into account many individual factors. As you read about the options for sexual expression in the pages ahead, use these questions to explore your feelings about what is normal for you. See the Assess Yourself box to examine your own feelings about sexual differences.

Options for Sexual Expression

The range of human sexual expression is virtually infinite. What you find enjoyable may not be an option for someone else. The ways you choose to meet your sexual needs today may be very different from how you meet them two years from now. Accepting yourself as a sexual person with individual desires and preferences is the first step in achieving sexual satisfaction.

Celibacy Celibacy is avoidance of or abstention from sexual activities with others. A completely celibate person also does not engage in masturbation (self-stimulation), whereas

Attitudes toward Sexual Differences

☀ my**health**lab

Fill out this assessment online at www.aw-bc.com/myhealthlab or www.aw-bc.com/donatelle

How comfortable would you be in the following situations? Why?

	Completely Comfortable			Not at All Comfortable	
1. Your close same-sex friend reveals to you her/his preference for same-sex partners.	1	2	3	4	5
2. Your roommate tells you that she/he likes sexual encounters that involve three or more partners at one time.	1	2	3	4	5
3. Your sister tells you that she would like to have a sex-change operation.	1	2	3	4	5
4. You visit a friend's house, and she/he shows you her/his sexual fantasy room that includes vibrators, sexually explicit magazines, and erotic videos.	1	2	3	4	5
5. Your close friend of another sex reveals to you her/his preference for same-sex partners.	1	2	3	4	5
6. Your 85-year-old grandfather reveals that he is sexually active with his 85-year-old female partner.	1	2	3	4	5
7. A male friend reveals that, although he is primarily heterosexual, he occasionally has sex with other men.	1	2	3	4	5
8. Your lab partner, who looks and acts like a man, reveals that he is really a transgendered woman.	1	2	3	4	5
9. Your blind date tells you that she/he occasionally likes to engage in sadomasochistic sexual play.	1	2	3	4	5
10. Two women from your health class invite you to attend their commitment ceremony at the end of the term.	1	2	3	4	5
11. Your best friend reveals that she/he has made a personal commitment not to engage in sexual activity until marriage.	1	2	3	4	5
12. Your best male friend tells you that he enjoys phone sex.	1	2	3	4	5
13. The person with whom you are romantically involved asks you to tell her/him your sexual fantasies.	1	2	3	4	5
14. You meet someone in an Internet chat room who wants to engage in cybersex.	1	2	3	4	5
15. Your divorced mother reveals that she is dating a man who is your age.	1	2	3	4	5

MAKE IT HAPPEN!

Use the results of this self-assessment to begin your behavior change program. Follow the steps and use the examples on page 181 to complete your Behavior Change Contract and use these resources to take action.

a partially celibate person avoids sexual activities with others but may enjoy autoerotic behaviors such as masturbation. Some people choose celibacy for religious or moral reasons. Others may be celibate for a period of time due to illness, the breakup of a long-term relationship, or lack of an acceptable partner. For some, celibacy is a lonely, agonizing state, but others find it an opportunity for introspection, values assessment, and personal growth.

Autoerotic Behaviors   **Autoerotic behaviors** involve sexual self-stimulation. The two most common are sexual fantasy and masturbation.

Sexual fantasies are sexually arousing thoughts and dreams. Fantasies may reflect real-life experiences, forbidden desires, or the opportunity to practice new or anticipated sexual experiences. The fact that you fantasize about a particular sexual experience does not necessarily mean that you want to, or have to, act that experience out. Sexual fantasies are just that—fantasy.

Masturbation is self-stimulation of the genitals. Although many people feel uncomfortable discussing masturbation, it is a common sexual practice across the life span. Masturbation is a natural, pleasure-seeking behavior in infants and children. It is a valuable and important means for adolescent males and females, as well as adults, to explore sexual feelings and responsiveness.

Kissing and Erotic Touching   Kissing and erotic touching are two very common forms of nonverbal sexual communication. Both males and females have **erogenous zones,** areas of the body that when touched lead to sexual arousal. Erogenous zones may include genital as well as nongenital areas, such as the earlobes, mouth, breasts, and inner thighs. Almost any area of the body can be conditioned to respond erotically to touch. Spending time with your partner to explore and learn about his or her erogenous areas is another pleasurable, safe, and satisfying means of sexual expression.

Autoerotic behaviors   Sexual self-stimulation.

Sexual fantasies   Sexually arousing thoughts and dreams.

Masturbation   Self-stimulation of genitals.

Erogenous zones   Areas of the body of both males and females that, when touched, lead to sexual arousal.

Cunnilingus   Oral stimulation of a female's genitals.

Fellatio   Oral stimulation of a male's genitals.

Vaginal intercourse   The insertion of the penis into the vagina.

Anal intercourse   The insertion of the penis into the anus.

Manual Stimulation   Both men and women can be sexually aroused and achieve orgasm through manual stimulation of the genitals by a partner. For many women, orgasm is more likely to be achieved through manual stimulation than through intercourse. *Sex toys* include a wide variety of objects that can be used for sexual stimulation alone or with a partner. Vibrators and dildos are two common types of toys and can be found in a variety of shapes, styles, and sizes. Sex toys can add zest to sexual experiences and, for women who may not reach orgasm by intercourse, may provide another option for satisfaction. Toys must be cleaned between uses.

Oral–Genital Stimulation   **Cunnilingus** refers to oral stimulation of a female's genitals, and **fellatio** to oral stimulation of a male's genitals. Many partners find oral–genital stimulation intensely pleasurable. Seventy percent of college-age men and women have had oral sex.[11] For some people, oral sex is not an option because of moral or religious beliefs.

Note that HIV and other sexually transmitted infections (STIs) can be transmitted via unprotected oral–genital sex just as through intercourse. Use of an appropriate barrier device is strongly recommended if either partner's health status is in question.

Vaginal Intercourse   The term *intercourse* generally refers to **vaginal intercourse** (*coitus,* or insertion of the penis into the vagina), which is the most frequently practiced form of sexual expression. Coitus can involve a variety of positions, including the missionary position (man on top facing the woman), woman on top, side by side, or man behind (rear entry). Many partners enjoy experimenting with different positions. Knowledge of yourself and your body, along with your ability to communicate effectively, will play a large part in determining the enjoyment and meaning of intercourse for you and your partner. Whatever your circumstance, you should practice safer sex to avoid disease and unwanted pregnancy.

Anal Intercourse   The anal area is highly sensitive to touch, and some couples find pleasure in the stimulation of this area. **Anal intercourse** is insertion of the penis into the anus. Sixteen percent of college-age men and women have had anal sex.[12] Stimulation of the anus by mouth or with the fingers is also practiced. As with all forms of sexual expression, anal stimulation or intercourse is not for everyone. If you do enjoy this form of sexual expression, remember to use condoms to avoid transmitting disease. Also, anything inserted into the anus should not be directly inserted into the vagina, as bacteria commonly found in the anus can cause vaginal infections.

Variant Sexual Behavior

Although attitudes toward sexuality have changed radically since the Victorian era, some people still believe that any sexual behavior other than heterosexual intercourse is abnormal or perverted. People who study sexuality prefer to use the neutral term **variant sexual behavior** to describe sexual behaviors that are not engaged in by most people; for example:

- *Group sex.* Sexual activity involving more than two people. Participants in group sex run a higher risk of exposure to AIDS and other sexually transmitted infections.
- *Transvestism.* Wearing the clothing of the opposite sex. Most transvestites are male, heterosexual, and married.
- *Fetishism.* Sexual arousal achieved by looking at or touching inanimate objects, such as underclothing or shoes.

Some variant sexual behaviors can be harmful to the individual, to others, or to both. Many of the following activities are illegal in at least some states.

- *Exhibitionism.* Exposing one's genitals to strangers in public places. Most exhibitionists are seeking a reaction of shock or fear from their victims. Exhibitionism is a minor felony in most states.
- *Voyeurism.* Observing other people for sexual gratification. Most voyeurs are men who attempt to watch women undressing or bathing. Voyeurism is an invasion of privacy and illegal in most states.
- *Sadomasochism.* Sexual activities in which gratification is received by inflicting pain (verbal or physical) on a partner or by being the object of such infliction. A sadist is a person who receives gratification from inflicting pain, and a masochist receives gratification from experiencing it.
- *Pedophilia.* Sexual activity or attraction between an adult and a child. Any sexual activity involving a minor, including possession of child pornography, is illegal.
- *Autoerotic asphyxiation.* The practice of reducing or eliminating oxygen to the brain, usually by tying a cord around one's neck while masturbating to orgasm. Tragically, asphyxiation is usually discovered when people accidentally hang themselves.

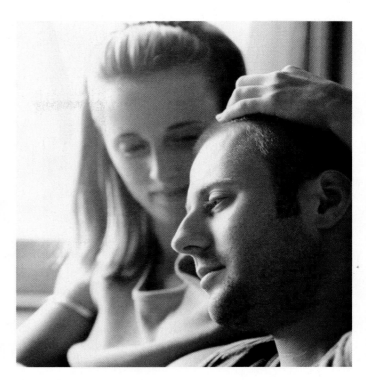

Sexual dysfunction can affect couples of any age. Communication is critical to resolving the problem.

other body system. Sexual dysfunction can be divided into five major classes: disorders of sexual desire, sexual arousal, orgasm, sexual performance, and sexual pain. All of them can be treated successfully. Figure 6.6 on page 178 reports the prevalence of sexual dysfunctions.

Sexual Desire Disorders

The most frequent reason why people seek out a sex therapist is **ISD**, or **inhibited sexual desire**.[13] ISD is the lack of a sexual appetite or simply a lack of interest and pleasure in sexual activity. In some instances, it can result from stress or boredom. **Sexual aversion disorder** is another type of desire dysfunction, characterized by sexual phobias (unreasonable fears) and anxiety about sexual contact. The psychological

---

What do you think?

How does our society define "normal" sexual behavior? ■ *What behaviors do you consider normal or abnormal?* ■ *Do you consider your own preferred forms of sexual expression to be normal? Why or why not?*

Difficulties That Can Hinder Sexual Function

Research indicates that **sexual dysfunction,** the term used to describe problems that can hinder sexual functioning, is quite common. Don't feel embarrassed if you experience sexual dysfunction at some point in your life. The sexual part of you does not come with a lifetime warranty. You can have breakdowns involving your sexual function just as in any

---

Variant sexual behavior A sexual behavior that is not engaged in by most people.

Sexual dysfunction Problems associated with achieving sexual satisfaction.

Inhibited sexual desire (ISD) Lack of sexual appetite or simply a lack of interest and pleasure in sexual activity.

Sexual aversion disorder Type of desire dysfunction characterized by sexual phobias and anxiety about sexual contact.

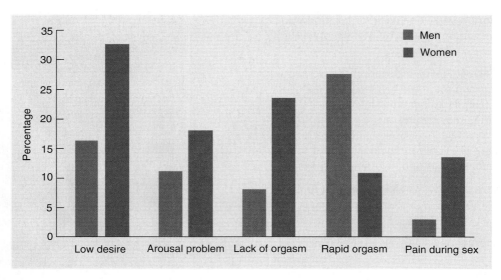

Figure 6.6

Prevalence of Sexual Problems in Men and Women

Source: Data from E. O. Laumann, et al., *The Social Organization of Sexuality: Sexual Practices in the United States* (Chicago, IL: University of Chicago Press, 1994). Reprinted in McAnulty and Burnette, *Exploring Human Sexuality,* Allyn & Bacon, Boston, MA. Copyright 1999.

stress of a punitive upbringing, a rigid religious background, or a history of physical or sexual abuse may be sources of these desire disorders.

Sexual Arousal Disorders

The most common disorder in this category is **erectile dysfunction (impotence)**—difficulty in achieving or maintaining a penile erection sufficient for intercourse. At some time in his life, every man experiences impotence. Causes are varied and include underlying diseases, such as diabetes or prostate problems; reactions to some medications (for example, drugs for high blood pressure); depression; fatigue; stress; alcohol; performance anxiety; and guilt over real or imaginary problems (such as when a man compares himself to his partner's past lovers).

Some 30 million men in this country, half of them under age 65, suffer from impotence. Impotence generally becomes more of a problem as men age, affecting one in four men over the age of 65.[14] The FDA has approved the drug Viagra (sildenafil citrate) to treat impotence. Taken by mouth one hour before sexual activity, Viagra is reported to manage erectile dysfunction successfully in 60 to 80 percent

of cases.[15] The medication is not, however, without risk. The most commonly reported side effects include headache, flushing, stomachache, urinary tract infection, diarrhea, dizziness, rash, and mild and temporary visual changes. In addition, there have been several deaths in the United States among Viagra users, prompting more caution in prescribing it to patients with known cardiovascular disease and those taking commonly prescribed short- and long-acting nitrates, such as nitroglycerin.[16]

Levitra and Cialis, other FDA-approved drug treatments for erectile dysfunction, work in the same way as Viagra. Levitra takes effect in about 30 minutes but works a bit longer than Viagra (about five hours as compared to four). Cialis takes a bit longer to work, but the effects may last as long as two to three days. Alprostadil can be given either as an injection or as a suppository placed into the opening at the tip of the penis. Alprostadil works in five to ten minutes. Another drug that can help prolong erection is Trazodone, an antidepressant. Several other Viagra-like drugs are being developed that will have different side effects. Another potential treatment is the internal penile pump, a soft fluid-filled (saline) device that expands and contracts. The pump transfers saline into the penis, causing an erection.

Orgasm Disorders

Premature ejaculation—ejaculation that occurs prior to or very soon after the insertion of the penis into the vagina—affects up to 50 percent of the male population at some time in their lives. Treatment for premature ejaculation first involves a physical examination to rule out organic causes. If the cause of the problem is not physiological, therapy is available to help a man learn how to control the timing of his

> **Erectile dysfunction (impotence)** Difficulty in achieving or maintaining a penile erection sufficient for intercourse.
>
> **Premature ejaculation** Ejaculation that occurs prior to or almost immediately following penile penetration of the vagina.

ejaculation. Fatigue, stress, performance pressure, and alcohol use can all contribute to orgasmic disorders in men.

In a woman, the inability to achieve orgasm is termed **female orgasmic disorder.** A woman with this disorder often blames herself and learns to fake orgasm to avoid embarrassment or preserve her partner's ego. Contributing to this response are the messages women have historically been given about sex as a duty rather than a pleasurable act. As with men who experience orgasmic disorders, the first step in treatment is a physical exam to rule out organic causes. However, the problem is often solved by simple self-exploration to learn more about what forms of stimulation are arousing enough to produce orgasm. Through masturbation, a woman can learn how her body responds sexually to various types of touch. Once she has become orgasmic through masturbation, she learns to communicate her needs to her partner.

Sexual Performance Anxiety

Both men and women can experience **sexual performance anxiety,** when they anticipate some sort of problem in the sex act. A man may become anxious and unable to maintain an erection, or he may experience premature ejaculation. A woman may be unable to achieve orgasm or to allow penetration because of the involuntary contraction of vaginal muscles. Both can overcome performance anxiety by learning to focus on immediate sensations and pleasures rather than on orgasm.

Sexual Pain Disorders

Two common disorders in this category are dyspareunia and vaginismus. **Dyspareunia** is pain experienced by a female during intercourse. This pain may be caused by diseases such as endometriosis, uterine tumors, chlamydia, gonorrhea, or urinary tract infections. Damage to tissues during childbirth and insufficient lubrication during intercourse may also cause discomfort. Dyspareunia can also be psychological

in origin. As with other sexual problems, dyspareunia can be treated with good results.

Vaginismus is the involuntary contraction of vaginal muscles, making penile insertion painful or impossible. Most cases of vaginismus are related to fear of intercourse or to unresolved sexual conflicts. Treatment involves teaching a woman to achieve orgasm through nonvaginal stimulation.

Seeking Help for Sexual Dysfunction

Many theories and treatment models can help people with sexual dysfunction. A first important step is choosing a qualified sex therapist or counselor. A national organization, the American Association of Sex Educators, Counselors, and Therapists (AASECT), has been in the forefront of establishing criteria for certifying sex therapists. These criteria include appropriate degree(s) in the helping professions, specialized coursework in human sexuality, and sufficient hours of practical therapy work under the direct supervision of a certified sex therapist. Lists of certified counselors and sex therapists, as well as clinics that treat sexual dysfunctions, can be obtained by contacting AASECT and SIECUS.

Female orgasmic disorder   The inability to achieve orgasm.

Sexual performance anxiety   A condition of sexual difficulties caused by anticipating some sort of problem with the sex act.

Dyspareunia   Pain experienced by women during intercourse.

Vaginismus   A state in which the vaginal muscles contract so forcefully that penetration cannot be accomplished.

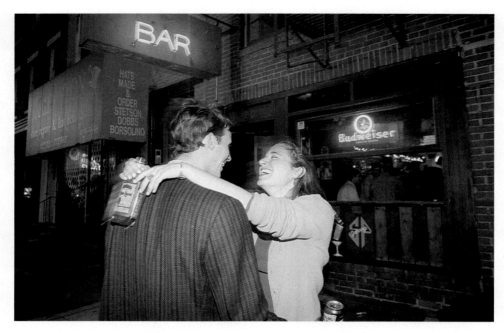

Alcohol and drug use can impair judgment and lead to sexual encounters that are later regretted.

Drugs and Sex

Because psychoactive drugs affect the entire physiology, it is only logical that they affect sexual behavior. Promises of increased pleasure make drugs very tempting to those seeking greater sexual satisfaction. Too often, however, drugs become central to sexual activities and damage the relationship. Drug use can also lead to undesired sexual activity.

Alcohol is notorious for reducing inhibitions and promoting feelings of well-being and desirability. At the same time, alcohol inhibits sexual response; thus, the mind may be willing, but not the body.

Perhaps the greatest danger associated with use of drugs during sex is the tendency to blame the drug for negative behavior. "I can't help what I did last night because I was drunk" is a statement that demonstrates sexual immaturity. A sexually mature person carefully examines risks and benefits and makes decisions accordingly. If drugs are necessary to increase erotic feelings, it is likely that the partners are being dishonest about their feelings for each other. Good sex should not depend on chemical substances.

"Date rape" drugs are a growing concern in recent years. They have become popular among college students and are often used in combination with alcohol.[17] Rohypnol ("roofies," "rope," "forget pill"), GHB (gamma-hydroxybutyrate, or "liquid X," "Grievous Bodily Harm," "easy lay,"

"Mickey Finn"), and ketamine ("K," "Special K," "cat valium") have been used to facilitate rape. GHB and Rohypnol are difficult-to-detect drugs that depress the central nervous system. Ketamine can cause dream-like states, hallucinations, delirium, amnesia, and impaired motor function. These drugs are often introduced to unsuspecting women through alcoholic drinks in order to render them unconscious and vulnerable to rape. This problem is so serious that the U.S. Congress passed the Drug-Induced Rape Prevention and Punishment Act of 1996 to provide increased federal penalties for using drugs to facilitate sexual assault. The dangers of these drugs are discussed in more detail in Chapter 4 (see the Reality Check: Drug-Facilitated Rapes box) and Chapter 14 (see the Club Drugs section).

What do you think?

Why do we find it so difficult to discuss sexual dysfunction in our society? ■ *Do you think it is more difficult for men than for women to talk about dysfunction?* ■ *Have you ever used alcohol or some other drug to enhance your sexual performance?* ■ *Why are "roofies" of major concern on college campuses?*

TAKING CHARGE

MAKE IT HAPPEN!

Assessment: The Assess Yourself box on page 175 asks you to consider your comfort level with a variety of sexual situations and preferences. If you were surprised or unhappy with any of your responses, you may want to consider how to change the attitudes that disturb you.

Making a Change: In order to change your behavior, you need to develop a plan. Follow these steps:

1. Evaluate your behavior, and identify patterns and specific things you are doing. What can you change now? What can you change in the near future?
2. Select one pattern of behavior that you want to change.
3. Fill out a Behavior Change Contract. It should include your long-term goal for change, your short-term goals, the rewards you'll give yourself for reaching these goals, potential obstacles along the way, and strategies for overcoming these obstacles. For each goal, list the small steps and specific actions that you will take.
4. Chart your progress in a journal. At the end of a week, consider how successful you were in following your plan. What helped you be successful? What made change more difficult? What will you do differently next week?

5. Revise your plan as needed: Are the short-term goals attainable? Are the rewards satisfying?

One Student's Plan: Jerome considered himself an open-minded and even experimental person. In fact, one of his goals in attending college was to meet people of all different types. Taking the self-assessment made him re-evaluate some of his assumptions about his comfort level when it came to sexual differences. He found that most of the situations described made him very uncomfortable. Although he was comfortable with his personal decisions about sexuality, he was unhappy to feel judgmental about others' choices. Jerome knew that there was a student group dedicated to representing gay, lesbian, and bisexual students. Among other activities, they sponsored speakers and lectures. Jerome checked their schedule and attended a talk about gay students' experiences on his campus. Later in the month, he signed up for a lecture by a transgender activist. His goal was not necessarily to change his beliefs about sexuality as much as to learn as much about its variations as possible, and then to accept his comfort level based on his increased understanding.

Summary

- Sexual identity is determined by a complex interaction of genetic, physiological, and environmental factors. Biological sex, gender identity, gender roles, and sexual orientation are all blended into our sexual identity.
- The major components of the female sexual anatomy include the mons pubis, labia minora and majora, clitoris, urethral and vaginal openings, vagina, cervix, uterine tubes, and ovaries. The major components of the male sexual anatomy are the penis, scrotum, testes, epididymides, ductus deferentia, ejaculatory ducts, and urethra.
- Physiologically, males and females experience four phases of sexual response: excitement/arousal, plateau, orgasmic, and resolution.

- Humans can express their sexual selves in a variety of ways, including celibacy, autoerotic behaviors, kissing and erotic touch, manual stimulation, oral–genital stimulation, vaginal intercourse, and anal intercourse. Sexual orientation refers to a person's enduring emotional, romantic, sexual, or affectionate attraction to other persons. Irrational hatred or fear of homosexuality or gay and lesbian persons is termed homophobia.
- Sexual dysfunctions can be classified into disorders of sexual desire, sexual arousal, orgasm, sexual performance anxiety, and sexual pain. Drug use can also lead to sexual dysfunction.

Questions for Discussion and Reflection

1. How have gender roles changed over the past 20 years? Do you view the changes as positive for both men and women?
2. Discuss the cycle of changes that occurs in our bodies in response to various hormones (for example, sexual differentiation while in the womb, secondary sex characteristics at puberty, menopause).
3. What is "normal" sexual behavior? What criteria should we use to determine healthful sexual practice?

4. If scientists finally establish the combination of factors that interact to produce homosexual, heterosexual, or bisexual orientation, will that put an end to antigay prejudice? Why or why not?
5. How can we remove the stigma that surrounds sexual dysfunction so that individuals feel more open to seeking help? Are men and women impacted differently by sexual dysfunction?

Accessing Your Health on the Internet

Visit the following Internet sites to explore further topics and issues related to personal health. To visit an organization's website, go to the Companion Website for *Access to Health, Ninth Edition* at www.aw-bc.com/donatelle, click on the book image, and select "Accessing Your Health on the Internet" from the navigation menu.

1. *American Association of Sex Educators, Counselors, and Therapists (AASECT).* Professional organization providing standards of practice for treatment of sexual issues and disorders.
2. *Bacchus and Gamma Peer Education Network.* Student-friendly source of information about sexual and other health issues.

3. *Go Ask Alice.* An interactive question-and-answer resource from the Columbia University Health Services. "Alice" is available to answer questions each week about any health-related issues, including relationships, nutrition and diet, exercise, drugs, sex, alcohol, and stress.
4. *Sexuality Information and Education Council of the United States (SIECUS).* Information, guidelines, and materials for advancement of healthy and proper sex education.
5. *Teen Sexual Health.* Current research and other resources dealing with sexual health for high school and college-age students.

Further Reading

Caron, S. L. *Sex Matters for College Students: Sex FAQ's in Human Sexuality.* Englewood Cliffs, NJ: Prentice Hall, 2002.

This is a brief, easy-to-read, and affordable paperback designed specifically to answer the basic sexual questions of today's young adults in a friendly and age-appropriate way.

Caster, W. *The Lesbian Sex Book: A Guide for Women Who Love Women,* 2nd ed. Alyson, 2003.

A handbook for lesbian sexual practices and health.

Goldstone, S. *The Ins and Outs of Gay Sex: A Medical Handbook for Men.* New York: Dell, 1999.

A comprehensive guide to the sexual and medical concerns of gay men.

Men's Health Books, ed. *The Complete Book of Men's Health: The Definitive, Illustrated Guide to Healthy Living, Exercise, and Sex.* Emmaus, PA: Rodale Press, 2000.

A comprehensive and lushly illustrated guide to information on healthy lifestyles for men.

Sexuality Information and Education Council of the United States (SIECUS) Report. 130 West 42nd Street, New York, NY 10036.

Highly acclaimed and readable bimonthly journal. Includes timely and thought-provoking articles on human sexuality, sexuality education, and AIDS.

Wingood, G. M. and R. DiClemente, eds. *Handbook of Women's Sexual and Reproductive Health.* Boston: Plenum Publishing, 2002.

Medical researchers, including those in behavioral sciences and health education, summarize in depth the epidemiology, social and behavioral factors, policies, and effective intervention and prevention strategies related to women's sexual and reproductive health.

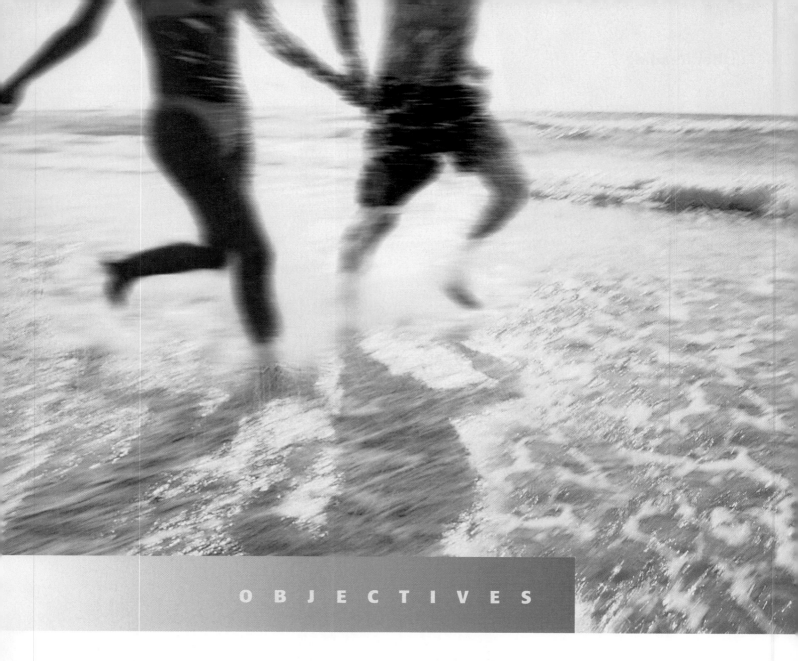

- Discuss the different types of contraceptive methods, and compare their effectiveness in preventing pregnancy and sexually transmitted infections.

- Summarize the legal decisions surrounding abortion and the various types of abortion procedures.

- Discuss key issues to consider when planning a pregnancy.

- Explain the importance of prenatal care and the physical and emotional aspects of pregnancy.

- Describe the basic stages of childbirth, methods of managing childbirth, and the complications that can arise during labor and delivery.

- Review primary causes of and possible solutions to infertility.

7

REPRODUCTIVE CHOICES

MAKING RESPONSIBLE DECISIONS

IN THE NEWS

F.D.A. Strengthens Warning on the Abortion Pill

By Gardiner Harris

The death of a California woman in January after she took an abortion pill prompted federal drug regulators on Monday to strengthen the warning label on the drug, RU-486, also known as mifepristone.

The death was the third in the United States that the Food and Drug Administration has linked to the pill since its approval in 2000.

The warnings, though largely present on the old labeling, will now be given added prominence, with physicians urged to redouble efforts at watching their patients carefully for signs of systemic bacterial infection, excessive vaginal bleeding and ectopic, or tubal, pregnancies.

Opponents of abortion say the latest death demonstrates that mifepristone is unsafe and should be withdrawn from the market. Abortion rights advocates, on the other hand, say that it has been used by nearly 360,000 women in the United States and that bad outcomes with it are exceptionally rare.

In the case of the latest death, though, the argument does not end there. Dr. Cynthia Summers, spokeswoman for mifepristone's American maker, Danco Laboratories, said she did not believe the fatality should be attributed to the drug, since the coroner's report said the woman had instead taken methotrexate, a cancer medication that has also been used to induce abortions.

Read the complete article online in the eThemes section of this book's website: www.aw-bc.com/donatelle.

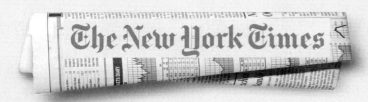

Today, we not only understand the intimate details of reproduction, but also possess technologies that can control or enhance our **fertility.** Along with information and technological advances comes choice, and choice goes hand in hand with responsibility. Choosing if and when to have children is one of our greatest responsibilities. A woman and her partner have much to consider before planning or risking a pregnancy. Children, whether planned or unplanned, change people's lives. They require a lifelong personal commitment of love and nurturing. Are you physically, emotionally, and financially prepared to care for another human being?

One measure of maturity is the ability to discuss reproduction and birth control with one's sexual partner before succumbing to sexual urges. Men often assume that their partners are taking care of birth control. Women often feel that bringing up the subject implies that they are promiscuous. Both may feel that this discussion interferes with romance and spontaneity. You will find embarrassment-free discussion a lot easier if you understand human reproduction and contraception and honestly consider your attitudes toward these matters before you find yourself in a compromising situation.

Methods of Fertility Management

Conception refers to the fertilization of an ovum by a sperm. The following conditions are necessary for conception:

1. A viable egg
2. A viable sperm
3. Access to the egg by the sperm

The term **contraception** (also called **birth control**) refers to methods of preventing conception. These methods offer varying degrees of control over when and whether pregnancy occurs. However, since people first associated sexual activity with pregnancy, society has searched for a sim-

ple, infallible, and risk-free way to prevent pregnancy. We have not yet found one.

To evaluate the effectiveness of a particular contraceptive method, you must be familiar with two concepts: perfect failure rate and typical use failure rate. *Perfect failure rate* refers to the number of pregnancies that are likely to occur in the first year of use (per 100 uses of the method during sexual intercourse) if the method is used absolutely perfectly, that is, without any error. The *typical use failure rate* refers to the number of pregnancies that are likely to occur in the first year of use with typical use, that is, with the normal number of errors, memory lapses, and incorrect or incomplete use. This information is much more practical for making informed decisions about contraceptive methods. See Table 7.1 for ratings of various contraceptive methods, many of which we'll discuss in this chapter. See the New Horizons in Health box on page 188 for an overview of new contraceptive options.

Many contraceptive methods can also protect, at least to some degree, against **sexually transmitted infections (STIs).** This is an important factor to consider in choosing a contraceptive. Table 7.1 compares the level of STI protection offered by various contraceptives; see Chapter 17 for more about specific STIs.

Present methods of contraception fall into several categories. **Barrier methods** use a physical or chemical block to prevent the egg and sperm from joining. Hormonal methods introduce synthetic hormones into the woman's system that prevent ovulation, thicken cervical mucus, or prevent a fertilized egg from implanting. Surgical methods can permanently prevent pregnancy. Other methods of contraception involve temporary or permanent abstinence or planning intercourse in accordance with fertility patterns. (See the Assess Yourself box on page 189 to determine what method is right for you and your partner.)

Barrier Methods

The Male Condom The **male condom** is a thin sheath designed to cover the erect penis and catch semen before it enters the vagina. The majority of male condoms are made of latex, although condoms made of polyurethane or lambskin are now available. This condom is the only temporary means of birth control available for men, and latex and polyurethane condoms are the only barriers that effectively prevent the spread of STIs and HIV. ("Skin" condoms, made from lamb intestines, are not effective against STIs.)

Condoms come in a wide variety of styles: colored, ribbed for "extra sensation," lubricated, nonlubricated, and with or without reservoirs at the tip. All may be purchased with or without spermicide in pharmacies, in some supermarkets and public bathrooms, and in many health clinics. A new condom must be used for each act of intercourse or oral sex.

In addition to helping to prevent some sexually transmitted infections, including genital herpes and HIV, condoms

---

Fertility A person's ability to reproduce.

Conception The fertilization of an ovum by a sperm.

Contraception (birth control) Methods of preventing conception.

Sexually transmitted infections (STIs) A variety of infections that can be acquired through sexual contact.

Barrier methods Contraceptive methods that block the meeting of egg and sperm by means of a physical barrier (such as condom, diaphragm, or cervical cap), a chemical barrier (such as spermicide), or both.

Male condom A single-use sheath of thin latex or other material designed to fit over an erect penis and to catch semen upon ejaculation.

Table 7.1
Contraceptive Effectiveness and STI Prevention

Number of Unintended Pregnancies per 100 Women during First Year of Use

Method	Typical Use[a]	Perfect Use[b]	Risk Reduction for Sexually Transmitted Infections (STIs)
Continuous Abstinence	0.00	0.00	Complete
Outercourse	N/A[c]	N/A	Some
Sterilization			
Men	0.15	0.1	None
Women	0.5	0.5	None
Depo-Provera Injection	0.3	0.3	None
IUD (intrauterine device)			
ParaGard (copper T 380A)	0.8	0.6	None
Mirena	0.1	0.1	None
Oral Contraceptives ("The Pill")			
Combination	5.0	0.1	None
Progestin-only	5.0	0.5	None
Male Condom	14.0	3.0	Good against HIV; reduces risk of others
Withdrawal	19.0	4.0	None
Diaphragm	20.0	6.0	Limited
Cervical Cap			
Women who have not given birth	20.0	9.0	Limited
Women who have given birth	40.0	30.0	Limited
Female Condom	21.0	5.0	Some
Predicting Fertility			
Periodic abstinence	20.0		None
Postovulation method		1.0	None
Symptothermal method		2.0	None
Cervical mucus (ovulation) method		3.0	None
Calendar method		9.0	None
Fertility Awareness Methods			
With male or female condom	N/A	N/A	None
With diaphragm or cap	N/A	N/A	None
With withdrawal or other methods	N/A	N/A	None
Spermicide	26.0	6.0	Limited
No Method	85.0	85.0	None

Emergency Contraception

Emergency contraception pills: Treatment initiated within 72 hours after unprotected intercourse reduces the risk of pregnancy by 75–89 percent (with no protection against STIs). Emergency IUD insertion: Treatment initiated within seven days after unprotected intercourse reduces the risk of pregnancy by more than 99 percent (with no protection against STIs).

a. "Typical Use" refers to failure rates for men and women whose use is not consistent or always correct.
b. "Perfect Use" refers to failure rates for those whose use is consistent and always correct.
c. N/A means that effectiveness rates are not available.

Source: Contraceptive Effectiveness Rates: R. Hatcher et al., *Contraceptive Technology,* 17th ed. (New York: Ardent Media, 1998). Reprinted by permission of Ardent Media.

News from the World of Contraceptives Research

The introduction of a new contraceptive may take years of research and clinical trials prior to approval by the U.S. Food and Drug Administration. However, it appears that within the next few years, our contraceptive options may be expanding. Here's a look at future contraceptives.

New Barrier Methods

- Lea's Shield is a one-size-fits-all silicon rubber device that covers the cervix. It has been approved by the FDA and is distributed through Planned Parenthood clinics.
- A new vaginal sponge, Protectaid, is made of polyurethane foam and contains a combination of chemicals that serve as spermicide and microbicide to protect against STIs. It is available in Canada. The original version of the sponge, the Today sponge, is in the final stages for FDA approval to be distributed in the United States.

- FemCap is a nonlatex device that covers the cervix and forms a seal against the vaginal wall. It is used with spermicide and contains a groove that traps sperm. Already in use in Europe, it was approved in 2003 by the FDA for use if fitted and prescribed by a physician. Distribution is not widespread.

Contraceptives for Men

- The oft-discussed "male pill" remains about five years away.
- An injectable contraceptive that stimulates the production of antibodies to male sex hormones is in the works and will be tested more extensively within the next few years.
- The Population Council has developed a synthetic testosterone that would be delivered via a skin implant. It is undergoing further tests to determine side effects.

Implant Refinements

- The Population Council is also working on a single-rod implant delivery system that would inhibit ovulation for two years. The implant contains Nesterone, a synthetic progestin.

- Also being studied are biodegradable implants containing progestin that would be implanted under the skin of the arm or the hip. The hormone is released gradually into the body for 12 to 18 months.

Injections and Vaccines for Women

- Oral or injectable vaccines could stimulate the immune system to create antibodies to a crucial protein molecule found on the head of sperm.

Unisex Contraception

- A new group of drugs known as gonadotropin-releasing hormone (GnRH) agonists can prevent the release of FSH and LH from the pituitary gland. Blocking these hormones will temporarily suppress fertility in men and women.

Sources: Population Council, "Biomedical Research and Products," 2004, www .popcouncil.org/biomed/contradev.html; J. Allen, "New Fit for U.S. Birth Control," *Los Angeles Times,* April 28, 2003; and Johns Hopkins University, "Reproductive Health Online," 2003, www.reproline. jhu.edu

---

may also slow or reduce the development of cervical abnormalities in women that can lead to cancer. A condom must be rolled onto the penis before the penis touches the vagina, and held in place when removing the penis from the vagina after ejaculation (Figure 7.1 on page 190). For greatest efficacy, they should be used with a spermicide containing nonoxynol-9, the same agent found in many of contraceptive foams and creams. If necessary or desired, users can lubricate their own condoms with contraceptive foams, creams, and jellies or other water-based lubricants, such as K-Y jelly, ForPlay Lubricants, Astroglide, or Wet or Aqua Lube, to name just a few. However, never use products such as baby oil, cold cream, petroleum jelly, vaginal yeast infection medications, or hand and body lotion with a condom. These products contain mineral oil and will make the latex begin to disintegrate within 60 seconds.

Condoms are less effective and more likely to break during intercourse if they are old or poorly stored. To maintain effectiveness, store them in a cool place (not in a wallet or hip pocket), and inspect them for small tears before use.

For some people, a condom ruins the spontaneity of sex. Stopping to put it on breaks the mood for them. Others report that the condom decreases sensation. These inconveniences contribute to improper use of the device. Partners who incorporate putting a condom on during foreplay are generally more successful with this form of birth control.

Foams, Suppositories, Jellies, and Creams Like condoms, jellies, creams, suppositories, and foam do not require a prescription. Chemically, they are referred to as **spermicides**—substances designed to kill sperm. Recent studies indicate that spermicides containing nonoxynol-9 (N-9) are not effective in preventing certain STIs such as gonorrhea,

Spermicides Substances designed to kill sperm.

Contraceptive Comfort and Confidence Scale

myhealthlab

Fill out this assessment online at www.aw-bc.com/myhealthlab or www.aw-bc.com/donatelle

These questions will help you assess whether the method of contraception you are using now or may consider using in the future will be effective for you.

Method of contraception you use now or are considering: _____

Length of time you used this method in the past: _____

Answer yes or no to the following questions:	Yes	No
1. Have I ever had problems using this method?	❑	❑
2. Have I ever become pregnant while using this method?	❑	❑
3. Am I afraid of using this method?	❑	❑
4. Would I really rather not use this method?	❑	❑
5. Will I have trouble remembering to use this method?	❑	❑
6. Will I have trouble using this method correctly?	❑	❑
7. Do I still have unanswered questions about this method?	❑	❑
8. Does this method make menstrual periods longer or more painful?	❑	❑
9. Does this method cost more than I can afford?	❑	❑
10. Could this method cause serious complications?	❑	❑
11. Am I opposed to this method because of any religious or moral beliefs?	❑	❑
12. Is my partner opposed to this method?	❑	❑
13. Am I using this method without my partner's knowledge?	❑	❑
14. Will using this method embarrass my partner?	❑	❑
15. Will using this method embarrass me?	❑	❑
16. Will I enjoy intercourse less because of this method?	❑	❑
17. If this method interrupts lovemaking, will I avoid using it?	❑	❑
18. Has a nurse or doctor ever told me not to use this method?	❑	❑
19. Is there anything about my personality that could lead me to use this method incorrectly?	❑	❑
20. Am I at risk of being exposed to HIV (the AIDS virus) or other sexually transmitted infections if I use this method?	❑	❑

Total number of yes answers: _____

INTERPRETING YOUR ANSWERS

Answering yes to any of these questions predicts potential problems. Most individuals will have a few yes answers. If you have more than a few yes responses, however, you may want to talk to a health care provider, counselor, partner, or friend to decide whether to use this method or how to use it so that it will really be effective. In general, the more yes answers you have, the less likely you are to use this method consistently and correctly with every act of intercourse.

Source: From R. A. Hatcher et al., *Contraceptive Technology,* 17th ed. (New York: Ardent Media, 1998).

MAKE IT HAPPEN!

Use the results of this self-assessment to begin your behavior change program. Follow the steps and use the examples on page 218 to complete your Behavior Change Contract, and use these resources to take action.

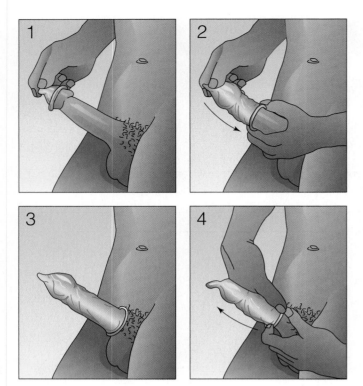

Figure 7.1
How to Use a Condom
The condom should be rolled over the erect penis before any penetration occurs. A small space (about 1/2 inch) should be left at the end of the condom to collect the semen after ejaculation. Hold the tip of the condom, and unroll it all the way to the base of the penis. Hold the base of the condom before withdrawal to avoid spilling any semen.

chlamydia, and HIV. In fact, frequent use of N-9 spermicides has been shown to cause irritation and breaks in the mucous layer or skin of the genital tract, creating a point of entry for viruses and bacteria that cause disease.[1] Although they are not recommended as the primary form of contraception, spermicides are often recommended for use with other methods and are most effective when used in conjunction with a condom.

Jellies and creams are packaged in tubes, and foams are available in aerosol cans. All have tubes designed for insertion into the vagina. They must be inserted far enough to cover the cervix, providing both a chemical barrier that kills sperm and a physical barrier that stops sperm from continuing toward an egg (Figure 7.2).

Female condom   A single-use polyurethane sheath for internal use by women.

Diaphragm   A latex, cup-shaped device designed to cover the cervix and block access to the uterus; should always be used with spermicide.

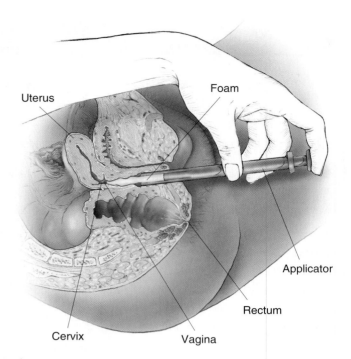

Figure 7.2
The Proper Method of Applying Spermicide within the Vagina

Suppositories are waxy capsules that are inserted deep in the vagina, where they melt. They must be inserted 10 to 20 minutes before intercourse to have time to melt but no longer than one hour prior to intercourse or they lose their effectiveness. Additional spermicide must be applied for each subsequent act of intercourse.

Vaginal contraceptive film is another method of spermicide delivery. A thin film infused with spermicidal gel is inserted into the vagina, so that it covers the cervix. The film dissolves into a spermicidal gel that is effective for up to three hours. As with other spermicides, a new film must be inserted for each act of intercourse.

The Female Condom   The **female condom** is a single-use, soft, loose-fitting polyurethane sheath meant for internal use by women. It is designed as one unit with two diaphragm-like rings. One ring, which lies inside the sheath, serves as an insertion mechanism and internal anchor. The other ring, which remains outside the vagina once the device is inserted, protects the labia and the base of the penis from infection. Many women like the female condom because it gives them more control than does the male condom. When used correctly, the female condom provides protection against HIV and STIs comparable to that of a latex male condom. The product's brand name, the Reality Condom, reflects the fact that it can also be used for male anal sex, not solely by women.

The Diaphragm, with Spermicidal Jelly or Cream   Invented in the mid-nineteenth century, the **diaphragm** was the first widely used birth control method for women. The device is a

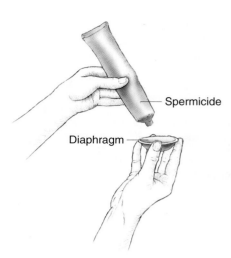
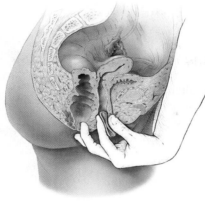
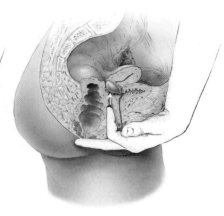

a. Place spermicide inside and around the rim of the diaphragm.

b. Insertion: squeeze rim together; insert with spermicide-side up.

c. Check placement, making certain cervix is covered.

Figure 7.3
The Proper Use and Placement of a Diaphragm

soft, shallow cup made of thin latex rubber. Its flexible, rubber-coated ring is designed to fit snugly behind the pubic bone in front of the cervix and over the back of the cervix on the other side. Diaphragms are manufactured in different sizes and must be fitted to the woman by a trained practitioner. The practitioner should also be certain that the user knows how to insert her diaphragm correctly before she leaves the practitioner's office.

Diaphragms must be used with spermicidal cream or jelly, which is applied to the inside of the diaphragm before insertion. The diaphragm holds the spermicide in place, creating a physical and chemical barrier against sperm. Additional spermicide must be applied before each subsequent act of intercourse, and the diaphragm must be left in place

for six to eight hours after intercourse to allow the chemical to kill any sperm remaining in the vagina. When used with spermicidal jelly or cream, it offers significant protection against gonorrhea and possibly chlamydia and human papilloma virus (HPV) (Figure 7.3).

Using a diaphragm during the menstrual period or leaving it in place longer than 24 hours slightly increases the user's risk of developing **toxic shock syndrome (TSS).** This condition results from the multiplication of bacteria that spread to the bloodstream and cause sudden high fever, rash, nausea, vomiting, diarrhea, and a rapid drop in blood pressure. If not treated, TSS can be fatal. The diaphragm (as well as tampons left too long in place) creates conditions conducive to the growth of these bacteria. To reduce the risk of TSS, women should wash their hands carefully with soap and water before inserting or removing the diaphragm.

Another problem with the diaphragm is that it can put undue pressure on the urethra, blocking urinary flow and predisposing the user to bladder infections. Inserting the device can be awkward, especially if the woman is rushed. When inserted incorrectly, diaphragms are much less effective.

The Cervical Cap, with Spermicidal Jelly or Cream One of the oldest methods used to prevent pregnancy, early cervical caps were made from beeswax, silver, or copper. Today's **cervical cap** is a small cup made of latex that fits snugly over

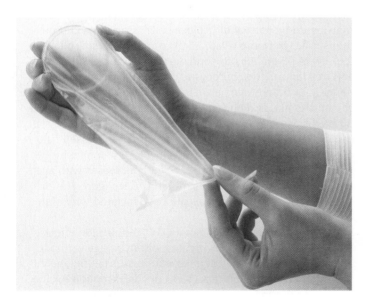

The Female Condom

> **Toxic shock syndrome (TSS)** A potentially life-threatening disease that occurs when specific bacterial toxins are allowed to multiply unchecked in wounds or through improper use of tampons or diaphragms.
>
> **Cervical cap** A small cup made of latex that is designed to fit snugly over the entire cervix.

the entire cervix. It must be fitted by a practitioner and is designed for use with contraceptive jelly or cream. It is somewhat more difficult to insert than a diaphragm because of its smaller size.

The cap works by blocking sperm from the uterus. It is held in place by suction created during application. Insertion may take place up to six hours prior to intercourse, and the device must be left in place for six to eight hours after intercourse. The maximum length of time the cap can be left on the cervix is 48 hours. If removed and cleaned, it can be reinserted immediately. The cervical cap may offer protection against some STIs but not HIV.

Some women report unpleasant vaginal odors after use. Because the device can become dislodged during intercourse, placement must be checked frequently. It cannot be used during the menstrual period or for longer than 48 hours because of the risk of TSS.

Hormonal Methods

Oral Contraceptives Oral contraceptive pills were first marketed in the United States in 1960. Their convenience quickly made them the most widely used reversible method of fertility control.

Most oral contraceptives work through the combined effects of synthetic estrogen and progesterone. Because the levels of estrogen in the pill are higher than those produced by the body, the pituitary gland is never signaled to produce follicle-stimulating hormone (FSH), without which ova will not develop in the ovaries. Progesterone in the pill prevents proper growth of the uterine lining and thickens the cervical mucus, forming a barrier against sperm.

Pills are meant to be taken in a cycle. At the end of each three-week cycle, the user discontinues the drug or takes placebo pills for one week. The resultant drop in hormones causes the uterine lining to disintegrate, and the user will have a menstrual period, usually within one to three days. The same cycle is repeated every 28 days. Menstrual flow is generally lighter than it is for women who don't use the pill because the hormones in the pill prevent thick endometrial buildup.

Today's pill is different from the one introduced more than four decades ago. The original pill contained large amounts of estrogen, which caused certain risks, whereas the current pill contains the minimal amount of estrogen necessary to prevent pregnancy.

Because the chemicals in oral contraceptives change the way the body metabolizes certain nutrients, women using the pill should check with their practitioners to see if dietary supplements are advisable, especially vitamins C,

---

Oral contraceptives Pills taken daily for three weeks of the menstrual cycle that prevent ovulation by regulating hormones.

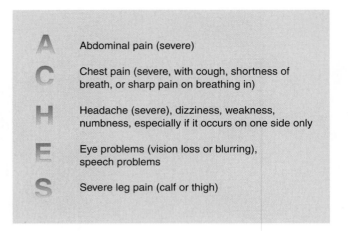

Figure 7.4
Early Warning Signs of Medical Complications for Pill Users

Source: Hatcher, R. A. et al. *Contraceptive Technology,* 17th ed. (New York: Ardent Media, 1998):457.

B_2 (riboflavin), B_6 (pyridoxine) and B_{12} (cobalamin). A nutritious diet that includes whole grains, fresh fruits and vegetables, lean meats, fish and poultry, and nonfat dairy products is important. Oral contraceptives can also interact negatively with other drugs. For example, some antibiotics diminish the pill's effectiveness and may require an adjustment in dosage. Someone taking tetracycline, for example, should use a backup contraceptive for the entire duration of treatment or 14 days, whichever is shorter, plus seven days.[2] Women in doubt should check with their practitioners or pharmacists.

Return of fertility may be delayed after discontinuing the pill, but the pill is not known to cause infertility. Women who had irregular menstrual cycles before going on the pill are more likely to have problems conceiving, regardless of pill use.

The pill is convenient and does not interfere with lovemaking, which can lead to enhanced sexual enjoyment. It may lessen menstrual difficulties, such as cramps and premenstrual syndrome (PMS). Oral contraceptives also lower the risk of several health conditions, including endometrial and ovarian cancers, fibrocystic breast disease, ectopic pregnancies, ovarian cysts, pelvic inflammatory disease, iron deficiency anemia, and endometriosis.[3] Possible serious health problems associated with the pill include blood clots, which can lead to strokes or heart attacks, and an increased risk of high blood pressure. The risk is low for most healthy women under 35 who do not smoke; it increases with age and especially with cigarette smoking. (See Figure 7.4 for early warning signs of complications associated with oral contraceptives.)

Outside of these risk factors and certain side effects associated with the pill, its greatest disadvantage is that it must be taken every day. If a woman misses taking one pill, she should use an alternative form of contraception for the remainder of that cycle. Another drawback is that the pill does not protect against STIs. Some teenagers report that the requirement to have a complete gynecological examination in order to get a prescription for the pill is a huge obstacle. Educating young women about what goes on in a gynecological exam would certainly help ease their anxiety. Finally, cost may be a problem for some women.

Progestin-Only Pills   Progestin-only pills (or minipills) contain small doses of progesterone. Women who feel uncertain about using estrogen pills, who suffer from side effects related to estrogen, or who are nursing may choose these medications rather than combination pills. There is still some question about how progestin-only pills work. Current thought is that they change the composition of the cervical mucus, thus impeding sperm travel. They may also inhibit ovulation in some women. The effectiveness rate of progestin-only pills is 96 percent, which is slightly lower than that of estrogen-containing pills. Also, their use usually leads to irregular menstrual bleeding. As with all oral contraceptives, the user has no protection against STIs.

Ortho Evra (The Patch)   A hormonal contraceptive patch, **Ortho Evra,** became available by prescription in 2002. The patch is worn for one week and replaced on the same day of the week for three consecutive weeks, with the fourth week patch-free. Ortho Evra is 99 percent effective and works by delivering continuous levels of estrogen and progestin through the skin and into the bloodstream. This new weekly patch is easy to apply and barely noticeable, with adhesive strong enough to even withstand swimming. The patch can be worn on one of four areas of the body: buttocks, abdomen, upper torso (front or back, excluding the breasts), or upper outer arm.

Ortho Evra contains hormones similar to those in birth control pills. Some women report experiencing breast symptoms, headache, application site reaction, nausea, upper respiratory infection, menstrual cramps, and abdominal pain. However, most side effects are not serious. Serious risks, which occur infrequently but can be life threatening, include blood clots, stroke, or heart attacks; tobacco use increases these risks. The patch does not protect against HIV or other STIs.

NuvaRing   Introduced in 2002, this effective contraceptive offers protection for four weeks at a time when used as prescribed. **NuvaRing** is a soft, flexible, transparent ring about two inches in diameter. The user inserts it into her vagina, leaves it in place for three weeks, and removes it for one week for her menstrual period. Once the ring is inserted, it continuously releases a steady flow of estrogen and progestin.

Advantages of NuvaRing include protection against pregnancy for one month; no pill to take daily; no need to be fitted by a clinician; does not require spermicide; and the ability to become pregnant returns quickly when use is stopped. Some of the disadvantages that women might

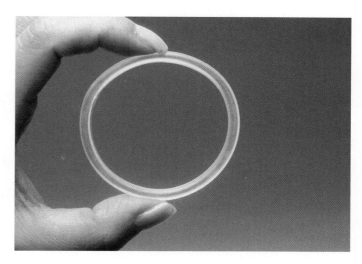

NuvaRing (actual size)

experience include increased vaginal discharge; vaginal irritation or infection; oil-based vaginal medicines to treat yeast infections cannot be used when the ring is in place; and a diaphragm or cervical cap cannot be used as a backup method for contraception.

Depo-Provera   **Depo-Provera** is a long-acting synthetic progesterone that is injected intramuscularly every three months. Researchers believe that the drug prevents ovulation. Depo-Provera allows sexual spontaneity because the user does not have to remember to take a pill or insert a device. There are fewer health problems associated with Depo-Provera than with estrogen-containing pills. The main disadvantage is irregular bleeding, which can be troublesome at first, but within a year, most women are amenorrheic (have no menstrual periods). Weight gain (an average of five pounds in the first year) is common. Other possible side effects include dizziness, nervousness, and headache. Unlike other methods of contraception, this method cannot be stopped immediately if problems arise. Also, women who wish to become pregnant may find that it takes up to a year after their last injection to succeed.

Lunelle and Norplant   Two other methods are currently off the market but could be reinstated. Lunelle is a monthly injection that contains the time-released synthetic forms of

---

Ortho Evra   A patch that releases hormones similar to those in oral contraceptives; each patch is worn for one week.

NuvaRing   A soft, flexible ring inserted into the vagina that releases hormones, preventing pregnancy.

Depo-Provera   An injectable method of birth control that lasts for three months.

estrogen and progestin. It was recalled from the market due to manufacturing problems that led to prefilled syringes containing less than the required amount of hormone.

Norplant is a set of six silicon capsules containing progestin that are surgically inserted under the skin of a woman's upper arm. The progestin works the same way that oral contraceptives do to suppress ovulation. Norplant was withdrawn from the market due to legal issues, but if they are resolved, it may become available again.

Surgical Methods

Sterilization has become the leading method of contraception for women (10.7 million women), closely followed by the oral contraceptive pill (10.4 million women).[4] Although newer surgical techniques make reversal of sterilization theoretically possible, anyone considering sterilization should assume that the operation is *not* reversible. Before becoming sterilized, people should think through possibilities such as divorce and remarriage or a future improvement in financial status that might make a larger family realistic.

Female Sterilization   **Tubal ligation** is one method of sterilization for females. In this surgical procedure, the uterine tubes are either tied shut or cut and cauterized (burned) at the edges to seal the tubes, blocking sperm's access to released eggs. The operation is usually done in a hospital on an outpatient basis. First, the abdomen is inflated with carbon dioxide gas through a small incision in the navel. The surgeon then inserts a *laparoscope* into another incision just above the pubic bone. This specially designed instrument has a fiber-optic light source that enables the physician to see the uterine tubes clearly.

A tubal ligation does not affect ovarian and uterine function. The woman's menstrual cycle continues, and released eggs simply disintegrate and are absorbed by the lymphatic system. As soon as her incision heals, the woman may resume sexual intercourse with no fear of pregnancy.

As with any surgery, there are risks. Although rare, the possible complications of a tubal ligation include infection, pulmonary embolism, hemorrhage, and ectopic pregnancy. Some patients are given general anesthesia, which itself presents a small risk; others receive local anesthesia. The procedure itself usually takes less than an hour, and the patient is generally allowed to return home within a short time after waking up. Women considering a tubal ligation should thoroughly discuss all the risks with their physician before the operation.

A **hysterectomy,** or removal of the uterus, is a method of sterilization requiring major surgery. It is usually done only when the patient's uterus is diseased or damaged.

Male Sterilization   Sterilization in men is less complicated than in women. The procedure, called a **vasectomy,** is frequently done on an outpatient basis, using a local anesthetic. The surgeon (generally a urologist) makes an incision on each side of the scrotum, locates the ductus deferens on each side, and removes a piece from each. The ends are usually tied or sewn shut.

In a small percentage of cases, complications occur: formation of a blood clot in the scrotum (which usually disappears without medical treatment), infection, or inflammatory reactions. Because sperm are stored in other areas of the reproductive system besides the ductus deferentia, couples must use alternative methods of birth control for at least one month after the vasectomy. The man must check with his physician (who will do a semen analysis) to determine when unprotected intercourse can take place. The pregnancy rate in women whose partners have had vasectomies is about 15 in 10,000.

Many men are reluctant to consider sterilization because they fear the operation will affect their sexual performance. However, a vasectomy in no way affects sexual response. Because sperm constitute only a small percentage of the semen, the amount of ejaculate is not changed significantly. The testes continue to produce sperm, but the sperm can no longer enter the ejaculatory duct. After a time, sperm production may diminish. Any sperm that are manufactured disintegrate and are absorbed into the lymphatic system.

Although a vasectomy should be considered permanent, surgical reversal can sometimes restore fertility successfully. Recent improvements in microsurgery techniques have resulted in annual pregnancy rates of 40 to 60 percent for women whose partners have had reversals. The two major factors influencing the success rate of reversal are the doctor's expertise and the time elapsed since the vasectomy.

Sterilization   Permanent fertility control achieved through surgical procedures.

Tubal ligation   Sterilization of the female that involves the cutting and tying off or cauterizing of the uterine tubes.

Hysterectomy   Removal of the uterus.

Vasectomy   Sterilization of the male that involves the cutting and tying off of both ductus deferentia.

What do you think?

Who do you think is responsible for deciding which method of contraception should be used in a sexual relationship? ■ *What are some examples of good opportunities for you and your partner to have a discussion about contraceptives?* ■ *What do you think are the biggest barriers in our society to the use of condoms?*

Table 7.2
Costs of Contraception

Method	Cost
Continuous abstinence	None
Outercourse (sex play without vaginal intercourse)	None
Withdrawal	None
Sterilization	
Tubal ligation: permanently blocks female's uterine tubes where sperm join egg	$1,500–$6,000
Vasectomy: permanently blocks male's ductus deferentia that carry sperm	$240–$1,000
Depo-Provera	$20–$40/visits to clinician; $50/injection
IUD (intrauterine device)	$175–$400/exam, insertion, and follow-up visit
Oral contraceptives	$15–$35/monthly pill–pack at drugstores, often less at clinics; $35–$125/exam
NuvaRing	$30–$35/ring; $35–$125/exam
Ortho Evra (patch)	$30–$35/monthly supply of patches; $35–$125/exam
Condoms/female condoms and spermicide	50¢ and up/condom—some family planning centers give them away or charge very little; $2.50/female condom; $8–$17/applicator kit of spermicide foam and jelly ($4–$8 refills); similar prices for creams, films, and suppositories
Diaphragm or cervical cap	$15–$75/diaphragm or cap; $50–$125/examination; $4–$8/supplies of spermicide jelly or cream
Fertility awareness methods	$10–$12 for temperature kits; free classes often available in health and church centers

Note: Some family planning clinics charge for services and supplies on a sliding scale according to income.

Source: Reprinted with permission from Planned Parenthood® Federation of America, Inc. © 2004 PPFA. All rights reserved.

Other Methods of Contraception

Intrauterine Devices   Women have been using **intrauterine devices (IUDs)** since 1909, but we still are not certain how they work. Although it was once thought that IUDs act by preventing implantation of a fertilized egg, most experts now believe that they interfere with the sperm's fertilization of the egg.

Two IUDs are currently available. ParaGard is a T-shaped plastic device with copper wrapped around the shaft. It does not contain any hormones and can be left in place for ten years before replacement. A newer IUD, Mirena, is effective for five years and releases small amounts of the progestin levonorgestrel.

A physician must fit and insert an IUD. For insertion, the device is folded and placed into a long, thin plastic applicator. The practitioner measures the depth of the uterus with a special instrument and then uses these measurements to place the IUD accurately so the arms of the T open out across the top of the uterus. One or two strings extend from the IUD into the vagina so the user can check to make sure that her IUD is in place. The device is removed by a practitioner when desired.

Disadvantages of IUDs include discomfort, cost of insertion, and potential complications. The device can cause heavy menstrual flow and severe cramps. Women using IUDs have a higher risk of uterine perforation, ectopic pregnancy,

pelvic inflammatory disease, infertility, and tubal infections. If a pregnancy occurs while the IUD is in place, the chance of miscarriage is 25 to 50 percent. The device should be removed as soon as possible. Doctors often offer therapeutic abortion to women who become pregnant while using an IUD because of the serious risks (including premature delivery, infection, and congenital abnormalities) associated with continuing the pregnancy.

For a comparison of this and other contraceptive option costs, see Table 7.2.

Withdrawal   This not very effective method of birth control is most commonly used by people who have not taken the time to consider alternatives. The **withdrawal** method involves withdrawing the penis from the vagina just prior to ejaculation. Because there can be up to half a million sperm in the drop of fluid at the tip of the penis before ejaculation, this method is unreliable. Timing withdrawal is also difficult,

> **Intrauterine device (IUD)**   A T-shaped device that is implanted in the uterus to prevent pregnancy.
>
> **Withdrawal**   A method of contraception that involves withdrawing the penis from the vagina before ejaculation. Also called coitus interruptus.

and males concentrating on accurate timing may not be able to relax and enjoy intercourse.

Emergency Contraceptive Pills   There are more than 2.7 million unintended pregnancies per year in the United States, and nearly half are due to contraceptive failure. According to the Centers for Disease Control and Prevention, more than 11 million American women report using contraceptive methods associated with high failure rates, including condoms, withdrawal, periodic abstinence, and diaphragms.

Emergency contraception can be used when a condom breaks, after a sexual assault, or any time unprotected sexual intercourse occurs. **Emergency contraceptive pills (ECPs)** are ordinary birth control pills containing estrogen and progestin. Although the therapy is commonly known as the "morning-after pill," the term is misleading; ECPs can be used up to 72 hours after intercourse and can reduce the risk of pregnancy by 75 percent.

Emergency contraceptives currently require a prescription, although the FDA is considering allowing it to be dispensed over the counter. The two FDA-approved products are Preven and Plan B. After a woman determines she is not already pregnant, by using the pregnancy test included in the kit, the first dose of two light blue emergency pills is taken as soon as possible, within 72 hours after intercourse. The second dose is taken 12 hours later.[5] The most common side effects related to ECPs are nausea, vomiting, menstrual irregularities, breast tenderness, headache, abdominal pain and cramps, and dizziness.

Emergency minipills contain progestin only. Like ECPs, minipills can be used up to 72 hours after unprotected intercourse. Emergency minipills are equally as effective as ECPs, but nausea and vomiting are far less common. Emergency minipills are an excellent alternative for most women who cannot use ECPs that contain estrogen.

Emergency contraceptive pills (ECPs)   Drugs taken within three days after intercourse to prevent fertilization or implantation.

Emergency minipills   Contraceptive pills containing only progestin that can be taken up to three days after unprotected intercourse.

Fertility awareness methods (FAMs)   Several types of birth control that require alteration of sexual behavior rather than chemical or physical intervention into the reproductive process.

Cervical mucus method   A birth control method that relies upon observation of changes in cervical mucus to determine when the woman is fertile so the couple can abstain from intercourse during those times.

Body temperature method   A birth control method in which a woman monitors her body temperature for the rise that signals ovulation in order to abstain from intercourse around this time.

Abstinence and "Outercourse"   Strictly defined, abstinence means deliberately avoiding intercourse. This strict definition would allow one to engage in such forms of sexual intimacy as massage, kissing, and solitary masturbation. However, many people today have broadened the definition of abstinence to include all forms of sexual contact, even those that do not culminate in sexual intercourse.

Couples who go a step further than massage and kissing and engage in activities such as oral–genital sex and mutual masturbation are sometimes said to be engaging in "outercourse." Like abstinence, outercourse can be 100 percent effective for birth control as long as the male does not ejaculate near the vaginal opening. Unlike abstinence, however, outercourse is not 100 percent effective against sexually transmitted infections (STIs). Oral–genital contact can transmit disease, although the practice can be made safer by using a condom on the penis or a dental dam on the vaginal opening.

Fertility Awareness Methods

Methods of fertility control that rely upon the alteration of sexual behavior are called **fertility awareness methods (FAMs).** These techniques require observing female fertile periods and abstaining from sexual intercourse (penis–vagina contact) during these fertile times.

Two decades ago, the rhythm method was ridiculed because of its low effectiveness rates. However, it was the only method of birth control available to women belonging to religious denominations that forbid the use of oral contraceptives, barrier methods, and sterilization. Our present reproductive knowledge enables women and their partners to use natural methods of birth control with less risk of pregnancy, although these methods remain far less effective than others.

Fertility awareness methods rely upon a knowledge of basic physiology (Figure 7.5.) A released ovum can survive for up to 48 hours after ovulation. Sperm can live for as long as five days in the vagina. Natural methods of birth control teach women to recognize their fertile times. Changes in cervical mucus prior to and during ovulation and a rise in basal body temperature are two frequently used indicators. Another method involves charting a woman's menstrual cycle and ovulation times on a calendar. Women may use any combination of these methods to determine their fertile times more accurately (Figure 7.6 on page 198).

Cervical Mucus Method   The **cervical mucus method** requires women to examine the consistency and color of their normal vaginal secretions. Prior to ovulation, vaginal mucus becomes gelatinous and stretchy, and normal vaginal secretions may increase. Sexual activity involving penis–vagina contact must be avoided while this mucus is present and for several days afterward.

Body Temperature Method   The **body temperature method** relies on the fact that the female's basal body temperature rises between 0.4 and 0.8 degrees after ovulation

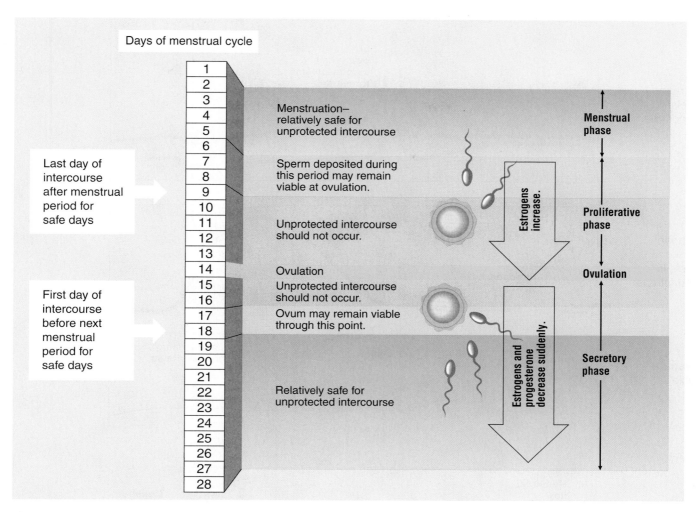

Figure 7.5
The Fertility Cycle
Fertility awareness methods (FAMs) can combine the use of a calendar, the cervical mucus method, and body temperature measurements to identify the fertile period. It is important to remember that most women do not have a consistent 28-day cycle.

has occurred. For this method to be effective, the woman must chart her temperature for several months to learn to recognize her body's temperature fluctuations. Abstinence from penis–vagina contact must be observed preceding the temperature rise until several days after the temperature rise was first noted.

The Calendar Method   The **calendar method** requires the woman to record the exact number of days in her menstrual cycle. Since few women menstruate with complete regularity, this involves keeping a record of the menstrual cycle for 12 months, during which time some other method of birth control must be used. The first day of a woman's period counts as day 1. To determine the first fertile, unsafe day of the cycle, she subtracts 18 from the number of days in the shortest cycle. To determine the last unsafe day of the cycle,

she subtracts 11 from the number of days in the longest cycle. This method assumes that ovulation occurs during the midpoint of the cycle. The couple must abstain from penis–vagina contact during the fertile time.

Women who wish to use fertility awareness methods of birth control are advised to take classes in their use. Women who are untrained in these techniques run a high risk of unwanted pregnancy.

Calendar method   A birth control method in which a woman's menstrual cycle is mapped on a calendar to determine presumed fertile times in order to abstain from penis–vagina contact during those times.

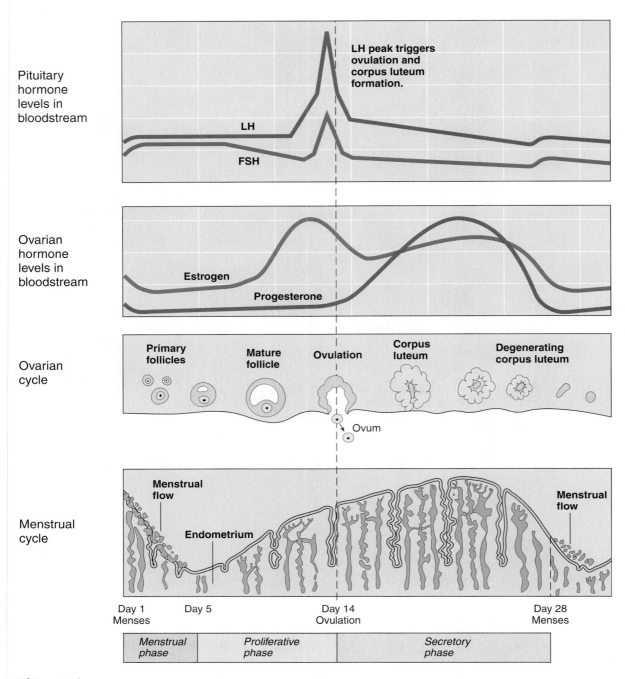

Figure 7.6
Changes during the Menstrual Cycle

Abortion

In 1973, the landmark U.S. Supreme Court decision in *Roe v. Wade* stated that the "right to privacy . . . founded on the Fourteenth Amendment's concept of personal liberty . . . is broad enough to encompass a woman's decision whether or not to terminate her pregnancy."[6] The decision maintained that during the first trimester of pregnancy, a woman and her practitioner have the right to terminate the pregnancy through **abortion** without legal restrictions. It allowed individual states to set conditions for second-trimester abortions. Third-trimester abortions were ruled illegal unless the mother's life or health was in danger.

Prior to the legalization of first- and second-trimester abortions, women wishing to terminate a pregnancy had to

Abortion   The medical means of terminating a pregnancy.

Facts about Abortion

Because abortion is an issue intensely debated in the media, most of us have heard numerous statements, opinions, and arguments about the subject. How well do the following facts match your understanding of the practice of abortion in the United States and abroad?

✔ Worldwide, more than a quarter of women who become pregnant have either an abortion or an unwanted child.

✔ Each year, an estimated 80,000 women die from complications of unsafe abortion, accounting for 13 percent of global maternal mortality.

✔ Seventy percent of U.S. abortions are obtained by white women, 20 percent by black women, and 10 percent by other women of color.

✔ Seven percent of abortions are performed in hospitals, 4 percent in private physicians' offices, and 89 percent in clinics.

✔ In the United States, 25 percent of women seeking an abortion must travel more than 50 miles.

✔ In 95 percent of rural U.S. counties, there is no abortion provider.

✔ The National Cancer Institute and the American Cancer Society have concluded that induced abortion *does not* increase the risk of breast cancer.

✔ Ninety percent of all abortions occur by the end of the first 12 weeks of pregnancy.

✔ Of the 46 million abortions that occur worldwide each year, roughly 20 million are performed under unsafe conditions because of poorly trained providers, unsanitary circumstances, and crude and dangerous methods of self-induction.

Sources: "Facts in Brief: Induced Abortion," Alan Guttmacher Institute, 1999, www.agi-usa.org/pubs/fb_0599.html; "Unsafe Abortion around the World," Planned Parenthood Fact Sheet, 2002 www.plannedparenthood.org/library/abortion/unsafeab.html; L. Ross, "Emergency Memorandum to Women of Color" in *From Abortion to Reproductive Freedom,* ed. M. G. Fried (Boston: South End Press, 1990): 149; S. K. Henshaw, "Abortion Incidence and Services in the United States, 1995–1996," *Family Planning Perspectives* 30, no. 6 (1998): 263–270; Abortion Access Project, brochure, 1999, www.abortionaccess.org; "Induced Abortion Does Not Increase the Risk of Breast Cancer," Fact Sheet No. 240, World Health Organization, June 2000, www.who.int/mediacentre/factsheets/fs240/en

---

travel to a country where the procedure was legal, consult an illegal abortionist, or perform their own abortions. Approximately 480,000 illegal abortions were performed in the United States each year, one-third of them on married women. These procedures led to death from hemorrhage or infection in some cases and to infertility from internal scarring in others.

People who oppose abortion believe that the embryo or fetus is a human being with rights that must be protected. The political debate continues as opponents of abortion pressure state and local governments to pass laws prohibiting the use of public funds for abortion and abortion counseling. In recent years, new legislation has given states the right to impose certain restrictions on abortions. Abortions cannot be performed in publicly funded clinics in some states, and other states have laws requiring parental notification before a teenager can obtain an abortion. In 2003 alone, states enacted 45 new anti-abortion measures.[7] On the federal level, the U.S. Congress recently banned access to abortion for virtually all women who receive health care through the federal government. This affects Medicaid recipients, women in the military, military dependents stationed overseas, women in federal prison, American Indian women, federal employees, and even Peace Corps volunteers. *Roe v. Wade* has not been overturned, but it faces many future challenges.

Although many opponents work through the courts and the political process, attacks on abortion clinics and on doctors who perform abortions are increasingly common. Nearly all clinics have faced some form of threats or acts of violence. Legal protection, such as the Freedom of Access to Clinic Entrance Act (FACE), offers some relief from the harassment and violence directed at abortion clinics. However, because of such acts, the biggest threat to a woman's access to an abortion now is finding a clinic rather than legal restrictions. See the Reality Check box for more information on abortion access and prevalence.

The best birth control methods can fail. Women may be raped. Pregnancies can occur despite every possible precaution. When an unwanted pregnancy does occur, the decision whether to terminate, carry to term and keep the baby, or carry to term and give the baby away must be made. This is a personal decision that each woman must make, based on her personal beliefs, values, and resources, after carefully considering all alternatives. For a discussion on how abortion is perceived in different countries, see the Health in a Diverse World box on page 200.

Methods of Abortion

The choice of abortion procedure is determined by how many weeks the woman has been pregnant. Length of pregnancy is calculated from the first day of her last menstrual period.

Surgical Abortions If performed during the first trimester of pregnancy, abortion presents a relatively low health risk to the mother. The most commonly used method of first-trimester

International Access to Abortion

The United States has had a long struggle over the issue of abortion. A review of laws and guidelines in other countries shows that different cultures have their own customs and beliefs about the practice of abortion. Here's a look at some international differences.

- Over 41 percent of the world's population live in countries that do not require women seeking abortion to meet specific reason requirements, meaning that they don't have to explain why they desire an abortion.
- Fourteen countries (including India, Great Britain, and Zimbabwe) have laws that instruct health care providers to consider a woman's economic or social situation in providing abortion services. Women who can show that carrying a baby to term would cause hardship are permitted abortions.
- Thirteen percent of the world's population (53 nations) permit abortion only when the pregnancy poses a threat to the woman's health or safety. Some countries have specific guidelines for determining threat, whereas others allow room for interpretation. For example, in Jamaica, a woman's mental health can be considered, but in Peru there must be a physical threat of permanent injury if the woman carries to term.
- The most stringent laws, those prohibiting abortion completely or allowing abortion only in cases where the mother's life is endangered, are in place in 74 nations (representing 21 percent of the world's population), mainly in Africa and Latin America. In these nations, there can be criminal penalties for both the woman and the abortion provider.
- Fourteen countries require a husband to provide authorization before his wife can receive abortion services. These countries include Japan, Syria, and Turkey.

Sources: From The Center for Reproductive Law and Policy, "Reproductive Rights 2000: Moving Forward," www.crlp.org/ pub_bo _rr2k.html; and A. Rahman, L. Katzive, and S. Fienshaw, "A Global Review of Laws on Induced Abortion, 1985–1997," *International Family Planning Perspectives* 24, no. 2 (1998): 56–64.

---

abortion is **vacuum aspiration.** The procedure is usually performed under a local anesthetic. The cervix is dilated with instruments or by placing *laminaria,* a sterile seaweed product, in the cervical canal. The laminaria is left in place for a few hours or overnight and slowly dilates the cervix. After it is removed, a long tube is inserted into the uterus through the cervix, and gentle suction removes fetal tissue from the uterine walls (Figure 7.7).

Pregnancies that progress into the second trimester can be terminated through **dilation and evacuation (D&E),** a procedure that combines vacuum aspiration with a technique called **dilation and curettage (D&C).** For this procedure, the cervix is dilated with laminaria for one to two days, and a combination of instruments and vacuum aspiration is used to empty the uterus. Second-trimester abortions may be done under general anesthetic. Both procedures can be performed on an outpatient basis (usually in the physician's office), with or without pain medication. Generally, however, the woman is given a mild tranquilizer to help her relax. Both procedures may cause moderate to severe uterine cramping and blood loss.

Two other methods used in second-trimester abortions, though less common than the D&E, are prostaglandin or saline **induction abortions**. Prostaglandin hormones or saline solution are injected into the uterus, which kills the fetus and initiates labor contractions. After 24 to 48 hours, the fetus and placenta are expelled from the uterus.

The **hysterotomy,** or surgical removal of the fetus from the uterus, may be used during emergencies, when the mother's life is in danger, or when other types of abortions are deemed too dangerous.

The risks associated with abortion include infection, incomplete abortion (when parts of the placenta remain in the uterus), missed abortion (when the fetus is not actually removed), excessive bleeding, and cervical and uterine trauma. Follow-up and attention to dangerous signs decrease the chances of long-term problems.

The mortality rate for first-trimester abortions averages one death per every 500,000 procedures at eight or fewer

---

Vacuum aspiration The use of gentle suction to remove fetal tissue from the uterus.

Dilation and evacuation (D&E) An abortion technique that combines vacuum aspiration with dilation and curettage; fetal tissue is both sucked and scraped out of the uterus.

Dilation and curettage (D&C) An abortion technique in which the cervix is dilated and the uterine walls scraped clean.

Induction abortion A type of abortion in which chemicals are injected into the uterus through the uterine wall; labor begins, and the woman delivers a dead fetus.

Hysterotomy The surgical removal of the fetus from the uterus.

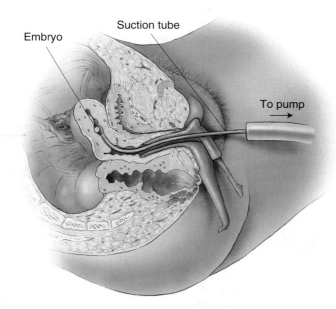

Figure 7.7
Vacuum Aspiration Abortion

induces abortion by blocking the action of progesterone, a hormone produced by the ovaries and placenta that maintains the lining of the uterus. Similar in structure to progesterone, mifepristone binds to cell receptor sites normally occupied by progesterone, causing the uterine lining to break down. As a result, the uterine lining and the embryo are expelled from the uterus, terminating the pregnancy.

Mifepristone's nickname, "the abortion pill," may imply an easy process. However, this treatment actually involves more steps than a clinical abortion, which takes approximately 15 minutes followed by a physical recovery of about one day. A first visit to the clinic involves a physical exam and a dose of three mifepristone tablets, which may cause minor side effects such as nausea, headaches, weakness, and fatigue. The patient returns two days later for a dose of prostaglandins (trade name: misoprostol), which cause uterine contractions that expel the fertilized egg. Women are required to stay under observation at the clinic for four hours.

Ninety-six percent of women who take mifepristone and prostaglandins during the first nine weeks of pregnancy will experience a complete abortion. A return visit is required 12 days later because the pills fail to induce expulsion of the fetus completely in 4 percent of cases. In such an event, a clinical abortion becomes necessary.[10]

The side effects of this treatment are similar to those reported during heavy menstruation and include cramping, minor pain, and nausea. Approximately 1 in 1,000 women requires a blood transfusion because of severe bleeding. The procedure does not require hospitalization; women may be treated on an outpatient basis.

Another drug that has been used to induce early-term medical abortions is methotrexate, although it is not approved by the FDA for this purpose. Typically a woman receives an injection from her clinician and, during an office visit three to seven days later, receives a prostaglandin dose. The pregnancy usually ends within four hours.

Emotional Aspects of Abortion

The emotional aftereffects of abortion have been the subject of much interest. Do women who have had abortions suffer symptoms similar to those of post-traumatic stress disorder? Are they forever haunted by the experience?

Although a variety of feelings, such as regret, guilt, sadness, relief, and happiness, are normal, no evidence has

weeks. The risk of death increases with the length of pregnancy. At 16 to 20 weeks, the mortality is 1 per 27,000, and at 21 weeks or more it increases to 1 per 8,000.[8] This higher rate later in the pregnancy is due to the increased risk of uterine perforation, bleeding, infection, and incomplete abortion due to the fact that the uterine wall becomes thinner as the pregnancy progresses.

One surgical method of performing abortion has been the subject of much controversy. **Intact dilation and extraction (D&X),** sometimes referred to by the nonmedical term *partial-birth abortion,* is used only in certain cases, such as when other abortion methods could injure the mother. The procedure generally involves repositioning the fetus to a breech (feet-first) position before extracting most of the body except for the head. The contents of the cranium are then aspirated, resulting in vaginal delivery of a dead but otherwise intact fetus.[9] Thirty-one states have passed legislation attempting to ban intact dilation and extraction. However, the wording of the legislation in many states has been so general that it could be used to ban all types of abortion. For this reason, such legislation has often been challenged, and currently only ten states fully enforce the laws as written. Professional organizations such as the American College of Obstetrics and Gynecology and the American Medical Association state that physicians, acting in the best interests of their patients, should choose the safest and most appropriate method of abortion in each individual case.

Medical Abortions Unlike surgical abortions, medical abortions are performed without entering the uterus. **Mifepristone,** formerly known as RU-486, is a steroid hormone that

---

Intact dilation and extraction (D&X) A late-term abortion procedure in which the body of the fetus is extracted up to the head and then the contents of the cranium are aspirated.

Mifepristone A steroid hormone that induces abortion by blocking the action of progesterone.

shown that an abortion causes long-term psychological trauma for a woman. In a longitudinal study of over 5,000 women who had had abortions, researchers found that the best predictor of a woman's emotional well-being following an abortion was her emotional well-being prior to the procedure. Even factors such as marital status or affiliation with a religion that is strongly antiabortion were found to have no effect on a woman's later sense of self-esteem and well-being.[11]

A small percentage of women who undergo abortions experience depressive symptoms similar to postpartum blues, but the vast majority express no regrets about their decision and state they would make the choice again if they found themselves in similar circumstances. Certainly the presence of a support network and the assistance of mental health professionals is helpful to any woman who is struggling with the emotional aspects of the abortion decision in her own life.

What do you think?

If you or your partner unexpectedly became pregnant, would you choose to terminate the pregnancy? ■ How might an abortion affect your relationship? ■ What factors would you consider in making your decision? ■ Why do you consider these factors important?

Planning a Pregnancy

The many methods available to control fertility give you choices that did not exist when your parents—and even you—were born. If you are in the process of deciding whether to have children, take the time to evaluate your emotions, finances, and health.

Emotional Health

First and foremost, consider why you want to have a child: To fulfill an inner need to carry on the family? To escape loneliness? Are there any other reasons? Can you care for this new human being in a loving and nurturing manner? Are you ready to make all the sacrifices necessary to bear and raise a child? If you feel, based on your self-evaluation, that you are ready to be a parent, you can prepare for this change in your life by reading about parenthood, taking classes, talking to parents of children of all ages, and joining a support group. If you choose to adopt, you will find many support groups available to you as well.

Preconception care   Medical care received prior to becoming pregnant that helps a woman assess and address potential maternal health.

Maternal Health

Before becoming pregnant, a woman should have a thorough medical examination. **Preconception care** should include assessment of potential complications. Medical problems such as diabetes and high blood pressure should be discussed, as should any genetic disorders that run in the family. Additional suggestions for a healthy pregnancy include:

- If you smoke or drink alcohol, stop.
- Reduce or eliminate caffeine intake.
- Avoid X rays and environmental chemicals, such as lawn and garden chemicals.
- Maintain a normal weight; lose weight if necessary.
- Take prenatal vitamins, which are especially important in providing adequate folic acid.
- Prior to becoming pregnant, get any dental X rays that will be needed for a checkup.

Paternal Health

It is common wisdom that pregnant women should steer clear of toxic chemicals that can cause birth defects. Even women who are trying to conceive are cautioned to avoid toxic environments, eat a nourishing diet, stop smoking and drinking alcohol, and avoid most medications. Now similar precautions are recommended for fathers-to-be. New research suggests that a man's exposure to chemicals influences not only his ability to father a child, but also the future health of his child.

Fathers-to-be have been overlooked in past preconception and prenatal studies for several reasons. Researchers assumed that the genetic damage leading to birth defects and other health problems occurred while a child was in the mother's womb. After all, they reasoned, that's where embryonic and fetal development take place. Conventional medical wisdom also held that defective-looking sperm (those with misshapen heads, crooked tails, or retarded swimming ability) were incapable of fertilizing an egg. However, scientists have recently discovered that how sperm look has little to do with how they act. Misshapen sperm can penetrate an egg, and they do not necessarily carry defective genetic goods. Moreover, sperm that look healthy and swim well can be the true genetic culprits. DNA fluorescent markers have identified normal-looking, yet genetically flawed, sperm that carry too many or too few chromosomes. Fathers contribute the extra chromosome 21 in about 6 percent of children with Down syndrome, which causes mental retardation; the extra X chromosome in 50 percent of boys with Klinefelter's syndrome, which causes abnormal sexual development; and the shortened chromosome 15 in about 85 percent of children with Prader-Willi syndrome, a disorder characterized by retardation and obesity.

Although some birth defects are caused by random errors of nature, it now appears that some disorders can be traced to sperm damaged by chemicals. Sperm are naturally vulnerable to toxic assault and genetic damage. Many drugs and ingested chemicals can readily invade the testes from the bloodstream; others ambush sperm after they leave the testes and pass through the epididymides, where they mature and are stored. By one route or another, half of 100 chemicals studied so far (including by-products of cigarette smoke) apparently harm sperm.

Some researchers believe that vitamin C is nature's way of protecting sex cells from damage. Bad diets, exposure to toxic chemicals, cigarette smoking, and not enough foods rich in vitamin C are probably the biggest culprits in sperm damage.[12]

Financial Evaluation

Another important consideration is finances. First check your medical insurance: Does it provide pregnancy benefits? If not, you can expect to pay between $1,500 and $5,000 for medical care during pregnancy and birth—and substantially more if complications arise. Both partners should investigate their employers' policies concerning parental leave, including length of leave available and conditions for returning to work.

The U.S. Department of Agriculture estimates that it can cost as much as $250,000 for a middle-class married couple to raise a child to the age of 17. (Housing costs and food are the two largest expenditures.)[13] That figure does not include college, which can now run up to $40,000 per year with room and board at a private institution. Can you afford to give your child the life you would like him or her to enjoy?

Also consider the cost and availability of quality child care. How much family assistance can you realistically expect with a new baby, and is nonfamily child care available? While you may be aware of the federal tax credit available for child care, you may not realize how little assistance it actually provides: between a maximum of $480 for one child in a family having income of over $28,000 to a maximum of $720 for one child in a family having income of under $10,000. A second child doubles the credit, but no further assistance is provided for a third child or more children. How much does full-time child care cost? Costs vary by region and type of care. In some areas the average monthly cost per child is $500 to $800, but in other areas, it may be as much as $1,200 or more per month.[14]

Contingency Planning

A final consideration is how to provide for the child should something happen to you and your partner. If both of you were to die while the child is young, do you have relatives or close friends who would raise the child? If you have more than one child, would they have to be split up or could they be kept together? Though unpleasant to think about, this sort of contingency planning is very important. Children who lose their parents are heartbroken and confused. A prearranged plan of action will smooth their transition into new families.

What do you think?

What factors will you consider in deciding whether or when to have children? ■ *Is there a certain age at which you feel you will be ready to be a parent?* ■ *What goals do you hope to achieve before undertaking parenthood?* ■ *What are your biggest concerns about parenthood?*

Pregnancy

Pregnancy is an important event in a woman's life. The actions taken before a pregnancy begins, as well as behaviors during pregnancy, can have a significant effect on the health of both infant and mother.

Prenatal Care

A successful pregnancy depends on the mother taking good care of herself and the fetus. It is essential to have regular medical checkups, beginning as soon as possible (certainly within the first three months). Early detection of fetal abnormalities and identification of high-risk mothers and infants are the major purposes of prenatal care. On the first visit, the practitioner should obtain a complete medical history of the mother and her family and note any hereditary conditions that could put a woman or her fetus at risk.

Regular checkups to measure weight gain and blood pressure and to monitor the size and position of the fetus continue throughout the pregnancy. This early care reduces infant mortality and low birth weight. A study group for the American College of Obstetricians and Gynecologists recommends seven or eight prenatal visits for women with low-risk pregnancies. Unfortunately, prenatal care is not available to everyone. Approximately 30 percent of pregnant teenagers and unmarried women do not receive adequate prenatal attention. Babies of mothers who received no prenatal care are about ten times more likely to die in the first month of life than babies of mothers who did get prenatal care.

Additional concerns include the mother's physical condition, her level of nutrition, her confidence in her ability to give birth, her use of drugs and medications, and the availability of a skilled practitioner who can oversee the pregnancy and delivery. A woman planning a pregnancy also needs a support system (spouse or partner, family, friends, community groups) willing to provide love and emotional support during and after her pregnancy.

Choosing a Practitioner A woman should carefully choose a practitioner to attend her pregnancy and delivery. If possible, this choice should be made before she becomes pregnant. Recommendations from friends are a good starting point. The woman's family physician may also be able to recommend a specialist.

When choosing a practitioner, parents should ask about credentials, professional qualifications, and experience. Besides this information, a pregnant woman must ask questions specific to her condition. Prospective parents should inquire about the practitioner's experience in handling various complications, commitment to being at the mother's side during delivery, and beliefs and practices concerning the use of anesthesia, fetal monitoring, induced labor, and forceps delivery. What are the practitioner's attitudes toward birth control, abortion, and alternative birthing procedures? The practitioner's approach to nutrition and medication during pregnancy should be similar to the woman's own. Finally, the parents must learn under what circumstances the practitioner would perform a cesarean section.

Two types of physicians can attend pregnancies and deliveries. The *obstetrician-gynecologist* (OB-Gyn) is a medical doctor who specializes in obstetrics (pregnancy and birth) and gynecology (care of women's reproductive organs). These practitioners are trained to handle all types of pregnancy- and delivery-related emergencies. A *family practitioner* is a licensed medical doctor who provides comprehensive care for people of all ages. The majority of family practitioners have obstetrical experience but will refer a patient to a specialist if necessary. Unlike the OB-Gyn, the family practitioner can serve as the baby's physician after attending the birth.

Midwives are also experienced practitioners who can attend both pregnancies and deliveries. *Certified nurse-midwives* are registered nurses having specialized training in pregnancy and delivery. Most midwives work in private practice or in conjunction with physicians. Those who work with physicians have access to traditional medical facilities to which they can turn in an emergency. *Lay midwives* may or may not have extensive training in handling an emergency. They may be self-taught or trained through formal certification procedures.

Alcohol and Drugs   A woman should avoid all types of drugs during pregnancy. Even common over-the-counter medications such as aspirin and beverages such as coffee and tea can damage a developing fetus.

During the first three months of pregnancy, the fetus is especially subject to the **teratogenic** (birth defect–causing) effects of some chemical substances. The fetus can also develop an addiction to or tolerance for drugs that the mother

takes. Medical professionals are especially concerned about the use of tobacco and alcohol during pregnancy.

Women who are heavy drinkers may have normal first babies but subsequently deliver children having fetal alcohol syndrome. The symptoms of **fetal alcohol syndrome (FAS)** include mental retardation, slowed nerve reflexes, and small head size. The exact amount of alcohol that causes FAS is not known, but researchers doubt that any alcohol is safe. Therefore, they recommend total abstinence from alcohol during pregnancy.

Smoking harms every phase of reproduction. Women who smoke have more difficulty becoming pregnant and have a higher risk of being infertile. Women who smoke during pregnancy have a greater chance of complications, premature births, low birth weight infants, stillbirth, and infant mortality.[15] Smoking restricts the blood supply to the developing fetus and thus limits oxygen and nutrition delivery and waste removal. It appears to be a significant factor in the development of cleft lip and palate, and a significant relationship has been shown for both smoking and "secondhand" smoke with sudden infant death syndrome.[16] Research on the fetal effects of secondhand, or sidestream, smoke (inhaling smoke produced by others) is inconclusive, but babies whose parents smoke can be twice as susceptible to pneumonia, bronchitis, and related illnesses as other babies. Recent statistics for the United States show that tobacco use among pregnant women has steadily fallen since 1989, when about 20 percent of pregnant women smoked. In 1998, that rate had declined to 12.9 percent.[17]

X rays   X rays present a clear danger to the fetus. Although most diagnostic tests produce minimal amounts of radiation, even low levels may cause birth defects or other problems, particularly if several low-dose X rays are taken over a short time period. Pregnant women are advised to avoid X rays unless absolutely necessary.

Nutrition and Exercise   Pregnant women need additional protein, calories, vitamins, and minerals, so their diets should be carefully monitored by a qualified practitioner. Special attention should be paid to getting enough folic acid (found in dark, leafy greens), iron (dried fruits, meats, legumes, liver, egg yolks), calcium (nonfat or low-fat dairy products, some canned fish), and fluids.

Vitamin supplements can correct some deficiencies, but there is no substitute for a well-balanced diet. Babies born to poorly nourished mothers run high risks of substandard mental and physical development. Folic acid, when consumed before and during early pregnancy, reduces the risk of spina bifida, a common disabling birth condition resulting from failure of the spinal column to close. Manufacturers of breads, pastas, rice, and other grain products are now required to add folic acid to their products to reduce neural tube defects in newborns.

Weight gain during pregnancy helps nourish a growing baby. For a woman of normal weight before pregnancy,

---

Midwives   Experienced practitioners who assist with pregnancy and delivery.

Teratogenic   Causing birth defects; may refer to drugs, environmental chemicals, X rays, or diseases.

Fetal alcohol syndrome (FAS)   A collection of symptoms, including mental retardation, that can appear in infants of women who drink too much alcohol during pregnancy.

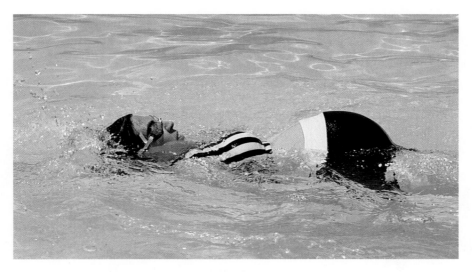

A doctor-approved exercise program during pregnancy can help manage weight, make delivery easier, and have a healthy effect on the fetus.

the recommended weight gain during pregnancy is 25 to 35 pounds. For obese or overweight women, 15 to 25 pounds are recommended. Underweight women can gain 28 to 40 pounds, and women carrying twins should gain about 35 to 45 pounds. Gaining too much or too little weight can lead to complications. With higher weight gains, women may develop gestational diabetes, hypertension, or increased risk of delivery complications. Gaining too little weight increases the chance of a low–birth weight baby.

Of the total number of pounds gained during pregnancy, about 6 to 8 are the baby. The baby's birth weight is important, since low weight can mean health problems during labor and the baby's first few months. Pregnancy is not the time to think about losing weight—doing so may endanger the fetus.[18]

As in all other stages of life, exercise is an important factor in weight control during pregnancy and overall maternal health. In one study, a balanced 45-minute exercise session three days per week was associated with heavier–birth weight babies, fewer surgical births, and shorter hospital stays after birth. Pregnant women should consult their physicians before starting any exercise program.

Other Factors   A pregnant woman should avoid exposure to toxic chemicals, heavy metals, pesticides, gases, and other hazardous compounds. She should not clean cat-litter boxes because cat feces can contain organisms that cause a disease called **toxoplasmosis.** If a pregnant woman contracts this disease, her baby may be stillborn or suffer mental retardation or other birth defects.

Before becoming pregnant, a woman should be tested to determine if she has had rubella (German measles). If she has not had rubella, she should be immunized for it and wait the recommended length of time before becoming pregnant.

A rubella infection can kill the fetus or cause blindness or hearing disorders in the infant. If the woman has ever had genital herpes, she should inform her physician. The physician may want to deliver the baby by cesarean section, especially if the woman has active lesions. Contact with an active herpes infection during birth can be fatal to the baby.

What do you think?

In looking at your current lifestyle, what behaviors (nutritional choices, fitness, etc.) would you cease or begin in order to promote a healthy pregnancy? ■ *What characteristics or skills would you look for in selecting a health care provider during your own or your partner's pregnancy?*

A Woman's Reproductive Years

More than half of the average American woman's expected life span is spent between menarche (first menses) and menopause (last menses), a period of approximately 40 years. Deciding if and when to have children, as well as how to prevent pregnancy when necessary, is a long-term concern.

Toxoplasmosis   A disease caused by an organism found in cat feces that, when contracted by a pregnant woman, may result in stillbirth or an infant with mental retardation or birth defects.

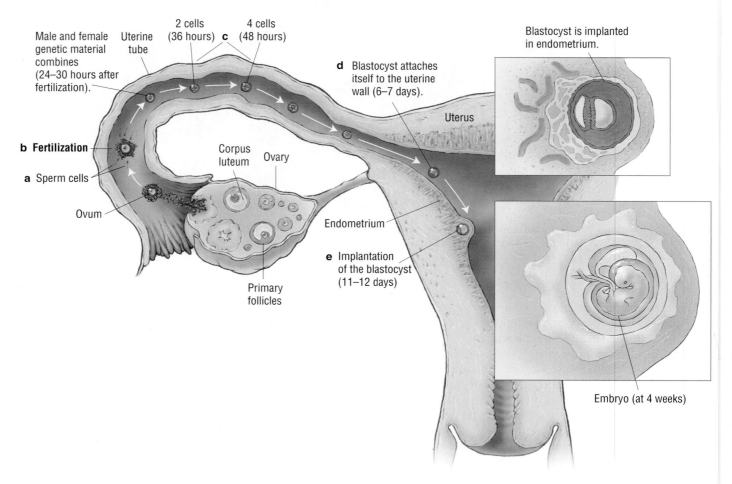

Figure 7.8

Fertilization

(a) The efforts of hundreds of sperm may allow one sperm to penetrate the ovum's corona radiata, an outer layer of cells, and then the zona pellucida, a thick inner membrane.
(b) The sperm nucleus fuses with egg nucleus at fertilization, which produces a zygote.
(c) The zygote divides first into two cells, then four cells, and so on. **(d)** The blastocyst attaches itself to the uterine wall. **(e)** The blastocyst implants itself in the endometrium.

Today, a woman over 35 who is pregnant has plenty of company. While births to women in their twenties are declining, the rate of first births to women between the ages of 30 and 39 has doubled in the past decade, and births to women over 39 have increased by more than 50 percent. Many women who wait until their thirties to consider having a child find themselves wondering, "Am I too old to have a baby?" Statistically, the chances of having a baby with birth defects do rise after the age of 35. Researchers believe that

there is a decline in both the quality and viability of eggs after this age.

Down syndrome, a condition characterized by mild to severe mental retardation and a variety of physical abnormalities, is the most common genetic condition. One in every 800 to 1,000 live births a year is a child with Down syndrome, representing approximately 5,000 births per year in the United States alone.

A common myth is that most children with Down syndrome have older parents. The truth is that 80 percent of these children are born to women younger than 35. However, the incidence does increase with age. The incidence of Down syndrome in babies born to a mother age 20 is 1 in 10,000 births; it rises to 1 in 400 by age 35, to 1 in 110 by age 40, and to 1 in 35 when she is 45.[19]

> **Down syndrome** A condition characterized by mental retardation and a variety of physical abnormalities.

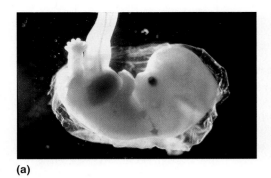
(a)

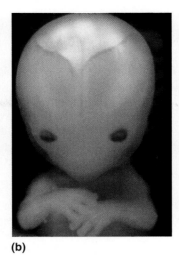
(b)

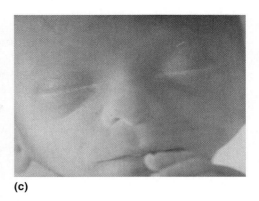
(c)

This series of fetoscopic photographs show the development of the fetus in the (a) first, (b) second, and (c) third trimesters of pregnancy.

Women who delay motherhood until their late thirties also worry about their physical ability to carry and deliver their babies. For these women, a comprehensive exercise program will assist in maintaining good posture and promoting a successful delivery.

Despite these concerns, there are some advantages to having a baby later in life. In fact, many doctors note that older mothers tend to be more conscientious about following medical advice during pregnancy and are more psychologically mature and ready to include an infant in their family than some younger women.

Pregnancy Testing

A woman may suspect she is pregnant before she has any pregnancy tests. A typical sign is a missed menstrual period, yet this is not always an accurate indicator. A woman can miss her period for a variety of reasons, including stress, exercise, and emotional upset. A pregnancy test scheduled in a medical office or birth control clinic will confirm the pregnancy. Women who wish to know immediately can purchase home pregnancy test kits, sold over the counter in drugstores. A positive test is based on the secretion of **human chorionic gonadotropin (HCG),** found in the woman's urine. Home test kits come equipped with a small sample of red blood cells coated with HCG antibodies to which the user adds a small amount of urine. If the concentration of HCG is great enough, it will clump together with the HCG antibodies, indicating that the user is pregnant.

Home pregnancy test kits are about 85 to 95 percent reliable. If done too early in the pregnancy, they may show a false negative. Other causes of false negatives are unclean test tubes, ingestion of certain drugs, and vaginal or urinary tract infections. Accuracy also depends on the quality of the test itself and the user's ability to perform it and interpret the results. Blood tests administered and analyzed by a medical laboratory are more accurate.

The Process of Pregnancy

Pregnancy begins the moment a sperm fertilizes an ovum in the uterine tubes (Figure 7.8). From there, the single cell multiplies, becoming a sphere-shaped cluster of cells as it travels toward the uterus, a journey that may take three to four days. Upon arrival, the embryo burrows into the thick, spongy endometrium and is nourished from this carefully prepared lining.

Early Signs of Pregnancy The first sign of pregnancy is usually a missed menstrual period (although some women "spot" in early pregnancy, which may be mistaken for a period). Other signs of pregnancy include breast tenderness, emotional upset, extreme fatigue, nausea, sleeplessness, and vomiting (especially in the morning).

Pregnancy typically lasts 40 weeks. The due date is calculated from the expectant mother's last menstrual period. Pregnancy is typically divided into three phases, or **trimesters,** of approximately three months each.

The First Trimester During the first trimester, few noticeable changes occur in the mother's body. The expectant mother may urinate more frequently and experience morning sickness, swollen breasts, or undue fatigue. These symptoms may not be frequent or severe, so she may not even realize she is pregnant unless she has a pregnancy test.

Human chorionic gonadotropin (HCG) Hormone detectable in blood or urine samples of a mother within the first few weeks of pregnancy.

Trimester A three-month segment of pregnancy; used to describe specific developmental changes that occur in the embryo or fetus.

Table 7.3
Common Emotions Experienced throughout the Pregnancy Process

First Trimester	Second Trimester	Third Trimester	Fourth Trimester
Disbelief that one is actually pregnant	Sense that the pregnancy feels "real"	Development of emotional relationship with baby—beginning to view baby as a person as more fetal movement occurs	Sense of being overwhelmed at new responsibility—"What do we do now?"
Fear of miscarriage	Less fear of miscarriage	Fear of labor, labor complications, possible defects	Difficulty in settling limits on friend and family visits; learning to negotiate everyone's roles in baby's life
Feeling of being overwhelmed by changes	Wonder at hearing the heartbeat, feeling movement, bulging tummy	Possible tiredness of pregnancy (Pregnancy seems to take over identity—"Is that all people want to talk about?")	Exhaustion and emotional vacillation due to sleep deprivation, breast-feeding
Tendency to be more emotional, (e.g., crying more easily)	Frustration when symptoms make fulfilling other responsibilities difficult	Impatience for due date to arrive, possible frustration with limited mobility	Surprise at how slow the physical healing process may be, impatient to get back to pre-pregnancy shape
Apprehension about upcoming decisions (screening tests, etc.)	Differing emotions about weight gain (some enjoy it; others struggle with it)	Interest in others' birth experiences (especially one's mother's) and parenting styles	Amazement at the birth process
Excitement about telling others about pregnancy if waiting until the end of first trimester	Excitement and anxiety in making plans for future	Excitement in making final preparations for baby; baby showers and other activities that make the event seem more real	Excitement about future; apprehension about postmaternity leave transition, if applicable—"How will I balance everything?"
Anxiety about being a parent	Anxiety about being a parent	Anxiety about being a parent	Anxiety about being a parent

Source: Information for second through fourth trimesters adapted from C. M. Peterson and N. L. Stotland, "Physical and Emotional Changes," *Lamaze Parents Magazine,* 2000 spring/summer issue. Reprinted by permission of Lamaze, Inc.

During the first two months after conception, the **embryo** differentiates and develops its various organ systems, beginning with the nervous and circulatory systems. At the start of the third month, the embryo is called a **fetus,** indicating that all organ systems are in place. For the rest of the pregnancy, growth and refinement occur in each major body system so that they can function independently, yet in coordination, at birth. The photos on the preceding page illustrate physical changes during fetal development.

The Second Trimester   At the beginning of the second trimester, physical changes in the mother become more visible.

Embryo   The fertilized egg from conception until the end of two months' development.

Fetus   The name given the developing baby from the third month of pregnancy until birth.

Placenta   The network of blood vessels, connected to the umbilical cord, that carries nutrients to the developing infant and carries wastes away.

Fourth trimester   The first six weeks of an infant's life outside the womb.

Her breasts swell, and her waistline thickens. During this time, the fetus makes greater demands upon the mother's body. In particular, the **placenta,** the network of blood vessels that carry nutrients and oxygen to the fetus and fetal waste products to the mother, becomes well established.

The Third Trimester   From the end of the sixth month through the ninth is the third trimester. This is the period of greatest fetal growth, when the fetus gains most of its weight. During the third trimester, the fetus must get large amounts of calcium, iron, and nitrogen from the food the mother eats. Approximately 85 percent of the calcium and iron the mother digests goes into the fetal bloodstream.

Although the fetus may live if it is born during the seventh month, it needs the layer of fat it acquires during the eighth month and time for the organs (especially the respiratory and digestive organs) to develop to their full potential. Infants born prematurely usually require intensive medical care.

Of course, the process of pregnancy involves much more than the changes in a woman's body. Many important emotional changes occur from the time a woman learns she is pregnant through the **"fourth trimester"** (the first six weeks of an infant's life outside the womb). Table 7.3

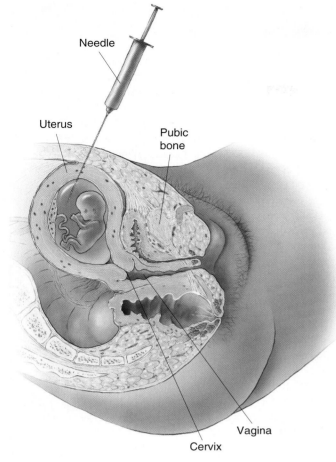

Needle

Uterus

Pubic
bone

Vagina

Cervix

Figure 7.9
Amniocentesis
The process of amniocentesis can detect certain congenital
problems as well as the sex of the fetus.

outlines common emotions and emotional challenges that
may arise over the course of pregnancy.

Prenatal Testing and Screening

Modern technology enables medical practitioners to detect
health defects in a fetus as early as the fourteenth to eighteenth weeks of pregnancy. One common testing procedure,
amniocentesis, which is strongly recommended for women
over age 35, involves inserting a long needle through the
mother's abdominal and uterine walls into the **amniotic sac,**
the protective pouch surrounding the fetus (Figure 7.9). The
needle draws out 3 to 4 teaspoons of fluid, which is analyzed
for genetic information about the baby. This test can reveal
the presence of 40 genetic abnormalities, including Down
syndrome, Tay-Sachs disease (a fatal disorder of the nervous
system common among Jewish people of Eastern European

descent), and sickle-cell anemia (a debilitating blood disorder
found primarily among blacks). Amniocentesis can also reveal gender, a fact many parents choose not to know until
the birth. Although widely used, amniocentesis is not without risk. Chances of fetal damage and miscarriage as a result
of testing are 1 in 400.

Another procedure, *ultrasound,* or *sonography,* uses
high-frequency sound waves to determine the size and
position of the fetus. Ultrasound can also detect fetal defects in the central nervous system and digestive system.
Knowing the position of the fetus assists practitioners in
performing amniocentesis and delivering the infant. New
three-dimensional ultrasound techniques clarify images
and improve doctors' efforts to detect and treat defects
prenatally.

A third procedure, *fetoscopy,* involves making a small
incision in the abdominal and uterine walls and inserting
an optical viewer into the uterus to view the fetus directly.
This device is used with ultrasound to determine fetal age
and location of the placenta. This method is still experimental and involves some risk. It causes miscarriage in approximately 5 percent of cases.

A fourth procedure, *chorionic villus sampling (CVS),* involves snipping tissue from the developing fetal sac. CVS can
be used at 10 to 12 weeks of pregnancy, and the test results
are available in 12 to 48 hours. CVS is an attractive option for
couples who are at high risk for having a baby with Down
syndrome or a debilitating hereditary disease.

If any of these tests reveals a serious birth defect, parents are advised to undergo genetic counseling. In the case
of a chromosomal abnormality such as Down syndrome, the
parents are usually offered the option of a therapeutic abortion. Some parents choose this option; others research the
disability and decide to go ahead with the birth.

Some prospective parents even undergo procedures
aimed at increasing the odds of having a baby of a particular gender; see the Health Ethics: Conflict and Controversy box.

What do you think?

What are your thoughts on prenatal testing?
■ *Would you want to know if you were carrying a
child with a genetic defect or other abnormality?
Why or why not?*

Amniocentesis   A medical test in which a small
amount of fluid is drawn from the amniotic sac to test for
Down's syndrome and other genetic diseases.

Amniotic sac   The protective pouch surrounding
the baby.

The Science of Sex Selection

Parents have wanted the ability to choose the gender of their child since prehistoric times, with intense interest in sex selection in early Chinese, Egyptian, and Greek cultures. Even in these high tech times, people try a variety of avenues, most based on folklore, to conceive a particular sex. From diet, sexual positioning, testicle temperature, and the phases of the moon, couples try to defy the odds of nature.

Now science may help couples have the baby they want. Choosing gender may obliterate one of the fundamental mysteries of procreation, but for people who have grown accustomed to seeing three-dimensional ultrasounds of fetuses, learning a baby's sex within weeks of conception, and scheduling convenient delivery dates, it's simply the next logical step.

Currently, an FDA clinical trial of sophisticated sperm-sorting technology is more than halfway to completion. Approval of the technique by the FDA would add it to the arsenal of couples intent on having a baby of a particular sex. The *MicroSort method* is an experimental technique that separates X (female) chromosomes from Y (male) chromosomes. Sperm are stained with a fluorescent dye that binds to the chromosomes. X chromosomes are bigger than Y and soak up more dye. The sperm are then zapped with a laser that illuminates the dye. X chromosomes have more dye and are brighter. Then the dyed sperm passes by an electrode that gives Xs a positive charge and Ys a negative one. Charged plates attract and separate the chromosomes, channeling them into separate receptacles. Separation is not absolutely perfect, but one sample is used to fertilize a woman's eggs, depending on the requested sex.

The *Ericsson method* has been used for about a decade. In this technique, sperm are poured into a viscous layer of fluid. The heavy head of the sperm makes them swim downward. Sperm carrying the Y (male) chromosomes swim faster than those with X chromosomes, reaching the bottom of the tube faster. They can then be extracted and used for insemination. This technique claims to have a 78 to 85 percent chance of producing a boy, although critics says the odds are not better than 50:50.

Preimplantation genetic diagnosis, the third technique, was originally used for detecting genetic diseases. Doctors remove eggs from the woman and fertilize them with sperm in the lab, creating embryos. After three days, technicians extract a cell from each embryo. They can differentiate male and female embryos by examining their chromosomes. After determining the sex of the embryos, doctors implant the desired ones. While more invasive and costly than other methods, success is virtually guaranteed.

Source: Adapted from Karen Springen "Brave New Babies," *Newsweek,* January 26, 2004, 45–53. © 2004 Newsweek, Inc. All rights reserved. Reprinted by permission.

Childbirth

Prospective parents need to make a number of key decisions long before the baby is born. These include where to have the baby, whether to use drugs during labor and delivery, choice of childbirth method, and whether to breast-feed or bottle-feed. Answering these questions in advance will ensure a smoother passage into parenthood.

Choosing Where to Have Your Baby

Today's prospective mothers have many delivery options, ranging from traditional hospital birth to home birth. Parental values are important. Many couples, for instance, feel that the modern medical establishment has dehumanized the birth process; thus they choose to deliver at home or at a *birthing center,* a homelike setting outside a hospital where women can give birth and receive postdelivery care by a team of professional practitioners, including physicians and registered nurses.

However, hospitals have responded to the desire for a more relaxed, less medically oriented birthing process. Many hospitals now offer labor–delivery–postpartum birthing rooms, which allow patients with noncomplicated deliveries to remain in one room during the entire process. In addition, "rooming-in," or keeping the baby in the same room with the mother at all times, is encouraged to facilitate bonding and breast-feeding. Partners are generally encouraged to room-in with mother and baby as well.

Labor and Delivery

The birth process has three stages (Figure 7.10). The exact mechanisms that initiate labor are unknown. During the last few weeks before delivery, the baby normally shifts and turns to a head-down position, and the cervix begins to dilate (widen). The junction of the pubic bones gradually loosens as the third trimester progresses to permit expansion of the pelvic girdle during birth.

In the first stage of labor, the amniotic sac breaks, causing a rush of fluid from the vagina (commonly referred to as "water breaking"). Contractions in the abdomen and lower back also signal the beginning of labor. Early contractions push the baby downward, putting pressure on the cervix and dilating it further. The first stage of labor may last from a couple of hours to more than a day for a first birth but is usually much shorter during subsequent births.

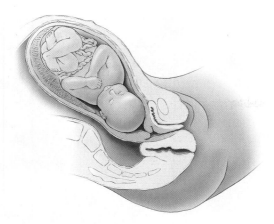

Dilation of the cervix

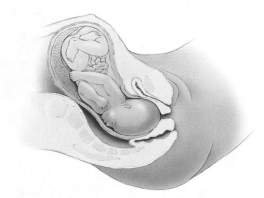

Transition ─────────────── **End of Stage I**

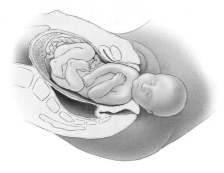

Birth of the baby (Expulsion) ───── **End of Stage II**

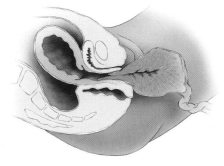

Delivery of the placenta ──────── **End of Stage III**

Figure 7.10
The Birth Process

The end of the first stage of labor, called **transition,** is the process during which the cervix becomes fully dilated and the baby's head begins to move into the vagina, or birth canal. Contractions usually come quickly during transition, which generally lasts 30 minutes or less.

The second stage of labor (the *expulsion stage*) follows transition, when the cervix has become fully dilated. Contractions become rhythmic, strong, and more painful as the uterus works to push the baby through the birth canal. The expulsion stage lasts one to four hours and concludes when the infant is finally pushed out of the mother's body. In some cases, the attending practitioner will do an **episiotomy,** a straight incision in the mother's perineum, to prevent the baby's head from tearing vaginal tissues and speed the baby's exit from the vagina. Sometimes women can avoid the need for an episiotomy by exercising and getting good nutrition throughout pregnancy, by trying different birth positions, or by having an attendant massage the perineal tissue. However, the skin's natural elasticity and the baby's size are limiting factors.

After delivery, the attending practitioner cleans the baby's mucus-filled breathing passages, and the baby takes its first breath, generally accompanied by a loud wail. (The traditional slap on the baby's buttocks, often depicted in old movies, is no longer a common practice because of the trauma associated with it.) The umbilical cord is then tied and severed. The stump of cord attached to the baby's navel dries up and drops off within a few days.

In the meantime, the mother continues into the third stage of labor, during which the placenta, or **afterbirth,** is expelled from the womb. This stage is usually completed within 30 minutes after delivery.

Most mothers prefer to have their new infants next to them following the birth. Together with their spouse or partner, they can share this time of bonding with their infant.

Managing Labor: Medical and Nonmedical Approaches

Because painkilling drugs given to the mother during labor can cause sluggish responses in the newborn and other complications, many women choose drug-free labor and delivery—but it is important to keep a flexible attitude about pain relief because each labor is different. Working in partnership with a health care provider to make the best decision for mother and baby is optimal. Use of painkilling medication during a delivery is not a sign of weakness. One person

Transition   The process during which the cervix becomes nearly fully dilated and the head of the fetus begins to move into the birth canal.

Episiotomy   A straight incision in the mother's perineum in the area between the vulva and the anus.

Afterbirth   The expelled placenta.

is not a "success" for delivering without medication while another is a "failure" for using medical measures. Remember, pain is to be expected. In fact, many experts say that the pain of labor is the most difficult in the human experience. There is no one right answer for managing that pain.

Birth Alternatives

Expectant parents have several options beyond the traditional hospital setting for the process of their infant's birth and their participation in it. Although several of these methods have decreased in popularity, all continue to be used.

The Lamaze method is the most popular birth alternative in the United States. Prelabor classes teach the mother to control her pain through special breathing patterns, focusing exercises, and relaxation. Lamaze births usually take place in a hospital or birthing center with a physician or midwife in attendance. The partner (or labor coach) assists by giving emotional support, physical comfort (massage and ice chips), and coaching for proper breath control during contractions. Lamaze proponents discourage the use of drugs.

Other methods that prospective parents can research include the Harris method, Childbirth without Fear, the Leboyer method, the Bradley method, and water birth. These vary in their philosophies regarding painkillers, partner participation, and other issues.

Breast-Feeding and the Postpartum Period

Although the new mother's milk will not begin to flow for two or more days, her breasts secrete a thick yellow substance called *colostrum*. Because this fluid contains vital antibodies to help fight infection, the newborn baby should be allowed to suckle.

The American Academy of Pediatrics strongly recommends that infants should be breast-fed for at least 6 months and ideally for 12 months. Scientific findings indicate there are many advantages to breast-feeding. Breast milk is perfectly suited to a baby's nutritional needs. Breast-fed babies have fewer illnesses and a much lower hospitalization rate because breast milk contains maternal antibodies and immunological cells that stimulate the infant's immune system. When breast-fed babies do get sick, they recover more quickly. They are also less likely to be obese than babies fed on formulas, and they have fewer allergies. They may even be more intelligent: a new study finds that the longer a baby was breast-fed, the higher the IQ in adulthood. Researchers theorize that breast milk contains substances that enhance brain development.[20]

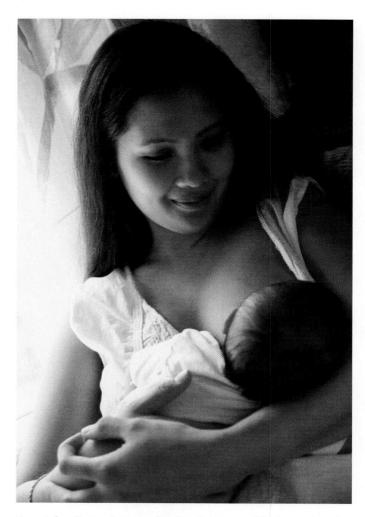

Breast-feeding enhances the development of intimate bonds between mother and child.

Another study found that women who were able to breast-feed successfully for longer periods of time generally viewed breast-feeding as more positive, had more knowledge about the process, and had higher self-efficacy in their ability to breast-feed.[21]

This does not mean that breast milk is the only way to nourish a baby. Some women are unable or unwilling to breast-feed. Prepared formulas can provide nourishment that allows a baby to grow and thrive. When deciding whether to breast- or bottle-feed, mothers need to consider their own desires and preferences too. Both feeding methods can supply the physical and emotional closeness so essential to the parent–child relationship.

The *postpartum period* lasts from four to six weeks after delivery. During this time, the mother's reproductive organs revert to a nonpregnant state. Many women experience energy depletion, anxiety, mood swings, and depression during this period. This experience, known as **postpartum depression,** appears to be a common end-product of the birth

Postpartum depression   The experience of energy depletion, anxiety, mood swings, and depression that women may feel during the postpartum period.

process. For most women, the symptoms gradually disappear as their bodies return to normal. For others, the symptoms, coupled with the stress of managing a new family, can cause more severe depression that lasts for several months.

Complications

Complications are a possibility during both pregnancy and the period of labor and delivery. **Preeclampsia** is a condition that is characterized by high blood pressure, protein in the urine, and edema (fluid retention), which usually causes swelling of the hands and face. This condition complicates approximately 10 percent of pregnancies and is responsible for 18 percent of U.S. maternal deaths each year. Symptoms may include sudden weight gain, headache, nausea or vomiting, changes in vision, racing pulse, mental confusion, and stomach or right shoulder pain. If preeclampsia is not treated, it can cause seizures, a condition called **eclampsia.** Potential problems can include liver and kidney damage, internal bleeding, stroke, poor fetal growth, and fetal and maternal death.

This condition tends to occur in the late second or third trimesters. The cause is not known; however, the incidence of preeclampsia is higher in first-time mothers, women over 40 or under 18 years of age, women carrying multiple fetuses, and women with a history of chronic hypertension, diabetes or kidney disorder, or previous history of preeclampsia. Family history of preeclampsia is also a risk factor, whether the history is on the male or female side. Treatment for preeclampsia ranges from bed rest and monitoring for those with mild cases, to hospitalization and close monitoring for more severe cases, which have the potential to be life-threatening for the woman and her fetus.

Problems and complications can also occur during labor and delivery, even following a successful pregnancy. The mother should discuss these possibilities with her practitioner prior to labor so she understands the medical procedures that may be necessary for her safety and that of her child. Although pregnancy still involves a certain amount of risk, the risk is lower than for many other common activities.

Cesarean Section (C-section)

If labor lasts too long or if a baby is presenting wrong (about to exit the uterus any way but head first), a **cesarean section (C-section)** may be necessary. This surgical procedure involves making an incision across the mother's abdomen and through the uterus to remove the baby. This operation is also performed if labor is extremely difficult, maternal blood pressure falls rapidly, the placenta separates from the uterus too soon, the mother has diabetes, or other problems occur. A C-section can be traumatic for the mother if she is not prepared for it. Risks are the same as for any major abdominal surgery, and recovery from birth takes considerably longer after a C-section.

The rate of delivery by C-section in the United States has increased from 5 percent in the mid-1960s to 26 percent in 2002.[22] Although necessary in certain cases, some

physicians and critics, including the Centers for Disease Control and Prevention (CDC), feel that C-sections are performed too frequently in this country. The CDC had hoped to lower the rate of cesareans in the United States to 15 per 100 births by the year 2000, a level the agency considers medically appropriate. Clearly, the goal has not been met.

Surgical techniques allow some women who have had a cesarean section to deliver later children vaginally. Guidelines published by the American College of Obstetricians and Gynecologists give an estimated 50 to 80 percent of women the option of a vaginal birth after cesarean (VBAC). Cesarean sections will still be necessary, however, if the original incision runs from the top to the bottom of the uterus (as opposed to across); if the baby is over 9 pounds; if the birth is multiple; or if the mother has a medical condition that would make vaginal delivery difficult or dangerous, such as a very small pelvis, chronic high blood pressure, or diabetes.

Miscarriage

One in ten pregnancies does not end in delivery. Loss of the fetus before it is viable is called a **miscarriage** (also referred to as *spontaneous abortion*). An estimated 70 to 90 percent of women who miscarry eventually become pregnant again.

Reasons for miscarriage vary. In some cases, the fertilized egg has failed to divide correctly. In others, genetic abnormalities, maternal illness, or infections are responsible. Maternal hormonal imbalance may also cause a miscarriage, as may a weak cervix or toxic chemicals in the environment. In most cases, the cause is not known.

A blood incompatibility between mother and father can cause **Rh factor** problems, sometimes resulting in miscarriage. Rh is a blood protein, and problems occur when the mother is Rh-negative and the fetus is Rh-positive. During a first birth, some of the baby's blood passes into the mother's bloodstream. An Rh-negative mother may manufacture antibodies to destroy the Rh-positive blood

---

Preeclampsia   A complication in pregnancy characterized by high blood pressure, protein in the urine, and edema.

Eclampsia   Untreated preeclampsia can develop into this potentially fatal complication that involves maternal strokes and seizures.

Cesarean section (C-section)   A surgical procedure in which a baby is removed through an incision made in the mother's abdominal and uterine walls.

Miscarriage   Loss of the fetus before it is viable; also called spontaneous abortion.

Rh factor   A blood protein related to the production of antibodies. If an Rh-negative mother is pregnant with an Rh-positive fetus, the mother will manufacture antibodies that can kill the fetus, causing miscarriage.

introduced into her bloodstream at the time of birth. Her first baby will be unaffected, but subsequent babies with positive Rh factor will be at risk for a severe anemia called *hemolytic disease* because the mother's Rh antibodies will attack the fetus's red blood cells.

If prenatal testing reveals Rh incompatibility, intrauterine transfusions can be given or an early delivery by C-section can be done. Prevention is preferable to treatment. All women with Rh-negative blood should be injected with a medication called RhoGAM within 72 hours of any birth, miscarriage, or abortion. This injection will prevent them from developing the Rh antibodies.

Another cause of miscarriage is **ectopic pregnancy,** or implantation of a fertilized egg outside the uterus. A fertilized egg may implant itself in the uterine tube or, occasionally, in the pelvic cavity. Because these structures are not capable of expanding and nourishing a developing fetus, the pregnancy cannot continue. Such pregnancies are surgically terminated. Most often, the affected uterine tube is also removed.

Ectopic pregnancy is generally accompanied by pain in the lower abdomen or aching in the shoulders as the blood flows up toward the diaphragm. If bleeding is significant, blood pressure drops and the woman can go into shock. If an ectopic pregnancy goes undiagnosed and untreated, the uterine tube will rupture, putting the woman at great risk of hemorrhage, peritonitis (infection in the abdomen), and even death.

Over the past 12 years, the incidence of ectopic pregnancy has tripled, and no one really understands why. We do know that ectopic pregnancy is a potential side effect of pelvic inflammatory disease (PID), which has become increasingly common in recent years. The scarring or blockage of the uterine tubes characteristic of this disease prevents the fertilized egg from passing to the uterus. About 50 percent of women who have had an ectopic pregnancy conceive again. But women who have had one ectopic pregnancy run a higher risk of having another.

Stillbirth is one of the most traumatic events a couple can face. A stillborn baby is born dead, often for no apparent reason. The grief experienced following a stillbirth is devastating. Nine months of happy anticipation have been thwarted. Family, friends, and other children may be in a state of shock, needing comfort and not knowing where to turn. The mother's breasts produce milk, and there is no infant to be fed. A room with a crib and toys is left empty.

The grief can last for years, and partners may blame themselves or each other. In many cases, no amount of reassurance from the attending physician, relatives, or friends can assuage the grief or guilt. Well-intentioned comments such as "Oh, you'll have another baby someday" may bring no comfort.

Some communities have groups called the Compassionate Friends to help parents and other family members through this grieving process. This nonprofit organization is for parents who have lost a child of any age for any reason.

Sudden Infant Death Syndrome (SIDS) The sudden death of an infant under one year of age, for no apparent reason, is called **sudden infant death syndrome (SIDS).** Though SIDS is the leading cause of death for children aged one month to one year, affecting about 1 in 1,000 infants in the United States each year, it is not a disease. Rather, it is ruled the cause of death after all other possibilities are ruled out. A SIDS death is sudden and silent; death occurs quickly, often associated with sleep and no signs of suffering.

Because SIDS is a diagnosis of exclusion, doctors do not know what causes it. However, research done in countries including England, New Zealand, Australia, and Norway has shown that placing children on their backs or sides to sleep cuts the rate of SIDS by as much as half. The American Academy of Pediatrics advises parents to lay infants on their backs and is a sponsor of the Back to Sleep educational campaign urging parents to position babies on their backs. Additional precautions against SIDS include having a firm surface for the infant's bed, not allowing the infant to become too warm, maintaining a smoke-free environment, having regular pediatric visits, breast-feeding, and seeking prenatal care.

What do you think?

What are your thoughts on medical versus natural management of labor and delivery?
■ *Do you have strong preferences for how you'd like to manage your own birthing process? If so, what are they?* ■ *What might be the advantages and disadvantages of breast-feeding?*

Infertility

An estimated one in six American couples experiences **infertility,** or difficulties in conceiving. Reasons include the trend toward delaying childbirth (as a woman gets older, she is less likely to conceive), endometriosis, and the rising incidence of pelvic inflammatory disease.

Ectopic pregnancy Implantation of a fertilized egg outside the uterus, usually in a uterine tube; a medical emergency that can end in death from hemorrhage for the mother.

Stillbirth The birth of a dead baby.

Sudden infant death syndrome (SIDS) The sudden death of an infant under one year of age for no apparent reason.

Infertility Difficulties in conceiving.

Causes in Women

Endometriosis is the leading cause of infertility in women in the United States. With this disorder, parts of the endometrial lining of the uterus implant themselves outside the uterus—in the uterine tubes, lungs, intestines, outer uterine walls or ovarian walls, and/or on the ligaments that support the uterus. The disorder can be treated surgically or with hormonal preparations. Success rates vary.

Another cause of infertility is **pelvic inflammatory disease (PID),** a serious infection that scars the fallopian tubes and blocks sperm migration. PID is a collective name for any extensive bacterial infection of the female pelvic organs, particularly the uterus, cervix, uterine tubes, and ovaries. PID often results from chlamydia or gonorrheal infections that spread to the uterine tubes or ovaries. Symptoms of PID include severe pain, fever, and sometimes vaginal discharge.

The past 30 years have brought a tremendous increase in the annual number of PID cases, from 17,800 to about 1 million per year. During the reproductive years, one in seven women reports having been treated for PID,[23] and tens of thousands have been rendered sterile. One episode of PID causes sterility in 10 to 15 percent of women, and 50 to 75 percent become sterile after three or four infections.[24]

Causes in Men

Among men, the single largest fertility problem is **low sperm count.** Although only one viable sperm is needed for fertilization, research has shown that all the other sperm in the ejaculate aid in the fertilization process. There are normally 60 to 80 million sperm per milliliter of semen. When the count drops below 20 million, fertility declines.

Low sperm count may be attributable to environmental factors such as exposure of the scrotum to intense heat or cold, radiation, or altitude, or even wearing excessively tight underwear or outerwear. However, other factors, such as the mumps virus, can damage the cells that make sperm. Varicose veins above one or both testicles can also render men infertile. Male infertility problems account for around 40 percent of infertility cases.

Treatment

For the couple desperately wishing to conceive, the road to parenthood may be frustrating. Fortunately, medical treatment can identify the cause of infertility in about 90 percent of cases. The chances of becoming pregnant range from 30 to 70 percent, depending on the reason for infertility. The countless tests and the invasion of privacy that characterize some couples' efforts to conceive can put stress on an otherwise strong, healthy relationship. Before starting fertility tests, couples should reassess their priorities. Some will choose to undergo counseling to help them clarify their feelings about the fertility process. A good physician or fertility team will take the time to ascertain the couple's level of motivation.

Fertility workups can be very expensive, and the costs are not usually covered by insurance companies. Fertility workups for men include a sperm count, a test for sperm motility, and analysis of any disease processes present. Such procedures should be undertaken only by a qualified urologist. Women are thoroughly examined by an obstetrician-gynecologist for the composition of cervical mucus and evidence of tubal scarring or endometriosis.

Complete fertility workups may take four to five months and can be unsettling. The couple may be instructed to have sex "by the calendar" to increase their chances of conceiving. Sometimes pregnancy can be achieved by collecting the man's sperm from several ejaculations and inseminating the woman at a later time. In some cases, surgery can correct structural problems such as tubal scarring. In others, administering hormones can improve the health of ova and sperm.

Fertility drugs such as Clomid and Pergonal stimulate ovulation in women who are not ovulating. Ninety percent of women who use these drugs will begin to ovulate, and half will conceive. Fertility drugs can have many side effects, including headaches, irritability, restlessness, depression, fatigue, edema (fluid retention), abnormal uterine bleeding, breast tenderness, vasomotor flushes (hot flashes), and visual difficulties. Women using fertility drugs are also at increased risk of developing multiple ovarian cysts (fluid-filled growths) and liver damage. The drugs sometimes trigger the release of more than one egg. Thus a woman treated with one of these drugs has a one in ten chance of having multiple births. Most such births are twins, but triplets and even quadruplets are not uncommon.

Alternative insemination of a woman with her partner's sperm is another treatment option. This technique has led to an estimated 250,000 births in the United States, primarily for couples in which the man is infertile. If this

---

Endometriosis   A disorder in which uterine lining tissue establishes itself outside the uterus; the leading cause of infertility in the United States.

Pelvic inflammatory disease (PID)   An infection that scars the uterine tubes and consequently blocks sperm migration, causing infertility.

Low sperm count   A sperm count below 60 million sperm per milliliter of semen; the leading cause of infertility in men.

Fertility drugs   Hormones that stimulate ovulation in women who are not ovulating; often responsible for multiple births.

Alternative insemination   Fertilization accomplished by depositing a partner's or a donor's semen into a woman's vagina via a thin tube; almost always done in a doctor's office.

procedure fails, the couple may choose insemination by an anonymous donor through a sperm bank. Many men sell their sperm to such banks. The sperm are medically screened, classified according to the physical characteristics of the donor (for example, blonde hair, blue eyes), and then frozen for future use. Frozen sperm can survive for up to five years. The woman being inseminated usually chooses sperm from a man whose physical characteristics resemble those of her partner or match her own personal preferences.

In the last few years, concern has been expressed about the possibility of transmitting the AIDS virus through alternative insemination. As a result, donors are routinely screened for the disease.

In vitro fertilization, often referred to as test tube fertilization, involves collecting a viable ovum from the prospective mother and transferring it to a nutrient medium in a laboratory, where it is fertilized with sperm from the woman's partner or a donor. After a few days, the embryo is transplanted into the mother's uterus, where, it is hoped, it will develop normally. Until 1984, in vitro fertilization was classified as experimental. Since then, it has moved into the mainstream of infertility treatments. Since 1984, the in vitro process has been responsible for an estimated 60,000 babies.

In **gamete intrafallopian transfer (GIFT),** the egg is harvested from the woman's ovary and placed in one of the uterine tubes with the man's sperm. Less expensive and time consuming than in vitro fertilization, GIFT mimics nature by allowing the egg to be fertilized in the uterine tube and migrate to the uterus according to the normal timetable.

Intracytoplasmic sperm injection (ICSI) was first performed successfully in 1992. In this procedure, a sperm cell is injected into an egg. This complex process required researchers to learn how to manipulate both egg and sperm without damaging them. This technique can help men with low sperm counts or motility, and even those who cannot ejaculate or have no live sperm in their semen as a result of vasectomy, chemotherapy, or a medical disorder. However, recent studies have found that infants conceived with the use of ICSI or in vitro fertilization have twice the risk of a major birth defect as those conceived naturally.[25]

In **nonsurgical embryo transfer,** a donor egg is fertilized by the man's sperm and implanted in the woman's uterus. This procedure may also be used to transfer an already fertilized ovum into the uterus of another woman. In **embryo transfer,** an ovum from a donor is artificially inseminated by the man's sperm, allowed to stay in the donor's body for a time, and then transplanted into the woman's body.

Some laboratories are experimenting with **embryo freezing,** in which a fertilized embryo is suspended in a solution of liquid nitrogen. When desired, it is gradually thawed and implanted into the prospective mother. The first U.S. birth of a frozen embryo was reported in 1986. In the future, this technique may make it possible for young couples to produce an embryo and save it for later implantation when they are ready to have a child, thus reducing the risks of fertilizing older eggs.

Infertile couples have another alternative—**embryo adoption programs.** The embryos are originally collected from couples who want children via in vitro fertilization. These couples often donate and freeze extra embryos in case the procedure fails or they want to have more children at a later time. These couples can now donate their unneeded embryos to others. The adopting couple can experience pregnancy and control prenatal care. The cost is approximately $4,000 dollars for the embryos to be thawed and transferred to an infertile woman's uterus or uterine tubes.

The ethical and moral questions surrounding experimental infertility treatments are staggering. Before moving forward with any of these treatments, individuals need to ask themselves a few important questions. Has infertility been absolutely confirmed? Are reputable infertility counseling services accessible? Have they explored all possible alternatives and considered potential risks? Have all parties examined their attitudes, values, and beliefs about conceiving a child in this manner? Finally, they need to consider what and how they will tell the child about their method of conception.

In vitro fertilization   Fertilization of an egg in a nutrient medium and subsequent transfer back to the mother's body.

Gamete intrafallopian transfer (GIFT)   Procedure in which an egg harvested from the female partner's ovary is placed with the male partner's sperm in her uterine tube, where it is fertilized and then migrates to the uterus for implantation.

Intracytoplasmic sperm injection (ICSI) Fertilization accomplished by injecting a sperm cell directly into an egg.

Nonsurgical embryo transfer   In vitro fertilization of a donor egg by the male partner's (or donor's) sperm and subsequent transfer to the female partner's or another woman's uterus.

Embryo transfer   Artificial insemination of a donor with the male partner's sperm; after a time, the embryo is transferred from the donor to the female partner's body.

Embryo freezing   The freezing of an embryo for later implantation.

Embryo adoption programs   A procedure whereby an infertile couple is able to purchase frozen embryos donated by another couple.

Surrogate Motherhood

Sixty to 70 percent of infertile couples are able to conceive after treatment. The rest decide to live without children, to adopt, or to attempt surrogate motherhood. In this option, the couple hires a woman to be alternatively inseminated by the male partner. The surrogate then carries the baby to term and surrenders it upon birth to the couple. Surrogate mothers are reportedly paid about $10,000 for their services and are reimbursed for medical expenses. Legal and medical expenses can run as high as $30,000 for the infertile couple.

Couples considering surrogate motherhood are advised to consult a lawyer regarding contracts. Most of these legal documents stipulate that the surrogate mother must undergo amniocentesis and that if the fetus is defective, she must consent to an abortion. In that case, or if the surrogate miscarries, she is reimbursed for her time and expenses. The prospective parents must also agree to take the baby if it is carried to term, even if it is unhealthy or has physical abnormalities.

Adoption

For couples for whom biological childbirth is not an option, adoption provides an alternative. Currently, about 50,000 children are available for adoption in the United States every year. This is far fewer than the number of couples seeking adoptions. By some estimates, only 1 in 30 couples receives the children they want. On average, couples spend two years and $100,000 on the adoption process.

In the early 1950s approximately 9 percent of unwed pregnant women gave their child up for adoption. Currently, approximately 2 percent of unmarried pregnant women place their children for adoption. The decline in the number of women placing their children for adoption results from a number of influences, including the decreased stigma of unwed motherhood, declining number of teens placing their children up for adoption, declining pregnancy rate, and the increased use of contraceptives. There is no research to show that women are choosing to abort their children rather than place them for adoption.

Women who place their children for adoption are likely to have greater educational and vocational goals for themselves than those who keep their children. Women who choose adoption come from families who are supportive of the adoption process. If you are pregnant and considering adoption, make sure you think through all the possibilities before you make your decision. Remember: adoption is permanent. People who can help you think though your options include your partner, friends, family, crisis centers, student health services, family planning clinic, family service agency, or adoption agency.

There are two types of adoption: *confidential* and *open*. In confidential adoption the birth parents and the adoptive parents never know each other. Adoptive parents are only given information about the birth parents that they need to take care of the child, such as medical information. In open adoption, birth parents and adoptive parents know something about each other. There are different levels of openness, ranging from the birth mother being able to pick from several possible families the one that sounds best for the child to the birth parents and adoptive parents staying in contact over the years. This might include visiting, calling, and writing each other. Both parties must agree to this plan, and it is not available in every state.

Because the number of American children available for adoption is limited, young women who consider placing their child for adoption have gained new leverage. Increasingly, couples wishing to adopt have turned to independent adoptions arranged by a lawyer, or they may directly negotiate with the birth mother. Independent adoptions now surpass those arranged by social service agencies.

Increasingly, couples are choosing to adopt children from other countries. In 2002, U.S. families adopted over 20,000 foreign-born children. The cost of intercountry adoption can range greatly, from approximately $10,000 to more than $30,000, including agency fees, dossier and immigration processing fees, and court costs. However, it may be a good alternative for many couples, especially those who want to adopt an infant.

> ### What do you think?
>
> *If you found that you or your partner had infertility problems, how much time and money would you be willing to invest in infertility treatments?* ■ *Do you think that single women and lesbians should have equal access to alternative methods of insemination? Why or why not?* ■ *Do you think single women or men and gay males or lesbians should have equal opportunities at adoption?* ■ *How do you think society views these types of adoptions? Why?*

MAKE IT HAPPEN!

Assessment: The Assess Yourself box on page 189 gave you the chance to assess your comfort and confidence with a contraceptive method you are using now or may use in the future. Depending on the results of the assessment, you may consider making a change in your birth control method.

Making a Change: In order to change your behavior, you need to develop a plan. Follow these steps:

1. Evaluate your behavior and identify patterns. What can you change now? What can you change in the near future?
2. Select one pattern of behavior that you want to change.
3. Fill out a Behavior Change Contract. It should include your long-term goal for change, your short-term goals, the rewards for reaching these goals, potential obstacles along the way, and strategies for overcoming these obstacles. For each goal, list the small steps and specific actions that you will take.
4. Chart your progress in a journal. At the end of a week, consider how successful you were in following your plan. What helped you be successful? What made change more difficult? What will you do differently next week?

5. Revise your plan as needed: Are the short-term goals attainable? Are the rewards satisfying?

One Student's Plan: Marissa had been using a diaphragm as her form of birth control; when she completed the self-assessment she discovered that there were several aspects of it that made her uncomfortable. The questions to which she answered "yes" showed that she sometimes forgot to bring her diaphragm with her when she planned to see her boyfriend, she disliked using it because it interrupted sexual activity, and she was embarrassed to use it. She decided she should investigate other birth control options and discuss them with her boyfriend. Her first step was to visit her student health center and, based on her likes and dislikes, choose one or two alternatives. Among the options suggested to her were the contraceptive patch (Ortho Evra) and the vaginal ring (NuvaRing), both of which she would not have to remember to bring or insert for each sexual encounter and would not interrupt sexual activity. Marissa's next step was to talk to her boyfriend about his preferences and then to make a final decision based on her confidence in the method, its convenience, and its cost.

Summary

- Latex condoms and the female condom, when used correctly for oral sex or intercourse, provide the most effective protection from sexually transmitted infections. Other contraceptive methods include abstinence, outercourse, oral contraceptives, foams, jellies, suppositories, creams, the diaphragm, the cervical cap, skin patches, the vaginal ring, intrauterine devices, withdrawal, and Depo-Provera. Fertility awareness methods rely on altering sexual practices to avoid pregnancy. Whereas all these methods of contraception are reversible, sterilization is considered permanent.
- Abortion is legal in the United States through the second trimester. Abortion methods include vacuum aspiration, dilation and evacuation (D&E), dilation and curettage (D&C), intact dilation and extraction (D&X), hysterotomy, induction abortion, mifepristone, and methotrexate.
- Parenting is a demanding job that requires careful planning. Emotional health, maternal health, paternal health, financial evaluation, and contingency planning all need to be taken into account.

- Prenatal care includes a complete physical exam within the first trimester and avoidance of alcohol and drugs, cigarettes, X rays, and chemicals having teratogenic effects. Full-term pregnancy covers three trimesters.
- Childbirth occurs in three stages. Partners should jointly choose a labor method early in the pregnancy to be better prepared for labor when it occurs. Complications of pregnancy and childbirth include miscarriage, ectopic pregnancy, preeclampsia, stillbirth, and cesarean section.
- Infertility in women may be caused by pelvic inflammatory disease or endometriosis. In men, it may be caused by low sperm count. Treatment may include alternative insemination, in vitro fertilization, gamete intrafallopian transfer, intracytoplasmic sperm injection, nonsurgical embryo transfer, and embryo transfer. Surrogate motherhood involves hiring a fertile woman to be alternatively inseminated by the male partner.

Questions for Discussion and Reflection

1. List the most effective contraceptive methods. What are their drawbacks? What medical conditions would keep a person from using them? What are the characteristics of the methods you think would be most effective for you, and why?
2. What are the various methods of abortion? What are the two opposing viewpoints concerning abortion? What is *Roe v. Wade,* and what impact has it had on the abortion debate?
3. What are the most important considerations in deciding whether the time is right to become a parent? What fac-tors will you consider regarding the number of children you will have?
4. Discuss the growth of the fetus through the three trimesters. What medical checkups or tests should be done during each trimester?
5. Discuss the emotional aspects of pregnancy. What types of emotional reactions are common in each trimester and in the postpartum period (the "fourth trimester")?
6. If you and your partner were unable to have children, what alternative methods of conception would you con-sider? Would you consider adoption?

Accessing Your Health on the Internet

Visit the following Internet sites to explore further topics and issues related to personal health. To visit an organization's website, go to the Companion Website for *Access to Health, Ninth Edition* at www.aw-bc.com/donatelle, click on the book image, and select "Accessing Your Health on the Internet" from the navigation menu.

1. ***The Alan Guttmacher Institute.*** This site focuses on sexual and reproductive health research, policy analysis, and public education.
2. ***The Answer Spot.*** This website enables you to ask health questions anonymously. It is designed to help visitors make informed decisions about all aspects of their health by providing nonjudgmental, science-based responses to their questions.
3. ***Baby Center.*** A complete online resource for new and expecting parents.
4. ***Planned Parenthood.*** This site offers a range of up-to-date information on sexual health issues, such as birth control, the decision of when and whether to have a child, and sexually transmitted infections and safer sex.
5. ***Sexuality Information and Education Council of the United States.*** Information, guidelines, and materials for the advancement of sexuality education. The site advocates the right of individuals to make responsible sexual choices.

Further Reading

Boston Women's Health Collective. *Our Bodies, Ourselves for the New Century: A Book by and for Women.* New York: Simon and Schuster, 1998.

Like its earlier editions, this volume contains information about women's health from a decidedly feminist angle. Every aspect of health is covered, including nutrition, emotional health, fitness, relationships, reproduction, contraception, and pregnancy.

Feldt, G. *The War on Choice.* New York: Bantam, 2004.

A history and analysis of threats to women's reproductive rights. Feldt describes political efforts to outlaw abortion and argues that women should mobilize to support pro-choice causes.

Hatcher, R. A., et al. *Contraceptive Technology,* 18th revised edition. New York: Ardent Media, 2004.

Perhaps the best primary reference concerning birth control for physicians, family planning centers, student health ser-vices, and educators. Contributors include staff members from the Centers for Disease Control and Prevention.

Kitzinger, S. *The Complete Book of Pregnancy and Childbirth,* 4th edition. New York: Knopf, 2003.

The books provides expectant mothers with new insights into having a healthy pregnancy and what happens in today's birthing rooms. Offers women and their partners an in-depth look at both the baby's and the mother's physical and emotional development during pregnancy.

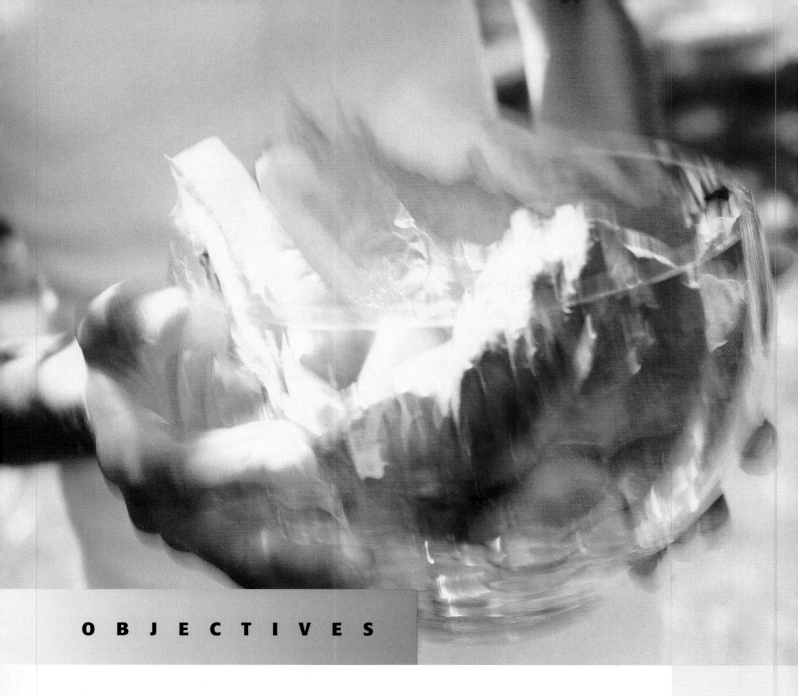

OBJECTIVES

- Examine the factors that influence dietary choices.

- Discuss how to change old eating habits, including how to use the Food Guide Pyramids, eat nutritious foods, and improve other behaviors.

- Summarize the major essential nutrients and their role in maintaining health.

- Discuss food as a form of medicine and the facts related to new trends in nutrition, food supplements, and their roles in health and well-being.

- Distinguish among the various forms of vegetarianism, discussing possible health benefits and risks from these dietary alternatives.

- Discuss issues surrounding gender, exercise, and nutrition.

- Discuss how unique situations in your life (pregnancy, stress, illness) can influence dietary needs.

- Discuss the unique problems that college students face when trying to eat healthy foods and the actions they can take to comply with the Food Guide Pyramids.

- Explain food safety concerns facing Americans and people in other regions of the world.

NUTRITION

EATING FOR OPTIMUM HEALTH

IN THE NEWS

It's Better to Be Whole Than Refined

By Marian Burros

In just a couple of years, low-carbohydrate diets have accomplished what the government has failed to do in decades of trying: convince the public that refined grains are bad actors and whole grains are good.

"Low-carb diets have steered people toward whole grains," said Bonnie Liebman, the director of nutrition for the Washington-based Center for Science in the Public Interest, "and made millions of people cut back on things made with white flour, like white bread, hamburger buns, megamuffins, 400-calorie bagels, pizza crusts, cakes, cookies, doughnuts and other sweets, even pasta and white rice.

"If you were asked to compare the impact of the South Beach diet with dietary guidelines, there would be no contest."

Now if only consumers could distinguish between grains that are refined and grains that are whole. Just because bread is brown and has specks of something in it does not mean it is whole grain.

Whole grains (and foods made from them) consist of the entire grain seed, usually referred to as the kernel. The kernel is made of three components: the bran, the germ and the endosperm.

Read the complete article online in the eThemes section of this book's website: www.aw-bc.com/donatelle.

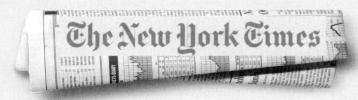

When was the last time you ate something without thinking about how much fat or carbohydrates it had? Did you wonder whether the calories would end up as fat on your hips or stomach, and whether the food was good or bad for you? Knowing what to eat, how much to eat, and how to choose foods that help prevent disease and promote health is not as easy as it was even 50 years ago. Today, we are bombarded with dietary regimens—from low carb to low fat to low glycemic index—that promise quick weight loss, more energy, decreased risk from disease, and other benefits. The tradeoff is giving up chocolate, substituting vegetable burgers for hamburgers, tossing high-carb pizza, pasta, and baked potatoes, or adding fiber-rich flax to just about everything we eat. And, if you aren't confused and frustrated enough by all of the claims about healthful and harmful foods, diets that promise too much, and an ever-increasing deluge of new food products, you must also be concerned about the safety of the foods you eat. Are they full of preservatives and chemicals, are there pathogens lurking in them, or can you contract deadly diseases from ingesting them?

Clearly, Americans are trying to heed expert advice about how to have a healthy diet. For example, in survey after survey, 60 to 80 percent of food shoppers say they read food labels before selecting products, yet these same surveys reveal frequent misunderstandings and confusion.[1] Nutritionists, fad diet advocates, and media reports of research studies offer an array of claims and warnings. The seemingly endless array of choices and conflicting reports has generated distrust in all dietary recommendations and a corresponding desire for nutrition information that is clear, authoritative, and easy to understand. Although efforts are being made to improve food labels, make guidelines clearer, and provide reliable information, these efforts are works in progress. What can you do now to insure that you are making wise dietary choices?

First, it is important to recognize that it takes effort, education, and reliable resources to be able to make informed decisions. Although the U.S. Food and Drug Administration (FDA) does a remarkable job in helping to protect us, it can't possibly regulate or control every dietary claim, every new food product, or every new nutritional term that comes into the market. That means that the responsibility for making wise dietary decisions and separating fact from fiction in your daily eating behaviors is largely your own. The good news is that according to the American Dietetic Association, more Americans are seeking information on food and nutrition and taking action to improve their habits than ever before.[2]

College students especially face nutritional challenges. Finding time to purchase and prepare meals, the cost of many high nutrient foods, and having a well-equipped kitchen to prepare meals are just three. In addition, some students grew up in homes where their parents did not cook or follow nutrition guidelines, leaving them without the experience needed to prepare healthy meals. Students often enter

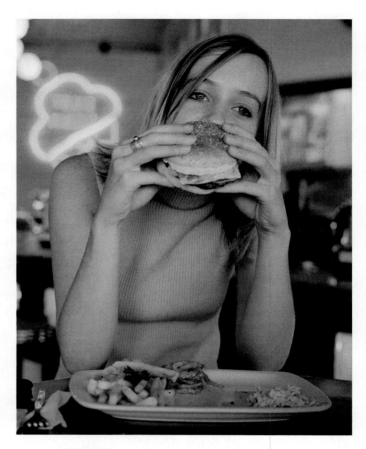

It takes information and planning to make smart menu choices, whether you are eating out, in your dining hall, or at home.

their adult years thinking that *homecooked meals* means instant macaroni and cheese dinners or other microwaveable foods.

Although numerous studies have pointed to the importance of diet in overall health, many people lack the motivation or knowledge to eat for health. Just how important is sound nutrition? As an example, a review of over 4,500 research studies concluded that widespread consumption of 5 to 6 servings of fruits and vegetables daily would lower cancer rates by over 20 percent in the global population.[3] Subsequent research has emphasized the role of diet and nutrition on cardiovascular disease, diabetes, and a host of other chronic and disabling conditions.[4]

It doesn't take a research study for each of us to know what it feels like to gain weight, to feel run down and listless, or to be unhappy with our body, our overall appearance, or our health. The next three chapters focus on fundamental principles designed to help you eat more healthy foods, avoid the problems that so many people face with their weight, and improve your general fitness. In this chapter, we will discuss basic nutrition science and apply sound principles to lifestyle behaviors. But first, it is important to gain an appreciation for why you eat as you do, the role of your family of origin and basic biology in determining your eating patterns and choices, and the resources that can help you change negative patterns while building on the healthy choices you are already making.

Assessing Eating Behaviors: Are You What You Eat?

True **hunger** occurs when there is a lack or shortage of basic foods needed to provide the energy and nutrients that support health.[5] When we are hungry, chemical messages in the brain, especially in the hypothalamus, initiate a physiological response that prompts us to seek food.[6] Although we have all experienced hunger before mealtime, few Americans have experienced the type of hunger that continues for days and threatens survival. Most of us do not eat to sustain physical survival. Instead, we eat because of our **appetite,** a learned desire to eat that may or may not have anything to do with feeling hungry. Time of day, the smell or sight of food, or other triggers often stimulate our appetite, even when we are actually full.

Many factors influence when we eat, what we eat, and how much we eat. Finding out which triggers influence each of us, and learning to balance eating to maintain body function (eating to live) with eating to satisfy appetite (living to eat), is a constant struggle for many of us. Typical influences that make us head to the kitchen or nearest restaurant include: [7]

- *Cultural and social meanings attached to food.* From our earliest days, we learn to celebrate our family's cultural heritage with special meals or food choices. For your author, spaghetti and meatball dinners were a weekly event, and other Italian foods were a form of comfort food that meant family gatherings and sharing. Cultural traditions and food choices give us many of our *food preferences.* We learn to like the tastes of certain foods, and a yearning for sweet, salty, and high-fat foods can evolve from our earliest days. People crave the foods they grew up eating, whether the bratwurst and beer of northern Wisconsin, the Creole and seafood of Louisiana, the hot peppers of Mexican cooking, or the curry spices of Indian dishes.
- *Convenience.* Smell it, see it, think about it, want to have it now.
- *Habit or custom.* Often we select foods because they are familiar and fit religious, political, or spiritual views.
- *Advertising.* You saw that juicy burger on TV and decide it looks really good. You've got to have it.
- *Availability.* You're driving by and it's right there, or it's the only convenient option.
- *Economy.* It seems like a good buy for the money, and you can afford it.
- *Emotional comfort.* Eating it makes you feel better—a form of reward and security. We derive pleasure or sensory delight from eating the foods.

- *Positive associations.* A certain food may be eaten by people you admire or be a status symbol.
- *Weight/body image.* You think a food will help you gain, maintain, or lose weight.
- *Social pressure.* It is offered/served, and you can't say no.
- *Regional/seasonal trends.* Some foods may be favored in your area by season or overall climate.
- *Nutritional value.* You think the food is good or bad for you. A new interest in **functional foods,** foods that are believed to enhance physiological function and improve health, motivates many people (see Chapter 23).
- *Environmental conditions.* People prefer hot foods in winter, cooler foods in summer.
- *Social interaction.* Eating out or having company over for a meal is an enjoyable social event.

With all of the factors that influence our dietary choices and the wide array of foods available, the challenge of eating for health increases daily. Fortunately, we have a wealth of solid information that serves as a foundation for our decisions. **Nutrition** is the science that investigates the relationship between physiological function and the essential elements of the foods we eat. With our country's overabundance of food and vast array of choices, media that "prime" us to want the tasty morsels shown in advertisements, and easy access to almost every type of **nutrient** (proteins, carbohydrates, fats, vitamins, minerals, and water), Americans should have few nutritional problems. However, these "diets of affluence" contribute to many major diseases, including obesity-related problems with heart disease, certain types of cancer, diabetes, hypertension (high blood pressure), cirrhosis of the liver, sleep apnea, varicose veins, gout, gallbladder disease, respiratory problems, abdominal hernias, flat feet, complications in pregnancy and surgery, and even higher accident rates, to name but a few.[8] Diabetes, in particular, has reached epidemic proportions in the United States and is largely a product of poor diet, excess weight, and lack of exercise. (See Chapters 9 and 18.) Put in perspective, a weight gain of 11 to 18 pounds increases a person's risk of developing diabetes to twice that of individuals who have not gained weight.[9]

Hunger   The physiological impulse to seek food, prompted by the lack or shortage of basic foods needed to provide the energy and nutrients that support health.

Appetite   The desire to eat; normally accompanies hunger but is more psychological than physiological.

Functional foods   Foods believed to be beneficial and/or to prevent disease.

Nutrition   The science that investigates the relationship between physiological function and the essential elements of foods eaten.

Nutrients   The constituents of food that sustain us physiologically: proteins, carbohydrates, fats, vitamins, minerals, and water.

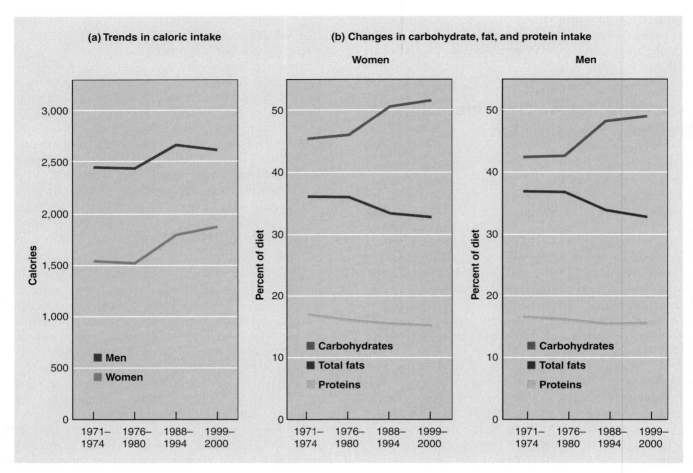

(a) Trends in caloric intake

(b) Changes in carbohydrate, fat, and protein intake

Figure 8.1
Trends in Caloric Intake and Carbohydrate, Fat, and Protein Intake

Source: J. D. Wright et al., "Trends in Intake of Energy and Macronutrients—United States 1971–2000," *Morbidity and Mortality Weekly Report,* February 6, 2004.

Eating for Health

Americans consume more calories per person than any other population in the world. Not coincidentally, we also have the highest rates of obesity. A **calorie** is a unit of measure that indicates the amount of energy we obtain from a particular food. Calories are eaten in the form of *proteins, fats,* and *carbohydrates,* three of the basic nutrients necessary for life. Three other nutrients—*vitamins, minerals,* and *water*—are necessary for bodily function but do not contribute any calories to our diets.

Recent research shows that our food choices rival transportation as the human activity with the greatest impact on the environment.[10] By 2020, people in developing countries will consume more than 39 kilograms (kg) of meat per person each year—twice as much as they did in the 1980s. People in industrial countries such as the United States will still consume the most meat (100 kg a year) the equivalent of a side of beef, 50 chickens, and 1 pig each.[11]

Excess consumption such as this is a factor in our tendency to be overweight. However, it is not so much the quantity of food we eat that is likely to cause weight problems as it is the poor nutritional content and lack of physical activity to burn the calories we consume. Nearly one-third of the calories we consume come from junk foods. Sweets and desserts, soft drinks, and alcoholic beverages made up 25 percent of those calories, and another 5 percent come from salty snacks and fruit-flavored drinks. In sharp contrast, healthy foods, such as vegetables and fruit, make up only 10 percent of our total calories.[12]

In a 30-year study of changes in consumption, women's overall caloric intake increased by 22 percent and men's by 7 percent[13] (Figure 8.1). When this increase is combined with

Calorie A unit of measure that indicates the amount of energy obtained from a particular food.

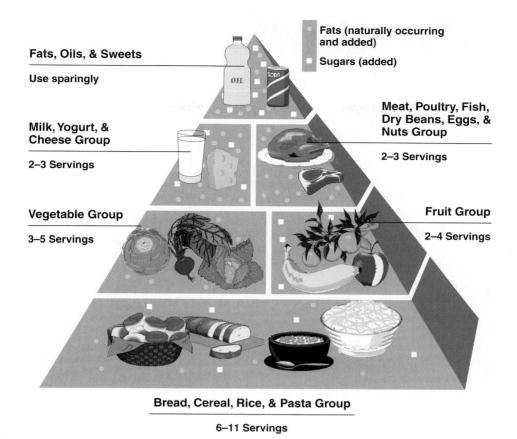

Figure 8.2

Food Guide Pyramid: A Guide to Daily Food Choices

Source: U.S. Department of Agriculture, "The Food Guide Pyramid," *Home and Garden Bulletin* no. 252 (1996).

our increasingly sedentary lifestyle, it is not surprising that we have seen a dramatic increase in obesity rates.

Americans typically get approximately 38 percent of their calories from fat, 15 percent from proteins, 22 percent from complex carbohydrates, and 24 percent from simple sugars.[14] New federal food guidelines recommend increasing complex carbohydrates to make up 48 percent of our total calories and reducing proteins to 12 percent, simple sugars to 10 percent, and fats to no more than 30 percent of our diets.

Sugar and carbohydrates, per se, are not inherently good or bad and are not conclusively linked to any one disease (simple sugars are linked to dental caries). Dr. Dean Ornish, clinical professor of medicine at UC–San Francisco and a leading advocate of carbohydrate-heavy diets, argues that it is simple carbohydrates, particularly those found in high-fructose corn syrups, that are responsible for our significant increases in calories in recent decades. He says that our goal should be to reduce simple carbs (and fat) in favor of complex carbohydrates and balance in our diets, and he is not alone. Currently, several federal agencies and professional groups are working on significant changes in national dietary recommendations that reflect these sentiments, including an

overhaul of the Food Guide Pyramid. While these changes are in the works, it is important that each of us keep on top of emerging information from reliable sources and assess our eating habits. How much do you know about nutrition and healthy eating? Find out by completing the quiz in the Assess Yourself box on page 226.

The Food Guide Pyramid: A Work in Progress

The Food Guide Pyramid, promoted by the United States Department of Agriculture (USDA) and several professional organizations since 1992, is designed to graphically illustrate the importance of grains, cereals, vegetables, and fruits compared to meat, fish, poultry, dairy products, and other foods. Figure 8.2 shows the Food Guide Pyramid with recommended servings and examples from each food group. However, the entire food guideline system, including the Food Guide Pyramid, is being reassessed to ensure that it reflects the latest nutritional science and helps us make healthier food choices.[15] The revision is being done in concert with

(text continues on page 228)

What's Your EQ (Eating Quotient)?

myhealthlab

Fill out this assessment online at www.aw-bc.com/myhealthlab or www.aw-bc.com/donatelle

Keeping up with the latest on what to eat—or not to eat—isn't easy. If you think a few facts might have slipped past you, this quiz should help. There's only one correct answer for each question.

	True	False
1. Fresh fruits and vegetables contain more nutrients than canned or frozen varieties.	❑	❑
2. While you are shopping, it makes a difference what area of the store you start in, in terms of keeping your foods safe.	❑	❑
3. Fruit drinks count as a serving from the fruit group in the Food Guide Pyramid.	❑	❑
4. Baked potatoes have a higher glycemic index (carbohydrate's ability to raise blood sugar levels quickly) than sweet potatoes or apples.	❑	❑
5. A late dinner is more likely to cause weight gain than eating the same meal earlier in the day.	❑	❑
6. Nuts are okay to eat if you are trying to stick to a low fat diet.	❑	❑
7. Certain foods, like grapefruit, celery, or cabbage soup, can burn fat and make you lose weight.	❑	❑

8. Which of the following has the most fiber?
   a. chuck roast
   b. dark meat chicken with skin
   c. skinless chicken wing
   d. They are all about the same.

9. Which of the following is the strongest predictor of obesity in America today?
   a. region of the country you live in
   b. ethnicity/culture
   c. lack of exercise
   d. socioeconomic status

10. When you eat a meal, how long does it take for your brain to get the message that you are full?
   a. 10 minutes
   b. 20 minutes
   c. at least an hour
   d. 2 hours or more

11. Which of the following are at the *top* of the list in bacteria levels among domestically grown vegetables?
   a. Green onions, cantaloupe, and cilantro
   b. Beets, potatoes, and summer squash
   c. Celery, leaf lettuce, and parsley
   d. Strawberries, apples, and tomatoes

12. Which of the following foods contains the most grams of fiber per serving?
   a. ½ cup of strawberries
   b. ½ cup of kidney beans
   c. 1 cup popcorn
   d. 1 medium banana

13. To insure that you are getting your antioxidants each day, which tip below would be most helpful?
   a. Eat several dark green vegetables and orange, red, and yellow fruits and vegetables.
   b. Eat at least two servings of lean red meat per day.
   c. Eat whole grain foods with at least 2 grams of fiber per serving.
   d. Eat several servings of tuna and salmon per week.

14. Olive oil, one of the heart-healthy monounsaturated fats, is a great source for antioxidants. To reap the most benefits from olive oil, which recommendation should you follow?
   a. Buy it only in amounts that you will use relatively quickly. Nutrients are lost quickly after 12 months sitting on the shelf.
   b. If you buy larger bottles, separate it into smaller bottles and keep the lid on tightly to reduce oxidation from air contact. Refrigerate if possible. Refrigeration causes cloudiness, but doesn't affect quality.
   c. Store it in opaque airtight glass bottles or metal tins away from heat and light.
   d. All of the above

15. Which strategy will help you identify high fiber breads to maximize your quality carbohydrate intake?
   a. Choose a whole grain bread that lists a whole grain as the first ingredient—preferably *all* the grain ingredients.

b. Try to purchase breads with 1 to 2 grams of fiber per slice.

c. Look for bread that is dark colored. The darker it is, the greater the chance that it has lots of good quality fiber in its recipe.

d. All of the above

ANSWERS

1. *False:* There is usually little difference, depending on how produce is handled and how quickly it reaches your supermarket. Canned and frozen produce is typically picked at its peak and may contain more nutrients than fresh produce that was picked over-ripe or too early, sat in a warehouse, spent days in transit, or sat at improper temperatures for prolonged periods. However, a downside is that canned or frozen fruits and vegetables may have added salt or sugar, sometimes at much higher levels than you might suspect. Be sure to check labels carefully. Whenever possible, buy local produce fresh from the fields or neighboring areas.

2. *True:* As a general rule, foods such as milk, meat, and other perishables that have been left at room temperature for more than two hours have a significant risk of conveying a food-borne illness. Thus, when you shop for groceries, be sure to factor in the time that you spend driving home from the store, time spent running any other errands on the way home, etc. It is best to start your shopping foray in the canned and non-refrigerated sections of the store and save your meat and dairy projects and frozen foods until last. Also, run your other errands before you shop for food; if you know it will take time to get home, bring along a cooler with ice.

3. *False:* Even if fruit juice is an actual ingredient (often it is not), most fruit drinks are primarily water and high fructose corn syrup or other sweeteners, colorings, and fruit flavoring. For the real deal, it is always better to eat the whole fruit, as you will get added fiber, more nutrients, and other benefits. Next best are 100 percent fruit juices, preferably with added vitamin C, and lowest on the nutrient quality list are the sweetened, flavored fruit drinks, which don't necessarily include any actual juice.

4. *True:* Unfortunately for those of us who've been substituting baked potatoes for fries, we'd probably be better off with a sweet potato or apple if we are trying to keep our blood sugar levels down or control diabetes. For more information, check the glycemic index reference books available at most bookstores or use the handy guide found at www.diabetesnet .com/diabetes_food_diet/glycemic_index.php

5. *False:* It's not when you eat, but what you eat that makes a difference in weight gain. If you ate a 500 calorie salad at 10 PM and it was your only meal, you wouldn't gain weight. However, a 5,000 calorie pizza eaten at breakfast (for those of you who like cold pizza in the morning) followed by a big lunch and dinner would provide enough total calories to bring on those love handles in the majority of people.

6. *True:* Although they are high in fat, nuts contain mostly unsaturated fat (a good fat) and are good sources of protein, magnesium, and the antioxidants vitamin E and selenium. Nuts are little bundles of nutrients, and their benefits outweigh their risks when they are eaten in moderation. Most people have trouble eating just one small handful. Dole out your portions carefully, and be mindful of how many calories you are eating.

7. *False:* No foods can burn fat. Some foods with caffeine may speed up your metabolism for a short time, but they do not cause weight loss.

8. *D:* There is no fiber in animal foods. Fiber is found only in plants and plant-based foods such as fruits, beans, whole grains, and vegetables.

9. *D:* While the other responses are all contributors to obesity, the greatest single predictor of obesity is low socioeconmic status. Although related factors such as education play a role in dietary behaviors, the poor nutritional quality of foods commonly eaten when people are forced to stretch their food budgets often results in increased risk for obesity. High-fat meats, hot dogs, inexpensive white breads and pastries, and high calorie, low fiber foods tend to be high on the list of those living at or below the poverty level.

10. *B:* It takes about 20 minutes for your brain to get the message that you are full. To make sure you don't gorge yourself, eat slowly, talk with others, put your fork down after taking a bite, take a drink of water, or do other things to delay your meal. Let your brain catch up to your fork, and slow it down!

11. *A:* The bad news is that in a recent government study of bacteria levels found in domestic produce, green onions, cantaloupe, and cilantro scored the highest in positive tests for two common bacteria: *Salmonella* or *Shigella*. The good news is that out of nearly 1,100 samples, only 2 to 3 percent of them were contaminated. It still means that washing your produce is a must. Running a heavy stream of water over the produce while rubbing the outside under the water may help protect you.

12. *B:* One-half cup of kidney beans provides 4.5 grams of fiber. The medium banana has 2 grams of fiber, while strawberries and popcorn each have 1 gram of fiber per serving.

13. *A:* Antioxidants, particularly vitamins C and E, the mineral selenium, and plant pigments known as carotenoids (which include beta-carotene) are found in green leafy vegetables and orange, yellow, and red vegetables and fruit. Eating several servings of these per day helps avoid risks from several health problems.

14. *D:* Although relatively resistant to outside forces, olive oil does lose nutrients over time, with one year being the

(continues)

general guesstimate of "use by" time. If the oil smells rancid or if you note mold or other discoloration, discard the bottle.

15. *A:* A true whole-grain bread clearly says so on the label (for example, "100% whole wheat" or "100% stone ground whole wheat") If all the ingredients aren't whole grain, then it's not a true whole-grain bread. The more fiber in each slice the better; the minimum you look for should be 3 grams. Color is not a good indicator of nutrient value. Dyes and coloring (such as caramel) may make even the whitest white bread turn brown.

ANALYZING YOUR SCORES

If you have answered all of the above correctly, congratulations! You clearly have a good sense of some of the current issues and facts surrounding dietary choices. If you missed one or more

questions, read the corresponding section of this chapter to find out more. Don't despair. Nutrition information changes rapidly and there is a wealth of information available. Check with your instructor to see if there are specific courses you can take to increase your nutritional knowledge. Review the resources that are recommended, and work hard to stay current.

MAKE IT HAPPEN!

Use the results of this self-assessment to begin your behavior change program. Follow the steps and use the examples on page 265 to complete your Behavior Change Contract, and use these resources to take action.

---

revisions of the *Dietary Guidelines for Americans* and the Dietary Reference Intake (DRI) recommendations, two more federally sponsored initiatives discussed later in this chapter. The USDA expects to release the new recommendations, including a revised pyramid and guidelines, early in 2005. These documents are the products of a careful review of nutrition and dietary science to insure that the Pyramid's daily food intake recommendations continue to meet current nutritional standards. In addition, the Pyramid may be redesigned to make it as easy to understand and use as possible. A variation of the pyramid, the Healthy Eating Pyramid, emphasizes not only dietary choices, but the importance of daily exercise and weight control (Figure 8.3)

Making the Pyramid Work for You

Many people are overwhelmed by their first glance at the Food Guide Pyramid because the number of servings per day in some groups is so high. However, look at what the USDA considers a serving: an ounce of ready-to-eat cereal, for example. A normal bowl of cereal contains three to four ounces of cereal. When was the last time you ate a quarter bowl of cereal? When you consider breakfast, lunch, dinner, and snacks, it is really quite easy to get all the servings in this group that you need.

Serving The amount of a given food recommended by materials such as the Food Guide Pyramid.

Portion The amount of a given food that you choose to eat at a particular time.

Portion Distortion: Understanding what a Serving Really Means How much is one serving? Is it different than one portion? While these two terms are often used interchangeably, they actually mean very different things, and it is important to understand the difference in order to be able to use the Pyramid and other nutrition guidelines effectively. A **serving** is the amount recommended in materials such as the Food Guide Pyramid, while a **portion** is the amount you choose to eat at any one time and may be more or less than a serving. Most of us select and eat portions that are much bigger than servings. According to a survey conducted by the American Institute for Cancer Research (AICR), respondents were asked to estimate the standard servings defined by the USDA Food Guide Pyramid for eight different foods, including pasta, green salad, beans, and mashed potatoes. Only 1 percent of those surveyed correctly answered all serving size questions, and nearly 65 percent answered five or more of them incorrectly.[16] In another national survey, more than half of Americans overestimated the serving size of cooked pasta and rice and took two times the amount that they should have.[17]

Unfortunately, we don't always get a clear picture from food producers and advertisers about what a serving really is. You may have looked at a bottle of soda and noted that it listed a serving size as 8 fluid ounces with a calorie listing of 100 calories—but a savvy consumer will note that the bottle holds 20 ounces and that drinking the entire bottle serves up a whopping 250 calories. Considering the "big gulps" and "super-sizing" going on in most fast-food settings, drinking these monster drinks could contribute over half of your caloric needs for the day! Because many consumer groups feel that labels should accurately reflect the calories, fats, carbohydrates, and so on for the entire container, new labeling will allow consumers to have a quicker fix on just what they

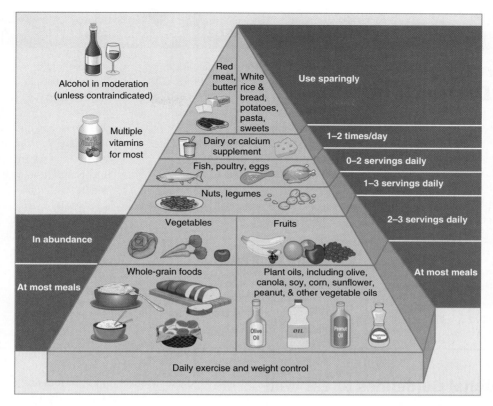

Figure 8.3
The Healthy Eating Pyramid

Source: Reprinted with the permission of Simon & Schuster Adult Publishing Group, from *Eat, Drink, and Be Healthy: The Harvard Medical School Guide to Healthy Eating* by Walter C. Willett, M.D., Copyright © 2001 by President and Fellows of Harvard College.

are consuming in the near future. See the Skills for Behavior Change box on page 230 for help on recognizing servings.

The amount of food that counts as one serving in the various food groups is listed below. If you eat a larger portion, count it as more than one serving. Be sure to eat at least the lowest number of servings from the major food groups; you need them for the nutrients they provide. (Some people need more servings from the milk, yogurt, and cheese group; teens and breast-feeding or pregnant women should get three servings, and pregnant or breast-feeding teens should get four.) No specific serving size is given for fats, oils, and sweets because they should be used sparingly.

Breads, Cereals, Rice, and Pasta Group
- 1 slice of bread or medium dinner roll
- 1/2 cup cooked rice, pasta, or other grains
- 1 ounce ready-to-eat cereal
- 3 cups popped popcorn

Fruit Group
- Whole fruit such as 1 medium apple, banana, or orange
- 1/2 cup of raw, cooked, or canned fruit
- 3/4 cup of fruit juice

- 1/2 cup canned fruit
- 1/4 cup dried fruit

Vegetable Group
- 1 cup leafy raw vegetables
- 1/2 cup chopped fresh, frozen, or canned vegetables

Meat, Poultry, Fish, Dry Beans, Eggs, and Nuts Group
- 2–3 ounces lean, trimmed, and baked or roasted meat, fish, or poultry.
  The following can substitute for 1 ounce of meat:
  - 2 tablespoons peanut butter or other nut or seed butter
  - 1/4 cup nuts1
  - 1/2 cup cooked legumes
  - 3 ounces tofu
  - 1 egg

Milk, Yogurt, and Cheese Group
- 1 cup milk or yogurt
- 1 1/2 ounces natural cheese
- 2 ounces processed cheese
- 1/2 cup cottage cheese
- 1 1/2 cups ice cream, ice milk, or frozen yogurt

Getting a Grip on Portion Distortion

One of the challenges of following a healthy diet is judging how big a portion size should be and how many servings you are really eating each time you put your hand in the potato chip bag or scoop some ice cream into a dish. The American Dietetic Association and other experts have developed some tips for getting a grip.

SERVING SIZES

- A deck of playing cards = 1 serving (3 ounces) of meat, poultry, or fish

(The palm of a woman's hand or a com-puter mouse can also be used, but mice and women's hands can vary in size.)
- Half a baseball (not a softball!) = 1 serving ($\frac{1}{2}$ cup) of fruit, vegetables, pasta, or rice
- Pair of dice = 1 serving (1 ounce) of cheese
- A tennis ball = 1 cup serving of yogurt or fresh greens

MANAGING YOUR PORTIONS

- Before eating, visualize the serving sizes recommended above. Putting one of these servings onto a smaller plate may help it look bigger.

- Don't eat out of a bag or a carton. There can be a lot hidden in there, and it's very difficult to compare it to a serving size.
- Use measuring cups or a small scale at home until you can accurately assess the size of a serving.
- Buffets and restaurant meals served "family style" make it difficult to gauge servings. Try to avoid these situations unless you can really pay attention to how much food ends up on your plate.

Using the National Guidelines to Eat Well

In addition to understanding the amount and size of servings, there are other factors to consider when planning your daily intake of nutrients. For several decades, the USDA and leading health and nutrition professional groups have worked together to develop dietary guidelines for optimal health. A comparison of how these guidelines have changed in response to national goals and objectives is reflected in Table 8.1. Changes include the growing recognition of physical activity as part of a healthy lifestyle, better understanding of the differences among fats, and increased concern over food safety. The most recent guidelines, published in 2000, responded in particular to our growing epidemics of obesity and diabetes. The latest guidelines, published in January 2005, are available at www.healthierus.gov/dietaryguidelines.

Know Your ABC's Current *Dietary Guidelines for Americans* use an easy-to-remember system to help you incorporate physical activity and appropriate dietary principles into your daily routine. Known as A, B, C's for good health, they suggest:

- *Aiming for Fitness.* Recommendations include aiming for a healthy weight and being physically active each day. Strive to be physically active for at least 30 minutes daily, preferably with moderate activity levels on most days. (Moderate activity is any activity that requires about as much energy as walking two miles in 30 minutes).
- *Building a Healthy Base.* Recommendations include using the Food Guide Pyramid to guide your choices, with plant foods (whole grains, fruits, and vegetables) serving as a foundation of your daily intake. This guideline also includes taking care of the unique nutrient needs of special age groups or circumstances, checking food labels,

exercising moderation with fats and sweets, aiming for variety, and making sure foods are safely and properly prepared and stored.
- *Choosing Sensibly.* Recommendations include choosing a diet that is low in saturated fat and cholesterol and moderate in total fat, knowing the differences between fats, choosing beverages and foods that limit intake of sugar, consuming less salt, and drinking alcohol in moderation, if at all.

Let the Pyramid Be Your Guide

- *Work to achieve adequacy.* Choose at least six servings from the bread, cereal, rice, and pasta group; three from the vegetable group; two from the fruit group; two from the meat, poultry, fish, dry bean, and nuts group; and two from the milk, yogurt, and cheese group. To remember these, think of the numbers, 6, 3, 2, 2, and 2.[18]
- *Eat a balanced diet in moderation.* Remember that grains form the foundation of the Pyramid and should make up the largest portion of your diet, followed by fruits and vegetables. Diets that suggest that you should eliminate grains and most fruits in favor of high fat or lean forms of protein will not achieve the appropriate balance. Also, keep in mind that moderation refers to numbers of servings, size of portions, and the total calories consumed, more than any one food category.[19]
- *Seek variety within groups.* Although the Pyramid may appear rigid, it is really quite flexible and encourages variety within categories. Meat alternatives and other products are encouraged; vegetarians have many options, and there are ample combinations that will meet recommended guidelines.[20]

Table 8.1
Dietary Guidelines for Americans, 1980–2000

1980 7 Guidelines	1985 7 Guidelines	1990 7 Guidelines	1995 7 Guidelines	2000 10 Guidelines
Eat a variety of foods	Eat a variety of foods	Eat a variety of foods	Eat a variety of foods	**Aim for Fitness**
Maintain ideal weight	Maintain desirable weight	Maintain healthy weight	Balance the food you eat with physical activity—maintain or improve your weight	Aim for a healthy weight Be physically active each day
				Build a Healthy Base
Avoid too much fat, saturated fat, and cholesterol	Avoid too much fat, saturated fat, and cholesterol	Choose a diet low in fat, saturated fat, and cholesterol		Let the Pyramid guide your food choices
Eat foods with adequate starch and fiber	Eat foods with adequate starch and fiber	Choose a diet with plenty of vegetables, fruits, and grain products	Choose a diet with plenty of grain products, vegetables, and fruits	Choose a variety of grains daily, especially whole grains Choose a variety of fruits and vegetables daily Keep food safe to eat
				Choose Sensibly
			Choose a diet low in fat, saturated fat, and cholesterol	Choose a diet low in saturated fat and cholesterol and moderate in total fat
Avoid too much sugar	Avoid too much sugar	Use sugars only in moderation	Choose a diet moderate in sugars	Choose beverages and foods to moderate your intake of sugars
Avoid too much sodium	Avoid too much sodium	Use salt and sodium only in moderation	Choose a diet moderate in salt and sodium	Choose and prepare foods with less salt
If you drink alcohol, do so in moderation	If you drink alcohol, do so in moderation	If you drink alcohol, do so in moderation	If you drink alcohol, do so in moderation	If you drink alcohol, do so in moderation

Note: Shading highlights how the order in which the guidelines are presented has changed over time. The 2005 guidelines are available at www.healthierus.gov/dietaryguidelines.

Eating Nutrient-Dense Foods

Although eating the proper number of servings from the Food Guide Pyramid is important, it is also important to recognize that there are large caloric, fat, and energy differences between food categories within Pyramid groups. For example, you might get the same number of calories from a glass of beer as you would from a glass of milk, but you would get many more nutrients from the milk. You may get a hefty dose of sugar and less nutrient value from a large glass of orange juice than from eating an orange. Likewise, fish and hot dogs provide vastly different fat and energy levels per ounce, with fish providing better energy and caloric value per serving. Nutrient density is even more important for someone who is ill and unable to keep food down. That is why nutrient supplements such as Ensure and others are often provided for cancer patients who need a nutrient "hit" in a small package.

What do you think?

Which food groups from the Food Guide Pyramid are you most likely to eat enough of during a typical day? ■ *Which ones are you most likely to skimp on?* ■ *What are some simple changes that you could make right now in your diet to help meet Pyramid recommendations?*

The Digestive Process

Food provides the chemicals we need for energy and body maintenance. Because our bodies cannot synthesize or produce certain essential nutrients, we must obtain them from the foods we eat. Even though we may take in adequate amounts of foods and nutrients, if our body systems are not functioning properly, much of the nutrient value in our food may be lost. Before foods can be utilized properly, the digestive system must break the larger food particles down into smaller, more usable forms. The process by which foods are broken down and either absorbed or excreted by the body is known as the **digestive process.**

Even before you take your first bite of pizza, your body has already begun a series of complex digestive responses. Your mouth prepares for the food by increasing production of **saliva.** Saliva contains mostly water, which aids in chewing and swallowing, but it also contains important enzymes that begin the process of food breakdown; for example, the enzyme amylase begins to break down carbohydrates. *Enzymes* are protein compounds that facilitate chemical reactions but are not altered in the process. From the mouth, the food passes down the **esophagus,** a 9- to 10-inch tube that connects the mouth and stomach. A series of contractions and relaxations by the muscles lining the esophagus gently move food to the next digestive organ, the **stomach.** Here food mixes with enzymes and stomach acids. Hydrochloric acid begins to work in combination with pepsin, an enzyme, to break down proteins. In most people, the stomach secretes enough mucus to protect the stomach lining from these harsh digestive juices.

Further digestive activity takes place in the **small intestine,** a 20-foot coiled tube containing three sections: the *duodenum, jejunum,* and *ileum.* Each section secretes digestive enzymes that, when combined with enzymes from the liver and the pancreas, further contribute to the breakdown of proteins, fats, and carbohydrates. These nutrients are absorbed into the bloodstream to supply body cells with energy. The liver is the major organ that determines whether nutrients are stored, sent to cells or organs, or excreted. Solid wastes consisting of fiber, water, and salts are dumped into the large intestine, where most of the water and salts are reabsorbed into the system, and the fiber is passed out through the anus. The entire digestive process takes approximately 24 hours.

Obtaining Essential Nutrients

Water: A Crucial Nutrient

If you were to go on a survival trip, which would you take with you—food or water? You may be surprised to learn that you could survive for much longer without food than you could without water. Even in severe conditions, the average person can go for weeks without certain vitamins and minerals before experiencing serious deficiency symptoms. **Dehydration,** however, can cause serious problems within a matter of hours; after a few days without water, death is likely.

Just what function does water serve in the body? Between 50 and 60 percent of our total body weight is water. The water in our system bathes cells, aids in fluid and electrolyte balance, maintains pH balance, and transports molecules and cells throughout the body. Water is the major component of our blood, which carries oxygen and nutrients to the tissues, removes metabolic wastes, and is responsible for maintaining cells in working order.

Individual needs for water vary drastically according to dietary factors, age, size, environmental temperature and humidity levels, exercise, and the effectiveness of the individual's system. Certain diseases, such as diabetes or cystic fibrosis, cause people to lose fluids at a rate necessitating a higher volume of fluid intake.

Judging by the large number of people sucking at water bottles today, many Americans seem to fear becoming dehydrated. They also seem to be trying to flush their systems with pure water to help organs function more efficiently and enhance their health. Bottled water has become a multimillion-dollar industry that rivals the soda industry. Is all this water consumption really necessary? See the New Horizons in Health box about ongoing research into how much water each of us truly needs.

Is bottled water better for you than tap water? In most instances, expensive "spring" and bottled water are no healthier than chlorinated and fluoride-containing city water. In fact, if you look closely at the labels, you'll find that most expensive little bottles don't contain pristine water from natural springs but rather, purified city water that has been subjected to reverse osmosis. Is it worth the extra cost? Most experts think not. If you are concerned about your current water source, have it tested. Otherwise, don't spend your money needlessly. In addition, if you refill and reuse those plastic bottles, you may cause yourself problems. Bacteria flourish in a warm, moist environment, and the bacteria from your saliva may turn your "pure" water into a teeming soup of disease-causing liquid.

Digestive process   The process by which foods are broken down and either absorbed or excreted by the body.

Saliva   Fluid secreted by the salivary glands; enzymes in the fluid aid in the breakdown of certain foods for digestion.

Esophagus   Tube that transports food from the mouth to the stomach.

Stomach   Large muscular organ that temporarily stores, mixes, and digests foods.

Small intestine   Muscular, coiled digestive organ; consists of the duodenum, jejunum, and ileum.

Dehydration   Abnormal depletion of body fluids; a result of lack of water.

How Much Water Do We Need?

How much water do we really need? According to a generation of health experts, we should drink eight 8-ounce glasses per day, not including caffeinated beverages. Not until recently had anyone really questioned what scientific evidence there was for that recommendation. That is when Dr. Heinz Valtin, professor emeritus at Dartmouth Medical School and an expert on how the body maintains fluid balance, began to assess the basis for the 64-ounce/day concept. He determined that the advice probably stems from a muddled interpretation of a 1945 Food and Nutrition Board report that said the body needs about 1 milliliter of water for each calorie consumed—almost 8 cups for a typical 2,000-calorie diet. That advice is probably sound; however, it does not account for the fact that most of this quantity is contained in prepared foods. (Fruits and vegetables are 80 to 95 percent water, meats contain over 50 percent water, and even dry bread and cheese are about 35 percent water.) Dr. Valtin was unable to determine how the report came

to be interpreted as recommending eight glasses of pure water per day. Nor did he find any supporting research showing that the average person needs 64 ounces of fluid from any source per day, whether it be from foods or beverages.

Another key finding of Dr. Valtin's group was that, contrary to popular opinion, caffeinated drinks don't dehydrate the person who consumes them; in fact, coffee, tea, and sodas are actually hydrating for people used to caffeine and, thus, should count toward overall fluid intake.

So, should you continue to pay for all those bottles of water? (See Chapter 21 for information on the environmental effect of the plastic from all those bottles.) If you're drinking water for the health benefits of those eight additional glasses per day, you may be disappointed. For most of us, adding that much water to what we are already getting just means more trips to the bathroom with little harm done—an expensive habit with few rewards. Furthermore, people with certain medical conditions can put undue stress on the bladder and other systems or can excrete more water soluble-vitamins than they would if they had not been drinking so much.

Healthy people who take Ecstasy, which increases thirst dramatically, can drink enough to suffer from *water intoxication*, which may lead to sodium depletion, cardiac arrhythmias, and other problems.

The Food and Nutrition Board has revised its recommendations, and new water-intake guidelines are available on its website at www.iom.edu/board.asp?id=3788. In the meantime, everyone agrees that drinking water is important. The question is whether or not you are already getting close to the right amount with food, juice, milk, soda, coffee, and other fluid sources. Students who aren't eating properly, those who exercise heavily and sweat profusely, and those who aren't getting adequate fluids to compensate for fluid losses may need to pay attention to this. Older people with diminished mental capacity or sensory acuity or those on diuretics for cardiac conditions can also become water depleted and experience serious consequences.

Source: H. Valtin, "Water Consumption Needs: A Look at the Accumulated Evidence," *American Journal of Physiology,* 283, no. 5 (2002): 88–94.

Proteins

Next to water, **proteins** are the most abundant substances in the human body. Proteins are major components of nearly every cell and have been called the "body builders" because of their role in developing and repairing bone, muscle, skin, and blood cells. Proteins are also the key elements of the antibodies that protect us from disease, of enzymes that control chemical activities in the body, and of hormones that regulate bodily functions. Moreover, proteins aid in the transport of iron, oxygen, and nutrients to all body cells and supply another source of energy to cells when fats and carbohydrates are not readily available. In short, adequate amounts of protein in the diet are vital to many body functions and ultimately to survival.

Whenever you consume proteins, your body breaks them down into smaller molecules known as **amino acids,** which link together like beads in a necklace to form 20 different combinations. Nine of these combinations are termed **essential amino acids,** meaning that the body must obtain them from the diet; the other 11 are produced by the body.

Dietary protein that supplies all of the essential amino acids is called **complete (high-quality) protein.** Typically, protein from animal products is complete. When we consume foods that are deficient in some of the essential amino acids, the total amount of protein that can be synthesized from the

Proteins The essential constituents of nearly all body cells; necessary for the development and repair of bone, muscle, skin, and blood; the key elements of antibodies, enzymes, and hormones.

Amino acids The building blocks of protein.

Essential amino acids Nine of the basic nitrogen-containing building blocks of protein that must be obtained from foods to ensure health.

Complete (high-quality) proteins Proteins that contain all of the nine essential amino acids.

A Consumer's Guide to Soy

Have you been hearing a lot about soy as a healthy protein alternative? Here's some information that will help you reduce the amount of saturated fat in your diet by increasing your soy intake. Substituting soy for animal-based protein in your diet is a healthy behavior change.

THE SKINNY ON SOY

Soy has hit mainstream America in a wave of soy milk, soy burgers, soy dogs, and cheeselike products, totaling nearly $3 billion per year. Interestingly, although touted as a great boon to health-conscious individuals, much of what we believe to be true about soy is still largely in question. Researchers still don't know which of several soybean components provide soy's important health benefits. To date, 70 to 80 percent of the health benefits we've seen from soy products appear to be attributable to *isoflavones.* These isoflavones are *phytoestrogens* (plant compounds with estrogen-like activity), which are thought to block human estrogens that may encourage the growth of hormone-sensitive cancers. However, be-

fore you run out and buy soy purely for anticancer benefits, it is important to note that phytoestrogens have been found to have both estrogenic and antiestrogenic effects. Researchers aren't sure why, but it may depend on when in life you consume them and in what quantity.

In conjunction with soy protein, iso-flavones also appear to reduce blood cholesterol and overall risk of heart disease, build bone, and protect against some cancers—particularly prostate cancer in men and breast cancer in women. Especially for postmenopausal women, soy seems to be a factor in decreased breast density, which may promote early detection of tumors. In general, soy foods naturally contain about two milligrams of isoflavones for every gram of soy protein.

OPTIONS FOR ADDING SOY TO YOUR DIET

Tofu: A soft, cheeselike food made by curdling soy milk that tends to take on the flavor of foods that it is cooked with. Use firm or extra-firm tofu if you want to chunk it for soups, stir fries, or grilling. Choose soft and silky tofu for blending and baking.

Soy nuts: Whole soybeans that have been soaked in water, drained, and baked, usually with salt added. These make great

substitutes for peanuts and are loaded with protein and isoflavones.

Tempeh: A tender cake, often a mixture of soybeans and other grains such as rice or millet, that has been fermented to have a smoky or nutty flavor. Can be used in soups, casseroles, or sandwiches.

Edamamé: Green soybeans in their pods or shells; often available frozen. Cook in boiling water and eat like other pea pods with a bit of salt.

Natto: Made of fermented, cooked whole soybeans. Cheeselike texture; best used as topping for rice, in soups, and with vegetables.

Soy milk: Soybeans are soaked, ground fine, and strained to produce a milklike fluid. Often flavored to enhance taste. Unlike milk, doesn't contain calcium (unless fortified).

Soy cheese and yogurt: Made from soy milk and may be substituted as desired.

Source: From "*EN* Presents a Buyer's Guide to Selected Soy Foods," by Julie Upton. Reprinted with permission from *Environmental Nutrition* (May 2002), 52 Riverside Drive, Suite 15A, New York, NY 10024. For subscription information, 800-829-5384; www.environmentalnutrition.com

other amino acids is decreased. For proteins to be complete, they must also be present in digestible form and in amounts proportional to body requirements.

What about plant sources of protein? Proteins from plant sources are often **incomplete proteins** in that they lack one or two of the essential amino acids. Nevertheless, it is relatively easy for the nonmeat eater to combine plant foods effectively and eat complementary sources of plant protein (Figure 8.4). An excellent example of this mutual supplementation process is eating peanut butter on whole-grain bread. Although each of these foods lacks certain essential amino acids, eating them together provides high-quality protein.

Incomplete proteins Proteins that are lacking in one or more of the essential amino acids.

Plant sources of protein fall into three general categories: *legumes* (beans, peas, peanuts, and soy products), *grains* (whole grains, corn, and pasta products), and *nuts and seeds.* Certain vegetables, such as leafy green vegetables and broccoli, also contribute valuable plant proteins. Mixing two or more foods from each of these categories during the same meal will provide all of the essential amino acids necessary to ensure adequate protein absorption. People who are not interested in obtaining all of their protein from plants can combine incomplete plant proteins with complete low-fat animal proteins such as chicken, fish, turkey, and lean red meat. Low-fat or nonfat cottage cheese, skim milk, egg whites, and nonfat dry milk all provide high-quality proteins and have few calories and little dietary fat. Soy provides an excellent option for many people and is growing in popularity as soy products become more flavorful. See the Skills for Behavior Change box above for ways to incorporate soy into your diet.

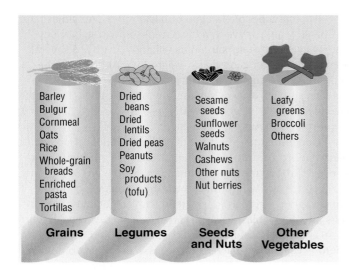

Figure 8.4
Complementary Proteins

Source: Adapted from J. Thompson and M. Manore, *Nutrition: An Applied Approach* (San Francisco: Benjamin Cummings, 2005).

You need to eat enough protein, but make sure you don't overdo it. Eating too much protein, particularly animal protein, can place added stress on the liver and kidneys. It also may increase calcium excretion in urine, which can elevate the risk of osteoporosis and bone fractures.[21]

Recently, several low-calorie diets that practically eliminate carbohydrates and focus on eating large quantities of protein have reemerged in the popular press. Diets that deviate from a balanced nutritional approach are almost certainly flawed. In particular, people who have kidney or liver problems or suffer from fluid imbalances should avoid such diets. For more information, see the following section on carbohydrates and Chapter 9 on weight management.

A person might need to eat extra protein if fighting off a serious infection, recovering from surgery or blood loss, or recovering from burns. In these instances, proteins that are lost to cellular repair need to be replaced. There is considerable controversy over whether someone in high-level physical training needs additional protein to build and repair muscle fibers or whether normal daily requirements should suffice.

Although protein deficiency continues to pose a threat to the global population, few Americans suffer from protein deficiencies. In fact, the average American consumes more than 100 grams of protein daily, and about 70 percent of this comes from high-fat animal flesh and dairy products.[22] The recommended protein intake for the average man is only 63 grams (g), and the average woman needs only 50 g. (As an example, a 6-ounce broiled sirloin steak contains about 53 g of protein.) The typical recommendation is that, in a 2,000-calorie diet, about 10 percent of calories should come from protein, 60 percent from carbohydrates, and less than

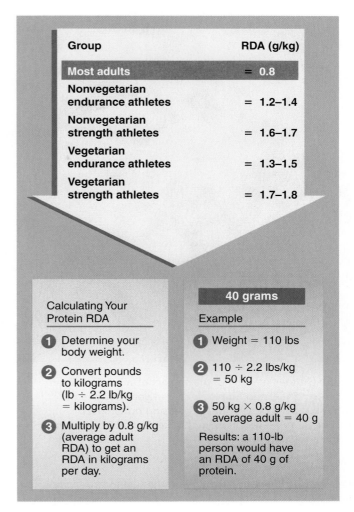

Figure 8.5
Calculating Your Protein RDA

Source: Adapted from J. Thompson and M. Manore, *Nutrition: An Applied Approach* (San Francisco: Benjamin Cummings, 2005).

30 percent from fat. The excess is stored as extra calories, leading to extra fat. See Figure 8.5 to determine your own Recommended Dietary Allowance (RDA) for protein.

Carbohydrates

Although the importance of proteins in the body cannot be underestimated, it is **carbohydrates** that supply us with the energy needed to sustain normal daily activity. Carbohydrates can actually be metabolized more quickly and efficiently than proteins and are a quick source of energy for the body,

> **Carbohydrates** Basic nutrients that supply the body with glucose, the energy form most commonly used to sustain normal activity.

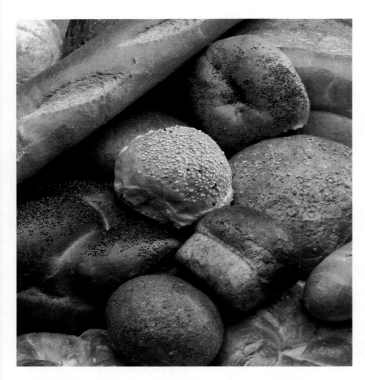

Carbohydrates have been the subject of much attention recently. Understanding their role in your body—and differences between whole grains and other sources of carbohydrates—will help you make decisions about your own eating patterns.

being easily converted to glucose, the fuel for the body's cells. These foods also play an important role in the functioning of internal organs, the nervous system, and the muscles. They are the best fuel for endurance athletics because they provide both an immediate and a time-released energy source as they are digested easily and then consistently metabolized in the bloodstream.

Simple sugar   A major type of carbohydrate, which provides short-term energy.

Complex carbohydrates   A major type of carbohydrate, which provides sustained energy.

Monosaccharide   A simple sugar that contains only one molecule of a simple sugar.

Disaccharide   A combination of two monosaccharides.

Polysaccharide   A complex carbohydrate formed by the combination of long chains of saccharides.

Cellulose   Fiber; a major form of complex carbohydrates.

Glycogen   The polysaccharide form in which glucose is stored in the liver and, to a lesser extent, in muscles.

For many people, a plate of pasta represents an attractive, healthy alternative to a fatty steak. However, carbohydrates have also been painted as villains recently in several popular diets promising quick weight loss. Although some studies seem to support the low carbohydrate, high protein and fat approach to weight loss, previous decades of research have consistently disagreed with these claims. See Chapter 9 for more information about these diets.

One issue that proponents of these diets overlook is that *not all carbohydrates are the same.* There are two major types of carbohydrates: **simple sugars,** which are found primarily in fruits, and **complex carbohydrates,** which are found in grains, cereals, dark green leafy vegetables, yellow fruits and vegetables (carrots, yams), *cruciferous* vegetables (such as broccoli, cabbage, and cauliflower), and certain tuberous vegetables, such as potatoes. Most of us do not get enough complex carbohydrates in our daily diets.

A typical American diet contains large amounts of simple sugars. The most common form is *glucose.* Eventually, the human body converts all types of simple sugars to glucose to provide energy to cells; glucose is the only energy form used by the brain. In its natural form, glucose is sweet and is obtained from substances such as corn syrup, honey, molasses, vegetables, and fruits. *Fructose* is another simple sugar found in fruits and berries. Glucose and fructose are **monosaccharides** that contain only one molecule of sugar. High-fructose corn syrup has come under sharp criticism recently for its massive overuse in our food supply and its contribution to dietary excess.

Disaccharides are combinations of two monosaccharides. Perhaps the best-known example is granulated table sugar (known as sucrose), which consists of a molecule of fructose chemically bonded to a molecule of glucose. Lactose, found in milk and milk products, is another form of disaccharide, formed by the combination of glucose and galactose (another simple sugar). Disaccharides must be broken down into simple sugars before they can be used by the body.

Controlling the amount of sugar in your diet can be difficult because sugar, like sodium, is often present in food products that you might not expect to contain it. Such diverse items as ketchup, Russian dressing, Coffee-mate, and Shake 'n' Bake derive 30 to 65 percent of their calories from sugar. Read food labels carefully before purchasing.

Polysaccharides are complex carbohydrates formed by long chains of saccharides. Like disaccharides, they must be broken down into simple sugars before the body can utilize them. There are two major forms of complex carbohydrates: *starches* and *fiber,* or **cellulose.**

Starches make up the majority of the complex carbohydrate group. Starches in our diets come from flours, breads, pasta, potatoes, and related foods. They are stored in body muscles and the liver in a polysaccharide form called **glycogen.** When the body requires a sudden burst of energy, it quickly uses up the available store of glucose and then breaks down glycogen into more glucose.

Carbohydrates and Athletic Performance   Over the past decade, carbohydrates have become the "health foods" of many athletes. Some fitness enthusiasts consume concentrated sugary foods or drinks before or during athletic activity, thinking that the sugars will provide extra energy. This may actually be counterproductive.

One possible problem involves the gastrointestinal tract. If your intestines react to activity (or the nervousness before competition) by moving material through the small intestine more rapidly than usual, undigested disaccharides and/or unabsorbed monosaccharides will reach the colon, which can result in an inopportune bout of diarrhea.

Consuming large amounts of sugar during exercise can also have a negative effect on hydration. Concentrations exceeding 24 g of sugar per 8 ounces of fluid can delay stomach emptying and hence absorption of water. Some fruit juices, fruit drinks, and other sugar-sweetened beverages have more than this amount of sugar. If you use these products, dilute them with ice cubes or water.

Marathon runners and other people who require reserves of energy for demanding tasks often attempt to increase stores of glycogen in the body by *carbohydrate loading*. This process involves modifying the nature of both workouts and diet, usually during the week or so before competition. The athletes train very hard early in the week while eating small amounts of carbohydrates. Right before competition, they dramatically increase their intake of carbohydrates to force the body to store more glycogen, which can then be used during endurance activities (such as the last miles of a marathon).

The Myth of Sugar and Hyperactivity   Contrary to early media reports, extensive research in recent years indicates that sugars *do not* cause hyperactivity.[23] In well-controlled dietary challenge studies, consumption of sugar has not been shown to have negative effects on motor activity, spontaneous behavior, performance in psychological tests, learning, memory, attention span, or problem-solving ability. In addition, sugar intake is not related to violence or criminal activity.

Is Sugar Addictive?   Another sugar-related controversy is whether sugar can be addictive. A recent report on this topic summarizes the accumulated research and concludes that there is little evidence to support an addiction. It might be more appropriate to say that your sweet tooth is a preference.[24]

According to the report, scientists agree that babies are born with a preference for sweet and salty tastes and a dislike for sour and bitter tastes. Some people are "supertasters," which means that they have more taste buds on the tip of the tongue (up to 1,100 taste buds per square centimeter) than medium, low, or nontasters (low tasters have around 40 taste buds in the same area). Low and nontasters require more sugar for taste and thus may have a stronger sweet tooth.

Preference for sweets is also a part of our cultural heritage, with indications that we develop a "taste" for sugar based on learned eating patterns, rather than as an addiction. Culture, genetics, and other factors appear to explain why some of us love sugar far too much. The keys are to monitor sugar intake and eat sweet foods in moderation.

Carbohydrates and Carcinogens   The World Health Organization recently labeled *acrylamide,* a compound found in plastics, as a "probable human carcinogen" because it has been shown to cause cancer, as well as genetic, neurological, and reproductive damage, in animals. While some of the concern arises from our use of plastics to cover food in microwaves, the larger issue arose because acrylamide is formed when starchy foods are cooked at high temperatures. University of Stockholm researchers found the highest concentrations of acrylamide in potato chips and crispbreads that were baked or fried, like French fries, crackers, and cereals.[25] Acrylamide was not found in raw foods, meats, or starchy foods that were boiled, such as rice or pasta.

Critics of the study say that too few samples were used and the amounts of acrylamide found were a thousandfold less than levels shown to cause cancer in mice. Follow-up research by the Center for Science in the Public Interest showed that a large order of French fries contained 39 to 82 micrograms (µg) of acrylamide, roughly 300 times what the U.S. Environmental Protection Agency allows in a glass of water.[26] At this writing, the FDA and other agencies are still deciding on a course of action or whether one is justified.

Fiber

Fiber, often referred to as "bulk" or "roughage," is the indigestible portion of plant foods that helps move foods through the digestive system, delays absorption of cholesterol and other nutrients, and softens stools by absorbing water. Fiber also helps to control weight by creating a feeling of fullness without adding extra calories and appears to reduce risk from heart disease.[27] In spite of all the fiber advocates, the average American consumes between 12 and 17 g of fiber a day, about half the recommended daily amount of 20 to 35 grams.[28]

Insoluble fiber, which is found in bran, whole-grain breads and cereals, and most fruits and vegetables, is associated with these gastrointestinal benefits and has also been found to reduce the risk for several forms of cancer. *Soluble fiber* appears to be a factor in lowering blood cholesterol levels and reducing risk for cardiovascular disease. Major sources of soluble fiber in the diet include oat bran, dried beans (such as kidney, garbanzo, pinto, and navy beans), and some fruits and vegetables.

Fiber   The indigestible portion of plant foods that helps move foods through the digestive system and softens stools by absorbing water.

There's More to Whole Grains Than Whole Wheat

It's hard to beat whole grains. They are packed with vitamins, minerals, and fiber that you just don't find in white bread, processed cereals, white rice, or even in many healthful-looking, enriched, "multigrain" breads. Plus, whole grains have a new health cachet, now that researchers have uncovered disease-fighting properties from the phytonutrients they contain.

Whole grains are also loaded with flavor and texture and add interest to meals. Here is a guide to some less traditional whole grains.

If you can't find these grains or flours in your local supermarket or health food store, try these mail-order sources:

- King Arthur Flour
  www.kingarthurflour.com
- True Foods Market
  www.truefoodsmarket.com

Grain	What It Is and Nutrients	Flavor Basics and Shopping Tips	Preparation and Serving Suggestions
Amaranth	A high-protein grain that's a good source of fiber and vitamin E. Rich in lysine, an amino acid often missing in grain foods. Tolerated by people sensitive to wheat or gluten-intolerant.	Amaranth seeds have a pleasant, peppery flavor.	• Boil and eat as cereal or use in soups and granolas. The seeds of some varieties can be popped like popcorn. • To prepare: Cook 1 cup amaranth in 3 cups water for ½ hour.
Kasha (buckwheat groats)	Technically, a fruit (the roasted seed of the buckwheat plant), but the food world classifies it as a grain. It's an excellent source of magnesium and a good source of copper and fiber. Like amaranth, it is rich in lysine. Tolerated by people sensitive to wheat or gluten-intolerant, though be careful of mixes that also contain wheat.	Kasha has a hearty, nutty flavor and chewy texture. Kasha comes in whole, coarse, medium, and fine consistencies. Also available as flour.	• Great when served as a hot cereal or as a hearty salad with vegetables and paired with a light soup. • Kasha makes an exceptionally flavorful pilaf; prepare with carmelized or browned onions and mushrooms. • Kasha flour makes flavorful, hearty pancakes and pasta. • To prepare: Simmer 1 part groats in 2 parts water for 15 minutes (medium and fine grades cook more quickly).

What's the best way to increase your intake of dietary fiber? Eat more complex carbohydrates, such as whole grains, fruits, vegetables, dried peas and beans, nuts, and seeds. As with most nutritional advice, however, too much of a good thing can pose problems. Sudden increases in dietary fiber may cause flatulence (intestinal gas), cramping, or a bloated feeling. Consume plenty of water or other liquids to reduce such side effects.

A few years ago, fiber was thought to be the remedy for just about everything. Much of this hope was probably unrealistic, although research does support many benefits of fiber, such as:[29]

- *Protection against colon and rectal cancer.* One of the leading causes of cancer deaths in the United States, colorectal cancer is much rarer in countries having diets high in fiber and low in animal fat. Several studies contributed to the theory that fiber-rich diets, particularly those including insoluble fiber, prevent the development of precancerous growths. It remained uncertain whether this was because more fiber helps to move foods through the colon faster, thereby reducing the colon's contact time with cancer-causing substances, or because insoluble fiber reduces bile acids and certain bacterial enzymes that may promote cancer. However, although research continues, the latest findings indicate that fiber may not be as protective against colon cancer as once believed.[30] Earlier studies failed to adequately control for other factors that may have caused an apparent protective effect. While fiber is still promoted for its possible benefits, more research is necessary.
- *Protection against breast cancer.* Research into the effects of fiber on breast cancer risk is inconclusive. However, some studies indicate that wheat bran (rich in insoluble fiber) reduces blood-estrogen levels, which may affect the risk for breast cancer. Another theory is that people who

Grain	What It Is and Nutrients	Flavor Basics and Shopping Tips	Preparation and Serving Suggestions
Quinoa (KEEN-wah)	A staple of ancient Incan culture. It is an excellent source of B vitamins, copper, iron, magnesium, and lysine. It provides a more complete protein than many other grains. A popular alternative for people sensitive to wheat or gluten-intolerant.	Quinoa has a mild flavor and a slightly crunchy texture. It comes in different colors, ranging from a pale yellow to red and black. Health food stores sell pasta and other products made from it.	• Quinoa flakes are seeds that have been steamed, rolled, then flaked to make an oatmeal-like hot cereal. • Rinse quinoa before cooking to remove its bitter natural coating. • To prepare: Cook 1 cup quinoa in 2 cups water for 20 minutes.
Spelt	Spelt, a distant cousin to wheat, is hearty and grows well without chemical fertilizers, pesticides, and herbicides and therefore is a commonly available organic grain. It is a good source of fiber and B vitamins.	Available as whole berries and whole or refined flour. Also found in bread and pastas in natural food stores.	• Use whole spelt berries as you would rice and barley, in hearty grain salads, pilafs, and fillings. • To prepare: Cook 1 cup berries in 4 cups water for 30–40 minutes.
Teff	This Ethiopian staple is the world's smallest grain and is less refined than many common grains. As a result, it's a nutritional powerhouse, especially rich in protein and calcium. Tolerated by people sensitive to wheat or gluten-intolerant.	Teff has a sweet, nutty flavor and comes in different colors, ranging from creamy white to reddish-brown.	• Serve as a hot breakfast cereal, sprinkled with cinnamon and brown sugar, maple syrup, raisins, or sliced fruit. • To prepare: Cook 1 cup teff in 3 cups water for 15–20 minutes; to add flavor, roast teff with cornmeal for 5 minutes before boiling.
Triticale (Tri-ti-CAY-lee)	This relatively young (only 200 years old) grain is a cross between wheat and rye. It is an excellent source of fiber, B vitamins, and magnesium, plus a good source of iron.	Triticale berries are gray-brown and oval shaped, similar to wheat berries but with a subtle rye flavor. Available as flour, flakes (for cereal), berries, and as part of muesli, granola, or whole-grain cereal combinations.	• Triticale makes wonderful sandwich bread, similar in taste to honey wheat bread. • Use triticale flakes like rolled oats to make a hot breakfast cereal. They cook in about 15 minutes. • To prepare: Cook 1 cup berries in 4 cups water for 1 hour.

Source: From "There's More to Whole Grains Than Whole Wheat," by Luanne Hughes. Reprinted with permission from *Environmental Nutrition* (October 2001), 52 Riverside Drive Suite 15A, New York, NY 10024. For subscription information 800-829-5384; www.environmentalnutrition.com

eat more fiber have proportionally less fat in their diets and this is what reduces overall risk.

- *Protection against constipation.* Insoluble fiber, consumed with adequate fluids, is the safest, most effective way to prevent or treat constipation. The fiber acts like a sponge, absorbing moisture and producing softer, bulkier stools that are easily passed. Fiber also helps produce gas, which in turn may initiate a bowel movement.

- *Protection against diverticulosis.* About one American in ten over the age of 40 and at least one in three over age 50 suffers from *diverticulosis,* a condition in which tiny bulges or pouches form on the large intestinal wall. These bulges can become irritated and cause chronic pain if under strain from constipation. Insoluble fiber helps to reduce constipation and discomfort.

- *Protection against heart disease.* Many studies have indicated that soluble fiber (as in oat bran, barley, and fruit

pectin) helps reduce blood cholesterol, primarily by lowering LDL ("bad") cholesterol. Whether this reduction is a direct effect or occurs instead through the displacement of fat calories by fiber calories or through intake of other nutrients, such as iron, remains in question.[31]

- *Protection against diabetes.* Some studies suggest that soluble fiber improves control of blood sugar and can reduce the need for insulin or medication in people with diabetes. Exactly why isn't clear, but soluble fiber seems to delay the emptying of the stomach and slow the absorption of glucose by the intestine. The significance of this effect has been downgraded in recent years, however.[32]

- *Protection against obesity.* Because most high-fiber foods are high in carbohydrates and low in fat, they help control caloric intake. Many take longer to chew, which slows you down at the table, and fiber stays in the digestive tract longer than other nutrients, making you feel full sooner.

Flaxseed: The Oat Bran of the Twenty-First Century?

Just as oat bran began to lose its luster as a fiber icon, a new version of good fiber in a small package started arriving in trendy specialty nutrition stores. The blue-flowered flax plant, cultivated since ancient times for its value in clothing (linen fabrics) is part of a growing food enthusiasm. Why all the interest? Largely because the tiny, shiny brown seeds with the mild, nutty flavor are rich in alpha-linolenic acid (ALA), an omega-3 fatty acid that helps reduce blood clotting, primes immune function, and helps prevent abnormal heart rhythms. The seeds are also rich in lignans, phytoestrogens that may hinder hormone-related cancers. The fiber in flax is mostly insoluble, which helps relieve constipation, and partly soluble, which helps lower cholesterol and balance blood sugars.

Although flax is available in pills and liquid form, its highest nutritive value is when it is in its ground, natural form. It is most easily digested and stores best in this medium, particularly when refrigerated, is less likely to become rancid, and, in general, offers consumers the best range of available benefits. Flax can be added to casseroles, meatloafs, and burgers or be mixed in yogurts and breakfast cereals, sprinkled on salads, or added to baked products. Increase your water consumption to assist in the digestive process. In short, flax is easy to obtain and appears to offer numerous benefits to the health-conscious consumer.

Source: From "Flaxseed Comes of Age: Good Nutrition in a Small Package," by Amy Aubertin, R.D. Reprinted with permission from *Environmental Nutrition* (August 2002), 52 Riverside Drive, Suite 15A, New York, New York 10024. For subscription information, 800-829-5384; www.environmentalnutrition.com

---

Most experts believe that Americans should double their current consumption of dietary fiber—to 20 to 35 g per day for most people and perhaps to 40 to 50 g for others. (A large bowl of high-fiber cereal with a banana provides close to 20 g of fiber.) Tips for increasing your fiber intake include:

- Whenever possible, select whole-grain breads, especially those that are low in fat and sugars. Look for the word "whole" on the package and the ingredient list, preferably among the first three ingredients.
- Choose breads with three or more grams of fiber per serving.
- Eat the fruits rather than the juices. Juices, such as orange or apple, tend to have concentrated sources of sugar and raise blood sugar levels quickly, while the fiber in the whole fruit tends to slow blood sugar increases by comparison.
- Whenever possible, eat the skin of fruits and vegetables. Apples, pears, and other fruits add fiber safely, as long as you wash them before eating.

- Substitute whole-grain pastas, bagels, and pizza crust for the refined, white flour versions.
- Add wheat crumbs or grains to meat loafs and burgers to increase fiber intake.
- Toast grains to bring out their nutty flavor and make foods more appealing.
- Remember that just because a bread or roll is brown does not guarantee that it is fiber-rich. Brown sugars, molasses, or dyes are sometimes used to make foods look healthy. Check the label!
- See the New Horizons in Health box for information on the benefits of flaxseed.

Fats

Fats (or *lipids*), another group of basic nutrients, are perhaps the most misunderstood of the body's required energy sources. Fats play a vital role in maintaining healthy skin and hair, insulating body organs against shock, maintaining body temperature, and promoting healthy cell function. Fats make foods taste better and carry the fat-soluble vitamins A, D, E, and K to the cells. They also provide a concentrated form of energy in the absence of sufficient carbohydrates.

So why, if fats perform all these functions, are we constantly urged to cut back on them? Although moderate consumption of fats is essential to health, overconsumption can be dangerous. **Triglycerides,** which make up about 95 percent of total body fat, are the most common form of fat circulating in the blood. When we consume too many calories, the liver converts the excess into triglycerides, which are stored throughout our bodies.

The remaining 5 percent of body fat is composed of substances such as **cholesterol,** which can accumulate on

---

Fats Basic nutrients composed of carbon and hydrogen atoms; needed for the proper functioning of cells, insulation of body organs against shock, maintenance of body temperature, and healthy skin and hair.

Triglycerides The most common form of fat in the body; excess calories consumed are converted into triglycerides and stored as body fat.

Cholesterol A form of fat circulating in the blood that can accumulate on the inner walls of arteries.

the inner walls of arteries, causing a narrowing of the channel through which blood flows. This buildup, called **plaque,** is a major cause of *atherosclerosis* (hardening of the arteries). At one time, the amount of circulating cholesterol in the blood was thought to be crucial. Current thinking is that the actual amount of circulating cholesterol itself is not as important as the ratio of total cholesterol to a group of compounds called **high-density lipoproteins (HDLs).** Lipoproteins are the transport facilitators for cholesterol in the blood. High-density lipoproteins are capable of transporting more cholesterol than are **low-density lipoproteins (LDLs).** Whereas LDLs transport cholesterol to the body's cells, HDLs apparently transport circulating cholesterol to the liver for metabolism and elimination from the body. People with a high percentage of HDLs therefore appear to be at lower risk for developing cholesterol-clogged arteries. Regular vigorous exercise plays a part in reducing cholesterol by increasing high-density lipoproteins.

PUFAs and MUFAs: Unsaturated "Good Guys"

Fat cells consist of chains of carbon and hydrogen atoms. Those that are unable to hold any more hydrogen in their chemical structure are labeled **saturated fats.** They generally come from animal sources, such as meats and dairy products, and are solid at room temperature. **Unsaturated fats,** which come from plants and include most vegetable oils, are generally liquid at room temperature and have room for additional hydrogen atoms in their chemical structure. The terms *monounsaturated fat (MUFA)* and *polyunsaturated fat (PUFA)* refer to the relative number of hydrogen atoms that are missing. Peanut and olive oils are high in monounsaturated fats, whereas corn, sunflower, and safflower oils are high in polyunsaturated fats.

There is currently a great deal of controversy about which type of unsaturated fat is most beneficial. Many believe that PUFAs may decrease beneficial HDL levels as well as the harmful LDL. PUFAs come in two forms: omega-3 fatty acids and omega-6 fatty acids. MUFAs, such as olive oil, seem to lower LDL levels and increase HDL levels and thus are currently the "preferred," or least harmful, fats. Nevertheless, a tablespoon of olive oil gives you a hefty 10 g of MUFAs. For a breakdown of the types of fats in common vegetable oils, see Figure 8.6.

Reducing Total Fat in Your Diet Want to cut the fat? These guidelines offer a good place to start:

- *Know what you are putting in your mouth.* Read food labels. Remember that no more than 10 percent of your total calories should come from saturated fat, and no more than 30 percent should come from all forms of fat.
- *Choose fat-free or low-fat versions of cakes, cookies, crackers, or chips.* (Remember, though, that calories still count. Don't eat *more* chips just because they're lower in fat.)

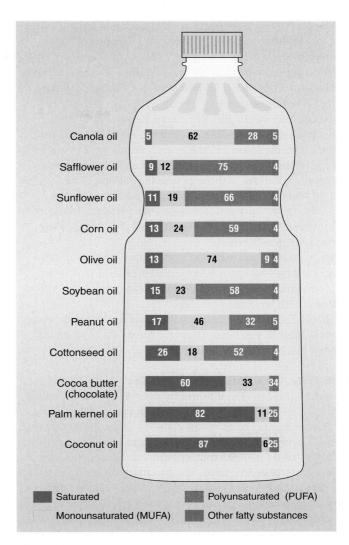

Figure 8.6
Percentages of Saturated, Polyunsaturated, and Monounsaturated Fats in Common Vegetable Oils

Plaque Cholesterol buildup on the inner walls of arteries, causing a narrowing of the channel through which blood flows; a major cause of atherosclerosis.

High-density lipoproteins (HDLs) Compounds that facilitate the transport of cholesterol in the blood to the liver for metabolism and elimination from the body.

Low-density lipoproteins (LDLs) Compounds that facilitate the transport of cholesterol in the blood to the body's cells.

Saturated fats Fats that are unable to hold any more hydrogen in their chemical structure; derived mostly from animal sources; solid at room temperature.

Unsaturated fats Fats that do have room for more hydrogen in their chemical structure; derived mostly from plants; liquid at room temperature.

- *Use olive oil for baking and sautéing.* Animal studies have shown that it doesn't raise cholesterol or promote the growth of tumors.
- *If you use margarine, use it in liquid, diet, or whipped forms.* These products have far less *trans* fatty acids than solid fat (see the next section).
- *Choose lean meats, fish, or poultry.* Remove skin. Broil or bake whenever possible. In general, the more well-done the meat, the fewer the calories. Drain off fat after cooking.
- *Choose fewer cold cuts, sausages, hot dogs, organ meats, and bacon.* Be careful of those products claiming to be "95 percent fat-free" as they may still have high levels of fat.
- *Select nonfat dairy products whenever possible.* Part-skim-milk cheeses such as mozzarella, farmer's, lappi, and ricotta are good choices.
- *When cooking, use substitutes for butter, margarine, oils, sour cream, mayonnaise, and salad dressings.* Chicken broth, wine, vinegar, and low-calorie dressings provide flavor with less fat.
- *Think of your food intake as an average over a day or a couple of days.* If you have a high-fat breakfast or lunch, balance it with a low-fat dinner.

Trans *Fatty Acids: Still Bad?* Since 1961, Americans have decreased their intake of butter by over 43 percent. Instead, they have substituted margarine, which became known as the "better butter" after reports labeled unsaturated fats the "heart-healthy" alternative. In response to a widely publicized landmark study in 1990 that questioned the benefits of margarine, experts investigated whether margarine was indeed less detrimental to cholesterol levels.[33] The culprits? **Trans fatty acids (*trans* fats),** fatty acids having unusual shapes, are produced when polyunsaturated oils are *hydrogenated,* a process in which hydrogen is added to unsaturated fats to make them more solid and resistant to chemical change.[34] Besides raising cholesterol levels, *trans* fats have been implicated in certain types of cancer.[35]

A more recent study found that the *trans* fats found in margarine may in fact pose an even greater risk for heart disease than the saturated fat in butter and lard[36]—but before you dash out and fill your refrigerator with butter, be aware that this research is controversial.

Keep in mind that *trans* fats, even monounsaturated acids, alter blood cholesterol the same way as some saturated fats; they raise LDL and lower HDL cholesterol.[37] The American Heart Association has steadfastly stated that because butter is rich in both saturated fat and cholesterol whereas margarine is made from vegetable fat with no dietary cholesterol, margarine is still preferable to butter.[38] Others disagree, claiming that the occasional use of butter is

preferable to margarine.[39] Most experts claim that the whole area of *trans* fats needs much more research.

The bottom line? Moderation in all fat intake continues to be the best rule of thumb.[40] Whenever possible, opt for other condiments on your bread, using jams, fat-free cream cheese, garlic, or other toppings. Today, several newer generation low- or no-*trans* fats options are available. While cost is an issue, they offer an alternative for those able to afford it. Some experts advocate using low-fat salad dressings as toppings for bread and pasta or using olive oil in moderation to add a bit of flavor. If you have high cholesterol, reducing all types of fat and cholesterol in the diet is still sound advice.

New Fat Advice: Is More Fat Ever Better? Although most of this chapter has promoted the age-old recommendation to reduce saturated fat, avoid *trans* fatty acids, and eat more monounsaturated fats, some researchers worry that we have gone too far in our antifat frenzy. In fact, according to some experts, our zeal to eat no-fat or low-fat foods may be one of the greatest causes of obesity in America today. According to the American Heart Association, eating fewer than 15 percent of our calories as fat (less than 34 g a day on a 2,000-calorie diet) can actually increase blood triglycerides to levels that promote heart disease, while lowering levels of protective HDLs. There is also a concern that such very-low-fat diets may lead to shortages of essential fatty acid (EFA) in the diet.[41] See Chapter 15 for new classifications of cholesterol levels.

Not all fat is bad. In addition to the benefits already mentioned, dietary fat supplies the two essential fatty acids that we must receive from our diets, *linoleic acid* and *alpha-linolenic acid.* These two fats are needed to make hormonelike compounds that control immune function, pain perception, and inflammation, to name a few key benefits.[42]

Although linoleic acid and alpha-linolenic acid are both polyunsaturated fats and have similar names, they are actually quite different in what they do. Linoleic acid, a member of the *omega-6* family of fats (found in soybeans, peanuts, corn, and sunflower seeds), reduces blood levels of total cholesterol and "bad" cholesterol (LDL) when consumed in reasonable amounts. Alpha-linolenic acid is part of the *omega-3* family of fats and is found in flax, canola oil, sardines, spinach, kale, green leafy vegetables, walnuts, and wheat germ. Alpha-linolenic acid is converted to two other beneficial omega-3 fats in the body, but you get a much bigger dose of those nutrients by eating cold water fish such as salmon and tuna that have abundant supplies of omega-3. Today, Americans eat 17 times more omega-6 than omega-3 fats, and most experts agree that we need a more balanced approach.[43]

While both of these essential fats are important, too much linoleic acid may promote blood clots and constrict arteries, leading to inflammation and damaged blood vessels. Recent research indicates that a form of linoleic acid known as conjugated linoleic acid (CLA) seems to be effective in inhibiting breast cancer and may, in fact, moderate the negative effects of high fat diets. CLA is found in minute

---

Trans fatty acids (*trans* fats) Fatty acids that are produced when polyunsaturated oils are hydrogenated to make them more solid.

---

quantities in meat and dairy products, so eating small portions of these foods as part of a mostly plant-based diet may provide the health benefits of CLA without the risks of consuming too much fat.[44] Consuming more alpha-linolenic acid reduces risks for blood clots and abnormal heart rhythms and may improve immune function. The best rule of thumb is to balance, using the following recommendations:[45]

- Eat fatty fish (bluefish, herring, mackerel, salmon, sardines, or tuna) at least twice weekly.
- Substitute soy and canola oils for corn, safflower, and sunflower. Keep using olive oil, too.
- Add healthy doses of green leafy vegetables, walnuts, walnut oil, and ground flaxseed to your diet to increase intake of alpha-linolenic acid.
- Limit processed and convenience foods, since they often contain harmful saturated and *trans* fats.
- Pick the MUFA or PUFA with the least amount of calories and most nutrients.

Vitamins

Vitamins are potent, essential, organic compounds that promote growth and help maintain life and health. Every minute of every day, vitamins help maintain nerves and skin, produce blood cells, build bones and teeth, heal wounds, and convert food energy to body energy—and they do all of this without adding any calories to your diet.

Age, heat, and other environmental conditions can destroy vitamins in food. Vitamins can be classified as either *fat soluble*, meaning that they are absorbed through the intestinal tract with the help of fats, or *water soluble*, meaning that they are easily dissolved in water. Vitamins A, D, E, and K are fat soluble; B complex vitamins and vitamin C are water soluble. Fat-soluble vitamins tend to be stored in the body, and toxic accumulations in the liver may cause cirrhosis-like symptoms. Water-soluble vitamins are generally excreted and cause few toxicity problems (Table 8.2 on page 244).

Despite media suggestions to the contrary, few Americans suffer from true vitamin deficiencies if they eat a diet containing all of the food groups at least part of the time. Nevertheless, Americans continue to purchase large quantities of vitamin supplements. For the most part, vitamin supplements are unnecessary and even, in certain instances, harmful. Overusing them can lead to a toxic condition known as **hypervitaminosis.**

Minerals

Minerals are the inorganic, indestructible elements that aid physiological processes within the body. Without minerals, vitamins could not be absorbed. Minerals are readily excreted and are usually not toxic. **Macrominerals** are those minerals that the body needs in fairly large amounts: sodium, calcium, phosphorus, magnesium, potassium, sulfur, and chloride. **Trace minerals** include iron, zinc, manganese, copper, and iodine. Only trace amounts of these minerals are needed, and serious problems may result if excesses or deficiencies occur (see Table 8.3 on page 246).

Although minerals are necessary for body function, there are limits on the amounts we should consume. Americans tend to overuse or underuse certain minerals.

Sodium Sodium is necessary for the regulation of blood and body fluids, transmission of nerve impulses, heart activity, and certain metabolic functions. However, we consume much more than we need. It is estimated that the average adult who does not sweat profusely needs only 500 milligrams (mg) of sodium (about 1/4 teaspoon) per day; yet the average American consumes 6,000 to 12,000 milligrams. Most professional groups recommend restricting sodium to 1,100 to 2,300 mg per day; less is better.[46]

The most common form of sodium in the American diet comes from table salt. However, table salt accounts for only 15 percent of sodium intake. The remainder comes from water and from highly processed foods that are infused with sodium to enhance flavor. Pickles, salty snack foods, processed cheeses, many breads and bakery products, and smoked meats and sausages often contain several hundred milligrams of sodium per serving. Many fast-food entrées and convenience entrees pack 500 to 1,000 mg of sodium per serving.

Many experts believe that there is a link between excessive sodium intake and hypertension (high blood pressure). Although this theory is controversial, researchers recommend that hypertensive Americans cut back on sodium to reduce their risk for cardiovascular disorders.[47] Osteoporosis researchers confirm that high sodium intake may increase calcium loss in urine, increasing your risk for debilitating fractures as you age.

Calcium The issue of calcium consumption has gained national attention with the rising incidence of osteoporosis among older adults. Although calcium plays a vital role in building strong bones and teeth, muscle contraction, blood clotting, nerve impulse transmission, regulating heartbeat, and fluid balance within cells, most Americans do not consume the 1,200 milligrams of calcium per day established by the RDA.

(Text continues on page 246)

Vitamins Essential organic compounds that promote growth and reproduction and help maintain life and health.

Hypervitaminosis A toxic condition caused by overuse of vitamin supplements.

Minerals Inorganic, indestructible elements that aid physiological processes.

Macrominerals Minerals that the body needs in fairly large amounts.

Trace minerals Minerals that the body needs in only very small amounts.

Table 8.2
A Guide to Vitamins

Vitamin	Best Sources	Chief Functions in the Body
Water-Soluble		
Thiamin RDA: 1.2 mg/day (men) 1.1 mg/day (women)	Meat, pork, liver, fish, poultry, whole-grain and enriched breads, cereals, pasta, nuts, legumes, wheat germ, oats	Helps enzymes release energy from carbohydrate; supports normal appetite and nervous system function
Riboflavin RDA: 1.3 mg/day (men) 1.1 mg/day (women)	Milk, dark green vegetables, yogurt, cottage cheese, liver, meat, whole-grain or enriched breads and cereals	Helps enzymes release energy from carbohydrate, fat, and protein; promotes healthy skin and normal vision
Niacin RDA: 16 mg/day (men) 14 mg/day (women)	Meat, eggs, poultry, fish, milk, whole-grain and enriched breads and cereals, nuts, legumes, peanuts, nutritional yeast, all protein foods	Helps enzymes release energy from energy nutrients; promotes health of skin, nerves, and digestive system
Vitamin B_6 RDA: 1.3 mg/day (men and women aged 19 to 50) 1.7 mg/day (men 51 and older) 1.5 mg/day (women 51 and older)	Meat, poultry, fish, shellfish, legumes, whole-grain products, green leafy vegetables, bananas	Protein and fat metabolism, formation of antibodies and red blood cells; helps convert tryptophan to niacin
Folate RDA: 400 µg/day (men and women)	Green leafy vegetables, liver, legumes, seeds	Red blood cell formation; protein metabolism; new cell division; prevents neural tube defects
Vitamin B_{12} RDA: 2.4 µg/day (men and women)	Meat, fish, poultry, shellfish, milk, cheese, eggs, nutritional yeast	Helps maintain nerve cells; red blood cell formation; synthesis of genetic material
Pantothenic acid AI: 5 mg/day (men and women)	Widespread in foods	Coenzyme in energy metabolism
Biotin AI: 30 µg/day (men and women)	Widespread in foods	Coenzyme in energy metabolism; fat synthesis; glycogen formation
Vitamin C RDA: 90 mg/day (men) 75 mg/day (women)	Citrus fruits, cabbage-type vegetables, tomatoes, potatoes, dark green vegetables, peppers, lettuce, cantaloupe, strawberries, mangos, papayas	Synthesis of collagen (helps heal wounds, maintains bone and teeth, strengthens blood vessels); antioxidant; strengthens resistance to infection; helps body's absorption of iron
Fat-Soluble		
Vitamin A RDA: 900 µg/day (men) 700 µg/day (women)	Retinal: fortified milk and margarine, cream, cheese, butter, eggs, liver Carotene: spinach and other dark leafy greens, broccoli, deep orange fruits (apricots, peaches, cantaloupe) and vegetables (squash, carrots, sweet potatoes, pumpkin)	Vision; growth and repair of body tissues; reproduction; bone and tooth formation; immunity; cancer protection; hormone synthesis
Vitamin D AI: 5 µg/day (men and women aged 19 to 50) 10 µg/day (men and women aged 51 to 70) 15 µg/day (men and women aged 71 and older)	Self-synthesis with sunlight, fortified milk, fortified margarine, eggs, liver, fish	Calcium and phosphorus metabolism (bone and tooth formation); aids body's absorption of calcium
Vitamin E RDA: 15 mg alpha-tocopherol/day (men and women)	Vegetable oils, green leafy vegetables, wheat germ, whole-grain products, butter, liver, egg yolk, milk fat, nuts, seeds	Protects red blood cells; antioxidant; stabilization of cell membranes
Vitamin K AI: 120 µg/day (men) 90 µg/day (women)	Liver; green, leafy, and cabbage-type vegetables; milk	Bacterial synthesis in digestive tract; synthesis of blood-clotting proteins and a blood protein that regulates blood calcium

Table 8.2
A Guide to Vitamins (continued)

Deficiency Symptoms	Toxicity Symptoms
Beriberi, edema, heart irregularity, mental confusion, muscle weakness, low morale, impaired growth	None known at this time
Skin disorders around nose and mouth, sore throat, anemia	None known at this time
Pellagra: skin rash on parts exposed to sun, loss of appetite, dizziness, weakness, irritability, fatigue, mental confusion, indigestion	Flushing, blurred vision, glucose intolerance, abnormal liver function
Nervous disorders, skin rash, muscle weakness, anemia, convulsions	Sensory neuropathy, skin lesions
Anemia, fatigue, headache, palpitations, neural tube defects in developing fetus	Neurological damage, may mask a vitamin B_{12} deficiency
Anemia, fatigue, tingling/numbness in extremities, dementia	None known at this time
Rare; sleep disturbances, nausea, fatigue	None known at this time
Depression, muscle pain, weakness, fatigue, rash, hallucinations	None known at this time
Scurvy, anemia, atherosclerotic plaques, depression, frequent infections, bleeding gums, loosened teeth, pinpoint hemorrhages, muscle degeneration, rough skin, bone fragility, poor wound healing, hysteria	Nausea, abdominal cramps, diarrhea, breakdown of red blood cells in persons with certain genetic disorders, deficiency symptoms may appear at first on withdrawal of high doses, kidney stones in those with kidney disease
Night blindness, rough skin, susceptibility to infection, eye problems leading to blindness, impaired growth, infertility	Miscarriage, birth defects in developing fetus, red blood cell breakage, nosebleeds, abdominal cramps, nausea, diarrhea, weight loss, blurred vision, irritability, loss of appetite, bone pain, dry skin, rashes, hair loss, cessation of menstruation, growth retardation liver and nervous system damage
Rickets in children; osteomalacia in adults; abnormal growth, joint pain, osteoporosis	Raised blood calcium, constipation, weight loss, irritability, weakness, nausea, kidney stones, mental and physical retardation, calcium deposits
Muscle wasting, weakness, red blood cell breakage, anemia, hemorrhaging, fibrocystic breast disease, leg cramps	Interference with anticlotting medication, intestinal discomfort, increased risk of stroke
Reduced ability to form blood clots, excessive bleeding and bruising	None known at this time

Note: RDA = Recommended Dietary Allowances. AI = Adequate Intakes. Values are for adults aged 19 and older, except as noted. Values increase among women who are pregnant or lactating.

Source: Adapted from J. Thompson and M. Manore, *Nutrition: An Applied Approach* (San Francisco: Benjamin Cummings, 2005). Reprinted by permission of Pearson Education, Inc.

Table 8.3
A Guide to Minerals

Mineral	Significant Sources	Chief Functions in the Body

Calcium
AI: 1,000 mg/day (men and women
    aged 19 to 50)
    1,200 mg/day (men and women
    over 50)
	Milk and milk products, small fish (with bones), tofu, greens, legumes	Principal mineral of bones and teeth; involved in muscle contraction and relaxation, nerve function, blood clotting, blood pressure

Phosphorus RDA: 700 mg/day (men and women)	All animal tissues	Part of every cell; involved in acid-base balance

Magnesium
RDA: 400 mg/day (men aged 19 to 30)
    420 mg/day (men 31 and older)
    310 mg/day (women aged 19 to 30)
    320 mg/day (women 31 and older)
	Nuts, legumes, whole grains, dark green vegetables, seafood, chocolate, cocoa	Involved in bone mineralization, protein synthesis, enzyme action, normal muscular contraction, nerve transmission

Sodium AI: 1.5 g/day (men and women)	Salt, soy sauce, processed foods (cured, canned, pickled) and many boxed foods	Helps maintain normal fluid and acid-base balance
Chloride AI: 2.3 g/day (men and women)	Salt, soy sauce, processed foods	Part of stomach acid, necessary for proper digestion, fluid balance
Potassium AI: 4.7 g/day (men and women)	All whole foods: meats, milk, fruits, vegetables, grains, legumes	Facilitates many reactions including protein synthesis, fluid balance, nerve transmission, and contraction of muscles
Iodine RDA: 150 µg/day (men and women)	Iodized salt, seafood	Part of thyroxine, which regulates metabolism

Iron
RDA: 8 mg/day (men)
    18 mg/day (women aged 19 to 50)
    8 mg/day (women 51 and older)
    27 mg/day (pregnant women)
	Beef, fish, poultry, shellfish, eggs, legumes, dried fruits	Hemoglobin formation; part of myoglobin; energy utilization

Zinc RDA: 11 mg/day (men) 8 mg/day (women)	Protein-containing foods: meats, fish, poultry, grains, vegetables	Part of many enzymes; present in insulin; involved in making genetic material and proteins, immunity, vitamin A transport, taste, wound healing, making sperm, normal fetal development
Copper RDA: 900 µg/day (men and women)	Meats, drinking water	Absorption of iron; part of several enzymes
Fluoride AI: 4 mg/day (men) 3 mg/day (women)	Drinking water (if naturally fluoride-containing or fluoridated), tea, seafood	Formation of bones and teeth; helps make teeth resistant to decay and bones resistant to mineral loss
Selenium RDA: 55 µg/day (men and women)	Seafood, meats, grains	Helps protect body compounds from oxidation

Chromium
AI: 35 µg/day (men aged 19 to 50)
    30 µg/day (men 51 and older)
    25 µg/day (women aged 19 to 50)
    20 µg/day (women 51 and older)
	Meats, unrefined foods, fats, vegetable oils of energy from glucose	Associated with insulin and required for the release

Molybdenum RDA: 45 mg/day (men and women)	Legumes, cereals, organ meats	Facilitates (with enzymes) many cell processes
Manganese AI: 2.3 mg/day (men) 1.8 mg/day (women)	Widely distributed in foods	Facilitates (with enzymes) many cell processes

Table 8.3
A Guide to Minerals (continued)

Deficiency Symptoms	Toxicity Symptoms
Stunted growth in children; bone loss (osteoporosis) in adults, heart failure, spasms	Mineral imbalances, shock, kidney failure, fatigue, mental confusion
Muscle weakness, bone pain, dizziness	Can create relative deficiency of calcium, spasms, convulsions
Weakness, confusion, muscle spasms, heart disease, high blood pressure, osteoporosis	Pharmacological overuse can cause nausea, cramps, dehydration, death
Muscle cramps, mental apathy, loss of appetite	Hypertension (in salt-sensitive persons), water retention, increased calcium loss
Dangerous changes in pH, irregular heartbeat	Vomiting
Muscle weakness, paralysis, confusion, can cause death, accompanies dehydration	Causes muscular weakness; triggers vomiting; if given into a vein, can stop the heart; irregular heartbeat
Goiter, cretinism, hypothyroidism	Goiter, enlargement of thyroid gland
Anemia: weakness, pallor, headaches, reduced resistance to infection, inability to concentrate	Nausea, vomiting, dizziness, rapid heartbeat, damage to organs, death
Growth failure in children, delayed development of sexual organs, loss of taste, poor wound healing, hair loss	Fever, nausea, vomiting, diarrhea, headaches, depressed immune function
Anemia, bone changes (rare in human beings)	Liver damage if a result of Wilson's disease, otherwise, nausea, diarrhea, vomiting
Susceptibility to tooth decay and bone loss	Fluorosis (discoloration of teeth), joint pain, stiffness
Keshan disease, Kashin-Ber disease, impaired immune function, infertility, depression, muscle pain	Vomiting, nausea, rash, brittle hair and nails, cirrhosis of liver
Diabetes-like condition marked by inability to use glucose normally, elevated blood lipid levels, damage to brain/nervous system	Unknown as a nutrition disorder. Occupational exposures damage skin and kidneys.
Unknown	Enzyme inhibition
Impaired reproduction and growth, reduced bone density, impaired glucose and lipid metabolism, rash	Nervous system disorders causing spasms and tremors

Note: RDA = Recommended Daily Allowance. AI = Adequate Intakes. Values are for adults aged 19 and older, except as noted.

Source: Adapted from J. Thompson and M. Manore, *Nutrition: An Applied Approach* (San Francisco: Benjamin Cummings, 2005). Reprinted by permission of Pearson Education, Inc.

Because calcium intake is so important throughout life for maintaining strong bones, it is critical to consume the minimum required amount each day. Over half of our calcium intake usually comes from milk, one of the highest sources. Calcium-fortified orange juice and soy milk provide a good way to get calcium if you do not drink dairy milk. Many green, leafy vegetables are good sources of calcium, but some contain oxalic acid, which makes their calcium harder to absorb. Spinach, chard, and beet greens are not particularly good sources of calcium, whereas broccoli, cauliflower, and many peas and beans offer good supplies (pinto beans and soybeans are among the best). Many nuts, particularly almonds, Brazil nuts, and hazelnuts, and seeds such as sunflower and sesame contain good amounts of calcium. Molasses is fairly high in calcium, and some fruits—citrus, figs, raisins, and dried apricots—have moderate amounts. Bone meal is not a recommended calcium source due to possible contamination.

Do you consume carbonated soft drinks? Be aware that the added phosphoric acid (phosphate) in these drinks can cause you to excrete extra calcium, which may result in calcium being pulled out of your bones. Calcium-phosphorus imbalance may lead to kidney stones and other calcification problems, as well as to increased atherosclerotic plaque.

We also know that sunlight increases the manufacture of vitamin D in the body and is therefore like having an extra calcium source because vitamin D improves absorption of calcium. Stress, on the other hand, depletes calcium. It is generally best to take calcium throughout the day, consuming it with foods containing protein, vitamin D, and vitamin C for optimum absorption. Experts vary on which type of supplemental calcium is most readily and efficiently absorbed, although aspartate and citrate salts of calcium are often recommended. As with all nutrients, the best way to obtain calcium is to consume it as part of a balanced diet.

Iron   Worldwide, iron deficiency is the most common nutrient deficiency, affecting more than 1 billion people. In developing countries, more than one-third of the children and women of childbearing age suffer from *iron-deficiency anemia*.[48] In the United States iron-deficiency anemia is less prevalent but still affects 10 percent of toddlers, adolescent girls, and women of childbearing age, making prevention a high priority.[49] In addition to suffering from **anemia,** a problem resulting from the body's inability to produce hemoglobin (the bright red, oxygen-carrying component of the

blood), people with iron-deficiency anemia may develop a condition known as **pica,** an appetite for ice, clay, paste, and other nonfood substances that do not actually contain iron and, in fact, may inhibit iron absorption.

How much iron do we need? Females aged 19 to 50 need about 18 mg per day, and males aged 19 to 50 need about 10 mg.

When iron deficiency occurs, body cells receive less oxygen, and carbon dioxide wastes are removed less efficiently. As a result, the iron-deficient person feels tired and run down. While iron deficiency in the diet is a common cause of anemia, it can also result from blood loss, cancers, ulcers, and other conditions. Generally, women are more likely to develop iron-deficiency problems because they typically eat less than men and their diets contain less iron. Women having heavy menstrual flow may be at greater risk.

Considerable research has linked iron to a host of problems. Iron deficiency may tax the immune system, causing it to function less effectively. Research suggesting a link between cardiovascular disease and elevated iron stores is inconclusive.[50] Likewise, although there appears to be a slight association between iron deficiency and cancer, the mechanism remains inconclusive.[51]

Iron overload (known as **hemochromatosis**), or iron toxicity due to ingesting too many iron-containing supplements, remains the leading cause of accidental poisoning in small children in the United States. Symptoms of toxicity include nausea, vomiting, diarrhea, rapid heartbeat, weak pulse, dizziness, shock, and confusion. As few as five iron tablets containing as little as 200 mg of iron have killed dozens of children.

Can Food Have Medicinal Value?

The old adage "you are what you eat" is indeed a motto to live by. Beneficial foods are termed *functional foods* based on the ancient belief that eating the right foods may not only prevent disease, but also actually cure it. This perspective is gaining credibility among the scientific community. (It is also important to be aware of potential interactions between the medications you take and the foods you eat; see Table 8.4.)

Two major studies, the *Dietary Approaches to Stop Hypertension (DASH) Study* and the *Dietary Intervention Study (DIS),* provide compelling evidence that diet may be as effective as drugs in bringing borderline hypertension back to the normal range. Diet may also play a role in reducing cholesterol and controlling type 1 (insulin-dependent) diabetes.[52] In these clinically controlled trials, subjects were assigned to two groups: treatment and control. In the treatment group, subjects had to follow recommended diets, which were low in fats and high in fiber and fruits. The control group followed typical American dietary intervention. In each study, subjects in the treatment groups showed significantly improved health indicators (blood pressure, cholesterol, and blood glucose in the DIS study), which reflected the potential

Anemia   Iron-deficiency disease that results from the body's inability to produce hemoglobin.

Pica   Iron-deficiency disease characterized by craving for certain foods and substances.

Hemochromatosis   Iron toxicity due to excess consumption.

Table 8.4
Common Food-Medication Interactions

Interactions are listed by drug category, followed by examples of specific medications (with generic and brand names). As always, alert your physician and pharmacist to any over-the-counter medications, herbal remedies, and supplements you are taking.

Medications	Interactions with Foods/Nutrients	What to Do
Antibiotics ciprofloxacin (Cipro) doxycycline (Vibramycin) minocycline (Minocin) tetracycline (Achromycin-V, Surrycin) penicillin (Ledercillin)	• Calcium and iron bind with these drugs, which inhibits absorption of the drug plus the calcium and iron. Results in less antibiotic effect, which risks the possibility that the bacteria causing the infection will not be killed. • Food slows down absorption of the drug.	• Do not take within three hours of taking calcium-containing antacids, iron supplements or multivitamin/minerals. • Do not take ciprofloxacin or tetracycline with foods rich in calcium, such as milk and other dairy products. • Take an hour before or two hours after eating.
Cardiovascular Medications ***ACE Inhibitors*** captopril (Capoten) enalapril (Vasotec) lisinopril (Prinivil, Zestril) moexipril (Univasc)	• Some ACE inhibitors cause hyperkalemia (elevated blood potassium). • Licorice can disrupt potassium balance. • Chili pepper worsens persistent cough side effect. • Food decreases absorption of captopril and moexipril.	• Limit potassium-rich foods and salt substitutes containing potassium. • Avoid natural licorice. • Avoid chili pepper. • Take captopril, moexipril an hour before or two hours after eating.
Blood Thinners warfarin (Coumadin)	• Vitamin K reduces the effectiveness of anticoagulants. If you maintain a consistent intake of vitamin K, your doctor can adjust your medication level accordingly.	• Keep a consistent intake of vitamin K–rich foods: broccoli, spinach, kale, turnip greens, Swiss chard, cauliflower, brussels sprouts, asparagus, beet, and chicken liver.
Calcium Channel Blockers amlodipine (Norvasc) felodipine (Plendil) nifedipine (Adalat, Procardia)	• Licorice can increase potassium excretion and sodium reabsorption and raise blood pressure. • Grapefruit can increase blood levels of these drugs up to twofold, which causes blood pressure to drop dangerously low.	• Avoid natural licorice. • Avoid grapefruit, grapefruit juice, and Seville oranges.
HMG-CoA Reductase Inhibitors ("statins") atorvastatin (Lipitor) lovastatin (Mevacor) simvastatin (Zocor)	• Grapefruit significantly increases blood levels of the drug, which causes more side effects or toxicity. • Soluble fiber inhibits absorption of lovastatin. • Lovastatin is best absorbed with a big meal containing fat. Works best when asleep.	• Avoid grapefruit, grapefruit juice, and Seville oranges. • Don't eat foods rich in fiber, oat bran, or pectin within several hours of taking lovastatin. • If taken once a day, take lovastatin with the evening meal.
Diuretics ***Potassium-Losing Diuretics*** furosemide (Lasix) hydrochlorothiazide (HydroDIURIL)	• Cause a loss of potassium and magnesium, which require extra potassium and magnesium in the diet or supplements. A potassium deficiency can trigger a heart attack. • Licorice can cause a loss of potassium.	• Eat plenty of potassium-rich foods; apricots, bananas, cantaloupe, dairy foods, dried beans, lentils, oranges, tomatoes. • Eat magnesium-rich foods: bananas, dried beans, lentils, nuts. • Avoid natural licorice.

(continues)

Note: oz = ounces, mg = milligram

Table 8.4
Common Food-Medication Interactions (continued)

Medications	Interactions with Foods/Nutrients	What to Do
Potassium-Sparing Diuretics spironolactone (Aldactone)	• Prevent kidneys from excreting potassium. Taking in too much potassium can cause irregular heartbeat. • Licorice can disrupt potassium balance.	• Don't overdo foods rich in potassium. • Avoid salt substitutes that contain potassium. • Avoid natural licorice.
Psychotherapeutic Medications buspirone (Buspar)—treats anxiety	• Grapefruit significantly increases blood levels of the drug.	• Avoid grapefruit, grapefruit juice, and Seville oranges.
Mononamine Oxidase Inhibitors (MAOIs) isocarboxazid (Marplan) phenelzine (Nardil) tranylcypromine (Parnate)	• Combining with too much caffeine, beer or wine (even alcohol-free) or foods rich in tyramine can lead to a dangerous increase in blood pressure.	• Avoid excessive caffeine; use with caution. • Avoid foods rich in tyramine: aged cheeses and meats, beer, fava beans, sauerkraut, soy sauce, wine. Use small amounts of beer (one or two 12-oz. bottles a day) and wine (2–4 oz. a day) with caution.
Other Medications cilostazol (Pletal)—treats circulatory conditions colchicine—treats gout levodopa (Dopar, Larodopa, Sinemet)—treats Parkinson's disease theophylline (Slo-bid, Theobid, Elixophyllin, Theo-Dur, Uniphyl)—treats asthma and other pulmonary disorders.	• Grapefruit significantly increases blood levels of the drug, which causes increased side effects or drug toxicity. • Grapefruit significantly increases blood levels of the drug. • Vitamin B_6 decreases effectiveness of the drug. Keep vitamin B_6 intake to less than 5 mg a day. • Caffeine increases theophylline's side effects: dizziness, nausea, vomiting, convulsions, or coma. • Black pepper and chili pepper increase drug blood levels. • Amount of protein and carbohydrate in diet can alter enzyme levels that affect theophylline breakdown.	• Avoid grapefruit, grapefruit juice, and Seville oranges. • Avoid grapefruit, grapefruit juice, and Seville oranges. • Limit foods rich in vitamin B_6: chicken, fish, pork, liver, and kidney. Go easy on legumes, nuts, and whole grains. • Avoid excessive caffeine (e.g., coffee, tea, cola). • Avoid excessive black pepper or chili pepper. • Keep intake of protein and carbohydrate consistent to keep drug levels consistent.

Note: oz. = ounces, mg = milligram

Sources: From "Foods Too, Can Interfere with Medications, If You're Not Careful," by Kerry Neville. Reprinted with permission from *Environmental Nutrition* (November 2001), 52 Riverside Drive, Suite 15A, New York, NY 10024. For subscription information, 800-829-5384; www.environmentalnutrition.com; data from *Food Medication Interactions,* 12th ed. (2002: available at 800-746-2324); Food & Drug Interactions (Food and Drug Administration with National Consumers League, 1998; online updated 2000, available at http://vm.cfsan.fda.gov/~lrd/fdinter.html); interviews with Zaneta Pronsky, MS, RD, FADA, Sr. Jeanne Crowe, Pharm D., RPh, and Dean Elbe, Bsc.

benefits of diet in improving health and treating disease. Today, the DASH diet is widely recommended as a plan for reducing hypertension. See the National Heart, Lung, and Blood Institute website (www.nhlbi.nih.gov) for information on the diet and ongoing clinical trials.

Antioxidants Substances believed to protect active people from oxidative stress and resultant tissue damage at the cellular level.

Antioxidants and Your Health

Many people today believe that **antioxidants** are wonder nutrients that will prevent just about anything. While these substances do appear to protect people from the ravages of oxidative stress and resultant tissue damage at the cellular level, you may want to take a step back and consider all of the evidence. First, it is important to understand what *oxidative stress* really is. This damage occurs in a complex process in which *free radicals* (molecules with unpaired electrons that

Vitamin E: Have We Jumped the Gun?

For the past several years, sales of vitamin E have soared. Why? Some studies indicated that it might reduce the risk of heart disease. Even food manufacturers have gotten into the act. Kraft, for example, markets a line of salad dressing, boasting that it is "rich in vitamin E—for a healthy body."

However, people began to question the effectiveness of vitamin E when a highly regarded study reported that vitamin E doesn't appear to provide any protection against heart troubles. Researchers from Ontario concluded this after following 9,500 people aged 55 and older who were at high risk for cardiovascular "events," such as heart attacks. For nearly five years, half of the group was given 400 international units (IU) of vitamin E daily, while the other half took a placebo. In the end, there was no difference in their rates

of heart attack, stroke, or death from heart disease. There was no difference, either, in the frequency of other cardiovascular problems such as unstable angina or heart failure.

The Heart Outcomes Prevention Evaluation Study, or HOPE, as it has been dubbed, casts doubt on previous research that pointed to vitamin E as a hedge against heart attack. Those earlier studies indicated that people who eat foods rich in antioxidants such as vitamin E—particularly nuts, oils, and some vegetables—appear to have lower rates of heart disease. Animal studies in which vitamin E appeared to slow the development of atherosclerosis have also been promising. Two large studies from Harvard University particularly boosted hopes when they revealed that people who reported taking 100 IU of vitamin E per day had lower rates of heart trouble and less advanced damage to arteries.

One other study, nicknamed CHAOS (The Cambridge Heart Antioxidant Study), used the same rigorous methods as the HOPE trial did and found that people tak-

ing 400 to 800 IU of vitamin E significantly reduced their risk of heart attack. However, the average length of the subjects' participation was barely a year and a half, and many of the participants dropped out before conclusive results could be obtained.

The jury is still out on vitamin E. Because people in the HOPE study already had severe heart disease, people questioned the study's results. However, in November 2004, researcher Edgar Miller of Johns Hopkins University and others summarized the results of 19 trials. In striking contrast to previous reports, Miller discovered that not only was vitamin E not helping people live longer, but it may increase the risk of cardiovascular events. Clearly, there is cause for concern and more investigation is needed.

Source: E. Miller et al., "Meta-analysis: High Dosage Vitamin E Supplementation May Increase All-Cause Mortality," *Annals of Internal Medicine* 142, no. 1 (2005): 1–11; *Tufts University Health and Nutrition Letter* 18, by Tufts University © 2000 and reproduced by permission of Tufts University Health & Nutrition Letter.

---

are produced in excess when the body is overly stressed through exposure to toxic substances or events) either damage or kill healthy cells, cell proteins, or genetic material in the cells. Antioxidants produce enzymes that destroy excess free radicals by scavenging free radicals, slowing their formation, and/or actually repairing oxidative stress damage. Thus, the theory goes that if you consume lots of antioxidants, you will nullify or greatly reduce the negative effects of oxidative stress. Among the more commonly cited nutrients touted as providing a protective effect are vitamin C, vitamin E, beta-carotene and other carotenoids, and the mineral selenium.

How valid is the theory? To date, researchers have identified possible links between oxidative stress and over 200 diseases, such as arthritis, cancers, cardiovascular disease, Alzheimer's disease, kidney disease, and diabetes. However, many claims about the benefits of antioxidants in reducing risks of heart disease, improving vision, and slowing or reversing the aging process have not been fully investigated and are inconclusive. The consensus among nutrition experts is that these results are only preliminary. Much of the evidence is from epidemiological or observational studies, which suggest interesting possibilities, but have no specific

implications for individuals.[53] Research on vitamin C and cancer is mixed; many studies indicate that when people's diets include foods rich in vitamin C, they seem to develop fewer cancers, but other studies detect no effect from dietary vitamin C.[54] Part of the problem is that in foods, vitamin C occurs along with several other nutrients, often in foods that are high in fiber and low in fat. Separating out the positive effects of just one vitamin found in a healthy package is difficult.

Possibilities of a positive effect from vitamin E are even more controversial. It has long been theorized that many cancers result from DNA damage; and since vitamin E appears to protect against DNA damage, it would also cause reduced cancer risk. However, the great majority of studies demonstrate no effect and more recent studies may indicate potential harm from vitamin E. (See the New Horizons in Health box.) In July 2004, the American Heart Association released an advisory cautioning people to get their antioxidants from a balanced diet, rather than from supplements in pill form.

Certain minerals, including selenium, copper, zinc, iron, and magnesium also have shown promising results in trials where they are linked to a variety of health benefits. Like their vitamin cousins, much of this research continues to be controversial.

Beta-carotene is one of the many compounds classified as **carotenoids.** Carotenoids are part of the red, orange, and yellow pigments found in fruits and vegetables. They are fat soluble, transported in the blood by lipoproteins, and stored in the fatty tissues of the body. Beta-carotene, the most researched carotenoid, is a precursor of vitamin A. This means that vitamin A can be produced in the body from beta-carotene; like vitamin A, beta-carotene has antioxidant properties.[55]

Although there are over 600 carotenoids in nature, two that have received the most attention are *lycopene* (found in tomatoes, papaya, pink grapefruit, and guava) and *lutein* (found in green leafy vegetables such as spinach, broccoli, kale, and brussels sprouts). Both are believed to be more beneficial than beta-carotene in preventing disease.

The National Cancer Institute and the American Cancer Society have endorsed lycopene as a possible factor in reducing the risk of cancer. A landmark study assessing the effects of tomato-based foods reported that men who ate 10 or more servings of lycopene-rich foods per week had a 45 percent reduced risk of prostate cancer.[56] Subsequent research has indicated positive benefits of lycopene on other cancers and on heart disease.[57]

Lutein is most often touted as a means of protecting the eyes, particularly from age-related macular degeneration (ARMD), a leading cause of blindness for people aged 65 and over. Although researchers don't know for sure what causes ARMD, they do know that older age, light-colored eyes, smoking, and exposure to sunlight increase the risk. They speculate that oxidative damage may be the crux of the problem, and thus antioxidants may be a means of prevention.[58] Researchers at the National Eye Institute found that those with the highest blood levels of lutein and other antioxidants found in foods were 70 percent less likely to develop ARMD than those with the lowest levels. Researchers in the Nurses Health study found that eating spinach more than five days a week lowered risk by 47 percent and also lowered risk of cataracts.[59]

Other research points to additional potential benefits from lutein. A recent study by Tufts University and Korean investigators revealed a dramatic 88 percent drop in breast cancer in women who had the highest blood concentration of lutein. Researchers at the University of Utah Medical School found that the highest consumers of lutein had the lowest risk of colon cancer. In animals, lutein slowed the growth of breast tumors and, in test tubes, it killed cancer cells. Preliminary research has also shown a possible reduction in artery clogging among those consuming the highest amounts of lutein.[60]

According to the experts, the answer is moderation. "Antioxidants should always be taken as part of a well-balanced mixture, either as a diet or as a supplement, and not singly," says Dr. John R. Smythies, a researcher at the University of California–San Diego and author of *Every Person's Guide to Antioxidants*.[61] Smythies, like many other experts, advocates for balance in intake and advises that adults take daily 500 mg of vitamin C and 400 to 800 international units (IU) of vitamin E, plus 10 mg of beta-carotene. Researchers agree that intake should vary based on physical activity levels and overall health. Dr. Balz Frei at the Linus Pauling Institute indicates that the "200 rule" might be the best option. This recommendation calls for fruits and vegetables in the diet and a supplement of 200 mg of vitamin C, 200 IU of vitamin E, and 200 µg of selenium, along with 400 µg of folate and 3 mg of vitamin B_6 (pyridoxine).[62] Until research conclusively proves the benefit or harm, a moderate intake as part of a vegetable- and fruit-rich diet is desirable.

To find the right balance, keep in mind the following:

- Keep your daily vitamin C intake (from both food and supplements) below 2,000 mg. Higher amounts may cause diarrhea. Vitamin C also enhances iron absorption, making iron overload likely in some people.
- The upper limit for vitamin E, based only on supplements, is 1,000 milligrams. That's roughly equivalent to 1,500 IU of D-alpha-tocopherol, sometimes labeled *natural vitamin E*. More than this could increase risk of stroke and uncontrolled bleeding. Vitamin E can also worsen autoimmune diseases, such as asthma or rheumatoid arthritis.
- The maximum intake level for selenium from both food and supplements is 400 µg per day. Taking more could cause *selenosis,* a toxic reaction marked by hair loss and brittle nails.

Folate

In 1998, the FDA began requiring folate fortification of all bread, cereal, rice, and pasta sold in the United States. This practice, which will boost folate intake by an average of about 100 µg daily, is expected to decrease the number of infants born with spina bifida and other neural tube defects.

Folate is a form of vitamin B that is believed to protect against cardiovascular disease and decrease blood levels of *homocysteine,* an amino acid that has been linked to vascular diseases. Homocysteine results from the breakdown of methionine, an amino acid found in meat and other protein-laden foods. Two B vitamins—folate and B_6—are believed to control homocysteine levels.[63] When intake of folate and B_6 is low, homocysteine levels rise in the blood. Recent studies indicate that when the level of homocysteine rises, arterial

---

Carotenoids Fat-soluble compounds with antioxidant properties.

Folate A type of vitamin B that is believed to decrease levels of homocysteine, an amino acid that has been linked to vascular diseases.

Adding More Salads to Your Diet

Salads and healthful salad toppings add variety to your diet and balance out the average American's meat-and-potatoes diet. Use this information to choose healthful salad greens and toppings.

NUTRITIONAL COMPARISON OF SALAD GREEN SERVINGS

Salad Green	Calories	Vitamin A (IU)	Vitamin C (mg)	Potassium (mg)	Calcium (mg)
Arugula (rocket, roquette)	5	480	3	74	32
Butterhead lettuce (Boston, Bibb)	7	534	4	141	18
Cabbage, red	19	28	40	144	36
Endive	8	1,025	3	157	26
Iceberg lettuce	7	182	2	87	10
Leaf lettuce	10	1,064	10	148	38
Romaine lettuce	8	1,456	13	162	20
Spinach	7	2,015	8	167	30*

Note: Serving size is one cup; IU = international units, mg = milligrams

*Much not available to body for use.

NUTRITIONAL COMPARISON OF HEALTHFUL SALAD TOPPINGS

Topping	Serving Size	Calories	Bonus Nutrients
Artichoke hearts, in olive oil	1 heart	40	Fiber, folate, potassium, calcium
Avocado, California	¼ of whole fruit	77	Monounsaturated fats, vitamin E, folate, fiber
Beets	½ cup boiled	37	Folate, potassium
Broccoli	½ cup raw	12	Vitamins A and C, calcium, potassium, fiber
Carrots	½ cup raw	31	Vitamin A, beta-carotene, fiber
Cauliflower	½ cup raw	13	Vitamin C
Celery	½ cup raw	6	Vitamin C, potassium
Chicken breast	3 ounces white meat	173	Protein, niacin, vitamin B_6
Chickpeas (garbanzo beans)	½ cup boiled or canned	135	Protein, folate, calcium, potassium, zinc, fiber
Egg	1 whole	78	Vitamins A, E, B_{12}, and D, riboflavin, folate, selenium, zinc. Limit to one egg.
Mushrooms	½ cup	9	Riboflavin, niacin, potassium, selenium
Olives	5 small	20	Monounsaturated fats
Peppers, red, yellow, orange	½ cup raw	14	Vitamins A and C, beta-carotene, fiber
Sunflower seeds	1 ounce	160	Vitamins E, B_6, niacin, folate, copper, magnesium, zinc, fiber, linoleic acid
Tofu, processed with calcium sulfate	½ cup	94	Protein, calcium, iron, manganese
Tomatoes	½ tomato	13	Vitamins A, C, potassium, lycopene
Tuna, canned in water	3 ounces	99	Protein, niacin, omega-3 fatty acids

Source: From *"Salads: Going Beyond the Green to Boost Nutrition,"* by Andrea Platzman and "Nutrition Comparison of Healthful Salad Toppings," by Andrea Platzman. Reprinted with permission from *Environmental Nutrition* (August 2002), 52 Riverside Drive, Suite 15A, New York, NY 10024. For subscription information, 800-829-5384; www.environmentalnutrition.com

walls and blood platelets become sticky, which encourages clotting. (*Note:* Homocysteine levels tend to rise with age, smoking, and menopause.) When clots develop in areas already narrowed by atherosclerosis, a heart attack or stroke can result.

Although the amount of folate needed to protect the heart has not been determined, many people have jumped on the folate bandwagon, taking daily folate supplements of up to 800 µg. Recently, a new *dietary folate equivalent (DFE)* was established to distinguish folate in food from its synthetic counterpart, *folic acid.* As a food additive or a supplement, folic acid is absorbed about twice as efficiently as folate. The DFE for folate in women aged 19 or over is approximately 400 µg, with higher levels for pregnant or lactating women. (See Table 8.2 for daily recommended amounts of other B vitamins.) Potential dangers of taking too much folate include masking of B_{12} (cobalamin) deficiencies and resulting problems, ranging from nerve damage, immunodeficiency problems, anemia, fatigue, and headache, to constipation, diarrhea, weight loss, gastrointestinal disturbances, and a host of neurological symptoms.[64]

Gender and Nutrition

Men and women differ in body size, body composition, and overall metabolic rates. Not surprisingly, they have differing needs for most nutrients throughout the life cycle and face unique difficulties in keeping on track with their dietary goals. We have already discussed some of these differences. However, there are some factors that need further consideration. Have you ever wondered why men can eat more than women without gaining weight? Although there are many possible reasons, one factor is that women have a lower ratio of lean body mass to adipose (fatty) tissue at all ages and stages of life. Also, after sexual maturation, the rate of metabolism is higher in men, meaning that they will burn more calories doing the same activities.

Different Cycles, Different Needs

In addition to these differences, women have many more "landmark" times in life when their nutritional needs vary significantly from requirements at other times. From menarche to menopause, women undergo cyclical physiological changes that can exert dramatic effects on metabolism and nutritional needs. For example, during pregnancy and lactation, women's nutritional requirements increase substantially. Those who are unable to follow the strict dietary recommendations of their doctors may find themselves gaining much more weight during pregnancy and retaining it afterwards. During the menstrual cycle, many women report significant food cravings. Later in life, with the advent of menopause, nutritional needs again change rather dramatically. With depletion of the hormone estrogen, the body's need for

calcium to ward off bone deterioration becomes pronounced. Women must pay closer attention to exercising and getting enough calcium through diet or dietary supplements, or they run the risk of osteoporosis (see Chapter 19).

Changing the "Meat-and-Potatoes" American

Since our earliest agrarian years, many Americans—especially men—have relied on a "meat-and-potatoes" diet. What's wrong with all those hot dogs, steaks, hamburgers, and french fries? Heart disease, stroke, and cancer are probably the greatest threats. Add increased risk for colon and prostate cancers, and the rationale for dietary change becomes even more compelling. Consider the following points:

- Heavy red meat eaters are more than twice as likely to get prostate cancer and nearly five times more likely to develop colon cancer.
- For every three servings of fruits or vegetables they consume per day, men can expect a 22 percent lower risk of stroke.
- Diets high in fruit and vegetables may lower the risk of lung cancer in smokers from 20 times the risk of nonsmokers to "only" 10 times the risk. They may also protect against oral, throat, pancreatic, and bladder cancers, all of which are more common among smokers.
- The fastest-rising malignancy in the United States is cancer of the lower esophagus, particularly among white men. Though obesity seems to be a factor, fruits and vegetables are the protectors. (The average American male eats fewer than three servings per day, although five to nine servings are recommended. Women average three to seven servings per day.)

Does something in meat make it inherently bad? The fat content of meat and fried potatoes and the potential carcinogenic substances produced through cooking have been implicated. Probably something more basic is also involved. By eating so much protein, a person fills up sooner and never gets around to the fruits and vegetables. Thus, the potential protective value of consuming these foods is lost. Use the information in the Skills for Behavior Change box on page 253 to incorporate more salads into a meat-and-potatoes diet.

What do you think?

Think about the women you know who seem to have weight problems. How old are they? ■ *What factors may have influenced them to have problems keeping weight off?* ■ *What factors do men have to deal with in controlling their eating and managing their weight?*

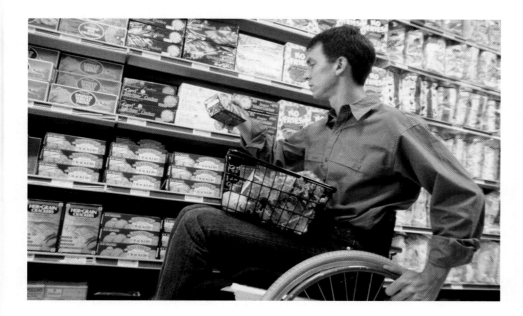

Reading food labels before you purchase products will help you understand your nutritional options.

Determining Your Nutritional Needs

Determining the right amount of a given nutrient can be a challenging task. Since the early 1940s, various committees have devised several standards for nutritional needs. These are constantly revised as the science changes, so consumers must continue to be informed. The most familiar dietary guidelines are:

Recommended Dietary Allowances (RDAs), which were originally established by the National Academy of Sciences' Food and Nutrition board in the early 1940s. First designed to prevent nutritional deficiencies, these standards have been revised periodically to reflect changes in nutrition science. In recent years, as deficiencies that lead to disease conditions have declined, the RDAs have taken on more of a prevention focus. For example, calcium requirements have steadily been increased to reflect concerns about osteoporosis. In the late 1990s, the Food and Nutrition board added these new mechanisms for assessing dietary needs:

Adequate Intake (AI) recommendations are a best estimate of what nutritional needs are likely to be for most people when there hasn't been enough research conducted to fully determine an RDA for a specific nutrient.

Tolerable Upper Intake Level (UL) is the highest amount of a nutrient that an individual can safely consume every day without risking adverse health effects.

After a careful analysis of RDAs and the new AI and UL values, Canadian and U.S. researchers developed the **Dietary Reference Intake (DRI),** a new, combined listing of over 26 essential vitamins and minerals.[65] Although you seldom see the DRI on labels, these are the guidelines recommended for healthy adults and are more comprehensive than RDAs

alone because they indicate likely recommendations for nutrients that are currently being studied. Essentially, DRI should be considered the umbrella guidelines under which RDA, AI, and UL will fall.[66]

Reading Labels for Health   To help consumers choose between similar types of food products that can be incorporated into a healthy diet, the FDA and the U.S. Department of Agriculture developed the **U.S. Recommended Daily Allowances (USRDA)** as a spin-off of RDA recommendations in 1973. The first voluntary food labels with USRDAs were a part of this action. Eventually, in response to consumer demand, the USDA issued mandatory guidelines for food labeling in 1993.[67] These new, mandatory guidelines generally

Recommended Dietary Allowances (RDAs)   The average daily intakes of energy and nutrients considered adequate to meet the needs of most healthy people in the United States under usual conditions.

Adequate Intake (AI)   Best estimates of nutritional needs.

Tolerable Upper Intake Level (UL)   The highest amount of a nutrient that an individual can safely consume every day without risking adverse health effects.

Dietary Reference Intake (DRI)   A new, combined listing of over 26 essential vitamins and minerals developed by Canadian and U.S. researchers.

U.S. Recommended Daily Allowances (USRDA) Dietary guidelines developed by the Food and Drug Administration (FDA) and the United States Department of Agriculture.

Nutrition Facts

Serving Size 1 cup (228g)
Servings Per Container 2

Amount Per Serving

Calories 250   Calories from Fat 110

% Daily Value*

Total Fat 12g	**18%**
Saturated Fat 3g	**15%**
Trans Fat 1.5g	
Cholesterol 30mg	**10%**
Sodium 470 mg	**20%**
Total Carbohydrate 31g	**10%**
Dietary Fiber 0g	**0%**
Sugars 5g	
Protein 5g	

Vitamin A	4%
Vitamin C	2%
Calcium	20%
Iron	4%

* Percent Daily Values are based on a 2,000 calorie diet.
Your Daily Values may be higher or lower depending on
your calorie needs:

	Calories:	2,000	2,500
Total Fat	Less than	65g	80g
Sat Fat	Less than	20g	25g
Cholesterol	Less than	300mg	300mg
Sodium	Less than	2,400mg	2,400mg
Total Carbohydrate		300g	375g
Dietary Fiber		25g	30g

Start here

Limit these
nutrients

Quick guide to % DV:
5% or less is low
20% or more is high

Get enough
of these
nutrients

Footnote

Figure 8.7
Reading a Food Label

Source: Center for Food Safety and Applied Nutrition, "Questions
and Answers about *Trans* Fat Nutrition Labeling," 2004,
www.cfsan.fda.gov/~dms/qatrans2.html

Reference Daily Intakes (RDIs)   Recommended
amounts of 19 vitamins and minerals, also known as micronutrients.

Daily Reference Values (DRVs)   Recommended
amounts for micronutrients such as total fat, saturated fat,
and cholesterol.

Daily Values (DVs)   The RDIs and DRVs together make
up the Daily Values seen on food and supplement labels.

Vegetarian   A term with a variety of meanings: vegans
avoid all foods of animal origin; lacto-vegetarians avoid
flesh foods but eat dairy products; ovo-vegetarians
avoid flesh foods but eat eggs; lacto-ovo-vegetarians avoid
flesh foods but eat both dairy products and eggs; pesco-
vegetarians avoid meat but eat fish, dairy products, and
eggs; semivegetarians eat chicken, fish, dairy products,
and eggs.

replaced USRDAs with **Reference Daily Intakes (RDIs)** and
Daily Reference Values (DRVs). RDIs are the recommended
amounts of 19 vitamins and minerals, also known as micronutrients, and DRVs are the recommended amounts for
macronutrients, such as total fat, saturated fat, cholesterol,
total carbohydrates, dietary fiber, sodium, potassium, and
protein.

Together, RDIs and DRVs make up the **Daily Values
(DV)** that you will find on food and supplement labels listed
as a percentage (% DV); see Figure 8.7 for an example.
When you look at a label with a % DV listing, you can tell
what percentage of a nutrient is found in a serving of food.
Although % DV has become widely accepted, it should be
noted that it is not as up to date as RDA or DRIs. Although
DVs will eventually be updated, they also do not reflect the
different needs of older adults, people with conditions such
as pregnancy, or gender differences. Advocates of the DV
system argue that there isn't enough room for such information on labels, and a basic, easy-to-understand system
works best.

Vegetarianism: Eating for Health

For ethical, economic, personal, health, cultural, or religious
reasons, some people choose specialized diets. Between
5 and 15 percent of all Americans today identify themselves
as vegetarians. Normally, vegetarianism provides a superb
alternative to our high-fat, high-calorie, meat-based cuisine,
but without proper information and food choices, vegetarians
can also develop serious dietary problems.

The term **vegetarian** means different things to different people. Strict vegetarians, or *vegans,* avoid all foods of
animal origin, including dairy products and eggs. Vegans
must be careful to obtain all of the necessary nutrients. Far
more common are *lacto-vegetarians,* who eat dairy products
but avoid flesh foods. Their diet can be low in fat and cholesterol but only if they consume skim milk and other low-fat or
nonfat products. *Ovo-vegetarians* add eggs to their diet, while
lacto-ovo-vegetarians eat both dairy products and eggs. *Pesco-
vegetarians* eat fish, dairy products, and eggs, while *semivegetarians* eat chicken, fish, dairy products, and eggs. Some
people in the semivegetarian category prefer to call themselves "non–red meat eaters."

Generally, people who follow a balanced vegetarian
diet weigh less and have better cholesterol levels, fewer
problems with irregular bowel movements (constipation and
diarrhea), and a lower risk of heart disease than do nonveg-
etarians. Some preliminary evidence suggests that vegetarians may also have a reduced risk for colon and breast
cancer.[68] Whether these lower risks are due to the vegetarian diet per se or to some combination of lifestyle variables
remains unclear.

Although in the past vegetarians often suffered from
vitamin deficiencies, the vegetarian of the new millennium

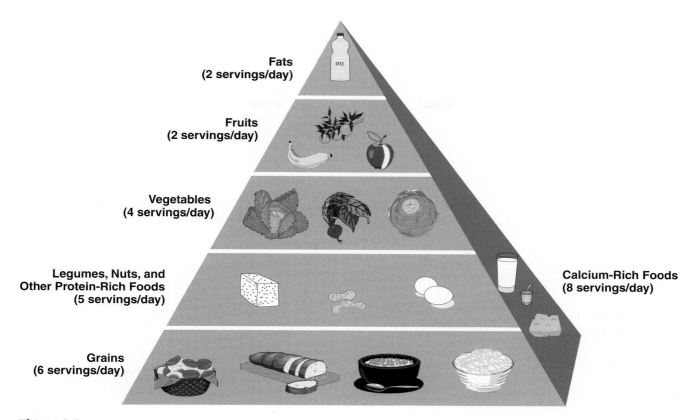

Figure 8.8

The Vegetarian Food Guide Pyramid

Vegetarians should eat the suggested number of servings from each group daily for a balanced diet.

Source: V. Messina, V. Melina, and A. R. Mangels, "A New Food Guide for North American Vegetarians," *Journal of the American Dietetic Association* 103, no. 6 (2003): 771. Reprinted with permission from American Dietetic Association.

is usually extremely adept at combining the right types of foods to ensure proper nutrient intake. People who eat dairy products and small amounts of chicken or fish are seldom nutrient-deficient; in fact, while vegans typically get 50 to 60 g of protein per day, lacto-ovo-vegetarians normally consume between 70 and 90 g per day, well beyond the RDA. Vegan diets may be deficient in riboflavin (vitamin B_2), B_{12}, and D. Riboflavin is found mainly in meat, eggs, and dairy products; but broccoli, asparagus, almonds, and fortified cereals are also good sources. Vitamins B_{12} and D are found only in dairy products and fortified products such as soy milk. Vegans are also at risk for deficiencies of calcium, iron, zinc, and other minerals but can obtain these nutrients from supplements. Strict vegans have to pay much more attention to what they eat than the average person does; but, by eating complementary combinations of plant products, they can receive adequate amounts of essential amino acids. Examples of complementary combinations are corn and beans, and peanut butter and whole-grain bread. Eating a full variety of grains, legumes, fruits, vegetables, and seeds each day will keep even the strictest vegetarian in excellent health.

Pregnant women, the elderly, the sick, and children who are vegans need to take special care to ensure that their diets are adequate. People who take part in heavy aerobic exercise programs (over three hours per week) may need to increase their protein consumption. In all cases, seek advice from a health care professional if you have questions.

The Vegetarian Pyramid

The American Dietetic Association has developed a food guide pyramid that conveys the essentials of a vegetarian diet (Figure 8.8). Modeled after the USDA Food Guide Pyramid discussed earlier in this chapter, the vegetarian version clarifies what people who don't eat meat need to do to stay healthy. The vegetarian pyramid defines the following categories. We include examples of single servings in each category:

Grains (6 servings/day)
- 1 slice bread
- 1 ounce cold cereal
- $1/2$ cup cooked cereal, rice, or pasta

**Legumes, nuts and other protein-rich foods
(5 servings/day)**

- ¹/₂ cup cooked dry beans, peas, or lentils
- 1 egg
- ¹/₂ cup bean curd or tofu
- 2 tablespoons peanut butter
- 1 ounce meat substitute
- ¹/₄ cup nuts

Vegetables (4 servings/day)

- ¹/₂ cup cooked vegetables
- 1 cup raw vegetables
- ¹/₂ cup vegetable juice

Fruits (2 servings/day)

- 1 medium whole piece of fruit
- ¹/₂ cup chopped or cooked fruit
- ¹/₂ cup fruit juice
- ¹/₄ cup dried fruit

Calcium-rich foods (8 servings/day)

- ¹/₂ cup fortified fruit juice
- 5 figs
- 1 cup cooked or 2 cups raw bok choy, broccoli, collards, Chinese cabbage, kale, mustard greens, or okra
- ¹/₂ cup fortified tomato juice
- ¹/₂ cup cow's milk, yogurt, or fortified soy milk
- ³/₄ ounce cheese
- ¹/₂ cup tempeh or calcium-set tofu
- ¹/₄ cup almonds
- 2 tablespoons almond butter or sesame tahini
- ¹/₂ cup cooked soy beans
- ¹/₄ cup soy nuts
- 1 ounce calcium-fortified cold cereal

Fats (2 servings/day)

- 1 teaspoon oil, mayonnaise, or soft margarine

What do you think?

Why are so many people today becoming vegetarians? ■ *How easy is it to be a vegetarian on your campus?* ■ *What concerns about vegetarianism would you be likely to have, if any?*

Improved Eating for the College Student

College students often face a challenge when trying to eat healthy foods. Some students live in dorms and do not have their own cooking or refrigeration facilities. Others live in crowded apartments where everyone forages in the refrigerator for everyone else's food. Still others eat at university food services where food choices may be limited. And nearly all

of them have financial and time constraints that make buying, preparing, and eating healthy food a difficult task. What's a student to do?

Fast Foods: Eating on the Run

If your campus is like many others, you've probably noticed a distinct move toward fast-food restaurants in your student unions so that they now resemble the food courts found in shopping malls. These new eating centers fit students' needs for a fast bite of food at a reasonable price between classes and also bring in money to your school. But many fast foods are high in fat and sodium. Are they all unhealthy?

Not all fast foods are created equal, and not all are bad for you. Even at the often-maligned burger chains, menus are healthier than ever before and offer excellent choices for the discriminating eater. The key word here is *discriminating.* It really is possible to eat healthy fast food if you follow these suggestions:

- Ask for nutritional analyses of items. Most fast-food chains now have them; check their websites, or ask at your local outlet.
- Avoid mayonnaise, sauces, and other add-ons. Some places even have fat-free mayonnaise if you ask. Put a hold on extra ketchup.
- Hold the cheese. This extra contributes substantially to total fat while not adding a lot to taste.
- Order single, small burgers rather than large, high-calorie, bacon- or cheese-topped choices. Put on your own ketchup, and keep portions small.
- Order salads and be careful how much dressing you put on. Many people think they are being health-smart by eating salad, only to load it with calorie- and fat-rich dressing. Try the vinegar and oil or low-fat alternative dressings. Stay away from eggs and other high-fat add-ons such as bacon bits.
- When ordering a chicken sandwich, order the skinless broiled version rather than the deep-fried version. Many people think that the deep-fried chicken sandwich is a more healthy choice when it really has more fat than the loaded double burger.
- Check to see what type of oil is used to cook fries if you must have them. Avoid lard-based or other saturated fat products.
- Order wheat buns or bread, and ask them to hold the butter.
- Avoid fried foods in general, including hot apple pies and other crust-based fried foods.
- Opt for places where foods tend to be broiled rather than fried.
- Avoid the giant sizes whenever possible and refrain from ordering extra sauces, bacon, and other extras that add additional calories and fat.

For more tips on healthy restaurant food, see the Reality Check box.

What's Good on the Menu?

While some restaurants offer hints for health-conscious diners, you're on your own most of the time. To help you order wisely, here are lighter options and high-fat pitfalls. "Best" choices contain fewer than 30 grams (g) of fat, a generous meal's worth for an active, medium-size woman. "Worst" choices have up to 100 g of fat.

FAST FOOD

Best	Grilled chicken sandwich Roast beef sandwich Single hamburger Salad with light vinaigrette
Worst	Bacon burger Double cheeseburger French fries Onion rings
Tips	Order sandwiches without mayo or "special sauce." Avoid deep-fried items like fish fillets, chicken nuggets, and French fries.

ITALIAN

Best	Pasta with red or white clam sauce Spaghetti with marinara or tomato-and-meat sauce
Worst	Eggplant parmigiana Fettuccine alfredo Fried calamari Lasagna
Tips	Stick with plain bread instead of garlic bread made with butter or oil. Ask for the waiter's help in avoiding cream- or egg-based sauces. Try vegetarian pizza, and don't ask for extra cheese.

MEXICAN

Best	Bean burrito (no cheese) Chicken fajitas
Worst	Beef chimichanga Chile relleno
	Quesadilla Refried beans
Tips	Choose soft tortillas (not fried) with fresh salsa, not guacamole. Special-order grilled shrimp, fish, or chicken. Ask for beans made without lard or fat and for cheeses and sour cream provided on the side or left out altogether.

CHINESE

Best	Hot-and-sour soup Stir-fried vegetables Shrimp with garlic sauce Szechuan shrimp Wonton soup
Worst	Crispy chicken Kung pao chicken Moo shu pork Sweet-and-sour pork
Tips	Share a stir-fry; help yourself to steamed rice. Ask for vegetables steamed or stir-fried with less oil. Order moo shu vegetables instead of pork. Avoid fried rice, breaded dishes, egg rolls and spring rolls, and items loaded with nuts. Avoid high-sodium sauces.

JAPANESE

Best	Steamed rice and vegetables Tofu as a substitute for meat Broiled or steamed chicken and fish
Worst	Fried rice dishes Miso (very high in sodium) Tempura
Tips	Avoid soy sauces. Use caution in eating sashimi and sushi (raw fish) dishes to avoid possible bacteria or parasites.

THAI

Best	Clear broth soups Stir-fried chicken and vegetables Grilled meats
Worst	Coconut milk Peanut sauces Deep-fried dishes
Tips	Avoid coconut-based curries. Ask for steamed, not fried, rice.

BREAKFAST

Best	Hot or cold cereal with 2% milk Pancakes or French toast with syrup Scrambled eggs with hash browns and plain toast
Worst	Belgian waffle with sausage Sausage and eggs with biscuits and gravy Ham and cheese omelette with hash browns and toast
Tips	Ask for whole-grain cereal or shredded wheat with 1% milk or whole-wheat toast without butter or margarine. Order omelettes without cheese, fried eggs without bacon or sausage.

SANDWICHES

Best	Ham and Swiss cheese Roast beef Turkey
Worst	Tuna salad Reuben Submarine
Tips	Ask for mustard; hold the mayo and cheese. See if turkey-ham is available.

SEAFOOD

Best	Broiled bass, halibut, or snapper Grilled scallops Steamed crab or lobster
Worst	Fried seafood platter Blackened catfish
Tips	Order fish broiled, baked, grilled, or steamed—not pan-fried or sauteed. Ask for lemon instead of tartar sauce. Avoid creamy and buttery sauces.

Sources: American Dietetic Association, 2002, www.eatright.org; *Health* 10 (November/December 1996): 79.

When Funds Are Short

Maintaining a nutritious diet within the confines of student life can be challenging. However, if you take the time to plan healthy meals, you will find that you are eating better, enjoying it more, and actually saving money. Follow these steps to ensure a healthy but affordable diet:

- Buy fruits and vegetables in season whenever possible for their lower cost, higher nutrient quality, and greater variety.
- Use coupons and specials to get price reductions.
- Shop at discount warehouse food chains; capitalize on volume discounts and no-frills products.
- Plan ahead to get the most for your dollar and avoid extra trips to the store; extra trips usually mean extra purchases. Make a list and stick to it.
- Purchase meats and other products in volume, freezing portions for future needs. Or purchase small amounts of meat and combine it with beans and plant proteins for lower cost, calories, and fat.
- Cook large meals, and freeze small portions for later.
- Drain off extra fat after cooking. Save juices/broths to use in soups and other dishes.
- If you find that you have no money for food, talk to staff at your county or city health department. They may know of ways for you to get assistance.

What do you think?

What problems cause you the most difficulty when you try to eat more healthful foods? ■ *Are these problems typical in your family, or are they unique to your current situation as a student?* ■ *What actions can you take to improve your current eating practices?*

Supplements: New Research on the Daily Dose

For years, health experts touted the benefits of eating a balanced diet over popping a vitamin and mineral supplement. In fact, we were told that supplements were rarely necessary in the United States and that if we chose to pop those pills, most of their water-soluble content would simply replenish the nutrient supplies of our underground sewer systems.

So eyebrows were raised when an article in the esteemed *Journal of the American Medical Association (JAMA)* broke with tradition and recommended that "a vitamin/mineral supplement a day just might be important in keeping the doctor away, particularly for some groups of people."[69] Essentially, the article indicated that elderly people, vegans, alcohol-dependent individuals, and patients with malabsorption problems may be at particular risk of deficiency of several vitamins. Although it acknowledged that there may be a risk if you overdose on fat-soluble vitamins, it noted that preliminary research has linked inadequate amounts of nutrients such as vitamins B_6, B_{12}, D, E, and lycopene to chronic diseases, including coronary heart disease, cancer, and osteoporosis. As a result of this study, *JAMA* indicated that all adults should take a basic multivitamin.

However, according to Dr. David Bender, writing in the *British Medical Journal*,[70] the *JAMA* review article produced little convincing evidence in favor of supplements. According to Dr. Bender, if our dietary intake is adequate, supplements will probably do us little good. Surely there will be much more controversy over supplement utilization in the future. If you are in doubt, make sure you eat from the food groups recommended in the Pyramid. If you are facing extreme stressors on the body from physical endurance events, illness, or other nutrient-depleting events, supplements might be beneficial, and in general, a multivitamin added to a balanced diet is likely to do more good than harm. In all cases, beware of megadoses and overdosing on ultravitamin supplements. Pick the least expensive brands, and aim to meet minimal levels.

Food Safety: A Growing Concern

As we become increasingly worried that the food we put in our mouths may be contaminated with bacteria, insects, worms, or other substances, the food industry has come under fire. To convince us that their products are safe, some manufacturers have come up with "new and improved" ways of protecting our foods. How well do they work?

Foodborne Illnesses

Are you concerned that the chicken you are buying doesn't look pleasingly pink, or that your "fresh" fish smells a little *too* fishy or has a grayish tinge? Are you *sure* that your apple juice is free of animal waste? You may have good reason to be worried. In increasing numbers, Americans are becoming sick from what they eat, and many of these illnesses are life threatening. Scientists estimate, based on several studies conducted over the past ten years, that foodborne pathogens sicken over 76 million people and cause some 325,000 hospitalizations and 5,200 deaths in the United States annually.[71] Because most of us don't go to the doctor every time we feel ill, we may not make a connection between what we eat and later symptoms.

Signs of foodborne illnesses vary tremendously and usually include one or several symptoms: diarrhea, nausea, cramping, and vomiting. Depending on the amount and virulence of the pathogen, symptoms may appear as early as 30 minutes after eating contaminated food or as long as several days or weeks later. Most of the time, symptoms occur five to eight hours after eating and last only a day or two. For certain populations, however, such as the very young, the elderly, or people with severe illnesses such as cancer, diabetes, kidney disease, or AIDS, foodborne diseases can be fatal.

Several factors may be contributing to the increase in foodborne illnesses. According to Michael T. Osterholm, PhD, state epidemiologist in Minneapolis,[72] the movement away from a traditional meat-and-potato American diet to "heart-healthy" eating—increasing consumption of fruits, vegetables, and grains—has spurred demand for fresh foods that are not in season most of the year. This means that we must import fresh fruits and vegetables, thus putting ourselves at risk for ingesting exotic pathogens or even pesticides that have been banned in the United States for safety reasons. Depending on the season, up to 70 percent of the fruits and vegetables consumed in the United States come from Mexico alone. The upshot is that a visit to developing countries isn't necessary to be stricken with foodborne "traveler's diarrhea" because the produce does the traveling.[73] Although we are told when we travel to developing countries, "boil it, peel it, or don't eat it," we bring these foods into our kitchens and eat them, often without even washing them.[74] Food can become contaminated by being watered with contaminated water, fertilized with "organic" fertilizers (animal manure), hand picked by people who have not washed their hands properly after using the toilet, or not subjected to the same rigorous pesticide regulations as American-raised produce. To give you an idea of the implications, studies have shown that *Escherichia coli* (*E. coli*, a lethal bacterial pathogen) can survive in cow manure for up to 70 days and can multiply in foods grown with manure unless heat or additives such as salt or preservatives are used to kill the microbes.[75] There are essentially no regulations that prohibit farmers from using animal manure to fertilize crops. Turkey manure, pig manure, and other agribusiness by-products are often sprayed on fields that ultimately grow foods for consumers. *E. coli* O157:H7 actually increases in summer months in cows awaiting slaughter in crowded, overheated pens. This increases the chances of meat coming to market already contaminated.[76]

Key factors associated with the increasing spread of foodborne diseases include:[77]

- *Globalization of the food supply.* Because food is distributed worldwide, the possibility of exposure to pathogens native to remote regions of the world is greater. For example, a large outbreak of *Shigella* occurred in Norway, Sweden, and the United Kingdom from lettuce that originated in southern Europe.
- *Inadvertent introduction of pathogens into new geographic regions.* Cholera may have been introduced into waters off the coast of the southern United States when a cargo ship discharged contaminated ballast as it came into harbor. Other pathogens may enter into aquatic life in a similar manner.
- *Exposure to unfamiliar foodborne hazards.* Travelers, refugees, and immigrants who move through foreign countries are exposed to foodborne hazards and bring them home.
- *Changes in microbial populations.* Changing microbial populations can lead to the evolution of new pathogens. As a result, old pathogens develop new virulence factors or become resistant to antibiotics, making diseases more difficult to treat.
- *Increased susceptibility of varying populations.* People are becoming more vulnerable to disease. The numbers of highly susceptible persons are expanding worldwide because of aging populations, HIV infection, and other underlying medical conditions, such as malnutrition and the compromised health status that results from the use of immunosuppressive drugs. High birth rates and increased longevity have increased the numbers of vulnerable populations at the margins.
- *Insufficient education about food safety.* Increased urbanization, industrialization, and travel, combined with more people eating out, raise the risk of unsafe food handling and illness.

Know what the typical foodborne hazards are, how you can contract them, and what you can do to prevent infection. Table 8.5 on page 262 lists common foodborne illnesses and their symptoms.

Responsible Use: Avoiding Risks in the Home

Part of the responsibility for preventing foodborne illness lies with consumers—over 30 percent of all such illnesses result from unsafe handling of food at home.

- When shopping, pick up packaged and canned foods first, and save frozen foods and perishables such as meat, poultry, and fish till last. Place these foods in separate plastic bags so drippings don't run onto other foods in your cart and contaminate them.
- Check for cleanliness at the salad bar and meat and fish counters. For instance, cooked shrimp lying on the same small bed of ice as raw fish can easily be contaminated.
- When shopping for fish, buy from markets that get their supplies from state-approved sources; stay clear of vendors who sell shellfish from roadside stands or the back of trucks. If you're planning to harvest your own shellfish, check the safety of the water in the area.
- Most cuts of meat, fish, and poultry should be kept in the refrigerator no more than one or two days. They shouldn't be in the grocery store meat counter beyond their dated shelf life, either. If your fish smells particularly "fishy" and your meat has a dark or greenish tinge to it, use caution. Check the shelf life of all products before buying. If expiration dates are close, freeze or eat the product immediately.
- Avoid preparing food if you are sick. Wear latex gloves if you have cuts or burns on your hands. Keep your hands away from your nose, mouth, and eyes. Thoroughly wash your hands after bathroom trips.
- Eat leftovers within three days.
- Keep hot foods hot and cold foods cold.
- Use a thermometer to ensure that meats are completely cooked. Beef and lamb steaks and roasts should be

Table 8.5
Recognizing the Common Foodborne Illnesses

Illness	Symptoms/Related Problems
Campylobacteriosis	Most common bacterial cause of diarrhea in the United States, affecting over 2 million people a year. Ranges from a mild illness with diarrhea lasting a day, to severe abdominal pain, severe diarrhea (sometimes bloody), sometimes accompanied by fever, occasionally lasting several weeks. Incubation period is 2–5 days, and illness usually lasts 2–10 days. Usually mild, but deaths have been noted among the very young, the very old, or the immunocompromised.
Clostridium perfringens	Typically occurs 6–24 hours after ingestion of food that bears large counts of this bacteria. Usually mild gastrointestinal distress lasting a day or so. Deaths are uncommon.
Escherichia coli O157:H7	Usually a mild gastrointestinal illness that occurs 3–5 days after eating contaminated foods. Severe complications, however, can arise. Hemorrhagic colitis is distinguished by the sudden onset of severe abdominal cramps, little or no fever, and diarrhea that may become grossly bloody. Fewer than 5 percent develop hemolytic uremic syndrome (HUS), a severe, life-threatening illness in which red blood cells are destroyed, kidneys fail, and neurologically based seizures and strokes occur.
Listeria monocytogenes	*Listeria* may be either mild or severe. Milder cases are characterized by sudden onset of fever, severe headache, vomiting, and other flulike symptoms. Listeriosis may appear mild in healthy adults and more severe in fetuses, older adults, those with kidney disease, users of glucocorticosteroids, and the immunocompromised. Women infected during pregnancy may transmit infection to the fetus, resulting in possible stillbirth or babies born with mental retardation. Over 2,500 people become seriously ill each year, leading to 500 deaths.
Salmonella	Usually occurs 6–72 hours after eating contaminated foods and lasts for a day or two. Nausea, diarrhea, stomach pain and vomiting are hallmark symptoms. There are over 40,000 reported cases each year (the actual incidence may be 20 times higher) and about 1,000 deaths.
Staphylococcus aureus	Usually occurs within 1–6 hours following consumption of the toxins produced by the bacteria but may occur within 30 minutes. Severe nausea and vomiting, cramps, and diarrhea are common. Although the illness generally doesn't last longer than 1–2 days, more serious symptoms may require hospitalization.
Toxoplasmosis	Mild flulike symptoms, or *no* symptoms. Undercooked meat or cat feces often the cause. Pregnant women may have stillbirths or babies born with birth defects ranging from hearing or visual impairments to mental retardation.

Source: Centers for Disease Control and Prevention, "Foodborne Illnesses," 2003, www.cdc.gov/health/foodill.htm

cooked to at least 145°F; ground meat, pork chops, ribs, and egg dishes to 160°F; ground poultry and hot dogs to 165°F; chicken and turkey breasts to 170°F; and chicken and turkey legs, thighs, and whole birds to 180°F.

- Fish is done when the thickest part becomes opaque and the fish flakes easily when poked with a fork. If you have any concerns, skip seafood such as sushi and raw oysters.
- Never leave cooked food standing on the stove or table for more than two hours. Disease-causing bacteria grow in temperatures between 40°F and 140°F. Cooked foods that have been left standing in this temperature range for more than two hours should be thrown away.
- Never bring your grilled meat into the house on the same plate you took it out on when it was uncooked. Raw meat juices are hotbeds for deadly bacteria.

- Never thaw frozen foods at room temperature. Put them in the refrigerator for a day to thaw or thaw in cold water, changing the water every 30 minutes.
- Wash your hands with soap and water between courses when preparing food, particularly after handling meat, fish, or poultry. Use warm (not hot) water and soap. Don't use antibacterial soap, which only contributes to antibacterial resistance. To wash, rub hands vigorously together for 15 to 20 seconds. Wash the countertop and all utensils before using them for other foods.

Food Irradiation: How Safe Is It?

Each year, thousands of people get sick from largely preventable diseases such as those caused by *E. coli* and other bacteria such as *Salmonella* and *Listeria*. In response to these concerns, in 2000 the USDA approved large-scale irradiation of beef, lamb, poultry, pork, and other raw animal foods.

Food irradiation is a process that involves treating foods with gamma radiation from radioactive cobalt, cesium,

Food irradiation Treating foods with gamma radiation from radioactive cobalt, cesium, or some other source of X rays to kill microorganisms.

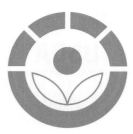

Figure 8.9
Label for Irradiated Foods
The "radura" indicates food that has been irradiated.

Source: Center for Food Safety and Applied Nutrition, "Food Safety A to Z Reference Guide," 2004, www.cfsan.fda.gov/~dms/a2z-i.html

or other sources of X rays. When foods are irradiated, they are exposed to low doses of radiation, or ionizing energy, which breaks chemical bonds in the DNA of harmful bacteria, destroying the pathogens and keeping them from replicating. The rays essentially pass through the food without leaving any radioactive residue.[78]

Some companies use cobalt-60, a radioactive substance, for irradiation, but others are beginning to use a new kind of irradiation that dispenses with radioactive compounds and uses electricity as the energy source instead. Thus, as foods pass along a conveyor belt, the energy used to kill bacteria comes from electron beams rather than gamma rays.[79] Irradiation lengthens food products' shelf life and prevents the spread of deadly microorganisms, particularly in high-risk foods such as ground beef and pork. Thus, the minimal costs of irradiation should result in lower overall costs to consumers, in addition to reducing the need for toxic chemicals now used to preserve foods and prevent contamination from external pathogens.

Food irradiation has been approved for potatoes, spices, pork carcasses, and fruits and vegetables since the mid-1980s. Some environmentalists and consumer groups have raised concerns, so irradiated products are not common fare. However, the facts appear to support the use of irradiation. Foods that have been irradiated are marked with the "radura" logo (Figure 8.9).

Food Additives

Additives (such as nitrates added to cured meats) generally reduce the risk of foodborne illness, prevent spoilage, and enhance the ways foods look and taste. Additives can also enhance nutrient value, especially to benefit the general public. A deficiency can be a terrible public health problem, and a solution is relatively easy to administer. Good examples include the fortification of milk with vitamin D and of grain products with folate. Although the FDA regulates additives according to effectiveness, safety, and ability to detect them in foods, questions have been raised about those additives put into foods intentionally and those that get in unintentionally before or after processing. Whenever such products are

added, consumers should take the time to determine what the substances are and if there are alternatives. As a general rule of thumb, the fewer chemicals, colorants, and preservatives, the better. Also, it should be noted that certain foods and additives can interact with medications (see Table 8.4). To be a smart consumer, be aware of these potential dietary interactions. Examples of common additives include:

- *Antimicrobial agents.* Substances such as salt, sugar, nitrates, and others that tend to make foods less hospitable for microbes.
- *Antioxidants.* Substances that preserve color and flavor by reducing loss due to exposure to oxygen. Vitamins C and E are among those antioxidants believed to reduce the risk of cancer and cardiovascular disease. BHA and BHT are additives that also are antioxidant in action.
- *Artificial colors.*
- *Nutrient additives.*
- *Flavor enhancers such as MSG (monosodium glutamate).*
- *Sulfites* Used to preserve vegetable color; some people have severe allergic reactions.
- *Substances that inadvertently get into food products from packaging and/or handling.*
- *Dioxins.* Found in coffee filters, milk containers, and frozen foods.
- *Methylene chloride.* Found in decaffeinated coffee.
- *Hormones.* Bovine growth hormone (BGH) is found in some animal meat.

Food Allergy or Food Intolerance?

At some point in time, nearly everyone will experience a *food allergy* or *food intolerance.* You eat something, develop gas or have an unpleasant visit to the bathroom, and then assume that it is a food allergy. One out of every three people today either say they have a food allergy or avoid something in their diet because they think they are allergic; in fact, only 3 percent of all children and 1 percent of all adults experience genuine allergic reactions to what they eat.[80] Surprised? Most people are when they hear this.

A **food allergy,** or hypersensitivity, is an abnormal response to a food that is triggered by the immune system. Reactions range from minor rashes to severe swelling in the mouth, tongue, and throat, to violent vomiting and diarrhea and occasionally death.

In adults, the most common foods to cause true allergic reactions are shellfish (such as shrimp, crayfish, lobster, and crab); peanuts, which can cause severe anaphylaxis, a sudden drop in blood pressure that can be fatal if not treated

Food allergies Overreaction by the body to normally harmless proteins, which are perceived as allergens. In response, the body produces antibodies, triggering allergic symptoms.

promptly; tree nuts such as walnuts; fish; and eggs. In children, food allergens that cause the most problems are eggs, milk, and peanuts.[81]

In contrast to allergies, in cases of **food intolerance** you may have symptoms of gastric upset, but they are not the result of an immune system response. Probably the best example of a food intolerance is *lactose intolerance,* a problem that affects about 1 in every 10 adults. Lactase is an enzyme in the lining of the gut that degrades lactose, which is in dairy products. If you don't have enough lactase, lactose cannot be digested and remains in the gut to be used by bacteria. Gas is formed, and you experience bloating, abdominal pain, and sometimes diarrhea. Food intolerance also occurs in response to some food additives, such as the flavor enhancer MSG, certain dyes, sulfites, gluten, and other substances. In some cases the food intolerance may have psychological triggers.

If you suspect that you have an actual allergic reaction to food, see an allergist to be tested to determine the source of the problem. Because there are several diseases that share symptoms with food allergies (ulcers and cancers of the gastrointestinal tract can cause vomiting, bloating, diarrhea, nausea, and pain), you should have persistent symptoms checked out as soon as possible. If particular foods seem to bother you consistently, look for alternatives or modify your diet. In true allergic instances, you may not be able to consume even the smallest amount safely. For example, people have had severe allergic reactions to peanuts from ingesting as little as a crumb or an airborne particle.

Is Organic for You?

Due to mounting concerns about food safety, many people refuse to buy processed foods and mass-produced agricultural products. Instead, they purchase foods that are **organically grown**—foods reported to be pesticide- and chemical-free. Less than a decade ago, buying organic foods meant going to a specialty store and paying premium prices for produce that was wilted, wormy, and smaller than its nonorganic alternative. These products also came with no guarantee that they were really grown in organic environments. People who bought

---

Food intolerance   Adverse effects resulting when people who lack the digestive chemicals needed to break down certain substances eat those substances.

Organically grown   Foods that are grown without use of pesticides or chemicals.

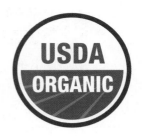

Figure 8.10

Label for Certified Organic Foods
This seal indicates that the product is at least 95 percent organic according to USDA guidelines.

Source: USDA Agriculture Marketing Program, The National Organic Program, "Organic Food Standards and Labels: The Facts," 2004, www.ams.usda.gov/nop

these foods did so out of a desire to eat "healthier" produce and avoid the chemicals that they were increasingly being told caused cancer, immune system problems, and a host of other ailments.

Enter the organics of the twenty-first century—larger, more attractive, and fresher looking but still carrying a hefty price tag. Is buying organic really better for you? Perhaps if we could put a group of people in a pristine environment and ensure that they never ate, drank, or were exposed to chemicals, we could test this hypothesis; however, it is difficult, if not impossible, to assess the overall impact of organic versus nonorganic food in terms of health outcomes. Nevertheless, the market for organics has been increasing by 15 to 20 percent per year—five times faster than food sales in general. Nearly 40 percent of U.S. consumers now reach occasionally for something labeled organic, with sales topping $11 billion per year.

As of 2002, any food sold as organic has to meet criteria set by the U.S. Department of Agriculture under the National Organic Rule and can carry a new USDA seal verifying that it is "certified organic" (Figure 8.10). Under this rule, something that is certified may carry one of the following terms: 100 Percent Organic (100 percent compliance with organic criteria), Organic (must contain at least 95 percent organic materials), Made with Organic Ingredients (must contain at least 70 percent organic ingredients), or Some Organic Ingredients (contains less than 70 percent organic ingredients—usually listed individually). In order to be certified and use any of the above terms, the foods must be produced without hormones, antibiotics, herbicides, insecticides, chemical fertilizers, genetic modification, or germ-killing radiation.

MAKE IT HAPPEN!

Assessment: The Assess Yourself box on page 226 gave you the chance to test your knowledge of the health effects of various foods. Now that you have considered these results, you can decide whether you need to do more to keep up on what to eat (and not eat) for long-tern health.

Making a Change: In order to change your behavior, you need to develop a plan. Follow these steps.

1. Evaluate your behavior, and identify patterns and specific things you are doing. What can you change now? What can you change in the near future?
2. Select one pattern of behavior that you want to change.
3. Fill out a Behavior Change Contract. It should include your long-term goal for change, your short-term goals, the rewards you'll give yourself for reaching these goals, potential obstacles along the way, and strategies for overcoming these obstacles. For each goal, list the small steps and specific actions that you will take.
4. Chart your progress in a journal. At the end of a week, consider how successful you were in following your plan. What helped you to be successful? What made change more difficult? What will you do differently next week?
5. Revise your plan as needed. Are the short-term goals attainable? Are the rewards satisfying?

One Student's Plan: Tara was surprised to see that she had very little idea about what foods to eat and to avoid. She decided to keep track of her normal diet for a week and then to evaluate it in light of some of the guidelines in this chapter.

She considered her diet fairly balanced and was surprised to find that she was eating less than 2 servings of vegetables a day, instead of the recommended 3 to 5. Tara looked at her eating patterns and saw several times during the week where she snacked on foods that could be replaced with other, healthier snacks. She decided to cut carrots up into sticks that she could toss into her backpack. They stayed fresh all day and made a good snack between classes instead of a candy bar from the vending machine. She also found that her favorite Mexican restaurant offered a vegetarian burrito full of black beans (not refried), squash, tomatoes, and other vegetables that was even tastier than her usual pork burrito. At the end of the first week, Tara and her friends decided to order pizza after a late night of studying. Instead of getting pepperoni or sausage, Tara suggested a pizza with green peppers, spinach, and onions as toppings. Tara did have a setback when she went to a baseball game and ate peanuts and hot dogs all day, but the next day she had a salad for lunch and saw that her vegetable consumption was almost at her goal.

Tara's goal for the next week is to continue to substitute healthy snacks and to look for healthier alternatives when she is eating out. When she is consistently eating the recommended servings of vegetables each week, she will start focusing on other parts of her diet that could use improvement. She is already thinking about how to replace some of the white bread and sugary breakfast cereals she eats now with more whole wheat and whole grains.

Summary

- Recognizing that we eat for more reasons than just survival is the first step toward changing our dietary habits.
- The Food Guide Pyramid provides guidelines for healthy eating.
- The major nutrients that are essential for life and health include water, proteins, carbohydrates, fiber, fats, vitamins, and minerals.
- Experts are interested in the role of food as medicine and in the benefits of "functional foods." These foods may play an important role in improving certain conditions, such as hypertension.
- Men and women have differing needs for most nutrients throughout the life cycle because of different body size and composition.
- Vegetarianism can provide a healthy alternative for those wishing to cut fat from their diets or reduce animal consumption. The vegetarian pyramid provides dietary guidelines to help vegetarians obtain needed nutrients.

- College students face unique challenges in eating healthfully. Learning to make better choices at fast-food restaurants, eat healthily when funds are short, and eat nutritionally in the dorm are all possible when you use the knowledge in this chapter.

- Foodborne illnesses, food irradiation, food allergies, organic foods, and other food safety and health concerns are becoming increasingly important to healthwise consumers. Recognizing potential risks and taking steps to prevent problems are part of a sound nutritional plan.

Questions for Discussion and Reflection

1. Which factors influence the dietary patterns and behaviors of the typical college student? What factors have been the greatest influences on your eating behaviors? Why is it important to recognize influences on your diet as you think about changing eating behaviors?
2. What are the six major food groups in the USDA Food Guide Pyramid? From which groups do you eat too few servings? What can you do to increase or decrease your intake of selected food groups to improve your health? How can you remember the six groups?
3. What are the major types of nutrients that you need to obtain from the foods you eat? What happens if you fail to get enough of some of them? Are there significant differences between the sexes in particular areas of nutrition?
4. Distinguish between the different types of vegetarianism. Which types are most likely to lead to nutrient deficien-

cies? What can be done to ensure that even the strictest vegetarian receives enough of the major nutrients?
5. What are functional foods? What are the major functional foods discussed in this chapter? What are their reported benefits, if any?
6. What are the major problems that many college students face when trying to eat the right foods? List five actions that you and your classmates could take immediately to improve your eating.
7. What are the potential benefits and risks of food irradiation? Why is it being used? What are the major risks for foodborne illnesses, and what can you do to protect yourself? How are food illnesses and food allergies different?

Accessing Your Health on the Internet

Visit the following Internet sites to explore further topics and issues related to personal health. To visit an organization's website, go to the Companion Website for *Access to Health, Ninth Edition* at www.aw-bc.com/donatelle, click on the book image, and select "Accessing Your Health on the Internet" from the navigation menu.

1. *American Dietetic Association (ADA).* Provides information on a full range of dietary topics, including sports nutrition, healthful cooking, and nutritional eating; also links to scientific publications and information on scholarships and public meetings.
2. *American Heart Association (AHA).* Includes information about a heart-healthy eating plan and an easy-to-follow guide to healthy eating.

3. *Food and Nutrition Information Center.* Offers a wide variety of information related to food and nutrition.
4. *National Institutes of Health: Office of Dietary Supplements.* Site of the International Bibliographic Database Information on Dietary Supplements (IBIDS), updated quarterly.
5. *U.S. Department of Agriculture (USDA).* Offers a full discussion of the USDA *Dietary Guidelines for Americans.*
6. *U.S. Food and Drug Administration (FDA).* Provides information for consumers and professionals in the areas of food safety, supplements, and medical devices and links to other sources of nutrition and food information.

Further Reading

Center for Science in the Public Interest. *Nutrition Action Healthletter.* Washington, DC.

This newsletter, published ten times a year, contains up-to-date information on diet and nutritional claims and current research issues. The newsletter can be obtained by writing to the Center for Science in the Public Interest, 1501 16th St. NW, Washington, DC 20036.

Nutrition Today. Baltimore, MD: Williams and Wilkins.

An excellent magazine for the interested nonspecialist. Covers controversial issues and provides a forum for conflicting opinions. Six issues per year. Order from Williams and Wilkins, 351 West Camden Street, Baltimore, MD 21201-2436.

Schlosser, E. *Fast Food Nation.* Boston: Houghton Mifflin, 2001.

Overview of the influence of the fast-food industry and its effect on health and well-being in America.

Thompson, J. and M. Manore, *Nutrition: An Applied Approach.* San Francisco: Benjamin Cummings, 2005.

An introductory college health text that provides an outstanding overview of nutritional information in a highly accessible, easy-to-read format.

Tufts University Health and Nutrition Letter. Medford, MA: Tufts University.

An excellent source for quick "fixes" on current nutritional topics. Reputable sources and information. E-mail: tufts@tiac.net Phone: (800) 274-7581. The Tufts Nutrition Navigator website (http://navigator.tufts.edu) rates nutrition-related websites for information and accuracy.

U.S. Department of Agriculture.

For information on the proper handling of meat and poultry and other information, call the USDA's Meat and Poultry Hot Line at the toll-free number 1-800-535-4555 between 10:00 AM and 4:00 PM on weekdays. Write to the Meat and Poultry Hot Line, USDA-FSIS, Room 1165-S, Washington, DC, 20250 for a new booklet, A Quick Consumer's Guide to Safe Food Handling.

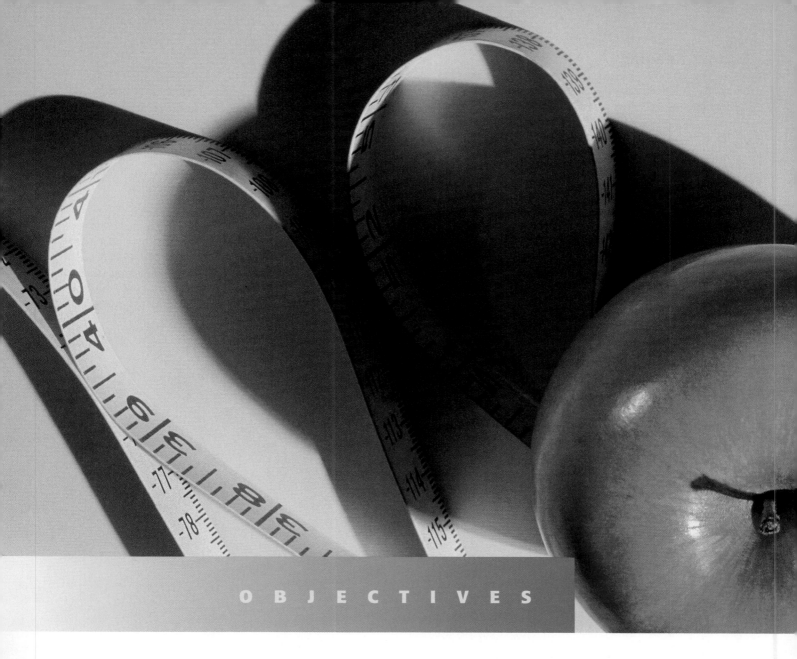

O B J E C T I V E S

- Explain why so many people are obsessed with body size and how to determine the right weight for you. Define *obesity*, and describe the current epidemic of obesity in the United States.

- Discuss reliable options for determining body fat content.

- Describe factors that place people at risk for problems with obesity. Distinguish between factors that can and cannot be controlled.

- Discuss the roles of exercise, dieting, nutrition, lifestyle modification, fad diets, and other strategies of weight

control. Describe the most effective methods of weight management.

- Describe major eating disorders, explain the health risks related to these conditions, and indicate the factors that make people susceptible to these disorders.

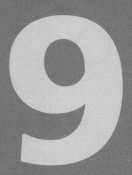

MANAGING YOUR WEIGHT

FINDING A HEALTHY BALANCE

IN THE NEWS

Sorry. Your Eating Disorder Doesn't Meet Our Criteria.

By Robin Marantz Henig

Imagine a 20-year-old woman who refuses to eat anything except carrots and toast because she is afraid of gaining weight, even though she is 5-foot-8 and weighs only 99 pounds. She exercises to the point of exhaustion five mornings a week because, though she is bone-thin, she thinks her thighs are too flabby. Her periods are irregular, but she has never gone more than three months without menstruating.

Another woman, who is also 20 and also 5-foot-8, has an opposite eating pattern. She goes without eating all day, and starting at 6 PM she eats nonstop, whatever she can get her hands on. Her favorite pastime is to sit in front of the television with a gallon of mocha-chip ice cream. She maintains a normal weight of 130 by occasionally forcing herself to vomit. But purging is not always easy in her college dormitory, with four young women sharing a single bathroom, so she ends up vomiting, on average, about once a week.

Everyone can agree that these women have some sort of disordered eating.

But psychiatrists would say that neither one falls into the strict definition of anorexia nervosa, the most severe eating disorder, or its relative, bulimia nervosa.

Read the complete article online in the eThemes section of this book's website: www.aw-bc.com/donatelle.

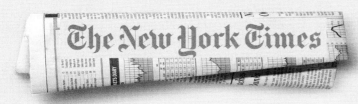

Over the past 20 years, the United States has become known as one of the fattest nations on earth. From young children who find it difficult to walk even short distances because of severe obesity to seniors who can't perform daily activities such as cleaning their homes because of crippling weight-related joint problems or obesity-related diseases, virtually no segment of the populace is immune to the epidemic of overweight and obesity. Soaring rates of obesity-related diseases such as hypertension and diabetes have caused health professionals to sound the alarm about potentially devastating individual and societal health care burdens that will result from our **obesogenic** society. Just how serious is the problem?

According to a national survey of health behaviors, the Behavioral Risk Factor Surveillance System, 34 percent of American adults are considered overweight and an additional 31 percent are obese.[1] While these high rates are disturbing, perhaps even more disturbing are the health-related problems that occur as obesity rates soar. For example, since 1990 there has been a 49 percent increase in the number of Americans who have diabetes, a major obesity-associated problem. About 27 percent of Americans reported that they did not engage in any physical activity, and only about 25 percent consumed the recommended five or more servings of fruits and vegetables each day.[2] Characteristics of those most prone to obesity indicated great disparities in level of risk by age, race, and other demographic characteristics (Table 9.1). Other reports by professional groups such as the *National Health and Nutrition Examination Survey, 1999–2002* confirmed that an estimated 64 percent of U.S. adults are either overweight or obese.[3]

What does all of this excess weight really mean to the health of our population? A recent government study discovered that obesity is fast approaching tobacco as the top underlying preventable cause of death in the United States.[4] According to recent assessments of contributors to death, obesity and physical inactivity caused up to 400,000 American deaths—second only to tobacco in terms of preventable causes of deaths. The worrisome part of these statistics is that while deaths from tobacco appear to be the same or declining slightly, obesity and inactivity seem to be making large gains. Importantly, like tobacco, obesity and inactivity increase the risks from three of our leading killers: heart disease, cancer, and cerebrovascular ailments, including strokes.[5] They also are strongly associated with diabetes risk, leading many experts to talk about the dual epidemics of obesity and diabetes in America today.

In addition to contributing to these diseases, increased obesity and physical inactivity have contributed to dramatic

Obesogenic   Society in which several factors make people more prone to obesity.

Table 9.1
Changes in Obesity Rates, 1991 to 2000

	Percent Obese	
	1991	**2000**
Men	11.7	20.2
Women	12.2	19.4
Age Groups		
18–29	7.1	13.5
30–39	11.3	20.2
40–49	15.8	22.9
50–59	16.1	25.6
60–69	14.7	22.9
>70	11.4	15.5
Race		
White, non-Hispanic	11.3	18.5
Black, non-Hispanic	19.3	29.3
Hispanic	11.6	23.4
Other	7.3	12.0
Education		
Less than high school	16.5	26.1
High school degree	13.3	21.7
Some college	10.7	19.5
College or above	8.0	15.2
Smoking Status		
Never smoked	12.0	19.9
Ex-smoker	14.0	22.7
Current smoker	9.9	16.3

Source: CDC Behavioral Risk Factor Surveillance System (BRFSS), "Prevalence of Obesity Among U.S. Adults, by Characteristics," 2001, www.cdc.gov/nccdphp/dnpa/obesity/trend/prev_char.htm

increases and bleak forecasts in the rates of several other diseases.

Associated health risks (Table 9.2) include coronary heart disease, hypertension, diabetes, gallstones, sleep apnea, osteoarthritis, and several cancers. For example, some experts predict that the numbers of Americans diagnosed with diabetes will increase by a whopping 165 percent, from 11 million in 2000 to 29 million in 2050.[6] In addition, the relationship between obesity and psychosocial development, including self-esteem, is believed to be significant.

The estimated annual cost of obesity in the United States exceeds $123 billion in medical expenses and lost productivity.[7] Much of this cost, over $75 billion in medical expenditures, is paid by states as they share the costs of obesity and overweight in Medicare and Medicaid populations. As the population ages, these costs will increase proportionately.[8] More than 500,000 lives are lost each year to conditions directly related to obesity, and many more deaths may be indirectly related to a history of obesity

Table 9.2
Selected Health Consequences of Overweight and Obesity

Premature Death

- Obese individuals have a 50–100% increased risk of death from all causes compared with people of normal weight. Among 25- to 35-year-olds, severe obesity increases the risk of death by a factor of 12.
- At least 300,000 deaths per year may be attributable to obesity.
- The risk of death rises with increasing weight.
- Even moderate excess weight (10–20 pounds for a person of average height) increases risk of death.

Cardiovascular Disease

- High blood pressure is twice as common in obese adults as it is for those who are at healthy weights.
- Incidence of all forms of heart disease is increased among overweight and obese people.
- Obesity is associated with elevated triglycerides and decreased HDLs ("good" cholesterol).

Diabetes

- A weight gain of 11–18 pounds increases a person's risk of developing type 2 diabetes to twice that of individuals who have not gained weight.
- More than 80% of people with diabetes are overweight or obese.

Cancer

- Overweight and obesity are associated with increased risk of endometrial, colon, gallbladder, prostate, kidney, and postmenopausal breast cancer.
- Women gaining more than 20 pounds between age 18 and midlife double their risk of postmenopausal breast cancer compared to women whose weight remains stable.

Additional Health Consequences

- Sleep apnea and asthma are both associated with obesity.
- For every 2-pound increase in weight, the risk of developing arthritis increases by 9–13%.
- Obesity-related complications during pregnancy include increased risk of fetal and maternal death, labor and delivery complications, and increased risk of birth defects.

Source: U.S. Department of Health and Human Services, "The Surgeon General's Call to Action to Prevent and Decrease Overweight and Obesity," 2001, www.surgeongeneral.gov/topics/obesity/calltoaction/fact _consequences.htm; D. Eberwine, "Globesity: The Crisis of Growing Proportions," *Perspectives in Health* 7, no. 3 (2003): 6–11.

throughout a person's life.[9] Of course, it is impossible to place a dollar value on a life lost prematurely due to diabetes, stroke, or heart attack or to assess the cost of social isolation and discrimination against obese and overweight individuals. Of growing importance is the recognition that obese individuals suffer significant disability during their lives, both in terms of mobility and activities of daily living.[10]

Many of us struggle to learn which foods are the most healthful, maintain healthy weight levels, and get adequate exercise. This chapter will help you understand why we have such a weight problem in America today and provide simple strategies to help you manage your weight. It will also help you understand what *underweight, normal weight, overweight,* and *obesity* really mean, and why managing your weight is essential to overall health and well-being.

To begin, answer the questions about readiness for weight loss in the Assess Yourself box. Your responses will help you obtain a better understanding of your own dietary habits.

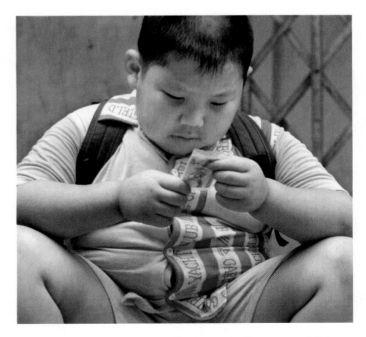

Obesity is increasing especially dramatically among children. Being overweight or obese from an early age can have devastating physical and emotional consequences.

Readiness for Weight Loss

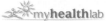

Fill out this assessment online at www.aw-bc.com/myhealthlab or www.aw-bc.com/donatelle

To see how well your attitudes equip you for a weight loss program, answer the questions that follow. For each question, circle the answer that best describes your attitude. As you complete each of the six sections, tally your score and analyze it according to the scoring guide.

PART I. GOALS, ATTITUDES, AND READINESS

1. Compared to previous attempts, how motivated are you to lose weight this time?

1	2	3	4	5
Not at all motivated	Slightly motivated	Somewhat motivated	Quite motivated	Extremely motivated

2. How certain are you that you will stay committed to a weight loss program for the time it will take to reach your goal?

1	2	3	4	5
Not at all motivated	Slightly motivated	Somewhat motivated	Quite motivated	Extremely motivated

3. Considering all outside factors at this time in your life—stress at work, family obligations, and so on—to what extent can you tolerate the effort required to stick to a diet?

1	2	3	4	5
Cannot tolerate	Can tolerate somewhat	Uncertain	Can tolerate well	Can tolerate easily

4. Think honestly about how much weight you hope to lose and how quickly you hope to lose it. Figuring a weight loss of one to two pounds per week, how realistic is your expectation?

1	2	3	4	5
Very unrealistic	Somewhat unrealistic	Moderately unrealistic	Somewhat realistic	Very realistic

5. While dieting, do you fantasize about eating a lot of your favorite foods?

1	2	3	4	5
Always	Frequently	Occasionally	Rarely	Never

6. While dieting, do you feel deprived, angry, and/or upset?

1	2	3	4	5
Always	Frequently	Occasionally	Rarely	Never

ANALYZING THIS SECTION

Scores of 6 to 16: This may not be a good time for you to start a diet. Inadequate motivation and commitment and unrealistic goals could block your progress. Think about what contributes to your unreadiness, and consider changing these factors before undertaking a diet.

Scores of 17 to 23: You may be close to being ready to begin a program but should think about ways to boost your readiness.

Scores of 24 to 30: The path is clear: you can decide how to lose weight in a safe, effective way.

PART II. HUNGER AND EATING CUES

	Never	Rarely	Occasionally	Frequently	Always
7. When food comes up in conversation or in something you read, do you want to eat, even if you are not hungry?	1	2	3	4	5
8. How often do you eat because of physical hunger?	1	2	3	4	5
9. Do you have trouble controlling your eating when your favorite foods are around the house?	1	2	3	4	5

ANALYZING THIS SECTION

Scores of 3 to 6: You might occasionally eat more than you should, but it does not appear to be due to high responsiveness to environmental cues. Controlling the attitudes that make you eat may be especially helpful.

Scores of 7 to 9: You may have a moderate tendency to eat just because food is available. Losing weight may be easier for you if you try to resist external cues and eat only when you are physically hungry.

Scores of 10 to 15: Some or much of your eating may be in response to thinking about food or exposing yourself to temptations to eat. Think of ways to minimize your exposure to temptations so you eat only in response to physical hunger.

PART III. CONTROL OVER EATING

If the following situations occurred while you were on a diet, would you be likely to eat more or less immediately afterward and for the rest of the day?

	Would eat much less	Would eat somewhat less	Would make no difference	Would eat somewhat more	Would eat much more
10. Although you planned on skipping lunch, a friend talks you into going out for a midday meal.	1	2	3	4	5
11. You "break" your plan by eating a fattening, "forbidden" food.	1	2	3	4	5
12. You have been following your diet faithfully and decide to test yourself by eating something you consider a treat.	1	2	3	4	5

ANALYZING THIS SECTION

Scores of 3 to 7: You recover rapidly from mistakes. However, if you frequently alternate between eating that is out of control and dieting very strictly, you may have a serious eating problem and should get professional help.

Scores of 8 to 11: You do not seem to let unplanned eating disrupt your program. This is a flexible, balanced approach.

Scores of 12 to 15: You may be prone to overeat after an event breaks your control or throws you off the track. Your reaction to these problem-causing events can be improved.

PART IV. BINGE EATING AND PURGING

13. Aside from holiday feasts, have you ever eaten a large amount of food rapidly and felt afterward that this eating incident was excessive and out of control?	2 Yes	0 No

14. If you answered yes to question 13, how often have you engaged in this behavior during the past year?

1	2	3	4	5	6
Less than once a month	About once a month	A few times a month	About once a week	About 3 times a week	Daily

15. Have you purged (used laxatives or diuretics; induced vomiting) to control your weight?	5 Yes	0 No

16. If you answered yes to question 15, how often have you engaged in this behavior during the past year?

1	2	3	4	5	6
Less than once a month	About once a month	A few times a month	About once a week	About 3 times a week	Daily

ANALYZING THIS SECTION

Scores of 0: It appears that binge eating and purging are not problems for you.

Scores of 2 to 11: Pay attention to these eating patterns. Should they arise more frequently, get professional help.

Scores of 12 to 19: You show signs of having a potentially serious eating problem. See a counselor experienced in evaluating eating disorders right away.

(continues)

PART V. EMOTIONAL EATING

	Never	Rarely	Occasionally	Frequently	Always
17. Do you eat more than you would like to when you have negative feelings such as anxiety, depression, anger, or loneliness?	1	2	3	4	5
18. Do you have trouble controlling your eating when you have positive feelings—do you celebrate feeling good by eating?	1	2	3	4	5
19. When you have unpleasant interactions with others in your life or after a difficult day at work, do you eat more than you'd like?	1	2	3	4	5

ANALYZING THIS SECTION

Scores of 3 to 8: You do not appear to let your emotions affect your eating.

Scores of 9 to 11: You sometimes eat in response to emotional highs and lows. Monitor this behavior to learn when and why it occurs, and be prepared to find alternate activities.

Scores of 12 to 15: Emotional ups and downs can stimulate your eating. Try to deal with the feelings that trigger the eating and find other ways to express them.

PART VI. EXERCISE PATTERNS AND ATTITUDES

20. How often do you exercise?

1	2	3	4	5
Never	Rarely	Occasionally	Frequently	Always

21. How confident are you that you can exercise regularly?

1	2	3	4	5
Not at all confident	Slightly confident	Somewhat confident	Highly confident	Completely confident

22. When you think about exercise, do you develop a positive or negative picture in your mind?

1	2	3	4	5
Completely negative	Somewhat negative	Neutral	Somewhat positive	Completely positive

23. How certain are you that you can work regular exercise into your daily schedule?

1	2	3	4	5
Not at all certain	Slightly certain	Somewhat certain	Quite certain	Extremely certain

ANALYZING THIS SECTION

Scores of 4 to 10: You're probably not exercising as regularly as you should. Determine whether attitude about exercise or your lifestyle is blocking your way, then change what you must and put on those walking shoes!

Scores of 11 to 16: You need to feel more positive about exercise so you can do it more often. Think of ways to be more active that are fun and fit your lifestyle.

Scores of 17 to 20: It looks as if the path is clear for you to be active. Now think of ways to get motivated.

After scoring yourself in each section of this questionnaire, you should be able to better judge your dieting strengths and weak-nesses. Remember that the first step in changing eating behavior is to understand the conditions that influence your eating habits.

MAKE IT HAPPEN!

Use the results of this self-assessment to begin your behavior change program. Follow the steps and use the examples on page 299 to complete your Behavior Change Contract, and use these resources to take action.

Source: Reprinted from "The Diet Readiness Test," in K. D. Brownell, "When and How to Diet," *Psychology Today,* June 1989, 41–46. Reprinted with permission from *Psychology Today* Magazine, copyright © 1989 (Sussex Publishers, Inc.). www.psychologytoday.com

Determining the Right Weight for You

What weight is right for you? Each person's optimal weight depends on a wide range of variables, including body structure, height, weight distribution, and the ratio of fat to lean tissue. In fact, your weight can be a deceptive indicator. Many extremely muscular athletes would be considered overweight based on traditional height-weight charts, while many young women think that they are the right weight based on charts, only to be shocked to discover that 35 to 40 percent of their weight is body fat!

In general, weights at the lower end of the range on traditional charts are recommended for individuals with a low ratio of muscle and bone to fat; those at the upper end are advised for people with more muscular builds. However, since actual body composition is hard to determine, most charts today simply give a general range for men and women.

Overweight or Obese?

Most of us cringe at the thought of being labeled with one of the "O" words. What is the distinction between the two? **Overweight** refers to increased body weight in relation to height, when compared to a standard such as the height–weight charts in Table 9.3. Historically, nutritionists have defined overweight as being 1 to 19 percent above one's ideal weight and obese as over 19 percent.

The most highly regarded measurement of overweight and obesity is a mathematical formula known as **body mass index (BMI),** which represents weight levels associated with the lowest overall risk to health (see the next section to calculate your BMI). Desirable BMI levels may vary with age.[11] You would be classified as being overweight if you have a BMI of 25.0 to 29.9. About 34 percent of all Americans fit this category, but it is important to remember that BMI is a good—but not perfect—indicator of a weight problem.

According to the standards, a person could be classified as overweight even if the weight gain is due to an increase in lean muscle mass. For example, as described above, an athlete may be very lean and muscular, with very little body fat, yet she may weigh a lot more than others of the same height who have little muscle tissue. Conversely, a person may proudly proclaim that he weighs the same amount that he did in high school but carry a much greater proportion of body fat, particularly in the hips, buttocks, or thighs, than he did at a younger age. Body weight alone may not be a good indicator of overall fitness.

Another problem with using BMI is that people who have lost muscle mass, such as older adults, people with anorexia, or those who are seriously disabled or bedridden, could be in the "healthy weight" range even though their nutritional reserves are dangerously low. Therefore, BMI is a useful guideline, but by itself is not diagnostic of a person's overall health status.[12] It remains the measurement

most commonly used by most health agencies and health professionals.

Obesity is defined as an excessively high amount of body fat or adipose tissue in relation to lean body mass or a BMI of 30 or more. Over 31 percent of all Americans are obese. It is important to consider both the distribution of fat throughout the body and the size of the adipose tissue deposits. Body fat distribution can be estimated by skinfold measures, waist-to-hip circumference ratios, or techniques such as ultrasound, computed tomography, magnetic resonance imaging, or others. Using traditional standards, people 20 to 40 percent above their ideal weight are labeled as *mildly obese* (90 percent of the obese fall into this category). Those 41 to 99 percent above their ideal weight are

Table 9.3
Healthy Weight Ranges*

Height without Shoes	Weight[†] without Clothes
4'10"	91–119
4'11"	94–124
5'0"	97–128
5'1"	101–132
5'2"	104–137
5'3"	107–141
5'4"	111–146
5'5"	114–150
5'6"	118–155
5'7"	121–160
5'8"	125–164
5'9"	129–169
5'10"	132–174
5'11"	136–179
6'0"	140–184
6'1"	144–189
6'2"	148–195
6'3"	152–200
6'4"	156–205
6'5"	160–211
6'6"	164–216

* Each data entry applies to both men and women.
† In pounds

Source: Center for Nutrition Policy and Promotion, "Dietary Guidelines for Americans, 2000," 2000, www.usda.gov/cnpp/Pubs/ DG2000

Overweight Increased body weight in relation to height.

Body mass index (BMI) A technique of weight assessment based on the relationship of weight to height.

Obesity A weight disorder generally defined as an accumulation of fat beyond that considered normal for a person based on age, sex, and body type.

described as *moderately obese* (about 7 to 8 percent of the obese fit into this category), and 2 to 3 percent are in the *severely, morbidly,* or *grossly obese* category, meaning that they are 100 percent or more above their ideal weight. In the last decade, more and more people are at the moderate and severe levels of obesity, meaning increased risks at all ages and stages of their lives.[13]

The difficulty with defining obesity lies in determining what is normal. To date, there are no universally accepted standards for the most desirable or ideal body weight or *body composition* (the ratio of lean body mass to fat body mass). While sources vary slightly, men's bodies should contain between 11 and 15 percent total body fat, and women should be within the range of 18 to 22 percent body fat. At various ages and stages of life, these ranges also vary, but generally, when men exceed 20 percent body fat, and women exceed 30 percent body fat, they have slipped into obesity.

Why the difference between men and women? Much of it may be attributed to the normal structure of the female body and to sex hormones. Lean body mass consists of the structural and functional elements in cells, body water, muscle, bones, and other body organs such as the heart, liver, and kidneys. Body fat is composed of two types: essential and storage fat. Essential fat is necessary for normal physiological functioning, such as nerve conduction. Essential fat makes up approximately 3 to 7 percent of total body weight in men and approximately 15 percent of total body weight in women. Storage fat, the part that many of us try to shed, makes up the remainder of our fat reserves. It accounts for only a small percentage of total body weight for very lean people and between 5 and 25 percent of body weight of most American adults. Female bodybuilders, who are among the leanest of female athletes, may have body fat percentages ranging from 8 to 13 percent, nearly all of which is essential fat.

Too Little Fat?

A certain amount of body fat is necessary for insulating the body, cushioning parts of the body and vital organs, and maintaining body functions. In men, this lower limit is approximately 3 to 4 percent. Women should generally not go below 8 percent. Excessively low body fat in females may lead to amenorrhea, a disruption of the normal menstrual cycle. The critical level of body fat necessary to maintain normal menstrual flow is believed to be between 8 and 13 percent, but there are many additional factors that affect the menstrual cycle. Under extreme circumstances, such as extreme diets and certain diseases, the body utilizes all available fat reserves and begins to break down muscle tissue as a last-ditch effort to obtain nourishment.

The fact is that too much fat and too little fat are both potentially harmful. The key is to find a healthy level at which you are comfortable with your appearance and your ability to be as active as possible. Many options are available for determining your body fat and weight.

Assessing Fat Levels

Today, most authorities believe that getting on the scale to determine your weight and then looking at where you fall on some arbitrary chart may not be helpful. A number of other measures exist for calculating body fat content, and some provide a very precise reading or calculation of body fat. They include body mass index, various measures of body fat, and waist-to-hip ratio.

Body Mass Index (BMI)

A useful index of the relationship between height and weight, BMI is the measurement of choice for obesity researchers and health professionals. It is not gender specific, and although it does not directly measure percentage of body fat, it does provide a more accurate measure of overweight and obesity than weight alone.[14]

We find BMI by dividing a person's weight in kilograms by height in meters squared. The mathematical formula is:

$$BMI = \text{weight (kg)} \div \text{height squared (m}^2)$$

To determine BMI using pounds and inches, multiply your weight in pounds by 704.5, then divide the result by your height in inches, and divide that result by your height in inches a second time. (The National Institutes of Health uses the multiplier 704.5. Other organizations, such as the American Dietetic Association, suggest multiplying by 700. The variation in outcomes between the two is insignificant, and 700 is easier for most people to remember.) For example, if you are 5 feet, 5 inches tall and weigh 145 pounds, you would follow these steps:

1. 145 (weight) × 704.5 = 102,152.5
2. 102,152.5 ÷ 65 (inches) = 1571.6
3. 1571.6 ÷ 65 = 24.1
4. Your BMI is 24.1

The BMI calculator also is available at the National Heart, Lung, and Blood Institute (NHLBI) website at http://nhlbisupport.com/bmi/bmicalc.htm or see Figure 9.1.

Healthy weights are defined as those associated with BMIs of 19 to 25, the range of lowest statistical health risk.[15] The desirable range for females falls between 21 and 23; for males, between 22 and 24.[16] A BMI greater than 25 indicates overweight and potentially significant health risks. A body mass index of 30 or more is considered obese.[17] Many experts believe that this number is too high, particularly for younger adults.

Calculating BMI is simple, quick, and inexpensive—but it does have limitations. One problem with using BMI as a measurement is that very muscular people may fall into the overweight category when they are actually healthy and fit. As well, certain population groups, such as Asians, tend to have higher-than-healthy body fat at normal BMI levels, while Polynesians have somewhat lower body fat than other populations at the same BMI.[18] Another problem is that, as

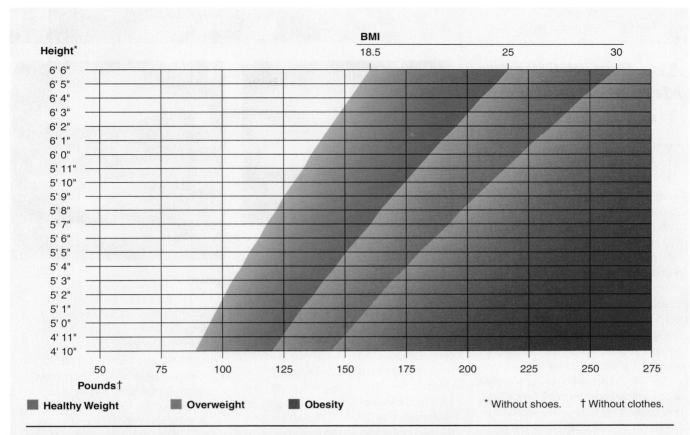

Figure 9.1

Body Mass Index: Are You at a Healthy Weight?

Source: Dietary Guidelines Advisory Committee, USDA Agricultural Research Service, "Dietary Guidelines for Americans," 2000, www.ars.usda.gov/dgac/2kdiet.pdf

previously described, people who have lost muscle mass such as older adults may be in the healthy weight category according to BMI, when they actually have reduced nutritional reserves.

These standards may seem almost impossible for people who consistently exceed the target weights and who have difficulty keeping off any lost weight. Constant failure may lead them to stop trying. The secret lies in establishing a healthful weight at a young age and maintaining it—a task easier said than done. The U.S. *Dietary Guidelines for Americans* encourage a weight gain of no more than ten pounds after reaching adult height and endorse small weight losses of one-half to one pound per week, if needed, as well as

smaller weight losses of 5 to 10 percent to make a difference toward health.[19]

Measuring Body Fat

There are numerous ways of assessing whether your body fat levels are too high besides BMI calculations. One low-tech way is simply to look in the mirror or consider how your clothes fit compared to how they fit the last season you wore them. Of course, we've all seen people who appear to have a disconnect between how they look and the size of clothing they are wearing or their body image. More accurate ways of determining body fat are available for those who really are interested in having a precise measurement.

Are Super-Sized Meals Super-Sizing Americans?

Today, super-sized meals are the norm at many restaurants. Biscuits and gravy, huge steaks, and plate-filling meals are popular fare. Consider the 25-ounce prime rib dinner served at a local steak chain. At nearly 3,000 calories and 150 grams of fat for the meat alone, this meal both slams shut arteries and adds on pounds. Add a baked potato with sour cream and/or butter, a salad loaded with creamy salad dressing, and fresh bread with real butter, and the meal may surpass the 5,000-calorie mark and ring in at close to 300 grams of fat. In other words, it exceeds what most adults should eat in two days!

And this is just the beginning. Soft drinks, once commonly served in 12-ounce sizes, now come in Big Gulps and 1-liter bottles. Cinnamon buns at local chains now come in giant, butter-laden, 700-calorie portions. What is the result? Super-sized portions consumed by super-sized Americans. A quick glance at the fattening of Americans provides growing evidence of a significant health problem. According to Donna Skoda, a dietitian and chair of the Ohio State University Extension Service, "People are eating a ton of extra calories. For the first time in history, more people are overweight in America than are underweight. Ironically, although the U.S. fat intake has dropped in the past 20 years from an average of 40 to 33 percent of calories, the daily calorie intake has risen from 1,852 calories per day to over 2,000 per day. In theory, this translates into a weight gain of 15 pounds a year." Skoda and others say that the main reason that Americans are gaining weight is that people no longer know what a normal serving size is. In a recent U.S. Department of Agriculture survey, only 1 percent of the respondents could correctly identify the serving sizes recommended in the Food Guide Pyramid, the visual dietary aid developed by the USDA.

The National Heart, Lung, and Blood Institute, part of the National Institutes of Health, has developed a "Portion Distortion"

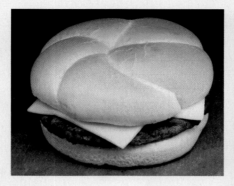

20 years ago

quiz that shows how today's portions compare to those of 20 years ago. Test yourself online at http://hin.nhlbi.nih.gov/portion to see if you can recognize the differences between today's super-sized meals and those once considered normal. Just one example is the difference between an average cheeseburger 20 years ago (left photo) and the typical cheeseburger of today (right).

According to Carrie Wiatt, a Los Angeles dietitian and author of the recently released book *Portion Savvy,* a telling marker of the big-food trend is that restaurant plates have grown from an average of 9 to 13 inches in the past decade. Studies show that people eat 40 to 50 percent more than they normally would now that large portions are available.

These statistics alone are alarming; however, they are made worse by a growing trend toward sedentary lifestyles, increased use of technology and gadgetry, and computer-gazing. The relationship between energy input and output is being knocked out of balance on both sides. Americans are taking in more calories and doing less to burn them off. Hence, an epidemic of obesity prevails and is getting worse. Younger and younger kids are eating more and more and picking up lifetime habits that will be hard to change. To reduce your own risk of super-sizing, follow these simple strategies:

✔ Avoid super-sizing anything. Order the smallest size available when dining out. Focus on taste, not quantity. Get used to eating less and enjoying what you are eating.

✔ Chew your food, and avoid the urge to wash it down with high-calorie drinks.

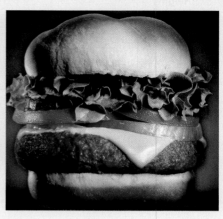

Today

✔ Serve food on a small or medium plate. Put those big platter-size dinner plates on the top shelf of your cupboard, and leave them there.

✔ Always order dressings, gravies, and sauces on the side. Sprinkle these added calories on carefully, rather than washing your foods down with them. Remember that a tablespoon of gravy could mean an hour on the treadmill to burn off its 200+ calories!

✔ If you order a large muffin or bagel, share it with a friend, or eat only half and wrap up the rest. Carry a small ziplock bag, and use it to take home part of those big portions for another day.

✔ Avoid appetizers in restaurants. They are expensive—in terms of money, calories, *and* fat content.

✔ Share your dinner with a friend, and order a side salad for each of you. Alternatively, eat only half of your dinner and save the rest for another day.

✔ Measure portions. Before ordering, ask for the size of servings, and always order a size smaller than you really want. When the server tells you it is a "rich dish" or "a lot of food," avoid it.

✔ Avoid buffets and all-you-can-eat establishments. Most of us can eat two to three times what we need—or more.

Source: Some statistics from J. Snow, "Are Super-Sized Meals Super-Sizing Americans?" *Akron Beacon Journal,* May 24, 2000. © 2004 Akron Beacon Journal. All rights reserved. Distributed by Knight Ridder Digital.

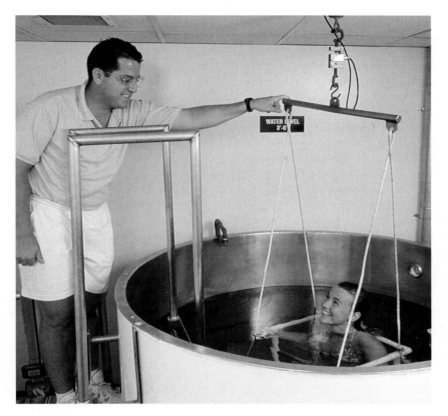

Hydrodensitometry weighing is one of the most accurate techniques for measuring body fat, although even more advanced techniques are being pursued.

One of the most accurate techniques is **hydrodensitometry weighing (underwater weighing).** This method measures the amount of water a person displaces when completely submerged. Because fat tissue is less dense than muscle or bone, a relatively accurate indication of actual body fat can be made by comparing a person's underwater and out-of-water weights. This method is not foolproof, however. Athletes tend to have denser bones and muscles than nonathletes, which may lead to an underestimation of body fat. People with osteoporosis may find their body fat levels are overestimated. Other factors such as the amount of air in your lungs when taking the test and water movement may also influence accuracy. Although this test is considered the gold standard, many people find it difficult and uncomfortable or find it impossible to hold their breath underwater while expelling all the air from their lungs. To insure accuracy in laboratory research, measures must be taken several times, and an average body fat is computed.

One of the most common methods of assessing body fat is the **skinfold caliper technique.** In this method a handheld caliper is used to measure the skinfold thickness at several points on the body (usually between 3 and 7 spots). The technician grasps the skin and underlying tissue, shakes it slightly to make sure that muscle is not part of the grab, and pinches the remaining skin and fat in the grips of the caliper, which provides a measure. Measurements are

added, and a percentage is calculated. This method assumes that that thickness of the subcutaneous fat under the skin is similar to fatness found in body cavities and other areas of the body. It is a good rough indicator of fatness, but the skill of the technician is key here. In general, the more overweight or obese a person is, the more difficult it is to get accurate measures. Sometimes calipers are not large enough to get a good measure. If you are using this technique, it's probably a good idea to have different technicians assess you and take their average.

Dual energy X-ray absorptiometry (DEXA) is one of the newer technologies available for assessing body fat. It is

Hydrodensitometry weighing (underwater weighing) Method of determining body fat by measuring the amount of water displaced when a person is completely submerged.

Skinfold caliper technique A method of determining body fat whereby folds of skin and fat at various points on the body are grasped between thumb and forefinger and measured with calipers.

Dual energy X-ray absorptiometry (DEXA) Technique using low-dose X rays that read bone and soft tissue mass at the same time.

also among the most accurate and precise. DEXA is based on a three-compartment model that divides the body into total body mineral, fat-free soft (lean) mass, and fat tissue mass. Essentially, DEXA is a whole body scanning technique that has two low dose X rays that read bone and soft tissue mass at the same time. DEXA scans are also used for assessing osteoporosis risk. It takes about 20 minutes to perform as the scanner slowly passes over your body while you lie on a table. DEXA is more precise than other methods and is relatively easy for anyone to have done. The downside is that it isn't as accurate for extremely obese individuals. Because of the high cost of the machines, it is one of the more costly techniques, and it isn't available everywhere. Many universities have DEXA machines in their exercise physiology or biomechanics labs. If you have one on your campus, you may be able to participate in a research study and obtain free testing for your willingness to participate.

Near-infrared interactance (NIR) is also a newer technique in which a fiber optic probe is connected to a digital analyzer that indirectly measures tissue composition (both fat and water). Usually, the biceps are used to assess fatness; once measures are taken, an equation that includes your height, weight, frame size, and level of activity is used to calculate body fat. Often you will see this technique used outside of the laboratory. It is relatively inexpensive and fast, but it is not nearly as accurate as the other methods described above. Very fat and very lean, muscular people are likely to have inaccurate measures. Numerous studies have indicated that more research must be done to determine if this technique is accurate and if it is better than caliper methods and other simple strategies.

Magnetic resonance imaging (MRI) is a technique that has been around for a long time, but its cost typically

prohibits its use for simple body fat calculations. MRI uses magnetic fields to accurately assess how much fat a person has and where it is deposited. If you were having a full body MRI for diagnosis of other illnesses, it is possible that you could ask the technician to determine your body fat.

Total body electrical conductivity (TOBEC) is another imaging technique much like an MRI in that a person lies in a cylinder that generates a very weak electromagnetic field. It is based on the assumption that lean tissue is a better conductor of electricity than fat; and, as it takes a series of readings, it provides data on fat versus lean tissue in your body. Like MRI, it is very expensive and not practical for many people.

Computed tomography (CT) provides a cross-sectional scan of the body, using radiation as in a typical X ray. This technique is good for assessing intraabdominal fat as compared to fat under the skin and in other body areas. Costs of this fat-assessing technique are also high, and the added risk of radiation exposure makes it less than desirable.

Bioelectrical impedance (BIA) is the only method based on measuring electrical signals as they pass through fat, lean mass, and water in the body, rather than estimating fat from other measures. Essentially, it is measuring how lean you are, rather than how fat you are, yet the net results are just as informative. BIA can be very accurate and is generally simple and easy to use. Its strength, however, is related to the sophistication of the machine doing the testing and the knowledge of the technician. Be wary of mail-order BIA equipment or very inexpensive offers.

Although most of these methods can be useful, they can also be inaccurate and even harmful unless the testers are skillful and well trained. Before undergoing any procedure, make sure you understand the expense, potential for accuracy, risks, and training of the tester.

Circumference and Ratio Measurements

The presence of excess body fat in the abdomen, when out of proportion to total body fat, is considered an independent predictor of risk factors and ailments associated with obesity. **Waist circumference measurement** is a useful tool for assessing abdominal fat. Research indicates that a waistline greater than 40 inches (102 cm) in men and 35 inches (88 cm) in women may indicate greater health risk. If a person has a short stature (under 5 feet tall) or has a BMI of 35 or above, waist circumference standards used for the general population might not apply.[20] Measure waist circumference by wrapping a tape measure comfortably around the smallest area below the rib cage and above the belly button.

Another useful measure is the **waist-to-hip ratio,** a measure of regional fat distribution. Research has shown that excess fat in the abdominal area poses a greater health risk than excess fat in the hips and thighs and is associated with a number of disorders, including high blood pressure, diabetes, heart disease, and certain cancers. A waist-to-hip ratio greater than 1.0 in men and 0.8 in women indicates increased health risks.[21] Therefore, knowing where your fat

---

Near-infrared interactance (NIR) Fiber optic measurement of tissue composition.

Magnetic resonance imaging (MRI) Diagnostic technique using magnetic fields, which can be used to measure body fat.

Total body electrical conductivity (TOBEC) Technique using an electromagnetic force field to assess relative body fat.

Computed tomography (CT) Use of X-ray for a cross section of the body, which can reveal intraabdominal fat.

Bioelectrical impedence analysis (BIA) A technique of body fat assessment in which electrical currents are passed though fat and lean tissue.

Waist circumference measurement Assessment of healthy weight by measurement of the circumference of the waist.

Waist-to-hip ratio Ratio that indicates increased risks due to an unhealthy weight distribution.

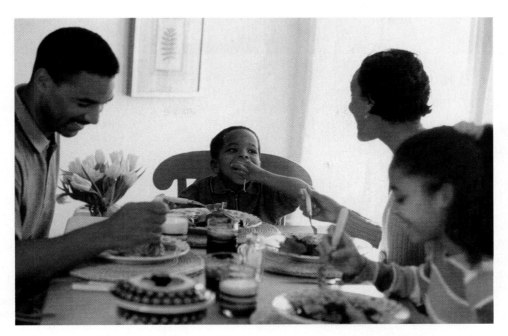

Many factors help determine body type, including heredity and genetic makeup, environmental factors, and learned eating patterns, many of which are connected to habits learned from family.

is carried may be more important than knowing your total fat content.

Men and postmenopausal women tend to store fat in the upper regions of their body, particularly in the abdominal area. Premenopausal women usually store their fat in lower regions of their bodies, particularly the hips, buttocks, and thighs.[22]

What do you think?

Calculate your BMI using the formula provided. Cross-check your results by using the calculator found at the NHLBI website. If possible, also try to have your percentage of body fat tested with calipers or one of the other methods listed. Which value is most important to you? Why? ■ *How are they similar?*

Risk Factors for Obesity

In spite of massive efforts to keep Americans fit and in good health, obesity is the most common nutritional disorder in the United States, with rates that have increased dramatically among children and adults in recent decades.[23] The prevalence of obesity and overweight (defined as a BMI of 25 or higher) is generally higher among minorities, especially minority women. For example, 77.3 percent of black females and 71.9 percent of Mexican American females are considered overweight or obese, while 57.3 percent of non-Hispanic white women fall into these categories. Among men, 74.7 percent of Mexican American men and 60.7 percent of black men are overweight or obese; 67.4 percent of white men are in these categories.[24] These rates are especially noteworthy when compared to obesity trends in the rest of the world (see the Health in a Diverse World box).

In a major report on strategies to combat overweight and obesity, the Surgeon General stated it quite plainly: "Overweight and obesity result from an energy imbalance. This means eating too many calories and not getting enough exercise."[25] However, many have criticized such a simplistic view. If it were that simple, many Americans would merely reevaluate their diets, reduce the amount they eat, and exercise more. Unfortunately, it's not that easy. In fact, there are probably many more factors conspiring to make us fat and keep us fat than we have even begun to fathom. Knowing what these factors are, recognizing how they specifically influence our own dietary patterns, and making conscious decisions to change specific lifestyle behaviors is an important first step in beating the "battle of the bulge." For those who don't currently have a weight problem, knowing how to maintain a healthy weight through a lifetime of temptations and metabolic changes is yet another important message to be retained.

What are some of these factors that influence our collective trends toward overweight and obesity? We know that body weight is a result of genes, metabolism, behavior, environment, culture, and socioeconomic status. Of these, behavior and environment are the easiest to change. Indeed, environmental factors play a large role, especially factors that favor increased energy intake (consuming too much) and decreased energy expenditure (too little physical activity).

Globesity: An Epidemic of Growing Proportions

It's not just Americans today who are bigger and less fit than at any time in history. A similar trend is emerging around the world in both developed and developing regions. In countries as diverse as the Czech Republic, Kuwait, and Jamaica, at least half of the population is overweight, and one in five is obese. The highest obesity rate is in Samoa, where two-thirds of all women and half of men are obese. Although rates in Canada and South America are slightly lower than in the United States, residents of the Americas as a whole are among the most overweight and obese in the world (see details by country in the figure).

While there is growing concern about the epidemic in adults, even more disturbing is the enormous jump in obesity rates among children. Rates of childhood obesity have increased 66 percent in the United States in past decades. If that isn't bad enough, the incidence has increased a whopping 240 percent during the same period in Brazil.

Among the consequences is the parallel rise in type 2 diabetes in the global population; it is now nearly five times more prevalent than it was 18 years ago. The dual impact of diabetes and obesity is sure to demand increasing attention to the global health consequences and disease burden.

Dietary excesses and sedentary lifestyles are key contributors to the increases in obesity. However, according to Donna Eberwine, editor of the Pan American Health Organization's *Perspectives in Health,* "The growing body of public health literature on the 'globesity' epidemic places the bulk of the blame not on individuals, but on globalization and development, with poverty as an exacerbating factor." As entire cultures move away from traditional diets, with raw fruits and vegetables and fewer fats, to diets heavy in highly processed, high fat, and high calorie fast food and packaged products, the same thing that happened to Americans during the move from the farms to cities is occurring. The world population is becoming super-sized along with the products we consume.

Another factor is the increasingly sprawling environment in which people travel only by car and walking or bicycling is difficult. Lack of health education about the risks of obesity also contributes to its increase.

The challenge is daunting. Nations must work together in the decades ahead to educate their populations, promote nutritious diets, and encourage physical activity.

Source: D. Eberwine, "Globesity: The Crisis of Growing Proportions," *Perspectives in Health* 7, no. 3 (2003): 6–11.

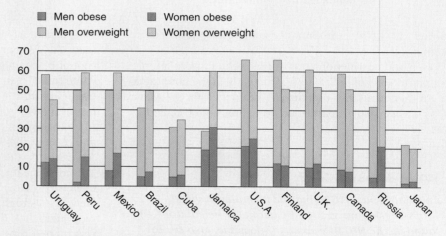

Percentage of Men and Women Who Are Overweight or Obese, by Country

Source: Figure reprinted with permission from *Perspectives in Health* 7, no. 3 © 2003 Pan American Health Organization.

Key Environmental Factors

There is a long list of environmental factors that encourage us to increase our consumption, including the following.

- Bombardment with advertising designed to increase energy intake—ads for high-calorie foods at a low price, marketing super-sized portions.[26] Prepackaged meals, fast food, and soft drinks are all increasingly widespread. High-calorie drinks such as coffee lattes and energy drinks add to daily caloric intake.[27]
- Changes in the number of working women, leading to greater use of restaurant meals, fast foods, and convenience foods. Women now consume, on average, nearly 350 calories per day more than they did in the 1970s.[28]
- Bottle-feeding of infants, which may increase energy intake relative to breast-feeding.[29]
- Misleading food labels that confuse consumers about portion and serving sizes.

Factors contributing to decreased energy expenditure include:

- The increasingly sedentary nature of many jobs.[30]
- Automated equipment and electronic communications, such as cell phones, remote controls, and other labor-saving devices.[31]

- Spending more time in front of the computer and TV and playing video games.[32]
- Fear of playing or being outside based on the threat of violence.
- Decline in physical education requirements in schools.[33]
- Lack of community resources for exercise.

What do you think?

In addition to those listed, can you think of other environmental factors that contribute to obesity?
■ *What actions could you take to reduce your risk for each of these factors?*

Heredity

Are some people born to be fat? Several factors appear to influence why one person becomes obese and another remains thin; genes seem to interact with many of these factors. In fact, over 430 gene markers, genes, and chromosomal markers have been linked to obesity.[34]

Body Type and Genes   In some animal species, the shape and size of the individual's body are largely determined by its parents' shape and size. Many scientists have explored the role of heredity in determining human body shape. You need only look at your parents and then glance in the mirror to see where you got your own body type. Children whose parents are obese also tend to be overweight. In fact, a family history of obesity has long been thought to increase one's chances of becoming obese by 25 to 30 percent.[35] Some researchers argue that obesity has a strong genetic determinant—it tends to run in families. They cite the statistic that 80 percent of children who have two obese parents are also obese.[36] Genes play a significant role in how the body balances calories and energy. Also, by influencing the amount of body fat and fat distribution, genes can make a person more susceptible to gaining weight.

Twin Studies   Early studies of identical twins who were separated at birth and raised in different environments have provided strong evidence that the genes a person inherits are a major factor determining overweight, leanness, or average weight. Whether raised in family environments with fat or thin family members, twins with obese natural parents tend to be obese in later life.[37] According to another study, sets of identical twins who were separated and raised in different families and who ate widely different diets still grew up to weigh about the same.[38]

Although the exact mechanism remains unknown, it is believed that genes set metabolic rates, influencing how the body handles calories. Some experts believe that this genetic tendency may contribute as much as 25 to 40 percent of the reason for being overweight.[39]

Specific Obesity Genes?   In the past decade, more and more research has pointed to the existence of a "fat gene." Rather than inheriting a particular body type that predisposes us to overweight, it may be that our genes predispose us toward certain satiety and feeding behaviors. This "I need to eat" gene may account for up to one-third of our risk for obesity.[40] The most promising candidate for such a gene is the *Ob* gene (for obesity), which is believed to disrupt the body's "I've had enough to eat" signaling system and may prompt individuals to keep eating past the point of being comfortably full. Research on Pima Indians, who have an estimated 75 percent obesity rate (nine out of ten are overweight), points to an *Ob* gene that is a "thrifty gene." It is theorized that because their ancestors struggled through centuries of famine, their basal metabolic rates slowed, allowing them to store precious fat for survival. Survivors may have passed these genes on to their children, which would explain the lower metabolic rates found in Pimas today and their tendency toward obesity.[41]

Scientists have found that they can manipulate mice genes and construct an *Ob* gene that invariably leads to fatness in mice and the development of type 2 diabetes. Many suspect a human counterpart to this gene, but it has yet to be found. In addition, the beta-3 adrenergic receptor gene has been identified and found in human beings and mice. When mutated, it is thought to impede the body's ability to burn fat.[42]

Endocrine Influence: The Hungry Hormones

Although the discovery of the *Ob* gene in mice has provided fertile ground for speculation, researchers have further refined their theories to focus on a protein that the *Ob* gene may produce, known as *leptin*, and a new leptin receptor in the brain. According to these studies, leptin is a hormone that signals the brain when you are full and need to stop eating.[43] If there are excess levels of leptin in the blood, appetite levels drop and calories are burned more rapidly.[44] Although obese people have adequate amounts of leptin and leptin receptors, they do not seem to work properly. It is believed that if we can enhance leptin levels in the blood, people may find it easier to control their hunger urges.

A hormone produced in the stomach known as *ghrelin* may be among the most important players in our collective difficulties in keeping weight off. Researchers at the University of Washington studied a small group of obese people who had lost weight over a six-month period.[45] They noted that ghrelin levels rose before every meal and fell drastically shortly afterward, suggesting that the hormone plays a role in appetite stimulation. People who lost large amounts of weight via gastric bypass surgery had ghrelin levels that were 72 percent lower than those who lost weight through traditional diets and 77 percent lower than those in a control group. While ghrelin doesn't seem to be a cause of obesity, researchers believe that it may make it more difficult to lose weight once you gain it due to its influence on appetite and eating cues. Subsequent studies will test the impact of ghrelin-blocking drugs in controlling appetite as a form of intervention.

Other scientists have isolated a protein called *GLP-1*, which is known to slow down the passage of food through the intestines to allow the absorption of nutrients. In early studies, when scientists injected GLP-1 into the brains of hungry rats, the rats stopped eating immediately.[46] Newer research suggests that the GLP-1 hormone may be a key factor in stimulating insulin production and may eventually be a key factor in diabetes and obesity prevention and control.[47]

It is speculated that leptin and GLP-1 might play complementary roles in weight control. Leptin and its receptors may regulate body weight over the long term, calling upon fast-acting appetite suppressants like GLP-1 when necessary.

Over the years, many people have attributed obesity to problems with their thyroid gland. They believed that an underactive thyroid impeded their ability to burn calories. However, most authorities agree that less than 2 percent of the obese population have a thyroid problem and can trace their weight problems to a metabolic or hormone imbalance.[48]

Hunger, Appetite, and Satiety

Theories abound concerning the mechanisms that regulate food intake. The hypothalamus (the part of the brain that regulates appetite) closely monitors levels of certain nutrients in the blood. When these levels fall, the brain signals us to eat. According to one theory, in the obese person the monitoring system does not work properly and the cues to eat are more frequent and intense than they are in people of normal weight.

Adaptive thermogenesis   Theoretical mechanism by which the brain regulates metabolic activity according to caloric intake.

Hunger   An inborn physiological response to nutritional needs.

Appetite   A learned response that is tied to an emotional or psychological craving for food and is often unrelated to nutritional need.

Satiety   The feeling of fullness or satisfaction at the end of a meal.

Hyperplasia   A condition characterized by an excessive number of cells.

Hypertrophy   The ability of cells to swell.

Setpoint theory   A theory of obesity causation that suggests that fat storage is determined by a thermostatic mechanism in the body that acts to maintain a specific amount of body fat.

Another theory is that thin people send more effective messages to the hypothalamus. This concept, known as **adaptive thermogenesis,** states that thin people can consume large amounts of food without gaining weight because the appetite center of their brains speeds up metabolic activity to compensate for the increased consumption.

Another hypothesis, that food tastes better to obese people, thus causing them to eat more, has largely been refuted.

Scientists distinguish between **hunger,** an inborn physiological response to nutritional needs, and **appetite,** a learned response to food that is tied to an emotional or psychological craving and is often unrelated to nutritional need. Obese people may be more likely than thin people to satisfy their appetite and eat for reasons other than nutrition.

In some instances, the problem with overconsumption may be more related to **satiety** than to appetite or hunger. People generally feel satiated, or full, when they have satisfied their nutritional needs and their stomach signals "no more." For undetermined reasons, obese people may not feel full until much later than thin people. The leptin and GLP-1 studies seem to support this theory.

Developmental Factors

Some obese people may have excessive numbers of fat cells. This type of obesity, **hyperplasia,** usually appears in early childhood and perhaps, due to the mother's dietary habits, even prior to birth. The most critical periods for the development of hyperplasia seem to be the last two to three months of fetal development, the first year of life, and between the ages of 9 and 13. Parents who allow their children to eat without restrictions and become overweight may be setting them up for a lifelong excess of fat cells. Central to this theory is the belief that the number of fat cells in a person's body does not increase appreciably during adulthood. However, the ability of each of these cells to swell (**hypertrophy**) and shrink does carry over into adulthood. Weight gain may be tied to both the number of fat cells in the body and the capacity of individual cells to enlarge.

An average-weight adult has approximately 25 billion to 30 billion fat cells, a moderately obese adult about 60 billion to 100 billion, and an extremely obese adult as many as 200 billion.[49] People who add large numbers of fat cells to their bodies in childhood may be able to lose weight by decreasing the size of each cell in adulthood, but the total number of cells will remain the same. With the next calorie binge, the cells swell and sabotage weight loss efforts (Figure 9.2). Additional research is needed to test these theories.

Setpoint Theory

Nutritional researchers William Bennett and Joel Gurin developed the **setpoint theory,** which stated that a person's body has a setpoint of weight at which it is programmed to be comfortable. If your setpoint is around 160 pounds, you will

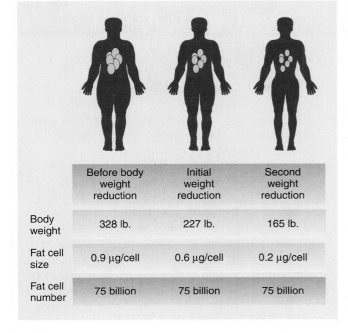

Figure 9.2
One Person at Various Stages of Weight Loss

	Before body weight reduction	Initial weight reduction	Second weight reduction
Body weight	328 lb.	227 lb.	165 lb.
Fat cell size	0.9 μg/cell	0.6 μg/cell	0.2 μg/cell
Fat cell number	75 billion	75 billion	75 billion

Note that, according to the hyperplasia theory, the number of fat cells remains constant but their size decreases when weight is lost.

gain and lose weight fairly easily within a given range of that point. For example, if you gain 5 to 10 pounds on vacation, it will be fairly easy to lose that weight and remain around the 160-pound mark. Through adaptive thermogenesis, the body actually tries to maintain this weight. Some people equate this point with the **plateau** that dieters sometimes reach after losing a certain amount of weight. The setpoint theory proposes that after losing a predetermined amount of weight, the body will actually sabotage additional weight loss by slowing down metabolism. In extreme cases, the metabolic rate will decrease to a point at which the body will maintain its weight on as little as 1,000 calories per day.

Can a person change this predetermined setpoint? Proponents of this theory argue that it is possible to raise one's setpoint over time by continually gaining weight and failing to exercise. Conversely, reducing caloric intake and exercising regularly can slowly decrease one's setpoint. Exercise seems to be the most critical factor in readjusting setpoint, although diet may also be important.

The setpoint theory remains controversial today, and many consider it superseded by research into hormonal and other factors. Perhaps its greatest impact was the sense of relief it provided for people who had lost weight, plateaued, and regained weight time and time again. It told them that their failure was not due to lack of willpower alone. The setpoint theory has also prompted nutritional experts to look more carefully at popular methods of weight loss. If it is correct, an extremely low-calorie diet isn't just dangerous; it may also cause the body to protect the dieter from "starvation" by slowing down metabolism, making weight loss even more difficult.

Psychosocial Factors

The relationship of weight problems to deeply rooted emotional insecurities, needs, and wants remains uncertain. Food is often used as a reward for good behavior in childhood. As adults face unemployment, broken relationships, financial uncertainty, fears about health and other problems, the bright spot in the day is often "what's on the table for dinner" or "we're going to that restaurant tonight." Again, the research underlying theories linking obesity with psychosocial factors is controversial. What is certain is that eating tends to be a focal point of people's lives, and the comfort foods of childhood may provide a salve for painful social pressures. Eating is essentially a social ritual associated with companionship, celebration, and enjoyment. For many people, the social emphasis on the eating experience is a major obstacle to successful dieting. Although some restaurants offer menu items designed to aid dieters, many people have difficulty choosing responsibly when confronted with an entire menu of delicious, fattening foods.

Some theorists contend that obese people ignore internal cues of hunger and are more likely to use the clock as a guide for "time to eat" than real hunger cues. Other studies refute this hypothesis.

Early Sabotage: Obesity in Youth

Another major factor is the pressure placed on us by the food industry's sophisticated marketing campaigns. There may be salad bars at the local fast-food joints, but customers have to run the gauntlet of starchy, beefy delights and high-fat fries to find them. The food and restaurant industries spend billions each year on ads to entice hungry people to forgo fresh fruit and sliced vegetables for Ring Dings and Happy Meals. Children are among the most vulnerable to these ads.

Children's impulses to eat junk food haven't changed much in recent decades. However, as noted earlier, they are eating larger portions. Social forces mentioned earlier, including the decline of home cooking, increased production of calorie- and fat-laden fast foods, and video technology that encourages kids to surf the Internet rather than ride their bicycles, have converged to increase the number of overweight young Americans. As a direct consequence, over 6 million American children are now fat enough to endanger their health. An additional 5 million are on the threshold, and the problem is growing more extreme daily. Obese children suffer both physically and emotionally throughout childhood, and those who stay heavy in adolescence tend to stay fat as adults.[50]

Plateau That point in a weight loss program at which the dieter finds it difficult to lose more weight.

From Atkins to the Glycemic Index: Getting the "Skinny" on Carbohydrates

Low carbohydrate diets have attracted millions of Americans with reports of massive, quick weight loss. Bookstores struggle to keep the latest editions of *The Atkins Diet, The South Beach Diet,* and other bestsellers on their shelves. Restaurants have added "low-carb" items to their menus and a multimillion dollar industry of low-carb food products has emerged. The promise? Eliminate nearly all of the bread, pasta, sweets, and high-carbohydrate foods from your diet, eat red meat and other high-protein, high-fat foods until you are satisfied, and lose weight.

Many health professionals have spent the past 20 years describing low-carb diets as foolish, dangerous, ineffective, and unhealthy for many dieters. The American Heart Association and the American Dietetic Association were just two of many professional health groups that issued warnings about the craze. Yet several well-designed clinical trials indicated that low-carbohydrate diets were as good as—and in many cases, better than—low-fat diets in helping very overweight people shed pounds.

In these studies, more people stayed with the low-carb diet than the low-fat one, and, although they ate more fat, they did not experience the harmful changes in blood cholesterol that many expected. In fact, their LDL ("bad") cholesterol and triglycerides were reduced and their HDL ("good") cholesterol increased.

However, these short-term benefits were soon outweighed by long-term results, as reports of problems with the diet began to surface. A study by the Stanford University Medical Center in conjunction with researchers at Yale University found that, although low-carbohydrate diets cause weight loss, it's the total calorie reduction and the duration of the reduction that causes the loss, not the reduction in carbohydrate intake per se. The take-home message was that any low-calorie diet that a person can stay on long enough will have similar results. Furthermore, people had difficulty in sticking to the rigid dietary requirements. When they lost weight, they began to gain it back nearly as quickly as they had lost it. People with diabetes had problems because whole grains, beans, and other fiber-rich foods were not allowed. Rather than remembering to cut back on saturated fats, people were gulping down bacon and eggs, eating huge steaks, and feeling good about the guilt-free diet.

A major problem with the Atkins and similar diets is that they assume that virtually any carbohydrate is bad for you. However, they do not account for the vast difference in nutrient value among carbohydrates and their *glycemic index,* a ranking of foods according to how quickly their sugars are released into the bloodstream. The body converts a food's sugars into glucose, which is released slowly or rapidly into the bloodstream. Insulin is secreted to counter glucose levels and return the body to healthy levels. Researchers at the University of Toronto discovered in the 1990s that some foods raise blood sugar faster and higher than others, placing greater demands on the insulin system. The research into the glycemic index eventually led to an even more useful measurement known as *glycemic load,* which considers both a food's glycemic index and how much carbohydrate the food delivers in one hit in a single serving.

Most fruits, vegetables, beans, and whole grains have low glycemic loads; their sugars enter the bloodstream gradually and trigger only a moderate rise in insulin. The more high-calorie sugars you consume, the higher your insulin levels rise, triggering a chain of reactions that ultimately make you sluggish, bloated, and

Dietary Myths and Misperceptions

A revealing study compared the self-reported and actual caloric intakes and amounts of exercise among a group of overweight adults. The researchers carefully followed obese people who had been unsuccessful on as many as 20 diets but claimed that they consumed fewer than 1,200 calories per day. They blamed their failure to lose weight on metabolism. It turned out that their metabolism levels were normal, but they were actually eating nearly twice as much as they thought they were and exercising only three-quarters as much as they reported.[51]

Does this mean that obesity is simply the result of gluttony and sloth? No. In fact, many studies have shown that obese individuals do not eat much more than their normal-weight counterparts. However, it should be noted that they do exercise less. The majority of overweight individuals are less active than nonobese people. Of course, it could be argued that their obesity leads to their sedentary lifestyle. Much more research is necessary before scientists have a clear profile of both the obese and nonobese.

Metabolic Rates and Weight

Even at rest, the body consumes a certain amount of energy. The amount of energy your body uses at complete rest is your **basal metabolic rate (BMR)**. About 60 to 70 percent of all the calories you consume on a given day go to support your basal metabolism: heartbeat, breathing, maintaining body temperature, and so on. So if you consume 2,000 calories per

Basal metabolic rate (BMR) The energy expenditure of the body under resting conditions at normal room temperature.

with a slower rate of calorie burning. They may also lead to feelings of hunger, driving you to eat more and continuing the cycle. For those who are overweight and inactive, high levels of insulin production often means that the body either begins to produce less insulin or the cells can't absorb it; ultimately, these high insulin levels can lead to diabetes.

Given this new understanding of carbohydrates, should you do what Atkins suggests, and follow a diet that avoids most carbs? No. The bulk of scientific evidence suggests that you should choose foods with low glycemic loads and continue to reduce your total caloric intake and saturated fat intake.

A few examples of the glycemic load of common foods demonstrates the range you may find in your daily diet: a serving of high quality orange juice has nearly three times the glycemic load (13) as an orange; a serving of cornflakes has five times the load (21) as a serving of All Bran (4). Listings for many foods can be found online, particularly in connection with diabetes resources.

However, instead of memorizing glycemic load values for all your favorite foods, try following these general guidelines:

- *Choose plants.* Pick the fruit rather than its sugar-laden juice counterpart. Eating the skin of apples adds fiber and

slows the entry of glucose into the bloodstream. If you must eat potatoes, eat them with the skin on and cut back on other starches. Instead of potatoes and corn, try sweet potatoes and yams.

- *Forgo meat in favor of beans.* It isn't necessary to cut all meat-based protein from your diet. However, when you eat meat, opt for the lean cuts and choose poultry over pork or beef. Learn to cook and flavor beans. They are high in protein and other nutrients and have very little effect on blood sugar and insulin.

- *Go nuts several times a week.* Contrary to what you may have heard, nuts are not little bundles of fatty calories. Almonds, hazelnuts, peanuts, pecans, and others are healthy low-carbohydrate alternatives for snacking on chips and desserts made from white flour. They are not calorie free, though, so manage your intake based on exercise patterns and caloric needs.

- *Mix your carbs with other foods.* Eating carbohydrates with other foods such as monounsaturated oils (olive or canola) can slow the rate of carbohydrate absorption. Milk or yogurt with cereal is one example; bananas and cottage cheese in cereal is another.

- *Make whole-grain breads a staple.* Avoid white bread and look for brown breads with 100 percent whole wheat

or other grains. Consider options such as substituting brown rice for white and using whole-wheat pizza dough and pasta. These are good choices for slowing your blood sugar rises.

- *Exercise regularly.* Most people would be shocked if they ate a normal meal, measured their blood sugar, then noted how dramatically their blood sugars go down after a 30-minute walk. It may seem simple, but one of the best ways to keep yourself healthy and still consume the carbs you want is through exercise.

These recommendations hold true no matter what low-fat, low-carb, low-calorie or other plan you choose to follow.

Sources: W. Willet and P. Skerrett, "Going Beyond Atkins," *Newsweek,* January 19, 2004, 46; S. Conner et al., "Should a Low-Fat, High-Carb Diet be Recommended for Everyone?" *New England Journal of Medicine* 350 (2004): 1691–1692; F. F. Samaha et al., "A Low-Carbohydrate as Compared with a Low-Fat Diet in Severe Obesity," *New England Journal of Medicine* 348, no. 21 (2003): 2074–2081; G. D. Foster et al., "A Randomized Trial of Low Carbohydrate Diet for Obesity," *New England Journal of Medicine* 348, no. 21 (2003):2082–2090; D. M. Bravata et al., "Efficacy and Safety of Low-Carbohydrate Diets," *Journal of the American Medical Association* 289, no. 14 (2003): 1837–1850.

day, between 1,200 and 1,400 of those calories are burned without your doing any significant physical activity. However, unless you exert yourself enough to burn the remaining 600 to 800 calories, you will gain weight.

Your BMR can fluctuate considerably, with several factors influencing whether it slows down or speeds up. In general, the younger you are, the higher your BMR, partly because in young people cells undergo rapid subdivision, which consumes a good deal of energy. BMR is highest during infancy, puberty, and pregnancy, when bodily changes are most rapid.

BMR is also influenced by body composition. Muscle tissue is highly active—even at rest—compared to fat tissue. In essence, the more lean tissue you have, the greater your BMR, and the more fat tissue you have, the lower your BMR. Men have a higher BMR than women do, at least partly because of their greater proportion of lean tissue. (This is another reason why developing muscular strength and

endurance is so important to weight loss and obesity reduction plans.[52])

Age is another factor. After age 30, BMR slows down by about 1 to 2 percent a year. Therefore, people over 30 commonly find that they must work harder to burn off an extra helping of ice cream than they did when in their teens. "Middle-aged spread," a reference to the tendency to put on weight later in life, is partly related to this change. A slower BMR, coupled with less activity, shifting priorities (family and career become more important than fitness), and loss in muscle mass, puts the weight of many middle-aged people in jeopardy.

In addition, the body has a number of self-protective mechanisms that signal BMR to speed up or slow down. For example, when you have a fever, the energy needs of your cells increase, which generates heat and speeds up your BMR. In starvation situations, the body protects itself by slowing down BMR to conserve precious energy. Thus, when people repeatedly resort to extreme diets, it is believed that their bodies reset their BMRs at lower rates. **Yo-yo diets,** in which people repeatedly gain weight and then starve themselves to lose it, are doomed to failure. When dieters resume eating after their weight loss, their BMR is set lower, making it almost certain that they will regain the pounds they just lost. After repeated cycles of dieting and regaining weight, these people find it increasingly hard to lose weight and increasingly easy to regain it, so they become heavier and heavier.

According to a recent study by Kelly Brownell of Yale University, middle-aged men who maintained a steady weight (even if they were overweight) had a lower risk of heart attack than men whose weight cycled up and down in a yo-yo pattern. Brownell found that small, well-maintained weight losses are more beneficial for reducing cardiovascular risk than large, poorly maintained weight losses.[53]

New research also supports the theory that by increasing your muscle mass, you will increase your metabolism and burn more calories each time you exercise (Chapter 10).

Lifestyle

Of all the factors affecting obesity, perhaps the most critical is the relationship between activity levels and calorie intake. Obesity rates are rising. But how can this be happening? Aren't more people exercising than ever before?

Though the many advertisements for sports equipment and the popularity of athletes may give the impression that Americans love a good workout, the facts are not so positive. Data from the National Health Interview Survey show that four in ten adults in the United States *never* engage in any exercise, sports, or physically active hobbies in their leisure time.[54] Women (43.2 percent) were somewhat more likely than men (36.5 percent) to be sedentary, a finding that was consistent across all age groups. Among both men and women, black and Hispanic adults were more sedentary than white adults.[55] Leisure-time physical activity was also strongly associated with level of education. About 72 percent of adults who never attended high school were sedentary, declining steadily to 45 percent among high school graduates and about 24 percent among adults with graduate-level college degrees.[56]

Do you know people who seemingly can eat whatever they want without gaining weight? With few exceptions, if you were to follow them around for a typical day and monitor the level and intensity of their activity, you would discover the reason. Even if their schedule does not include jogging or intense exercise, it probably includes a high level of activity. Walking up a flight of stairs rather than taking the elevator, speeding up the pace while mowing the lawn,

getting up to change the TV channel rather than using the remote, and doing housework all burn extra calories.

Actually, it may even go beyond that. In studies of calorie burning by individuals placed in a controlled respiratory chamber environment where calories consumed, motion, and overall activity were measured, it was found that some people are better fat burners than others. It is possible that low fat burners may not produce as many of the enzymes needed to convert fat to energy. Or they may not have as many blood vessels supplying fatty tissue, making it tougher for them to deliver fat-burning oxygen. Or perhaps in subtle ways, these people burn more calories through extra motions. Clearly, any form of activity that burns additional calories helps maintain weight.

Smoking Women who smoke tend to weigh six to ten pounds less than nonsmokers. After quitting, weight generally increases to the level found among nonsmokers. Weight gain after smoking cessation may be partly due to nicotine's ability to raise metabolic rate. When smokers stop, they burn fewer calories. Another reason former smokers often gain weight is that they generally eat more after they quit in order to satisfy free-floating cravings.[57]

Gender and Obesity

Throughout our lives, issues of appearance and attractiveness are constantly in the foreground. Only recently have researchers begun to understand just how significant, especially for women, the quest for beauty and the perfect body really is.

Researchers have determined that being severely overweight in adolescence may influence one's social and economic future—particularly for females.[58] Researchers found that obese women complete about half a year less schooling, are 20 percent less likely to get married, and earn thousands less on average per year than their slimmer counterparts. Obese women also have rates of household poverty 10 percent higher than those of women who are not overweight. In contrast, the study found that overweight men are 11 percent less likely to be married than thinner men but suffer few adverse economic consequences.

It may be that women suffer such negative consequences because the social stigma of being overweight is more severe for women than for men. Women are also disadvantaged biologically when it comes to losing weight.

Yo-yo diets Cycles in which people repeatedly gain weight, and then starve themselves to lose weight. This lowers their BMR, which makes regaining weight even more likely.

Compared to men, they have a lower ratio of lean body mass to fatty mass, in part due to differences in bone size and mass, muscle size, and other variables. Muscle uses more energy than fat does. Because men have more muscle, they burn 10 to 20 percent more calories than women do during rest.[59] (See Chapter 10 for an overview of the role that increased muscle mass has on weight reduction.) After sexual maturity, men have higher metabolic rates, making it easier for them to burn off excess calories. Women also face greater potential for weight fluctuation due to hormonal changes, pregnancy, and other conditions that increase the likelihood of weight gain. Also, as a group, men are more socialized into physical activity from birth. Strenuous work and play are encouraged for men, whereas women's roles have typically been more sedentary and required a lower level of caloric expenditure.

Not only are women more vulnerable to weight gain, but also pressures to maintain and/or lose weight make them more likely to take dramatic measures to lose weight. For example, eating disorders are more prevalent among women, and more women than men take diet pills.

However, males experience these pressures, too. The male image is becoming more associated with the body-builder shape and size, and men are becoming more preoccupied with their own physical form. Thus eating disorders, exercise addictions, and other maladaptive responses are on the increase among men as well.

Of increasing interest is an emerging problem seen in both young men and women, known as **social physique anxiety (SPA),** in which the desire to "look good" has a destructive and sometimes disabling effect on one's ability to function effectively in relationships and interactions with others. People suffering from SPA may spend a disproportionate amount of time fixating on their bodies, working out, and performing tasks that are ego-centered and self-directed, rather than focusing on interpersonal relationships and general tasks.[60] Incessant worry about their bodies and their appearance permeates their lives. Overweight and obesity are clear risks for these people, and experts speculate that this anxiety may contribute to eating-disordered behaviors.

Individuality

Although researchers have learned a great deal in recent years about the factors that predispose people to gain or lose weight, controversy remains. Perhaps the most overlooked element is the individual. Just as no two people are exactly alike physiologically, we are not psychologically identical. Each person is a unique result of genetic background, environment, lifestyle, and emotional responses to a lifetime of experiences.

It is highly possible that the causes of obesity are as varied as the people who are obese. If this is so, there can be no universal cure for weight problems. Instead, we must look for a mechanism of prevention or intervention for each individual that is based upon appropriate cultural, social, environmental, and other factors.

Managing Your Weight

At some point in our lives, almost all of us will decide to go on a diet, and many will meet with mixed success. The problem is probably related to the fact that we think in terms of dieting rather than adjusting lifestyle and eating behaviors. It has been well documented that hypocaloric (low-calorie) diets produce only temporary losses and may actually lead to disordered binge eating or related problems. While repeated bouts of restrictive dieting may be physiologically harmful, the sense of failure that we get each time we try and fail can exact far-reaching psychological costs. Drugs and intensive counseling can contribute to positive weight loss, but even then, many people regain weight after treatment.

Keeping Weight Control in Perspective

Although experts say that losing weight simply requires burning more calories than are consumed, putting this principle into practice is far from simple. According to William W. Hardy, MD, president of the Michigan-based Rochester Center for Obesity, to say weight control is simply a matter of pushing away from the table is ludicrous. Nature is a cheat. Sure, calories in minus calories out equals weight, but people of the same age, sex, height, and weight can have differences of as much as 1,000 calories a day in resting metabolic rate—this may explain why one person's gluttony is another's starvation, even if it results in the same readout on the scale. And while people of normal weight average 25 to 35 billion fat cells, obese people can inherit a billowing 135 billion. A roll of the genetic dice adds more variety: hundreds of genes can affect weight.[61] Other factors such as depression, stress, culture, and available foods can also play a role.

Weight loss is more difficult for some people and may require supportive friends, relatives, and community resources, plus extraordinary efforts to prime the body for burning extra calories. Being overweight does not mean people are weak-willed or lazy. As scientists unlock the many secrets of genetic messengers that influence body weight

Social physique anxiety (SPA) A desire to look good that has a destructive effect on a person's ability to function effectively socially.

Tips for Sensible Weight Management

Rather than thinking about the best diet, the key to successful weight management is finding a sustainable way to control food that will work for you. Combine the following strategies with a Behavior Change Contract to develop a weight management plan that is right for you. Remember, you are not going on a diet that you will quit someday. You are making life-long changes that will result in weight loss.

MAKING A PLAN

- *Think of it as a way of life.* This is a way of improving your body and your health rather than a punishment or a diet.
- *Assess where you are.* Monitor your eating habits for two to three days, taking careful note of the good things you are doing and the things that need improvement.
- *Set realistic goals.* No matter what you do, you may not have a perfect body. Realistically, how do you want to look and feel? Set either a weight or a BMI that you want to achieve. Establish short-term goals on the way to the final goal.
- *Establish a plan.* What are three dietary changes you can make today? What exercise will you do tomorrow, the next day, and sustain for one week? Once you do one week, plot a course for two weeks. Jot down how you feel after each week's activity.
- *Be consistent.* Make a number of small changes in what you regularly eat and drink and in your daily activity levels. Make changes that you can stick with and that are comfortable for you (parking farther from a destination and walking, eating cereal and juice for breakfast, walking three days per week, and so on). Set a schedule and try to stick to it, with an alternative time each day in case your plans change. Always

have a fallback option for your scheduled exercise.
- *Look for balance in what you do.* Remember that it's more about balance than about giving things up. If you must have that piece of pizza or chocolate cake, have it, but then be responsible for doing the extra exercise it takes to burn off the calories or for limiting caloric intake the next day. Remember that it's calories taken in and burned over time that makes the difference.
- *Stay positive.* Focus on the positive steps you are taking and the healthy things you do each week rather than the less healthy things.
- *Be patient and persistent.* You didn't develop a weight problem overnight. Don't expect instant results. Assess other gains that you make each week: gains in energy level, the fit of your clothes, and how you feel in your body.
- *Reward successes.* Set short-term goals and reward yourself when you've reached them—new shoes, a new CD, whatever it takes to keep you motivated.

CHANGING YOUR DIET

- *Be adventurous.* Expand your usual meals and snacks to enjoy a wide variety of different options. Focus on the quality of the food rather than the amount you get. Avoid buffets that allow you to replenish your plate several times.
- *Do not constantly deprive yourself of favorite foods or set unrealistic guidelines.* If you slip and eat something you know you shouldn't, just be more careful the next day. Balance over a week's time is important. Allow slips and reward successes.
- *Be sensible with your knife and fork.* Enjoy all foods, just don't overdo. When you eat out, eat slowly, cut food into smaller pieces, and think about taking some home for tomorrow's lunch or dinner. Share entrées with a friend and order salads with dressings on the side.
- *Eat on a regular schedule.* Do not skip meals or let yourself get too hungry.

- *Eat breakfast.* This will prevent you from being too hungry and overeating at lunch.
- *Plan ahead and be prepared for when you might get hungry.* Always have good food available when and where you get hungry.

CHANGING YOUR LEVEL OF ACTIVITY

- *Be active and slowly increase activity.* If you stick to something, it will gradually take less and less effort to walk that mile, for example. Gradually increase your speed and/or distance (see Chapter 10). Move more, sit less. Remember, every step counts. Purchasing an inexpensive pedometer and recording your daily steps is an excellent way to monitor and improve your level of activity.
- *Be creative with your physical activity.* Find activities that you really love and stick to them. If you hate to walk in the rain but love to shop, walk in a covered mall, and then shop! Try things you haven't tried before. Today, options such as yoga, Pilates, dancing, swimming, skiing, and gardening are available.
- *Pick an activity that is inexpensive and does not require fancy equipment.* This means you will maintain your fitness program even when you are traveling away from home.
- *Find an exercise partner to help you stay motivated.* Don't pick your fittest friend. Find someone who is patient, understanding, and supportive. Choose people who need help and commit to helping them. It will also help you get through the difficult days until exercise is part of your lifestyle.

Source: Adapted in part from M. Manore and J. Thompson, "Table 15.3: Techniques to Help an Active Individual Identify and Maintain a Healthy Body Weight Throughout the Life Cycle" in *Sport Nutrition for Health and Performance* (Champaign, IL: Human Kinetics Publishing, 2000), 417.

and learn more about the role of certain foods in the weight loss equation, dieting may not be the same villain in the future that it is today.

To reach and maintain the weight at which you will be healthy and feel best, you need to develop a program of exercise and healthy eating behaviors that will work for you now and in the long term. See the Skills for Behavior Change box for strategies to make your weight management program succeed. To become a wise food consumer, you also need to become familiar with important concepts in weight control.

Understanding Calories

A **calorie** is a unit of measure that indicates the amount of energy we obtain from a particular food. One pound of body fat contains approximately 3,500 calories. So each time you consume 3,500 calories more than your body needs to maintain weight, you gain a pound. Conversely, each time your body expends an extra 3,500 calories, you lose a pound. So if you drink an extra can of Coca-Cola or Pepsi (140 calories) every day and make no other changes in diet or activity, you would gain a pound in 25 days (3,500 calories ÷ 140 calories/day = 25 days). Conversely, if you walk for half an hour each day at a pace of 15 minutes per mile (172 calories burned), you would lose a pound in 20 days (3,500 calories ÷ 172 calories/ day = 20.3 days). Remember, too, that the number of calories you burn is also related to your weight. The heavier you are, the more energy (calories) it takes to move you.

The two ways to lose weight, then, are to lower caloric intake (through better eating habits) and to increase exercise (thereby expending more calories). Don't forget, it took time to gain weight; it will take time to lose it. The best strategy is to go slow, set short-term goals, and stick to them.

Adding Exercise

Approximately 90 percent of the daily caloric expenditures of most people occurs as a result of the **resting metabolic rate (RMR).** Slightly higher than the BMR, the RMR includes the BMR plus any additional energy expended through daily sedentary activities such as food digestion, sitting, studying, or standing. The **exercise metabolic rate (EMR)** accounts for the remaining 10 percent of all daily caloric expenditures; it refers to the energy expenditure that occurs during physical exercise. For most of us, these calories come from light daily activities, such as walking, climbing stairs, and mowing the lawn. If we increase the level of physical activity to moderate or heavy, however, our EMR may be 10 to 20 times greater than typical resting metabolic rates and can contribute substantially to weight loss.

Increasing BMR, RMR, or EMR levels will help burn calories. Any increase in the intensity, frequency, and duration of daily exercise levels can have a significant impact on total calorie expenditure.

Physical activity makes a greater contribution to BMR when it involves large muscle groups. The energy spent on physical activity is the energy used to move the body's muscles—the muscles of the arms, back, abdomen, legs, and so on—and the extra energy used to speed up heartbeat and respiration rate. The number of calories spent depends on three factors:

1. The amount of muscle mass moved
2. The amount of weight moved
3. The amount of time the activity takes

An activity involving both the arms and legs burns more calories than one involving only the legs, an activity performed by a heavy person burns more calories than one performed by a lighter individual, and an activity performed for 40 minutes requires twice as much energy than one performed for only 20 minutes. Thus, obese persons walking for one mile burn more calories than slim people walking the same distance. It may also take overweight people longer to walk the mile, which means that they are burning energy for a longer time and therefore expending more overall calories than the thin walkers.

Improving Your Eating Habits

At any given time, many Americans are trying to lose weight. Given the hundreds of different diets and endless expert advice available, why do we find it so difficult?

Determining What Triggers an Eating Behavior Before you can change a behavior, you must first determine what causes it.

Many people have found it helpful to keep a chart of their eating patterns: when they feel like eating, where they are when they decide to eat, the amount of time they spend eating, other activities they engage in during the meal (watching television or reading), whether they eat alone or with others, what and how much they consume, and how they felt before they took their first bite. If you keep a detailed daily log of the triggers listed in Figure 9.3 on page 292 for at least a week, you will discover useful clues about what in your environment or your emotional makeup causes you to want food. Typically, these dietary triggers center on problems in everyday living rather than on real hunger pangs. Many people find that they eat compulsively when stressed or when they have problems in their relationships. For other people, the same circumstances diminish their appetite, causing them to lose weight.

Changing Your Triggers Once you recognize the factors that cause you to eat, removing the triggers or substituting other

---

Calorie A unit of measurement indicating the energy obtained from a particular food.

Resting metabolic rate (RMR) The energy expenditure of the body under BMR conditions plus other daily sedentary activities.

Exercise metabolic rate (EMR) The energy expenditure that occurs during exercise.

What Triggers Your "Eat" Response?		What Stops Your "Eat" Response?

What Triggers Your "Eat" Response?

- Time of day
- Mood
- Boredom

- Nervousness/anxiety/stress
- Hormonal fluctuations
- Peer/family pressure
- Inattentiveness
- Habit
- Hunger/appetite
- Low self-esteem
- Environment
- Sight and smell of favorite foods

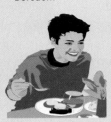

What Stops Your "Eat" Response?

- Acting responsibly in assessing foods
- Practicing stress management
- Breaking the habit
- Remaining active
- Analyzing emotional problems
- Making a conscious effort
- Recognizing true hunger
- Avoiding environment that causes "eat" response

- Selecting alternatives
- Recognizing triggers
- Planning

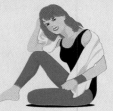

Figure 9.3
The "Eat" Response
Learn to understand what triggers and stops your "eat" response by keeping a daily log.

activities for them will help you develop more sensible eating patterns. Here are some examples of substitute behaviors:

- When eating dinner, turn off all distractions, including the television and radio.
- Replace snack breaks or coffee breaks with exercise breaks.
- Instead of gulping your food, chew each bite slowly and savor it.
- Vary the time of day when you eat. Instead of eating by the clock, do not eat until you are truly hungry. Allow yourself only a designated amount of time for eating—but do not rush. Try to become more aware of true feelings of hunger.
- If you find that you generally eat all that you can cram on a plate, use smaller plates. Put your dinner plates away, and use the salad plates instead.
- Stop buying high-calorie foods that tempt you to snack, or store them in an inconvenient place. (Having to run upstairs for the potato chips will force you to think twice before munching them.)

These are just suggestions. After recording your daily intake for a week, you will be able to devise a list of substitutes that are geared toward your particular eating behaviors. You will find more weight management tips in the Skills for Behavior Change box on page 290.

What do you think?

If you wanted to lose weight, what strategies would you most likely choose? ■ *Which strategies offer the lowest health risk and the greatest chance for success?* ■ *What factors might serve to support or sabotage your weight loss efforts?*

Selecting a Nutritional Plan

Once you have discovered what factors tend to sabotage your weight loss efforts, you will be on your way to healthy weight management. To succeed, however, you must plan for success. By setting goals that are unrealistic or too far in the future, you will doom yourself to failure. Do not try to lose 40 pounds in two months. Try, instead, to lose a healthy one to two pounds during the first week, and stay with this slow and easy regimen. Reward yourself when you lose pounds, and if you binge and go off your nutrition plan, get right back on it the next day. Remember that you did not gain 40 pounds in eight weeks, so it is unrealistic to punish your body by trying to lose that amount of weight in such a short time.

Seek assistance from reputable sources in selecting a dietary plan that is nutritious and easy to follow. Registered dietitians, some physicians (not all physicians have a strong background in nutrition), health educators and exercise physiologists with nutritional training, and other health professionals can provide reliable information. Beware of people who call themselves "nutritionists." There is no such official designation, leaving the door open for just about anyone to call himself or herself a nutritional expert. Avoid weight loss programs that promise quick, miracle results. They are expensive, and most people regain the weight soon after completing the program.

For any weight loss program, ask about the credentials of the adviser, assess the nutrient value of the prescribed diet, verify that dietary guidelines are consistent with reliable nutrition research, and analyze the suitability of the diet to your tastes, budget, and lifestyle. Any diet that requires radical behavior changes is doomed to failure. The most successful plans allow you to make food choices and do not ask you to sacrifice everything you enjoy (see the Reality Check box on page 294 for an analysis of popular diets).

Ultimately, the decision to practice responsible weight management is yours. To be successful, choose a combination of exercise and eating that fits your needs and lifestyle. Find a workable plan, stick to it, and you will succeed.

Considering Drastic Weight Loss Measures

When nothing seems to work, people often become willing to take significant risks in order to lose weight. Dramatic weight loss may be recommended in high-risk cases of hypertension, cardiac strain, imperiled lung capacity, gastrointestinal difficulties, crippling strain on bones and joints, surgical risk, and other problems. Even in such situations, drastic dietary, pharmacological, or surgical measures should be considered carefully and discussed with several knowledgeable health professionals and with full awareness of potential adverse effects.

"Miracle" Diets   Fasting, starvation diets, and other forms of **very low-calorie diets (VLCDs)** have been shown to cause significant health risks. Typically, depriving the body of food for prolonged periods forces it to make adjustments to prevent the shutdown of organs. The body depletes its energy reserves to obtain necessary fuels. One of the first reserves the body turns to in order to maintain its supply of glucose is lean, protein tissue. As this is consumed, weight is lost rapidly because protein contains only half as many calories per pound as fat. At the same time, significant water stores are lost. Over time, the body begins to run out of liver tissue, heart muscle, and so on, as these readily available substances are burned to supply energy. Only after depleting the readily available proteins from these sources does the body begin to burn fat reserves. In this process, known as **ketosis,** the body adapts to prolonged fasting or carbohydrate deprivation by converting body fat to ketones, which can be used as fuel for some brain cells. Within about ten days after the typical adult begins a complete fast, the body will have used many of its energy stores, and death may occur.

In VLCDs, powdered formulas are usually given to patients under medical supervision. These formulas have daily values of 400 to 700 calories plus vitamin and mineral supplements. Although these diets may be beneficial for people who have failed at all conventional weight loss methods and who face severe health risks due to obesity, they should never be undertaken without strict medical supervision. Problems associated with fasting, VLCDs, and other forms of severe caloric deprivation include blood sugar imbalance, cold intolerance, constipation, decreased BMR, dehydration, diarrhea, emotional problems, fatigue, headaches, heart irregularity, ketosis, kidney infections and failure, loss of lean body tissue, weakness, and eventual weight gain due to the yo-yo effect and other variables.

Drug Treatment   Experts reason that if obesity is a chronic disease, it should be treated as such, and the treatment for most chronic diseases includes drugs.[62] The challenge is to develop an effective drug that can be used over time without adverse effects or abuse, and no such drug currently exists.

A classic example of supposedly safe drugs that later were found to have dangerous side effects were Pondimen and Redux, known as *fen-phen* (from their chemical names fenfluramine and phentermine), two of the most widely prescribed diet drugs in U.S. history.[63] When they were found to damage heart valves and contribute to pulmonary hypertension, a massive recall and lawsuit occurred.

Other diet drugs that you should view with caution include:

- *Sibutramine (MERIDIA):* Suppresses appetite by inhibiting the uptake of serotonin. It works best with a reduced calorie diet and exercise, but side effects are not to be taken lightly. They include dry mouth, headache, constipation, insomnia, and high blood pressure. As many obese people already have high blood pressure, this is an obvious concern.
- *Orlistat (Xenical):* Works by inhibiting the action of lipase, an enzyme that helps digest fats. About 30 percent of fats consumed pass through the system undigested, leading to reduced overall caloric intake. Known side effects include oily spotting; gas with watery fecal discharge; fecal urgency; oily stools; frequent, often unexpected, bowel movements; and possible deficiencies of fat-soluble vitamins.[64]
- *Over-the-counter (OTC) drugs:* Only one OTC medication to help with weight loss has FDA approval. It contains *benzocaine* (in candy or gum form), which anesthetizes the tongue, reducing taste sensation. In 2000, the FDA asked drug companies to reformulate any diet aids containing *phenylpropanolamine,* an appetite suppressant, due to problems with rapid pulse, insomnia, hypertension, irregular heartbeats, and kidney failure.[65]
- *Herbal weight-loss aids:* St. John's wort (SJW) and other substances that enhance serotonin and suppress appetite have been widely marketed for weight loss. Be aware that SJW is often combined with *ephedrine,* a stimulant found in certain cold and allergy pills and believed to cause heart attacks, seizures, and strokes.[66] Before you take any herbal medication, make sure you know its possible ingredients and their risks (see Chapter 23).

Surgery   When all else fails, a relatively permanent, yet risky, solution may lie in surgically stapling or tying off the stomach, known as *gastric bypass.* This procedure effectively

---

Very low calorie diets (VLCDs)   Diets with a daily caloric value of 400 to 700 calories.

Ketosis   A condition in which the body adapts to prolonged fasting or carbohydrate deprivation by converting body fat to ketones, which can be used as fuel for some brain activity.

Analyzing Popular Diets

In our ongoing quest to find an effective way to lose weight, Americans consider many seemingly reputable options. Are any of these diet plans really the "miracles" they often claim to be? Don't count on it.

Some are quite good, but others produce no long-term effects and may even be dangerous. Each year, "new and improved" versions of the same old dietary ploys surface in bookstores, where they sell millions of copies. Then there are reports of successes and dangers and finally professional groups jump into the fray to label these diets as ineffective or dangerous. Just

when we think we've seen the last of a fad, its authors reinvent themselves and capture our interest yet again. Dr. Kelly Brownell, noted obesity researcher at Yale University, describes this pattern: "When I get calls about the latest diet fad, I imagine a trick birthday cake candle that keeps lighting up and we have to keep blowing it out over and over again."

Book/Program and Author	Premise of the Diet	How It Claims to Work	Experts' Opinions	Comments
The Atkins Diet, Robert Atkins, MD	Says overweight people eat too many carbohydrates. High protein diet allows you to eat all the protein you want (meat, eggs, cheese, and more) and restricts refined sugar, milk, white rice, and white flour.	Restrict carbohydrates and body goes into ketosis. In ketosis, body gets energy from ketones, little carbon fragments that are the fuel created by breakdown of fat stores. You feel less hungry.	Highly controversial. Low intake of fruits and vegetables a problem.	Possible side effects: nausea, fatigue, low blood pressure, elevated uric acid/kidney problems, bad breath, constipation, fetal harm if pregnant.
Dean Ornish Diet, Dean Ornish, MD	Diet and exercise are important. Watch what you eat; there are foods you should eat all of the time, some of the time, and none of the time. Less than 10% of your calories should come from fat. Eat lots of little meals.	Metabolism is inherited from our ancestors. We need to change old metabolic patterns. Meditation is a part of this: when your soul is fed, you have less need to overeat.	Mostly positive for highly restrictive diet and healthy lifestyle regimen. Documented studies show heart blockage reversal. Drawbacks are that is tough to stick to this diet and new eating patterns must be learned. Only the most committed will stick to this rigid diet.	May be tough for all but strict vegans to adhere to this plan. Eating smaller, more frequent meals may be difficult. Otherwise a good model.
Eating Well for Optimum Health, Andrew Weil, MD	Eat less, exercise more. Take a more Eastern than Western approach. Avoid quick fixes and set realistic goal of 1–2 pounds of weight loss per week. Balance the amount and type of food. Describes meats as "flesh foods." Minimize dairy, and take a Mediterranean dietary approach.	Keeps it simple. Criticizes high protein diets because of rise in cholesterol and calcium depletion. Moderation is key.	A more holistic approach to dieting than most. Considers exercise and stress as factors.	May not be sustainable for those who are used to diets high in dairy or meat. Nutrition experts support this common-sense approach. Vegetarian emphasis substantiated as healthy by numerous studies.
The Pritikin Principle, Robert Pritikin	Concern not for calories, but for density of calories. Eat more foods that are not calorie-dense, such as apples and oatmeal.	Fill up on foods that have fewer calories. Large volume of fiber and water will keep you full. Emphasis on vegetables, fruits, beans, unprocessed grains; exercise strongly recommended.	Weight loss will occur but so will frequent feelings of hunger. Weight will usually creep back. Low in fat so healthy in general, except when taken to extreme or for certain groups of people.	Strict limitations of animal products a plus. Incorporates exercise and stress management. Not an easy plan to stick to.
The South Beach Diet, Arthur Agatston, MD	Similar to other low carb diets but with more emphasis on glycemic index.	Carbohydrates lead to overeating and cravings. Advocates combining small amounts of undesirable carbs with vegetables and proteins.	As with other low carb diets, research is still being conducted into effectiveness of this style of dieting.	Does not include recommendations to incorporate exercise into program, a key to any weight loss. Less restrictive on portion sizes than other diets.

Virtually anyone can write a book making diet claims. Even if the authors have PhDs, MDs, or other credentials, they may not have expertise in the area that they write about. If they do have the expertise, they may base their arguments on unproven science or faulty scientific reasoning. Although health claims should only be published after solid research has proven the results repeatedly with different populations, this happens all too infrequently.

Here we summarize some of the most popular diets and the consensus opinions of the U.S. Department of Agriculture, the American Heart Association, the Center for Science in the Public Interest, and several other professional groups and individuals regarding effectiveness and safety. For a detailed discussion of recent research into low carbohydrate diets, see the New Horizons in Health box on page 286.

Source: United States Department of Agriculture, "The Great Nutrition Debate," 2000, www.usda.gov/cnpp/publications.html

Book/Program and Author	Premise of the Diet	How It Claims to Work	Experts' Opinions	Comments
Sugar Busters, H. Leighton Steward, Morrison Bethea, MD, Samuel Andrews, MD, and Luis Balart, MD	Cut sugar to trim fat. Pay attention to portion size. Eliminate potatoes, corn, rice, bread, carrots, refined sugar, honey, colas, and beer.	Glucose, insulin production theory: the more insulin produced, the more fat.	Most don't like this diet. When you gain weight, it doesn't matter where calories come from; it is total calorie intake that is most important.	You'll lose weight due to decreased calorie intake, but this is not a good long-term strategy.
Weight Watchers	Eat from food groups, tally points to monitor intake. Based on weight and dietary goals. Eat what you want, but use discretion in amount.	Based on calories in and calories out. Includes exercise and social support.	Life focus rather than diet focus. Has support of most national organizations. One of the most highly recommended diets.	Works well for many people, particularly those for whom social support is important.
The Zone, Barry Sears, PhD	Offers a wellness philosophy to develop a metabolic state in which the body works efficiently. Recommends eating different calories than you do now and a small amount of protein. Identifies favorable vs. unfavorable carbohydrates.	Claims that his percentages of fat, protein, and carbohydrates are the best ratios for health.	Superiority of given ratios is unsubstantiated by research. Mixed reviews from experts: easy to follow, but don't count on results. Some recommendations (eating high-fat ice cream) are questionable.	Not a lot of do's and don'ts. Dieters may find it easy to follow.

reduces stomach size to hold only a few tablespoons of food. Patients can't eat enough calories, so they lose weight. Make no mistake about it, this procedure should be reserved only for the morbidly obese who face imminent health risks. Complications are many, and include infections, nausea, vomiting, vitamin and mineral deficiencies, and dehydration. (Imagine really being thirsty and only being able to drink a few tablespoons of water at a time). Lifelong medical and sometimes psychological monitoring is necessary for those who have this procedure. Because it is costly to undergo and difficult to undo, it should be considered only when all other avenues have been exhausted. For those who successfully lose weight with this procedure, however, the health benefits are clear. Drastic reductions in cardiovascular disease risk factors, including blood glucose, blood pressure, total cholesterol, HDL cholesterol, and triglycerides were seen in patients in one recent study.[67]

Liposuction is another surgical procedure for spot reducing. Although this technique has garnered much attention, it, too, is not without risk: infections, severe scarring, and even death have resulted. In many cases, people who have liposuction regain fat in those areas or require multiple surgeries to repair lumpy, irregular surfaces from which the fat was removed.

Trying To Gain Weight

Although trying to lose weight poses a challenge for many, a smaller group of Americans, for a variety of metabolic, hereditary, psychological, and other reasons, inexplicably start to lose weight or can't seem to gain weight no matter how hard they try. If you are one of these individuals, the first priority is to determine why you cannot gain weight.

Positive Steps in the War Against Obesity

Although there is much that you can do in managing your weight, one thing is true. Individuals are up against powerful forces that have economic motives to encourage you to eat, eat, eat. While it may seem that the challenges of weight management often overshadow positive actions, there are positive actions being taken every day in our battle with the bulge.

When consumer groups actively pursued the fast-food industry and threatened lawsuits for super-sizing Americans, several fast-food chains responded. McDonalds stopped pushing super-sized burgers and fries (although they are still available on the menu). Other chains began adding salads and fruit options. Choices for more healthy entrées increased. Restaurant chains, notably Ruby Tuesdays, began putting nutrient values on their menus. Now, if you choose the triple burger with bacon, cheese, and other add-ons, the total calories, fats and carbohydrates are clearly there for you to see.

The U.S. Food and Drug Administration is working to force changes that will help consumers. Some likely to happen in the very near future include:

- Going beyond making calories more prominent on food labels. Bigger font sizes and more distinctive coloring are also under consideration.
- Being clearer about the number of calories in a package. For example, you may pick up a standard candy bar and see that there are 175 calories per serving. You eat the whole candy bar, thinking that that neat little package is one serving. However, on further reading, you might find that the serving size is only one-third of the bar. Multiplied by three, the entire bar is over 500 calories, nearly one-third of what many people should consume in an entire day.
- Setting standards for what terms such as "low carb" and "net carb" mean.

- Creating a plan to address label violations. Who punishes manufacturers if they misrepresent nutrient values on labels? What about those who don't even put the information on labels, and tell consumers to call in to obtain the information? The Federal Trade Commission is considering standards, penalties, and enforcement issues.
- Improving consumer education. The Food Guide Pyramid is being revised and reissued in response to criticisms, in a new version intended to address major concerns and be more readily understandable to the general public.
- Requiring restaurants and other food sellers to publish nutrient values on their menus. You can help by asking restaurants to supply this information and supporting those that do.

Do you believe restaurants and other food providers should be required to provide healthy options? Whose responsibility is it to choose nutritious meals?

For example, among older adults, senses of taste and smell may decline, which makes food taste differently and be less pleasurable. Visual problems and other disabilities may make food more difficult to prepare, and dental problems may make eating certain foods more difficult. People who engage in extreme sports that require extreme nutritional supplementation may be at risk for nutritional deficiencies, which can lead to immune system problems and organ dysfunction, weakness that leads to falls and fractures, slower recovery from diseases, and a host of other problems.

Once you know what is causing a daily caloric deficit, there are steps you can take to gain extra weight:

- Eat at regularly scheduled times, whether hungry or not.
- Eat more. Obviously, you are not taking in enough calories to support whatever is happening in your body. Eat more frequently, spend more time eating, eat the high-calorie foods first if you fill up fast, and always start with the main course. Take time to shop, to cook, to eat slowly. Put extra spreads such as peanut butter, cream cheese, or cheese on your foods. Make your sandwiches with extra-thick slices of bread, and add more filling. Take seconds whenever possible, and eat high-calorie snacks during the day.

- Supplement your diet. Add high-calorie drinks that have a healthy balance of nutrients.
- Try to eat with people you are comfortable with. Avoid people who you feel are analyzing what you eat or make you feel like you should eat less.
- If you are sedentary, be aware that exercise can increase appetite. If you are exercising or exercising to extremes, moderate your activities until you've gained some weight.
- Avoid diuretics, laxatives, and other medications that cause you to lose body fluids and nutrients.
- Relax. Many people who are underweight operate at high gear most of the time. Slow down, get more rest, and control stress.

Thinking Thin: Body Image and Eating Disorders

Most of us think of the obsession with weight control as a recent phenomenon. Beginning with supermodel Twiggy in the 1960s and continuing with supermodel Kate Moss in the early 2000s, the thin look has dominated fashion and the

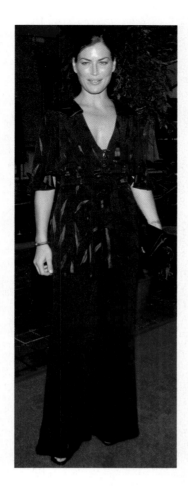

Model Carre Otis struggled with eating disorders for many years. Ironically, now that she is at a healthy weight, she is considered a "plus-size" model.

media. However, an obsession with being thin has long been part of our culture. During the Victorian era, women wore corsets to achieve unrealistically tiny waists. By the 1920s, it was common knowledge that obesity was linked to poor health. The American Tobacco Company coined the phrase "reach for a Lucky instead of a sweet" to promote the idea that cigarettes dulled appetite.

Today more than ever before, underweight models and celebrities exemplify desirability and success, delivering the subtle message that thin is in. Public health warnings that being overweight increases risk for heart disease, certain cancers, and a number of other disorders can send a panic through people when their weight isn't what they think it should be. Some of these distorted views of self-image arise from misinterpreting height–weight charts, making some people strive for the lower readings stipulated for a light-boned person when determining their own normal weight. Increasing numbers of adolescents, teens, and adults are so preoccupied with trying to be like the size 4 models that they make themselves ill. Being overweight has become socially unacceptable in many circles, and obese people are increasingly stigmatized in our society.[68] Americans are looking for fast answers: Should we count calories or carbohydrates? Is dietary fat your biggest enemy? Is Pritikin, Atkins, Weight Watchers, or something else your best weight control strategy? Sadly, many people end up answering these questions with disordered eating patterns such as anorexia, bulimia, and binge-eating.

Eating Disorders

For an increasing number of people, particularly young women, an obsessive relationship with food develops into **anorexia nervosa,** a persistent, chronic eating disorder characterized by deliberate food restriction and severe, life-threatening weight loss. **Bulimia nervosa** involves frequent bouts of binge eating followed by purging (through self-induced vomiting or laxative abuse) or excessive exercise. A variation known as **binge eating disorder (BED)** includes occasional bouts of binge eating but not the purging behavior. In the United States, more than 10 million people, 90 percent of whom are women, meet the established criteria for one of these disorders, and their numbers appear to be increasing.[69] Many more suffer from lesser forms of these conditions—not enough for a true diagnosis, but dangerously close to the precipice that will ultimately lead to life-threatening results (Table 9.4 on page 298).

Anorexia involves self-starvation motivated by an intense fear of gaining weight along with an extremely distorted body image. When anorexia occurs in childhood, failure to gain weight in a normal growth pattern may be the key indicator; later, anorexia typically results in actual weight loss. Nearly 1 percent of girls in late adolescence meet the full criteria for anorexia; many others suffer from significant symptoms.

Initially, most people with anorexia lose weight by reducing total food intake, particularly of high-calorie foods, eventually leading to restricted intake of almost all foods. What they do eat, they often purge through vomiting or using laxatives. Although they lose weight, people with anorexia never seem to feel "thin enough" and constantly identify body parts that are "too fat."

People with bulimia often binge and then take inappropriate measures, such as secret vomiting, to lose the calories they have just acquired. Up to 3 percent of adolescents and young female adults are bulimic, with male rates being about 10 percent of the female rate. People with bulimia are also

Anorexia nervosa Eating disorder characterized by excessive preoccupation with food, self-starvation, and/or extreme exercising to achieve weight losses.

Bulimia nervosa Eating disorder characterized by binge eating followed by inappropriate measures to prevent weight gain.

Binge eating disorder (BED) Eating disorder characterized by recurrent binge eating, without excessive measures to prevent weight gain.

Table 9.4
DSM-IV Eating Disorder Criteria

Anorexia

According to the American Psychiatric Association's *Diagnostic and Statistical Manual of Mental Disorders,* 4th edition *(DSM-IV)*, people who meet the criteria for anorexia nervosa experience all of the following symptoms:

- Refusal to maintain the minimum body weight for one's height and age
- Intense fear of gaining weight even though underweight
- Disturbed perception of one's body weight or size
- In postpubescent women, the absence of at least three consecutive menstrual cycles (in some women, the loss of periods precedes any significant weight loss)

Disordered Eating

People with unhealthy or disordered eating patterns may show some or all of these signs:

- Excessive weight loss; preoccupation with food; intense fear of weight gain
- Obsession with clothing size, scales, and mirrors
- Refusal to eat with others; ritualistic eating
- Excessive exercise
- Moodiness; social withdrawal

Bulimia

People with bulimia experience all of the following:

- Recurrent episodes of consuming a much larger amount of food than most people would during a similar time period (this is usually about two hours) and a sense of loss of control over eating during each episode
- Accompanying attempts to compensate for eating binges by vomiting, abusing laxatives or other drugs, or by fasting or excessive exercise
- Both the binge eating and purging occur at least twice a week for three months
- A negative perception of one's shape and weight
- Frequent vomiting or use of laxatives
- Absent or irregular menstruation
- Excessive facial and body hair; hair loss
- Swollen salivary glands
- Broken blood vessels in the eyes

Sources: Reprinted with permission from the *Diagnostic and Statistical Manual of Mental Disorders,* 4th ed., Text Revision. Copyright 2000 American Psychiatric Association; E. Sohn, "The Roots of Anorexia," *U.S. News and World Report Guide to Family Health,* July 1, 2003 © 2003 *U.S. News & World Report,* L. P. Reprinted with permission.

obsessed with their bodies, weight gain, and how they appear to others. Unlike those with anorexia, people with bulimia are often hidden from the public eye because their weight may vary only slightly or fall within a normal range. Also, treatment appears to be more effective for bulimia than for anorexia.

Individuals with binge eating disorder also binge like their bulimic counterparts but do not take excessive measures to lose the weight that they gain. Often they are clinically obese, and they tend to binge much more often than the typical obese person, who may consume too many calories but spaces his or her eating over a more normal daily eating pattern.

Who's at Risk?

There's no simple explanation for why intelligent, often highly accomplished people spiral downward into the destructive behaviors associated with eating disorders. Obsessive-compulsive disorder, depression, and anxiety can all play a role, as can a desperate need to win social approval or gain control of their lives through food.

Sufferers tend to be women from white middle-class or upper-class families in which there is undue emphasis on achievement, body weight, and appearance. Contrary to popular thinking, however, eating disorders span social class, gender, race, and ethnic backgrounds and are present in countries throughout the world.

Once believed to be primarily a female issue, eating disorders are on the rise among young men. While it is true that females between ages 12 and 25 make up 85 to 90 percent of people with eating disorders, some 15 percent of people affected are males.[70] Certain athletic competitions appear to put males at much greater risk. Jockeys, bodybuilders, wrestlers, dancers, swimmers, rowers, gymnasts, and runners are at highest risk. At the other end of the continuum of men and women who are so obsessed with bulking up and obtaining "six-pack abs" that they are willing to do just about anything to get "the look."

Some studies have shown possible associations between identical twins, and others point to the large numbers of eating disordered persons who have a mother or sister with the disease. Many people with disordered eating patterns also suffer from other problems: many are clinically depressed, suffer from obsessive-compulsive disorder, and have other health problems.

Treatment for Eating Disorders

Because eating disorders result from many factors, spanning many years of development, there are no quick or simple solutions. Treatment often focuses first on reducing the threat to life; once the patient is stabilized, long-term therapy involves family, friends, and other significant people in the individual's life. Therapy focuses on the psychological, social, environmental, and physiological factors that have led to the problem. Finding a therapist who really understands the multidimensional aspects of the problem is a must. Therapy allows the patient to focus on building new eating behaviors, recognizing threats, building self-confidence, and finding other ways to deal with life's problems. Support groups often help the family and the individual gain understanding and emotional support and learn self-development techniques designed to foster positive reactions and actions. Treatment of underlying depression may also be a focus.

TAKING CHARGE

MAKE IT HAPPEN!

Assessment: The Assess Yourself box on page 272 identifies six areas of importance in determining your readiness for weight loss. If you think you should lose weight to improve your health, understanding your attitudes about food and exercise will help you succeed.

Making a Change: In order to change your behavior, you need to develop a plan. Follow these steps.

1. Evaluate your behavior, and identify patterns and specific things you are doing. What can you change now? What can you change in the near future?
2. Select one pattern of behavior that you want to change.
3. Fill out a Behavior Change Contract. It should include your long-term goal for change, your short-term goals, the rewards you'll give yourself for reaching these goals, potential obstacles along the way, and strategies for overcoming these obstacles. For each goal, list the small steps and specific actions that you will take.
4. Chart your progress in a journal. At the end of a week, consider how successful you were in following your plan. What helped you to be successful? What made change more difficult? What will you do differently next week?
5. Revise your plan as needed. Are the short-term goals attainable? Are the rewards satisfying?

One Student's Plan: Shannon had gained the "freshman 15" and wanted to put together a weight management plan. She assessed her readiness for weight loss and saw that her scores in certain areas highlighted areas that she needed to be aware of to succeed. She had never binged and purged

(Part IV), she had strong motivation (Part I), and she already had an enjoyable, regular exercise program (Part VI). However, Shannon also saw that she was not always aware of the eating cues and emotions that caused her to overeat (Parts II, III, and V). Although she hadn't realized it, she tended to do most of her snacking while she was studying at night. No matter what else she had eaten during the day, she would end up eating candy and chips from the vending machines. Especially when she was anxious about an upcoming test or bored by her reading, she would eat even though she was already full.

Shannon made a plan for herself that would help her manage her snacking. She wanted to become aware of what she was eating and how it was contributing to her weight gain. Her first step was to buy study snacks that were healthier choices than chips and candy, such as grapes and low fat granola. Her next step was to make a commitment to think about how hungry she was before automatically starting to snack when she was studying. If she was snacking because she was bored or anxious, she would try to restrict her snack to a predetermined amount or wait until she really was hungry. Shannon tried this plan for two weeks. At the end of two weeks she saw that she had lost four pounds. She decided she wanted to address another of her eating habits, which was ordering pizza with her roommates when they watched their favorite TV shows during the week. Even when she had had a full dinner, Shannon found herself eating two or three pieces of pizza in front of the TV. Shannon suggested to her roommates that, if they had already had dinner, they pop some popcorn to eat instead. Not only was this healthier, but it cost less than having a pizza delivered.

Summary

- Overweight, obesity, and weight-related problems are on the rise in the United States. Obesity is now defined in terms of fat content rather than in terms of weight alone.
- There are many different methods of assessing body fat. Body mass index (BMI) is one of the most commonly accepted measures of weight based on height. Body fat percentages more accurately indicate how fat or lean a person is.
- Many factors contribute to one's risk for obesity, including genetics, developmental factors, setpoint, endocrine influences, psychosocial factors, eating cues, lack of awareness, metabolic changes, lifestyle, and gender. Women often have considerably more difficulty with losing weight.
- Exercise, dieting, diet pills, and other strategies are used to maintain or lose weight. However, sensible eating behavior and adequate exercise probably offer the best options.
- Eating disorders consist of severe disturbances in eating behaviors, unhealthy efforts to control body weight, and abnormal attitudes about body and shape. Anorexia nervosa, bulimia nervosa, and binge eating disorder are the three main eating disorders. Though prevalent among white women of upper- and middle-class families, eating disorders affect women of all backgrounds as well as men.

Questions for Discussion and Reflection

1. Discuss the pressures, if any, you feel to improve your personal body image. Do these pressures come from media, family, friends, and other external sources, or from concern for your personal health?
2. What type of measurement would you choose in order to assess your fat levels? Why?
3. List the risk factors for obesity. Evaluate which seem to be most important in determining whether you will be obese in middle age.
4. Create a plan to help someone lose the "freshman 15" over the summer vacation. Assume that the person is male, 180 pounds, and has 15 weeks to lose the excess weight.
5. Differentiate among the three eating disorders. Then give reasons why females might be more prone to anorexia and bulimia than males are.

Accessing Your Health on the Internet

Visit the following Internet sites to explore further topics and issues related to personal health. To visit an organization's website, go to the Companion Website for *Access to Health, Ninth Edition* at www.aw-bc.com/donatelle, click on the book image, and select "Accessing Your Health on the Internet" from the navigation menu.

1. *American Dietetic Association.* Recommended dietary guidelines and other current information about weight control.
2. *Duke University Diet and Fitness Center.* Information about one of the best programs in the country focused on helping people live healthier, fuller lives through weight control and lifestyle change.
3. *Helping to End Eating Disorders (HEED).* The website of an organization dedicated to fighting eating disorders and helping individuals through the ordeal. Includes a chatroom for people to exchange thoughts and share support.
4. *Mayo Health O@sis.* Summary of many weight control issues and concerns.
5. *Shape Up America.* Strategies and ideas for getting in shape and staying at your optimal weight.

Further Reading

Brownell, K. and K. Horgen, *Food Fight The Inside Story of America's Obesity Crisis—and What We Can Do about It.* New York: McGraw-Hill, 2003.

Director of the Yale Center for Eating and Weight Disorders, Brownell critiques the way that food is marketed and sold to children, placing much of the blame for childhood obesity on advertising and unhealthy foods being offered in schools.

Gaesser, G. *Big Fat Lies.* New York: Fawcett Columbine Press, 1997.

Excellent overview of leading theories on fat, obesity, and a host of related problems and issues. Also discusses potential weight loss strategies that are "keepers" for life.

Piscatella, J. *The Fat-Gram Guide to Restaurant Food,* 3rd ed. New York: Workman Press, 2000.

Useful guide to fast foods and restaurant fat content.

U.S. Department of Agriculture, "The Great Nutrition Debate," 2000 (www.usda.gov/cnpp).

An online transcript of a day of presentations and panel discussions by leading obesity experts and authors of fad diet books.

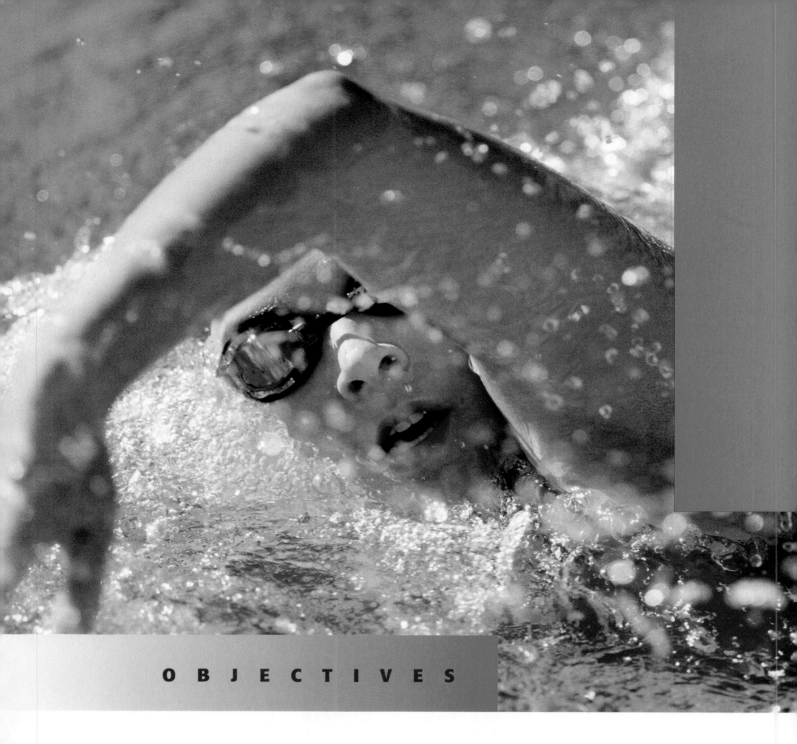

OBJECTIVES

- Describe the benefits of regular physical activity, including improved cardio-respiratory fitness, muscular fitness, bone mass, weight control, stress management, mental health, and life span.

- Define physical activity and exercise as they relate to health and fitness.

- Explain the components of an aerobic exercise program and how to determine the best frequency, intensity, and duration of exercise.

- Discuss different stretching and strength exercises designed to improve strength and flexibility.

- Compare the various types and benefits of resistance exercise programs.

- Summarize ways to prevent and treat common fitness injuries.

- Discuss the factors that contribute to obsessive exercise patterns, and suggest strategies for preventing them.

- Summarize the key components of a personal fitness program, and develop your own fitness program.

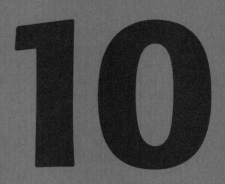

10

PERSONAL FITNESS

IMPROVING HEALTH THROUGH EXERCISE

IN THE NEWS

Pudgy Pooches and Owners Can Shed Pounds Together

By Anahad O'Connor

Couples who exercise together, experts have always said, are more likely to stick to a fitness plan than those who go it alone. But a new study, offering a twist on the old-fashioned buddy system, has found that people looking for a sidekick need look no further than their pets.

In perhaps the first experiment of its kind, researchers showed that overweight owners and their pudgy pooches could lose weight and successfully stay trim by joining a diet and exercise program together. The owners shed as many pounds as a control group of people without pets, while the dogs fared even better, dropping a greater percentage of body weight. The findings of the study, financed by Hill's Pet Nutrition, a pet food company, were presented last week at the national obesity conference in Las Vegas.

"We're always looking for creative ways to help people manage their weight so they find it fun and rewarding," said Dr. Robert Kushner, the medical director of the Wellness Institute at Northwestern Memorial Hospital and the lead author of the study. "We are facing a dual obesity epidemic in this country among people and their pets, and the idea came about to tackle both problems together."

Read the complete article online in the eThemes section of this book's website: www.aw-bc.com/donatelle.

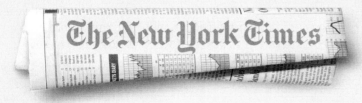

The New York Times

A century ago in the United States, simple survival required performing heavy physical labor on a daily basis. A trip to the store meant hitching up the horses or walking, without the benefit of special walking shoes; in fact, long walks were often taken barefoot or in hand-me-down shoes. Today, taking a walk is something we do for recreation rather than necessity. Motorized vehicles provide our transportation, and even bicycles are designed to minimize effort by the person riding them.

Science and technology have transformed our lives but made us more physically inactive than ever. Inactivity contributes to all causes of mortality, increases the risk of cardiovascular disease (CVD), diabetes, obesity (see Chapter 9), colon cancer, high blood pressure, osteoporosis, depression, and anxiety.[1] Consider the following facts about the U.S. population in the early twenty-first century:[2]

- Roughly 13.5 million people have coronary heart disease, and about 1.5 million suffer a heart attack in any given year.
- Some 8 million people have type 2 diabetes.
- Over 60 million people are overweight, and 44 million are obese.
- About 95,000 new cases of colon cancer are diagnosed each year.
- Fifty million people have high blood pressure.
- 14 million men and 30 million women have low bone mass and an increased risk for fractures.
- 18 million American adults suffer from depressive disorders, and 1 in 6 suffer from anxiety disorders.[3]

Even though these disease statistics look grim, there is something that can improve them. Decades of research show that physical activity has tremendous health-promoting and disease-preventing benefits. Unfortunately, most Americans do not take advantage of this. According to the 2000 Behavioral Risk Factor Surveillance System (BRFSS), a nationwide survey conducted by the Centers for Disease Control and Prevention (CDC), only 26 percent of adults engage in the recommended amounts of physical activity and over 25 percent reported doing no physical activity at all.[4]

Physical activity   Any bodily movement that is produced by the contraction of skeletal muscles and that substantially increases energy expenditure.

Exercise   Planned, structured, and repetitive bodily movement done to improve or maintain one or more components of physical fitness.

Physical fitness   The ability to perform moderate-to-vigorous levels of physical activity on a regular basis without excessive fatigue.

Physical Fitness, Activity, and Exercise

Physical activity is defined as any bodily movement that is produced by the contraction of skeletal muscles and that substantially increases energy expenditure.[5] Physical activities can be done in leisure-time, at work, or even for transportation. Walking, swimming, heavy lifting, and housework are all examples of physical activity. Physical activities also may vary by intensity. For example, walking to class may require little effort but walking to class up a hill while carrying a heavy backpack makes the activity more intense.

The term *exercise* is a bit more specific than physical activity. Exercise is defined as planned, structured, and repetitive bodily movement done to improve or maintain one or more components of physical fitness, such as endurance, flexibility, and strength.[6] **Physical fitness** is the ability to perform moderate-to-vigorous levels of physical activity on a regular basis without excessive fatigue. Table 10.1 identifies the major health-related components of physical fitness.

The recommendations for physical activity and exercise vary by their goal. Because research shows numerous health benefits from becoming more physically active, the CDC and American College of Sports Medicine (ACSM) recommend that adults engage in moderate-intensity physical activities for at least 30 minutes on most days of the week.[7] This amount of physical activity will not prepare you for running a marathon, but because many Americans find intense exercise difficult, it is a realistic goal for everyone. The ACSM and CDC recommend that if you want to improve your cardiorespiratory fitness, you need to perform vigorous physical activities (for example, jogging/running, walking hills, circuit weight training, singles tennis) at least three days per week for at least 20 minutes at a time.

Some people have limitations that make achieving these recommendations difficult, but they can still be physically active and reap the benefits of a regular exercise program. For example, a woman with arthritis in the knee and hip joints might not be able to jog without extreme pain, but she can engage in water exercise in a swimming pool. The water will help relieve much of the stress on her joints and she can improve her range of motion. Similarly, a man who uses a wheelchair may be unable to walk or run, but he can stay physically fit by playing wheelchair basketball.

Benefits of Regular Physical Activity

Regular physical activity has been shown to improve more than 50 different physiological, metabolic, and psychological aspects of human life. There is no better time than now to develop an exercise plan that will enable you to reap these benefits.[8]

Table 10.1
Major Components of Physical Fitness

Cardiorespiratory fitness	Ability to sustain moderate-intensity whole-body activity for extended time periods
Flexibility	Range of motion at a joint or series of joints
Muscular strength and endurance	Maximum force applied with single muscle contraction; ability to perform repeated high-intensity muscle contractions
Body composition	A composite of total body mass, fat mass, fat-free mass, and fat distribution

Source: American College of Sports Medicine, "ACSM Position Stand on the Recommended Quantity and Quality of Exercise for Developing and Maintaining Cardiorespiratory and Muscular Fitness and Flexibility in Adults," *Medicine and Science in Sports and Exercise* 30 (1998): 975–991. http://lww.com

Improved Cardiorespiratory Fitness

Cardiorespiratory fitness refers to the ability of the circulatory and respiratory systems to supply oxygen to the body during sustained physical activity.[9] Regular exercise makes these systems more efficient by enlarging the heart muscle, enabling more blood to be pumped with each stroke, and increasing the number of *capillaries* (small blood vessels that allow gas exchange between blood and surrounding tissues) in trained skeletal muscles, which supply more blood to working muscles. Exercise also improves the respiratory system by increasing the amount of oxygen that is inhaled and distributed to body tissues.[10]

Reduced Risk of Heart Disease Your heart is a muscular organ made up of highly specialized tissue. Because muscles become stronger and more efficient with use, regular exercise strengthens the heart, enabling it to pump more blood with each beat. This increased efficiency means that the heart requires fewer beats per minute to circulate blood throughout the body. A stronger, more efficient heart is better able to meet the ordinary demands of life.

Prevention of Hypertension *Blood pressure* refers to the force exerted by blood against blood vessel walls, generated by the pumping action of the heart. Hypertension, the medical term for abnormally high blood pressure, is a significant risk factor for cardiovascular disease and stroke. Hypertension is particularly prevalent in adult African Americans. Over 30 percent report having high blood pressure, compared with 23 percent of whites and 18 percent of Hispanics.[11] People with consistently elevated blood pressure are two to four times more susceptible to heart disease as are people

with normal blood pressure.[12] Studies report that moderate exercise can reduce both diastolic and systolic blood pressure by 7 mmHg.[13] See Chapter 15 for the newest blood pressure guidelines.)

Improved Blood Lipid and Lipoprotein Profile Lipids are fats that circulate in the bloodstream and are stored in various places in the body. Regular exercise is known to reduce the levels of low-density lipoproteins (LDLs, or "bad" cholesterol) while increasing the number of high-density lipoproteins (HDLs, or "good" cholesterol) in the blood. Higher HDL levels are associated with lower risk for arterial disease because they remove some of the "bad" cholesterol from arterial walls and hence reduce clogging. The bottom line: regular exercise lowers the risk of cardiovascular disease. (For more on cholesterol and blood pressure, see Chapter 15.)

Reduced Cancer Risk

Regular physical activity has been associated with reduction in a person's risk for some types of cancer. There is strong evidence that physical activity reduces the risks of breast[14] and colon cancer.[15] For example, experts say that because physical activity makes food move more quickly through your digestive system, there is less time for the body to absorb any potential carcinogens and for potential carcinogens to be in contact with the digestive tract. Physical activity also decreases the levels of prostaglandins, substances found in cells of the large intestine that are implicated in cancer.[16]

Improved Bone Mass

A common affliction among older adults is **osteoporosis,** a disease characterized by low bone mass and deterioration of bone tissue, which increase fracture risk. Osteoporosis currently affects 20 to 25 million Americans, 90 percent of them women. About 50 percent of all women eventually develop osteoporosis. Men are not immune; nearly 2 million men have the disease.

Osteoporosis is more common among women than among men for at least three reasons: women live longer, they have lower peak bone mass than men, and they lose bone mass at a faster rate after menopause as their estrogen levels decrease. Thus, the incidence of osteoporosis and fractures increases substantially with age in both women and men. Over 300,000 Americans aged 45 years and older are

Cardiorespiratory fitness The ability of the heart, lungs, and blood vessels to supply oxygen to skeletal muscles during sustained physical activity.

Osteoporosis A disease characterized by low bone mass and deterioration of bone tissue, which increase risk of fracture.

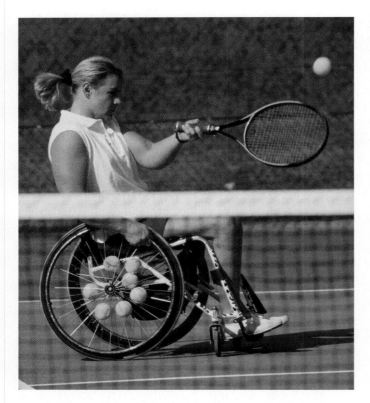

Everyone can attain cardiovascular fitness and muscular strength.

A recent meta-analysis challenges the commonly held view that exercise alone is not a useful strategy for obesity reduction. Moderately obese white men who participated in daily exercise of moderate intensity (brisk walking) for 45 to 60 minutes per day, without decreasing their caloric intake, lost weight and made rapid improvements in cardiovascular fitness.[23] However, remember that if you want to lose weight only through physical activity, you will have to spend more time exercising than if you reduce your calories at the same time.

Improved Health and Life Span

Prevention of Diabetes   Noninsulin-dependent diabetes (type 2 diabetes) is a complex disorder that affects millions of Americans, many of whom have no idea that they have the disease (see Chapter 18). Risk factors for diabetes include obesity, high blood pressure, and high cholesterol, as well as a family history of the disease.[24] Physicians suggest exercise combined with weight loss and healthy diet to help prevent diabetes. A recent large study found that for every 2,000 calories of energy expended during leisure-time activities, the incidence of diabetes was reduced by 24 percent. Perhaps the most encouraging finding was that the protective effect of exercise was greatest among those individuals who were at the highest risk.[25] Exercise also helps manage the disease. It is reported that walking 30 to 60 minutes a day lowers a diabetic's risk of dying from heart disease by 40 to 50 percent.[26]

Longer Life Span   Several large studies that followed groups of people over time found that those who exercised or were more fit lived longer.[27] In one study, capacity for exercise was a better predictor of whether a man would die in the next few years than were high blood pressure, high cholesterol, or smoking.[28]

Improved Immunity to Disease   Regular, consistent exercise promotes a healthy immune system. Research shows that moderate exercise gives the immune system a temporary boost in the production of the cells that attack bacteria.[29] While moderate amounts of exercise can be beneficial, extreme exercise may actually be detrimental. For example, athletes engaging in marathon-type events or very intense physical training have an increased risk of colds and flu.[30]

Just how exercise alters immunity is not well understood. We do know that brisk exercise temporarily increases the number of white blood cells (WBCs), the blood cells responsible for fighting infection. Generally speaking, the less fit the person and the more intense the exercise, the greater the increase in WBCs.[31] Studies on the influence of moderate exercise training on immune function have shown that near-daily brisk walking compared with inactivity reduced the number of sickness days by half over a 12- to 15-week period.[32]

admitted to hospitals each year with osteoporosis-related hip fractures.[17] Because the population is aging, the annual cost of medical care related to hip fractures in the United States may exceed $240 billion by the mid-twenty-first century.[18]

Bone, like other human tissues, responds to the demands placed upon it. Women (and men) have much to gain by remaining physically active as they age—bone mass levels are significantly higher among active than among sedentary women.[19] New research indicates that by "surprising" bone (by jumping and other sudden activities), young children may improve their bone density.[20] Regular weight-bearing exercise, when combined with a balanced diet containing adequate calcium, helps keep bones healthy.[21]

Improved Weight Control

Many people start exercising because they want to lose weight. Level of physical activity has a direct effect upon metabolic rate and can raise it for several hours following a vigorous workout. An effective method for losing weight combines regular endurance-type exercises with a moderate decrease in food intake. The ACSM recommends 30 minutes of moderate physical activity daily with an intake between 1500 to 2000 calories per day.[22] Cutting daily caloric intake beyond this range ("severe dieting") actually decreases metabolic rate by up to 20 percent and makes weight loss more difficult.

Exercise Benefits Your Brain and Your Body

It's not just our heart and muscles that benefit from a good workout—our brains get a boost, too. New evidence shows that exercise improves mental function, can deter some neurological disease, and can improve cognitive functions. The cognitive abilities of 6,000 women aged 65 and older were tested over six to eight years. Only 17 percent of the physically active women had significant declines in their test scores, whereas 24 percent of the inactive women experienced significant cognitive decline. In a study investigating the effects of exercise on depression, researchers found significant improvements in the cognitive ability of patients who began an exercise program. Improvements occurred in higher mental processes of memory and the so-called executive functions, which include planning, organization, and the ability to juggle different intellectual tasks at the same time. In another study, older adults who walked briskly for 45 minutes three times a week improved in their performance on computer decision-making tasks.

It's not just aerobic exercise that may give you a mental boost. A smaller study of 442 people aged 65 to 95 looked at resistance training and memory. After participating in a program for one year, measurements indicated that those with an increase in strength also had greater memory recall and recognition.

Why does exercise help improve the way we think? The exact mechanisms are unknown, but there are several theories. It is believed that the improved flow of oxygen-rich blood to specific regions of the brain enhances function. Just as exercise improves muscle tone and function, it may have similar effects on the brain. Another theory is more psychological. For older adults, the self-confidence that comes with exercising may have an effect on mental function. The increased motivation and self-confidence could be responsible for staying physically, socially, and mentally active and being self-reliant, all of which contribute to cognitive functioning.

Memory test scores aren't the only thing that may improve with exercise. The physiology of the brain may change as well. Imaging studies shows that there are actual anatomical differences in the brains of physically fit versus less fit older adults. This research has led neuroscientists to investigate whether exercise can help prevent neurological diseases such as Alzheimer's or Parkinson's disease. So far, rats who exercise and are exposed to a toxin that causes Parkinson's show a dramatic reduction in neurological symptoms.

It will take a few years to see if these findings translate to humans, but data collected from the Harvard Alumni Study already indicate a correlation between exercise and a reduction in Parkinson's disease.

The connection between exercise and brain function has been demonstrated by several studies but not consistently enough to say that regular workouts will help you on your biology final. Even so, with the many other physical and mental benefits of exercise, it can't hurt to add a brisk walk to your study regime!

Sources: J. A. Blumenthal, et al. "Effects of Exercise Training on Older Patients with Major Depression," *Archives of Internal Medicine* 159, no. 19 (1999): 2349–2356; E. McAuley, A. F. Kramer, and S. J. Colcombe, "Cardiovascular Fitness and Neurocognitive Function in Older Adults: A Brief Review," *Brain, Behavior, and Immunity* 18, no. 3 (2004): 214–220; P. Perrig-Chiello, et al. "The Effects of Resistance Training on Well-Being and Memory in Elderly Volunteers," *Age and Ageing* 27, no. 4 (1998): 469–475; A. D. Smith and M. J. Zigmond, "Can the Brain Be Protected Through Exercise? Lessons from an Animal Model of Parkinsonism," *Experimental Neurology* 184, no. 1 (2003): 31–39; K. Yaffe, et al. "A Prospective Study of Physical Activity and Cognitive Decline in Elderly Women: Women Who Walk," *Archives of Internal Medicine* 161, no. 14 (2001): 1703–1708.

Improved Mental Health and Stress Management

People who engage in regular physical activity also notice psychological benefits (see the New Horizons in Health box). Regular vigorous exercise has been shown to "burn off" the chemical by-products released by the nervous system during normal response to stress. This reduces stress levels by accelerating the body's return to a balanced state. Regular exercise improves physical appearance by toning and developing muscles and reducing body fat. Feeling good about personal appearance boosts self-esteem. At the same time, as people come to appreciate the improved strength, conditioning, and flexibility that accompany fitness, they often become less obsessed with physical appearance.[33] They learn new skills and develop increased abilities in favorite recreational activities, which also raise self-esteem. For some, however, the quest for fitness can lead to obsessive exercise patterns, such as the female athlete triad (see the Women's Health/Men's Health box).

What do you think?

Among the many benefits to be derived from physical activity, which two are most important to you? Why? ■ *After exercising regularly for several weeks, what benefits do you notice?*

The Female Athlete Triad: When Exercise Becomes Obsession

In a quest to be thin and achieve the ideal body, many women, particularly those who are physically active, are at risk for a group of symptoms called the female athlete triad. This often unrecognized disorder is a combination of conditions: disordered eating, amenorrhea (lack of menstrual periods), and osteoporosis.

Disordered eating behaviors (anorexia, bulimia, or other forms of binging, purging, or restricted eating) combined with excessive exercise can alter normal body functions. If the disordered eating is prolonged or without effective intervention, serious calcium depletion, changes in body hormones, and other negative effects may cause weakening of bone and other problems. Severe cases can lead to disability or even death.

Although men can suffer from many of these symptoms, the problem tends to be much more common in females, particularly those in highly competitive sports that value self-discipline and perfection. Gymnasts, ice skaters, cross country runners, swimmers, and ballet dancers are at the highest risk for the female athlete triad.

PHYSICAL WARNING SIGNS

- Fatigue
- Anemia
- Tendency toward stress fractures and injury
- Cold intolerance
- Sore throat
- Erosion of dental enamel from frequent vomiting
- Abdominal pain and bloating
- Constipation
- Dry skin
- Lightheadedness/fainting
- Chest pain
- Irregular or absent menstrual periods
- Lanugo (fine, downy hair covering the body)
- Changes in endurance, strength, or speed

BEHAVIORAL WARNING SIGNS

- Use of weight-loss products and/or laxatives
- Depression
- Decreased ability to concentrate
- Excessive and compulsive exercise
- Preoccupation with food and weight
- Trips to bathroom during or after eating
- Increasing self-criticism and hostility to self

The American College of Sports Medicine (ACSM) and other groups are noticing a growing incidence of the female athlete triad in physically active girls and women who don't compete athletically but want to look and feel their best. A key is to pay attention and notice what is happening. If you wonder whether a friend or family member may be experiencing the symptoms of the female athlete triad, ask her about her behavior. If symptoms are present, a multidisciplinary approach involving parents, coaches, friends, physicians, dietitians, and mental health professionals is warranted.

Sources: Brown University Health Education Office, "Nutrition: Eating Concerns: The Female Athlete Triad," 2002, www.brown .edu/Student_Services/Health_Services; Nebraska Cooperative Extension, "NEB Facts: The Female Athlete Triad," 1998, www.ianr.unl.edu/pubs/foods/nf361.htm

Improving Cardiorespiratory Fitness

There are many options for improving cardiorespiratory fitness. Swimming, jogging, cycling, and in-line skating are just a few of the choices. These types of exercise are **aerobic.** *Aerobic* means "with oxygen" and describes any type of exercise, typically performed at moderate levels of intensity for extended periods of time, that increases your heart rate. A person said to be in good shape has an above-average **aerobic capacity**—a term used to describe the functional status of the cardiorespiratory system (heart, lungs, blood vessels). Aerobic capacity (commonly written as VO_{2max}) is defined as the maximum volume of oxygen consumed by the muscles during exercise.

To measure your maximal aerobic capacity, an exercise physiologist or physician will typically have you exercise on a treadmill. He or she will initially ask you to walk at an easy pace, and then, at set time intervals during this **graded exercise test,** gradually increase the workload (the combination of running speed and the angle of incline of the treadmill). Generally, the higher your cardiorespiratory endurance level, the more oxygen you can transport to exercising muscles and the longer you can exercise without becoming exhausted. In other words, the higher the VO_{2max} value, the higher your level of aerobic fitness.

Aerobic exercise Any type of exercise that increases heart rate.

Aerobic capacity The current functional status of a person's cardiovascular system; measured as VO_{2max}.

Graded exercise test A test of aerobic capacity administered by a physician, exercise physiologist, or other trained person; two common forms are the treadmill running test and the stationary bike test.

Evaluating your Cardiorespiratory Endurance

☀ my**health**lab

Fill out this assessment online at www.aw-bc.com/myhealthlab or www.aw-bc.com/donatelle

After you have exercised regularly for several months, you might want to assess your cardiorespiratory endurance level. Find a local track, typically one quarter mile per lap, to perform your test. You may either run or walk for 1.5 miles and measure how long it takes to reach that distance, or run or walk for 12 minutes and determine the distance you covered in that time. Use the chart below to estimate your cardiorespiratory fitness level based upon your age and sex. Note that women have lower standards for each fitness category because they have higher levels of essential fat than men do.

Age*	1.5-Mile Run (min:sec)		12-Minute Run (miles)	
	Women (min:sec)	Men (min:sec)	Women (miles)	Men (miles)
	Good			
15–30	<12:00	<10:00	>1.5	>1.7
35–50	<13:30	<11:30	>1.4	>1.5
55–70	<16:00	<14:00	>1.2	>1.3
	Adequate for most activities			
15–30	<13:30	<11:50	>1.4	>1.5
35–50	<15:00	<13:00	>1.3	>1.4
55–70	<17:30	<15:30	>1.1	>1.3
	Borderline			
15–30	<15:00	<13:00	>1.3	>1.4
35–50	<16:30	<14:30	>1.2	>1.3
55–70	<19:00	<17:00	>1.0	>1.2
	Need extra work on cardiovascular fitness			
15–30	>17:00	>15:00	<1.2	<1.3
35–50	>18:30	>16:30	<1.1	<1.2
55–70	>21:00	>19:00	<0.9	<1.0

*Cardiorespiratory fitness declines with age.

If you are now at the Good level, congratulations! Your emphasis should be on maintaining this level for the rest of your life. If you are currently at lower levels, set realistic goals for improvement.

MAKE IT HAPPEN!

Use the results of this self-assessment to begin your behavior change program. Follow the steps and use the examples on page 328 to complete your Behavior Change Contract and use these resources to take action.

Source: From Edward T. Howley and B. Don Franks, *Fitness Leader's Handbook,* 2nd ed., "Checklist for the Fitness Tester." © 1992 by E. T. Howley and B. D. Franks. Reprinted with permission from Human Kinetics, Champaign, IL.

You can test your own aerobic capacity by using either the 1.5-mile run or the 12-minute run endurance test described in the Assess Yourself box. However, do not take these endurance-run tests if you are just starting to exercise.[34] Progress slowly through a walking/jogging program at low intensities before measuring your aerobic capacity with one of these tests. If you're new to exercise or have any medical conditions such as asthma, diabetes, heart disease, or obesity, consult your physician before beginning any exercise program.

Aerobic Fitness Programs

The most beneficial aerobic exercises are total body activities involving all the large muscle groups of your body; for example, swimming, cross-country skiing, and rowing. If you have been sedentary for quite a while, simply initiating a physical activity program may be the hardest task you'll face. Don't be put off by the next-day soreness you are likely to feel. The

Adults should strive to meet either of the physical activity recommendations:

• Adults should engage in moderate-intensity physical activities for at least 30 minutes on five or more days of the week (CDC/ACSM)

• Adults should engage in vigorous-intensity physical activity three or more days per week for 20 or more minutes per occasion (*Healthy People 2010*)

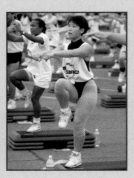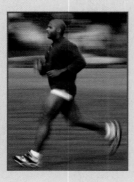

Figure 10.1
Guidelines for Physical Activity

Source: National Center for Chronic Disease Prevention and Health Promotion, "Physical Activity Recommendations," 2003, www.cdc .gov/nccdphp/dnpa/physical/recommendations/index.htm

key is to begin at a very low intensity, progress slowly, and stay with it!

There are three main components of an aerobic exercise program: frequency, intensity, and duration. The characteristics of these components vary by individual exercise goal and beginning fitness level. You can remember them with the acronym FIT (frequency, intensity, and time/duration).

Determining Exercise Frequency   In order to best improve your cardiovascular endurance, you will need to vigorously exercise at least three times a week. If you are a newcomer to exercise, you can still make improvements by doing less intense exercise but doing it more days a week, following the ACSM and CDC recommendations for moderate physical activity five days a week (Figure 10.1).

Determining Exercise Intensity   There are several ways of measuring exercise intensity. One of the main ways is using your **target heart rate.** To calculate target heart rate, start by

---

> **Target heart rate**   Calculated as a percentage of maximum heart rate (220 minus age); heart rate (pulse) is taken during aerobic exercise to check if exercise intensity is at the desired level (e.g., 60 percent of maximum heart rate).

subtracting your age from 220 to find your maximum heart rate. Your target heart rate is a desired percentage of this maximum heart rate, often 60 percent. Thus, if you are a 20-year-old female, your 60 percent target heart rate would be (220 – 20) x 0.60, or 120 beats per minute (bpm).

For moderate-intensity physical activity, you should work out at 50 to 70 percent of your maximum heart rate. For more vigorous activities (such as running), you should work within 70 to 85 percent of your maximum heart rate. People in poor physical condition should set a target heart rate between 40 and 50 percent of maximum. As your condition improves, you can gradually increase your target heart rate. Increases should be made in small increments, from 40 to 45 percent, then from 45 to 50 percent.

Heart rate reserve is another way to determine target heart rate. First, subtract your resting heart rate (bpm taken after 10 minutes of complete rest) from your maximum heart rate. This is your heart rate reserve. Then take a percentage of this figure (often 60 percent) and add it to your resting heart rate. The result is your target heart rate.

Once you know your target heart rate, you can take your pulse to determine how close you are to this value during your workout. As you exercise, lightly place your index and middle fingers (don't use your thumb) on your radial artery (inside your wrist, on the thumb side). Using a watch or clock, take your pulse for six seconds and multiply this number by 10 (just add a zero to your count) to get the number of beats per minute. Your pulse should be within a range of 5 bpm above or below your target heart rate. If necessary, adjust the pace or intensity of your workout to achieve your target heart rate.

Another way of determining intensity is to use the Borg rating of perceived exertion (RPE) scale, as shown in Figure 10.2. Perceived exertion is how hard you feel you are working, based on your heart rate, increased breathing rate, sweating, and muscle fatigue. This scale uses a rating from 6 (no exertion at all) to 20 (maximal exertion). This method corresponds to heart rate for most people. Experts agree that RPE ratings of 12 to 14 correspond to moderate intensity activity and 15 to 17 for vigorous activity.

A final way to measure exercise intensity is by metabolic equivalent, or MET level. This unit is used to estimate the amount of oxygen used by the body during exercise. For example, one MET equals the energy (oxygen) used by the body as you sit quietly. The harder your body works, the higher the MET level. An activity in the 3 to 6 MET range is considered moderate-intensity, and an activity that is greater than 6 METs is vigorous.[35]

The easiest, but least, scientific method of measuring exercise intensity is the "talk test." If you are exercising moderately, you should be able to carry on a conversation comfortably. If you are too out of breath to carry on a conversation, you are exercising vigorously.

Determining Exercise Duration   Duration refers to the number of minutes of activity performed during any one session. It is recommended that vigorous activities be performed for

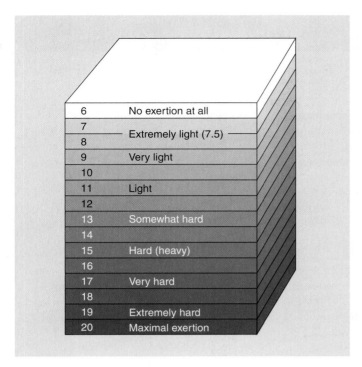

Figure 10.2
Rating of Perceived Exertion (RPE) Scale

Source: G. Borg, *Borg's Perceived Exertion and Pain Scales* (Champaign, IL: Human Kinetics, 1998), 47. Used with permission of Borg Products USA, Inc.

at least 20 minutes at a time, and moderate activities for at least 30 minutes at a time.

The lower the intensity of your activity, the longer the duration you'll need to get the same caloric expenditure. For example, a 120-pound woman will burn 180 calories walking for 30 minutes at 4.0 miles per hour but will burn 330 calories if she jogs for 30 minutes at a pace of 6.0 miles per hour. A 180-pound man will expend 210 calories per hour downhill skiing but about 700 calories cross-country skiing for an hour.[36] Aim to expend 300 to 500 calories per exercise session, with an eventual weekly goal of 1,500 to 2,000 calories. As you progress, add to your exercise load by increasing duration or intensity but not both at the same time. From week to week, don't increase duration or intensity by more than 10 percent.

A program of repeated sessions of exercise over several months or years—exercise training—changes the way your cardiovascular system meets your body's oxygen requirements at rest and during exercise. Many of the health benefits associated with cardiorespiratory fitness (such as lower blood pressure) may take several months to achieve; however, any physical activity of low-to-moderate intensity will benefit your overall health almost from the start (Figure 10.3).

Are you having trouble getting started? See the Skills for Behavior Change boxes in this chapter for strategies.

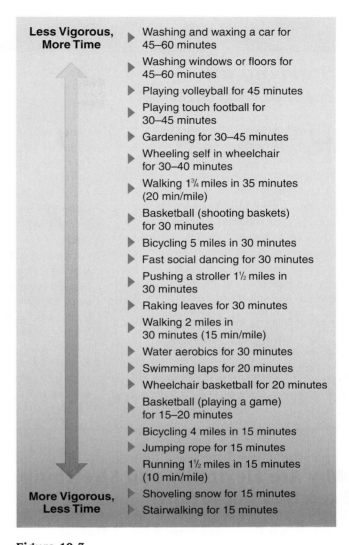

Figure 10.3
Levels of Physical Activity
A moderate amount of physical activity is roughly equivalent to physical activity that uses approximately 150 calories of energy per day, or 1,000 calories per week. Some activities can be performed at various intensities; the suggested durations correspond to expected intensity of effort.

Source: U.S. Department of Health and Human Services, *Physical Activity and Health: A Report of the Surgeon General* (Washington, DC: USDHHS, 1996).

What do you think?

Calculate your maximum heart rate. Pick an intensity of exercise that suits your fitness level, for example, 60 or 70 percent of your maximum heart rate. Using a familiar physical activity and monitoring your pulse, experiment by exercising at three different intensities. Did you notice any difference in the way you felt while exercising? ■ *Afterward?*

Starting an Exercise Routine

Beginners often start their exercise programs too rigorously. The most successful exercise program is one that is realistic and appropriate for your skill level and needs. Be realistic about the amount of time you will need to get into good physical condition. Perhaps the most significant factor early on in an exercise program is personal comfort. Experiment and find an activity that you truly enjoy. Be open to exploring new activities and new exercise equipment.

- *Start slow.* For the sedentary, first-time exerciser, any type and amount of physical activity will be a step in the right direction. If you are extremely overweight or out of condition, you might only be able to walk for five min-

utes at a time. Don't be discouraged; you're on your way!
- *Make only one life change at a time.* Success with one major behavioral change will encourage you to make other positive changes.
- *Set reasonable expectations for yourself and your fitness program.* Many people become exercise dropouts because their expectations were too high to begin with. Allow sufficient time to reach your fitness goals.
- *Choose a specific time to exercise, and stick with it.* Learning to establish priorities and keeping to a schedule are vital steps toward improved fitness. Experiment by exercising at different times of the day to learn what schedule works best for you.
- *Exercise with a friend.* It's easier to keep your exercise commitment if you exercise with someone else. Partners can motivate and encourage each

other, provided they remember that the rate of progress will not be the same for them both.
- *Make exercise a positive habit.* Usually, if you are able to practice a desired activity for three weeks, you will be able to incorporate it into your lifestyle.
- *Keep a record of your progress.* Include various facts about your physical activities (duration, intensity) and chronicle your emotions and personal achievements as you progress.
- *Reward yourself!* Think about an incentive to use to help you stick to your exercise program.
- *Take lapses in stride.* Physical deconditioning—a decline in fitness level—occurs at about the same rate as physical conditioning. Renew your commitment to fitness, and then restart your exercise program.

Why Are Flexibility and Stretching Exercises Important?

Stretching Exercises and Well-Being

Who would guess that improved flexibility can give you a sense of well-being, help you cope with stress, and stop your joints from hurting as much as they used to? But that's just what people who have improved their flexibility are saying. Stretching exercises have become the main highway to improved flexibility. Today, they are extremely popular, both because they work and because people can begin them at virtually any age and enjoy them for a lifetime. We'll look at three especially popular forms of exercise that focus on stretching and developing core muscle strength: yoga, tai chi, and Pilates.

A major objective of stretching exercises is to improve **flexibility,** a measure of the range of motion, or the amount of movement possible, at a particular joint. Improving the range of motion enhances efficiency, extent of movement,

and posture. Flexibility exercises also have been shown to be effective in reducing the incidence and severity of lower back problems and muscle or tendon injuries that can occur during sports and everyday physical activities.[37] Improved flexibility also means less tension and pressure on joints, resulting in less joint pain and joint deterioration.

Flexibility is enhanced by the controlled stretching of muscles and muscle attachments that act on a particular joint. Each muscle involved in a stretching exercise is attached to our skeleton by tendons. Figure 10.4 illustrates an example of the connection between muscle, bone, and tendons. The goal of stretching is to decrease the resistance of a muscle and its tendons to tension, that is, to reduce resistance to being stretched. Stretching exercises gradually result in greater flexibility. They involve stretching a muscle or group of muscles to a point of slight discomfort and holding that position for 20 to 30 seconds or more. For many people a regular program of stretching exercises enhances psychological as well as physical well-being.

Types of Stretching Exercises

In the language of exercise science, all commonly practiced stretching exercises fall into two major categories: static stretching and proprioceptive neuromuscular facilitation.[38]

Flexibility The measure of the range of motion, or the amount of movement possible, at a particular joint.

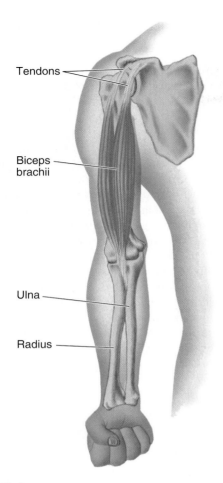

Figure 10.4
Muscles, Bones, and Tendons

Source: S. A. Plowman and D. L. Smith, *Exercise Physiology for Health, Fitness, and Performance,* 2nd ed. (San Francisco: Benjamin Cummings, 2003).

Static stretching techniques involve the slow, gradual stretching of muscles and their tendons, then holding them at a point. During this holding period—the stretch—participants may feel mild discomfort and a warm sensation in the stretched muscles. Static stretching exercises involve specialized tension receptors in our muscles. When done properly, it slightly lessens the sensitivity of tension receptors, which allows the muscle to relax and be stretched to greater length.[39] The stretch is followed by a slow return to the starting position. The physical aspect of yoga and tai chi is largely composed of static techniques, as are some of the exercises in Pilates programs.

The second major type of stretching exercise, **proprioceptive neuromuscular facilitation (PNF),** is a technique that uses various patterns of movement such as contraction of a muscle followed by a stretch. While PNF techniques have been shown to be superior for improving flexibility, they are, unfortunately, quite complex in their original form. A certified athletic trainer or physical therapist may be

required to help in performing PNF exercises correctly; however, several have been simplified to the point that they can be performed with an exercise partner or even alone.

There is a third type of stretching, *ballistic,* which involves repeated bouncing motions during which the muscle and tendon are rapidly stretched and returned to resting length. This process can be likened to taking a rubber band between two fingers, rapidly pulling it apart, and then releasing the tension, again and again. And just as a rubber band can snap in your fingers if you apply too much tension, the rapid movements of ballistic stretching can tear muscle fibers. The risk of injury is so high that ballistic stretching is no longer recommended.

Yoga, Tai Chi, and Pilates

Three major styles of exercise that include stretching have become widely practiced in the United States and other Western countries: yoga, tai chi, and Pilates. All three emphasize a joining of mind and body as a result of intense concentration on breathing and body position.

Yoga   One of the most popular fitness and static stretching activities, **yoga** originated in India about 5,000 years ago. Yoga blends the mental and physical aspects of exercise, a union of mind and body that participants find relaxing and satisfying. Done regularly, its combination of mental focus and physical effort improves flexibility, vitality, posture, agility, and coordination.

The practice of yoga focuses attention on controlled breathing as well as purely physical exercise. In addition to its mental dimensions, yoga incorporates a complex array of static stretching exercises expressed as postures (*asanas*). Over 200 postures exist, but only about 50 are commonly practiced. During a session, participants move to different asanas and hold them for 30 seconds or more. Yoga not only enhances flexibility, it has the great advantage of being flexible itself. Asanas and combinations of asanas can be changed and adjusted for young and old and to accommodate people with physical limitations or disabilities. Asanas can also be combined to provide even conditioned athletes with challenging sessions.

Static stretching   Techniques that gradually lengthen a muscle to an elongated position (to the point of discomfort) and hold that position for 10 to 30 seconds.

Proprioceptive neuromuscular facilitation (PNF) stretching   Techniques that involve the skillful use of alternating muscle contractions and static stretching in the same muscle.

Yoga   A variety of Indian traditions geared toward self-discipline and the realization of unity; includes forms of exercise widely practiced in the West today that promote balance, coordination, flexibility, and meditation.

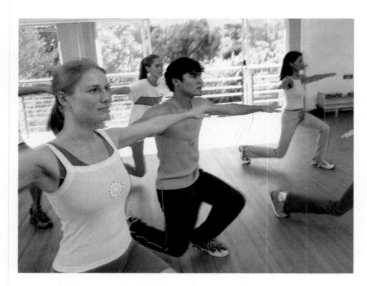

Yoga and other styles of exercise that strengthen core body muscles also enhance flexibility and lower stress levels.

A typical yoga session will move the spine and joints through their full range of motion. Yoga postures lengthen, strengthen, and balance musculature, leading to increased flexibility, stamina, and strength—and many people report a psychological sense of general well-being too.

There are many styles of yoga. Here are three of the most popular:

- *Iyengar yoga* focuses on precision and alignment in the poses. Standing poses are basic to this style, and poses are often held longer than in other styles.
- *Ashtanga yoga* in its pure form is based on a specific flow of poses with an emphasis on strength and agility that creates internal heat. Power yoga, a style growing in popularity, is a derivative of ashtanga yoga.
- *Bikram's yoga,* or hot yoga, is similar to power yoga but does not incorporate a specific flow of poses. Literally the hottest yoga going, it is performed in temperatures of 100°F, or even a bit higher. Proponents say that the heat increases the body's ability to move and stretch without injury.

Tai chi   Tai chi is an ancient Chinese form of exercise that, like yoga, combines stretching, balance, coordination, and meditation. It is designed to increase range of motion and

Tai chi   An ancient Chinese form of exercise widely practiced in the West today that promotes balance, coordination, stretching, and meditation.

Pilates   Exercise programs that combine stretching with movement against resistance, aided by devices such as tension springs and heavy bands.

flexibility while reducing muscular tension. Based on Chi Kung, a Taoist philosophy dedicated to spiritual growth and good health, tai chi was developed about 1000 AD by monks to defend themselves against bandits and warlords. It involves a series of positions called *forms* that are performed continuously. Both yoga and tai chi are excellent for improving flexibility and muscular coordination.

Pilates   Compared to yoga and tai chi, **Pilates** is the new kid on the exercise block. It was developed by Joseph Pilates, who came from Germany to New York City in 1926. Shortly after his arrival, he introduced his exercise methodology, which emphasizes flexibility, coordination, strength, and tone. Pilates combines stretching with movement against resistance, which is aided by devices such as tension springs or heavy rubber bands.

Pilates differs in part from yoga and tai chi because it includes a component designed to increase strength. The method consists of a sequence of carefully performed movements. Some are carried out on specially designed equipment, while others are performed on mats. Each exercise stretches and strengthens the muscles involved and has a specific breathing pattern associated with it. A Pilates class focuses on strengthening specific muscle groups, using equipment that provides resistance.

What do you think?

Why is it so important to have good flexibility throughout life? ■ *Describe some situations in which improved flexibility would help you perform daily activities with less effort.* ■ *What actions can you take to become more flexible?*

Designing Your Own Stretching Exercise Program: General Guidelines

If formal exercise classes aren't for you, you can easily design your own stretching exercise program. Figure 10.5 shows a selection of exercises that will stretch the major muscle groups of your body and which can be used as a warm-up for other activities such as jogging and tennis.

A program of regular stretching exercise doesn't require a lot of time or expensive equipment. You can reap the benefits of stretching with just two or three 10-minute sessions per week. Start off slowly with a five-minute session for the first week, then add a five-minute session each week, until you reach a schedule and comfort level that suit you. A hefty program would consist of five 30-minute sessions each week. Sessions get longer as you slowly increase the time you hold a particular stretch and how many times you repeat each type of stretch.

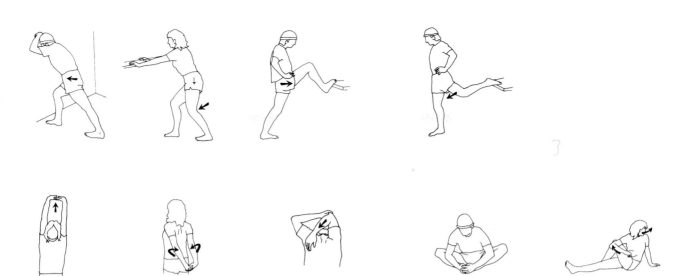

Figure 10.5
Stretching Exercises to Improve Flexibility
These diagrams show how simple stretching can be. Use these stretches as part of your warm-up and cool-down. Hold each one for 10 to 30 seconds, and repeat four times on each side. After only a few weeks of regular stretching, you'll begin to have more flexibility.

Source: Excerpted from *Stretching, 20th Anniversary Revised Edition.* © 2000 Shelter Publications, Box 279, Bolinas, CA 94924. Used by permission.

Improving Muscular Strength and Endurance

To get a sense of what resistance training is about, do a resistance exercise. Start by holding your right arm straight down by your side, then turn your hand palm up and bring it up toward your shoulder. That's a resistance exercise, using a muscle (your biceps) to move a resistance (in this case, just the weight of your hand)—not very much resistance. (Refer again to Figure 10.4.) Resistance training usually involves more weight or tension than this; unlike flexibility training, resistance training is usually equipment intense. You don't get to look like Arnold Schwarzenegger doing these exercises empty handed. Free weights such as dumbbells and barbells and all sorts of tension-producing machines are usually part of resistance training. It's not just bodybuilding that uses this type of exercise, either. Fitness programs and many sports employ resistance training to improve strength and endurance, and many rehabilitation programs for recovery from muscle and joint injuries are designed around resistance exercises.

Strength and Endurance

In the field of resistance training, **muscular strength** refers to the amount of force a muscle or group of muscles is capable of exerting. The most common way to assess strength in a resistance exercise program is to measure the **one repetition maximum (1 RM),** which is the maximum amount of weight a person can move one time (and no more) in a

particular exercise. For example, 1 RM for the simple exercise done at the beginning of this section is the maximum weight you lift to your shoulder one time. **Muscular endurance** is the ability of muscle to exert force repeatedly without fatiguing. If you can perform the exercise described earlier holding a five-pound weight in your hand and lifting 10 times, you will have greater endurance than someone who attempts that same exercise but is only able to lift the weight seven times.

Some resistance programs are designed primarily for increasing strength; others are aimed more at increasing endurance. Winning an Olympic weight-lifting event depends on the amount of weight that is lifted in just a few seconds. Endurance doesn't play a large role. Conversely, a soccer event lasts much longer and requires enormous endurance but less strength. In football, strength and endurance are both important. Training for endurance uses smaller weights but repeats an exercise more times than training for strength. If you were endurance training for performing our

Muscular strength The amount of force that a muscle is capable of exerting.

One repetition maximum (1 RM) The amount of weight/resistance that can be lifted or moved once, but not twice; a common measure of strength.

Muscular endurance A muscle's ability to exert force repeatedly without fatiguing.

hand-to-shoulder exercise (called a curl), you might hold a five-pound weight in each hand and curl 15 times per exercise segment. In training for strength, 40-pound weights might be used to curl five times.

Principles of Strength Development

An effective **resistance exercise program** involves three key principles: tension, overload, and specificity of training.[40]

The Tension Principle   The key to developing strength is to create tension within a muscle or group of muscles. Tension is created by resistance provided by weights such as barbells or dumbbells, specially designed machines, or the weight of the body.

The Overload Principle   The overload principle is the most important of our three key principles. Overload doesn't mean forcing a muscle or group of muscles to do too much, which could result in injuries. Rather, overload in resistance training requires muscles to do more than they are used to. Everyone begins a resistance training program with an initial level of strength. To become stronger, you must regularly create a degree of tension in your muscles that is greater than you are accustomed to. This overload will cause your muscles to adapt to a new level. As your muscles respond to a regular program of overloading by getting larger, they become stronger.

Remember that resistance training exercises cause microscopic damage (tears) to muscle fibers, and the rebuilding process that increases the size and capacity of the muscle takes about 24 to 48 hours. Thus resistance training exercise programs should include at least one day of rest and recovery between workouts before overloading the same muscles again.

The Specificity-of-Training Principle   According to the specificity principle, the effects of resistance exercise training are specific to the muscles being exercised. Only the muscle or muscle group that you exercise responds to the demands placed upon it. For example, if you regularly do curls, the muscles involved—your biceps—will become larger and stronger, but the other muscles in your body won't change. It is important to note that exercising only certain muscle groups may put adjacent muscle groups at a mechanical disadvantage, leading to possible injury.

Gender Differences in Weight Training   The results of resistance training in men and women are quite different. Women don't normally develop muscle to the same extent that men do. The main reason for this difference is that men and women have different levels of the hormone testosterone in their blood. Before puberty, testosterone levels are similar for both boys and girls. During adolescence, testosterone levels in boys increase dramatically, about tenfold, while testosterone levels in girls remain unchanged. Muscles will become larger (**hypertrophy**) as a result of resistance training exercise, but typically this change is less dramatic in women. To enhance muscle bulk, some bodybuilders (both men and women) take synthetic hormones (anabolic steroids) that mimic the effects of testosterone. However, using anabolic steroids is a dangerous and illegal practice. (See Chapter 14.)

Types of Muscle Activity

Your skeletal muscles act in three different ways: isometric, concentric, and eccentric.[41] In **isometric muscle action** (Figure 10.6a), force is produced through tension and muscle contraction, not movement. A **concentric muscle action** (Figure 10.6b) causes joint movement and a production of force while the muscle shortens. The empty-hand curl we did at the beginning of this section is a concentric exercise, with joint movement occurring at the elbow. In general, concentric muscle actions produce movement in a direction opposite to the downward pull of gravity.

Eccentric muscle action describes the ability of a muscle to produce force while lengthening. Typically, eccentric muscle actions occur when movement is in the same direction as the pull of gravity; see Figure 10.6c. Once you've brought a weight up during a curl, an eccentric muscle action would be to lower your hand and the weight back to their original position.

Methods of Providing Resistance

There are four commonly used resistance exercise methods: body weight resistance and fixed, variable, and accommodating resistance devices.

Body Weight Resistance (Calisthenics)   Strength and endurance training doesn't have to rely on equipment. You can use your own body weight to develop skeletal muscle fitness. Calisthenics (such as push-ups and chin-ups) use part or all of your body weight to offer resistance during exercise. While less effective than other resistance methods in developing

---

Resistance exercise program   A regular program of exercises designed to improve muscular strength and endurance in the major muscle groups.

Hypertrophy   Increased size (girth) of a muscle.

Isometric muscle action   Force produced without any resulting joint movement.

Concentric muscle action   Force produced while the muscle is shortening.

Eccentric muscle action   Force produced while the muscle is lengthening.

(a) Isometric contraction
Muscle contracts
but does not shorten

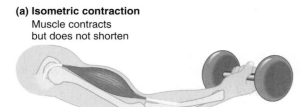

No movement

(b) Concentric contraction

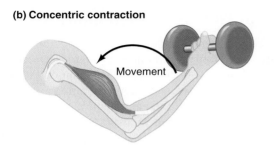

Movement

(c) Eccentric contraction

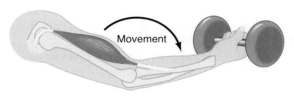

Movement

Figure 10.6
Isometric, Concentric, and Eccentric Muscle Actions

Source: S. Powers and E. Howley, *Exercise Physiology: Theory and Application to Fitness and Performance* (Madison, WI: Brown and Benchmark, 1997).

large muscle mass and strength, calisthenics are quite adequate for improving general muscular fitness and generally sufficient to improve muscle tone and maintain a level of muscular strength.

Fixed Resistance   Fixed resistance exercises provide a constant amount of resistance throughout the full range of movement. Barbells, dumbbells, and some machines provide fixed resistance because their weight, or the amount of resistance, does not change during an exercise. Fixed resistance equipment has the potential to strengthen all the major muscle groups in the body.

One advantage of dumbbells and barbells is that they are relatively inexpensive. Fixed resistance exercise machines are commonly available at college recreation/fitness facilities, health clubs, and many resorts and hotels.

Variable Resistance   Variable resistance equipment alters the resistance encountered by a muscle during a movement, so that the effort by the muscle is more consistent throughout the full range of motion. Variable resistance machines,

such as Nautilus and Bowflex, are typically single-station devices; a person stays on the same machine throughout the whole series of exercises. Other types of machines, such as Soloflex, have multiple stations and the person using them moves from one machine to another. While some of these machines are expensive and too big to move easily, others are affordable and more portable. Many forms of variable resistance devices are sold for home use.

Accommodating Resistance Devices   These machines adjust the resistance according to the amount of force generated by the person using the equipment. The exerciser performs at maximal level of effort, while the device controls the speed of the exercise. The machine is set to a particular speed, and muscles being exercised must move at a rate faster than or equal to that speed in order to encounter resistance.[42]

Benefits of Strength Training

Does strength training offer any benefits beyond simply getting stronger? Indeed, regular strength training can reduce the occurrence of lower back pain and joint and muscle injuries. It can also postpone loss of muscle tissue due to aging and a sedentary lifestyle and help prevent osteoporosis.

Strength training enhances muscle definition and tone and improves personal appearance. This, in turn, enhances self-esteem. Strength training even has a hidden benefit: muscle tissue burns calories faster than most other tissues, even when it is resting. So, increasing your muscle mass can help boost your metabolism and maintain a healthy weight.

Getting Started

When beginning a resistance exercise program, always consider your age, fitness level, and personal goals. Strength training exercises are done in a *set,* or a single series of multiple repetitions using the same resistance. For both men and women under the age of 50, the American College of Sports Medicine recommends working major muscle groups with one set of 8 to 10 different exercises two to three days per week. Weight loads should be at a level to allow up to 8 to 12 repetitions. Table 10.2 on page 318 presents essential information for a program to build muscular strength and endurance. Remember, experts suggest allowing at least one day of rest and recovery between workouts.

What do you think?

What types of resistance equipment can you currently access? ■ *Based on what you've read, what actions can you take to increase your muscular strength?* • *Muscular endurance?* ■ *How would you measure your improvement?*

Table 10.2
Resistance Training Program Guidelines

- Resistance training should be an integral part of an adult fitness program and be of sufficient intensity to enhance strength and muscular endurance and to maintain fat-free mass.
- Resistance training should be progressive in nature, individualized, and provide a stimulus (overload) to all major muscle groups in the body.
- The exercise sequence should include large before small muscle group exercises, multiple-joint exercises before single-joint exercises, and higher intensity before lower intensity exercises.
- Performing a minimum of 8 to 10 exercises that train the major muscle groups two to three days per week is recommended.
- The amount of weight used and number of repetitions vary by individual's target goal, physical capacity, and training status.

Source: W. J. Kraemer, et al. "American College of Sports Medicine Position Stand on Progression Models in Resistance Training for Healthy Adults," *Medicine and Science in Sports and Exercise* 3, no. 2 (2002): 364–380. http://lww.com

Body Composition

Body composition is the fourth and final component of a comprehensive fitness program. Body composition parameters that can be influenced by regular physical activity include total body mass, fat mass, fat-free mass, and regional fat distribution.[43] Body composition is significantly different between women and men, since women have a higher percentage of body fat and a significantly lower percentage of fat-free mass (such as muscle and bone) and bone mineral density.[44] As discussed earlier, changing your body composition by losing weight is more effective if an increase in physical activity is combined with changes in your diet.

Fitness Injuries

Overtraining is the most frequent cause of injuries associated with fitness activities, affecting up to 20 percent of all athletes. Enthusiastic but out-of-shape beginners can injure themselves by doing too much too soon. Experienced athletes can develop *overtraining syndrome* by engaging in systematic and progressive increases in training without getting enough rest and recovery time. Eventually, performance declines and training sessions become increasingly difficult.

Overuse injuries   Injuries that result from the cumulative effects of day-after-day stresses placed on tendons, muscles, and joints.

Traumatic injuries   Injuries that are accidental in nature, which occur suddenly and violently (including fractured bones, ruptured tendons, and sprained ligaments).

Adequate rest, good nutrition and rehydration are important to sustain or improve fitness levels.

Pay attention to your body's warning signs. To avoid injuring a particular muscle group or body part, vary your fitness activities throughout the week to give muscles and joints a rest. Set appropriate short-term and long-term training goals. Establishing realistic but challenging fitness goals can help you stay motivated without overdoing it.

Causes of Fitness-Related Injuries

There are two basic types of injuries stemming from fitness-related activities: overuse and traumatic injuries. **Overuse injuries** occur because of cumulative, day-after-day stresses placed on tendons, bones, and ligaments during exercise. These injuries occur most often in repetitive activities like swimming, running, bicycling, and step aerobics. The forces that occur normally during physical activity are not enough to cause a ligament sprain or muscle strain, but when these forces are applied on a daily basis for weeks or months, they can result in an injury. Common sites of overuse injuries are the leg, knee, shoulder, and elbow joints. However, use common sense, pay attention to your body's signals and you're likely to remain injury-free.

Traumatic injuries occur suddenly and violently, typically by accident. Typical traumatic injuries are broken bones, torn ligaments and muscles, contusions, and lacerations. Some traumatic injuries occur quickly and are difficult to avoid—for example, spraining your ankle by landing on another person's foot after jumping up for a rebound in basketball. If your traumatic injury causes a noticeable loss of function and immediate pain or pain that does not go away after 30 minutes, you should have a physician examine it.

Prevention

Your exercise clothing is more than a fashion statement—smart choices can help you prevent injuries. For some physical activities, you need clothing that allows body heat to dissipate—for example, light-colored nylon shorts and mesh tank top while running in hot weather. For other activities, you need clothing that retains body heat without getting you sweat-soaked—for example, layers of polypropylene and/or wool clothing while cross-country skiing. Today, there are many high-tech fabrics on the market that can help you stay cool, stay warm, or stay dry. Appropriate, quality exercise clothing is a good investment.

Appropriate Footwear   Shoes are made to protect the foot from sport-specific movements. *Proper footwear* can decrease the likelihood of foot, knee, or back injuries. When you purchase running shoes, look for several key components. Biomechanics research has revealed that running is a "collision" sport—that is, the runner's foot collides with the ground with a force three to five times the runner's body weight with each stride.[45] The 150-pound runner who takes 1,000 strides per mile applies a cumulative force to his or her body of

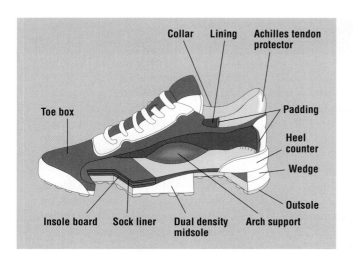

Figure 10.7
Anatomy of a Running Shoe

Source: Reprinted with permission of the American Council on Exercise, www.ACEFitness.org

450,000 pounds per mile. The force not absorbed by the running shoe is transmitted upward into the foot, leg, thigh, and back. Our bodies are able to absorb forces such as these but may be injured by the cumulative effect of repetitive impacts (such as running 40 miles per week). Therefore, the ability of running shoes to absorb shock is critical. Proper fit is also important.

The midsole of a running shoe must absorb impact forces but must also be flexible (see Figure 10.7). To evaluate the flexibility of the midsole, hold the shoe between the index fingers of your right and left hand. When you push on both ends of the shoe with your fingers, the shoe should bend easily at the midsole. If the force exerted by your index fingers cannot bend the shoe, its midsole is probably too rigid and may irritate your Achilles tendon, among other problems.[46] Other basic characteristics of running shoes include a rigid plastic insert within the heel of the shoe (known as a heel counter) to control the movement of your heel; a cushioned foam pad surrounding the heel of the shoe to prevent Achilles tendon irritation; and a removable thermoplastic innersole that customizes the fit of the shoe by using your body heat to mold it to the shape of your foot. Shoes are the runner's most essential piece of equipment, so carefully select appropriate footwear before you start a running program.

Shoe companies also sell cross-training shoes to combat the high cost of having to buy separate pairs of running shoes, tennis shoes, weight-training shoes, and so on. Although the cross-training shoe can be used for several different fitness activities by the novice or recreational athlete, a distance runner who runs 25 or more miles per week needs a pair of specialty running shoes to prevent injury.

Basketball, tennis, and other sport enthusiasts can also buy shoes specific to their sport. Whatever type of shoe you

are buying, keep in mind factors like distance, speed, style, surface, your body weight, and type of stride or movement. If unsure about proper fit, go to a specialty shoe store where knowledgeable staff can make recommendations.

Appropriate Exercise Equipment Some activities require special protective equipment to reduce chances of injury. Eye injuries can occur in virtually all fitness-related activities, although some are more risky than others. As many as 90 percent of the eye injuries resulting from racquetball and squash could be prevented by wearing appropriate eye protection—for example, goggles with polycarbonate lenses.[47] Nearly 100 million people in the United States ride bikes for pleasure, fitness, or competition. Eighty-five percent of all fatal bicycle accidents were due to head or brain injuries. Riding without a bicycle helmet significantly increases the risk of sustaining a head injury in the event of a crash. Non-helmeted riders are 14 times more likely to be involved in a fatal crash than helmeted riders.[48] Look for helmets that meet the standards established by the American National Standards Institute (ANSI) and the Snell Memorial Foundation (SNELL). See the Reality Check box on page 320 for advice on selecting equipment and evaluating health clubs.

What do you think?

Given your activity level, what injury risks are you exposed to on a regular basis? ■ *What changes can you make in your equipment and clothing to reduce these risks?*

Common Overuse Injuries

Three of the most common overuse injuries are plantar fasciitis, shin splints, and runner's knee.

Plantar Fasciitis Plantar fasciitis is an inflammation of the plantar fascia, a broad band of dense, inelastic tissue (fascia) that runs from the heel to the toe on the bottom of the foot. The main function of the plantar fascia is to protect the nerves, blood vessels, and muscles of the foot from injury. Repetitive weight-bearing fitness activities such as walking and running can inflame the plantar fascia. Common symptoms are pain and tenderness under the ball of the foot, at the heel, or at both locations.[49] The pain of plantar fasciitis is particularly noticeable during the first steps out of bed in the morning. If not treated properly, this injury may progress to the point that weight-bearing exercise is too painful to endure. Uphill running is not advised, since each uphill stride severely stretches (and thus irritates) the already inflamed plantar fascia.

This injury can often be prevented by regularly stretching the plantar fascia prior to exercise and by wearing

Avoiding the Muscle Hustle: Tips for Buying Exercise Equipment and Choosing a Health Club

If you have a treadmill that you use as a clothes hanger or belong to a gym you haven't visited in months, you are not alone. Many people buy great equipment and don't get motivated to get moving, but others buy services and equipment that don't have a ghost's chance of being useful.

Evaluate advertising claims for fitness products carefully. For example, the Federal Trade Commission (FTC) has sued marketers of electronic abdominal exercise belts for claiming that users could get "six-pack abs" and lose inches in a short time. The FDA has never approved any kind of electronic muscle stimulator for weight loss, for losing your double chin, or similar results. The FTC advises consumers to do the following:

✔ Ignore claims that an exercise machine or device can provide lasting, "no sweat" results in a short time. These claims are false. To get results, you must exercise.

✔ Disbelieve claims that a product can burn fat off a particular part of the body. Achieving a major change in body contour or appearance requires sensible eating and regular exercise that works the whole body and causes caloric deficiencies that affect the entire body.

✔ Read the fine print. Advertised results may be based on more than just using a machine; they may also be based on caloric restriction.

✔ Be skeptical of testimonials and before and after pictures from "satisfied" customers.

✔ Get details on warranties, guarantees, and return policies.

✔ Check out the company's customer support and service sections. Call the number to see how helpful the person on the other end really is.

EXERCISE EQUIPMENT

You should shop around and think carefully before investing in any fitness equipment, even products with proven benefits. Here are some consumer tips:

Heart Rate Monitors

Over the last few years these monitors have become popular among runners, bikers, and aerobicizers. Fitness enthusiasts use them to become aware of their heart rate and training intensity and push performance to the next level. These monitors usually have a strap with a sensor for placing around the chest and a watch-like readout on the wrist. Monitors cost between $50 and $200 and can provide instant feedback about the intensity of your workouts. If you want a more technical way to measure heart rate than fingers-to-the-wrist method, a heart rate monitor is for you.

Pedometers

Using a pedometer can help maintain motivation. Pedometers monitor your calories, number of steps, distance, and speed. They are usually small, easy to use, and can help you figure out how far you've gone on your daily walk/run or measure how many steps you take on an average day. Before you buy a pedometer, make sure it's simple to use and has an easy-to-read display. The unit should be accurate in its count when you wear it correctly— you may have to experiment with where to wear it. Distance accuracy depends on setting your stride length correctly. Some pedometers even come with a computer program to upload your step and distance records. Prices range from $20 to $100.

Exercise Balls

These balls are for more than playing with! Stabilizing yourself on a ball strengthens core muscles. If you sit on the ball and do arm or shoulder exercises, you work your abdominals as well as your arms and shoulders. Researchers at San Diego State University claim that doing "crunches" on the ball is one of the top three exercises to work the abdominal muscles. High quality balls are made of burst-resistant vinyl and are independently tested to withstand as much as 600 pounds while still retaining their shape and usefulness. Read the package carefully to be certain that if the ball is punctured, it will not drop you to the ground. (High quality balls are designed to deflate slowly if punctured to minimize the risk of injury.) Also, do not forget to inflate it to the right height and use it properly for safety reasons and to ensure maximum workout results. Cost is $25 to $50.

Balance Boards

By doing strengthening moves on the balance board, your core muscles contract, thus it works your abs as well as other

---

athletic shoes with good arch support and shock absorbency. Stretch the plantar fascia by slowly pulling all five toes upward toward your head, holding for 10 to 15 seconds. Repeat this three to five times on each foot prior to exercise.

Shin Splints   A general term for any pain that occurs below the knee and above the ankle is *shin splints*. This broad description includes more than 20 different medical conditions. Problems range from stress fractures of the tibia (shinbone) to severe inflammation in the muscles of the lower leg, which can interrupt the flow of blood and nerve supply to the foot. The most common type of shin splints occurs along the inner side of the tibia and is usually a combination of muscle irritation and irritation of the tissues that attach the muscle groups. Athletes who regularly train with balance boards develop propriocepter reaction and ankle strength. This greatly decreases the risk of ankle injury during play, while improving coordination and overall athletic ability. For less athletic-types, working out on the balance board can reduce your chances of tripping and falling in everyday life. The cost is $40 to $80.

Step Benches

Step workouts have been popular for over a decade. The step can provide a great aerobic workout that also sculpts your lower body. Routines can be as simple as an up-and-down cadence to more complex steps, lunges, and squats. Many steps come with variable risers so that beginners can start out low, increasing the height as fitness levels increase. The cost is $80 to $100.

Resistance Bands

Bands are usually rubber or elastic material with handles that can be used to work the muscles without weights. The bands can provide various ways to improve muscular endurance and strength, flexibility, and range of motion. They are lightweight, portable, and can add variety to gym workouts. They are also compact and easy to pack when traveling. You can buy bands in varying degrees of resistance, depending on your fitness level or exercise goal, for $5 to $15.

Weight Vests

These vests are used for aerobic conditioning and strength exercise programs. The vests concentrate weight to the upper body and chest area so when your core muscles work, you burn additional calories and build strength. Because vests work on the overload principle, they have been used in osteoporosis research. Researchers have used the vests to help people increase bone density. Most vests come with variable weights, so you can begin with just 2 percent of your body weight in the vest and gradually work up to 10 percent as your musculoskeletal system becomes stronger. Before purchasing, make sure the vest is snug fitting and comfortable. Breathable material on the vest is a plus. The cost is $150 to $300.

HEALTH CLUBS

While there are some excellent facilities and well-trained fitness trainers out there, carefully check the staff's credentials to ensure that your trainer is offering scientifically solid, safe advice. Tour the facilities before signing up, and ask lots of questions.

✔ Ask about the training that a person must have to advise you about use of machines and fitness programs in a particular club. Sometimes staff members take only a one- or two-week training class from club managers or outside trainers.

✔ Look for trainers who have graduated with majors in exercise physiology, nutrition, athletic training, physical education, health education, or other health-related disciplines. The higher the degree, the better.

✔ Look for trainers with American College of Sports Medicine (ACSM) certification. These individuals must pass a national exam to verify their knowledge of basic physiology and performance.

✔ Ask the trainer about his or her basic first aid and CPR certifications. Are they current? What emergency plans are in place in case someone is injured in the club?

✔ What are the fees to join and monthly fees? What do they entitle you to? Will you get individual attention and specialized training?

✔ When are the machines the busiest? Can you pay a reduced fee to come at nonpeak times?

✔ What are their provisions for family members? Guests?

✔ How regularly are the machines and mats cleaned with antibiotic washes and cleansers?

✔ Avoid the hot tubs and whirlpools unless users are required to shower to get rid of sweat, makeup, and other body debris before hopping in. One of the most germ-laden spots you'll ever encounter is a whirlpool where a bunch of sweaty exercisers have jumped in to refresh themselves after a heavy workout.

✔ If you do use the whirlpools or hot tubs, find out how often the water is completely changed, who monitors the chemicals in the water, and so on.

✔ If there is a pool on site, ask who monitors the number of people who can use the pool per hour, who regulates the chemicals, how often the water is changed, what the policies are about showering before entry, and similar issues.

✔ Check on the frequency of machine repairs and maintenance policies.

✔ What are the locker rooms like? Are they clean and odor-free? What are the club's policies about footwear and swimwear?

Source: Federal Trade Commission, Bureau of Consumer Protection, "FTC Consumer Alert," May 2002, www.ftc.gov

---

muscles to the bone in this region. Typically, there is pain and swelling along the middle third of the posteromedial tibia in the soft tissues, not the bone.

Sedentary people who start a new weight-bearing exercise program are at the greatest risk for shin splints, though well-conditioned aerobic exercisers who rapidly increase their distance or pace may also develop them.[50] Running is the most frequent cause of shin splints, but those who do a great deal of walking (such as mail carriers and restaurant workers) may also develop this injury.

To help prevent shin splints, wear athletic shoes with good arch support and shock absorbency. Also, gradually increase training intensity and vary your routine. If the pain continues, see your physician. You may be advised to

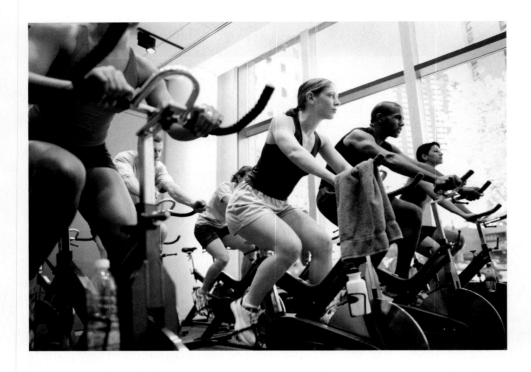

Spinning is just one of many activities that can improve fitness and provide health benefits.

substitute a nonweight-bearing activity such as swimming during your recovery period.

Runner's Knee *Runner's knee* describes a series of problems involving the muscles, tendons, and ligaments about the knee. Women experience such knee problems more often than men do. The most common condition identified as runner's knee is abnormal movement of the kneecap, which irritates the cartilage on the back side of the kneecap as well as nearby tendons and ligaments.[51]

The main symptom of this kind of runner's knee is the pain experienced when downward pressure is applied to the kneecap after the knee is straightened fully. Additional symptoms may include swelling, redness, tenderness around the kneecap, and a dull, aching pain in the center of the knee.[52] If you have these symptoms, your physician will probably recommend that you stop running for a few weeks and reduce activities that compress the kneecap (for example, exercise on a stair-climbing machine or doing squats with heavy resistance) until you no longer feel any pain.

Treatment

First-aid treatment for virtually all personal fitness injuries involves **RICE: r**est, **i**ce, **c**ompression, and **e**levation. *Rest,* the first component of this treatment, is required to avoid

---

RICE Acronym for the standard first-aid treatment for virtually all traumatic and overuse injuries: rest, ice, compression, and elevation.

---

further irritation of the injured body part. *Ice* is applied to relieve pain and constrict the blood vessels to stop any internal or external bleeding. Never apply ice cubes, reusable gel ice packs, chemical cold packs, or other forms of cold directly to your skin. Instead, place a layer of wet toweling or elastic bandage between the ice and your skin. Ice should be applied to a new injury for approximately 20 minutes every hour for the first 24 to 72 hours. *Compression* of the injured body part can be accomplished with a 4- or 6-inch-wide elastic bandage; this applies indirect pressure to damaged blood vessels to help stop bleeding. Be careful, though, that the compression wrap does not interfere with normal blood flow. A throbbing, painful hand or foot indicates that the compression wrap should be loosened. *Elevation* of the injured extremity above the level of your heart also helps to control internal or external bleeding by making the blood flow uphill to reach the injured area.

Exercising in the Heat

Heat stress, which includes several potentially fatal illnesses resulting from excessive core body temperatures, is a concern when exercising in warm, humid weather. In these conditions, your body's rate of heat production can exceed its ability to cool itself.

You can help prevent heat stress by following certain precautions. First, proper acclimatization to hot and/or humid climates is essential. The process of heat acclimatization, which increases your body's cooling efficiency, requires about 10 to 14 days of gradually increased activity in the hot environment. Second, avoid dehydration by replacing the fluids you lose during and after exercise. Third, wear clothing appropriate for your activity and the environment. And finally, use common sense—for example, on an 85°F, 80 percent humidity day, postpone your usual lunchtime run until the cool of evening.

The three different heat stress illnesses are progressive in severity. **Heat cramps** (heat-related muscle cramps), the least serious problem, can usually be prevented by warm-ups, adequate fluid replacement, and a diet that includes the electrolytes lost during sweating (sodium and potassium). (For general information on cramps, see page 326.) **Heat exhaustion** is caused by excessive water loss resulting from prolonged exercise or work. Symptoms of heat exhaustion include nausea, headache, fatigue, dizziness and faintness, and, paradoxically, "goosebumps" and chills. If you are suffering from heat exhaustion, your skin will be cool and moist. Heat exhaustion is actually a mild form of shock, in which the blood pools in the arms and legs away from the brain and major organs of the body, causing nausea and fainting.[53] **Heatstroke,** often called sunstroke, is a life-threatening emergency with a 20 to 70 percent death rate.[54] Heat stroke occurs during vigorous exercise when the body's heat production significantly exceeds its cooling capacities. Body core temperature can rise from normal (98.6°F) to 105°F to 110°F within minutes after the body's cooling mechanism shuts down. With no cooling taking place, rapidly increasing core temperatures can cause brain damage, permanent disability, and death. Common signs of heat stroke are dry, hot, and usually red skin; very high body temperature; and a very rapid heart rate.

If you experience any of the symptoms mentioned here, stop exercising immediately. Move to the shade or a cool spot to rest and drink large amounts of cool fluids. Be aware that heat stress can strike in situations in which the danger is not obvious. Serious or fatal heat stroke may result from prolonged sauna or steam baths, prolonged total immersion in a hot tub or spa, or exercising in a plastic or rubber head-to-toe "sauna suit."[55]

Remember that dehydration of "only" 1 to 2 percent of body weight quickly affects physiological function and performance. Dehydration of greater than 3 percent of body weight increases the risk of heat cramps, heat exhaustion, and heat stroke.[56] The ACSM, along with the National Athletic Trainers Association, recommend being well-hydrated before you start to exercise. Two hours prior to exercise, you should drink 14 to 22 ounces of fluid.

Drinking fluids during exercise is also important. For intense exercise, you should drink about 6 to 12 ounces per 15 to 20 minutes. What are the best fluids to drink? In comparing participants' performance during exercise sessions lasting less than one hour, the ACSM found little difference between plain water and sport drinks (drinks containing carbohydrates and electrolytes).[57] If your exercise session exceeds one hour, beverages containing carbohydrates in

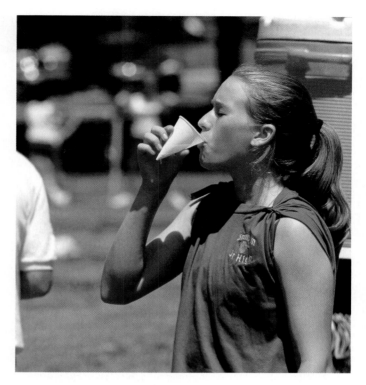

Avoiding dehydration is important when exercising in hot and cold weather, whether to avoid heat exhaustion, heat stroke, or hypothermia.

concentrations of 4 to 8 percent are recommended. Electrolytes aren't really depleted until after about three hours of intense exercise; however, sport drinks that contain sodium taste better, which promotes overall fluid consumption. It is recommended that athletes such as marathon runners use sports drinks to maintain their electrolyte balance. The over-consumption of plain water can dilute the sodium concentration in the blood with fatal results, an effect called *hyponatremia.* Fluid intake *following* physical activity is also important to prevent dehydration—be sure to drink at least a pint of fluid for every pound of body weight lost during your exercise session.[58]

Heat cramps   Muscle cramps that occur during or following exercise in warm or hot weather.

Heat exhaustion   A heat stress illness caused by significant dehydration resulting from exercise in warm or hot conditions; frequent precursor to heat stroke.

Heat stroke   A deadly heat stress illness resulting from dehydration and overexertion in warm or hot conditions; can cause body core temperature to rise from normal to 105°F to 110°F in just a few minutes.

Overcoming Obstacles to Physical Activity

There are many reasons why people do not exercise. These reasons range from personal ("I don't have time") to environmental ("I don't have a safe place to exercise"). You may be reluctant to start exercising if you are overweight or out of shape. Overcoming these barriers is an important part of starting and maintaining a regular exercise program. Take this quiz to determine what factors are undermining your ability to make regular physical activity a priority. After you calculate your score, look at the chart to find ideas on how to overcome the barriers that affect you the most.

WHAT KEEPS YOU FROM BEING MORE ACTIVE?

Directions: Listed below are reasons that people give to describe why they do not get as much physical activity as they think they should. Read each statement, and circle a number to indicate how likely you are to say each statement.

How likely are you to say:	Very likely	Somewhat likely	Somewhat unlikely	Very unlikely
1. My day is so busy now, I just don't think I can make the time to include physical activity in my regular schedule.	3	2	1	0
2. None of my family members or friends like to do anything active, so I don't have a chance to exercise.	3	2	1	0
3. I'm just too tired after work to get any exercise.	3	2	1	0
4. I've been thinking about getting more exercise, but I just can't seem to get started.	3	2	1	0
5. I'm getting older so exercise can be risky.	3	2	1	0
6. I don't get enough exercise because I have never learned the skills for any sport.	3	2	1	0
7. I don't have access to jogging trails, swimming pools, bike paths, etc.	3	2	1	0
8. Physical activity takes too much time away from other commitments—time, work, family, etc.	3	2	1	0
9. I'm embarrassed about how I will look when I exercise with others.	3	2	1	0
10. I don't get enough sleep as it is. I just couldn't get up early or stay up late to get some exercise.	3	2	1	0
11. It's easier for me to find excuses not to exercise than to go out to do something.	3	2	1	0
12. I know of too many people who have hurt themselves by overdoing it with exercise.	3	2	1	0
13. I really can't see learning a new sport at my age.	3	2	1	0
14. It's just too expensive. You have to take a class or join a club or buy the right equipment.	3	2	1	0
15. My free times during the day are too short to include exercise.	3	2	1	0
16. My usual social activities with family or friends do not include physical activity.	3	2	1	0
17. I'm too tired during the week, and I need the weekend to catch up on my rest.	3	2	1	0
18. I want to get more exercise, but I just can't seem to make myself stick to anything.	3	2	1	0

	Very likely	Somewhat likely	Somewhat unlikely	Very unlikely
19. I'm afraid I might injure myself or have a heart attack.	3	2	1	0
20. I'm not good enough at any physical activity to make it fun.	3	2	1	0
21. If we had exercise facilities and showers at work, then I would be more likely to exercise.	3	2	1	0

Interpreting Your Scores

Follow these instructions to score yourself:

- Enter the circled number in the space for each question, putting together the number for statement 1 on line 1, statement 2 on line 2, and so on.
- Add the three numbers for your score in each category of obstacle. A score of 5 or above in any category shows that this is an important barrier for you to overcome.

_____ + _____ + _____ = _____
(1)   (8)   (15)   Lack of time

_____ + _____ + _____ = _____
(2)   (9)   (16)   Social influence

_____ + _____ + _____ = _____
(3)   (10)   (17)   Lack of energy

_____ + _____ + _____ = _____
(4)   (11)   (18)   Lack of willpower

_____ + _____ + _____ = _____
(5)   (12)   (19)   Fear of injury

_____ + _____ + _____ = _____
(6)   (13)   (20)   Lack of skill

_____ + _____ + _____ = _____
(7)   (14)   (21)   Lack of resources

HOW CAN YOU OVERCOME THESE OBSTACLES?

Obstacles to Physical Activity	Possible Solutions
Lack of Time	• Take a good look at your schedule. Can you find three 30-minute time slots in your week? • Multitask. Read while riding an exercise bike or listen to lecture tapes while walking. • Exercise during your lunch breaks or between classes. • Select activities that require minimal time, such as brisk walking or jogging.
Social Influence	• Invite family and friends to exercise with you. • Join a class to meet new people who share your exercise interests. • Explain the importance of exercise to people who may not support your efforts.
Lack of Energy	• Schedule your workouts when you feel most energetic. • Remind yourself that exercise can give you more energy.
Lack of Motivation/Willpower	• Write your planned workout time in your schedule book. • Enlist the help of an exercise partner to make you accountable for working out. • Give yourself an incentive.
Fear of Injury	• Warm up and cool down. • Don't start off too vigorously. • Choose activities with minimum risk. • Remember that without becoming active now, you have a good chance of getting injured in later years due to poor muscle strength, weak bones, and low endurance.
Lack of Skill	• Select activities such as walking that require no new skills. • Exercise with friends who are at the same level. • Take a class, read a book, or watch a video on skills required to perform the desired activity.
Lack of Resources	• Select an activity that requires minimal equipment such as walking, jogging, jumping rope, or calisthenics. • Identify inexpensive resources on campus or in the community.

Source: National Center for Chronic Disease Prevention and Health Promotion, "How Can I Overcome Barriers to Physical Activity?" 2003, www.cdc.gov/nccdphp/dnpa/physical/life/overcome.htm

Exercising in the Cold

When you exercise in cool weather, especially in windy conditions, your body's rate of heat loss is frequently greater than its rate of heat production. These conditions may lead to **hypothermia**—a potentially fatal condition resulting from abnormally low body core temperature, which occurs when body heat is lost faster than it is produced. Temperatures need not be frigid for hypothermia to occur; it can also result from prolonged, vigorous exercise (as in snowboarding or rugby) in 40°F to 50°F temperatures, particularly if there is rain, snow, or a strong wind.

In mild cases of hypothermia, as body core temperature drops from the normal 98.6°F to about 93.2°F, you will begin to shiver. Shivering—the involuntary contraction of nearly every muscle in the body—increases body temperature by using the heat given off by muscle activity. During this first stage of hypothermia, you may also experience cold hands and feet, poor judgment, apathy, and amnesia.[59] Shivering ceases in most hypothermia victims as body core temperatures drop to between 87°F and 90°F, a sign that the body has lost its ability to generate heat. Death usually occurs at body core temperatures between 75°F and 80°F.

To prevent hypothermia, follow these commonsense guidelines:

- Analyze weather conditions and your risk of hypothermia before you undertake an outdoor physical activity. Remember that wind and humidity are as significant as temperature.
- Use the "buddy system"—have a friend join you for cold weather outdoor activities.
- Wear layers of appropriate clothing to prevent excessive heat loss (polypropylene or woolen undergarments, a windproof outer garment, and wool hat and gloves).
- Finally, don't allow yourself to become dehydrated.[60]

Cramps: Taking Action to Prevent Problems

Although most of us have experienced the quick, intense pain of muscle cramps, they are poorly understood. According to the overexertion theory of muscle cramps, when a muscle gets tired, the numerous muscle fibers that comprise it fail to contract in a synchronized rhythm, probably due to overstimulation from the nerves that trigger the muscles to contract.[61] Previous theories related cramping to fluid loss and electrolyte imbalance, but these theories have not held

up. For example, musicians, who do not often get sweaty, complain of muscle cramps.[62] Dietary insufficiencies can also be to blame for electrolyte imbalances—and don't require the person to do any sweating. The rate of calcium reuptake during muscle activity is often credited with causing cramps. Other electrolytes (including sodium and potassium) may be affected by dietary intake. Dehydration may also occur without sweating simply if someone doesn't consume sufficient liquids to compensate for loss in urine and evaporative loss of moisture (without obvious sweating). Hyponatremia, hypokalemia (low potassium), and hyperkalemia also can cause muscle weakness and paralysis.

Even if dehydration is not the only cause, it is clearly a problem for those who exercise and perspire heavily. Drinking enough fluids before, during, and after such activity is important. On a daily basis, drink enough fluid so you have to urinate every two to four hours. Your urine should be pale and there should be lots of it.[63]

Although calcium plays a role in muscle contraction and people with a tendency to have cramps are often calcium deficient, exercise physiologists question the validity of the low-calcium theory. However, because calcium has many health benefits, experts continue to recommend it for anyone who has a tendency toward cramping.

Lack of sodium is another possible factor. If you exercise a lot and perspire heavily, you will lose sodium through sweat and may develop a sodium imbalance and experience cramps. This is most likely to occur in extreme sports such as Ironman triathlons or 100-mile trail runs, particularly in athletes who have consumed only plain water (not sodium-containing food or beverages) during the event.[64] Many health-conscious athletes restrict their salt intake on a regular basis in an attempt to keep blood pressure under control, but clearly there is a risk in doing so. For the average exerciser, sodium intake and sodium replacement is usually not a concern, but for elite athletes or those participating in endurance events such as triathalons or marathons, sodium-infused drinks may deter muscle cramps and delay dehydration.

Although paying attention to the above nutrients is important to avoid cramping, it is probably more important to make sure your muscles are warmed up and not strained beyond their limit.

If you get cramps, what should you do? Generally massage, stretching, putting pressure on the muscle that is cramping, and deep breathing are useful remedies.

Hypothermia   Potentially fatal condition caused by abnormally low body core temperature.

What do you think?

Given what you've read about the symptoms of common fitness injuries, are you currently developing any overuse injuries? ■ *If so, what can you do to prevent these problems from getting more serious?*

Table 10.3
Picking Your Workout Machine

Machine	Workout	For the Best Workout
Exercise Rider	Upper body: Fair Lower body: Fair Learning curve: Easy	Experiment with seat heights until you find one that's comfortable. Make sure your legs don't bend more than 90 degrees at the bottom phase of the motion, which can be hard on the knees. Then, as you straighten, don't arch your spine backward; that stresses your lower back.
Rowing	Upper body: Excellent Lower body: Excellent Learning curve: Hard	Don't hyperextend your back as you finish your stroke. Keep your elbows tight to your body to best strengthen your arms.
Ski-Simulator	Upper body: Excellent Lower body: Excellent Learning curve: Hard	Perfect arm movements first, then the leg actions, then put it all together; it usually takes a few sessions. One habit to avoid: constantly leaning against the hop pad to hold yourself upright.
Stair-Climber	Upper body: Poor Lower body: Excellent Learning curve: Hard	Keep your posture upright, your steps shallow (no deeper than 6 inches), and your weight off your arms.
Treadmill	Upper body: Poor Lower body: Excellent Learning curve: Easy	Start on the flat as a warm-up, gradually increase speed and incline (to 10 percent), then wind down to a slow, flat walk.
Stationary Bike	Upper body: Poor Lower body: Excellent Learning curve: Easy	Adjust the seat so your leg is almost fully extended when the pedal is at its lowest. Then just start pumping.

Source: Adapted by permission of Time Inc. Health from Karmen Butterer, "Picking Your Dream Machine," *Health* (September 1995): 48. © 1995.

Creating Your Own Fitness Program

Identify Your Fitness Goals

Before you develop your own fitness program, analyze your personal needs, limitations, physical activity preferences, and daily schedule. Do you want to improve your quality of life? Lose weight? Lower your risk of health problems? Your specific goal may be to achieve (or maintain) healthy levels of body fat, cardiovascular fitness, muscular strength and endurance, or flexibility and mobility.

Once you become committed to regular physical activity and exercise, you will observe gradual improvements in your functional abilities and note progress toward your goals. Perhaps your most vital goal will be to become committed to fitness for the long haul—to establish a realistic schedule of diverse exercise activities that you can maintain and enjoy throughout your life.

Design Your Program

What type of fitness program is best suited to your needs? The amount and type of exercise required to yield beneficial results vary with the age and physical condition of the exerciser.

Men over age 40 and women over age 50 should consult their physicians before beginning any fitness program.

Good fitness programs are designed to improve or maintain cardiorespiratory fitness, flexibility, muscular strength and endurance, and body composition. A comprehensive program could include a warm-up period of easy walking followed by stretching activities to improve flexibility, then selected strength development exercises, followed by an aerobic activity for 20 minutes or more, and concluding with a cool-down period of gentle flexibility exercises.

The greatest proportion of exercise time should be spent developing cardiovascular fitness, but don't exclude the other components. Choose an aerobic activity you think you will like. Many people find cross training—alternate-day participation in two or more aerobic activities (i.e., jogging and swimming)—less monotonous and more enjoyable than long-term participation in only one activity. Cross training is also beneficial because it strengthens a variety of muscles, thus helping you avoid overuse injuries to muscles and joints.

Jogging, walking, cycling, rowing, step aerobics, and cross-country skiing are all excellent activities for developing cardiovascular fitness. Most colleges and universities have recreation centers where students can use stair-climbing machines, stationary bicycles, treadmills, rowing machines, and ski-simulators. Table 10.3 describes various workout machines and provides tips for using them.

MAKE IT HAPPEN!

Assessment: Complete the Assess Yourself box on page 309 to determine your current cardiorespiratory endurance level. Your results may indicate that you should take steps to improve this component of your physical fitness.

Making a Change: In order to change your behavior, you need to develop a plan. Follow these steps.

1. Evaluate your behavior, and identify patterns and specific things you are doing. What can you change now? What can you change in the next month? Next semester?
2. Select one pattern of behavior that you want to change.
3. Fill out a Behavior Change Contract. It should include your long-term goal for change, your short-term goals, the rewards you'll give yourself for reaching these goals, potential obstacles along the way, and strategies for overcoming these obstacles. (See Skills for Behavior Change box on page 324 for ideas on overcoming barriers.) For each goal, list the small steps and specific actions that you will take.
4. Chart your progress in a journal. At the end of a week, consider how successful you were in following your plan. What helped you be successful? What made change more difficult? What will you do differently next week?
5. Revise your plan as needed. Are the short-term goals attainable? Are the rewards satisfying?

One Student's Plan: Chris decided to measure how long it took him to run 1.5 miles around the school track to determine his level of cardiorespiratory endurance. It took him 14.5 minutes, which, as a 20-year-old, put him into the "borderline" category. Chris had played sports in high school and considered himself in good physical shape. However, he realized he had stopped exercising regularly in his freshman year when he didn't make the baseball team.

Chris decided to start by incorporating more activity into his daily routine. He tended to drive even to places that he could walk or bicycle to as easily. His friends had invited him to join in the pick-up basketball games they played on Saturday afternoons, but he had turned them down in order to play Playstation with his roommate. Chris filled out a Behavior Change Contract with a goal of riding his bicycle the three miles to and from campus three times a week and to play basketball every Saturday. If he did this consistently every week, he would reward himself with a new CD. After a month of this increased activity, Chris was already feeling more fit and was ready to add another aerobic activity. With winter weather coming, he thought he should add an indoor activity and started swimming laps at the school pool. He realized he was making excuses not to go, though, because he found swimming boring. Chris switched to using a stair-climbing machine, which he could do while reading Sports Illustrated or watching ESPN. He was able to stick to doing this three times a week and made a commitment to go a fourth time whenever he missed his Saturday basketball game.

Summary

- The physiological benefits of regular physical activity include (1) reduced risk of heart attack, some cancers, hypertension, and diabetes and (2) improved blood profile, skeletal mass, weight control, immunity to disease, mental health and stress management, and physical fitness. Regular physical activity can also increase life span. For general health benefits, it is recommended that every adult participate in moderate-intensity activities for 30 minutes at least 5 days a week. For improvements in cardiorespiratory fitness, you should work out aerobically for at least 20 minutes, a minimum of 3 days per week. The longer the exercise period, the more calories burned and the bigger improvement in cardiovascular fitness.
- Flexibility exercises should involve static stretching exercises performed in sets of four or more repetitions held for 10 to 30 seconds, at least two to three days a week. Popular forms of stretching exercise include yoga, tai chi, and Pilates.
- The key principles for developing muscular strength and endurance are the tension principle, the overload principle, and the specificity-of-training principle. The different types of muscle actions include isometric, concentric, and eccentric. Resistance training programs include body weight resistance (calisthenics), fixed resistance, variable resistance, and use of accommodating resistance devices.
- Fitness injuries are generally caused by overuse or trauma; the most common are plantar fasciitis, shin splints, and runner's knee. Proper footwear and equipment can help prevent injuries. Exercise in the heat or cold requires special precautions.
- Planning a fitness program involves setting goals and designing a program to achieve these goals.

Questions for Discussion and Reflection

1. How do you define physical fitness? What are the key components of a physical fitness program? What might you need to consider when beginning a fitness program?
2. How would you determine the proper intensity and duration of an exercise program? How often should exercise sessions be scheduled?
3. Why is stretching vital to improving physical flexibility?
4. Identify at least four physiological and psychological benefits of physical fitness. How would you promote these benefits to nonexercisers?
5. Describe the different types of resistance employed in an exercise program. What are the benefits of each type of resistance?
6. Your roommate has decided to start running first thing in the morning in an effort to lose weight, tone muscles, and improve cardiorespiratory fitness. What advice would you give to make sure your roommate gets off to a good start and doesn't get injured?
7. What key components would you include in a fitness program for yourself?

Accessing Your Health on the Internet

Visit the following Internet sites to explore further topics and issues related to personal health. To visit an organization's website, go to the Companion Website for *Access to Health, Ninth Edition* at www.aw-bc.com/donatelle, click on the book image, and select "Accessing Your Health on the Internet" from the navigation menu.

1. *ACSM Online.* A link with the American College of Sports Medicine and all its resources.
2. *American Council on Exercise.* Information on exercise and disease prevention.
3. *The American Medical Association's Health Insight.* Provides a fitness assessment and guidelines to help you develop your own fitness program.
4. *Just Move.* The American Heart Association's fitness website has the latest information on heart disease and exercise, plus a guide to local, regional, and national fitness events.
5. *Centers for Disease Control and Prevention. National Center for Chronic Disease Prevention and Health Promotion, Division of Nutrition and Physical Activity.* A resource for current information on exercise and health.
6. *National Strength and Conditioning Association.* A resource for personal trainers and others interested in conditioning and fitness.

Further Reading

Fahey, T. D. *Super Fitness for Sports, Conditioning, and Health.* Boston: Allyn & Bacon, 2000.

A brief guide to developing fitness that emphasizes training techniques for improving sports performance.

Powers, S. K, S. L. Dodd, and V. J. Noland. *Total Fitness and Wellness,* 4th ed. San Francisco: Benjamin Cummings, 2005.

A complete guide to improving all areas of fitness, including being a smart health consumer, interviews with fitness specialists, and the links between nutrition and fitness.

Schlosberg, S. *The Ultimate Workout Log: An Exercise Diary and Fitness Guide.* Boston: Houghton Mifflin, 1999.

A six-month log that also provides fitness definitions, training tips, and motivational quotes.

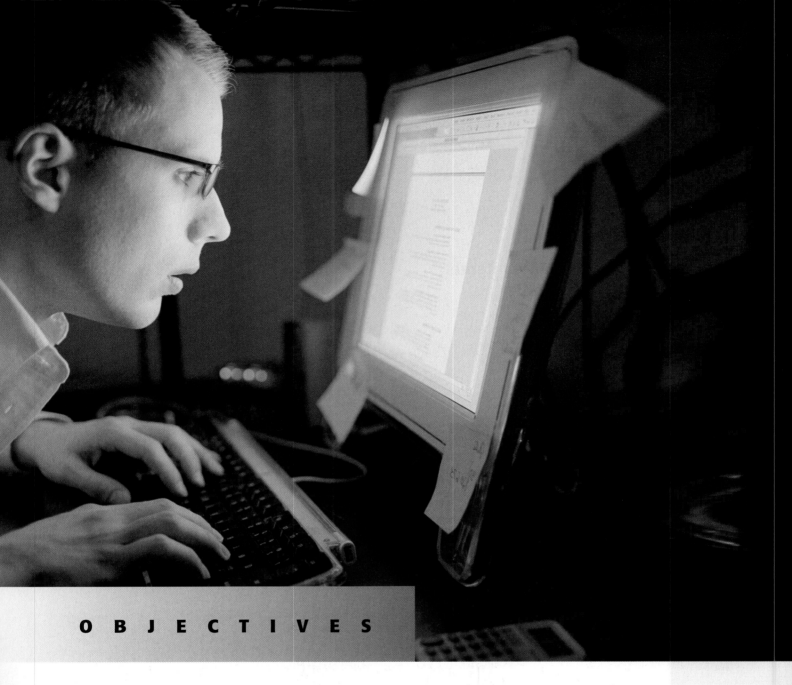

OBJECTIVES

- Define *addiction*.

- Distinguish addictions from habits, and identify the signs of addiction.

- Discuss the addictive process, the physiology of addiction, and the biopsychosocial model of addiction.

- Describe types of addictions, including money, work, exercise, sexual, and Internet addictions, as well as codependence.

- Evaluate treatment and recovery options for addicts, including individual therapy, group therapy, family therapy, and 12-step programs.

ADDICTIONS AND ADDICTIVE BEHAVIOR

THREATS TO WELLNESS

IN THE NEWS

Addiction: A Gene for Getting Hooked

By John O'Neil

Teenagers whose bodies clear nicotine unusually slowly from their systems became addicted to cigarettes at more than twice the rate of their peers, a study has concluded.

In recent years, researchers have come to believe that genetic factors make some people more susceptible to addiction to tobacco, alcohol and other drugs, along with well-established social and environmental factors, said the study's lead researcher, Dr. Jennifer Lee O'Loughlin of McGill University in Montreal.

The study, released last week, focused on genetic defects that have moderate or severe effects on the liver's ability to metabolize nicotine, the addictive stimulant in tobacco.

The study, published in *Tobacco Control,* a British journal, involved 281 seventh graders who had begun to smoke but were not yet considered addicted. Thirteen percent had one of the defective versions of the gene.

Over five years, 25 percent of the teenagers who were the slowest to process nicotine increased their smoking to the point of dependence, compared with 9 percent of those with normal nicotine metabolism and 10 percent who were slightly impaired, the study found.

Read the complete article online in the eThemes section of this book's website: www.aw-bc.com/donatelle.

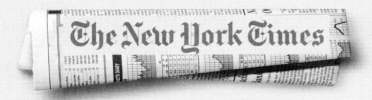

It isn't difficult these days to find high-profile cases of compulsive and destructive behavior. Stories of celebrities and politicians struggling with addictions to alcohol, drugs, and sex are splashed in the headlines and profiled on television news programs. But millions of "everyday" people throughout the world are staging their own battles with addiction as well. (See the Health in a Diverse World box.) Addictions can be perplexing, since many potentially addictive activities may actually enhance the lives of those who engage in them moderately. In addition to alcohol and drugs, the most commonly recognized objects of addiction include food, sex, relationships, spending money, work, exercise, gambling, and using the Internet.

Defining Addiction

Addiction is continued involvement with a substance or activity despite ongoing negative consequences. Addictive behaviors initially provide a sense of pleasure or stability that is beyond the addict's power to achieve in other ways. Eventually, the addicted person needs to be involved in the behavior in order to feel normal.

In this chapter, *addiction* is used interchangeably with *physiological addiction*. However, physiological dependence is only one indicator of addiction. Psychological dynamics play an important role, which explains why behaviors not related to the use of chemicals—gambling, for example—may also be addictive. A person who possesses a strong desire to continue engaging in a particular activity is said to have developed a psychological dependence. In fact, psychological and physiological dependence are so intertwined that it is not really possible to separate the two. For every psychological state, there is a corresponding physiological state. In other words, everything you feel is tied to a chemical process occurring in your body.[1] Thus, addictions once thought to be entirely psychological in nature are now understood to have physiological components.

To be addictive, a behavior must have the potential to produce a positive mood change. Chemicals are responsible for the most profound addictions, not only because they produce dramatic mood changes, but also because they cause cellular changes to which the body adapts so well that it eventually requires the chemical in order to function normally. Yet other behaviors, such as gambling, spending money, working, and sex, also create changes at the cellular

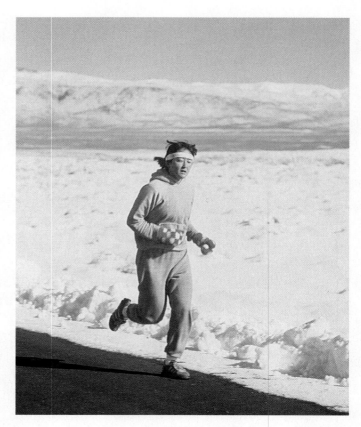

Obsession with a substance or behavior, even a generally positive activity such as exercise, can eventually develop into an addiction.

level along with positive mood changes. Although the mechanism is not well understood, all forms of addiction probably reflect dysfunction of certain biochemical systems in the brain.[2]

Traditionally, diagnosis of an addiction was limited to drug addiction and was based on three criteria: (1) the presence of an abstinence syndrome, or **withdrawal**—a series of temporary physical and psychological symptoms that occurs when the addicted person abruptly stops using the drug; (2) an associated pattern of pathological behavior (deterioration in work performance, relationships, and social interaction); and (3) **relapse,** the tendency to return to the addictive behavior after a period of abstinence.

Furthermore, until recently, health professionals were unwilling to diagnose an addiction until medical symptoms appeared in the patient. Now we know that although withdrawal, pathological behavior, relapse, and medical symptoms are valid indicators of addiction, they do not characterize all addictive behavior.

Habit versus Addiction

How do we distinguish between a harmless habit and an addiction? The stereotypical image of the addict is of someone desperately seeking a fix 24 hours a day. People have the

---

Addiction   Continued involvement with a substance or activity despite ongoing negative consequences.

Withdrawal   A series of temporary physical and biopsychosocial symptoms that occur when the addict abruptly abstains from an addictive chemical or behavior.

Relapse   The tendency to return to the addictive behavior after a period of abstinence.

Addiction across Cultures

Although alcohol is considered the typical drug of addiction in the United States, many countries are struggling with epidemic rates of dependence on other drugs. In fact, demand for addiction treatment services is increasing in many nations. Here's a look at some current drug addiction treatment data from around the world:

- The health impact of addiction, as measured by demand for treatment services, is highest for opiates. The most serious global drug problem, opiates account for 70 percent of drug treatment in Asia, 64 percent in Europe, and 62 percent in Australia.

- In European nations, opiates, primarily heroin, are the drug of choice for nearly three-quarters of individuals seeking treatment.
- In the Americas as a whole, cocaine and cocaine derivatives account for almost 60 percent of the demand for drug treatment.
- Political upheaval and the resulting disintegration of the family appear to be strongly related to rising drug abuse. A study in Ireland found that as many as 10 percent of young people (aged 15–20) in Dublin were addicted to heroin.
- Amphetamine use is higher in Nordic nations such as Sweden and Finland, where it accounts for 20 percent and 40 percent of treatment needs, respectively.

- Treatment for cannabis (marijuana, hashish) dependence is much higher in the Caribbean, including Jamaica, where it accounts for over 50 percent of treatment demand.

Sources: United Nations Office for Drug Control and Crime Prevention, "2004 World Drug Report," 2004, www.unodc.org /unodc/en/world_drug_report.html; United Nations Office for Drug Control and Crime Prevention, "The Social Impact of Drug Abuse," 1995 www.unodc.org/unodc/en /publications/technical_series_1995-03-01.html; United Nations Office for Drug Control and Crime Prevention, "Global Illicit Drug Trends," 2003, www.unodc.org/unodc /global_illicit_drug_trends.html.

---

notion that if you aren't doing the behavior every day, you're not addicted. The reality is somewhere between these two extremes.

Addiction certainly involves elements of **habit,** a repeated behavior in which the repetition may be unconscious. A habit can be annoying, but it can be broken without too much discomfort by simply becoming aware of its presence and choosing not to do it. Addiction also involves repetition of a behavior, but the repetition occurs by **compulsion,** and considerable discomfort is experienced if the behavior is not performed. An addiction is a habit that has gotten out of control and has negative health effects.

To understand addiction, we need to look beyond the amount and frequency of the behavior, for what happens when a person is involved in the behavior is far more meaningful. For example, someone who drinks only rarely, and then in moderation, may experience personality changes, blackouts (drug-induced amnesia), and other negative consequences (for example, failing a test, missing an important appointment, getting into a fight) that would never have occurred had the person not taken a few drinks. On the other hand, someone who has a few martinis every evening may never do anything out of character while under the influence of alcohol but may become irritable, manipulative, and aggressive without those regular drinks. For both of these people, alcohol appears to perform a function (mood control) that people should be able to perform without the aid of chemicals, which is a possible sign of addiction. Habits are behaviors that occur through choice and typically do not cause negative health consequences. In contrast, no one

decides to become addicted, even though people make choices that contribute to the development of an addiction.

Signs of Addiction

If you asked ten people to define addiction, you would quite possibly get ten different responses. Studies show that all animals share the same basic pleasure and reward circuits in the brain that turn on when they come into contact with addictive substances or engage in something pleasurable, such as eating or orgasm. We all engage in potentially addictive behaviors to some extent because some are essential to our survival and are highly reinforcing, such as eating, drinking, and sex. At some point along the continuum, however, some individuals are not able to engage in these or other behaviors moderately and become addicted.

Although different opinions exist as to the cause of addiction, most experts agree on some universal signs of it. All addictions are characterized by four common symptoms: (1) compulsion, which is characterized by **obsession,** or

---

Habit A repeated behavior in which the repetition may be unconscious.

Compulsion Obsessive preoccupation with a behavior and an overwhelming need to perform it.

Obsession Excessive preoccupation with an addictive object or behavior.

excessive preoccupation with the behavior and an overwhelming need to perform it; (2) **loss of control,** or the inability to predict reliably whether any isolated occurrence of the behavior will be healthy or damaging; (3) **negative consequences,** such as physical damage, legal trouble, financial problems, academic failure, and family dissolution, which do not occur with healthy involvement in any behavior; and (4) **denial,** or the inability to perceive that the behavior is self-destructive.

These four components are present in all addictions, whether chemical or behavioral.

What do you think?

Have you ever seen signs of addiction in a friend or family member? ■ *What types of negative consequences have you witnessed?* ■ *Can you think of any habits you have that could potentially become addictive?*

The Addictive Process

Addiction is a process that evolves over time. It begins when a person repeatedly seeks the illusion of relief to avoid unpleasant feelings or situations. This pattern is known as **nurturing through avoidance** and is a maladaptive way of taking care of emotional needs. As a person becomes increasingly dependent on the addictive behavior, there is a corresponding deterioration in relationships with family, friends, and coworkers; in performance at work or school; and in personal life. Eventually, addicts do not find the addictive behavior

Loss of control Inability to predict reliably whether a particular instance of involvement with the addictive object or behavior will be healthy or damaging.

Negative consequences Physical damage, legal trouble, financial problems, academic failure, family dissolution, and other severe problems associated with addiction.

Denial Inability to perceive or accurately interpret the effects of the addictive behavior.

Nurturing through avoidance Repeatedly seeking the illusion of relief to avoid unpleasant feelings or situations, a maladaptive way of taking care of emotional needs.

Neurotransmitters Biochemical messengers that exert influence at specific receptor sites on nerve cells.

Tolerance Phenomenon in which progressively larger doses of a drug or more intense involvement in a behavior is needed to produce the desired effects.

pleasurable but consider it preferable to the unhappy realities they are seeking to escape. Figure 11.1 illustrates the cycle of psychological addiction.

The Physiology of Addiction

Virtually all intellectual, emotional, and behavioral functions occur as a result of biochemical interactions between nerve cells in the body. Biochemical messengers, called **neurotransmitters,** exert their influence at specific receptor sites on nerve cells. Drug use and chronic stress can alter these receptor sites and cause the production and breakdown of neurotransmitters.

Mood-altering chemicals, for example, fill up the receptor sites for the body's natural "feel-good" neurotransmitters (endorphins) so that nerve cells are fooled into believing they have enough neurotransmitters and shut down production of these substances temporarily. When the drug use stops, those receptor sites empty, resulting in uncomfortable feelings that remain until the body resumes neurotransmitter production or the person consumes more of the drug. Some people's bodies always produce insufficient quantities of these neurotransmitters, so they naturally seek out chemicals such as alcohol as substitutes or pursue behaviors such as exercise that increase natural production. Thus, we may be "wired" to seek out substances or experiences that increase pleasure or reduce discomfort.

Mood-altering substances and experiences produce **tolerance,** a phenomenon in which progressively larger doses of a drug or more intense involvement in an experience are needed to obtain the desired effects. All of us develop some degree of tolerance to any mood-altering experience. But because addicts tend to seek intense mood-altering experiences, they eventually increase the amount and intensity to the point of causing negative side effects.

Withdrawal is another phenomenon associated with mood-altering experiences. The drug or activity replaces or causes an effect that the body should normally provide on its own. If the experience is repeated often enough, the body adjusts: it starts to require the drug or experience to obtain the effect it used to be able to produce itself but no longer can. Stopping the behavior will therefore cause a withdrawal syndrome.

Withdrawal symptoms of chemical dependencies are generally the opposite of the effects of the drug being withdrawn. For example, a cocaine addict experiences a characteristic "crash" (depression and lethargy), while a barbiturate addict experiences trembling, irritability, and convulsions upon withdrawal. Withdrawal symptoms for addictive behaviors are usually less dramatic. They usually involve psychological discomfort such as anxiety, depression, irritability, guilt, anger, and frustration, with an underlying preoccupation with or craving for another exposure to the behavior.

Withdrawal syndromes range from mild to severe. The most severe form of withdrawal syndrome is delirium tremens (DTs), which occurs in approximately 5 percent of dependent individuals withdrawing from alcohol.

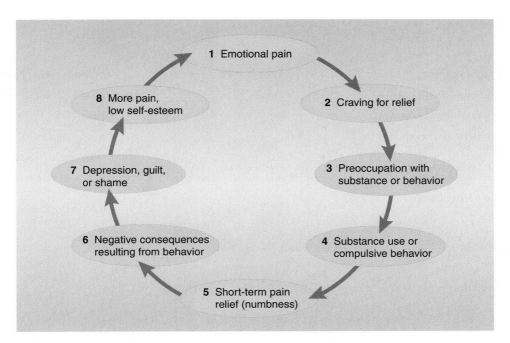

Figure 11.1
Cycle of Psychological Addiction

Source: From R. Goldberg, *Drugs Across the Spectrum,* 3rd edition. Copyright 2000. Reprinted with permission of Brooks/Cole, a division of Thomson Learning: www.thomsonrights.com. Fax 800-730-2215.

A Model of Addiction

Theories abound concerning the cause of addictions, and most of them focus on a single causative factor. Biological or disease models have been proposed since ancient times. However, it has become clear through time that psychological and environmental factors may also be involved in the development of addiction. The most effective treatment today is being provided by those who rely on the **biopsychosocial model of addiction,** which proposes that addiction is caused by a variety of factors operating together, thereby lending credibility to all the other theories. The biopsychosocial model is not a compromise solution to a theoretical controversy. Rather, it represents a reasonable comprehension of all that we have learned about addiction.

Biological or Disease Influences   Studies show that people addicted to mood-altering substances metabolize these substances differently than nonaddicted people do. For example, studies of adult children of alcoholics have found that these people have abnormal concentrations or activity of various neurotransmitters related to mood—specifically norepinephrine, serotonin, endorphin, and enkephalin.[3] Abnormal levels of any of these neurotransmitters may create a biochemically based mood disorder. To obtain relief from the disorder, people may turn to mood-altering chemicals or behaviors.

Studies also support a genetic influence on addiction. It has been known for centuries that alcoholism runs in families. Research on family members and twins has repeatedly

confirmed the existence of a genetic factor in alcoholism. In the past decade, other studies have shown that the children of drug-addicted parents are more likely to engage in addictive behaviors than are the children of nonaddicted parents. These findings hold true whether or not the children lived with their addicted parents.[4]

Environmental Influences   Cultural expectations and mores help determine whether people engage in certain behaviors. For example, although many native Italians use alcohol abundantly, there is a low incidence of alcoholism in this culture. Low rates of alcoholism typically exist in cultures such as Italy, where children are gradually introduced to alcohol in diluted amounts, on special occasions, and within a strong family group. There is deep disapproval of intoxication, which is not viewed as socially acceptable, stylish, or funny.[5] Such cultural traditions and values are less widespread in the United States, where the incidence of alcohol addiction and alcohol-related problems is very high.

Societal attitudes and messages also influence addictive behavior. The media's emphasis on appearance and the

> **Biopsychosocial model of addiction**   Theory of the relationship between an addict's biological (genetic) nature and psychological and environmental influences.

Biological Factors

- Unusual early response to the substance or experience (e.g., easy development of tolerance to alcohol)
- Attention deficit/hyperactivity disorder and other learning disabilities
- Biologically based mood disorders (depression and bipolar disorders)
- Addiction among biological family members

Psychological Factors

- Low self-esteem
- External locus of control (looking outside oneself for solutions)
- Passivity
- Post-traumatic stress disorders (victims of abuse or other trauma)

Environmental Factors

- Ready access to the substance or experience
- Abusive or neglectful home environment
- Peer norms
- Misperception of peer norms
- Membership in an alienated, oppressed, or marginalized group
- Life events, including chronic or acute stressors

Figure 11.2
Risk Factors for Addiction

ideal body plays a significant role in exercise addiction. Societal glorification of money and material achievement can lead to work addiction, which is often admired. Societal changes, in turn, influence individual norms. People living in cities characterized by rapid social change or social disorganization often feel less connected to social, religious, and civic institutions. The resulting disenfranchisement leads to increased destructive behaviors, including addiction.[6]

Social learning theory proposes that people learn behaviors by watching role models—parents, caregivers, and significant others. The effects of modeling, imitation, and identification with behavior from early childhood on are well documented. Modeling is especially influential when it involves behavior that is mood-altering. Many studies show that modeling by parents and by idolized celebrities exerts a profound influence on young people.[7]

On an individual level, major stressful life events, such as marriage, divorce, change in work status, and death of a loved one, may trigger addictive behaviors. The death of a spouse is the most common trigger event for excessive drinking among the elderly. Traumatic events in general often instigate addictive behaviors, as traumatized people seek to medicate their pain—pain they may not even be aware of because they've repressed it. One thing that makes addictive behaviors so powerfully attractive is that they reliably alleviate personal pain, at least for a short time. However, this relief of pain from addictive behaviors is only temporary; addictive behaviors actually cause more pain than they relieve. Family members whose needs for love,

security, and affirmation are not consistently met; who are refused permission to express their feelings, desires, or needs; and who frequently submerge their personalities to "keep the peace" are prone to addiction. Children whose parents are not consistently available to them (physically or emotionally); who are subjected to sexual abuse, physical abuse, neglect, or abandonment; or who receive inconsistent or disparaging messages about their self-worth may experience psychosocial or physical illness and addiction in adulthood.

Psychological Factors

A person's individual psychological makeup also factors into the potential for addiction. People with low self-esteem, a tendency toward risk-taking behavior, or poor coping skills are more likely to develop addictive patterns of behavior. Individuals who consistently look outside themselves (who have an external locus of control) for solutions and explanations for life events are more likely to experience addiction.[8]

The complexity of addiction and consistent evidence of multiple contributing factors lead us to conclude that addiction is not the result of a single influence, but rather of a variety of influences working together. Biological, psychological, and environmental factors all contribute to its development. Although one factor may play a larger role than another in a specific individual, a single factor is rarely sufficient to explain an addiction. Figure 11.2 lists risk factors for addiction.

Social learning theory Theory that people learn behaviors by watching role models—parents, caregivers, and significant others.

What do you think?

Which factors discussed in this section do you think play the biggest role in addiction? ■ *Do you think some addictions have a biological basis? Why?*

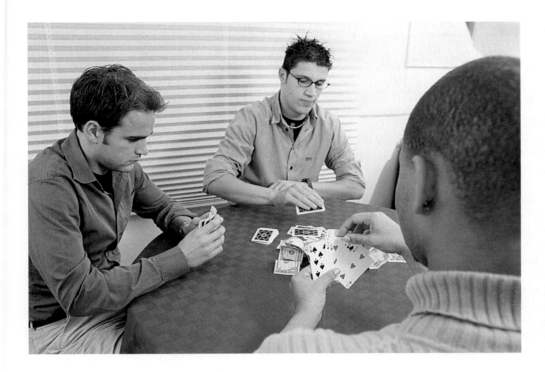

Though many people gamble occasionally as a form of recreation, others become addicted and may face grave financial and personal consequences.

Types of Addiction

It is difficult to document the incidence of addictions of any kind because involvement with a chemical or a behavior does not, by itself, indicate addiction. Nevertheless, many studies on morbidity and mortality associated with a substance or behavior provide reasonable estimates. Another indication of the possible prevalence of addictions is that an estimated 10 million people are actively involved in self-help groups in the United States,[9] although, of course, not all of these groups address addiction.

Clearly, tobacco, alcohol, and other drugs are addictive, and addictions to these drugs create multiple problems for addicted individuals as well as their families and society. Later chapters in this book will discuss specific substance-related addictions. In this chapter we examine the fundamental concepts and process of addiction, as well as its associated problems. We will also look at what are commonly called **process addictions**—behaviors known to be addictive because they are mood-altering. Examples include money, work, exercise, Internet, and sexual addictions.

Money Addictions

Money addictions include compulsive gambling, spending, and borrowing. Research has shown that, among susceptible individuals, the various money addictions produce profound mood elevations resulting from synthesis of the neurotransmitters that regulate stimulation, excitement, and pleasure.[10] Money addicts develop tolerance and also experience the phenomenon of withdrawal. Withdrawal symptoms include extreme restlessness, agitation, insomnia, depression, anxiety,

and anger.[11] Money addictions are common to both genders and across all ages, races, religions, and socioeconomic groups.

Compulsive Gambling Gambling is a healthy form of recreation and entertainment for millions of Americans. Most people who gamble do so casually and moderately to experience the excitement of anticipating a win.

But over 3 million Americans are **compulsive gamblers** (addicted to gambling), and 15 million more are considered to be at risk for developing a gambling addiction.[12]

Men are more likely to have gambling problems than women are. Gambling prevalence is also higher among lower-income individuals, those who are divorced, African Americans, older adults, and individuals residing within 50 miles of a casino. Residents of southern states, where opportunities to gamble have increased significantly in the past 20 years, also have higher problem gambling rates.[13] College students who identify themselves as problem gamblers are also much more likely to be regular tobacco and marijuana users and heavy drinkers, and to report negative consequences related to alcohol consumption.[14] For these people, gambling is a compulsion that rules, and often ruins, their lives (see

> **Process addictions** Behaviors such as money addictions, work addiction, exercise addiction, and sex addictions that are known to be addictive because they are mood-altering.
>
> **Compulsive gambler** A person addicted to gambling.

Gambling and College Students

The Final Four, the Super Bowl, Saturday college football games—there are numerous opportunities for gambling, and recent trends tell us that many college students are taking part. The National Collegiate Athletic Association (NCAA) estimates that during March Madness (the men's college basketball tournament) each year, there are over 1.2 million active gambling pools, with over $2.5 billion gambled. More and more of these dollars come from the pockets of college students. There is growing evidence, in fact, that betting on college campuses is interfering with some students' financial and academic futures. Consider the following:

✔ Almost 80 percent of college students have participated in most forms of gambling, including casino gambling, lottery tickets, racing, and sports betting.

✔ At least 78 percent of youths have placed a bet by the age of 18.

✔ Roughly 8 to 20 percent of college students have experienced a gambling problem and about 4.8 percent have gambled compulsively.

✔ Student athletes have come under increased scrutiny for their association with gambling. Student athletes who report having gambled also report risk-taking behaviors.

✔ The three most common reasons college students give for gambling are risk, excitement, and the chance to make money.

Although most college students who gamble are able to do so without developing a problem, warning signs of problem gambling include:

✔ Missing class or work to participate in gambling

✔ Spending more money than intended on bets

✔ Lying to roommates, friends, and family about betting, amounts spent, and losses

✔ Using tuition money, savings, or money set aside for living expenses to bet

✔ Taking cash advances on credit cards or dipping into savings for betting money

Source: T. J. Knapp, "Sports Betting by College Students: Who Bets and How Often?," *College Student Journal* 32, no. 2; Penn State University, "Survey on College Gambling," November 1999, www.sa.psu.edu /sara/pulse/64-gamble.PDF; "I Can Make That Shot!" *The Wager* 7, no. 2 (March 6, 2002), www.thewager.org

---

the Reality Check box). While casual gamblers can stop anytime they wish and are capable of seeing the necessity to do so, compulsive gamblers are unable to control the urge to gamble even in the face of devastating consequences: high debt, legal problems, and the loss of everything meaningful, including homes, families, jobs, health—and even their lives. Cardiovascular problems affect 38 percent of compulsive gamblers, and their suicide rate is 20 times higher than that of the general population.

Compulsive Shopping and Borrowing   Although compulsive spending has been a pervasive problem in the United States for some time, a more insidious form of the addiction lurks in the new "plastic generation." Credit card companies entice you with fantasies of having it all, right now—whether or not you can afford it.

The credit card companies seem to be succeeding. There are 400 million MasterCards and Visas out there. Add to that cable shopping stations, catalog shopping, and shopping over the Internet, and the opportunity to overspend is greater than ever before. The resulting debt from all this spending is phenomenal. Bankruptcies, formerly a last resort, have become almost run of the mill—almost 1.3 million were recorded for 2000. On average, compulsive spenders are $23,000 in debt, usually in the form of credit card debt or mortgages against their homes.[15]

Although most people can manage debt with careful planning, some spend money to meet emotional needs they can't fulfill elsewhere. Anxiety, self-doubt, and anger all lead to spending as a way of coping with daily stressors. College students may be particularly vulnerable to spending problems because advertisers and credit card companies heavily target them.

Compulsive gambling and shopping can frequently lead to compulsive borrowing to help support the addiction. Irresponsible investments and purchases lead to debts that the addict tries to repay by borrowing more. Compulsive debtors borrow money repeatedly from family, friends, or institutions in spite of the problems this causes. While most people incur overwhelming debt through a combination of hardship and ignorance about financial management, compulsive debtors incur debt primarily as a result of buying or gambling behaviors in which they have engaged to relieve painful feelings.

Work Addiction

In order to understand work addiction, we need to understand the concept of healthy work. Healthy work provides a sense of identity, helps develop our strengths, and is a means of satisfaction, accomplishment, and mastery of problems.

Healthy workers may work passionately for long hours. Although they have occasional projects that keep them away from family, friends, and personal interests for short periods of time, they generally maintain balance in their lives and full control of their schedules. Healthy work does not "consume" the worker.

Conversely, **work addiction** is the compulsive use of work and the work persona to fulfill needs of intimacy, power, and success. It is characterized by obsession, perfectionism, rigidity, fear, anxiety, feelings of inadequacy, low self-esteem, and alienation. Work addiction is more than being unable to relax when not doing something considered "productive." It is the pursuit of the "work persona"—the image that work addicts wish to project onto others. Work addiction is found among all age, racial, and socioeconomic groups, but it typically develops in people in their forties and fifties. Male work addicts outnumber female work addicts, but women are catching up fast as they gain more equality in the workforce.

Although work addicts tend to be admired in our society, the effects on individuals and those around them are far reaching. Work addiction is a major source of marital discord and family breakup. In fact, most work addicts come from homes that were alcoholic, rigid, violent, or otherwise dysfunctional. A survey of grandchildren of alcoholics revealed that 64 percent identified work addiction as the most common compulsion in one or both of their parents.[16]

Whether or not they lose their families, work addicts do compromise their emotional and physical health. They may become emotionally crippled, losing the communication and human interaction skills critical to living and working with other people. They are often riddled with guilt and chronic fear—of failure, boredom, laziness, persecution, or being found out. Because they are unable to relax and play, they commonly suffer from chronic fatigue. The excessive pumping of adrenaline that is part of the addiction causes fatigue, hypertension and other cardiovascular diseases, nervousness, trembling, and increased sweating. Work addicts commonly suffer from disorders of the gastrointestinal tract, and they often report a feeling of pressure in the chest, constricted breathing, dizziness, and lightheadedness. Figure 11.3 identifies other typical signs of work addiction.

Exercise Addiction

It may seem odd that a personal health text that advocates exercise would also identify it as a potential addiction. Yet, as a powerful mood enhancer, exercise can be addictive. Statistics on the incidence of this addiction are not available, but one indication of its prevalence is that a large portion of America's 2 million people with anorexia and/or bulimia use exercise to purge instead of or in addition to self-induced vomiting.

Addictive exercisers abuse exercise in the same way that alcoholics abuse alcohol or addictive spenders abuse money. They use it compulsively to try to meet needs that

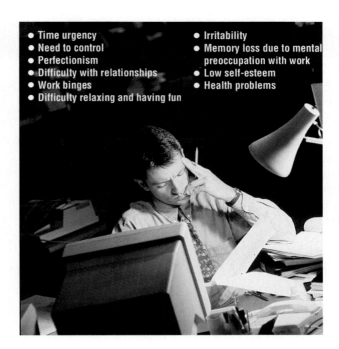

- Time urgency
- Need to control
- Perfectionism
- Difficulty with relationships
- Work binges
- Difficulty relaxing and having fun
- Irritability
- Memory loss due to mental preoccupation with work
- Low self-esteem
- Health problems

Figure 11.3
Signs of Work Addiction

cannot truly be met by an object or activity: nurturance, intimacy, self-esteem, and self-competency. As a result, addictive exercise results in negative consequences similar to those found in other addictions: alienation of family and friends, injuries from overdoing it, and a craving for more.

Traditionally, women have been perceived as more at risk for exercise addiction. However, evidence is growing that more men are developing unhealthy exercise patterns. Media images promoting "six-pack abs" and lean, muscular male bodies have influenced society's view of the masculine ideal. However, that body type is as unrealistic for most men as the stick-thin fashion model figure is for most women. Meanwhile, more men are abusing steroids and overexercising to attain the desired frame. **Muscle dysmorphia,** sometimes referred to as "bigarexia," is a pathological preoccupation with being larger and more muscular.[17] Sufferers view themselves as small and weak even though they may

Work addiction   The compulsive use of work and the work persona to fulfill needs for intimacy, power, and success.

Addictive exercisers   People who exercise compulsively to try to meet needs of nurturance, intimacy, self-esteem, and self-competency.

Muscle dysmorphia   Sometimes referred to as "bigarexia," a pathological preoccupation with being larger and more muscular, which can lead to exercise addiction.

Are You Addicted to the Internet?

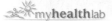 myhealthlab

Fill out this assessment online at www.aw-bc.com/myhealthlab or www.aw-bc.com/donatelle

Internet addiction is not simply a matter of time spent online. Some people indicate they are addicted with only 20 hours of Internet use, while others who spend much more time online insist it is not a problem for them. It's more important to measure how your Internet use affects your life. Have any conflicts emerged in family, relationships, work, or school?

Circle the answer that most closely describes your behavior:

This simple exercise will help you in two ways: (1) if you already know or strongly believe you are addicted to the Internet, this guide will assist you in identifying the areas in your life most impacted by your excessive Net use; and (2) if you're not sure whether you are addicted, this will help you determine the answer and assess the damage. When answering, consider only the time you spend online for nonacademic or non-job-related purposes.

	Rarely	Occasionally	Frequently	Often	Always
1. How often do you find that you stay online longer than you intended?	1	2	3	4	5
2. How often do you neglect household chores to spend more time online?	1	2	3	4	5
3. How often do you prefer the excitement of the Internet to intimacy with your partner?	1	2	3	4	5
4. How often do you form new relationships with fellow online users?	1	2	3	4	5
5. How often do others in your life complain to you about the amount of time you spend online?	1	2	3	4	5
6. How often do your grades or school work suffer because of the amount of time you spend online?	1	2	3	4	5
7. How often do you check your e-mail before something else that you need to do?	1	2	3	4	5
8. How often does your job performance or productivity suffer because of the Internet?	1	2	3	4	5
9. How often do you become defensive or secretive when anyone else asks you what you do online?	1	2	3	4	5
10. How often do you block out disturbing thoughts about your life with soothing thoughts about the Internet?	1	2	3	4	5

be quite the opposite.[18] Consequences of muscle dysmorphia include excessive weight lifting and exercising as well as steroid or supplement abuse.

Internet Addiction

There are enormous numbers of Internet users in the United States, with virtually unlimited access to all types of information.[19] It is no wonder that Internet use is becoming a serious

Internet addiction Compulsive use of computer activities such as fantasy games, online shopping, and chat rooms.

problem for some people. **Internet addiction** is a blanket term that encompasses various compulsive behaviors related to computer use. They include viewing sexually explicit materials, playing fantasy games or other computer games, online stock trading, and spending hours in chat rooms or on discussion boards.

Current research indicates that the Internet can be addictive for several reasons:[20]

- *It is accessible.* A person doesn't have to travel or leave the house to chat with people, shop, trade, or play games.
- *It provides control.* A person can trade stocks without a broker, and online auction sites allow users to bid on

	Rarely	Occasionally	Frequently	Often	Always
11. How often do you find yourself anticipating when you will go online again?	1	2	3	4	5
12. How often do you fear that life without the Internet would be boring, empty, and joyless?	1	2	3	4	5
13. How often do you snap, yell, or act annoyed if someone bothers you while you are online?	1	2	3	4	5
14. How often do you lose sleep to late-night log-ons?	1	2	3	4	5
15. How often do you feel preoccupied with the Internet when offline or fantasize about being online?	1	2	3	4	5
16. How often do you find yourself saying "just a few more minutes" when online?	1	2	3	4	5
17. How often do you try to cut down the amount of time you spend online and fail?	1	2	3	4	5
18. How often do you try to hide how long you've been online?	1	2	3	4	5
19. How often do you choose to spend more time online over going out with others?	1	2	3	4	5
20. How often do you feel depressed, moody, or nervous when you are offline? Do these feelings go away once you are back online?	1	2	3	4	5

INTERPRETING YOUR SCORES

After you have answered all the questions, add the numbers you selected for each response to obtain a final score. The higher your score, the greater your level of addiction and the problems your Internet usage causes.

20–49 points: You are an average Internet user. You may surf the Web a bit too long at times, but you have control over your usage.

50–79 points: You are experiencing occasional or frequent problems because of the Internet. You should consider the Internet's full impact on your life.

80–100 points: Your Internet usage is causing significant problems in your life. You should evaluate the impact of the Internet on your life and address the problems directly caused by your Internet usage.

MAKE IT HAPPEN!

Use the results of this self-assessment to begin your behavior change program. Follow the steps and use the examples on page 346 to complete your Behavior Change Contract, and use these resources to take action.

Source: Reprinted by permission of Dr. Kimberly S. Young, director of Center for Online Addiction, 2004, www.netaddiction.com

items without an auctioneer. The Internet also provides the illusion of privacy, meaning that people feel more comfortable having open or explicit conversations that they might not have face to face.

- *It is exciting.* Placing the winning bet, watching stocks rise, winning a fantasy game, and making the highest bid all provide a rush of excitement that reinforces the behavior.

Psychologists and other treatment professionals report an increase in the number of clients who exhibit symptoms of Internet addiction and experience subsequent problems in their relationships, work, and other areas of their lives.[21] See the Assess Yourself box to analyze your Internet use.

Sexual Addiction

Everyone needs love and intimacy, but the sexual practices of people addicted to sex involve neither. In **sexual addiction,** people confuse the intensity of physical arousal with intimacy.[22] They do not feel nurtured by the person with whom they have sex but by the activity itself. Likewise, they are incapable of nurturing another because sex, not

> **Sexual addiction** Compulsive involvement in sexual activity.

the person, is the object of their affection. In fact, people with sexual addictions do not necessarily seek partners to obtain sexual arousal; they may be satisfied by masturbation, whether alone or during phone sex or while reading or watching erotica. They may participate in a wide range of sexual activities, including affairs, sex with strangers, prostitution, voyeurism, exhibitionism, cross-dressing, rape, incest, and pedophilia.

People addicted to sex frequently experience crushing episodes of depression and anxiety, fueled by the fear of discovery. Suicide is high among people who have problems with sexual control. The toll that these addictions exacts is most clearly seen in loss of intimacy with loved ones, which frequently leads to family disintegration.

No group of people is more or less likely than another to become involved in sexual addictions. They affect men and women of all ages, including married and single people, and people of any sexual preference. Most people with sexual addictions share a similar background: a dysfunctional childhood family, often characterized by chemical dependency or other addictions. Many were physically and emotionally abused. People addicted to sex tend to have a history of sexual abuse.

Multiple Addictions

Treatment centers for addiction often find that addicts depend on more than one chemical and/or behavior. Though they tend to have a drug of choice or a behavior of choice, one that they prefer because it is more effective at meeting their needs, as many as 60 percent of people in treatment have problems with more than one addiction. The figure may be as high as 75 percent for people addicted to chemicals. For example, alcohol addiction and eating disorders are commonly paired in women. Both chemically dependent women and men frequently resort to compulsive eating to keep themselves abstinent from drugs. One study showed

---

that 49 percent of compulsive gamblers are also alcoholics.[23] While multiple addictions certainly complicate recovery, they do not make it impossible. As with single addictions, recovery begins with the recognition that there is a problem.

How Addiction Affects Family and Friends

The family and friends of an addicted person also suffer many negative consequences. Often they struggle with **codependence,** a self-defeating relationship pattern in which a person is "addicted to the addict." It is the primary outcome of dysfunctional relationships or families.

Codependence is not accurately defined by isolated incidents, but rather by a pattern of behavior. Codependents find it hard to set healthy boundaries and often live in the chaotic, crisis-oriented mode that naturally occurs around addicts. They assume responsibility for meeting others' needs to the point that they subordinate or even cease being aware of their own needs. They may be unable to perceive their needs because they have repeatedly been taught that their needs are inappropriate or less important than someone else's. Their behavior goes far beyond performing kind services for another person. Codependents feel less than human if they fail to respond to the needs of someone else, even when their help was not requested. Although the term *codependent* is used less frequently today, treatment professionals still recognize the importance of helping addicts recognize how their behavior affects those around them and of working with family and friends to establish healthier relationships and boundaries.

Family and friends can play an important role in getting an addict to seek treatment. They are most helpful when they refuse to be enablers. **Enablers** are people who knowingly or unknowingly protect addicts from the natural consequences of their behavior. If they don't have to deal with the consequences, addicts cannot see the self-destructive nature of their behavior and will therefore continue it. Codependents are the primary enablers of their addicted loved ones, although anyone who has contact with an addict can be an enabler and thus contribute (perhaps powerfully) to continuation of the addictive behavior. Enablers are generally unaware that their behavior has this effect. In fact, enabling is rarely conscious and certainly not intentional.

> ### What do you think?
>
> *We have used a broad definition of the concept of addiction in this text. Do you think any behavior can be addictive?* ■ *Can one be a chocolate addict or a study addict?* ■ *What potential dangers lie in using the term addiction too loosely?*

Codependence   A self-defeating relationship pattern in which a person is "addicted to the addict."

Enablers   People who knowingly or unknowingly protect addicts from the natural consequences of their behavior.

> ### What do you think?
>
> *Why do we tend to protect others from the natural consequences of their destructive behaviors?* ■ *Have you ever confronted someone you were concerned about? If so, was the confrontation successful?* ■ *What tips would you give someone who wants to confront a loved one about an addiction?*

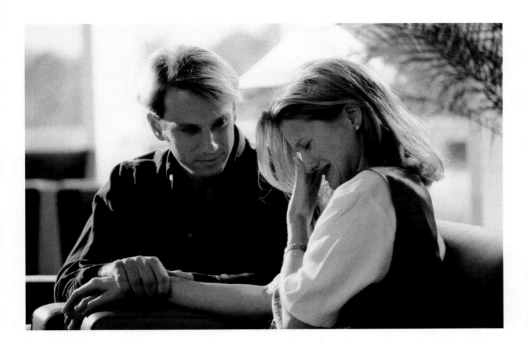

The process of acknowledging and overcoming an addiction is a long and difficult journey for everyone involved.

Treatment for and Recovery from Addiction

A key step in the recovery process is to recognize the addiction. This can be difficult because of the power of denial. Denial—the inability to see the truth—is the hallmark of addiction. It can be so powerful that intervention is sometimes necessary to break down the addict's denial system.

Intervention

Intervention is a planned process of confrontation by people who are important to the addict, including spouse, parents, children, boss, and friends. Its purpose is to break down the denial compassionately so that the addict can see the destructive nature of the addiction. It is not enough to get the person to admit that he or she is addicted. The addict must come to perceive that the addiction is destructive and requires treatment.

Individual confrontation is difficult and often futile. However, an addict's defenses generally crumble when significant others collectively share their observations and concerns about the addict's behavior. It is critical that those involved in the intervention clarify how they plan to end their enabling. For example, a wife may state that she will no longer cover bounced checks or make excuses for her money-addicted husband's antisocial behavior. She may even close their joint account and open a personal account so she will not be legally responsible for his irresponsible acts. All parties involved in the intervention must choose consequences they are ready to actually follow in the event

that the addict refuses treatment. Significant others must also be ready to give support if the addict is willing to begin a recovery program.

Components of effective intervention include the following:

- Emphasizing care and concern for the addicted person
- Describing the behavior that is the cause for concern
- Expressing how the behavior affects the addict, each person taking part in the intervention, and others
- Outlining specifically what you would like to see happen

Intervention is a serious step toward helping someone who probably does not want help. It should therefore be well planned and rehearsed. Most addiction treatment centers have specialists on staff who can help plan an intervention. In addition, books on the subject are available for families and friends who are concerned about someone who may be addicted. Once the problem has been recognized, recovery can begin.

Treatment

Treatment and recovery for any addiction generally begin with **abstinence**—refraining from the addictive behavior. While literal abstinence is possible for people addicted to chemicals, it obviously is not for people addicted to behaviors

> **Intervention** A planned process of confronting an addict; carried out by significant others.
>
> **Abstinence** Refraining from an addictive behavior.

like work and sex. For these addicts, abstinence means restoring balance to their lives through noncompulsive engagement in the behaviors, such as avoiding certain activities.

Detoxification refers to the early abstinence period during which an addict adjusts physically and cognitively to being free from the influence of the addiction. It occurs in virtually every recovering addict; and, whereas it is uncomfortable for them all, it can be dangerous for some. This is primarily true for those addicted to chemicals, especially alcohol, heroin, and painkillers such as OxyContin. For these people, early abstinence may involve profound withdrawal symptoms that require medical supervision. Therefore, most inpatient treatment programs provide a pretreatment component of supervised detoxification to achieve abstinence safely before treatment begins.

Abstinence alone does little to change the psychological, biological, and environmental dynamics that underlie the addictive behavior. Without recovery, an addict is apt to relapse time and again or simply to change addictions. Recovery involves learning new ways of looking at oneself, others, and the world. It may require exploring a traumatic past so that psychological wounds can be healed. It also involves learning interdependence with significant others and new ways of taking care of oneself, physically and emotionally—and it involves developing communication skills and new ways of having fun.

Recovery programs are the fuel that gives addicts the energy to resist relapsing. For a large number of addicts, recovery begins with a period of formal treatment. A good treatment program includes the following characteristics:

- Professional staff familiar with the specific addictive disorder for which help is being sought
- A flexible schedule of both inpatient and outpatient services
- Access to medical personnel who can assess the addict's health and treat all medical concerns as needed
- Medical supervision of addicts who are at high risk for a complicated detoxification
- Involvement of family members in the treatment process
- A team approach to treating addictive disorders (for example, medical personnel, counselors, psychotherapists, social workers, clergy, educators, dietitians, and fitness counselors)
- Both group and individual therapy options

Detoxification The early abstinence period during which an addict adjusts physically and cognitively to being free from the influences of the addiction.

- Peer-led support groups that encourage the addict to continue involvement after treatment ends
- Structured aftercare and relapse-prevention programs
- Accreditation by the Joint Commission on Accreditation of Healthcare Organizations (JCAHO) and a license from the state in which it operates

Most programs apply a combination of family, individual, and group counseling, supplemented with attendance at a 12-step support group. Individuals may also wish to explore alternatives to 12-step groups. Organizations such as Rational Recovery and the Secular Organization for Sobriety provide support without the spiritual emphasis of 12-step groups such as Alcoholics Anonymous.

Choosing a Treatment The National Institute on Alcohol Abuse and Alcoholism (NIAAA) completed Project MATCH (Matching Alcoholism Treatment to Client Heterogeneity), a large-scale study designed to determine if certain types of patients respond better to particular treatments.

The investigators studied three strategies: cognitive-behavior therapy, motivational psychology, and a facilitated 12-step program with sessions run by a therapist. Results showed that patients did equally well in each of the treatment approaches. This outcome was somewhat surprising, given that it has been common practice for treatment professionals to match patients to certain approaches. Researchers concluded that the focus, therefore, should simply be on selecting a competently run treatment program. Large-scale studies on other addictions have yet to occur.[24]

The Women's Health/Men's Health box describes factors that are important to address when treating female addicts.

Relapse

Relapse is an isolated occurrence of or full return to addictive behavior. It is one of the defining characteristics of addiction. A person who does not relapse or have powerful urges to do so was probably not addicted in the first place. Relapse is proof that a person is addicted and has abandoned the practice of an ongoing recovery program. Addicts are set up to relapse long before they actually do so because of their tendency to meet change and other forms of stress in their lives with the same kind of denial they once used to justify their addictive behavior (for example, "I don't have a problem, I can handle this"). This sets off a series of events involving immediate or gradual abandonment of structured recovery plans. For example, the addict may quit attending support group meetings and slip into situations that previously triggered the addictive behavior.

Addiction Treatment for Women: Still Confronting Barriers

The addiction treatment industry has been based on a male model and has only recently begun to address the unique needs of women. Studies support the need for greater prevention efforts targeted specifically at women at risk and gender-specific treatment for drug and alcohol dependence. Unfortunately, significant barriers remain for women seeking addiction treatment.

Although women entering treatment generally have fewer addiction-related legal problems (arrests for public intoxication or drug dealing, for example) than men do, they face more psychological issues and family, financial, and medical problems. Studies consistently indicate that the two primary barriers women face in successfully completing treatment are child care and transportation. One study found that women who were able to bring their children to inpatient treatment were more likely to remain healthy at six months after treatment. Additional barriers for women seeking addiction treatment include the following factors.

INDIVIDUAL

- Lack of insurance or inadequate coverage
- Fear of losing child custody
- Low self-esteem
- Low feelings of self-efficacy

FAMILY

- Too many responsibilities
- Lack of family support for treatment
- Abuse in the family environment

COMMUNITY

- Lack of support from employer
- Lack of gender-sensitive treatment options

A "women-friendly" treatment center should offer the following:

- Educational programs on self-worth, assertiveness, family issues, parenting, and anger management
- Women-only groups, especially for addressing issues of rape, incest, and abuse
- Networking with and support from other women in recovery
- Housing and day care

Clearly, many women have different treatment needs than men do. Finding a program that addresses these needs improves the likelihood of long-term success and recovery.

Sources: W. Weschberg, S. Craddock, and R. Hubbard, "How Are Women Who Enter Substance Abuse Treatment Different Than Men? A Gender Comparison from the Drug Abuse Treatment Outcome Study," In *Women and Substance Abuse: Gender Transparency,* eds. S. Stevens and H. Wexler (New York: Haworth, 1998); C. A Hernandez-Avila, B. J. Rounsaville, and H. R. Kranzler, "Opioid-, Cannabis-, and Alcohol-Dependent Women Show More Rapid Progression to Substance-Abuse Treatment," 74, no. 3 (2004): 265–272.

Because treatment programs recognize this strong tendency to relapse, they routinely teach clients and significant others concepts of relapse prevention. Relapse prevention teaches people to recognize the signs of imminent relapse and to develop a plan for responding to these signs. Without such a plan, recovering addicts are likely to relapse more frequently, more completely, and perhaps more permanently.

Relapse should not be interpreted as failure to change or lack of desire to stay well. The appropriate response to relapse is to remind addicts that they are addicted and to redirect them to the recovery strategies that have previously worked for them.

In addition to teaching skills, relapse prevention may involve aftercare planning such as connecting the recovering person with support groups, career counselors, or community services.

What do you think?

Why do you think people with addictions resist seeking treatment, even when they may admit they have a problem? ■ *What factors need to be considered in helping addicted individuals prevent relapse?*

TAKING CHARGE

MAKE IT HAPPEN!

Assessment: The Assess Yourself box on page 340 describes signs of Internet addiction. Depending on your results, you may need to take steps toward changing certain behaviors that may be detrimental to your health.

Making a Change: In order to change your behavior, you need to develop a plan. Follow these steps.

1. Evaluate your behavior, and identify patterns. What can you change now? What can you change in the near future?
2. Select one pattern of behavior that you want to change.
3. Fill out a Behavior Change Contract. It should include your long-term goal for change, your short-term goals, the rewards for reaching these goals, potential obstacles along the way, and strategies for overcoming these obstacles. For each goal, list the small steps and specific actions that you will take.
4. Chart your progress in a journal. At the end of a week, consider how successful you were in following your plan. What helped you be successful? What will you do differently next week?
5. Revise your plan as needed: Are the short-term goals attainable? Are the rewards satisfying?

One Student's Plan: Taylor is a freshman living on campus. He came to school from out of state and has not really developed a close group of friends or even met many of the students living in his dorm. He does not have a roommate, which he likes because it allows him to do whatever he wishes when he wishes. However, Taylor was surprised to score 90 points on the Internet addiction self-assessment. He had been spending many hours online and in chat rooms but had never realized how much time out of his day and nights it was consuming. Taylor also admitted that rather than study or socialize with other students he preferred being online. His grades and social life had deteriorated from his high school days, however, and he decided one cure was to spend less time on the Internet.

Taylor decided to develop a plan to cut back on his Internet use and to give himself some rewards for staying offline He also decided to anticipate and write down some times that might make it difficult to stay off the Internet (when he was feeling lonely, for example) and some strategies for those situations (meeting other students on the hall or going to a location away from his computer to study). Taylor also decided to keep a log of the time he was on the computer and set a daily time limit. He would also record when he went over the time limit and consider how to avoid the situation the next time. Over time, Taylor spent much less time online and developed friendships with other students living in his dorm.

Summary

- Addiction is the continued involvement with a substance or activity despite ongoing negative consequences.
- Habits are repeated behaviors whereas addiction is behavior resulting from compulsion; without the behavior, the addict experiences withdrawal. All addictions share four common symptoms: compulsion, loss of control, negative consequences, and denial.
- Addiction is a process, evolving over time through a pattern known as nurturing through avoidance. Mood-altering substances and experiences produce biochemical reactions that make the body feel good; when absent, the person feels a withdrawal effect. The biopsychosocial model of addiction takes into account biological (genetic) factors as well as psychological and environmental influences in understanding the addiction process.
- Addictions include money addictions (compulsive gambling, spending, and borrowing), work addiction, exercise addiction, sexual addiction, Internet addiction, and codependence. Codependents are "addicted to the addict." These behaviors are all addictive because they are mood-altering.
- Treatment begins with abstinence from the addictive behavior or substance, usually instituted through intervention by significant others. Treatment programs may include individual, group, or family therapy, as well as 12-step programs.

Questions for Discussion and Reflection

1. What factors distinguish a habit from an addiction? Is it possible for you to tell whether someone else is really addicted?
2. Explain why the biopsychosocial model of addiction is a more effective model for treatment than a single-factor model.
3. Explain the potential genetic, environmental, and psychological risk factors for addiction.
4. Discuss how addiction affects family and friends. What role do family and friends play in helping the addict get help and maintain recovery?
5. What are some key components of an effective treatment program? Do the components vary for men and women? Why or why not?

Accessing Your Health on the Internet

Visit the following Internet sites to explore further topics and issues related to various forms of addiction and treatment. Many offer self-assessment profiles designed to give you more information about your own health practices. To visit an organization's website, go to the Companion Website for *Access to Health, Ninth Edition* at www.aw-bc.com/donatelle, click on the book image, and select "Accessing Your Health on the Internet" from the navigation menu.

1. **Behavioral Health Online.** A comprehensive addiction site with information on Internet, gambling, eating, and other addiction issues. Includes news briefs, features, and Ask an Expert.
2. **Center for Online Addiction.** Information and assistance for those dealing with Internet addiction.
3. **The Wager.** A weekly research report on compulsive gambling. Summarizes current research and resources pertaining to gambling.
4. **Web of Addiction.** A comprehensive listing of various resources related to self-help, treatment, and policy.

Further Reading

Elster, J. (ed.). *Addiction: Entries and Exits.* New York: Russell Sage Foundation, 2000.

Addresses current addiction controversies from an international perspective, with authors from the United States and Norway. Topics include whether addicts have a choice in their behavior and current addiction theories.

Hurley, J. (ed.). *Addiction: Opposing Viewpoints.* San Diego: Greenhaven Press, 2000.

Part of the Opposing Viewpoints series; addresses addiction theories, treatment approaches, and risk factors, among other topics.

Nakken, C. *The Addictive Personality.* Center City, MN: Hazelden, 1996.

A very down-to-earth overview of addiction, including non-substance addictions.

Peele, S. *The Meaning of Addiction: An Unconventional View.* San Francisco: Jossey-Bass, 1998.

One of the leading critics of the disease-view of addictions provides an alternative model of addiction.

Stevens, S. and H. Wexler (eds.). *Women and Substance Abuse: Gender Transparency.* New York: Haworth, 1998.

A collection of the most current research pertaining to women and substance abuse.

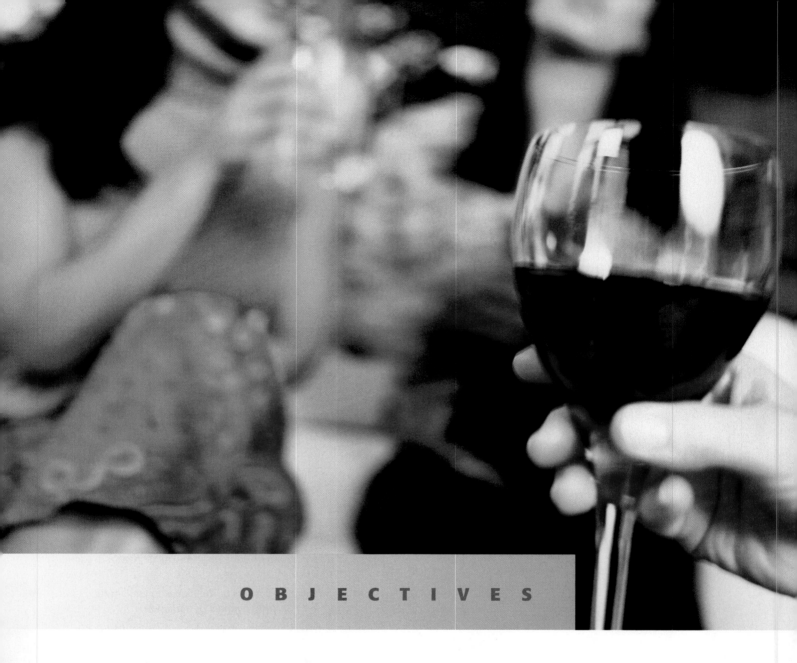

OBJECTIVES

- Summarize the alcohol use patterns of college students, and discuss overall trends in consumption.

- Explain the physiological and behavioral effects of alcohol, including blood alcohol concentration, absorption, metabolism, and immediate and long-term effects of alcohol consumption.

- Explain the symptoms and causes of alcoholism, its cost to society, and its effects on the family.

- Explain the treatment of alcoholism, including the family's role, varied treatment methods, and whether or not alcoholics can be cured.

12

DRINKING RESPONSIBLY

A LIFESTYLE CHALLENGE ON CAMPUS

Drinking Deaths Draw Attention to Old Campus Problem

By Mindy Sink

Lynn G. Bailey, 18, a freshman at the University of Colorado here, spent his last night chugging whiskey and wine as part of an initiation ceremony with his fraternity brothers. Left by his friends to sleep it off, he died from alcohol poisoning.

Less than two weeks earlier and an hour's drive away, Samantha Spady, 19, a sophomore at Colorado State University in Fort Collins, died of alcohol poisoning after an evening out with friends in which she drank the equivalent of 30 to 40 beers and shots.

In the aftermath of these deaths this fall, university officials and community leaders are joining forces, rather than pointing fingers, and are looking at how they can take responsibility together to prevent alcohol abuse.

"It was the straw that broke the camel's back," said a Boulder city councilman and the deputy mayor, Tom Eldridge, of the back-to-back deaths and years of tension built up in neighborhoods adjacent to the campus.

Read the complete article online in the eThemes section of this book's website: www.aw-bc.com/donatelle.

Original article published November 9, 2004. Copyright © 2004 *The New York Times.* Reprinted with permission.

The consumption of alcoholic beverages is interwoven with many traditions. Moderate use of alcohol can enhance celebrations or special times. Research shows that very low levels of drinking may actually lower some health risks. We may also consume alcohol to help ease the pain caused by rejection or loss. We are certainly not unique in this regard; people all over the world and throughout history have used alcohol for everything from social gatherings to religious ceremonies.

However, always remember that alcohol is a chemical substance that affects your physical and mental behavior. The fact is, alcohol is a drug, and if it is not used responsibly, it can become dangerous. In this chapter we will discuss the composition of alcohol and its effects on the body. We will also look at the hallmarks of responsible consumption, signs of alcohol dependency, and the health risks of irresponsible use.

Alcohol: An Overview

An estimated 65 percent of Americans consume alcoholic beverages regularly, though consumption patterns are unevenly distributed throughout the drinking population. Ten percent are heavy drinkers, and they account for half of all the alcohol consumed. The remaining 90 percent of the drinking population are infrequent, light, or moderate drinkers.

Alcohol and College Students

Alcohol is the most widely used (and abused) recreational drug in our society. It is also the most popular drug on college campuses, where approximately 83 percent of students consume alcoholic beverages.[1] About one-third of college students are classified as heavy drinkers, meaning that they consume large amounts of alcohol per drinking occasion. Therefore, students who might go out and drink only once a week are considered heavy drinkers if they consume a great deal of alcohol. In a new trend on college campuses, women's consumption of alcohol is close to equaling men's.

Colleges and universities have been described as "alcohol-drenched institutions." Every year, America's 12 million undergraduates drink 4 billion cans of beer, averaging 55 six-packs apiece, and spend $446 each on alcoholic beverages—more than they spend on soft drinks and textbooks combined.[2] Despite these figures, fewer students are drinking alcohol than in the past. In 1980, 9.5 percent of students nationwide said they abstained from alcohol; in 2001, 19 percent were abstainers.[3] (Exactly how much does a typical college student consume? See the Reality Check box.) According to the University of Michigan's Institute for Social Research, the percentage of students who report drinking daily also has declined, from 6.5 percent in 1980 to 5 percent in 2003.[4]

College is a critical time to become aware of and responsible for drinking. There is little doubt that drinking is a part of campus culture and tradition. Many students are away from home, often for the first time, and are excited by their newfound independence. For some students, this independence and the rite of passage into the college culture are symbolized by the use of alcohol. It provides the answer to one of the most commonly heard statements on any college campus: "There is nothing to do." Additionally, many students say they drink to have fun. Having fun, which often means drinking simply to get drunk, may really be a way of coping with stress, boredom, anxiety, or pressures created by academic and social demands.

Statistics about college students' drinking may not always reflect actual consumption. Students consistently report that their friends drink much more than they do and that average drinking within their own social living group is higher than actual self-reports. Such misinformation may promote or be used to excuse excessive drinking practices. In a survey of students at a large midwestern university, 42 percent reported not having a hangover in the past six months. Yet that same group of surveyed students believed that only 3 percent of their peers had not had a hangover in the past month.

Many colleges are working to change misperceptions of normal drinking behavior. An example of such a "social norms" campaign is Oregon State University's Just the Facts program, which publicizes the fact that the majority of the

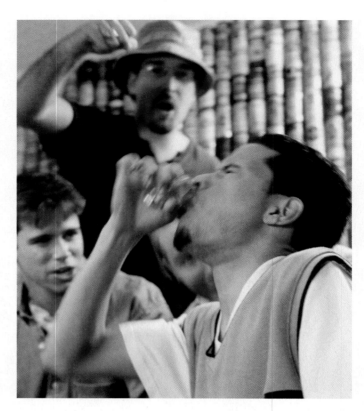

Deciding when to drink, and how much, is no small matter. Irresponsible consumption of alcohol can easily result in disaster.

The Facts about College Students and Drinking

Perhaps you've heard conflicting reports in the media about the prevalence and effects of drinking on campus. What are the facts? The following statistics reveal the scope of the problem.

✔ Alcohol kills more people below age 21 than cocaine, marijuana, and heroin combined.

✔ Half a million students between ages 15 and 24 are unintentionally injured each year while intoxicated.

✔ One night of heavy drinking can impair the ability to think abstractly for up to 30 days, limiting a student's ability to understand a professor's lecture or to think through a football play.

✔ College administrators estimate that alcohol is involved with 29 percent of dropouts, 38 percent of academic failures, and 64 percent of violent behaviors.

✔ Over the past decade, there has been a threefold increase in the number of college women who report having been drunk on ten or more occasions in the previous month.

✔ Areas of a college campus offering cheap beer prices have more crime, including trouble between students and police or other campus authorities, arguments, physical fighting, property damage, false fire alarms, and sexual misconduct.

✔ Alcohol is involved in more than two-thirds of suicides among college students, 90 percent of campus rapes and sexual assaults, and 95 percent of violent crime on campus.

✔ Seventy-five percent of male students and 55 percent of female students involved in acquaintance rape had been drinking or using drugs at the time.

✔ The likelihood that a woman will be raped is far greater on campuses with a high rate of binge drinking.

✔ Each year, more than 100,000 students between the ages of 18 and 24 report having been too intoxicated to know if they consented to having sex.

✔ College binge drinking occurs more often among male students, students who reside on campus, intercollegiate athletes, and members of fraternities and sororities. Approximately 40 percent of fraternity and sorority members report being frequent binge drinkers, and college athletes are 50

percent more like to binge drink than nonathletes.

✔ Rates of binge drinking among high-risk students (younger, white males) are lower on more diverse college campuses. When high-risk students are together to the exclusion of other groups, there are fewer role models for lighter or nondrinking behavior.

✔ College students under the age of 21 are more prone to binge drinking and pay less for their alcohol than their older classmates do. Though underage students drink less often, they consume more per occasion than students age 21 and older who are allowed to drink legally.

Source: Data were compiled from the numerous studies cited throughout this chapter and from M. Mohler-Kuo, et al., "College Rapes Linked to Binge-Drinking Rates," *Journal of Studies on Alcohol* 65, no. 1 (2004); H. Weschler, "Watering Down the Drinks: The Moderating Effect of College Demographics on Alcohol Use in High Risk Groups," *American Journal of Public Health* 93, no. 11 (2003): 1929–1933; T. F. Nelson, et al., "Alcohol and Collegiate Sports Fans," *Addictive Behaviors* 28, no. 1 (2003): 1–11; R. W. Hingson et al., "Magnitude of Alcohol-Related Mortality and Morbidity among U.S. College Students Aged 18–24," *Journal of Studies on Alcohol* 63, no. 2 (2002): 136–144.

university's students are responsible and moderate drinkers. Students are often surprised to learn that 87 percent of their peers have never driven a car while under the influence of alcohol, and 89 percent have never passed out from drinking. Almost 90 percent have never performed poorly on a test or important project due to their alcohol use, and 77 percent have never missed a class because of drinking. Approximately 75 percent consume only zero to four drinks per week, and 60 percent had four or fewer drinks the last time they went to a party. Clearly there are many students who use alcohol responsibly and in moderation.

Binge Drinking and College Students

There are, however, some students who indulge in heavy episodic, or **binge, drinking.** This is defined as having five drinks in a row for men or four in a row for women on a

single occasion. The stakes of binge drinking are high because of the increased risk for alcohol-related injuries and death. An estimated 50 students die each year from alcohol poisoning. In one month, five college students died in alcohol-related accidents in the state of Virginia alone.

A 2001 study by the Harvard School of Public Health found that 44.8 percent of students were binge drinkers, and, of those, 22.8 percent were frequent bingers (people who binge drink three times or more in a two-week period).[5]

Binge drinking Drinking for the express purpose of becoming intoxicated; five drinks in a single sitting for men and four drinks in a sitting for women.

Table 12.1
The Frequency and Effects of Binge-Drinking among College Students

College Students' Patterns of Alcohol Use, 2001

Category	Total (%)	Men (%)	Women (%)
Abstainer (past year)	19.3	20.1	18.7
Nonbinge drinker	36.3	31.3	40.4
Occasional binge drinker	21.6	23.4	20.0
Frequent binge drinker	22.8	25.2	20.9

Alcohol-Related Problems among Students in Different Binge-Drinking Categories

Problem Reported	Nonbinge Drinkers (%)	Frequent Binge Drinkers (%)
Did something regrettable	18	62
Missed a class	9	63
Forgot where they were or what they did	10	54
Got behind in schoolwork	10	46
Argued with friends	10	43
Got hurt or injured	4	27
Damaged property	2	23
Engaged in unplanned sexual activities	8	42
Drove after drinking	19	57

Secondhand Effects of Binge Drinking

Secondary Effect	Percentage
Experienced unwanted sexual advances	19.5
Had your studying/sleeping interrupted	60
Had to take care of a drunken fellow student	48
Been insulted or humiliated	29

Sources: H. Wechsler, et al., "Trends in College Binge Drinking during a Period of Increased Prevention Efforts: Findings from Four Harvard School of Public Health College Study Surveys: 1993–2001," *Journal of American College Health* 50, no. 5 (2002): 207. H. Wechsler, et al., "College Binge Drinking in the 1990s: A Continuing Problem," *Journal of American College Health* 48 (2002): 207. Reprinted with permission of Helen Dwight Reid Educational Foundation. Published by Heldref Publications, 1319 18th St NW, Washington, D.C. 20036. Copyright 2002.

(See Table 12.1.) Compared with nonbingers, frequent binge drinkers are 16 times more likely to miss class, 8 times more likely to get behind in their school work, and more apt to get into trouble with campus or local police.[6] Unfortunately, recent studies confirm what students have been experiencing for a long time—binge drinkers cause problems not only for themselves, but also for those around them.

Although everyone is at some risk for alcohol-related problems, college students seem to be particularly vulnerable for the following reasons:

- Alcohol exacerbates their already high risk for suicide, automobile crashes, and falls.
- Many college and university customs, norms, traditions, and mores encourage certain dangerous practices and patterns of alcohol use.
- University campuses are heavily targeted by advertising and promotions from the alcoholic beverage industry.
- It is more common for college students than their noncollegiate peers to drink recklessly and to engage in drinking games and other dangerous drinking practices.

- College students are particularly vulnerable to peer influence and have a strong need to be accepted by their peers.
- There is institutional denial by college administrators that alcohol problems exist on their campuses.

A recent study shows that 6 percent of college students meet the criteria for a diagnosis of alcohol dependence (also referred to as alcoholism), and 31 percent meet the criteria for alcohol abuse. Students who attend colleges with heavy drinking environments are more likely to be diagnosed with abuse or dependence. Those students at most risk are the frequent bingers, and male students are generally at greater risk than females. Nearly one in 10 college men under age 24 meet the criteria for alcohol dependence, compared to one in 20 college women. Despite the prevalence of alcohol disorders on campus, very few students seek treatment.[7]

To prevent alcohol abuse, many colleges and universities are instituting strong policies against drinking. University presidents have formed a leadership group to help curb the problem of alcohol abuse. Many fraternities have elected to

Should Colleges Call Parents without Student Consent?

Students' right to privacy versus parents' right to know is at the heart of a debate over a federal law that allows school administrators to disclose a student's academic or probationary record to parents without the student's consent. In 1999, Congress amended the Family Educational Rights and Privacy Act of 1974 as a means of reducing drug and alcohol abuse on college campuses. The revised law gives universities the option of telling a student's parents about underage drinking and illicit drug violations. Some college officials are taking a wait-and-see approach whereas others are embracing the law, saying it gives them a chance to respond to early warning signs to curb alcohol and drug abuse on campus.

What is your campus's policy on parental notification? What are some of the issues surrounding this amendment? Do you think this is a good idea? Explain your answer.

---

have dry houses. At the same time, colleges and universities are making more help available to students with drinking problems. Today, both individual and group counseling are offered on most campuses, and more attention is being directed toward the prevention of alcohol abuse. Student organizations such as BACCHUS (Boost Alcohol Consciousness Concerning the Health of University Students) promote responsible drinking and party hosting. See the Health Ethics box on another aspect of colleges' response to alcohol.

Trends in Consumption

In general, alcohol consumption levels among Americans have declined steadily since the late 1970s. In 2000, the estimated per capita consumption was the equivalent of 2.2 gallons of pure alcohol per person.[8] This represents a substantial decline from 2.64 gallons in 1977. (This measure indicates the amount of alcohol that a person would obtain by drinking approximately 50 gallons of beer, 20 gallons of wine, or more than 4 gallons of distilled spirits.)

This downward trend has been tied to a growing attention to weight, personal health, and physical activity. The alcohol industry has responded by introducing beer and wines with fewer calories and carbohydrates and with reduced alcohol content.

Physiological and Behavioral Effects of Alcohol

The Chemical Makeup of Alcohol

The intoxicating substance found in beer, wine, liquor, and liqueurs is **ethyl alcohol,** or **ethanol.** It is produced during a process called **fermentation,** whereby yeast organisms break down plant sugars, yielding ethanol and carbon dioxide. Fermentation continues until the solution of plant sugars (called mash) reaches a concentration of 14 percent alcohol. At this point, the alcohol kills the yeast and halts the chemical reactions that produce it.

For beers and ales, which are fermented from malt barley, manufacturers then add other ingredients that dilute the alcohol content of the beverage. Other alcoholic beverages are produced through further processing called **distillation,** during which alcohol vapors are released from the mash at high temperatures. The vapors are then condensed and mixed with water to make the final product.

The **proof** of an alcoholic drink is a measure of the percentage of alcohol in the beverage. "Proof" comes from "gunpowder proof," a reference to the gunpowder test, whereby

---

What do you think?

Why do some college students drink excessive amounts of alcohol? ■ *Are there particular traditions or norms related to when and why students drink on your campus?* ■ *Have you ever had your sleep or studies interrupted or have you had to baby-sit a roommate or friend because he or she had been drinking?* ■ *Did you say anything about it to your friend or roommate?* ■ *How did the person respond?*

Ethyl alcohol (ethanol)   An addictive drug produced by fermentation and found in many beverages.

Fermentation   The process whereby yeast organisms break down plant sugars to yield ethanol.

Distillation   The process whereby mash is subjected to high temperatures to release alcohol vapors, which are then condensed and mixed with water to make the final product.

Proof   A measure of the percentage of alcohol in a beverage.

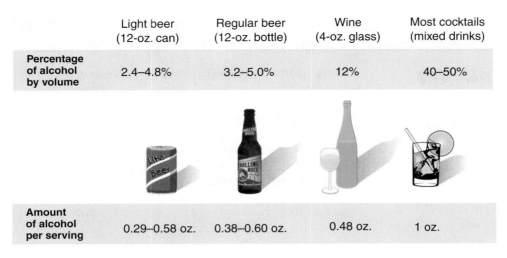

	Light beer (12-oz. can)	Regular beer (12-oz. bottle)	Wine (4-oz. glass)	Most cocktails (mixed drinks)
Percentage of alcohol by volume	2.4–4.8%	3.2–5.0%	12%	40–50%
Amount of alcohol per serving	0.29–0.58 oz.	0.38–0.60 oz.	0.48 oz.	1 oz.

Figure 12.1
Alcoholic Beverages and Their Alcohol Equivalencies

potential buyers would test the distiller's product by pouring it on gunpowder and attempting to light it. If the alcohol content was at least 50 percent, the gunpowder would burn; otherwise the water in the product would put out the flame. Thus, alcohol percentage is 50 percent of the given proof. For example, 80 proof whiskey or scotch is 40 percent alcohol by volume, and 100 proof vodka is 50 percent alcohol by volume. The proof of a beverage indicates its strength. Lower-proof drinks will produce fewer alcoholic effects than the same amount of higher-proof drinks.

Most wines are between 12 and 15 percent alcohol, and ales are between 6 and 8 percent. The alcoholic content of beers is between 2 and 6 percent, varying according to state laws and type of beer (Figure 12.1).

Behavioral Effects

Blood alcohol concentration (BAC) is the ratio of alcohol to total blood volume. It is the factor used to measure the physiological and behavioral effects of alcohol. Despite individual differences, alcohol produces some general behavioral effects depending on BAC (Table 12.2). At a BAC of 0.02, a person feels slightly relaxed and in a good mood. At 0.05, relaxation increases, there is some motor impairment, and a willingness to talk becomes apparent. At 0.08, the person feels euphoric, and there is further motor impairment. At 0.10, the depressant effects of alcohol become apparent, drowsiness sets in, and motor skills are further impaired, followed by a

> **Blood alcohol concentration (BAC)** The ratio of alcohol to total blood volume; the factor used to measure the physiological and behavioral effects of alcohol.
>
> **Learned behavioral tolerance** The ability of heavy drinkers to modify behavior so that they appear to be sober even when they have high BAC levels.

loss of judgment. Thus, a driver may not be able to estimate distance or speed, and some drinkers lose their ability to make value-related decisions and may do things they would not do when sober. As BAC increases, the drinker suffers increased physiological and psychological effects. All these changes are negative. Alcohol ingestion does not enhance any physical skills or mental functions.

People can acquire physical and psychological tolerance to the effects of alcohol through regular use. The nervous system adapts over time, so greater amounts of alcohol are required to produce the same physiological and psychological effects. Some people can learn to modify their behavior so that they appear to be sober even when their BAC is quite high. This ability is called **learned behavioral tolerance.**

Absorption and Metabolism

Unlike the molecules found in most other ingestible foods and drugs, alcohol molecules are sufficiently small and fat-soluble to be absorbed throughout the entire gastrointestinal system. A negligible amount of alcohol is absorbed through the lining of the mouth. Approximately 20 percent of ingested alcohol diffuses through the stomach lining into the bloodstream, and nearly 80 percent passes through the linings of the upper third of the small intestine. Absorption into the bloodstream is rapid and complete.

Several factors influence how quickly your body will absorb alcohol: the alcohol concentration in your drink, the amount of alcohol you consume, the amount of food in your stomach, pylorospasm (spasm of the pyloric valve in the digestive system), your metabolism, weight and body mass index, and your mood. The higher the concentration of alcohol in your drink, the more rapidly it will be absorbed in your digestive tract. As a rule, wine and beer are absorbed more slowly than distilled beverages. Carbonated alcoholic beverages—such as champagne and carbonated wines—are absorbed more rapidly than those containing no sparkling

Table 12.2
Psychological and Physical Effects of Various Blood-Alcohol Concentration Levels*

Number of Drinks[†]	Blood Alcohol Concentration (%)	Psychological and Physical Effects
1	0.02–0.03	No overt effects, slight mood elevation
2	0.05–0.06	Feeling of relaxation, warmth; slight decrease in reaction time and in fine-muscle coordination
3	0.08–0.09	Balance, speech, vision, and hearing slightly impaired; feelings of euphoria, increased confidence; loss of motor coordination
	0.10	Legal intoxication in most states; some have lower limits
4	0.11–0.12	Coordination and balance becoming difficult; distinct impairment of mental faculties, judgment
5	0.14–0.15	Major impairment of mental and physical control; slurred speech, blurred vision, lack of motor skills
7	0.20	Loss of motor control—must have assistance in moving about; mental confusion
10	0.30	Severe intoxication; minimal conscious control of mind and body
14	0.40	Unconsciousness, threshold of coma
17	0.50	Deep coma
20	0.60	Death from respiratory failure

*For each hour elapsed since the last drink, subtract 0.015 percent blood alcohol concentration, or approximately one drink.
†One drink = one beer (4 percent alcohol, 12 ounces), one highball (1 ounce whiskey), or one glass table wine (5 ounces).
Source: Modified from data given in Ohio State Police Driver Information Seminars and the National Clearinghouse for Alcohol and Alcoholism Information, Rockville, MD.

additives, or fizz. Carbonated beverages and drinks served with mixers cause the pyloric valve—the opening from the stomach into the small intestine—to relax, thereby emptying the contents of the stomach more rapidly into the small intestine. Since the small intestine is the site of the greatest absorption of alcohol, carbonated beverages increase the rate of absorption. On the other hand, if your stomach is full, absorption slows because the surface area exposed to alcohol is smaller. A full stomach also retards the emptying of alcoholic beverages into the small intestine.

In addition, the more alcohol you consume, the longer absorption takes. Alcohol can irritate the digestive system, causing a spasm in the pyloric valve (pylorospasm). When the pyloric valve is closed, nothing can move from the stomach to the upper third of the small intestine, which slows absorption. If the irritation continues, it can cause vomiting.

Mood is another factor, since emotions affect how long it takes for the contents of the stomach to empty into the intestine. Powerful moods, such as stress and tension, are likely to cause the stomach to dump its contents into the small intestine. That is why alcohol is absorbed much more rapidly when people are tense than when they are relaxed.

Alcohol is metabolized in the liver, where it is converted by the enzyme alcohol dehydrogenase to acetaldehyde. It is then rapidly oxidized to acetate, converted to carbon dioxide and water, and eventually excreted from the body. Acetaldehyde is a toxic chemical that can cause immediate symptoms

such as nausea and vomiting, as well as long-term effects such as liver damage. A very small portion of alcohol is excreted unchanged by the kidneys, lungs, and skin.

Like food, alcohol contains calories. Proteins and carbohydrates (starches and sugars) each contain 4 kilocalories (kcal) per gram. Fat contains 9 kcal per gram. Alcohol, although similar in structure to carbohydrates, contains 7 kcal per gram. The body uses the calories in alcohol in the same manner it uses those found in carbohydrates: for immediate energy or for storage as fat if not immediately needed.

When compared to the variable breakdown rates of foods and other beverages, the breakdown of alcohol occurs at a fairly constant rate of 0.5 ounce per hour. This amount of alcohol is equivalent to 12 ounces of 5 percent beer, 8 ounces of malt liquor, 4 ounces of 12 percent wine, or 1.5 ounces of 40 percent (80 proof) liquor. Legal limits of BAC for operating motor vehicles vary from state to state. Most states set the legal limit at 0.08 to 0.10 percent. A driver whose level of BAC exceeds the state's legal limit is considered legally intoxicated.

A drinker's BAC depends on weight and body fat, the water content in body tissues, the concentration of alcohol in the beverage consumed, the rate of consumption, and the volume of alcohol consumed. Heavier people have larger body surfaces through which to diffuse alcohol; therefore, they have lower concentrations of alcohol in their blood than do thin people after drinking the same amount. Since alcohol does not diffuse as rapidly into body fat as into water, the BAC is higher in a person with more body fat. Because a woman is likely to have more body fat and less water in her body tissues than a man of the same weight, she will be more intoxicated than a man after drinking the same amount of alcohol.

Alcohol Poisoning Alcohol poisoning occurs much more frequently than people realize, and all too often it can be fatal. Drinking large amounts of alcohol in a short period of time can cause the blood alcohol level to reach the lethal range relatively quickly. Alcohol, used either alone or in combination with other drugs, is probably responsible for more toxic overdose deaths than any other substance.

Death from alcohol poisoning can be caused by either central nervous system and respiratory depression or the inhalation of vomit or fluid into the lungs. The amount of alcohol it takes for a person to become unconscious is dangerously close to the lethal dose. Signs of alcohol poisoning include the following: being unable to be aroused; a weak, rapid pulse; an unusual or irregular breathing pattern; and cool (possibly damp), pale, or bluish skin. If you are with someone who has been drinking heavily and who exhibits these conditions, or if you are unsure about the person's condition, call 911 for emergency help right away.

What do you think?

Have you noticed that some types of alcoholic beverages affect people more quickly than others? ■ *What factors affect BAC levels?* ■ *Are these factors different for men and women? If so, how?*

Women and Alcohol Body fat is not the only contributor to the differences in alcohol's effects on men and women. Compared to men, women appear to have half as much alcohol hydrogenase, the enzyme that breaks down alcohol in the stomach before it has a chance to get to the bloodstream and the brain. Therefore, if a man and a woman drink the same amount of alcohol, the woman's BAC will be approximately 30 percent higher than the man's, leaving her more vulnerable to slurred speech, dangerous driving, and other drinking-related impairments.

Hormonal differences can also affect a woman's BAC. Specifically, one week prior to menstruating, women maintain the peak level of intoxication for longer periods of time than menstruating or postmenstruating women do. Women

---

Dehydration Loss of fluids from body tissues.

Cerebrospinal fluid Fluid within and surrounding the brain and spinal cord tissues.

---

who are using oral contraceptives are also likely to maintain peak intoxication for longer periods of time than they would otherwise. This prolonged peak appears to be related to estrogen levels.

Women who consume alcohol need to pay close attention to how much they consume. It is possible that a woman matching her male friend drink per drink could become twice as intoxicated. For example, if a 180-pound college-age man and a 120-pound college-age woman each have three drinks, the BAC for the male would be 0.06 and for the female 0.11, almost double that of her male friend. Table 12.3 compares blood alcohol levels by sex, weight, and consumption. Although this table can provide an estimate of probable BAC levels, many additional factors may cause considerable variation in these rates.

Breathalyzer and Other Tests The Breathalyzer tests used by law enforcement officers determine BAC based on the amount of alcohol exhaled in the breath. Urinalysis can also yield a BAC based on the concentration of unmetabolized alcohol in the urine. Both breath analysis and urinalysis are used to determine whether a driver is legally intoxicated, but blood tests are more accurate measures. An increasing number of states are requiring blood tests for people suspected of driving under the influence of alcohol. In some states, refusal to take the breath or urine test results in immediate revocation of the person's driver's license.

Immediate Effects

The most dramatic effects produced by ethanol occur within the central nervous system (CNS). The primary action of the drug is to reduce the frequency of nerve transmissions and impulses at synaptic junctions. This depresses CNS functions, with resulting decreases in respiratory rate, pulse rate, and blood pressure. As CNS depression deepens, vital functions become noticeably depressed. In extreme cases, coma and death can result.

Alcohol is a diuretic, causing increased urinary output. Although this effect might be expected to lead to automatic **dehydration** (loss of water from body tissues), the body actually retains water, most of it in the muscles or in cerebral tissues. This is because water is usually pulled out of the **cerebrospinal fluid** (fluid within the brain and spinal cord), leading to what is known as mitochondrial dehydration at the cellular level within the nervous system. Mitochondria are miniature organs within cells that are responsible for specific functions, and they rely heavily upon fluid balance. When mitochondrial dehydration occurs from drinking, the mitochondria cannot carry out their normal functions, resulting in symptoms that include the "morning-after" headaches suffered by some drinkers.

Alcohol irritates the gastrointestinal system and may cause indigestion and heartburn if taken on an empty stomach. Long-term consumption causes repeated irritation that has been linked to cancers of the esophagus and stomach. In

Table 12.3
Calculation of Estimated Blood Alcohol Concentration for Women and Men

Drinks*	90	100	120	140	160	180	200	220	240	
Women										
0	.00	.00	.00	.00	.00	.00	.00	.00	.00	Only safe driving limit
1	**.05**	**.05**	**.04**	.03	.03	.03	.02	.02	.02	Impairment begins
2	.10	.09	.08	**.07**	**.06**	.05	.05	.04	.04	**Driving skills**
3	.15	.14	.11	.10	**.09**	**.08**	.07	.06	.06	**significantly affected**
4	.20	.18	.15	.13	.11	.10	.09	**.08**	**.08**	**Possible criminal**
5	.25	.23	.19	.16	.14	.13	.11	.10	**.09**	**penalties**
6	.30	.27	.23	.19	.17	.15	.14	.12	.11	
7	.35	.32	.27	.23	.20	.18	.16	.14	.13	Legally intoxicated
8	.40	.36	.30	.26	.23	.20	.18	.17	.15	
9	.45	.41	.34	.29	.26	.23	.20	.19	.17	Criminal penalties
10	.51	.45	.38	.32	.28	.25	.23	.21	.19	
Men										
0		.00	.00	.00	.00	.00	.00	.00	.00	Only safe driving limit
1		**.04**	.03	.03	.02	.02	.02	.02	.02	Impairment begins
2		**.08**	**.06**	**.05**	**.05**	**.04**	**.04**	.03	.03	**Driving skills**
3		.11	**.09**	**.08**	**.07**	**.06**	**.06**	.05	.05	**significantly affected**
4		.15	.12	.11	**.09**	**.08**	**.08**	.07	.06	
5		.19	.16	.13	.12	.11	.09	**.09**	**.08**	**Possible criminal**
6		.23	.19	.16	.14	.13	.11	.10	**.09**	**penalties**
7		.26	.22	.19	.16	.15	.13	.12	.11	Legally intoxicated
8		.30	.25	.21	.19	.17	.15	.14	.13	
9		.34	.28	.24	.21	.19	.17	.15	.14	Criminal penalties
10		.38	.31	.27	.23	.21	.19	.17	.16	

Note: Blood alcohol percentages above bold values indicate beginning impairment; all percentages below bold values indicate legal intoxication with criminal penalty.

Subtract 0.01% for each 40 minutes elapsed since drinking.

*One drink is 1.25 oz. of 80-proof liquor, 12 oz. of beer, or 4 oz. of table wine.

Source: Data supplied by the Pennsylvania Liquor Control Board.

addition, people who engage in brief drinking sprees during which they consume unusually high amounts of alcohol put themselves at risk for irregular heartbeat or even total loss of heart rhythm, which can disrupt blood flow and damage the heart muscle.

A **hangover** is often experienced the morning after a drinking spree. The symptoms of a hangover are familiar to most people who drink: headache, muscle aches, upset stomach, anxiety, depression, diarrhea, and thirst. **Congeners** are thought to play a role in the development of a hangover. Congeners are forms of alcohol that are metabolized more slowly than ethanol and are more toxic. The body metabolizes the congeners after the ethanol is gone from the system, and their toxic by-products may contribute to the hangover. Alcohol also upsets water balance in the body, resulting in excess urination and thirst the next day. Increased production of hydrochloric acid can irritate the stomach lining and cause nausea. It usually takes 12 hours to recover from a hangover. Bed rest, solid food, and aspirin may help relieve its discomforts, but nothing cures it but time.

Drug Interactions When you use any drug (and alcohol is a drug), you need to be aware of its possible interactions with other drugs, whether prescription or over-the-counter. Table 12.4 on page 358 summarizes possible interactions. Note that alcohol may cause a negative interaction even with aspirin.

Long-Term Effects

Alcohol is distributed throughout most of the body and may affect many different organs and tissues. Problems associated with long-term, habitual abuse of alcohol include diseases of the cardiovascular system, nervous system, and liver, and some cancers.

Hangover The physiological reaction to excessive drinking, including symptoms such as headache, upset stomach, anxiety, depression, diarrhea, and thirst.

Congeners Forms of alcohol that are metabolized more slowly than ethanol and produce toxic by-products.

Table 12.4
Drugs and Alcohol: Actions and Interactions

Drug Class/Trade Name(s)	Effects with Alcohol
Antialcohol: Antabuse	Severe reactions to even small amounts; headache, nausea, blurred vision, convulsions, coma, possible death.
Antibiotics: penicillin, Cyantin	Reduced therapeutic effectiveness.
Antidepressants: Elavil, Sinequan, Tofranil, Nardil, Prozac, Zoloft	Increased central nervous system (CNS) depression, blood pressure changes. Combined use of alcohol and MAOIs, SSRIs, specific types of antidepressants can trigger massive increases in blood pressure, even brain hemorrhage and death.
Antihistamines: Allerest, Dristan	Drowsiness and CNS depression. Driving ability impaired.
Aspirin: Anacin, Excedrin, Bayer	Irritates stomach lining. May cause gastrointestinal pain, bleeding.
Depressants: Valium, Ativan, Placidyl	Dangerous CNS depression, loss of coordination, coma. High risk of overdose and death.
Narcotics: heroin, codeine, Darvon	Serious CNS depression. Possible respiratory arrest and death.
Stimulants: caffeine, cocaine	Masks depressant action of alcohol. May increase blood pressure, physical tension.

Source: Reprinted by permission from *Drugs and Alcohol: Simple Facts about Alcohol and Drug Combinations* (Phoenix: DIN Publications, 1988), no. 121.

Effects on the Nervous System   The nervous system is especially sensitive to alcohol. Even people who drink moderately experience shrinkage in brain size and weight and a loss of some degree of intellectual ability. The damage that results from alcohol use is localized primarily in the left side of the brain, which is responsible for written and spoken language, logic, and mathematical skills. The degree of shrinkage appears to be directly related to the amount of alcohol consumed. In terms of memory loss, the evidence suggests that having one drink every day is better than saving up for a binge and consuming seven or eight drinks in a night. The amount of alcohol consumed at one time is critical. Alcohol-related brain damage can be partially reversed with good nutrition and staying sober.

Cardiovascular Effects   Alcohol affects the cardiovascular system in a number of ways. Numerous studies have associated light-to-moderate alcohol consumption (no more than two drinks a day) with a reduced risk of coronary artery disease. Several mechanisms have been proposed to explain how this might happen. The strongest evidence favors an increase in high-density lipoprotein (HDL) cholesterol, which is known as the "good" cholesterol. Studies have shown that drinkers have higher levels of HDL. Another factor that might help is an *antithrombotic effect*. Alcohol consumption is associated with a decrease in clotting factors that contribute to the development of atherosclerosis.

However, this does not mean that alcohol consumption is recommended as a preventive measure against heart disease—it causes many more cardiovascular health hazards than benefits. Alcohol contributes to high blood pressure and slightly increased heart rate and cardiac output. Those who report drinking three to five drinks a day, regardless of race or sex, have higher blood pressure than those who drink less.

Liver Disease   One of the most common diseases related to alcohol abuse is **cirrhosis** of the liver. It is among the top ten causes of death in the United States. One result of heavy drinking is that the liver begins to store fat—a condition known as fatty liver. If there is insufficient time between drinking episodes, this fat cannot be transported to storage sites, and the fat-filled liver cells stop functioning. Continued drinking can cause a further stage of liver deterioration called fibrosis, in which the damaged area of the liver develops fibrous scar tissue. Cell function can be partially restored at this stage with proper nutrition and abstinence from alcohol. If the person continues to drink, however, cirrhosis results. At this point, the liver cells die and the damage becomes permanent.

Alcoholic hepatitis is a serious condition resulting from prolonged use of alcohol. A chronic inflammation of the liver develops, which may be fatal in itself or progress to cirrhosis.

Cirrhosis   The last stage of liver disease associated with chronic heavy use of alcohol during which liver cells die and damage becomes permanent.

Alcoholic hepatitis   Condition resulting from prolonged use of alcohol in which the liver is inflamed. It can result in death.

Cancer The repeated irritation caused by long-term use of alcohol has been linked to cancers of the esophagus, stomach, mouth, tongue, and liver. There is substantial evidence that breast cancer risk is elevated for women consuming high levels of alcohol (more than three drinks per day) compared with abstainers.[9] A Harvard Medical School study of male drinkers showed an increased cancer risk of 12 percent for those who had only one drink a day and 123 percent for those who had two drinks a day. It is unclear how alcohol exerts its carcinogenic effects, though it is thought that it inhibits the absorption of carcinogenic substances, permitting them to be taken to sensitive organs.

Other Effects An irritant to the gastrointestinal system, alcohol may cause indigestion and heartburn if ingested on an empty stomach. It also damages the mucous membranes and can cause inflammation of the esophagus, chronic stomach irritation, problems with intestinal absorption, and chronic diarrhea.

Alcohol abuse is a major cause of chronic inflammation of the pancreas, the organ that produces digestive enzymes and insulin. Chronic abuse of alcohol inhibits enzyme production, which further inhibits the absorption of nutrients. Drinking alcohol can block the absorption of calcium, a nutrient that strengthens bones. This should be of particular concern to women, for as women age their risk for osteoporosis (bone thinning and calcium loss) increases. Heavy consumption of alcohol worsens this condition.

Evidence also suggests that alcohol impairs the body's ability to recognize and fight foreign bodies such as bacteria and viruses. The relationship between alcohol and AIDS is unclear, especially since some of the populations at risk for AIDS are also at risk for alcohol abuse. But any stressor like alcohol, with a known effect on the immune system, would probably contribute to the development of the disease.

Alcohol and Pregnancy

Recall from Chapter 7 that *teratogens* are substances that cause birth defects. Of the 30 known teratogens in the environment, alcohol is one of the most dangerous and common. Alcohol can harm fetal development.

More than 10 percent of all children have been exposed to high levels of alcohol in utero. All will suffer varying degrees of effects, ranging from mild learning disabilities to major physical, mental, and intellectual impairment. It takes very little alcohol to cause serious damage. Research has shown that even a single exposure to high levels of alcohol can cause significant brain damage in the infant.[10] A disorder called **fetal alcohol syndrome (FAS)** is associated with alcohol consumption during pregnancy. Alcohol consumed during the first trimester poses the greatest threat to organ development; exposure during the last trimester, when the brain is developing rapidly, is most likely to affect CNS development. FAS is the third most common birth defect and the

second leading cause of mental retardation in the United States. The incidence of FAS is estimated to be 1 to 2 of every 1,000 live births. It is the most common preventable cause of mental impairment in the Western world.

FAS occurs when alcohol ingested by the mother passes through the placenta into the infant's bloodstream. Because the fetus is so small, its BAC will be much higher than that of the mother. Among the symptoms of FAS are mental retardation, small head, tremors, and abnormalities of the face, limbs, heart, and brain. Children with FAS may experience the following problems:[11]

- Difficulty in structuring work time
- Poor memory and impaired learning
- Trouble in generalizing behaviors and information
- Reduced attention span or distractible behavior
- Impulsive behaviors, fearlessness, and unresponsive reactions to verbal cautions
- Poor social judgment
- Inability to handle money in an age-appropriate manner
- Trouble with internalizing modeled behaviors
- Differences in sensory awareness (hyposensitive or hypersensitive)
- Language production higher than comprehension
- Poor problem-solving strategies

Children with a history of prenatal alcohol exposure but with fewer than the full physical or behavioral symptoms of FAS may be categorized as having **fetal alcohol effects (FAE).** FAE is estimated to occur three to four times more often than FAS, although it is much less recognized. The signs of FAE in newborns are low birthweight and irritability, and there may be permanent mental impairment. Infants whose mothers habitually consumed more than three ounces of alcohol (approximately six drinks) in a short time period when pregnant are at high risk for FAS. Risk levels for babies whose mothers consume smaller amounts are uncertain.

Alcohol can also be passed to a nursing baby through breast milk. For this reason, most doctors advise nursing mothers not to drink for at least four hours before nursing their babies and preferably to abstain altogether.

Fetal alcohol syndrome (FAS) A disorder that may affect the fetus when the mother consumes alcohol during pregnancy. Among its effects are mental retardation, small head, tremors, and abnormalities of the face, limbs, heart, and brain.

Fetal alcohol effects (FAE) A syndrome describing children with a history of prenatal alcohol exposure but without all the physical or behavioral symptoms of FAS. Among its symptoms are low birthweight, irritability, and possible permanent mental impairment.

Drinking and Driving

Traffic accidents are the leading cause of death for all age groups from 5 to 45 years old (including college students). Approximately 41 percent of all traffic fatalities in 2002 were alcohol related.[12] Unfortunately, college students are over-represented in alcohol-related crashes. The College Alcohol Study findings indicated that 20 percent of nonbingers, 43 percent of occasional bingers, and 59 percent of frequent bingers reported driving while intoxicated.[13] Furthermore, it is estimated that three out of every ten Americans will be involved in an alcohol-related accident at some time in their lives.[14] Studies show that those involved in car crashes after drinking have a 40 to 50 percent higher chance of dying than nondrinkers involved in car crashes.

In 2003, there were 17,013 alcohol-related traffic fatalities (ARTFs), a 5 percent reduction from the ARTF data reported in 1982.[15] Over the past 20 years, intoxication rates (BAC of 0.10 percent or greater) decreased for drivers of all age groups involved in fatal crashes (Figure 12.2). This number represents an average of one alcohol-related fatality approximately every 30 minutes.[16] The highest intoxication rates in fatal crashes were recorded for drivers 21 to 24 years old (33 percent), followed by ages 25 to 34 (28 percent) and 35 to 44 (26 percent). In the most current data reported, approximately 1.4 million drivers were arrested in 2001 for driving under the influence of alcohol or drugs. This is an arrest rate of 1 for every 137 licensed drivers in the United States.[17]

Several factors probably contributed to these reductions in ARTFs: laws that raised the drinking age to 21; stricter law enforcement; increased emphasis on zero tolerance (laws prohibiting those under 21 from driving with *any* detectable BAC); and educational programs designed to discourage drinking and driving. Most states have set 0.10 percent as the BAC at which drivers are considered to be legally drunk (see Table 12.3 on page 357). However, several states have lowered the standard to 0.08 percent, and others are likely to follow.

Laboratory and test track research shows that the vast majority of drivers, even experienced drinkers, are impaired at 0.08 with regard to critical driving tasks. Braking, steering, lane changing, judgment, and divided attention, among other measures, are all affected significantly at 0.08 BAC. National groups such as MADD (Mothers Against Drunk

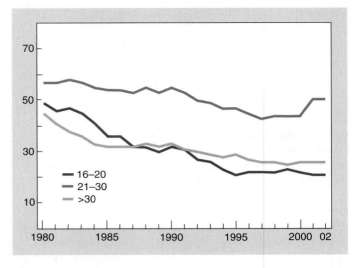

Figure 12.2

Percentage of Fatally Injured Passenger Vehicle Drivers with BACs > 0.10 Percent, by Driver Age

Source: Insurance Institute for Highway Safety, "Fatality Facts: Alcohol 2002," 2003, www.iihs.org

Driving), started by a woman whose child was killed by a drunk driver, go as far as tracking drunk driving cases through the court systems to ensure that drunk drivers are punished. Members of the high school group SADD (Students Against Destructive Decisions) educate their peers about the dangers of drinking and driving.

Despite all these measures, the risk of being involved in an alcohol-related automobile crash remains substantial. Researchers have shown a direct relationship between the amount of alcohol in a driver's bloodstream and the likelihood of a crash. A driver with a BAC level of 0.10 percent is approximately ten times more likely to be involved in a car accident than a driver who has not been drinking. At a BAC of 0.15 on weekend nights, the likelihood of dying in a single-vehicle crash is more than 380 times higher than for nondrinkers. Alcohol involvement is highest during nighttime (9:00 PM to 6:00 AM) single-vehicle crashes, in which 67 percent of fatally injured passenger-vehicle drivers in 2002 had BACs at or over 0.08 percent. Only 26 percent of fatally injured drivers involved in nighttime single-vehicle crashes had no alcohol in their blood.[18]

Not only does the time of day increase risk of being involved in an alcohol-related crash, but it also makes a difference whether it is a weekday or weekend. In 2002, 25 percent of all fatal crashes during the week were alcohol-related, compared with 45 percent on weekends.[19]

Alcohol Abuse and Alcoholism

Alcohol use becomes **alcohol abuse** when it interferes with work, school, or social and family relationships or when it entails any violation of the law, including driving under the influence (DUI). **Alcoholism,** or **alcohol dependency,** results when personal and health problems related to alcohol use are severe and stopping alcohol use results in withdrawal symptoms; some six million Americans can be described as alcoholics.

Identifying a Problem Drinker

As in other drug addictions, tolerance, psychological dependence, and withdrawal symptoms must be present to qualify a drinker as an addict. Addiction results from chronic use over a period of time that may vary from person to person. Irresponsible and problem drinkers, such as people who get into fights or embarrass themselves or others when they drink, are not necessarily alcoholics. The stereotype of the alcoholic on skid row applies to only 5 percent of the alcoholic population. The remaining 95 percent live in some type of extended family unit. Alcoholics can be found at all socioeconomic levels and in all professions, ethnic groups, geographical locations, religions, and races.

Studies suggest that the lifetime risk of alcoholism in the United States is about 10 percent for men and 3 percent for women. Moreover, almost 25 percent of the American population (50 million people) is affected by the alcoholism of a friend or family member. The 2003 National Survey on Drug Use and Health found that 6.8 percent of Americans were heavy drinkers and 22.6 percent were binge drinkers.[20]

Recognizing and admitting the existence of an alcohol problem are often extremely difficult. Alcoholics themselves deny their problem, often making statements such as "I can stop any time I want to. I just don't want to right now." Their families also tend to deny the problem, saying things like "He really has been under a lot of stress lately. Besides, he only drinks beer." The fear of being labeled a "problem drinker" often prevents people from seeking help.

Alcoholics tend to have a number of symptoms in common. The Assess Yourself box on the next page lists several. People who recognize one or more of these behaviors in themselves may wish to seek professional help to determine whether alcohol has become a controlling factor in their lives. You may also feel that you wish to moderate the amount of alcohol that you drink. See the Skills for Behavior Change box on page 363 for some tips to accomplish this.

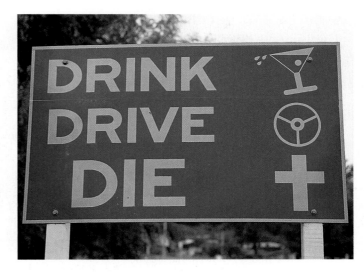

All too often, drinking and driving can be a deadly combination. Approximately 40 percent of U.S. traffic fatalities are alcohol related.

Women are the fastest-growing population of alcohol abusers. They tend to become alcoholic at a later age and after fewer years of heavy drinking than do male alcoholics. Women at highest risk for alcohol-related problems are those who are unmarried but living with a partner, are in their twenties or early thirties, or have a husband or partner who drinks heavily.

The Causes of Alcohol Abuse and Alcoholism

We know that alcoholism is a disease with biological and social/environmental components, but we do not know what role each component plays in the disease.

Biological and Family Factors   Research into the hereditary and environmental causes of alcoholism has found higher rates of alcoholism among family members of alcoholics. In fact, according to researchers, alcoholism is four to five times more common among children of alcoholics than in the general population.

Alcohol abuse   Use of alcohol that interferes with work, school, or personal relationships or that entails violations of the law.

Alcoholism (alcohol dependency)   Condition when personal and health problems related to alcohol use are severe and stopping alcohol use results in withdrawal symptoms.

Alcohol Abuse and Alcoholism: Common Questions

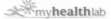

Fill out this assessment online at www.aw-bc.com/myhealthlab or www.aw-bc.com/donatelle

Although many people think that they have a clear understanding of alcoholism, much remains in question. Answering the following questions will indicate your own level of knowledge about the disease. For further information about alcohol use on college campuses, check out the National Institute of Alcohol Abuse and Alcoholism's website (www.niaaa.nih.gov).

1. Alcoholism is a disease characterized by what four symptoms?
   a.
   b.
   c.
   d.

2. Is alcoholism an inherited trait?
   Yes
   Probably
   No

3. Do you have to be an alcoholic to experience alcohol-related problems?
   Yes
   No

4. What groups of individuals tend to have the most problems with alcoholism?

ANSWERS

1. The four symptoms of alcoholism include:
   a. Craving (a strong need or urge to drink alcohol)
   b. Loss of control (not being able to stop drinking once drinking begins)
   c. Physical dependence (withdrawal symptoms, such as nausea, sweating, shakiness, and anxiety after stopping drinking)
   d. Tolerance (the need to drink greater amounts of alcohol for the same effect)
   (For more information, see the *Diagnostic and Statistical Manual of Mental Disorders IV* published by the American Psychological Association.)

2. Probably yes. The risk for developing alcoholism does indeed run in families. However, lifestyle is also a major factor. Currently, researchers are trying to locate the actual genes that put you at risk. Your friends, the amount of stress in your life, and how readily available alcohol is are also factors that increase risk. Remember that risk is not destiny. A child of an alcoholic won't automatically become an alcoholic, while others develop alcoholism even though no one in their family is an alcoholic. If you know you are at risk, you can take steps to protect yourself.

3. No. Alcoholism is only one type of alcohol problem. Alcohol abuse can be just as harmful. A person can abuse alcohol without being an alcoholic—that is, he or she may drink too much, too often and still not be dependent on alcohol. Some of the problems of alcohol abuse include: not being able to meet work, school, or family responsibilities; drunk driving arrests and car crashes; and drinking-related medical conditions. Under some circumstances, even social or moderate drinking is dangerous—for example, when driving, during pregnancy, or when taking certain medications.

4. Alcohol abuse and alcoholism cut across gender, race, and nationality. Nearly one in three adults abuse alcohol in the United States today. In general, more men than women are alcohol dependent or have alcohol problems. Alcohol problems are highest among young adults aged 18–29, and lowest among adults aged 65 and older. We also know that the younger you start the more likely that you will have a problem.

MAKE IT HAPPEN!

Use the results of this self-assessment to begin your behavior change program. Follow the steps and use the examples on page 369 to complete your Behavior Change Contract and use these resources to take action.

Source: National Institute on Alcohol Abuse and Alcoholism, "College Drinking: FAQ's on Alcohol Abuse and Alcoholism," 2004, www.collegedrinkingprevention.gov/facts/faq.aspx

How to Cut Down on Your Drinking

Are you concerned about your drinking? You can improve your life and health by cutting back. Start with these steps:

1. Write your reasons for cutting down or stopping.
2. Set a drinking goal. Choose a limit for how much you will drink each day.
3. Keep a diary of your drinking for a month. This will show you how much you drink and when, as well as how much money you spend. You may be surprised to see how much you spend each month.

To moderate your drinking, follow these tips.

1. Decide what you want from drinking alcohol.
   - Think about the pros and cons (short- and long-term) for moderating your use versus maintaining the status quo.
   - Also consider what you absolutely want to avoid when you drink.
2. Set drinking limits.
   - What's your upper limit on the number of drinks you consume per week?
   - At what point do you decide you've had enough?
   - What's the maximum number of days for drinking you will choose to give yourself?
   - Use standard guidelines to determine what constitutes one drink.
3. Count your drinks and monitor your drinking behavior.
   - Try it! Most people are surprised by what they learn when they actually count how much they drink.
   - Simply observe your behavior—this is like standing outside yourself and watching how you are acting when you are drinking.
4. Alter how and what you drink.
   - Switch to drinks that contain less alcohol (such as light beers).
   - Slow down your pace of drinking.
   - Space drinks farther apart.
   - Alternate drinking nonalcoholic beverages with alcoholic drinks.
5. Manage your drinking in the moment.
   - Stay awake and on top of how you drink and what you're drinking when you're at a party.
   - Choose what's right for you.

Sources: L. A. Dimeff, J. S. Baer, D. R. Kivlahan, and G. A. Marlatt, *Brief Alcohol Screening and Intervention for College Students (BASICS): A Harm Reduction Approach* (New York: Guilford Press, 1999), 166; reprinted with permission of The Guilford Press; National Institute on Alcohol Abuse and Alcoholism, "How to Cut Down on Your Drinking" (NIH Publication no. 96-3770), 2003, www.niaaa.nih.gov/publications/handout.htm

---

Male alcoholics, especially, are more likely than nonalcoholics to have alcoholic parents and siblings. Two distinct subtypes of alcoholism have provided important information about the inheritance of alcoholism. *Type 1 alcoholics* are drinkers who had at least one parent of either sex who was a problem drinker and who grew up in an environment that encouraged heavy drinking. Their drinking is reinforced by environmental events during which there is heavy drinking. Type 1 alcohol abusers share certain personality characteristics. They avoid novelty and harmful situations and are concerned about the thoughts and feelings of others. *Type 2 alcoholism* is seen in males only. These alcoholics are typically the biological sons of alcoholic fathers who have a history of both violence and drug use. Type 2 alcoholics display the opposite characteristics of Type 1 alcoholics. They do not seek social approval, they lack inhibition, and they are prone to novelty-seeking behavior.[21]

One study found a strong relationship between alcoholism and alcoholic patterns within the family.[22] Children with one alcoholic parent had a 52 percent chance of becoming alcoholics themselves. With two alcoholic parents, the chances of becoming alcoholic jumped to 71 percent.

Because the effects of heredity and environment are so difficult to separate, some scientists have examined the problem through twin and adoption studies.[23] So far, these studies have produced inconclusive results, although a slightly higher rate of similar drinking behaviors has been demonstrated among identical twins. Moreover, sons living away from their alcoholic parents tend to more closely resemble them in drinking behavior than they do their adoptive or foster parents.

Social and Cultural Factors Although a family history of alcoholism may predispose a person to problems with alcohol, numerous other factors may mitigate or exacerbate that tendency. Social and cultural factors may trigger the affliction for many people who are not genetically predisposed to alcoholism. Some people begin drinking as a way to dull the

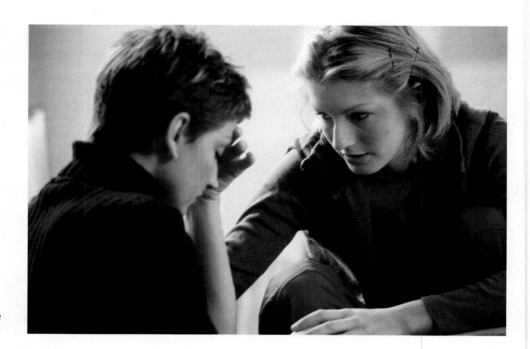

Often, family members or friends have to confront the alcohol-dependent person to help them take the first steps toward recovery.

pain of an acute loss or an emotional or social problem. For example, college students may drink to escape the stress of college life, disappointment over unfulfilled expectations, difficulties in forming relationships, or loss of the security of home, loved ones, and close friends. Involvement in a painful relationship, death of a family member, and other problems may trigger a search for an anesthetic. Unfortunately, the emotional discomfort that causes many people to turn to alcohol also ultimately causes them to become even more uncomfortable as the depressant effect of the drug begins to take its toll. Thus, the person who is already depressed may become even more depressed, antagonizing friends and other social supports until they turn away. Eventually, the drinker becomes physically dependent on the drug.

Family attitudes toward alcohol also seem to influence whether or not a person will develop a drinking problem. It has been clearly demonstrated that people who are raised in cultures in which drinking is a part of religious or ceremonial activities or in which alcohol is a traditional part of the family meal are less prone to alcohol dependency. In contrast, in societies in which alcohol purchase is carefully controlled and drinking is regarded as a rite of passage to adulthood, the tendency for abuse appears to be greater.

Certain social factors have been linked with alcoholism as well. These include urbanization, the weakening of links to the extended family and a general loosening of kinship ties, increased mobility, and changing religious and philosophical values. Apparently, then, some combination of heredity and environment plays a decisive role in the development of alcoholism. Certain ethnic and racial groups also have special alcohol abuse problems.

Effects of Alcoholism on the Family

Only recently have we recognized that it is not only the alcoholic, but the alcoholic's entire family that suffers. Although most research focuses on family effects during the late stages of alcoholism, the family unit actually begins to react early on as the person starts to show symptoms of the disease.

An estimated 76 million Americans (about 43 percent of the U.S. adult population) have been exposed to alcoholism in the family.[24] Twenty-two million members of alcoholic families are age 18 or older, and many have carried childhood emotional scars into adulthood. Approximately one in four children under age 18 lives in an atmosphere of anxiety, tension, confusion, and denial.[25]

In dysfunctional families, children learn certain rules from a very early age: don't talk, don't trust, and don't feel. These unspoken rules allow the family to avoid dealing with real problems and real issues. Family members unconsciously adapt to the alcoholic's behavior by adjusting their own behavior. Unfortunately, these behaviors actually help keep the alcoholic drinking. Children in such dysfunctional families generally assume at least one of the following roles:

- *Family hero.* Tries to divert attention from the problem by being too good to be true.
- *Scapegoat.* Draws attention away from the family's primary problem through delinquency or misbehavior.
- *Lost child.* Becomes passive and quietly withdraws from upsetting situations.
- *Mascot.* Disrupts tense situations by providing comic relief.

For children in alcoholic homes, life is a struggle. They have to deal with constant stress, anxiety, and embarrassment. Because the alcoholic is the center of attention, the children's wants and needs are often ignored. It is not uncommon for these children to be victims of violence, abuse, neglect, or incest. As we have seen, when such children grow up, they are much more prone to alcoholic behaviors themselves than are children from nonalcoholic families.

In the past decade, we have come to recognize the unique problems of adult children of alcoholics whose difficulties in life stem from a lack of parental nurturing during childhood. Among these problems are difficulty in developing social attachments, a need to be in control of all emotions and situations, low self-esteem, and depression. Fortunately, not all individuals who have grown up in alcoholic families are doomed to have lifelong problems. As many of these people mature, they develop a resiliency in response to their families' problems. They thus enter adulthood armed with positive strengths and valuable career-oriented skills, such as the ability to assume responsibility, strong organizational skills, and realistic expectations of their jobs and others.

Costs to Society

The entire society suffers the consequences of individuals' alcohol abuse. Close to half of all traffic fatalities are attributable to alcohol—and these fatalities include those in other vehicles that were struck by drunk drivers. According to the National Institute on Alcohol Abuse and Alcoholism, in 1998, alcohol-related costs to society were at least $184.6 billion when health insurance, criminal justice costs, treatment costs, and lost productivity were factored in. Reportedly, alcoholism is directly and indirectly responsible for over 25 percent of the nation's medical expenses and lost earnings. Well over 50 percent of all child abuse cases are the result of alcohol-related problems. Finally, the costs in emotional health are impossible to measure.[26]

Women and Alcoholism

In the past, women have consumed less alcohol and have had fewer alcohol-related problems than have men. But now, greater percentages of women, especially college-age women, are choosing to drink and are drinking more heavily.

Studies indicate that there are now almost as many female as male alcoholics. Women get addicted faster with less alcohol use and then suffer the consequences more profoundly. Women alcoholics have death rates 50 to 100 percent higher than male alcoholics, including deaths from suicide, alcohol-related accidents, heart disease and stroke, and cirrhosis.

Risk factors for drinking problems among *all women* include:

- A family history of drinking problems
- Pressure to drink from a peer or spouse
- Depression
- Stress

Risk factors among *young women* include:

- College attendance: women in college drink more, and more frequently, than they do after they graduate
- Nontraditional, low-status, and part-time jobs, and unemployment
- Being single, divorced, or separated

Among the risk factors for *middle-aged women* are:

- Loss of social roles (such as through divorce or children growing up and leaving the home)
- Abuse of prescription drugs
- Heavy drinking by spouse
- Presence of other disorders, such as depression

Risk factors among *older women* include:

- Heavy- or problem-drinking spouse
- Retirement, with a loss of social networks centered on the workplace

Drinking patterns among women in *different age groups* also differ in these ways:

- Younger women drink more overall, drink more often, and experience more alcohol-related problems, such as drinking and driving, assaults, suicide attempts, and difficulties at work.
- Middle-aged women are more likely to develop drinking problems in response to a traumatic or life-changing event, such as divorce, surgery, or death of a significant other.
- Older women are more likely than older men to have developed drinking problems within the past ten years.[27]

It is estimated that only 14 percent of women who need treatment get it. In one study, women cite potential loss of income, not wanting others to know they may have a problem, inability to pay for treatment, and fear that treatment would not be confidential as reasons for not seeking treatment.[28] Another major obstacle is child care. Most residential treatment centers do not allow women to bring their children with them.

Despite growing recognition of our national alcohol problem, fewer than 10 percent of alcoholics in the United States receive any care. Factors contributing to this low figure include an inability or unwillingness to admit to an alcohol problem; the social stigma attached to alcoholism; breakdowns in referral and delivery systems (failure of physicians or psychotherapists to follow up on referrals, client failure to follow through with recommended treatments, or failure of rehabilitation facilities to give quality care); and failure of the professional medical establishment to recognize and diagnose alcoholic symptoms among patients.

What do you think?

Why do you think women appear to be drinking more heavily today than they did in the past? ■ *Does society look at men's and women's drinking habits in the same way?* ■ *Can you think of ways to increase support for women in their recovery process?*

Recovery

Most alcoholics and problem drinkers who seek help have experienced a turning point: a spouse walks out, taking children and possessions; the boss issues an ultimatum to dry out or ship out. The alcoholic ready for treatment has, in most cases, reached a low point. Devoid of hope, physically depleted, and spiritually despairing, the person has finally recognized that alcohol controls his or her life. The first step on the road to recovery is to regain that control and assume responsibility for personal actions.

The Family's Role

Members of an alcoholic's family sometimes take action before the alcoholic does. They may go to an organization or a treatment facility to seek help for themselves and their relative.

As we saw in Chapter 11, *intervention*—a planned confrontation with the alcoholic that involves several family members and professional counselors—is an effective

method of helping an alcoholic to recognize the problem. Family members express their love and concern, telling the alcoholic that they will no longer refrain from acknowledging the problem and affirming their support for appropriate treatment. A family intervention is the turning point for a growing number of alcoholics. If you feel that you need to talk to a friend or family member about their drinking, see the Skills for Behavior Change box for some guidelines for this challenging task.

Treatment Programs

The alcoholic who is ready for help has several avenues of treatment: psychologists and psychiatrists specializing in the treatment of alcoholism, private treatment centers, hospitals specifically designed to treat alcoholics, community mental health facilities, and support groups such as Alcoholics Anonymous.

Private Treatment Facilities   Private treatment facilities have made concerted efforts to attract patients through radio and television advertising. Upon admission to the treatment facility, the patient receives a complete physical exam to determine whether underlying medical problems will interfere with treatment.

Alcoholics who decide to quit drinking will experience withdrawal symptoms such as hyperexcitability, confusion and agitation, sleep disorders, convulsions, tremors of the hands, depression, headache, and seizures. For a small percentage of people, alcohol withdrawal results in a severe syndrome known as **delirium tremens (DTs).** Delirium tremens is characterized by confusion, delusions, agitated behavior, and hallucinations.

For any long-term addict, medical supervision is usually necessary. *Detoxification,* the process by which addicts end their dependence on a drug, is commonly carried out in a medical facility, where patients can be monitored to prevent fatal withdrawal reactions. Withdrawal takes 7 to 21 days. Shortly after detoxification, alcoholics begin their treatment for psychological addiction. Most treatment facilities keep their patients from three to six weeks. Treatment at private treatment centers costs several thousand dollars, but some insurance programs or employers will assume most of this expense.

Family Therapy, Individual Therapy, and Group Therapy
In family therapy, the person and family members gradually examine the psychological reasons underlying the addiction. In individual and group therapy with fellow addicts, alcoholics learn positive coping skills for situations that have regularly caused them to turn to alcohol. On some college campuses, the problems associated with alcohol abuse are so great that student health centers are opening their own treatment programs.

Delirium tremens (DTs)   A state of confusion brought on by withdrawal from alcohol. Symptoms include hallucinations, anxiety, and trembling.

Talking to a Friend about Alcohol Use

It's difficult to know when to say something when you're worried about a friend's alcohol use. Ask yourself …

HOW DOES IT AFFECT YOU?

- Have you lost time from classes, studying, or a job in order to help your friend cope with problems caused by her drinking?
- Is your friend's drinking making you unhappy in any aspect of your life?
- Is your friend's behavior affecting your reputation in a way you don't like?
- Have you ever felt embarrassed or hurt by something he said or did while intoxicated?
- Have you ever had to take care of your friend because of his alcohol use?

HOW DOES IT AFFECT YOUR FRIEND?

- Does your friend drink in order to get drunk?
- Is your friend doing dangerous things because of alcohol?
- Has your friend ever wanted to cut down on drinking?
- Does your friend "slam" drinks?
- Does your friend ever have to drink to steady his nerves or get rid of a hangover?
- Has your friend ever been in trouble because of drinking?
- Does your friend find it necessary to drink or get high to enjoy a party?
- Is alcohol affecting your friend's academic performance?
- Does your friend drink to escape from or cope with problems or stress? Does she use drugs or alcohol to avoid painful feelings?
- Has your friend even been unable to remember things she said or did while drinking (blacked out)?
- Is your friend annoyed when people criticize his drinking?

- Has your friend ever received medical care for something related to drinking?
- Have you noticed a decline in his personal health or appearance?

The more questions you answer yes to, and the more frequently each factor is true, the more likely it is that your friend has a problem. A caring conversation will help your friend learn how his behavior affects others and can help him get the help he needs. Some people just need the wake-up call of your honest opinion; others can benefit from professional help to make changes or maintain abstinence.

BEFORE YOU TALK TO YOUR FRIEND

- Learn about alcohol abuse.
- Prepare a list of specific problems that have occurred because of your friend's drinking or drug use. Keep these items as concrete as possible. "You're so antisocial when you drink" will not mean as much as, "When you were drunk, you made fun of me and were mean to me. You hurt me." Bring the list with you and keep the conversation focused.
- Choose a private location where you can talk without embarrassment or interruption.

HOW TO TALK TO YOUR FRIEND

- Talk to your friend when she is sober. The sooner you can arrange this after a bad episode, the better.
- Restrict your comments to what you feel and what you have experienced of your friend's behavior. Express statements that cannot be disputed. Remarks like, "Everyone's disgusted with you," or, "Lily thinks you have a real problem," will probably lead to arguments about Lily's problems or who "everyone" is. Avoid such generalizations.
- Convey your concern for your friend's well being with specific statements. "I want to talk to you because I am worried about you," or "Our friendship

means a lot to me. I don't like to see what's been happening."
- It is important to openly discuss the negative consequences of your friend's drinking or drug use. Use concrete examples from your list. "At the party I was left standing there while you threw up. The next day you were too hung over to write your paper. It makes me sad that these things are happening in your life."
- Emphasize the difference between sober behavior that you like and drinking behavior that you dislike. "You have the most wonderful sense of humor, but when you drink it turns into cruel sarcasm, and you're not funny any more. You're mean."
- Be sure to distinguish between the person and the behavior. "I think you're a great person, but the more alcohol you drink, the less you seem to care about anything."
- Encourage your friend to consult with a professional to talk about his/her alcohol problem. You can offer to help them find resources or to go with them to an appointment.
- Talk to people you trust (other friends or relatives) about your concerns. Their involvement may help.

WHAT *NOT* TO DO

- Don't accuse or argue.
- Don't lecture or moralize. Remain factual, listen, and be nonjudgmental.
- Don't give up. If your friend seems resistant, you can bring it up later or let them know you're there for them if they ever want to talk.

Source: Brown University Health Education, "Talking To A Friend About Drinking Or Drug Use," 2004, www.brown.edu /Student_Services/Health_Services /Health_Education/atod/helpafriend.htm

Other Types of Treatment Two other treatments are drug therapy and group support. Disulfiram (trade name: Antabuse) is the drug of choice for treating alcoholics. If alcohol is consumed, the drug causes unpleasant effects such as headache, nausea, vomiting, drowsiness, and hangover. These symptoms discourage the alcoholic from drinking.

Alcoholics Anonymous (AA) is a private, nonprofit, self-help organization founded in 1935. The organization, which relies upon group support to help people stop drinking, currently has branches all over the world and more than 1 million members. At meetings, last names are never used, and no one is forced to speak. Members are taught to believe that their alcoholism is a lifetime problem and that they may never use alcohol again. They share their struggles with each other and talk about the devastating effects alcoholism has had on their personal and professional lives. All members are asked to place their faith and control of the habit into the hands of a "higher power." The road to recovery is taken one step at a time. AA offers specialized meetings for Spanish-speakers, gays, atheists, people with HIV, and a variety of other people with alcohol problems.

Alcoholics Anonymous also has auxiliary groups to help spouses or partners, friends, and children of alcoholics. *Al-Anon* is the group dedicated to helping adult relatives and friends of alcoholics understand the disease and how they can contribute to the recovery process. Spouses and other adult loved ones often play an unwitting role in perpetuating the alcoholic's problems. For example, they may call the alcoholic's boss and lie about why the alcoholic missed work. At Al-Anon, these people examine their roles in their loved one's drinking and explore alternative behaviors.

Alateen, another AA-related organization, helps adolescents live with alcoholic parents. They are taught that they are not at fault for their parents' problems. They develop their self-esteem to overcome their guilt and function better socially.

The support gained from talking with others who have similar problems is one of the greatest benefits derived from self-help groups. Many members learn to exert greater control over their own lives and rid themselves of the guilt they feel about their participation in their loved one's alcoholism.

Alcoholics Anonymous (AA) An organization whose goal is to help alcoholics stop drinking; includes auxiliary branches such as Al-Anon and Alateen.

Other self-help groups include Women for Sobriety and Secular Organizations for Sobriety (SOS). Women for Sobriety addresses the differing needs of female alcoholics, who often have more severe problems than males. Unlike AA meetings, where attendance can be quite large, each group has no more than 10 members. Secular Organizations for Sobriety was founded to help people who are uncomfortable with AA's spiritual emphasis.

Relapse

Success in recovery varies with the individual. A return to alcoholic habits often follows what appears to be a successful recovery. Some alcoholics never recover. Some partially recover and improve other parts of their lives but remain dependent on alcohol. Many alcoholics refer to themselves as "recovering" throughout their lifetime; they never use the word *cured.*

Roughly 60 percent of alcoholics relapse (resume drinking) within the first three months of treatment. Why is the relapse rate so high? Treating an addiction requires more than getting the addict to stop using a substance; it also requires getting the person to break a pattern of behavior that has dominated his or her life.

People who are seeking to regain a healthy lifestyle must not only confront their addiction, but also guard against the tendency to relapse. Drinkers with compulsive personalities need to learn to understand themselves and take control. Others need to view treatment as a long-term process that takes a lot of effort beyond attending a weekly self-help group meeting. In order to work, a recovery program must offer the alcoholic ways to increase self-esteem and resume personal growth.

Can Recovering Alcoholics Take a Drink? During the 1970s, some scientists believed that recovering alcoholics could return to drinking on a limited social basis. Several studies supported this notion, but they have since been refuted. Research conducted over a period of five to ten years has shown that fewer than 1 percent of recovering alcoholics are able to resume drinking on a limited basis. To prevent the return to the bottle, abstinence is the safest and sanest path.

A comprehensive approach that includes drug therapy, group support, family therapy, and personal counseling designed to improve living and coping skills is usually the most effective course of treatment. The alcoholics most likely to recover completely are those who developed their dependencies after the age of 20, those with intact and supportive family units, and those who have reached a high level of personal disgust coupled with strong motivation to recover.

TAKING CHARGE

MAKE IT HAPPEN!

Assessment: The Assess Yourself box on page 362 gave you the chance to test your knowledge about alcoholism. If you couldn't answer some of the questions, or were surprised by some of the answers, you may want to take steps to learn more or to change your behavior.

Making a Change: In order to change your behavior, you need to develop a plan. Follow these steps.

1. Evaluate your behavior, and identify patterns and specific things you are doing. What can you change now? What can you change in the near future?
2. Select one pattern of behavior that you want to change.
3. Fill out a Behavior Change Contract. It should include your long-term goal for change, your short-term goals, the rewards you'll give yourself for reaching these goals, potential obstacles along the way, and strategies for overcoming these obstacles. For each goal, list the small steps and specific actions that you will take.
4. Chart your progress in a journal. At the end of a week, consider how successful you were in following your plan. What helped you be successful? What made change more difficult? What will you do differently next week?
5. Revise your plan as needed. Are the short-term goals attainable? Are the rewards satisfying?

One Student's Plan: After completing the Assess Yourself box, Mark was surprised to discover that he had several misperceptions about alcohol abuse. In particular, he was surprised to realize that he exhibited one of the symptoms that characterize alcoholism. During his three years in college, Mark realized that he had developed a tolerance to alcohol that caused him to drink more to achieve the same effect. He decided to address his concerns about his alcohol use in several steps.

First, Mark kept a log of his alcohol consumption over two weeks. He saw that he was drinking almost every night of the week. Mark decided he wanted to reduce his drinking and set two goals: taking a break from drinking altogether for three weeks, and after that, drinking only on Friday and Saturday nights for the rest of the semester. Mark explained to his friends that he was taking a break and invited them to go with him on hikes, to the movies, and to other alcohol-free environments. After successfully taking this break, Mark decided to set some goals and limits for himself on the alcohol he would consume in the future. He went to a fraternity party on a Friday night and drank two beers, his predetermined limit. He was happy to realize when he woke up the next morning that he felt refreshed, not hung over. When he went out for dinner with his friends Saturday night, they wanted to go barhopping afterwards. He volunteered to be the designated driver, and the bar gave him free sodas for the night. The next weekend, Mark found he had extra money that he hadn't spent on beer during the week and bought himself a new DVD.

Summary

- Alcohol is a central nervous system depressant used by 70 percent of all Americans and 83 percent of all college students; 44 percent of college students are binge drinkers. While consumption trends are slowly creeping downward, college students are under extreme pressure to consume alcohol.
- Alcohol's effect on the body is measured by the blood alcohol concentration (BAC), the ratio of alcohol to total blood volume. The higher the BAC, the greater the impaired judgment and coordination and drowsiness.

- Negative consequences associated with alcohol use and college students are lower grade-point averages, academic problems, dropping out of school, unplanned sex, hangovers, and injury. Long-term effects of alcohol overuse include damage to the nervous system, cardiovascular damage, liver disease, and increased risk for cancer. Drinking during pregnancy can cause fetal alcohol effects (FAE) or fetal alcohol syndrome (FAS). Alcohol is also a causative factor in traffic accidents.

- Alcohol use becomes alcoholism when it interferes with school, work, or social and family relationships or entails violations of the law. Causes of alcoholism include biological, family, social, and cultural factors. Alcoholism has far-reaching effects on families, especially on children. Children of alcoholics have problematic childhoods and may take those problems into adulthood.

- Recovery is problematic for alcoholics. Most alcoholics do not admit to a problem until reaching a major life crisis or having their families intervene. Treatment options include detoxification at private medical facilities, therapy (family, individual, or group), and self-help programs such as Alcoholics Anonymous. Most alcoholics relapse (60 percent within three months) because alcoholism is a behavioral addiction as well as a chemical addiction.

Questions for Discussion and Reflection

1. When it comes to drinking alcohol, how much is too much? How can you avoid drinking amounts that will affect your judgment? When you see a friend having "too many" drinks at a party, what actions do you normally take? What actions could you take?
2. What are some of the most common negative consequences college students experience as a result of drinking? What are secondhand effects of binge drinking? Why do students tolerate negative behaviors of students who have been drinking?
3. Determine what your BAC would be if you drank four beers in two hours (assume they are spaced at equal intervals). What physiological effects will you feel after each drink? Would a person of similar weight show greater effects after having four gin and tonics instead of beer? Why or why not? At what point in your life should you start worrying about the long-term effects of alcohol abuse?
4. Describe the difference between a problem drinker and an alcoholic. What factors can cause someone to slide from responsibly consuming alcohol to becoming an alcoholic? What effect does alcoholism have on an alcoholic's family?
5. Does anyone ever recover from alcoholism? Why or why not? Do you think society's views on drinking have changed over the years? Explain your answer.

Accessing Your Health on the Internet

Visit the following Internet sites to explore further topics and issues related to personal health. To visit an organization's website, go to the Companion Website for *Access to Health, Ninth Edition* at www.aw-bc.com/donatelle, click on the book image, and select "Accessing Your Health on the Internet" from the navigation menu.

1. *College Drinking: Changing the Culture.* This online resource center is based on a series of reports published by the Task Force of the National Advisory Council on Alcohol Abuse and Alcoholism. It targets three audiences: the student population as a whole; the college and its surrounding environment; and the individual at-risk or alcohol-dependent drinker.

2. *Had Enough.* This entertaining website is designed for college students who have suffered the secondhand effects (baby-sitting a roommate who has been drinking, having sleep interrupted, etc.) of other students' drinking. It offers suggestions for taking action and being proactive about policy issues on your campus.

3. *Higher Education Center for Alcohol and Other Drug Prevention.* This website is funded through the U.S. Department of Education and provides information relevant to colleges and universities. A specific site exists for students who are seeking information regarding alcohol.

Further Reading

Jersild, Devon. *Happy Hours: Alcohol in a Woman's Life.* New York: HarperCollins, 2001.

This book, a combination of cutting-edge research and personal stories of women who have struggled with alcohol problems, examines the role that alcohol plays in women's lives.

Kuhn, C., S. Swartzwelder, W. Wilson, J. Foster, and L. Wilson. *Buzzed: The Straight Facts,* National Institute on Alcohol Abuse and Alcoholism (NIAAA), *Research Monographs.* Washington, DC: U.S. Department of Health and Human Services.

A series of publications containing the results of a number of studies conducted by research scientists under the auspices of NIAAA through 2002. These monographs address issues such as alcohol use among older adults, occupational alcoholism, social drinking, and the relationship between heredity and alcoholism.

Nuwer, H. *Wrongs of Passage: Fraternities, Sororities, Hazing, and Binge Drinking.* Bloomington: Indiana University Press, 1999.

A comprehensive exposé on the continuing crisis of death and injury among fraternity and sorority pledges. The book provides an overview of Greek customs and demands that encouraged hazing as well as the recent deaths of students at some of the nation's most prestigious universities. The author argues that we need to control the Greek system as well as other organizations that employ similar, sometimes deadly, hazing practices.

Sperber, M. *Beer and Circus: How Big Time College Sports is Crippling Undergraduate Education.* New York: Henry Holt, 2000.

Sperber's book is an indictment of the attraction of undergraduates to schools based on the school's sports success and party reputations. He links student drinking behaviors to sports programs and argues that such an atmosphere shortchanges undergraduates of their education.

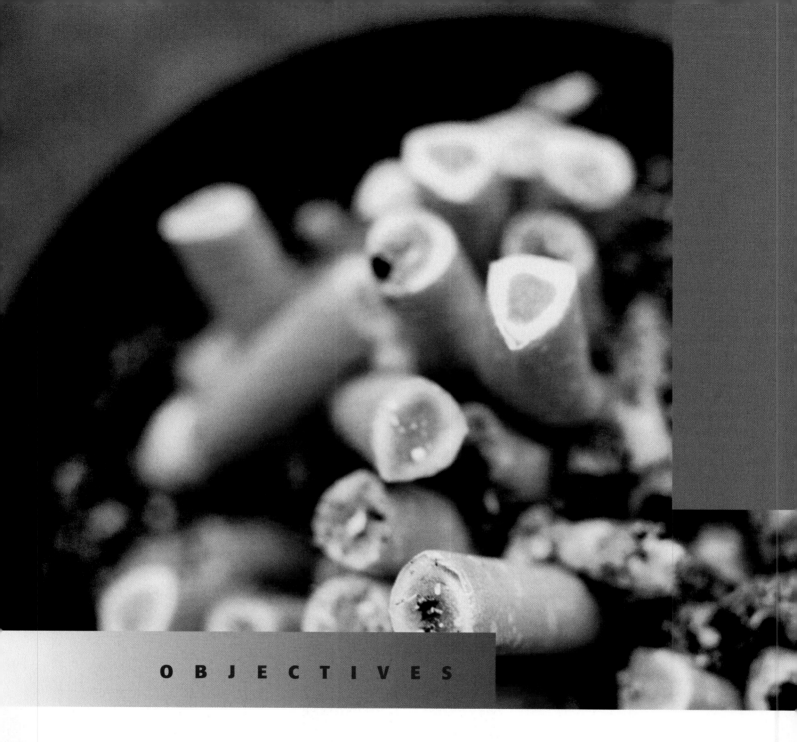

- Discuss the social issues involved in tobacco use, including advertising and medical costs.

- Explain how the chemicals in tobacco products affect a smoker's body.

- Review how smoking affects a smoker's risk for cancer, cardiovascular disease, and respiratory diseases and how it adversely affects a fetus's health.

- Discuss the risks associated with using smokeless tobacco.

- Evaluate the risks to nonsmokers associated with environmental tobacco smoke.

- Discuss the role of politics in regulating tobacco products.

- Describe strategies people adopt to quit using tobacco products, including strategies aimed at breaking the nicotine addiction, as well as habit.

- Compare the benefits and risks associated with caffeine, and summarize the health consequences of long-term caffeine use.

TOBACCO AND CAFFEINE

DAILY PLEASURES, DAILY CHALLENGES

IN THE NEWS

Habits: For Nicotine, a Too Happy Home

By Eric Nagourney

Why is it so hard to quit smoking cigarettes? One reason may be that nicotine acts on the same brain system in humans as heroin and morphine, a new study has found.

Earlier studies in animals had found that nicotine could set off the release of brain chemicals called opioids, which play a role in suppressing pain and causing pleasurable feelings. The new study is the first to establish that the same process occurs in people, the researchers said.

To prove that opioids were involved, the researchers first had to figure out a way to use positron emission tomography or PET

scanners to measure opioid brain activity. They also had to persuade officials at the University of Michigan to waive the no-smoking rules and allow their volunteers to smoke in the hospital's scanner. (They solved the problem by figuring out a way to vent the smoke to the outside.)

The study, led by David J. Scott, a graduate student, found that smokers appeared to have an increased flow of opioids in the brain all the time. After they smoked a cigarette, there was even more opioid activity in the parts of the brain involved in emotion and desire. The findings were presented last week at a meeting of the Society for Neuroscience.

Read the complete article online in the eThemes section of this book's website: www.aw-bc.com/donatelle.

Original article published November 2, 2004. Copyright © 2004 *The New York Times*. Reprinted with permission.

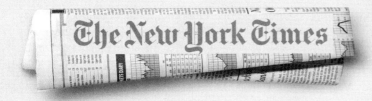

Tobacco use is the single most preventable cause of death in the United States.[1] While tobacco companies continue to publish full-page advertisements refuting the dangers of smoking, nearly 440,000 Americans die each year of tobacco-related diseases[2] (Figure 13.1). This is 50 times as many as will die from all illegal drugs combined. In addition, 10 million people will suffer from disorders caused by tobacco. To date, tobacco is known to cause about 25 diseases, and one in every five deaths in the United States is smoking related. About half of all regular smokers die of smoking-related diseases. Therefore, any contention by the tobacco industry that tobacco use is not dangerous is irresponsible and ignores the scientific evidence.

Our Smoking Society

In 1991, the Youth Risk Assessment Survey (YRAS), which includes only middle and high school students, indicated that 27.5 percent of teenagers smoked; by 2001, 28.5 percent were current smokers. The most recent survey of adolescent smokers has shown a downward trend from the 1999 peak (Figure 13.2). Currently, the percentage of teenage males and females who smoke is equal, at approximately 28.5 percent.[3] The number of teenagers who become daily smokers before the age of 18 is estimated to be more than 3,000 per day. Every day another 6,000 teens under the age of 18

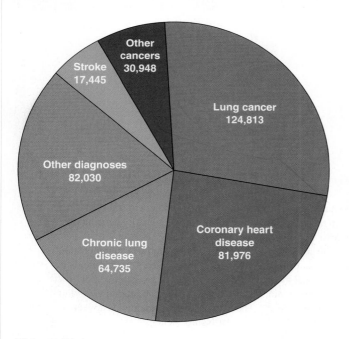

Figure 13.1
Annual Deaths Attributable to Smoking in the United States

Source: Centers for Disease Control and Prevention, "Annual Smoking-Attributable Mortality, Years of Potential Life Lost, and Economic Costs," *Morbidity and Mortality Weekly Report* 51, no. 14 (2002): 300–303.

Table 13.1
Percentage of Population That Smokes (age 18 and older) among Select Groups in the United States

	Percentage
United States overall	22.5
Race	
American Indian/Alaska Native	40.8
Asian/Pacific Islander	13.3
Black	22.4
Hispanic	16.7
White	23.6
Age	
18–24	28.5
25–44	25.7
45–64	22.7
>64	9.3
Sex	
Male	25.2
Female	20.0
Education	
>12 years	12.1
12 years	25.6
<12 years	31.0
Income Level	
Below poverty level	32.9
At or above poverty level	22.2

Source: Centers for Disease Control, "Cigarette Smoking Among Adults—United States 2002," *Morbidity and Mortality Weekly Report* 53, no. 20 (2004): 427–431.

smoke their first cigarette. The increase in cigarette use is attributed in part to the ready availability of tobacco products through vending machines and the aggressive drive by tobacco companies to entice young people to smoke.

Cigarette smoking results in untold loss of human potential, with thousands of Americans dying prematurely each year. As you can see in Table 13.1, the age groups with very similar rates of smoking are the 18- to 24-year-old age group and the 25- to 44-year-old age group. While the 18- to 24-year-old age group has been heavily targeted by cigarette promotions and advertising, the 25- to 44-year-olds developed their habits as adolescents 10 to 20 years ago, when the practice of smoking was more common.

Tobacco and Social Issues

The production and distribution of tobacco products in the United States and abroad involve many political and economic issues. Tobacco-growing states derive substantial income from tobacco production, and federal, state, and local governments benefit enormously from cigarette taxes.

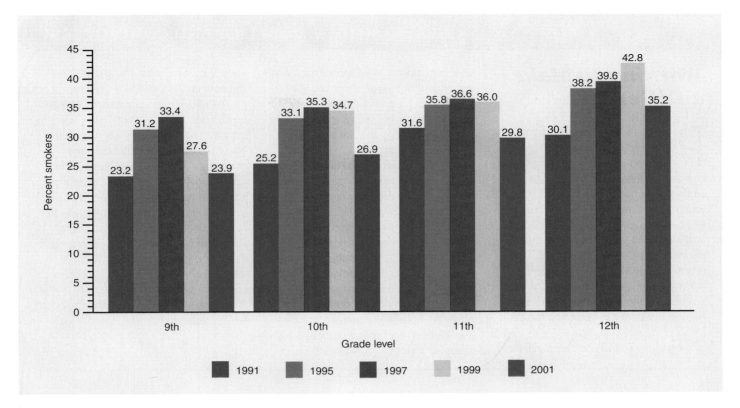

Figure 13.2
Cigarette Smoking by Grade Level

Source: Centers for Disease Control and Prevention, "Youth Risk Behavior Survey," *Morbidity and Mortality Weekly Report* 51, no. 19 (2002).

More recently, nationwide health awareness has led to a decrease in the use of tobacco products among U.S. adults. To compensate for revenue losses, many major tobacco companies have merged with or purchased other corporations that market food and beverage products and have aggressively expanded their marketing worldwide.

Advertising According to estimates, the tobacco industry spends $18 million per day on advertising and promotional materials. With the number of smokers declining by about 1 million each year, the industry must actively recruit new smokers. Campaigns are directed at all age, social, and ethnic groups, but because children and teenagers constitute 90 percent of all new smokers, much of the advertising has been directed toward them. Evidence of product recognition among underage smokers is clear: 86 percent of underage smokers prefer one of the three most heavily advertised brands—Marlboro, Newport, or Camel. One of the most blatant campaigns aimed at young adults was the popular Joe Camel ad campaign. After R. J. Reynolds introduced the cartoon figure, Camel's market share among underage smokers jumped from 3 to 13.3 percent in three years.

Advertisements in women's magazines imply that smoking is the key to financial success, independence, and

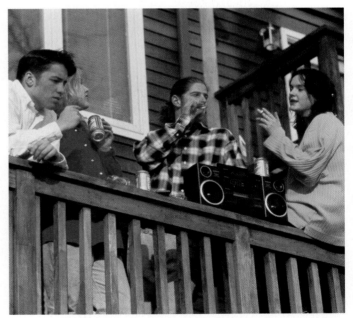

Despite all we know about the long-term effects of smoking, young people continue to put their health at risk. Why?

Working to Make a Difference

Philip Morris is the world's largest producer and marketer of consumer packaged goods and the largest food company in the nation. It is also the world's largest and most profitable tobacco corporation. To many Americans, Philip Morris, which owns Kraft Foods, is firmly linked to the more than 400,000 people in the United States and 3.4 million worldwide who die each year from smoking-related illnesses. This company has also led the way, in the United States and internationally, in spreading the tobacco epidemic, in particular to girls and women in regions where they traditionally have not smoked. In addition, Philip Morris and other tobacco companies have been convicted of lying, deliberately deceiving the public regarding the safety of tobacco, and creating and marketing a chemical addiction for profit.

However, a visit to the Philip Morris headquarters in New York paints a different picture. The company aggressively promotes its charitable work, in particular its youth smoking-prevention program. It houses the Whitney Museum exhibit of an Indian artist and sponsors the Thurgood Marshall Scholars. Furthermore, Philip Morris employees are involved in efforts to fight hunger and combat domestic violence. The company donates $60 million a year to charity and spends another $100 million in advertising to inform the public about its good deeds. The advertising campaign is a concerted strategy to improve Philip Morris's corporate image and build credibility. In addition to the advertising campaign, the company has established a speakers' bureau where top company executives go on the road to address PTA meetings and other groups about the company's charitable work.

What is a tobacco company's ethical obligation to society? Do you think Philip Morris is attempting to do the right thing, or are these initiatives a public relations effort? Consider that smokers choose to start smoking. Is it fair to blame Philip Morris if they develop tobacco-related health problems?

---

social acceptance. Many brands also have thin spokeswomen pushing "slim" and "light" cigarettes to cash in on women's fear of gaining weight. These ads have apparently been working. From the mid-1970s through early 2000s, cigarette sales to women increased dramatically. Not coincidentally, by 1987 cigarette-induced lung cancer had surpassed breast cancer as the leading cancer killer among women.

Women are not the only targets of gender-based cigarette advertisements. Males are depicted in locker rooms, charging over rugged terrain in off-road vehicles, or riding stallions into the sunset in blatant appeals to a need to feel and appear masculine. Minorities also are often targeted.

Apparently, 18- to 24-year-olds have become the new target for tobacco advertisers. The tobacco industry has set up aggressive marketing promotions at bars, music festivals, and the like, specifically targeted to this age group. Additionally, modeling and peer influence have an impact on smoking initiation. This potential impact is heightened by the fact that, although over half of campuses are considered smoke-free, they do permit smoking in residence hall rooms, student centers, and cafeterias, and many sell tobacco products in campus stores and student lounges.

See the Health Ethics box for more on the tobacco industry.

Financial Costs to Society   The use of tobacco products is costly to all of us in terms of lost productivity and lost lives. Estimates show that tobacco use caused over $157 billion in annual health-related economic losses from 1995 to 1999. The economic burden of tobacco use totaled more than $75.5 billion in medical expenditures (these costs include hospital, physician, and nursing home expenditures; prescription drugs; and home health care expenditures) and $89.1 billion in indirect costs (absenteeism, added cost of fire insurance, training costs to replace employees who die prematurely, disability payments, and so on). The economic costs of smoking are estimated to be about $3,391 per smoker per year.[4]

College Students and Smoking

College students are especially vulnerable when they are placed in a new, often stressful social and academic environment. For many, the college years are their initial taste of freedom from parental supervision. Smoking may begin earlier, but most university students are a part of the significant age group in which people start smoking and become hooked.

Cigarette smoking among U.S. college students increased by 32 percent between 1991 and 1999. In 1999, researchers surveyed more than 14,000 students from 119 U.S. colleges. This poll took into account all types of tobacco use, including cigars, smokeless tobacco, and pipe smoking, as well as cigarettes. Researchers found that more than 60 percent of college students had tried some tobacco product. One-third of students had used tobacco in the month before the study, and just under half had used tobacco in the past year; however, they did not consider themselves "smokers." Among current smokers, the survey found a wide range of smoking behaviors: Thirty-two percent smoked less than a

Are You Nicotine Dependent?

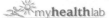

Fill out this assessment online at www.aw-bc.com/myhealthlab or www.aw-bc.com/donatelle

No one who starts smoking intends to become hooked. Imagine making a conscious decision to reduce your oxygen intake and deposit gooey tar on your lungs. It wouldn't be a very wise decision, would it? Smoking usually begins innocently enough, as an experiment or a dare or perhaps an attempt to fit in. Could you give it up right now without any problem? Or do you have a dependency? Take the following test to see.

		0 Points	1 Point	2 Points	3 Points
1.	How soon after you wake up do you smoke your first cigarette?	After 60 minutes	31–60 minutes	6–30 minutes	Within 5 minutes
2.	Do you find it difficult to refrain from smoking in places where it is forbidden?	No	Yes	—	—
3.	Which cigarette would you hate most to give up?	The first one in the morning	Any other		
4.	How many cigarettes a day do you smoke?	10 or less	11–20	21–30	31 or more
5.	Do you smoke more frequently during the first hours after awakening than during the rest of the day?	No	Yes	—	—
6.	Do you smoke if you are so ill that you are in bed most of the day?	No	Yes	—	—

INTERPRETING YOUR SCORE

If you scored over 7 points, your level of nicotine dependence is high. You and your doctor should consider various medications to help you stop smoking.

If you scored under 4 points, you probably will be able to succeed in stopping smoking without medication.

MAKE IT HAPPEN!

Use the results of this self-assessment to begin your behavior change program. Follow the steps and use the examples on page 393 to complete your Behavior Change Contract and use these resources to take action.

Source: T. F. Heatherton, L. T. Kozlowski, R. C. Frecker, K. O. Fagerstrom, "The Fagerstrom Test for Nicotine Dependence: A Revision of the Fagerstrom Tolerance Questionnaire," *British Journal of Addictions* 86 (1991): 1119–1127. Reprinted by permission of Dr. Karl Fagerstrom.

cigarette a day, while 13 percent smoked a pack or more per day. Furthermore, the study found students who used tobacco products were more likely to smoke marijuana, binge drink, have multiple sex partners, earn lower grades, rate parties as more important than academic activities, and spend more time socializing with friends.[5]

A common perception is that students do not want to stop smoking. However, a recent study reported that 70 percent of cigarette smokers had tried to quit smoking. Unfortunately, three out of four were still smokers.[6] It is important that colleges and universities engage in antismoking efforts, strictly control tobacco advertising, provide smoke-free residence halls, and offer greater access to smoking cessation programs. See the Assess Yourself box to determine whether you are dependent on tobacco.

What do you think?

Have you noticed an increase in the number of your friends who have become smokers or occasional smokers? ■ *How many of them smoked prior to coming to college, and how many picked up the habit at college?* ■ *What are their reasons for smoking?* ■ *What barriers keep your friends from quitting?*

Tobacco and Its Effects

The chemical stimulant **nicotine** is the major psychoactive substance in all tobacco products. In its natural form, nicotine is a colorless liquid that turns brown upon oxidation (removal of electrons, often by exposure to oxygen). When tobacco leaves are burned in a cigarette, pipe, or cigar, nicotine is released and inhaled into the lungs. Sucking or chewing a quid (a pinch of snuff typically tucked between the gum and lower lip) of tobacco releases nicotine into the saliva, and the nicotine is then absorbed through the mucous membranes in the mouth.

Smoking is the most common form of tobacco use. Smoking delivers a strong dose of nicotine to the user, along with an additional 4,700 chemical substances (Table 13.2). Among these chemicals are various gases and vapors that carry particulate matter in concentrations that are 500,000 times greater than those of the most air-polluted cities in the world.[7]

Particulate matter condenses in the lungs to form a thick, brownish sludge called **tar.** Tar contains various carcinogenic (cancer-causing) agents such as benzo[a]pyrene and chemical irritants such as phenol. Phenol has the potential to combine with other chemicals to contribute to the development of lung cancer.

In healthy lungs, millions of tiny hairlike tissues called cilia sweep foreign matter back toward the throat, to be expelled from the lungs by coughing. Nicotine impairs the cleansing function of the cilia by paralyzing them for up to one hour following the smoking of a single cigarette. This allows tars and other solids in tobacco smoke to accumulate and irritate sensitive lung tissue.

Tar and nicotine are not the only harmful chemicals in cigarettes. In fact, tars account for only 8 percent of tobacco smoke. The remaining 92 percent consists of various gases, the most dangerous of which is **carbon monoxide.** In tobacco smoke, the concentration of carbon monoxide is 800 times higher than the level considered safe by the U.S. Environmental Protection Agency (EPA). In the human body, carbon monoxide reduces the oxygen-carrying capacity of the red blood cells by binding with the receptor sites for oxygen. Carbon monoxide binds better than oxygen and is more difficult to remove, so carbon monoxide in the blood causes oxygen deprivation in many body tissues.

The heat from tobacco smoke, which can reach 1,616°F, is also harmful. Inhaling hot gases exposes sensitive

Nicotine   The primary stimulant chemical in tobacco products.

Tar   A thick, brownish substance condensed from particulate matter in smoked tobacco.

Carbon monoxide   A gas found in cigarette smoke that binds at oxygen receptor sites in the blood.

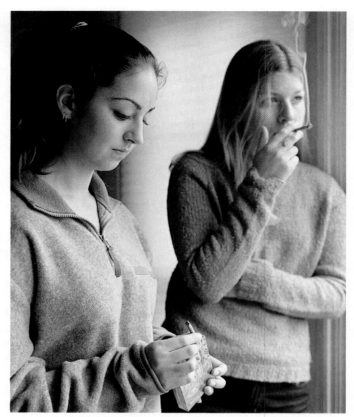

Bidis are becoming increasingly popular among teens and college students. They are equally or more dangerous to your health as cigarettes, yet they are easier to obtain.

mucous membranes to irritating chemicals that weaken the tissues and contribute to cancers of the mouth, larynx, and throat.

Tobacco Products

Tobacco comes in several forms. Cigarettes, cigars, pipes, and bidis are used for burning and inhaling tobacco. Smokeless tobacco is inhaled or placed in the mouth.

Cigarettes   Filtered cigarettes designed to reduce levels of gases such as hydrogen cyanide and hydrocarbons may actually deliver more hazardous carbon monoxide to the user than do nonfiltered brands. Some smokers use low-tar and low-nicotine products as an excuse to smoke more cigarettes. This practice is self-defeating because they wind up exposing themselves to more harmful substances than they would with regular-strength cigarettes. People smoking low-tar cigarettes also tend to inhale more often and more deeply than people smoking regular cigarettes.

Clove cigarettes contain about 40 percent ground cloves (a spice) and about 60 percent tobacco. Many users mistakenly believe that these products are made entirely of ground cloves and that smoking them eliminates the risks associated with tobacco. In fact, clove cigarettes contain higher levels of

Table 13.2
What's in Cigarette Smoke?

Cigarette smoke contains more than 4,000 chemicals, including these:

Cancer-Causing Agents	Metals		Other Chemicals
Benzo[a]pyrene	Aluminum	Acetic acid (vinegar)	Hydrogen cyanide (gas chamber poison)
beta-Naphthylamine	Copper	Acetone (nail polish remover)	Methane (swamp gas)
Cadmium	Gold	Ammonia (floor/toilet cleaner)	Methanol (rocket fuel)
Crysenes	Lead	Arsenic (poison)	Naphthalene (mothballs)
Diberiz acidine	Magnesium	Butane (cigarette lighter fluid)	Nicotine (insecticide/addictive drug)
Nickel	Mercury	Cadmium (rechargeable batteries)	Nitrobenzene (gasoline additive)
Nitrosamines	Silicon	Carbon monoxide (car exhaust fumes)	Nitrous oxide phenols (disinfectant)
N-nitrosonornicotine	Silver	DDT/dieldrin (insecticides)	Stearic acid (candle wax)
PAHs*	Titanium	Ethanol (alcohol)	Toluene (industrial solvent)
Polonium 210	Zinc	Formaldehyde (preserver of body tissue and fabric)	Vinyl chloride (makes PVC)
Toluidine		Hexamine (barbecue lighter)	

*PAH = polycyclic aromatic hydrocarbon

tar, nicotine, and carbon monoxide than do regular cigarettes. In addition, the numbing effect of eugenol, the active ingredient in cloves, allows smokers to inhale the smoke more deeply.

Cigars Those big stogies that we see celebrities and government figures puffing on these days are nothing more than tobacco fillers wrapped in more tobacco. Since 1991, cigar sales in the United States have increased dramatically. The fad, especially popular among young men and women, is fueled in part by the willingness of celebrities to be photographed puffing on one. Among some women, cigar smoking symbolizes an impulse to be slightly outrageous and liberated. Many people believe that cigars are safer than cigarettes, when in fact nothing could be further from the truth.[8] Cigar smoke contains 23 poisons and 43 carcinogens. As shown in Table 13.3, any argument about the safety of cigars is, well, a smokescreen.

Smoking as little as one cigar per day can increase the risk of several cancers, including cancer of the oral cavity (lip, tongue, mouth, and throat), esophagus, larynx, and lungs. Daily cigar smoking, especially for people who inhale the smoke, also increases the risk of heart disease (cigar smokers double their risk of heart attack and stroke) and a type of lung disease known as chronic obstructive pulmonary disease (COPD). Former president Bill Clinton, a regular cigar smoker, recently underwent quadruple bypass surgery necessitated in part due to his habit. Smoking one or two cigars daily doubles the risk for oral cancers and esophageal cancer, compared with the risk for someone who has never smoked. The risks increase with the number of cigars smoked per day.

Table 13.3
Comparing Cigarettes and Cigars

	Filter Cigarette	Regular Cigar
Weight	Approx. 0.68 g	Approx. 0.8 g
Nicotine	0.5–1.4 mg	1.7–5.2 mg
Tar	0.5–18 mg	16–110 mg
Carbon monoxide	0.5–18 mg	90–120 mg

Source: Downloaded from www.ymn.org, "No Such Thing as a Safe Smoke!" (1998). Reprinted by permission of Youth Media Network.

A common question is whether cigars are addictive. Most cigars contain as much nicotine as several cigarettes, and nicotine is highly addictive. When cigar smokers inhale the smoke, nicotine is absorbed as rapidly as it is with cigarettes. For those who don't inhale, nicotine is still absorbed through the mucous membranes in the mouth.

Bidis Bidis are small hand-rolled, flavored cigarettes, generally made in India or Southeast Asia. They come in a variety of flavors, such as vanilla, chocolate, and cherry, and cost $2 to $4 for a pack of 20. Bidis resemble a marijuana joint or a clove cigarette and have become increasingly popular with college students, who view them as safer, cheaper, and easier to obtain than cigarettes. However, they are far more toxic

Bidis Hand-rolled flavored cigarettes.

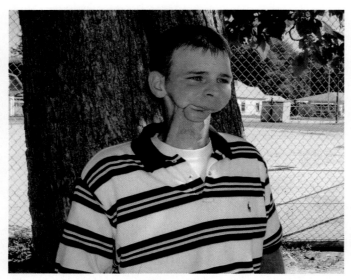

This 25-year-old cancer survivor has undergone almost 30 disfiguring surgeries. One operation removed half his neck muscles, lymph nodes, and tongue. He first tried smokeless tobacco at age 13; by age 17, he was diagnosed with squamous cell carcinoma. He now speaks out about the dangers of smokeless tobacco.

who are often emulating a professional sports figure or family member. There are two types of smokeless tobacco—chewing tobacco and snuff.

Chewing tobacco is placed between the gums and teeth for sucking or chewing. It comes in three forms: loose leaf, plug, or twist. Chewing tobacco contains tobacco leaves treated with molasses and other flavorings. The user places a "quid" of tobacco in the mouth between the teeth and gums and then sucks or chews the quid to release the nicotine. Once the quid becomes ineffective, the user spits it out and inserts another. **Dipping** is another method of using chewing tobacco. The dipper takes a small amount of tobacco and places it between the lower lip and teeth to stimulate the flow of saliva and release the nicotine. Dipping releases nicotine rapidly into the bloodstream.

Snuff is a finely ground form of tobacco that can be inhaled, chewed, or placed against the gums. It comes in dry or moist powdered form or sachets (tea bag–like pouches). Usually snuff is placed inside the cheek.

Smokeless tobacco is just as addictive as cigarettes because of its nicotine content. There is nicotine in all tobacco products, but smokeless tobacco contains even more than cigarettes. Holding an average-sized dip or chew in the mouth for 30 minutes delivers as much nicotine as smoking four cigarettes. A two-can-a-week snuff dipper gets as much nicotine as a one-and-a-half-pack-a-day smoker. Smokeless tobacco contains 10 times the amount of cancer-producing substances found in cigarettes and 100 times more than the U.S. Food and Drug Administration allows in foods and other substances used by the public.

A major risk of chewing tobacco is **leukoplakia,** a condition characterized by leathery white patches inside the mouth that are produced by contact with irritants in tobacco juice. Between 3 and 17 percent of diagnosed leukoplakia cases develop into oral cancer.

It is estimated that 75 percent of the 28,260 oral cancer cases in 2003 resulted from either smokeless tobacco or cigarettes.[10] Users of smokeless tobacco are 50 times more likely to develop oral cancers than are nonusers. Warning signs include lumps in the jaw or neck; color changes or lumps inside the lips; white, smooth, or scaly patches in the mouth or on the neck, lips, or tongue; a red spot or sore on the lips or gums or inside the mouth that does not heal in two weeks; repeated bleeding in the mouth; and difficulty or abnormality in speaking or swallowing.

The lag time between first use and contracting cancer is shorter for smokeless tobacco users than for smokers because absorption through the gums is the most efficient route of nicotine administration. A growing body of evidence suggests that long-term use of smokeless tobacco also increases the risk of cancer of the larynx, esophagus, nasal cavity, pancreas, kidney, and bladder. Moreover, many smokeless tobacco users eventually "graduate" to cigarettes and further increase their risk for developing additional problems.

The stimulant effects of nicotine may create the same circulatory and respiratory problems for chewers as for

than cigarettes. A study by the Massachusetts Department of Health found that bidis produced three times more carbon monoxide and nicotine and five times more tar than cigarettes. The tendu leaf wrappers are nonporous, meaning that smokers have to pull harder to inhale and inhale more often to keep the bidi lit. During testing, it took an average of 28 puffs to smoke a bidi, compared to only 9 puffs for a regular cigarette. This results in much more exposure to the higher amounts of tar, nicotine, and carbon monoxide, and bidis lack any sort of filter to lessen the levels. Research clearly indicates that bidi smokers are at the same, if not higher, risk for coronary heart disease and cancer due to smoking.[9]

Smokeless Tobacco   Approximately 5 million U.S. adults use smokeless tobacco. Most of them are teenage (20 percent of male high school students) and young adult males,

---

Chewing tobacco   A stringy type of tobacco that is placed in the mouth and then sucked or chewed.

Dipping   Placing a small amount of chewing tobacco between the lower lip and front teeth for rapid nicotine absorption.

Snuff   A powdered form of tobacco that is sniffed and absorbed through the mucous membranes in the nose or placed inside the cheek and sucked.

Leukoplakia   A condition characterized by leathery white patches inside the mouth; produced by contact with irritants in tobacco juice.

A Sweet but Deadly Addiction in India

Promoted by a slick advertising campaign, *gutka*, an indigenous form of smokeless tobacco, has become a fixture in the mouths of millions of Indians over the last two decades. It has spread through the subcontinent and even to South Asians in England. But what prompts particular concern is the popularity that gutka—as portable as chewing gum and sometimes as sweet as candy—has gained during the last ten years with Indian children.

Young people have become gutka consumers in large numbers, and they have become an alarming avant-garde in what doctors say is an oral cancer epidemic.

That, among other factors, has prompted the state of Mahārāshtra, which includes Bombay, to take an unusual step. It enacted a five-year ban, the longest permitted by law, on the production, sale, transport and possession of gutka, a $30 million business in the state. The ban started in 2002, but gutka is still available on the black market. Several other states have undertaken similar bans, although some have been stayed by the courts, leaving Mahārāshtra one of the few states to implement a ban.

It is easy, on the streets of Bombay, to find young men like Raga Vendra, a 19-year-old railway worker who began using gutka at age 11. It is also easy to find gutka sellers, like Ahmed Maqsood, who say they have had customers as young as 6.

Dr. Surendra Shastri, the head of preventive oncology at Tata Memorial Hospital, noticed about five years ago that his patients were getting younger, by about eight to ten years. "High school and college students were coming in with precancerous lesions," he says. "Usage was starting much earlier."

India has 75,000 to 80,000 new cases of oral cancer a year—the world's highest incidence—and about 2,000 deaths a day are tobacco related.

A 1998 survey of 1,800 boys ages 13 to 15 from a wide range of socioeconomic groups found that up to 20 percent were already using three to five packets of gutka daily. The price is low: sometimes less than two cents a packet. The contents, a mixture of ingredients including tobacco, are usually placed inside the cheek, savored, then expelled.

Gutka was the product of a packaging revolution that made an Indian tradition portable and cheap. Many Indians have long chewed *paan*, a betel leaf wrapped around a mixture of lime paste, spices, areca nut, and often tobacco. But obtaining paan required a visit to a *paanwallah*—it was too messy to be transported.

All of that changed with gutka, a dried version of the concoction minus the betel leaf, preserved and perfumed with chemicals and sealed in a plastic or foil pack. Gutka could be used at will, at work or at home or at school, and it was used, in very large quantities. Sales of gutka and its tobacco-less counterpart, paan masala, are now more than $1 billion a year, having quintupled during the past decade.

"What caused this boom of oral cancers was this packaging of tobacco," says

Dr. A. K. D'Cruz, the lead head-and-neck surgeon at Tata Memorial Hospital. "Convenience got them hooked."

Many consumers say they welcome the ban because they see no other way to curb their addiction. Even some vendors like Mr. Maqsood have embraced it, saying they felt they were trading in toxins. "The chemicals used in gutka were poisonous," he says. "I have seen some customers who can't open their mouth."

Doctors view gutka as particularly insidious because it is inexpensive and contains many unhealthful additives such as magnesium carbonate. For children and teenagers, smoking cigarettes remains taboo. Gutka has no social stigma among peers, and it is easy to hide from parents.

Padmini Samini, who started an anti-tobacco advocacy group after her father developed oral cancer, knows of gutka makers who give free samples to children after school. Sometimes it is sweetened to mask the harsh tobacco taste, until the children consider it candy.

About 30 percent of the cancers in India are located in the head and neck, compared with 4.5 percent in the West. Furthermore, Dr. D'Cruz adds, "Most of our cancers come a decade earlier than the West." They occur in the cheek and jaw, often preceded by submucosal fibrosis, a hardening of the palate that can make it almost impossible to open the mouth.

Source: A. Waldman, "Sweet but Deadly Addiction Is Seizing the Young in India," *The New York Times,* August 13, 2002. Copyright 2002 by The New York Times Co. Reprinted by permission.

smokers. Chronic smokeless tobacco use also delays wound healing and promotes peptic ulcers.

Like smoked tobacco, smokeless tobacco impairs the senses of taste and smell, causing the user to add salt and sugar to food, which may contribute to high blood pressure and obesity. Some smokeless tobacco products contain high levels of sodium (salt), which also promotes high blood pressure. Dental problems are common among users of smoke-less tobacco. Contact with tobacco juice causes receding gums, tooth decay, bad breath, and discolored teeth. Damage to both the teeth and jawbone can contribute to early loss of teeth. Users of any tobacco products may not be able to absorb the vitamins and other nutrients in food effectively.

See the Health in a Diverse World box to read about the development of a new form of smokeless tobacco.

What do you think?

Should smokeless tobacco be banned in all venues that also ban smoking? ■ *What is attractive about the use of smokeless tobacco?* ■ *Why do you think that it is popular with many athletes and males?*

Physiological Effects of Nicotine

Nicotine is a powerful central nervous system stimulant that produces a variety of physiological effects. In the cerebral cortex, its stimulant action produces an aroused, alert mental state. Nicotine also stimulates the adrenal glands, increasing the production of adrenaline. The physical effects of nicotine stimulation include increased heart and respiratory rate, constricted blood vessels, and subsequent increased blood pressure because the heart must work harder to pump blood through the narrowed vessels.

Nicotine decreases blood sugar levels and the stomach contractions that signal hunger. These factors, along with decreased sensation in the taste buds, reduce appetite. For this reason, many smokers eat less than nonsmokers do and weigh, on average, seven pounds less than nonsmokers.

Beginning smokers usually feel the effects of nicotine with their first puff. These symptoms, called **nicotine poisoning,** include dizziness, lightheadedness, rapid and erratic pulse, clammy skin, nausea, vomiting, and diarrhea. The effects of nicotine poisoning cease as soon as tolerance to the chemical develops. Medical research indicates that tolerance develops almost immediately in new users, perhaps after the second or third cigarette. In contrast, tolerance to most other drugs, such as alcohol, develops over a period of months or years. Regular smokers often do not experience the "buzz" of smoking. They continue to smoke simply because stopping is too difficult.

Tobacco Addiction

Smoking is a complicated behavior. Somewhere between 60 and 80 percent of people have tried or taken at least a puff on a cigarette. Why is it that some walk away from cigarettes while most get hooked? For one thing, smoking is a very efficient drug delivery system. It gets the drug to the brain in just a few seconds, much faster than it would travel if injected. A pack-a-day smoker experiences 300 "hits," or

Nicotine poisoning   Symptoms often experienced by beginning smokers, including dizziness, diarrhea, lightheadedness, rapid and erratic pulse, clammy skin, nausea, and vomiting.

Pairings   Paired associations (such as coffee and a cigarette) that trigger cravings.

pairings, a day, or 109,500 pairings per year. In pairing, an environmental cue triggers a craving for nicotine.[11] Simple pairings, such as drinking a cup of coffee, sitting in a car, finishing a meal, or sipping a beer, induce nicotine craving. Even college students who only smoke occasionally can find it hard to quit because of these paired associations. The brain gets used to these pairings and cries out in displeasure when the association is missing. It is easy to see how stopping even occasional use can be very difficult.

Why does this association occur? One explanation might lie in a person's genes. Two different twin studies found genetic factors to be more influential than environmental factors in smoking initiation and nicotine dependence. Two specific genes may influence smoking behavior by affecting the action of the brain chemical dopamine.[12] Understanding the influence of genetics on nicotine addiction will be crucial to developing more effective treatments for smoking cessation.

What do you think?

Because nicotine is highly addictive, should it be regulated as a controlled substance? ■ *How could tobacco be regulated effectively?* ■ *Should more resources be used for research into nicotine addiction? Why or why not?*

Health Hazards of Smoking

Cigarette smoking adversely affects the health of every person who smokes. Each day cigarettes contribute to over 1,000 deaths from cancer, cardiovascular disease, and respiratory disorders.

Cancer

The American Cancer Society estimates that tobacco smoking causes 85 to 90 percent of all cases of lung cancer—fewer than 10 percent of these cases occur among nonsmokers.[13] Lung cancer is the leading cause of cancer deaths in the United States. There were an estimated 173,700 *new* cases of lung cancer in the United States in 2004 alone, and an estimated 160,440 Americans died of the disease in 2004.[14] Figure 13.3 illustrates how tobacco smoke damages the lungs.

Lung cancer can take 10 to 30 years to develop, and the outlook for its victims is poor. Most lung cancer is not diagnosed until it is fairly widespread in the body; at that point, the five-year survival rate is only 13 percent. When a malignancy is diagnosed and recognized while still localized, the five-year survival rate rises to 47 percent. If you are a smoker, your risk of developing lung cancer depends on several factors. First, the number of cigarettes you smoke per day is important. Someone who smokes two packs a day is 15 to 25 times more likely to develop lung cancer than a

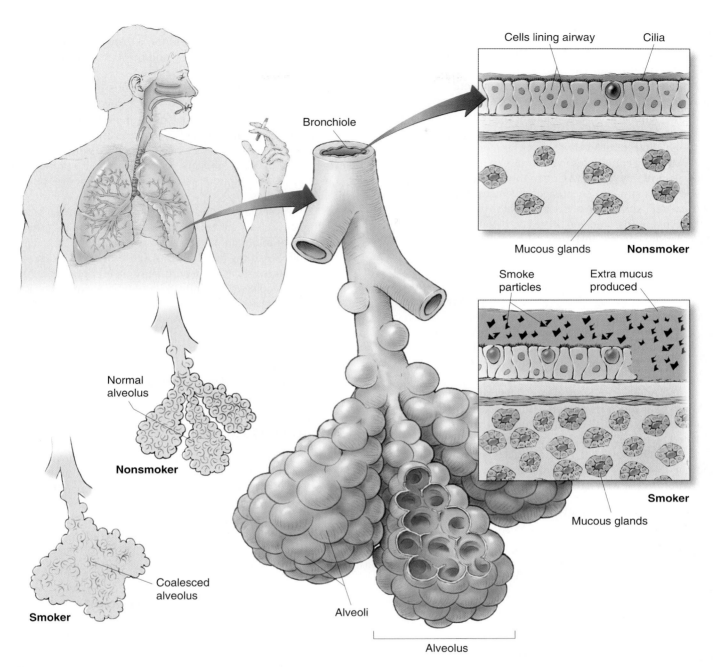

Figure 13.3

How Cigarette Smoking Damages the Lungs

Smoke particles irritate the lung pathways, which causes mucus production. They also indirectly destroy the walls of the lungs' alveoli, which coalesce. Both factors reduce lung efficiency. In addition, tar in tobacco smoke has a direct cancer-causing action.

nonsmoker. If you started smoking in your teens, you have a greater chance of developing lung cancer than people who started later. If you inhale deeply when you smoke, you also increase your chances. Occupational or domestic exposure to other irritants, such as asbestos and radon, will also increase your likelihood of developing lung cancer.

Tobacco is linked to other cancers as well. The rate of pancreatic cancer is more than twice as high for smokers as

nonsmokers. Typically, people diagnosed with pancreatic cancer live about 3 months after their diagnosis. Smokers can reduce those odds by 30 percent if they quit for 11 years or more.[15] Cancers of the lip, tongue, salivary glands, and esophagus are five times more likely to occur among smokers than among nonsmokers. Smokers are also more likely to develop kidney, bladder, and larynx cancers.

Cardiovascular Disease

Half of all tobacco-related deaths occur as a result of some form of heart disease.[16] Smokers have a 70 percent higher death rate from heart disease than nonsmokers do, and heavy smokers have a 200 percent higher death rate than moderate smokers. In fact, smoking cigarettes poses as great a risk for developing heart disease as high blood pressure and high cholesterol levels do.

Smoking contributes to heart disease by adding the equivalent of ten years of aging to the arteries.[17] One explanation is that smoking encourages atherosclerosis, the buildup of fatty deposits in the heart and major blood vessels. For unknown reasons, smoking decreases blood levels of HDLs (high-density lipoproteins), the "good" cholesterol that helps protect against heart attacks. Smoking also contributes to **platelet adhesiveness,** the sticking together of red blood cells that is associated with blood clots. The oxygen deprivation associated with smoking decreases the oxygen supplied to the heart and can weaken tissues. Smoking also contributes to irregular heart rhythms, which can trigger a heart attack. Both carbon monoxide and nicotine in cigarette smoke can precipitate angina attacks (pain spasms in the chest when the heart muscle does not get the blood supply it needs).

The number of years a person has smoked does not seem to bear much relation to cardiovascular risk. If a person quits smoking, the risk of dying from a heart attack is reduced by half after only one year without smoking and declines steadily thereafter. After about 15 years without smoking, the ex-smoker's risk of cardiovascular disease is similar to that of people who have never smoked.

Stroke Smokers are twice as likely to suffer strokes as nonsmokers are. A stroke occurs when a small blood vessel in the brain bursts or is blocked by a blood clot, denying oxygen and nourishment to vital portions of the brain. Depending on the area of the brain supplied by the vessel, stroke can result in paralysis, loss of mental function, or death. Smoking contributes to strokes by raising blood pressure, thereby increasing the stress on vessel walls. Platelet adhesiveness contributes to clotting. However, 5 to 15 years after they stop smoking, the risk of stroke for ex-smokers is the same as that for people who have never smoked.

Respiratory Disorders

Smoking quickly impairs the respiratory system. Smokers can feel its impact in a relatively short period of time—they are more prone to breathlessness, chronic cough, and excess phlegm than nonsmokers their age. Smokers tend to miss work one-third more often than nonsmokers do, primarily because of respiratory diseases, and they are up to 18 times more likely to die of lung disease.

Chronic bronchitis is the presence of a productive cough that persists or recurs frequently. It may develop in smokers because their inflamed lungs produce more mucus and constantly try to rid themselves of this mucus and foreign particles. This results in "smoker's hack," the persistent cough experienced by most smokers. Smokers are more prone than nonsmokers to respiratory ailments such as influenza, pneumonia, and colds.

Emphysema is a chronic disease in which the alveoli (the tiny air sacs in the lungs) are destroyed, impairing the lungs' ability to obtain oxygen and remove carbon dioxide. As a result, breathing becomes difficult. Whereas healthy people expend only about 5 percent of their energy in breathing, people with advanced emphysema expend nearly 80 percent of their energy. A simple movement such as rising from a seated position becomes painful and difficult for the emphysema patient. Since the heart has to work harder to do even the simplest tasks, it may become enlarged, and the person may die from heart damage. There is no known cure for emphysema. Approximately 80 percent of all cases are related to cigarette smoking.

Sexual Dysfunction

Despite attempts by tobacco advertisers to make smoking appear sexy, research shows just the opposite: it can cause impotence in men. A number of recent studies have found that male smokers are about two times more likely than nonsmokers to suffer from some form of impotence. Toxins in cigarette smoke damage blood vessels, reducing blood flow to the penis and leading to an inadequate erection. It is thought that impotence could indicate oncoming cardiovascular disease.

Other Health Effects of Smoking

Gum disease is three times more common among smokers than among nonsmokers, and smokers lose significantly more teeth.[18] Nicotine and the other ingredients in cigarettes also interfere with the metabolism of drugs: nicotine speeds up the process by which the body uses and eliminates drugs, so that medications become less effective. There are also health effects of special concern to women (see the Women's Health/Men's Health box).

Platelet adhesiveness   Stickiness of red blood cells associated with blood clots.

Emphysema   A chronic lung disease in which the tiny air sacs in the lungs are destroyed, making breathing difficult.

What do you think?

Most people are very aware of the long-term hazards associated with tobacco use, yet despite prevention efforts, people continue to smoke. Why do you think this is so? ■ *What strategies might be effective to reduce the number of people who begin smoking?*

Women and Smoking

For more than 50 years, tobacco company advertisements have enticed women to smoke cigarettes. Though their messages have glamorized smoking, the real-life results are not glamorous at all: women who smoke have an increased risk of developing cancer, heart disease, and problems associated with the reproductive organs. The risk of cervical cancer, for instance, is higher among women who smoke than among those who don't. A woman reduces her risk dramatically when she quits.

According to a recent study, cigarettes are even more dangerous for women than for men; women are more likely to develop lung cancer and to do so with fewer cigarettes. Already lung cancer deaths have surpassed breast cancer deaths for women. The risk of heart disease for women smokers who smoke more than 25 cigarettes per day is 500 percent higher than it is for nonsmokers. Even smoking one to four cigarettes per day doubles a woman's risk for heart attack. It makes no difference if she smokes low- or high-nicotine cigarettes.

Smoking appears to send women into menopause one to two years early. (Smokers who quit start menopause at about the same age as women who have never smoked.) Smoking also contributes to osteoporosis, a condition involving bone loss that particularly afflicts women. Current female smokers age 35 and older are more than ten times as likely to die of emphysema or chronic bronchitis than male smokers.

Women smokers who take birth control pills greatly increase their risk of heart attack. In a recent study, the risk for a heart attack was shown to be 20 times higher for pill users who smoked ten or more cigarettes per day than it was for women who did not smoke and did not use the pill. Oral contraceptives increase the risk of developing blood clots, which can block the already narrowing arteries of women with atherosclerosis, another disease with an increased risk for smokers. Smoking while taking oral contraceptives also increases the risk of peripheral vascular disease and stroke.

Although cigarette smoking is dangerous for all women, it presents special risks for pregnant women and their fetuses. Each year in the United States, approximately 50,000 miscarriages are attributed to smoking during pregnancy. On average, babies born to mothers who smoke weigh less than those born to nonsmokers, and low birth weight is correlated with many developmental problems. Pregnant women who stop smoking in the first three or four months of their pregnancies give birth to higher–birth weight babies than do women who smoke throughout their pregnancies. Prenatal exposure to smoking has been linked with impairments in memory, learning, cognition, and perception in the growing child. Infant mortality rates are also higher among babies born to smokers.

Maternal smoking has long been linked to increased risk of sudden infant death syndrome (SIDS). SIDS, or "crib death," occurs when an infant, usually less than one year of age, dies during its sleep for no apparent reason. The more the mother smokes, the greater the risk. Passive smoke has also been associated with SIDS. This risk is increased in normal-weight infants, about twofold with passive smoke exposure, and about threefold when the mother smokes both during the pregnancy and after the baby is born. Infants who are born to mothers who smoke during pregnancy have more episodes of apnea and excessive sweating. It has been suggested that smoking may influence the development of the infant's nervous system.

One study found that daughters of women who smoked during pregnancy are four times more likely to begin smoking during adolescence and to continue smoking than the daughters of nonsmoking women. The study suggests that nicotine, which crosses the placental barrier, may affect the fetus during an important period of development so as to predispose the brain to the addictive influence of nicotine more than a decade later.

Sources: "Tobacco Smoke and Women: A Special Vulnerability?" *Harvard Women's Health Watch,* May 2000, 1; WHO Collaborative Study of Cardiovascular Disease and Steroid Hormone Contraception, "Acute Myocardial Infarction and Combined Oral Contraceptives: Results of an International Multicentre Case-Control Study," *The Lancet* April 26, 1997, 1202–1209; "Nicotine Conference Highlights Research Accomplishments and Challenges," *NIDA Notes,* September/October 1995, 11–12; "Women and Smoking: A Report of the Surgeon General, Executive Summary," *Morbidity and Mortality Weekly Report,* 51 (August 30, 2002): 1–30.

Environmental Tobacco Smoke (ETS)

Although fewer than 30 percent of Americans are smokers, air pollution from smoking in public places continues to be a problem. **Environmental tobacco smoke (ETS)** is divided into two categories: mainstream and sidestream smoke (commonly called secondhand smoke). **Mainstream smoke** refers to smoke drawn through tobacco while inhaling; **secondhand smoke** refers to smoke from the burning end

Environmental tobacco smoke (ETS) Smoke from tobacco products, including secondhand and mainstream smoke.

Mainstream smoke Smoke that is drawn through tobacco while inhaling.

Secondhand smoke (sidestream smoke) The cigarette, pipe, or cigar smoke breathed by nonsmokers.

of a cigarette or smoke exhaled by a smoker. People who breathe smoke from someone else's smoking product are said to be *involuntary*, or *passive*, smokers. Nearly nine out of ten nonsmoking Americans are exposed to environmental tobacco smoke.

Risks from ETS

Although involuntary smokers breathe less tobacco than active smokers do, they still face risks from exposure to tobacco smoke. Secondhand smoke actually contains more carcinogenic substances than the smoke that a smoker inhales. According to the American Lung Association, secondhand smoke has about 2 times more tar and nicotine, 5 times more carbon monoxide, and 50 times more ammonia than mainstream smoke. Every year, ETS is estimated to be responsible for approximately 3,000 lung cancer deaths, 35,000 cardiovascular disease deaths, and 13,000 deaths from other cancers.[19] The Environmental Protection Agency (EPA) has designated secondhand tobacco smoke a *group A cancer-causing agent* that is even worse than other group A threats such as benzene, arsenic, and radon. There is also evidence that secondhand smoke poses an even greater risk for death due to heart disease than for death due to lung cancer.[20]

Secondhand smoke is estimated to cause more deaths per year than any other environmental pollutant. The risk of dying because of exposure to passive smoking is 100 times greater than the risk that requires the EPA to label a pollutant as carcinogenic and 10,000 times greater than the risk that requires the labeling of a food as carcinogenic.[21]

Lung cancer and heart disease are not the only dangers involuntary smokers face. Exposure to ETS among children increases their risk of infections of the lower respiratory tract. An estimated 300,000 children are at greater risk of pneumonia and bronchitis as a result.[22] Children exposed to secondhand smoke have a greater chance of developing other respiratory problems such as coughing, wheezing, asthma, and chest colds, along with a decrease in lung function. The greatest effects of secondhand smoke are seen in children under the age of five. Children exposed to secondhand smoke daily in the home miss 33 percent more school days and have 10 percent more colds and acute respiratory infections than those not exposed.

A recent study found that 31.2 percent of children are exposed to cigarette smoke daily in the home. This study found wide regional, income, and education differences: children of high-income, high-education-level parents in California are exposed far less than are children of low-income, low-education-level parents in the Midwest.[23]

Cigarette, cigar, and pipe smoke in enclosed areas presents other hazards. Ten to 15 percent of nonsmokers are extremely sensitive (hypersensitive) to cigarette smoke. These people experience itchy eyes, difficulty in breathing, painful headaches, nausea, and dizziness in response to minute amounts of smoke. The level of carbon monoxide in cigarette smoke contained in enclosed places is 4,000 times higher than that allowed in the clean air standard recommended by the EPA.

Efforts to reduce the hazards associated with passive smoking have gained momentum in recent years. Groups such as GASP (Group Against Smokers' Pollution) and ASH (Action on Smoking and Health) have been working since the early 1970s to reduce smoking in public places. In response to their efforts, some 44 states have enacted laws restricting smoking in public places such as restaurants, theaters, and airports. The federal government has restricted smoking in all government buildings. Hotels and motels now set aside rooms for nonsmokers, and car rental agencies designate certain vehicles for nonsmokers. Since 1990, smoking has been banned on all domestic and many international flights.

What do you think?

What rights, if any, should smokers have with regard to smoking in public places? ■ *Does your campus allow smoking in residence halls?* ■ *Does your community have nonsmoking restaurants, or does it only have nonsmoking sections?* ■ *Do you think your community would support non-smoking restaurants and bars? Why or why not?*

Tobacco and Politics

It has been nearly 40 years since the government began warning that tobacco use was hazardous to the health of the nation. Today the tobacco industry is under fire—46 states have sued to recover health care costs related to treating smokers.

In 1998, the tobacco industry reached a Master's Settlement Agreement with these states. Key provisions include the following:

- The tobacco payments will total approximately $206 billion to be paid over 25 years nationwide.
- The industry will pay $1.5 billion over ten years to support antismoking measures, including education and advertising. An additional $250 million will fund research to determine the most effective ways to stop kids from smoking.
- The industry is barred from billboard advertising, including advertisements on transit systems. In-store ads are still permitted but will be limited in size.
- All outdoor advertising is banned, including billboards, signs, and placards larger than a poster in arenas, stadiums, shopping malls, and video arcades.
- The agreement bans youth access to free samples, proof-of-purchase gifts, and sale and distribution of "branded" merchandise, such as T-shirts, hats, and other items bearing tobacco brand names or logos.
- There is a ban on the use of cartoon characters in advertising. (Such advertising is considered particularly appealing to young children.)

- Tobacco company sponsorship of concerts, athletic events, or any event in which a significant portion of the audience is young people is forbidden.
- The industry agreed not to market cigarettes to children and not to misrepresent the health effects of cigarettes.

However, funds from the settlement that were supposed to add a strong kick to antismoking initiatives have had trouble doing so. The majority of the funding, $8.7 billion in 2003 alone, is not being spent on anything related to smoking; facing budget woes, many states have drastically cut spending on antismoking programs.[24]

Many states and communities are advocating stricter tobacco control. A number of states have imposed extra taxes on cigarette sales in an effort to discourage use. The monies are then used for various purposes, including prevention and cessation programs and school health programs. Two community-based programs, ASSIST (American Stop Smoking Intervention Study) and IMPACT (Initiatives to Mobilize for the Prevention and Control of Tobacco Use), are tobacco control initiatives focused on creating legislation to prohibit the sale of tobacco to minors and to assist with enforcement.

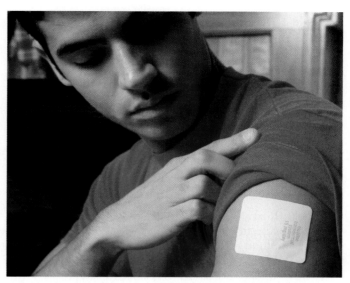

Among the products available for people trying to quit tobacco use are nicotine replacement products such as patches, inhalers, and gum. Nevertheless, most smokers succeed by going "cold turkey."

Quitting

Quitting smoking isn't easy. Smokers must break the physical addiction to nicotine—and they must break the habit of lighting up at certain times of the day.

From what we know about successful quitters, quitting is often a lengthy process involving several unsuccessful attempts before success is finally achieved. Even successful quitters suffer occasional slips, emphasizing the fact that stopping smoking is a dynamic process that occurs over time.

Approximately one-third of smokers attempt to quit each year. Unfortunately, 90 percent or more of those attempts fail. The person who wishes to quit smoking has several options. Most people who are successful at quitting quit "cold turkey"—that is, they decide simply not to smoke again. Over 90 percent of former smokers report that they quit by stopping or slowly decreasing the amount they smoked.[25] Others resort to short-term programs, such as those offered by the American Cancer Society, which are based on behavior modification and a system of self-rewards. Still others turn to treatment centers that are part of large franchises or a local medical clinic's community outreach plan. Finally, some people work privately with their physicians to reach their goal.

Prospective quitters must decide which method or combination of methods will work best for them. Programs that combine several approaches have shown the most promise. Financial considerations, personality characteristics, and level of addiction are all factors to consider.

Breaking the Nicotine Addiction

Nicotine addiction may be one of the toughest addictions to overcome. Smokers' attempts to quit lead to withdrawal symptoms. Symptoms of **nicotine withdrawal** include irritability, restlessness, nausea, vomiting, and intense cravings for tobacco.

Nicotine Replacement Products Nontobacco products that replace depleted levels of nicotine in the bloodstream have helped some people stop using tobacco (Table 13.4 on page 388). The two most common are nicotine chewing gum and the nicotine patch, both of which are available over the counter. The FDA has also approved a nicotine nasal spray and a nicotine inhaler.

Some patients use Nicorette, a prescription chewing gum containing nicotine, to reduce nicotine consumption over time. Under the guidance of a physician, the user chews 12 to 24 pieces of gum per day for up to six months. Nicorette delivers about as much nicotine as a cigarette does; but, because it is absorbed through the mucous membrane of the mouth, it doesn't produce the same rush. Users experience no withdrawal symptoms and fewer cravings for nicotine as the dosage is reduced until they are completely weaned.

Some controversy surrounds the use of nicotine replacement gum. Opponents believe that it substitutes one addiction for another. Successful users counter that it is a valid way to help break a deadly habit without suffering the unpleasant cravings that often lead to relapse.

The nicotine patch, first marketed in 1991, is generally used in conjunction with a comprehensive smoking-behavior

---

Nicotine withdrawal Symptoms, including nausea, headaches, and irritability, suffered by addicted smokers who cease using tobacco.

Table 13.4
Recommended Therapies for Smoking Cessation

Therapy	Duration	Approximate Cost per Day (in 2000)
Buproprion (Zyban) A nonnicotine based antidepressant, this drug can help reduce nicotine withdrawal symptoms and the urge to smoke. Some common side effects are dry mouth, difficulty sleeping, dizziness, and skin rash. Contraindicated if smoker has a history of seizures. *Availability:* Prescription only with a doctor consultation	7–12 weeks; maintenance up to 6 months; start 1–2 weeks before the quit date	$3.33
Nicotine Gum This chewing gum releases nicotine into the bloodstream through the lining of the mouth, but it might not be appropriate for people with temporomandibular joint disease or for those with dentures or other dental work. Up to 2 mg dose if less than 25 cigarettes/day; 4 mg dose if ≥ 25 cigarettes/day *Availability:* Over the counter (OTC)	Up to 12 weeks	$6.25 for 10 (2-mg pieces); $6.87 for 10 (4-mg pieces)
Nicotine Inhaler This device delivers a vaporized form of nicotine to the mouth through a mouthpiece attached to a plastic cartridge. Most of the nicotine travels to the mouth and throat, where it is absorbed through the mucous membranes. Common side effects include throat and mouth irritation and coughing. Anyone with bronchial problems should use caution. *Availability:* Prescription only with a doctor consultation	Up to 6 months	$10.94 for 10 cartridges
Nicotine Nasal Spray The spray comes in a pump bottle containing nicotine that tobacco users can inhale when they have an urge to smoke. This product is not recommended for people with nasal or sinus conditions, allergies, or asthma, nor is it recommended for young tobacco users. *Availability:* Prescription only with a doctor consultation	3–6 months	$5.40 for 12 doses
Nicotine Patch Patch supplies a steady amount of nicotine to the body through the skin, and it is sold in varying strengths as an 8-week smoking cessation treatment. Nicotine doses can be regularly lowered as the treatment progress or given as a steady dose during treatment. The nicotine patch may not be a good choice for people with skin problems or allergies to adhesive tape. *Availability:* Either OTC or by prescription with a doctor consultation	4 weeks; then 2 weeks; then 2 weeks (8 weeks total)	$4.22

Notes: This table contains brief descriptions and was adapted from published medical articles. Prices were based on retail prices at a national chain pharmacy located in Madison, Wisconsin, April 2000.

Source: "Recommended Therapies for Smoking Cessation" from American Cancer Society. *Cancer Facts and Figures 2004.* For complete data, see American Cancer Society website www.cancer.org. Used by permission of the American Cancer Society.

cessation program. A small, thin, 24-hour patch placed on the smoker's upper body delivers a continuous flow of nicotine through the skin, helping to relieve cravings. The patch is worn for 8 to 12 weeks under the guidance of a clinician. During this time, the dose of nicotine is gradually reduced until the smoker is fully weaned from the drug. Occasional side effects include mild skin irritation, insomnia, dry mouth, and nervousness. The patch costs less than a pack of cigarettes—about four dollars—and some insurance plans will pay for it.

The nasal spray, which requires a prescription, is much more powerful and delivers nicotine to the bloodstream faster than gum or the patch. Patients are warned to be careful not to overdose; as little as 40 milligrams of nicotine taken at once could be lethal. The spray is somewhat unpleasant to use. The FDA has advised that it should be used for no more than three months and never for more than six months so that smokers don't find themselves as dependent on nicotine in spray form as they were on cigarettes. The FDA also advises that no one who experiences nasal or sinus problems, allergies, or asthma should use it.

The nicotine inhaler, which also requires a prescription, consists of a mouthpiece and cartridge. By puffing on the mouthpiece, the smoker inhales air saturated with nicotine,

Developing a Plan to Kick the Habit

There is no magic cure that can help you stop. Take the first step by answering this question: Why do I want to stop smoking?

Write your reasons in the space below. Once you have prepared your list, carry a copy of it with you. Memorize it. Every time you are tempted to smoke, go over your reasons for stopping.

MY REASONS FOR STOPPING

1. _____
2. _____
3. _____
4. _____
5. _____

DEVELOP A PLAN; CHANGE SOME HABITS

Over time, smoking becomes a strong habit. Daily events such as finishing a meal, talking on the phone, drinking coffee, and chatting with friends trigger the urge to smoke. Breaking the link between the trigger and the smoking will help you stop. Think about the times and places you usually smoke. What could you do instead of smoking at those times?

THINGS TO DO INSTEAD OF SMOKING

1. _____
2. _____
3. _____

THE BOTTOM LINE: COMMIT YOURSELF

There comes a time when you have to say good-bye to your cigarettes.

- Pick a day to stop smoking.
- Fill out the Behavior Change Contract.
- Have a family member or friend sign the contract.

THEN

- Throw away all your cigarettes, lighters, and ashtrays at home and at work. You will not need them again.
- Be prepared to feel the urge to smoke. The urge will pass whether or not you smoke. Use the four Ds to fight the urge:
  Delay
  Deep breathing
  Drink water
  Do something else
- Keep "mouth toys" handy: Lifesavers, gum, straws, and carrot sticks can help.
- If you've had trouble stopping before, ask your doctor about nicotine chewing gum, patches, nasal sprays, inhalers, or pills.
- Tell your family and friends that you've stopped smoking.
- Put "no smoking" signs in your car, work area, and house.
- Give yourself a treat for stopping. Go to a movie, go out to dinner, or buy yourself a gift.

FOCUS ON THE POSITIVES

Now that you have stopped smoking, your mind and your body will begin to feel better. Think of the good things that have happened since you stopped. Can you breathe more easily? Do you have more energy? Do you feel good about what you've done?

Use the space below to list the good things about not smoking. Carry a copy with you, and look at it when you have the urge to smoke.

_____
_____
_____
_____
_____
_____

Source: From *Smart Move! A Stop Smoking Guide.* © 1996, American Cancer Society, Inc.

---

which is absorbed through the lining of the mouth, not the lungs. This nicotine enters the body much more slowly than the nicotine in cigarettes does. Using the inhaler mimics the hand-to-mouth actions used in smoking and causes the back of the throat to feel as it would when inhaling tobacco smoke. Each cartridge lasts for 80 long puffs, and each cartridge is designed for 20 minutes of use.

Approved in 1997 by the FDA, Zyban, the smoking cessation pill, offers hope to many who thought they could never quit. Zyban is thought to work on dopamine and norepinephrine receptors in the brain to decrease craving and withdrawal symptoms. Because of the way this prescription medication works, it is important to start the pills one to two weeks before the targeted quit date; it requires planning ahead.

How effective are these therapies? The evidence is strong that consistent pharmacological treatments can help a smoker quit, with estimated abstinence after use ranging from 17 to 30 percent.[26]

Breaking the Habit

For some smokers, the road to quitting includes antismoking therapy. Two common techniques are operant conditioning and self-control therapy. Pairing the act of smoking with an external stimulus is a typical example of an operant strategy. For example, one technique requires smokers to carry a timer that sounds a buzzer at different intervals. When the buzzer sounds, the patient is required to smoke a cigarette. Once the smoker is conditioned to associate the buzzer with smoking, the buzzer is eliminated, and, one hopes, so is the smoking. Self-control strategies view smoking as a learned habit associated with specific situations. Therapy is aimed at identifying these situations and teaching smokers the skills necessary to resist smoking.

The Skills for Behavior Change box presents one of the American Cancer Society's approaches.

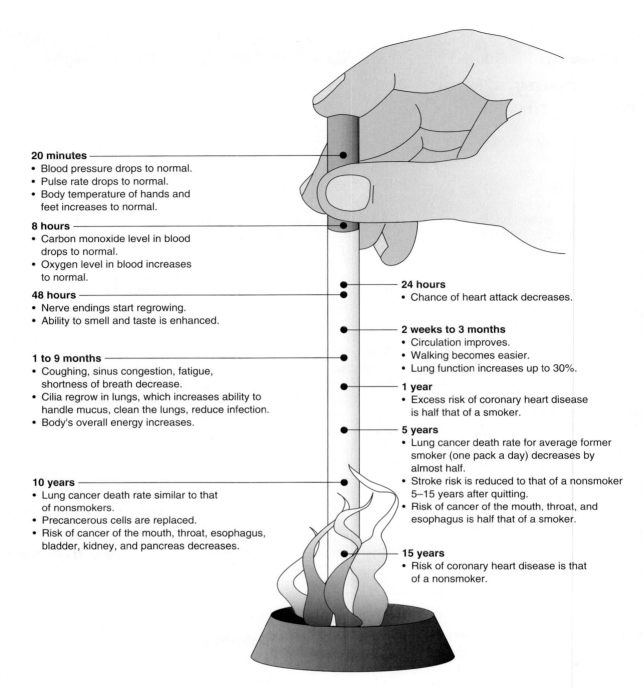

20 minutes
- Blood pressure drops to normal.
- Pulse rate drops to normal.
- Body temperature of hands and feet increases to normal.

8 hours
- Carbon monoxide level in blood drops to normal.
- Oxygen level in blood increases to normal.

48 hours
- Nerve endings start regrowing.
- Ability to smell and taste is enhanced.

1 to 9 months
- Coughing, sinus congestion, fatigue, shortness of breath decrease.
- Cilia regrow in lungs, which increases ability to handle mucus, clean the lungs, reduce infection.
- Body's overall energy increases.

10 years
- Lung cancer death rate similar to that of nonsmokers.
- Precancerous cells are replaced.
- Risk of cancer of the mouth, throat, esophagus, bladder, kidney, and pancreas decreases.

24 hours
- Chance of heart attack decreases.

2 weeks to 3 months
- Circulation improves.
- Walking becomes easier.
- Lung function increases up to 30%.

1 year
- Excess risk of coronary heart disease is half that of a smoker.

5 years
- Lung cancer death rate for average former smoker (one pack a day) decreases by almost half.
- Stroke risk is reduced to that of a nonsmoker 5–15 years after quitting.
- Risk of cancer of the mouth, throat, and esophagus is half that of a smoker.

15 years
- Risk of coronary heart disease is that of a nonsmoker.

Figure 13.4

When Smokers Quit

Within 20 minutes of smoking that last cigarette, the body begins a series of changes that continues for years. However, by smoking just one cigarette a day, the smoker loses all these benefits, according to the American Cancer Society.

Source: G. Hanson and P. Venturelli, *Drugs and Society,* 5th ed. (Sudbury, MA: Jones and Bartlett, 1998). © Jones and Bartlett, www.jbpub.com. Reprinted with permission.

Benefits of Quitting

According to the American Cancer Society, many tissues damaged by smoking can repair themselves. As soon as smokers stop, the body begins the repair process (Figure 13.4). Within eight hours, carbon monoxide and oxygen levels return to normal, and "smoker's breath" disappears. Often, within a month of quitting, the mucus that clogs airways is broken up and eliminated. Circulation and the senses of taste and smell improve within weeks. Many ex-smokers say they have more energy, sleep better, and feel more alert. By the end of one year, the risk for lung cancer and stroke decreases. In addition, ex-smokers reduce considerably their risk of developing cancers of the mouth, throat, esophagus, larynx, pancreas, bladder, and cervix. They also cut their risk of peripheral arterial disease, chronic obstructive lung disease, coronary heart disease, and ulcers. Women are less likely to bear babies with low birthweight. Within two years, the risk for heart attack drops to near normal. At the end of ten smoke-free years, the ex-smoker can expect to live out his or her normal life span.

What do you think?

Do you know people who have tried to quit smoking? ■ *What was this experience like for them?* ■ *Were they successful?* ■ *If not, what factors contributed to relapse?*

Caffeine

What is the most popular and widely consumed drug in the United States? Caffeine. Almost half of all Americans drink coffee every day, and many others use caffeine in some other form, mainly for its well-known "wake-up" effect. Drinking coffee is legal, even socially encouraged. Many people believe caffeine is not a drug and not really addictive. Coffee, soft drinks, and other caffeine-containing products seem harmless; with no cream or sugar added, many are calorie-free and therefore a good way to fill up if you are dieting. If you share these attitudes, you should think again, because research in the past decade has linked caffeine to certain health problems.

Caffeine is a drug derived from the chemical family called **xanthines.** Two related chemicals, *theophylline* and *theobromine,* are found in tea and chocolate, respectively. The xanthines are mild central nervous system stimulants that enhance mental alertness and reduce feelings of fatigue. Other stimulant effects include increased heart muscle contractions, oxygen consumption, metabolism, and urinary output. These effects are felt within 15 to 45 minutes of ingesting a product that contains caffeine.

Side effects of the xanthines include wakefulness, insomnia, irregular heartbeat, dizziness, nausea, indigestion,

Table 13.5
Caffeine Content of Various Products

Product	Caffeine Content (Average mg per Serving)
Coffee (5-oz. cup)	
Regular brewed	65–115
Decaffeinated brewed	3
Decaffeinated instant	2
Tea (6-oz. cup)	
Hot steeped	36
Iced	31
Bottled (12 oz.)	15
Soft Drinks (12-oz. servings)	
Jolt Cola	100
Dr. Pepper	61
Mountain Dew	54
Coca-Cola	46
Pepsi Cola	36–38
Chocolate	
1 oz. baking chocolate	25
1 oz. chocolate candy bar	15
½ cup chocolate pudding	4–12
Over-the-Counter Drugs	
No-Doz (2 tablets)	200
Excedrin (2 tablets)	130
Midol (2 tablets)	65
Anacin (2 tablets)	64

Source: Office of Department of Health and Welfare, October 2001.

and sometimes mild delirium. Some people also experience heartburn. As with some other drugs, the user's psychological outlook and expectations will influence the effects.

Different products contain different concentrations of caffeine. A five-ounce cup of coffee contains anywhere from 65 to 115 milligrams of caffeine. Caffeine concentrations vary with the brand of the beverage and the strength of the brew. Small chocolate bars contain up to 15 milligrams of caffeine and theobromine. Table 13.5 compares various caffeine-containing products.

Caffeine Addiction

As the effects of caffeine wear off, users may feel let down—mentally or physically depressed, exhausted, and weak. To counteract this, they commonly choose to drink another cup

---

Caffeine   A stimulant found in coffee, tea, chocolate, and some soft drinks.

Xanthines   The chemical family of stimulants to which caffeine belongs.

---

of coffee. Habitually engaging in this practice leads to tolerance and psychological dependency. Until the mid-1970s, caffeine was not medically recognized as addictive. Chronic caffeine use and its attendant behaviors were dismissed as "coffee nerves." This syndrome is now recognized as *caffeine intoxication,* or **caffeinism.**

Symptoms of caffeinism include chronic insomnia, jitters, irritability, nervousness, anxiety, and involuntary muscle twitches. Withdrawing the caffeine may compound the effects and produce severe headaches. (Some physicians ask their patients to take a simple test for caffeine addiction: don't consume anything containing caffeine, and if you get a severe headache within four hours, you are addicted.) Because caffeine meets the requirements for addiction— tolerance, psychological dependency, and withdrawal symptoms—it can be classified as addictive.

Although you would have to drink 67 to 100 cups of coffee in a day to produce a fatal overdose of caffeine, you may experience sensory disturbances after consuming only ten cups of coffee within a 24-hour period. These symptoms include tinnitus (ringing in the ears), spots before the eyes, numbness in arms and legs, poor circulation, and visual hallucinations. Because ten cups of coffee is not an extraordinary amount to drink in one day, caffeine use clearly poses health threats.

The Health Consequences of Long-Term Caffeine Use

Long-term caffeine use has been suspected of being linked to a number of serious health problems, ranging from heart disease and cancer to mental dysfunction and birth defects. However, no strong evidence exists to suggest that moderate caffeine use (less than 300 milligrams daily, approximately three cups of coffee) produces harmful effects in healthy, nonpregnant people.

It appears that caffeine does not cause long-term high blood pressure, and it has not been linked to strokes. Nor is there any evidence of a relationship between coffee and heart disease.[27] However, people who suffer from irregular heartbeat are cautioned against using caffeine because the resultant increase in heart rate might be life-threatening. Both decaffeinated and caffeinated coffee products contain ingredients that can irritate the stomach lining and be harmful to people with stomach ulcers.

For years, caffeine consumption was linked with fibrocystic breast disease, a condition characterized by painful, noncancerous lumps in the breast. Although these conclusions have been challenged, many clinicians advise patients with mammillary cysts to avoid caffeine. In addition, some reports indicate that very high doses of caffeine given to pregnant laboratory animals can cause stillbirths or offspring with low birthweights or limb deformations. Studies have found that moderate consumption of caffeine (less than 300 milligrams per day) did not significantly affect human fetal development.[28] However, women are usually advised to avoid or at least reduce caffeine use during pregnancy.

Caffeinism Caffeine intoxication brought on by excessive use; symptoms include chronic insomnia, irritability, anxiety, muscle twitches, and headaches.

What do you think?

How much caffeine do you consume? ■ *What is your pattern of caffeine consumption for the day?* ■ *Why do you consume it?* ■ *Have you ever experienced any ill effects after going without caffeine for a period of time?*

TAKING CHARGE

MAKE IT HAPPEN!

Assessment: The Assess Yourself box on page 377 gave you the chance to test your knowledge of nicotine dependence. If you feel that nicotine is more important to you than you would like it to be, you may want to take steps to change your behavior.

Making a Change: In order to change your behavior, you need to develop a plan. Follow these steps.

1. Evaluate your behavior, and identify patterns and specific things you are doing. What can you change now? What can you change in the near future?
2. Select one pattern of behavior that you want to change.
3. Fill out a Behavior Change Contract. It should include your long-term goal for change, your short-term goals, the rewards you'll give yourself for reaching these goals, potential obstacles along the way, and strategies for overcoming these obstacles. For each goal, list the small steps and specific actions that you will take.
4. Chart your progress in a journal. At the end of a week, consider how successful you were in following your plan. What helped you to be successful? What made change more difficult? What will you do differently next week?
5. Revise your plan as needed. Are the short-term goals attainable? Are the rewards satisfying?

One Student's Plan: After completing the Assess Yourself box, Jana was surprised to find that her score for nicotine dependence was 10 points. She had convinced herself over the past few semesters that her cravings for cigarettes really

were not harmful, but her score made her stop and think. Reflecting back over the last couple of years, she realized her smoking had progressed from occasional cigarettes with friends when they went out to having one or two while studying, to now pretty much smoking throughout the day. Knowing the health risks associated with smoking and the hassle of hiding her habit from family and friends, Jana decided it was time to quit.

First, Jana kept a daily journal for two weeks to record when and where she smoked and who she was with at the time. She wrote down how she felt and how important the cigarette was to her at the time on a scale of one to five. Then she decided to set some goals. The first goal was the date she would begin tapering off her cigarettes, and the second goal was a quit date. She outlined potential obstacles for achieving each goal and ways she could overcome the obstacles. For example, during the tapering phase, Jana decided she would buy only packs of cigarettes, instead of a carton. To assist her after her quit date, she decided she would tell her friends she was quitting and needed their support. She included all of this in her Behavior Change Contract.

Jana kept up her journal throughout her quitting process. She kept track of difficult moments and ways that were helpful to her in overcoming those moments. Also built into her contract were weekly rewards for her success. Jana would go out for dinner with friends or purchase new clothes with the money she was saving by not buying cigarettes.

Summary

- The use of tobacco involves many social issues, including advertising targeted at youth and women, the fastest growing populations of smokers. Health care and lost productivity resulting from smoking cost the nation as much as $157 billion per year.
- Tobacco is available in smoking and smokeless forms, both containing addictive nicotine (a psychoactive substance). Smoking also delivers 4,000 other chemicals to the lungs of smokers.
- The health hazards of smoking include markedly higher rates of cancer, heart and circulatory disorders, respira-

tory diseases, and gum diseases. Smoking while pregnant presents risks for the fetus, including miscarriage and low birth weight.
- Smokeless tobacco contains more nicotine than do cigarettes and dramatically increases risks for oral cancer and other oral problems.
- Environmental tobacco smoke (secondhand smoke) puts nonsmokers at risk for elevated rates of cancer and heart disease.
- For almost 40 years the government has been warning consumers of the dangers associated with tobacco use. In

a landmark legal settlement, the tobacco industry agreed to reimburse states for health care costs related to smoking and to finance various antismoking initiatives. Further legal battles are pending.

■ Quitting is complicated by the dual nature of smoking: smokers must kick a chemical addiction as well as a habit. Nicotine replacement products or Zyban can help wean smokers off nicotine. Therapy methods can also help smokers break the habit.

■ Caffeine is a widely used central nervous system stimulant. No long-term ill-health effects have been proven, although chronic users who try to quit may experience withdrawal.

Questions for Discussion and Reflection

1. New research suggests that genetic factors might be more influential than environmental factors in smoking initiation and nicotine dependence. How might this information change current prevention efforts? How would you design smoking prevention strategies targeted at adolescents?
2. Discuss the varied ways in which tobacco is used. Is any method less addictive or hazardous to health than another?
3. Discuss short-term and long-term health hazards associated with smoking. How will increased tobacco use among adolescents and college students impact the medical system in the future? Who should be responsible for the medical expenses of smokers? Insurance companies? Smokers themselves?

4. Do you believe that the tobacco companies could develop a "safe" cigarette? What would it take for you to consider a cigarette "safe"? Consider the claims for safety previously made by tobacco companies as you give your answer.
5. Discuss the various risks of smokeless tobacco use.
6. Restrictions on smoking are increasing in our society. Do you think these restrictions are fair? Do they infringe on people's rights? Are the restrictions too strict or not strict enough?
7. Describe the pros and cons of each method of quitting smoking. Which would be most effective for you? Explain why.
8. Discuss problems related to the ingestion of caffeine. How much caffeine do you consume? Why?

Accessing Your Health on the Internet

Visit the following Internet sites to explore further topics and issues related to tobacco and health. To visit an organization's website, go to the Companion Website for *Access to Health, Ninth Edition* at www.aw-bc.com/donatelle, click on the book image, and select "Accessing Your Health on the Internet" from the navigation menu.

1. *American Lung Association.* This site offers a wealth of information regarding smoking trends, environmental smoke, and advice on smoking cessation.
2. *ASH (Action on Smoking and Health).* The nation's oldest and largest antismoking organization, ASH regularly takes hard-hitting legal actions and does other work to fight smoking and protect the rights of nonsmokers. ASH provides nonsmokers with legal forms and valuable information about protecting their rights and about the problems and costs of smoking to nonsmokers. ASH's actions have helped prohibit cigarette commercials; ban smoking on planes, buses, and in many public places; and lower insurance premiums for nonsmokers.
3. *TIPS (Tobacco Information and Prevention Source).* This website provides access to a variety of information regarding tobacco use in the United States, with specific information for and about young people.

Further Reading

Glantz, S. A. and E. D. Balbach. *The Tobacco War: Inside the California Battles.* Berkeley: University of California Press, 2000.

Charts the dramatic and complex history of tobacco politics in California over the past quarter century. Shows how the accomplishments of tobacco-control advocates have changed how people view the tobacco industry and its behavior.

Kluger, R. *Ashes to Ashes: America's Hundred-Year Cigarette War, the Public Health, and the Unabashed Triumph of Philip Morris.* New York: Vintage Books, 1997.

A definitive history of America's controversial tobacco industry, focusing on Philip Morris. Traces the development of the cigarette, revelations of its toxicity, and the impact of political and corporate shenanigans on the battle over smoking.

Whelan, E. *Cigarettes: What the Warning Label Doesn't Tell You—The First Comprehensive Guide to the Health Consequences of Smoking.* New York: Prometheus Books, 1997.

From impotence to diabetes, cataracts to psoriasis, the proven dangers of smoking go well beyond heart and lung disease. This book details all the known health threats of smoking. Twenty-one experts explain how smoking can affect the body.

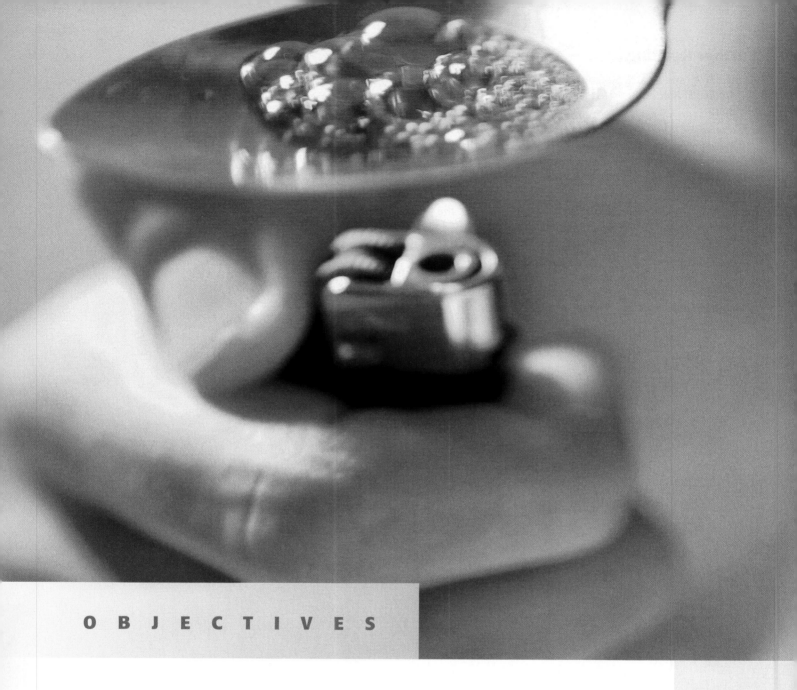

- Discuss the six categories of drugs, and explain their routes of administration.

- Discuss patterns of illicit drug use, including who uses illicit drugs and why.

- Discuss the use and abuse of controlled substances, including cocaine, amphetamines, marijuana, opiates, hallucinogens, designer drugs, inhalants, and steroids.

- Profile illegal drug use in the United States, including frequency, financial impact, arrests for drug offenses, and impact on the workplace.

ILLICIT DRUGS

USE, MISUSE, AND ABUSE

IN THE NEWS

This Is Your Brain on Meth: A 'Forest Fire' of Damage

By Sandra Blakeslee

People who do not want to wait for old age to shrink their brains and bring on memory loss now have a quicker alternative—abuse methamphetamine for a decade or so and watch the brain cells vanish into the night.

The first high-resolution M.R.I. study of methamphetamine addicts shows "a forest fire of brain damage," said Dr. Paul Thompson, an expert on brain mapping at the University of California, Los Angeles. "We expected some brain changes but didn't expect so much tissue to be destroyed."

The image, published in the June 30 issue of *The Journal of Neuroscience,* shows the brain's surface and deeper limbic system. Red areas show the greatest tissue loss.

The limbic region, involved in drug craving, reward, mood and emotion, lost 11 percent of its tissue. "The cells are dead and gone," Dr. Thompson said. Addicts were depressed, anxious and unable to concentrate.

The brain's center for making new memories, the hippocampus, lost 8 percent of its tissue, comparable to the brain deficits in early Alzheimer's. The methamphetamine addicts fared significantly worse on memory tests than healthy people the same age.

Read the complete article online in the eThemes section of this book's website: www.aw-bc.com/donatelle.

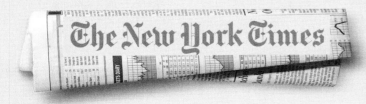

D rug misuse and abuse are problems of staggering proportions in our society. Each year drug and alcohol abuse contributes to the deaths of over 120,000 Americans. They also cost taxpayers more than $294 billion in preventable health care costs, extra law enforcement, auto crashes, crime, and lost productivity.[1] It's impossible to put a dollar amount on the pain, suffering, and dysfunction that drugs cause in our everyday lives. While overall use of drugs in the United States has fallen by 50 percent in the last 20 years, the past 10 years have shown an increase in the use of certain drugs by adolescents.[2]

It is important to understand how these drugs work and why people use them. Human beings appear to have a need to alter their consciousness, or mental state. We like to feel good, to escape and feel different. Consciousness can be altered in many ways: children spinning until they become dizzy and adults enjoying the rush of thrilling high-intensity activities are examples. To change our awareness, many of us listen to music, skydive, ski, read, daydream, meditate, pray, or have sexual relations. Others turn to drugs to alter consciousness.

Drug Dynamics

Drugs work because they physically resemble the chemicals produced naturally within the body (Figure 14.1). For example, many painkillers resemble the endorphins (meaning "morphine within") that are manufactured in the body. Most bodily processes result from chemical reactions or from changes in electrical charge. Because drugs possess an electrical charge and a chemical structure similar to those of chemicals that occur naturally in the body, they can affect physical functions in many different ways.

A current explanation of drug actions is the *receptor site theory*, which states that drugs bind to specific **receptor sites** in the body. These sites are specialized cells to which, because of their size, shape, electrical charge, and chemical properties, drugs can attach themselves. Most drugs bind to multiple receptor sites located throughout the body in places such as the heart and blood system and the lungs, liver, kidneys, brain, and gonads (testicles or ovaries).

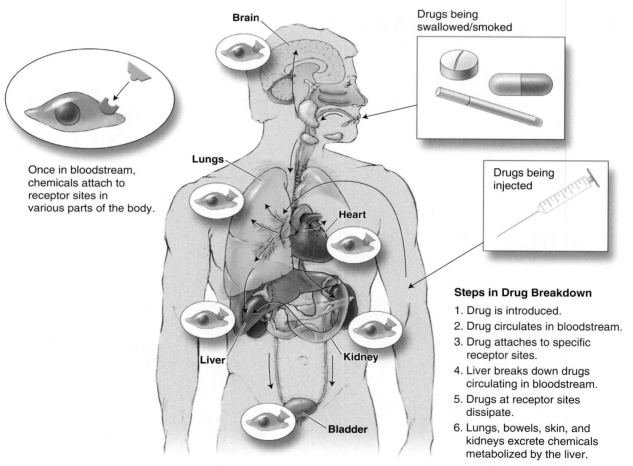

Brain

Drugs being swallowed/smoked

Once in bloodstream, chemicals attach to receptor sites in various parts of the body.

Lungs

Drugs being injected

Heart

Steps in Drug Breakdown

1. Drug is introduced.
2. Drug circulates in bloodstream.
3. Drug attaches to specific receptor sites.
4. Liver breaks down drugs circulating in bloodstream.
5. Drugs at receptor sites dissipate.
6. Lungs, bowels, skin, and kidneys excrete chemicals metabolized by the liver.

Liver

Kidney

Bladder

Figure 14.1
How the Body Metabolizes Drugs

Types of Drugs

Scientists divide drugs into six categories: prescription, over-the-counter (OTC), recreational, herbal, illicit, and commercial drugs. These classifications are based primarily on drug action, although some are based on the source of the chemical in question. Each category includes some drugs that stimulate the body, some that depress body functions, and others that produce hallucinations, images (auditory or visual) that are perceived but are not real. Each category also includes **psychoactive drugs,** which have the potential to alter a person's mood or behavior.

- **Prescription drugs** can be obtained only with the written prescription of a licensed physician. More than 10,000 types of prescription drugs are sold in the United States.
- **Over-the-counter (OTC) drugs** can be purchased without a prescription. Each year, Americans spend over $14 billion on OTC products, and the market is increasing at the rate of 20 percent annually. More than 300,000 OTC products are available through stores, pharmacies, and the Internet. An estimated three out of four people routinely self-medicate with them.
- **Recreational drugs** belong to a somewhat vague category whose boundaries depend upon how you define *recreation*. Generally, these substances contain chemicals used to help people relax or socialize. Most of them are legally sanctioned even though they are psychoactive. Alcohol, tobacco, coffee, tea, and chocolate products are usually included in this category.
- **Herbal preparations** form another vague category. Included among these approximately 750 substances are herbal teas and other products of botanical origin that are believed to have medicinal properties.
- **Illicit (illegal) drugs** are the most notorious type of drug. Although laws governing their use, possession, cultivation, manufacture, and sale differ from state to state, illicit drugs are generally recognized as harmful. All of them are psychoactive.
- **Commercial preparations** are the most universally used yet least commonly recognized chemical substances having drug action. More than 1,000 of these substances exist, including seemingly benign items such as perfumes, cosmetics, household cleansers, paints, glues, inks, dyes, gardening chemicals, pesticides, and industrial by-products.

Routes of Administration of Drugs

Route of administration refers to the way in which a given drug is taken into the body. Common routes are oral ingestion, injection, inhalation, inunction, and suppository.

    Oral ingestion is the most common route of administration. Drugs that are swallowed include tablets, capsules, and liquids. Oral ingestion generally results in relatively slow absorption compared to other methods of administration because the drug must pass through the stomach, where digestive juices act upon it, and then move on to the small intestine before it enters the bloodstream.

    Many oral preparations are coated to keep them from being dissolved by corrosive stomach acids before they reach the intestine and to protect the stomach lining from irritating chemicals in the drugs. A stomach that contains food slows the absorption of drugs. Some drugs must not be taken with certain foods because the food will inhibit their action, while others should be taken with food to prevent stomach irritation.

    Depending on the drug and the amount of food in the stomach, drugs taken orally produce their effects within 20 minutes to 1 hour after ingestion. The only exception is alcohol, which takes effect sooner because some of it is absorbed directly into the bloodstream from the stomach.

    Injection, another common form of drug administration, involves using a hypodermic syringe to introduce a drug into the body. **Intravenous injection,** or injection directly into a vein, puts the chemical in its most concentrated form directly into the bloodstream. Effects will be felt within three minutes, making this route extremely effective, particularly in medical emergencies. However, injection of many

---

Receptor sites   Specialized cells to which drugs can attach themselves.

Psychoactive drugs   Drugs that have the potential to alter mood or behavior.

Prescription drugs   Medications that can be obtained only with the written prescription of a licensed physician.

Over-the-counter (OTC) drugs   Medications that can be purchased without a physician's prescription.

Recreational drugs   Drugs that contain chemicals that help people relax or socialize; most, but not all, drugs in this category are legal.

Herbal preparations   Substances of plant origin that are believed to have medicinal properties.

Illicit (illegal) drugs   Drugs whose use, possession, cultivation, manufacture, and/or sale are against the law because they are generally recognized as harmful.

Commercial preparations   Commonly used chemical substances including cosmetics, household cleaning products, and industrial by-products.

Route of administration   The manner in which a drug is taken into the body.

Oral ingestion   Intake of drugs through the mouth.

Injection   The introduction of drugs into the body via a hypodermic needle.

Intravenous injection   The introduction of drugs directly into a vein.

substances into the bloodstream may cause serious or even fatal reactions, and some serious diseases, such as hepatitis and AIDS, can be transferred in this way. For this reason, intravenous injection can be one of the most dangerous routes of administration.

Intramuscular injection places the hypodermic needle into muscular tissue, usually in the buttocks or the back of the upper arm. Normally used to administer antibiotics and vaccinations, this route of administration results in much slower absorption than intravenous injection but ensures slow and consistent dispersion of the drug into body tissues.

Subcutaneous injection puts the drug into the layer of fat directly beneath the skin. Its common medical uses include administration of local anesthetics and insulin replacement therapy. A drug injected subcutaneously will circulate even more slowly than an intramuscularly injected drug because it takes longer to be absorbed into the bloodstream.

Inhalation refers to administration of drugs through the nostrils or mouth. This method transfers the drug rapidly into the bloodstream through the alveoli (air sacs) in the lungs. Examples of illicit inhalation include cocaine sniffing; inhaling aerosol sprays, gases, or fumes from solvents; and smoking marijuana. Effects are frequently immediate but do not last as long as effects associated with slower routes of administration because only small amounts of a drug can be absorbed and metabolized in the lungs.

Inunction introduces chemicals into the body through the skin. A common example is the small adhesive patch that is used to alleviate motion sickness. This patch, which contains a prescription medicine, is applied to the skin behind one ear, where it slowly releases its chemicals to provide relief for nauseated travelers.

Suppositories are drugs that are mixed with a waxy medium designed to melt at body temperature. The most common type is inserted into the anus past the rectal sphincter muscles, which hold the suppository in place. As the wax melts, the drug is released and absorbed through the rectal walls into the bloodstream. Since this area contains many blood vessels, the effects are usually felt within 15 minutes. Other types of suppositories are for use in the vagina. Vaginal suppositories usually release drugs, such as antifungal agents, that treat problems in the vagina itself rather than drugs meant to travel in the bloodstream.

Using, Misusing, and Abusing Drugs

Although drug abuse is usually referred to in connection with illicit psychoactive drugs, many people abuse and misuse prescription and OTC medications. **Drug misuse** involves the use of a drug for a purpose for which it was not intended. For example, taking a friend's high-powered prescription painkiller for your headache is a misuse of that drug. This is not too far removed from **drug abuse,** or the excessive use of any drug. The misuse and abuse of drugs may lead to *addiction,* the habitual reliance on a substance or behavior to produce a desired mood. Both risks and benefits are involved in the use of any type of chemical substance. Intelligent decision making requires a clear-headed evaluation of these risks and benefits. If, after considering all the facts, you feel that the benefits outweigh the potential problems associated with a particular drug, you may decide to use it—but sometimes unforeseeable reactions or problems arise even after the most careful deliberation.

Illicit Drugs

While some people become addicted to prescription drugs and painkillers, others use **illicit drugs**—those drugs that are illegal to possess, produce, or sell. The problem of illicit drug use touches us all. We may use illicit substances ourselves, watch someone we love struggle with drug abuse, or become the victim of a drug-related crime. At the very least, we are forced to pay increasing taxes for law enforcement and drug rehabilitation. An estimated 9.4 percent of full-time employees in the U.S. workforce is under the influence of illicit substances or alcohol on any given day.[3] When our coworkers use drugs, the effectiveness of our own work is diminished. If the car we drive was assembled by drug-using workers at the plant, we are in danger. A drug-using bus driver, train engineer, medical professional, or pilot jeopardizes our safety.

The good news is that the use of illicit drugs has declined significantly in recent years in most segments of society. Use of most drugs increased from the early 1970s to the late 1970s, peaked between 1979 and 1986, and declined until 1992, from which point it has not changed. In 2003, an estimated 19.2 million Americans were illicit drug users, about three-quarters the 1979 peak level of 25 million users. Among youth, however, illicit drug use, notably of marijuana, has been rising in recent years.[4]

Intramuscular injection   The introduction of drugs into muscles.

Subcutaneous injection   The introduction of drugs into the layer of fat directly beneath the skin.

Inhalation   The introduction of drugs through the nostrils.

Inunction   The introduction of drugs through the skin.

Suppositories   Mixtures of drugs and a waxy medium designed to melt at body temperature that are inserted into the anus or vagina.

Drug misuse   The use of a drug for a purpose for which it was not intended.

Drug abuse   The excessive use of a drug.

Illicit drugs   Drugs that are illegal to possess, produce, or sell.

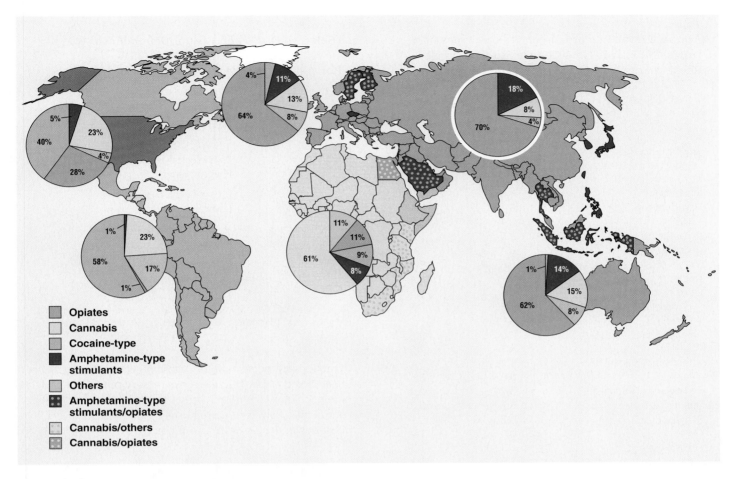

Figure 14.2

Global Use of Illicit Drugs, 2003

The main problem drugs in the world, as reflected in demand for treatment, remain the opiates, followed by cocaine. Reports of demand are based on an average from most, but not all, countries in a region over a period of years.

Source: United Nations Office on Drugs and Crime, "Executive Summary: Global Illicit Drug Trends: 2003," 2004, www.unodc.org/unodc/en/global_illicit_drug_trends.html

Who Uses Illicit Drugs?

While many of us have stereotypes in our minds of who uses illicit drugs, it is difficult to generalize. Illicit drug users span all age groups, ethnicities, occupations, and socioeconomic groups. What can be said is that illicit drug use has a devastating effect on users and their families in the United States and in many other countries (Figure 14.2).

After more than a decade of declining use on American college campuses, illicit drugs have reappeared. In 2003, the number of college students nationwide who had tried any drug stood at almost 52 percent; over a third had smoked pot in the past year, and 20 percent had done so in the past month. Daily use of marijuana was at its highest point since 1989.[5] Cocaine use is down sharply, but LSD use has more than doubled. These figures vary from school to school.

Patterns of drug use vary considerably by age. For example, a nationwide study of college campuses reported that approximately 30.7 percent of students had tried marijuana during the previous year[6] (Table 14.1 on page 402). In contrast, only 9 percent of all Americans used marijuana during that time. Approximately 4.8 percent of college students surveyed reported using cocaine in the past year, whereas only 2.2 percent of all Americans said they had used cocaine during the previous year.

Most antidrug programs have not been effective because they have focused on only one aspect of drug abuse, rather than examining all factors that contribute to the problem. The pressures to take drugs are often tremendous, and the reasons for using them are complex. People who develop drug problems generally begin with the belief that they can control their drug use. Initially, they often view taking drugs

Table 14.1
Annual Prevalence of Use for Various Types of Drugs, 2002: Full-Time College Students vs. Respondents 1–4 Years beyond High School

	Full-Time College (%)	Others (%)
Any illicit drug	37.0	39.6
Any illicit drug other than marijuana	16.6	23.0
Marijuana	34.7	36.3
Inhalants	2.0	2.8
Hallucinogens	6.3	7.1
LSD	2.1	3.3
Cocaine	4.8	9.6
Crack	0.4	2.6
MDMA (Ecstasy)	6.8	9.3
Heroin	0.1	0.4
Other narcotics	5.9	7.4
OxyContin	1.5	3.3
Vicodin	6.9	12.9
Amphetamines, adjusted	7.0	9.6
Ritalin	5.7	2.5
Methamphetamine	1.2	5.4
Ice	0.8	3.5
Sedatives (barbiturates)	3.7	6.7
Tranquilizers	6.7	10.8
Rohypnol	0.7	0.2
GHB	0.6	1.2
Ketamine	1.3	1.3
Alcohol	82.9	80.1
Cigarettes	38.3	47.7
Approximate weighted N =	1,260	880

Source: Monitoring the Future Study (Ann Arbor: MI: The University of Michigan, 2003).

Table 14.2
Selected Drugs and Risk of Dependence

Drug	Risk of Dependence
Cocaine	Psychological: high Physical (especially crack): moderate
Amphetamines	Psychological: high Physical: high
Marijuana	Psychological: moderate Physical: varies
Opiates	Psychological: high Physical: high
Hallucinogens	Psychological: low Physical: varies
Inhalants	Psychological: high Physical: moderate

Source: American College Health Association, "Alcohol and Other Drugs: Risky Business" (Baltimore, MD: ACH, 2001).

as a fun and manageable pastime. Peer influence is a strong motivator, especially among adolescents, who greatly fear not being accepted as part of the group. Other people use drugs to cope with feelings of worthlessness and despair or to battle depression and anxiety. Since most illegal drugs produce physical and psychological dependency, it is unrealistic to think that a person can use them regularly without becoming addicted. Table 14.2 gives a summary of the risk of dependence of selected illicit drugs. Consider whether you are controlled by drugs or a drug user by answering the questions in the Assess Yourself box.

Controlled Substances

To counteract the increased use of illegal drugs and the overuse of certain prescription drugs, Congress passed the Controlled Substances Act of 1970 (Public Law 91-513). This law created categories for both prescription and illegal substances that the federal government felt required strict regulation. The Drug Enforcement Agency (DEA) was founded within the Department of Justice to administer the law.

The law classified drugs into five schedules, or categories, based on their potential for abuse, their medical uses, and accepted standards of safe use (Table 14.3 on page 404). Schedule I drugs, those with the highest potential for abuse, are considered to have no valid medical uses. Although Schedule II, III, IV, and V drugs have known and accepted medical applications, many of them present serious threats to health when abused or misused. Penalties for illegal use are tied to the drugs' schedule level. Despite the 1970 law, however, manufacturing of and trafficking in illegal drugs in the United States have not diminished.

Hundreds of illegal drugs exist. For general purposes, they can be divided into seven categories: stimulants, such as cocaine; marijuana and its derivatives; depressants, such as the opiates; hallucinogens/psychedelics; designer drugs; inhalants; and steroids.

What do you think?

What factors do you believe influence trends of illicit drug use in the United States? ■ *What is the attitude toward drug use on your college campus?* ■ *Are some drugs considered more acceptable than others?* ■ *Is drug use considered more acceptable at certain times or occasions? Explain your answer.*

Recognizing a Drug Problem

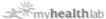

Fill out this assessment online at www.aw-bc.com/myhealthlab or www.aw-bc.com/donatelle

ARE YOU CONTROLLED BY DRUGS?

How do you know whether you are chemically dependent? A dependent person can't stop using drugs. This abuse hurts the user and everyone around him or her. Take the following assessment. The more "yes" checks you make, the more likely you have a problem.

		Yes	No
1.	Do you use drugs to handle stress or escape from life's problems?	❑	❑
2.	Have you unsuccessfully tried to cut down on or quit using your drug?	❑	❑
3.	Have you ever been in trouble with the law or been arrested because of your drug use?	❑	❑
4.	Do you think a party or social gathering isn't fun unless drugs are available?	❑	❑
5.	Do you avoid people or places that do not support your usage?	❑	❑
6.	Do you neglect your responsibilities because you'd rather use your drug?	❑	❑
7.	Have your friends, family, or employer expressed concern about your drug use?	❑	❑
8.	Do you do things under the influence of drugs that you would not normally do?	❑	❑
9.	Have you seriously thought that you might have a chemical dependency problem?	❑	❑

ARE YOU CONTROLLED BY A DRUG USER?

Is your life controlled by a chemical abuser? Your love and care (codependence) may actually be enabling the person to continue the abuse, hurting you and others. Try this assessment; the more "yes" checks you make, the more likely there's a problem.

		Yes	No
1.	Do you often have to lie or cover up for the chemical abuser?	❑	❑
2.	Do you spend time counseling the person about the problem?	❑	❑
3.	Have you taken on additional financial or family responsibilities?	❑	❑
4.	Do you feel that you have to control the chemical abuser's behavior?	❑	❑
5.	At the office, have you done work or attended meetings for the abuser?	❑	❑
6.	Do you often put your own needs and desires after the user's?	❑	❑
7.	Do you spend time each day worrying about your situation?	❑	❑
8.	Do you analyze your behavior to find clues to how it might affect the chemical abuser?	❑	❑
9.	Do you feel powerless and at your wit's end about the abuser's problem?	❑	❑

MAKE IT HAPPEN!

Use the results of this self-assessment to begin your behavior change program. Follow the steps and use the examples on page 420 to complete your Behavior Change Contract, and use these resources to take action.

Table 14.3
How Drugs Are Scheduled

Schedule	Characteristics	Examples
Schedule I	High potential for abuse and addiction; no accepted medical use	Amphetamine Heroin Phencyclidine (PCP) LSD Marijuana GHB
Schedule II	High potential for abuse and addiction; restricted medical use	Cocaine Codeine* Methadone Morphine Opium OxyContin Vicodin
Schedule III	Some potential for abuse and addiction; currently accepted medical use	Anabolic steroids Nalorphine Noludar
Schedule IV	Low potential for abuse and addiction; currently accepted medical use	Rohypnol Xanax Minor tranquilizers
Schedule V	Lowest potential for abuse; accepted medical use	Robitussin AC OTC preparations

*Can also be Schedule III or Schedule IV, depending on use.

Source: National Institute on Drug Abuse, "Commonly Abused Drugs," 2003, www.drugabuse.gov/DrugPages/DrugsofAbuse.html

Stimulants

Cocaine   A white crystalline powder derived from the leaves of the South American coca shrub (not related to cocoa plants), **cocaine** ("coke") has been described as one of the most powerful naturally occurring stimulants.

Methods of Cocaine Use   Cocaine can be taken in several ways. The powdered form of the drug is "snorted" through the nose. When cocaine is snorted, it can damage mucous membranes in the nose and cause sinusitis. It can destroy the user's sense of smell, and occasionally it even eats a hole through the septum.

Smoking (known as *freebasing*) and intravenous injections are even more dangerous means of taking cocaine. Freebasing has become more popular than injecting in recent years because people fear contracting diseases such as AIDS and hepatitis by sharing contaminated needles. But freebasing involves other dangers. Because the volatile mixes

it requires are very explosive, some people have been killed or seriously burned. Smoking cocaine can also cause lung and liver damage.

Many cocaine users still occasionally "shoot up," which introduces large amounts into the body rapidly. Within seconds, a sense of euphoria sets in. This intense high lasts for 15 to 20 minutes, and then the user heads into a "crash." To prevent the unpleasant effects of the crash, users must shoot up frequently, which can severely damage veins. Injecting users place themselves at risk not only for AIDS and hepatitis, but also for skin infections, inflamed arteries, and infection of the lining of the heart.

Physical Effects of Cocaine   The effects of cocaine are felt rapidly. Snorted cocaine enters the bloodstream through the lungs in less than one minute and reaches the brain in less than three minutes. When cocaine binds at its receptor sites in the central nervous system, it produces intense pleasure. The euphoria quickly abates, however, and the desire to regain the pleasurable feelings makes the user want more cocaine (Figure 14.3).

Cocaine is both an anesthetic and a central nervous system stimulant. In tiny doses, it can slow heart rate. In larger doses, the physical effects are dramatic: increased

---

Cocaine   A powerful stimulant drug made from the leaves of the South American coca shrub.

Women and Drug Abuse

Almost half of all women age 15 to 44 will have used drugs at least once in their lives. Of these women, nearly 2 million have used cocaine and more than 6 million have used marijuana in the past year. Some 3.7 million women have taken prescription drugs for nonmedical purposes. Most women who abuse drugs abuse more than one drug.

Today, approximately 28,000 (70 percent) of AIDS cases among U.S. women are related either to injecting drugs or to having sex with a man who injects drugs; consequently, AIDS is now the fourth leading cause of death among women of childbearing age.

Many women who use drugs have had troubled lives. Studies show that at least 70 percent of them have been sexually abused by the age of 16. Most of them had at least one parent who abused alcohol or drugs. Furthermore, they often have little self-esteem or self-confidence. They frequently feel lonely, powerless, and isolated from support networks.

Unfortunately, many female drug users are unable to seek help. Some may be unable to find or afford child care during a course of treatment, while others worry that the courts will take away their children once the drug problem is known. Others may fear violence from their husbands, boyfriends, or partners.

Research has shown that female drug abusers have a better chance of recovery when treatment takes care of their basic needs. Some women need the basic services of food, shelter, and clothing. Others also need transportation, child care, and training in parenting. The most successful treatments also teach reading, basic education, and the skills needed to find a job. As a woman's self-esteem increases, so do her chances of remaining drug-free.

Source: National Institute on Drug Abuse, "Women and Drug Abuse," downloaded September 8, 2004. www.nida.nih.gov/womendrugs/women-drugabuse.html

---

heart rate and blood pressure, loss of appetite that can lead to dramatic weight loss, convulsions, muscle twitching, irregular heartbeat, and even eventual death due to overdose. Other effects of cocaine include temporary relief of depression, decreased fatigue, talkativeness, increased alertness, and heightened self-confidence. However, as the dose increases, users become irritable and apprehensive, and their behavior may turn paranoid or violent.

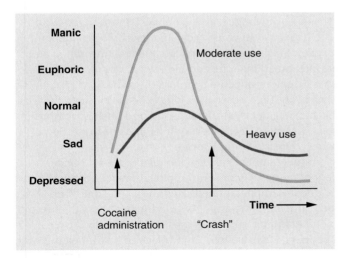

Figure 14.3

Ups and Downs of a Typical Dose of Cocaine

Source: C. Levinthal, *Drugs, Behavior, and Modern Society,* 2nd ed. (Boston: Allyn & Bacon, 1999). © Pearson Education. Reprinted by permission of the publisher.

Cocaine-Affected Babies Because cocaine rapidly crosses the placenta (as virtually all drugs do), the fetus is vulnerable when a pregnant woman uses cocaine. It is estimated that 2.4 to 3.5 percent of pregnant women between the ages of 12 and 34 abuse cocaine. It is difficult to gauge how many newborns have been exposed to cocaine because pregnant users are reluctant to discuss their drug habit with health care providers for fear of prosecution. The most threatening problem during pregnancy is the increased risk of a miscarriage. (See the Women's Health/Men's Health box.)

Fetuses exposed to cocaine in the womb are more likely to suffer a small head, premature delivery, reduced birthweight, increased irritability, and subtle learning and cognitive deficits. Research suggests that a significant number of these children develop problems with learning and language skills that require remedial attention.[7] It is critical to identify these children early so they can receive immediate intervention. For both financial and humane reasons, prenatal care and education programs for mothers at risk should be a priority for state and local government.[8]

Types of Cocaine Freebase is a form of cocaine that is more powerful and costly than powder or crack. Street cocaine (cocaine hydrochloride) is converted to pure base by using ether to remove the hydrochloride salt and many of the "cutting agents" used to dilute the drug. (The use of ether, which is flammable, adds to the danger.) The end product, freebase, is smoked through a water pipe.

Freebase The most powerful distillate of cocaine.

Because freebase cocaine reaches the brain within seconds, it is more dangerous than snorted cocaine. It produces a quick, intense high that disappears quickly, leaving an intense craving for more. Freebasers typically increase the amount and frequency of the dose. They often become severely addicted and experience serious health problems.

Side effects of freebasing cocaine include weight loss, increased heart rate and blood pressure, depression, paranoia, and hallucinations. Freebase is an extremely dangerous drug and is responsible for a large number of cocaine-related hospital emergency-room visits and deaths.

The street name **crack** is given to freebase cocaine processed from cocaine hydrochloride by using ammonia or sodium bicarbonate (baking soda), water, and heat to remove the hydrochloride. The mixture (90 percent pure cocaine) is then dried. The soapy-looking substance that results can be broken into "rocks" and smoked. These rocks are approximately five times as strong as cocaine. Crack gets its name from the popping noises it makes when burned.

Crack is also sometimes called "rock," which is not the same as rock cocaine. Rock cocaine is a cocaine hydrochloride substance that is primarily sold in California. White in color, it is about the shape of a pencil eraser and is typically snorted.

Because crack is such a pure drug, it takes much less time to achieve the desired high. One puff of a pebble-size rock produces an intense high that lasts for approximately 20 minutes. The user can usually get three or four hits off a rock before it is used up. Crack is typically sold in small vials, folding papers, or heavy tinfoil containing two or three rocks, and costing between $10 and $20.

A crack user can become addicted quickly. Addiction is accelerated by the speed at which crack is absorbed through the lungs (it hits the brain within seconds) and by the intensity of the high. It is not uncommon for crack addicts to spend over $1,000 a day on the habit.

Cocaine Addiction and Society   Cocaine addicts often suffer both physiological damage and serious disruption in lifestyle, including loss of employment and self-esteem. It is estimated that the annual cost of cocaine addiction in the United States exceeds $3.8 billion. However, there is no way to measure the cost in wasted lives. An estimated 5 million Americans from all socioeconomic groups are addicted,

and 1,160,000 new users try cocaine or crack every year. National surveys on drug use estimate that 5.9 million people used the drug at least once in the past year. Experts suggest that 10 percent of recreational users will go on to heavy use.[9]

Cocaine has been called unpredictable by drug experts, deadly by coroners, dangerous by former users, and disastrous by the media. Yet to date, there has not been a successful weapon to combat its use in the United States. Apparently, the risks do not override users' desire to experience its effects.

Because cocaine is illegal, a complex underground network has developed to manufacture and sell the drug. Buyers may not always get the product they think they are purchasing. Cocaine marketed for snorting may be only 60 percent pure. Usually, it is mixed, or "cut," with other white powdery substances such as mannitol or sugar, though occasionally it is cut with arsenic or other cocaine-like powders that may themselves be highly dangerous.

What do you think?

Have all segments of society been affected by crack use? If not, which segments of the U.S. population experience the greatest impact from crack use? Why might this be the case? ■ *Is there a difference in the profile of a person who uses crack rather than cocaine? Explain your answer.*

Amphetamines   The **amphetamines** include a large and varied group of synthetic agents that stimulate the central nervous system. Small doses of amphetamines improve alertness, lessen fatigue, and generally elevate mood. With repeated use, however, physical and psychological dependence develops. Sleep patterns are affected (insomnia) and heart rate, breathing rate, and blood pressure increase. Restlessness, anxiety, appetite suppression, and vision problems are common. High doses over long time periods can produce hallucinations, delusions, and disorganized behavior. Abusers become paranoid, fearing everything and everyone. Some become aggressive or antisocial.

Amphetamines for recreational use are sold under a variety of names: "Bennies" (amphetamine/Benzedrine), "dex" (dextroamphetamine/Dexedrine), and "meth" or "speed" (methamphetamine/Methedrine). Other street terms for amphetamines are "cross tops," "uppers," "wake-ups," "lid poppers," "cartwheels," and "blackies." Amphetamines do have therapeutic uses (see Chapter 22) in the treatment of attention deficit/hyperactivity disorder in children (Ritalin, Cylert) and of obesity (Pondimin).

Methamphetamine and Ice   An increasingly common form of amphetamine, **methamphetamine** is a powerfully addictive drug that strongly activates certain areas of the brain

---

Crack   A distillate of powdered cocaine that comes in small, hard "chips" or "rocks"; not the same as rock cocaine.

Amphetamines   A large and varied group of synthetic agents that stimulate the central nervous system.

Methamphetamine   A powerfully addictive drug that strongly activates certain areas of the brain and affects the central nervous system.

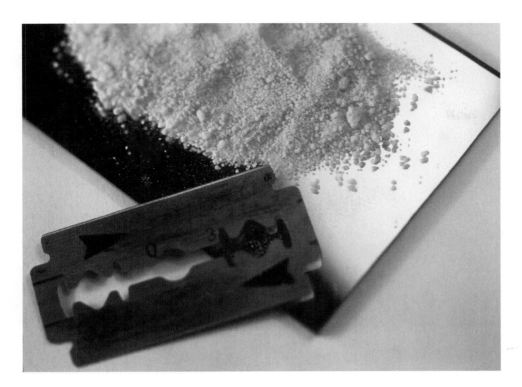

Methamphetamine is powerfully addictive and increasing in prevalence.

and affects the central nervous system in general. Methamphetamine is closely related chemically to amphetamine, but its central nervous system effects are greater.

Methamphetamine is relatively easy to make. People nicknamed "cookers" produce methamphetamine batches using cookbook-style recipes that often include common over-the-counter ingredients such as ephedrine and pseudoephedrine. Laws have strengthened the penalties associated with manufacturing methamphetamine.

The effects of the drug last six to eight hours, considerably longer than those produced by crack and cocaine. The immediate effects can include irritability and anxiety; increased body temperature, heart rate, and blood pressure; and possible death. The high state of irritability and agitation has been associated with violent behavior among some users.

Ice is a potent methamphetamine that is imported primarily from Asia, particularly from South Korea and Taiwan. It is purer and more crystalline than the version manufactured in many large U.S. cities. Because it is odorless, public use of ice often goes unnoticed.

Typically, ice quickly becomes addictive. Some users have reported severe cravings after using it only once. The effects of ice are long lasting. They include wakefulness, mood elevation, and excitability, all of which appeal to work-addicted young adults, particularly those who must put in long hours in high-stress jobs. Because the drug is inexpensive and produces such an intense high (lasting from 4 to 14 hours), it has become popular among young people looking for a quick high. However, as is true of other methamphetamines, the "down" side of this drug is devastating.

Prolonged use can cause fatal lung and kidney damage as well as long-lasting psychological damage. In some instances, major psychological dysfunction can persist as long as two and a half years after last use.

Marijuana

Although archaeological evidence documents the use of **marijuana** ("grass," "weed," "pot") as far back as 6,000 years, the drug did not become popular in the United States until the 1960s. Marijuana receives less media attention today than it did then, but it still is the illicit drug used most frequently by far. Nearly one of every three Americans over the age of 12 has tried marijuana at least once. Some 12 million Americans have used it; more than 1 million cannot control their use.

Physical Effects of Marijuana Marijuana is derived from either the *Cannabis sativa* or *Cannabis indica* (hemp) plants. Current American-grown marijuana is a turbocharged version of the hippie weed of the late 1960s. Developed using crossbreeding, genetic engineering, and American farming ingenuity, top-grade cannabis packs a punch very similar to

---

Ice A potent, inexpensive methamphetamine that has long-lasting effects.

Marijuana Chopped leaves and flowers of the *Cannabis indica* or *Cannabis sativa* plants (hemp); a psychoactive stimulant that intensifies reactions to environmental stimuli.

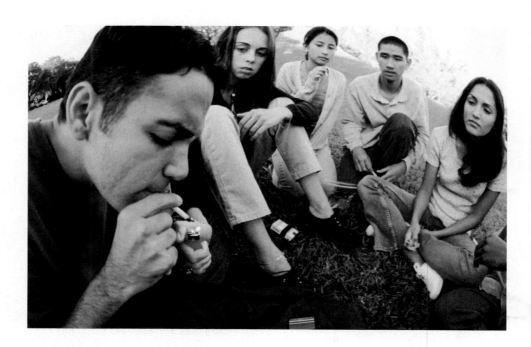

Marijuana is the most commonly used illicit drug.

that of hashish. **Tetrahydrocannabinol (THC)** is the psycho-active substance in marijuana and the key to determining how powerful a high it will produce. Whereas a marijuana cigarette three decades ago averaged 10 mg of THC, a current cigarette may contain around 150 mg of THC. Thus the modern-day marijuana user may be exposed to doses of THC many times greater than were users in the 1960s and 1970s.[10]

Hashish, a potent cannabis preparation derived mainly from the thick, sticky resin of the plant, contains high concentrations of THC. Hash oil, a substance produced by percolating a solvent such as ether through dried marijuana to extract the THC, is a tarlike liquid that may contain up to 300 mg of THC in a dose.

Most of the time, marijuana is rolled into cigarettes (joints) or smoked in a pipe or water pipe (bong). Effects are generally felt within 10 to 30 minutes and usually wear off within three hours.

The most noticeable effect of THC is the dilation of the eyes' blood vessels, which produces the characteristic bloodshot eyes. Smokers of the drug also exhibit coughing, dry mouth and throat ("cotton mouth"), increased thirst and appetite, lowered blood pressure, and mild muscular weakness, primarily exhibited in drooping eyelids. Users can also experience severe anxiety, panic, paranoia, and psychosis.

Users may have intensified reactions to various stimuli; colors, sounds, and the speed at which things move may seem altered. High doses of hashish may produce vivid visual hallucinations.

Effects of Chronic Marijuana Use   Because marijuana is illegal in most parts of the United States and has been widely used only since the 1960s, long-term studies of its effects have been difficult to conduct. Also, studies conducted in the 1960s involved marijuana with THC levels constituting only a fraction of today's plant levels, so their results may not apply to the stronger forms available today.

Most current information about chronic marijuana use comes from countries such as Jamaica and Costa Rica, where the drug is not illegal. These studies of long-term users (for ten or more years) indicate that it causes lung damage comparable to that caused by tobacco smoking. Indeed, smoking a single joint may be as bad for the lungs as smoking three tobacco cigarettes. Inhalation of marijuana transfers carbon monoxide to the bloodstream. Because the blood has a greater affinity for carbon monoxide than it does for oxygen, this diminishes the oxygen-carrying capacity of the blood. The heart must work harder to pump the vital element to oxygen-starved tissues. Furthermore, the tar from cannabis contains higher levels of carcinogens than does tobacco smoke. Smoking marijuana results in three times as much tar inhalation and retention in the respiratory tract than tobacco use.

Other risks associated with marijuana include suppression of the immune system, blood pressure changes, and impaired memory function. Recent studies suggest that pregnant women who smoke marijuana are at a higher risk for stillbirth or miscarriage and for delivering low–birth weight babies and babies with abnormalities of the nervous system. Babies born to marijuana smokers are five times more likely to have features similar to those exhibited by children with fetal alcohol syndrome.

Tetrahydrocannabinol (THC)   The chemical name for the active ingredient in marijuana.

Hashish   The sticky resin of the *Cannabis* plant, which is high in THC.

Medicinal Use of Marijuana: Legal Challenges Continue

For years, marijuana's legal status for medicinal purposes has been hotly debated. Currently, 30 states and the District of Columbia have laws that recognize marijuana's medical value. Eleven states with Therapeutic Research Program laws are nevertheless unable to give patients legal access to medical marijuana because of federal laws. Nine states and the District of Columbia have symbolic laws that recognize marijuana's medical value but fail to protect patients from arrest for possession of an illegal drug. Voters in Alaska, California, Colorado, Hawaii, Maine, Oregon, Nevada, Vermont, and Washington state have chosen to legalize marijuana for medicinal use (see the accompanying figures). These new state laws, however, conflict with federal laws against the possession of marijuana and have led to new, as yet unresolved, battles in court.

Source: Marijuana Policy Project, "State by State Medical Marijuana Laws: How to Remove the Threat of Arrest," 2004, www.mpp.org/statelaw/index.html; copyright 2004.

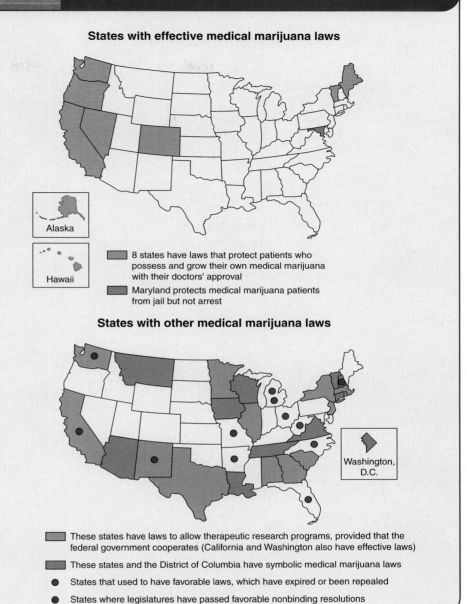

States with effective medical marijuana laws

Alaska

Hawaii

■ 8 states have laws that protect patients who possess and grow their own medical marijuana with their doctors' approval

■ Maryland protects medical marijuana patients from jail but not arrest

States with other medical marijuana laws

Washington, D.C.

■ These states have laws to allow therapeutic research programs, provided that the federal government cooperates (California and Washington also have effective laws)

■ These states and the District of Columbia have symbolic medical marijuana laws

● States that used to have favorable laws, which have expired or been repealed

● States where legislatures have passed favorable nonbinding resolutions

---

Debates concerning the effects of marijuana on the re-productive system have yet to be resolved. Studies conducted in the mid-1970s suggested that marijuana inhibited testosterone (and thus sperm) production in males and caused chromosomal breakage in both ova and sperm. Subsequent research in these areas is inconclusive. The question of whether the high-level THC plants currently available will increase the risks associated with this drug is, as yet, unanswered.

Marijuana and Medicine   Although recognized as a dangerous drug by the U.S. government, marijuana has several medical purposes. It helps control the side effects (such as severe nausea and vomiting) produced by chemotherapy (chemical treatment for cancer). It improves appetite and forestalls the loss of lean muscle mass associated with AIDS-wasting syndrome (previously known as AIDS-related complex or ARC). Marijuana reduces the muscle pain and spasticity caused by diseases such as multiple sclerosis. It also temporarily relieves the eye pressure of glaucoma, although it is unclear whether it is more effective than legal glaucoma drugs.[11] Marijuana's legal status for medicinal purposes continues to be hotly debated (see the New Horizons in Health box).

Marijuana and Driving   Marijuana use presents clear hazards for drivers of motor vehicles as well as others on the road. The drug substantially reduces a driver's ability to react and make quick decisions. Studies reveal that 60 to 80 percent of marijuana users sometimes drive while high.[12] Studies of automobile accident victims show that 6 to 12 percent of nonfatally injured drivers and 4 to 16 percent of fatally injured drivers had THC in their bloodstreams. Perceptual and other performance deficits resulting from marijuana use may persist for some time after the high subsides. Users who attempt to drive, fly, or operate heavy machinery often fail to recognize their impairment.

What do you think?

Why do you think that marijuana is the most popular illicit drug on college campuses? ■ *How widespread is marijuana use on your campus?*

Opiates

Among the oldest pain relievers known to humans, opiates cause drowsiness, reduce pain, and induce euphoria. A type of **narcotic,** opiates are derived from the parent drug **opium,** a dark, resinous substance made from the milky juice of the opium poppy. Other opiates include morphine, codeine, heroin, and black tar heroin.

The word *narcotic* comes from the Greek word for "stupor" and is generally used to describe sleep-inducing substances. Until the early twentieth century, many patent medicines contained opiates and were advertised as cures for everything from menstrual cramps to teething pains. More powerful than opium, **morphine** (named after Morpheus, the Greek god of sleep) was widely used as a painkiller during the Civil War. **Codeine,** a less powerful analgesic (pain reliever) derived from morphine, also became popular.

Narcotic   Drugs that induce sleep and relieve pain; primarily the opiates.

Opium   The parent drug of the opiates; made from the seedpod resin of the opium poppy.

Morphine   A derivative of opium; sometimes used by medical practitioners to relieve pain.

Codeine   A drug derived from morphine; used in cough syrups and certain painkillers.

Heroin   An illegally manufactured derivative of morphine, usually injected into the bloodstream.

Black tar heroin   A dark brown, sticky form of heroin.

As opiates became more common, physicians noted that patients tended to become dependent on them. Growing concern about addiction led to government controls of narcotic use. The Harrison Act of 1914 prohibited the production, dispensation, and sale of opiate products unless prescribed by a physician. Subsequent legislation required physicians prescribing opiates to keep careful records. Physicians are still subject to audits of their prescriptions.

Some opiates are still used today for medical purposes. Morphine is sometimes prescribed for severe pain, and codeine is found in prescription cough syrups and other painkillers. Several prescription drugs, including Percodan, Demerol, and Dilaudid, contain synthetic opiates. Although all opiate use is strictly regulated, illicit use of OxyContin, another powerful opiate, has increased dramatically in recent years (see the Reality Check box).

Physical Effects of Opiates   Opiates are powerful depressants of the central nervous system. In addition to relieving pain, these drugs lower heart rate, respiration, and blood pressure. Side effects include weakness, dizziness, nausea, vomiting, euphoria, decreased sex drive, visual disturbances, and lack of coordination. Of all the opiates, heroin has the greatest notoriety as an addictive drug. The following section discusses the progression of heroin addiction; addiction to any opiate follows a similar path.

Heroin Addiction   **Heroin** is a white powder derived from morphine. **Black tar heroin** is a sticky, dark brown, foul-smelling form of heroin that is relatively pure and inexpensive. Once considered a cure for morphine dependency, heroin was later discovered to be even more addictive and potent than morphine. Today, heroin has no medical use.

Authorities fear that the United States is at the beginning of a new heroin epidemic. It is estimated that 810,000 Americans are addicted to heroin, with men outnumbering women addicts by three to one.[13] There is concern that this epidemic will be worse than previous ones because the drug is now two to three times more available than ever before. The contemporary version of heroin is so potent that users can get high by snorting or smoking the drug rather than by injecting it and putting themselves at risk for AIDS (see Chapter 17), although many addicts continue to inject the drug. Once an inner-city drug, heroin use is now becoming more widespread among middle-class people who tend to try whatever is new and trendy. Many people have switched from cocaine to heroin because heroin is less stimulating and less expensive.

Heroin is a depressant that produces drowsiness and a dreamy, mentally slow feeling. It can cause drastic mood swings, with euphoric highs followed by depressive lows. Heroin also slows respiration and urinary output and constricts the pupils of the eyes. In fact, pupil constriction is a classic sign of narcotic intoxication; hence, the stereotype of the drug user hiding behind a pair of dark sunglasses. Symptoms of tolerance and withdrawal can appear within three weeks of first use.

OxyContin: A New and Dangerous Opiate Threat

OxyContin, a prescription central nervous system depressant in the opiate drug family, has catapulted to the top of the drug abuse scene in the United States. Since its 1995 approval as a painkiller by the FDA, it has become a major contributor to adult drug abuse, causing the diversion of pills and theft of prescriptions in many regions of the country. According to a National Drug and Intelligence Center (NDIC) drug threat survey and the DEA, reporting in 2002, OxyContin has become the drug of choice in many eastern states and has now hit midwestern and western states at an epidemic pace. Some 2 percent of all high school seniors reported using OxyContin without a prescription in 2003.

OxyContin is the brand name for *oxycodone hydrochloride,* one of a large group of pain relief products commonly prescribed for people suffering chronic pain. Other drugs in this category include Percocet, Percodan, Vicodin, and other high-strength painkillers, and most are highly addictive if taken for prolonged periods of time. Most of these drugs only contain 2.5–5 mg of oxycodone. In contrast,

OxyContin is marketed in doses of 10, 20, 40, 80 and even 160 mg tablets. The strength, duration, and known dosage of OxyContin make it a powerful painkiller but also make it extremely attractive to abusers. OxyContin has become a substitute for heroin for some addicts who find pharmaceutical drugs to be purer and cheaper than street drugs.

Due to OxyContin's widespread availability, the crimes, addictions, and fatal overdoses associated with it have skyrocketed—many people have no idea of the risks they take when abusing the drug. Although exact numbers of deaths are unavailable, it is likely that there are hundreds every year among unsuspecting young adults. Formulated as a 12-hour time release pill, OxyContin has a low addiction rate among those who take it as prescribed for the most acute pain of cancer or injury. However, abusers "disable" the time release structure of the pill by chewing it, crushing it, or dissolving the pill into liquid form and then eating, snorting, or injecting the solution. When taken orally or injected in this form, the user experiences a rush similar to heroin. The mind and body easily become obsessed with this pleasurable rush and a physical craving can develop, causing addiction. Chronic use results in increasing tolerance so that more of the drug is needed to feel

the same effects that smaller doses once provided. Often the user is unaware this is happening and goes from using two pills a day, to two pills an hour, to two pills every fifteen minutes as drug tolerance builds rapidly. Self-control in using the drug is lost as the brain becomes dependent.

Because many OxyContin abusers do not know of its dangers, they may make the situation even more risky by drinking alcohol or taking sleeping pills and over-the-counter pain medications with it. These drug interactions have caused many serious side effects, even coma and death.

The good news is that complete recovery from addiction is possible, but addicted users cannot do it on their own. Medical supervision and appropriate therapeutic techniques are necessary to ensure recovery.

Sources: L. D. Johnston, P. M. O'Malley, and J. G. Bachman, *Monitoring the Future National Survey Results on Drug Use, 1975–2003. Volume I: Secondary School Students* (Bethesda, MD: National Institute on Drug Abuse, 2004); Drug Enforcement Administration, "OxyContin: Pharmaceutical Diversion," 2002, www.dea.gov; Center for Drug Education and Research, "OxyContin: Questions and Answers," 2002, http://www.fda.gov/cder/drug/infopage/oxycontin/oxycontin-qa.htm

---

The most common route of administration for heroin addicts is "mainlining"—intravenous injection of powdered heroin mixed in a solution. Many users describe the "rush" they feel when injecting themselves as intensely pleasurable, whereas others report unpredictable and unpleasant side effects. The temporary nature of the rush contributes to the drug's high potential for addiction—many addicts shoot up four or five times a day. Mainlining can cause veins to scar and eventually collapse. Once a vein has collapsed, it can no longer be used to introduce heroin into the bloodstream. Addicts become expert at locating new veins to use: in the feet, the legs, even the temples. When they do not want their needle tracks (scars) to show, they inject themselves under the tongue or in the groin.

The physiology of the human body could be said to encourage opiate addiction. Opiate-like substances called

endorphins are manufactured in the body and have multiple receptor sites, particularly in the central nervous system. When endorphins attach themselves at these points, they create feelings of painless well-being. Medical researchers refer to them as "the body's own opiates." When endorphin levels are high, people feel euphoric. Long-distance runners, for example, experience "runner's high" from elevated endorphin levels. The same euphoria occurs when opiates or related chemicals are active at the endorphin receptor sites.

Endorphins Opiate-like hormones that are manufactured in the human body and contribute to natural feelings of well-being.

Treatment for Heroin Addiction Programs to help heroin addicts kick the habit have not been very successful. The rate of *recidivism* (tendency to return to previous behaviors) is high. Some addicts resume drug use even after years of drug-free living because the craving for the injection rush is very strong. It takes a great deal of discipline to seek alternative, nondrug highs.

Heroin addicts experience a distinct pattern of withdrawal. They begin to crave another dose four to six hours after their last dose. Symptoms of withdrawal include intense desire for the drug, yawning, a runny nose, sweating, and crying. About 12 hours after the last dose, addicts experience sleep disturbance, dilated pupils, loss of appetite, irritability, goose bumps, and muscle tremors. The most difficult time in the withdrawal process occurs 24 to 72 hours following last use. All of the preceding symptoms continue, along with nausea, abdominal cramps, restlessness, insomnia, vomiting, diarrhea, extreme anxiety, hot and cold flashes, elevated blood pressure, and rapid heartbeat and respiration. Once the peak of withdrawal has passed, all these symptoms begin to subside. Still, the recovering addict has many hurdles to jump.

Methadone maintenance is one treatment available for people addicted to heroin or other opiates. Methadone is a synthetic narcotic that blocks the effects of opiate withdrawal. It is chemically similar enough to the opiates to control the tremors, chills, vomiting, diarrhea, and severe abdominal pains of withdrawal. Methadone dosage is decreased over a period of time until the addict is weaned off the drug.

Methadone maintenance is controversial because of the drug's own potential for addiction. Critics contend that the program merely substitutes one addiction for another. Proponents argue that people on methadone maintenance are less likely to engage in criminal activities to support their habits than heroin addicts are. For this reason, many meth-adone maintenance programs are financed by state or federal government and are available to clients free of charge or at reduced cost.

A number of new drug therapies for opiate dependence are emerging. Naltrexone (Trexan), an opiate antagonist, has been approved as a treatment. While on naltrexone, recovering addicts do not have the compulsion to use heroin, and if they do use it, they don't get high, so there is no point in using the drug. More recently, researchers have reported promising results with Temgesic (buprenorphine) a mild, nonaddicting synthetic opiate, which, like heroin and methadone, bonds to certain receptors in the brain, blocks pain messages, and persuades the brain that its cravings for heroin have been satisfied. Addicts report that while they are taking buprenorphine, they do not crave heroin anymore.

Hallucinogens (Psychedelics)

Hallucinogens are substances that are capable of creating auditory or visual hallucinations. These types of drugs are also known as **psychedelics,** a term adapted from the Greek phrase meaning "mind manifesting." Hallucinogens are a group of drugs whose primary pharmacological effect is to alter feelings, perceptions, and thoughts in a user. The major receptor sites for most of these drugs are in the part of the brain that is responsible for filtering extraneous or irrelevant outside stimuli before allowing these signals to travel to other parts of the brain. This area, the **reticular formation,** is located in the brain stem at the upper end of the spinal cord (Figure 14.4). When a hallucinogen is present at a reticular formation site, messages become scrambled, and the user may see wavy walls instead of straight ones or may smell colors and hear tastes. This mixing of sensory messages is known as **synesthesia.** In addition to synesthetic effects, users may become less inhibited or recall events long buried in the subconscious mind.

The most widely recognized hallucinogens are LSD, mescaline, psilocybin, and PCP. All are illegal and carry severe penalties for manufacture, possession, transportation, or sale.

LSD Of all the psychedelics, **lysergic acid diethylamide (LSD)** is the most notorious. First synthesized in the late 1930s by Swiss chemist Albert Hoffman, LSD resulted from experiments to derive medically useful drugs from the ergot fungus found on rye and other cereal grains. Because LSD seemed capable of unlocking the secrets of the mind, psychiatrists initially felt it could be beneficial to patients unable to remember suppressed traumas. From 1950 through 1968, the drug was used for such purposes.

Media attention focused on LSD in the 1960s. Young people used the drug to "turn on" and "tune out" the world that gave them the war in Vietnam, race riots, and political assassinations. In 1970, federal authorities, under intense pressure from the public, placed LSD on the list of controlled substances (Schedule I). LSD's popularity peaked in 1972,

---

Methadone maintenance A treatment for people addicted to opiates that substitutes methadone, a synthetic narcotic, for the opiate of addiction.

Hallucinogens Substances capable of creating auditory or visual distortions and heightened states.

Psychedelics Drugs that distort the processing of sensory information in the brain.

Reticular formation An area in the brain stem that is responsible for relaying messages to other areas in the brain.

Synesthesia A (usually) drug-created effect in which sensory messages are incorrectly assigned—for example, the user hears a taste or smells a sound.

Lysergic acid diethylamide (LSD) Psychedelic drug causing sensory disruptions; also called *acid.*

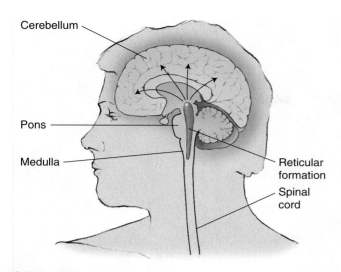

Cerebellum

Pons

Medulla

Reticular formation

Spinal cord

Figure 14.4
The Reticular Formation

then tapered off, primarily because of users' inability to control dosages accurately.

Because of the recent wave of nostalgia for the 1960s, this dangerous psychedelic drug has been making a comeback. Known on the street as "acid," LSD is now available in virtually every state. Over 11 million Americans, most of them under age 35, have tried LSD at least once. LSD especially attracts younger users. Approximately 3.5 percent of high school seniors report having tried it at least once in the past year.[14] A national survey of college students showed that 2 percent had used the drug in the past year.[15]

An odorless, tasteless, white crystalline powder, LSD is most frequently dissolved in water to make a solution that can be used to manufacture the street forms of the drug. The most common form is blotter acid—small squares of blotter-like paper that have been impregnated with the liquid. The blotter is swallowed or chewed briefly. LSD also comes in tiny thin squares of gelatin called windowpane and in tablets called microdots, which are less than an eighth of an inch across (it would take ten or more to add up to the size of an aspirin tablet). Microdots and windowpane are just a sideshow; blotter is the medium of choice. As with any illegal drug, purchasers run the risk of buying an impure product.

One of the most powerful drugs known to science, LSD can produce strong effects in doses as low as 20 micrograms (µg). (To give you an idea of how small a dose this is, the average postage stamp weighs approximately 60,000 µg.) The potency of the typical dose currently ranges from 20 to 80 µg, compared to 150 to 300 µg commonly used in the 1960s.

Despite its reputation as primarily a psychedelic, LSD produces a number of physical effects, including increased heart rate, elevated blood pressure and temperature, goose flesh (roughened skin), increased reflex speeds, muscle tremors and twitches, perspiration, increased salivation,

chills, headaches, and mild nausea. Since the drug also stimulates uterine muscle contractions, it can lead to premature labor and miscarriage in pregnant women. Research into long-term effects has been inconclusive.

The psychological effects of LSD vary. The mindset of the user and setting in which the drug is used are influential factors. Euphoria is the common psychological state produced by the drug, but *dysphoria* (a sense of evil and foreboding) may also be experienced. The drug also shortens attention span, causing the mind to wander. Thoughts may be interposed and juxtaposed, so the user experiences several different thoughts simultaneously. Synesthesia occurs occasionally. Users become introspective and suppressed memories may surface, often taking on bizarre symbolism. Many more effects are possible, including decreased aggressiveness and enhanced sensory experiences.

LSD causes distortions of ordinary perceptions, such as the movement of stationary objects. "Bad trips," the most publicized risk of LSD, are commonly related to the user's mood. The person, for example, may interpret increased heart rate as a heart attack (a "bad body trip"). Often bad trips result when a user confronts a suppressed emotional experience or memory (a "bad head trip").

While there is no evidence that LSD creates physical dependency, it may well create psychological dependence. Many LSD users become depressed for one or two days following a trip and turn to the drug to relieve this depression. The result is a cycle of LSD use to relieve post-LSD depression, which often leads to psychological addiction.

What do you think?

Are people today using LSD for the same reasons it was used in the 1960s? ■ *What are the perceived attractions and the real dangers of LSD use?*

Mescaline Mescaline is one of hundreds of chemicals derived from the **peyote** cactus, a small, buttonlike cactus that grows in the southwestern United States and Latin America. Natives of these regions have long used the dried peyote buttons for religious purposes. In fact, members of the Native American Church (a religion practiced by thousands of North American Indians) have been granted special permission to use the drug during religious ceremonies in some states.

Users normally swallow 10 to 12 dried peyote buttons. These buttons taste bitter and generally induce immediate

Mescaline   A hallucinogenic drug derived from the peyote cactus.

Peyote   A cactus with small "buttons" that, when ingested, produce hallucinogenic effects.

nausea or vomiting. Longtime users claim that the nausea becomes less noticeable with frequent use.

Those who are able to keep the drug down begin to feel the effects within 30 to 90 minutes, when mescaline reaches maximum concentration in the brain. (It may persist for up to nine or ten hours.) Mescaline is a powerful hallucinogen. It is also a central nervous system stimulant.

Products sold on the street as mescaline are likely to be synthetic chemical relatives of the true drug. Street names of these products include DOM, STP, TMA, and MMDA. Any of these can be toxic in small quantities.

Psilocybin Psilocybin and *psilocin* are the active chemicals in a group of mushrooms sometimes called "magic mushrooms." Psilocybe mushrooms, which grow throughout the world, can be cultivated from spores or harvested wild. Because many mushrooms resemble the psilocybe variety, people who use wild mushrooms for any purpose should be certain of what they are doing. Mushroom varieties can easily be misidentified, and mistakes can be fatal. Psilocybin is similar to LSD in its physical effects, which generally wear off in four to six hours.

PCP Phencyclidine, or **PCP**, is a synthetic substance that became a black-market drug in the early 1970s. PCP was originally developed as a dissociative anesthetic, which means that patients administered this drug could keep their eyes open, apparently remain conscious, and feel no pain during a medical procedure. Afterward, they would experience amnesia for the time the drug was in their system. Such a drug had obvious advantages as an anesthetic, but its unpredictability and drastic effects (postoperative delirium, confusion, and agitation) made doctors abandon it, and it was withdrawn from the legal market.

On the illegal market, PCP is a white, crystalline powder that users often sprinkle onto marijuana cigarettes. It is dangerous and unpredictable regardless of the method of administration. Common street names for PCP are "angel dust" for the crystalline powdered form and "peace pill" and "horse tranquilizer" for the tablet form. (It was used as a veterinary anesthetic for a time.)

The effects of PCP depend on the dosage. A dose as small as 5 mg will produce effects similar to those of strong central nervous system depressants—slurred speech, impaired coordination, reduced sensitivity to pain, and reduced heart and respiratory rate. Doses between 5 and 10 mg

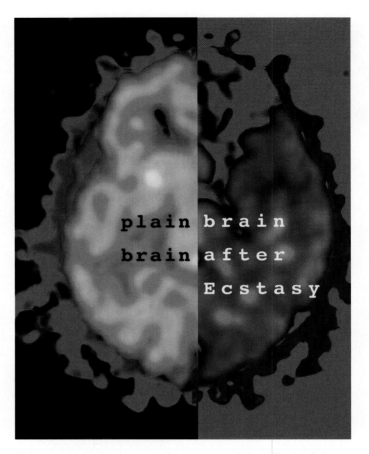

This composite brain scan shows some of the effects of the drug Ecstasy. The left side shows healthy serotonin sites. The dark sections on the right are serotonin sites no longer present even after three weeks without Ecstasy. Serotonin helps regulate mood, learning, and sleep.

cause fever, salivation, nausea, vomiting, and total loss of sensitivity to pain. Doses greater than 10 mg result in a drastic drop in blood pressure, coma, muscular rigidity, violent outbursts, and possible convulsions and death.

Psychologically, PCP may produce either euphoria or dysphoria. It is also known to produce hallucinations as well as delusions and overall delirium. Some users experience a prolonged state of "nothingness." The long-term effects of PCP use are unknown.

Designer Drugs (Club Drugs)

Designer drugs are produced in chemical laboratories, often manufactured in homes, and sold illegally. These drugs are easy to produce from available raw materials. The drugs themselves were once technically legal because the law had to specify the exact chemical structure of an illicit substance. However, there is now a law in place that bans all chemical cousins of illegal drugs.

Psilocybin The active chemical found in psilocybe mushrooms; it produces hallucinations.

Phencyclidine (PCP) A drug, commonly called "angel dust," that causes hallucinations, delusions, and delirium.

Club Drugs on Campus

Every era seems to have its hot drug. At one point it was Valium, then LSD, and then crack. Currently the so-called club drugs are popular on college campuses. Three of note include Rohypnol (flunitrazepam), also called "ropies" or "roofies"; GHB (gamma hydroxybutyrate), or as it is known on the street, "grievous bodily harm"; and Special K (ketamine).

Rohypnol is a potent tranquilizer similar in nature to Valium, but many times stronger. The drug produces a sedative effect, amnesia, muscle relaxation, and slowed psychomotor responses. Commonly known as the "date rape drug," Rohypnol has gained notoriety as a growing problem on college campuses. The drug has been added to punch and other drinks at fraternity parties and college social gatherings, where it is reportedly given to female partiers in hopes of lowering their inhibitions and facilitating potential sexual conquests. The manufacturer changed the formula to give the drug a bright blue color that would make it easy to detect in most drinks, so would-be perpetrators are turning to blue tropical drinks and punches to disguise the drug. While "ropie" fervor has subsided somewhat, it continues to be a concern. See the Reality Check box in Chapter 4 on strategies to protect yourself from being dosed with Rohypnol.

Rohypnol has been joined by a newer, liquid substance called GHB, or gamma-hydroxybutyrate. GHB is used as an aphrodisiac to increase one's sense of touch and sexual prowess, as a muscle builder, and as a tranquilizer. GHB is an odorless, tasteless fluid that can be made easily at home or in a chemistry lab. Like Rohypnol, GHB has been slipped into drinks without being detected, resulting in loss of memory, unconsciousness, amnesia, and even death. Other side effects of GHB include nausea, vomiting, seizures, memory loss, hallucinations, coma, and respiratory distress. During the 1980s, GHB was available in U.S. health food stores. Concerns about its use led the FDA to ban OTC sales in 1990, and GHB is now a Schedule I controlled substance.

The Special K we're referring to is not the breakfast cereal, but rather ketamine, used as an anesthetic in many hospital and veterinary clinics. On the street, Special K is most often diverted in liquid form from veterinary offices or medical suppliers. Dealers dry the liquid (usually by cooking it) and grind the residue into powder. Special K causes hallucinations as it inhibits the relay of sensory input; the brain fills the resulting void with visions, dreams, memories, and sensory distortions. The effects of Special K are not as severe as those of Ecstasy, so it has grown in popularity among people who have to go to work or school after a night of partying.

Sources: U.S. Department of Health and Human Services, "Ketamine: A Fact Sheet," downloaded September 9, 2004, www.health.org/nongovpubs/ketamine; Office of National Drug Control Policy, "Rohypnol Fact Sheet," February 2003, www.whitehousedrugpolicy.gov/publications/factsht/rohypnol; Office of National Drug Control Policy, "Gamma-Hydroxybutyrate (GHB) Fact Sheet," November 2002, www.whitehousedrugpolicy.gov.publications/factsht/gamma; T. Nordenberg, "The Death of the Party: All the Rave, GHB's Hazards Go Unheeded," *FDA Consumer Magazine*, March–April 2000, www.fda.gov/fdac/200_toc.html

---

Collectively known as **club drugs,** these dangerous substances include Ecstasy, GHB, Special K, and Rohypnol. Although users may think them harmless, research has shown that club drugs can produce a range of unwanted effects, including hallucinations, paranoia, amnesia, and in some cases, death. Some club drugs work on the same brain mechanisms as alcohol and can dangerously boost the effects of both substances. Since the drugs are odorless and tasteless, people can easily slip them into drinks. Some of them have been associated with sexual assault and for that reason are referred to as "date rape drugs" (see the Reality Check box above).

Ecstasy (methylene dioxymethylamphetamine, or MDMA), once dubbed the "LSD of the 80s," has had a resurgence of popularity on many college campuses. Almost one of every four students at some universities report having used it. Ecstasy creates feelings of openness and warmth, combined with the mind-expanding characteristics of hallucinogens. Effects begin within 30 minutes and can last for four to six hours. Young people may use Ecstasy initially to improve mood or get energized so they can keep dancing; it also increases heart rate and blood pressure and may raise body temperature to the point of kidney and/or cardiovascular failure. Chronic use appears to damage the brain's ability to think and to regulate emotion, memory, sleep, and pain. Combined with alcohol, Ecstasy can be extremely dangerous and sometimes fatal. Recent studies indicate that Ecstasy

---

Designer drug or **club drug**　A synthetic analog (a drug that produces similar effects) of an existing illicit drug.

Ecstasy　A club drug that creates feelings of openness and warmth but also raises heart rate and blood pressure.

Should We "Protect" Illicit Drug Users?

Recently, three young people died in Chicago after taking tablets they thought contained Ecstasy. One young woman ingested what she thought was "Mitsubishi," a potent version of Ecstasy. Within a few hours, she was rushed to the hospital. There she lapsed into a coma, and her body temperature rose quickly to 108°F. She was bleeding from her mouth and stomach and began having seizures. By the following afternoon, she was dead. Instead of taking Ecstasy (methylene dioxymethamphetamine or MDMA,

the chemical found in unadulterated Ecstasy) she had unknowingly swallowed paramethoxymethamphetamine (PMA). PMA is cheaper and easier to manufacture than Ecstasy, but far more dangerous.

Contaminated illegal drugs have never been a big issue in the United States, but if the use of Ecstasy continues to rise, as some researchers speculate it will, more and more dealers may start substituting deadly substances like PMA for less potent substances like MDMA, speed, cocaine, caffeine, PCP, Valium, ketamine, or a variety of other drugs. To deal with this potential danger, on-site pill testing has become available at some raves run by Dance Safe (a nonprofit organization promoting health and safety within the rave and nightclub

community). Also available are pill-testing kits, which can be purchased on the Internet, that allow people to test their own Ecstasy pills. Alternatively, they can send pills to a laboratory for testing.

Do you believe that such pill-testing services should be readily available? Why or why not? What ethical issues do such harm-reduction services raise? What benefits do they offer? Would you advocate an increase in such services? What other programs are you familiar with that aim to reduce the harm caused by drug use and abuse?

Source: T. Oehmke, "Ecstasy: The Poisoning of Suburbia," *Icon*, July 27, 2000, pp. 7–8.

---

may cause long-lasting neurotoxic effects by damaging brain cells that produce serotonin, and it is unknown whether these brain cells will regenerate.[16] (See the Health Ethics box for more on Ecstasy.)

Inhalants

Inhalants are chemicals that produce vapors which, when inhaled, can cause hallucinations and create intoxicating and euphoric effects. Not commonly recognized as drugs, inhalants are legal to purchase and universally available but dangerous when used incorrectly. They generally appeal to young people who can't afford or obtain illicit substances.

Some of these agents are organic solvents representing the chemical by-products of the distillation of petroleum products. Rubber cement, model glue, paint thinner, lighter fluid, varnish, wax, spot removers, and gasoline belong to this group. Most of these substances are sniffed by users in search of a quick, cheap high.

Because they are inhaled, the volatile chemicals in these products reach the bloodstream within seconds. An inhaled substance is not diluted or buffered by stomach acids or other body fluids and thus is more potent than it would be

if swallowed. This characteristic, along with the fact that dosages are extremely difficult to control because everyone has unique lung and breathing capacities, makes inhalants particularly dangerous.

The effects of inhalants usually last for fewer than 15 minutes. Users may experience dizziness, disorientation, impaired coordination, reduced judgment, and slowed reaction times. Signs of inhalant use include the following: unjustifiable collection of glues, paints, lacquer thinner, cleaning fluid, and ether; sniffles similar to those produced by a cold; and a smell on the breath similar to the inhalable substance. The effects of inhalants resemble those of central nervous system depressants, and combining inhalants with alcohol produces a synergistic effect. In addition, combining these substances can cause severe liver damage that can be fatal.

An overdose of fumes from inhalants can cause unconsciousness. If the user's oxygen intake is reduced during the inhaling process, death can result within five minutes. Whether a user is a first-time or chronic user, sudden sniffing death (SSD) syndrome can be a fatal consequence. This syndrome can occur if a user inhales deeply and then participates in physical activity or is startled.

Amyl Nitrite Sometimes called "poppers" or "rush," **amyl nitrite** is packaged in small, cloth-covered glass capsules that can be crushed to release the active chemical. The drug is often prescribed to alleviate chest pain in heart patients because it dilates small blood vessels and reduces blood pressure. Dilation of blood vessels in the genital area is thought to enhance sensations or perceptions of orgasm. It also produces fainting, dizziness, warmth, and skin flushing.

Inhalants Products that are sniffed or inhaled in order to produce highs.

Amyl nitrite A drug that dilates blood vessels and is properly used to relieve chest pain.

Nitrous Oxide Nitrous oxide is sometimes used as an adjunct to dental anesthesia or minor surgical anesthesia. It is also a propellant chemical in aerosol products such as whipped toppings. Users experience a state of euphoria, floating sensations, and illusions. Effects also include pain relief and a "silly" feeling, demonstrated by laughing and giggling (hence its nickname "laughing gas"). Regulating dosages of this drug can be difficult. Sustained inhalation can lead to unconsciousness, coma, and death.

Steroids

Public awareness of **anabolic steroids** has been heightened by media stories about their use by amateur and professional athletes, including Arnold Schwarzenegger during his competitive bodybuilding days. Anabolic steroids are artificial forms of the male hormone testosterone that promote muscle growth and strength. These **ergogenic drugs** are used primarily by young men who believe the drugs will increase their strength, power, bulk (weight), speed, and athletic performance.

Most steroids are obtained through the black market. It was once estimated that approximately 17 to 20 percent of college athletes used them. Now that stricter drug-testing policies have been instituted by the NCAA, reported use of anabolic steroids among intercollegiate athletes has dropped to 1.1 percent. However, a recent survey among high school students found a significant increase in the use of anabolic steroids since 1991. Few data exist on the extent of steroid abuse by adults. It has been estimated that hundreds of thousands of people age 18 and older abuse anabolic steroids at least once a year. Among both adolescents and adults, steroid abuse is higher among males than females. However, steroid abuse is growing most rapidly among young women.[17]

Steroids are available in two forms: injectable solutions and pills. Anabolic steroids produce a state of euphoria, diminished fatigue, and increased bulk and power in both sexes. These qualities give steroids an addictive quality. When users stop, they can experience psychological withdrawal and sometimes severe depression, in some cases leading to suicide attempts. If untreated, depression associated with steroid withdrawal has been known to last for a year or more after steroid use stops.

Men and women who use steroids experience a variety of adverse effects. These drugs cause mood swings (aggression and violence), sometimes known as "'roid rage"; acne; liver tumors; elevated cholesterol levels; hypertension; kidney disease; and immune system disturbances. There is also a danger of transmitting AIDS and hepatitis (a serious liver disease) through shared needles. In women, large doses of anabolic steroids may trigger the development of masculine attributes such as lowered voice, increased facial and body hair, and male pattern baldness; they may also result in an enlarged clitoris, smaller breasts, and changes in or absence of menstruation. When taken by healthy males, anabolic steroids shut down the body's production of testosterone, causing men's breasts to grow and testicles to atrophy.

To combat the growing problem of steroid use, the U.S. Congress passed the Anabolic Steroids Control Act (ASCA) of 1990. This law makes it a crime to possess, prescribe, or distribute anabolic steroids for any use other than the treatment of specific diseases. Anabolic steroids are now classified as a Schedule III drug. Penalties for their illegal use include up to five years' imprisonment and a $250,000 fine for the first offense and up to ten years' imprisonment and a $500,000 fine for subsequent offenses.

A new and alarming trend is the use of other drugs to achieve the effects of steroids. The two most common steroid alternatives are gamma hydroxybutyrate (GHB) and clenbuterol. GHB is a deadly, illegal drug that is a primary ingredient in many "performance-enhancing" formulas. GHB does not produce a high. It does, however, cause headaches, nausea, vomiting, diarrhea, seizures, and other central nervous system disorders, and possibly death. Clenbuterol is used in some countries for veterinary treatments but is not approved for any use—in animals or humans—in the United States.

New attention was drawn to the issue of steroids and related substances when St. Louis Cardinals slugger Mark McGwire admitted to using a supplement containing androstenedione ("andro"), an adrenal hormone that is produced naturally in both men and women. Andro raises levels of the male hormone testosterone, which helps build lean muscle mass and promotes quicker recovery after injury. McGwire had done nothing illegal, as the supplement could be purchased over the counter (with sales estimated at $800 million a year) and its use was legal in baseball, although banned by the NFL, NCAA, and International Olympic Committee. A recent study found that when men take 100 milligrams of andro three times daily, it increases estrogen levels by up to 80 percent, enlarges the prostate gland, and increases heart disease risk by 10 to 15 percent. Major league baseball banned its use in 2004.

Visits to the locker rooms of many sports teams would disclose large containers of other alleged muscle-building supplements, such as creatine. Although they are legal, questions remain whether enough research has been done concerning the safety of these supplements. Some

---

Nitrous oxide The chemical name for "laughing gas," a substance properly used for surgical or dental anesthesia.

Anabolic steroids Artificial forms of the hormone testosterone that promote muscle growth and strength.

Ergogenic drug Substance that enhances athletic performance.

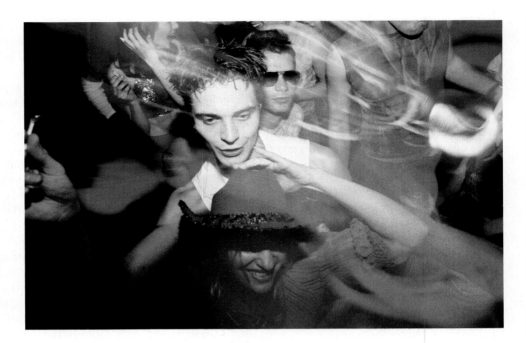

Beware of claims that the latest club drugs are "totally harmless" or "all natural." Such substances can be hazardous.

experts worry that they may bring consequences similar to those of steroids, such as liver damage and heart problems. Some of these performance-enhancing supplements are discussed further in Chapter 23, Complementary and Alternative Medicine.

What do you think?

Would you consider using supplements for the sole purpose of increasing your body build and potentially your athletic performance? ■ *Are steroid users stigmatized in our society in the same way as users of other illicit drugs?* ■ *Do you think they should be? Why or why not?*

Illegal Drug Use in the United States

Stories of people who have tried illegal drugs, enjoyed them, and suffered no consequences may tempt you to try them yourself. You may tell yourself it's "just this once," convincing yourself that one-time use is harmless. Given the dangers surrounding these substances, however, you should think twice. The risks associated with drug use extend beyond the personal. The decision to try any illicit substance encourages illicit drug manufacture and transport, thus contributing to the national drug problem. The financial burden of illegal drug use on the U.S. economy is staggering, with an estimated economic cost of around $160 billion.[18] This estimate includes costs associated with substance abuse treatment and prevention, health care, reduced job productivity and lost earnings, and social consequences such as crime and social welfare.

In addition, roughly half of all expenditures to combat crime are related to illegal drugs. The burden of these costs is absorbed primarily by the government (46 percent), followed by those who abuse drugs and members of their households (44 percent). One study found that Americans spend $64 billion on illicit drugs annually. These numbers break down as follows: $35 billion on cocaine, $10 billion each on marijuana and heroin, and $5 billion on methamphetamines. This is eight times what the federal government spends on research on HIV/AIDS, cancer, and heart disease put together.[19]

Drugs in the Workplace

The National Institute of Drug Abuse (NIDA) estimates that 8.5 percent of all U.S. workers use dangerous drugs on the job at some time. With approximately 70 to 75 percent of drug users in the United States employed to some degree, the cost to American business soars into the billions of dollars annually.[20] These costs reflect reduced work performance and efficiency, lost productivity, absenteeism and turnover, increased use of health benefits, accidents, and indirect losses stemming from impaired judgment.

The highest rates of illicit drug use among workers exist in the construction, food preparation, restaurant, transportation, and material-moving industries. Workers who require a considerable amount of public trust, such as police officers, teachers, and child-care workers, report the lowest use. In addition, younger employees (18 to 24 years old) are more likely to report drug use than employees aged 25 and older. Drug users are 1.6 times more likely than nonusers to quit their jobs or be fired and are 1.5 times more likely to be disciplined by their supervisor.[21]

Many companies have instituted drug testing for their employees. Mandatory drug urinalysis is controversial. Critics argue that such testing violates Fourth Amendment rights of protection from unreasonable search and seizure. Proponents believe the personal inconvenience entailed in testing pales in comparison to the problems caused by drug use in the workplace. Several court decisions have affirmed the right of employers to test their employees for drug use. They contend that Fourth Amendment rights pertain only to employees of government agencies, not to those of private businesses. Most Americans apparently support drug testing for certain types of jobs.

Drug testing is expensive, with costs running as high as $100 per test. Moreover, some critics question the accuracy and reliability of the results. Both false positives and false negatives can occur. As drug testing becomes more common in the work environment, it is gaining greater acceptance by employees, who see testing as a step to improving safety and productivity.

What do you think?

What do you believe are the moral and ethical issues surrounding drug testing? ■ *Are you in favor of drug testing?* ■ *Should all employees be subjected to drug tests or just those in high-risk jobs?* ■ *Is it the employer's right to conduct drug testing at the work site? Explain your answer.*

Solutions to the Problem

Americans are alarmed by the increasing use of illegal drugs. Respondents in public opinion polls feel that the most important strategy for fighting drug abuse is educating young people. They also endorse strategies such as stricter border surveillance to reduce drug trafficking, longer prison sentences for drug dealers, increased government spending on prevention, enforcing antidrug laws, and greater cooperation between government agencies and private groups and individuals providing treatment assistance. All of these approaches will probably help up to a point, but they do not offer a total solution to the problem. Drug abuse has been a part of human behavior for thousands of years, and it is not likely to disappear in the near future. For this reason, it is necessary to educate ourselves and to develop the self-discipline necessary to avoid dangerous drug dependence.

For many years, the most popular antidrug strategies were total prohibition and "scare tactics." Both approaches proved ineffective. Prohibition of alcohol during the 1920s created more problems than it solved, as did prohibition of opiates in 1914. Outlawing other illicit drugs has neither eliminated them nor curtailed their traffic across U.S. borders.

In general, researchers in the field of drug education agree that a multimodal approach is best. Students should be taught the difference between drug use and abuse. Factual information that is free of scare tactics must be presented; lecturing and moralizing do not work. Emphasis should be placed on things that are important to young people. Telling adolescent males that girls will find them disgusting if their breath stinks of cigarettes or pot will get their attention. Likewise, lecturing on the negative effects of drug use is a much less effective deterrent than teaching young people how to negotiate the social scene. Drug Abuse Resistance Education, commonly called DARE, is one program intended to educate students but has been largely ineffective. Education efforts need to focus on achieving better outcomes for preventing drug use.

We must also study at-risk groups so we can better understand the circumstances that make them susceptible to drug use. Time, money, and effort by educators, parents, and policy makers are needed to ensure that today's youth receive the love and security essential for building productive and meaningful lives and rejecting drug use.

What do you think?

Do you feel the public has a social responsibility to fight drug abuse? ■ *What is the cost society pays for drug use?* ■ *Have you ever personally known someone who has suffered because of addiction to drugs?* ■ *How did you respond?*

MAKE IT HAPPEN!

Assessment: The Assess Yourself box on page 403 describes signs of being controlled by drugs or by a drug user. Depending on your results, you may need to take steps toward changing certain behaviors that may be detrimental to your health.

Making a Change: In order to change your behavior, you need to develop a plan. Follow these steps.

1. Evaluate your behavior and identify patterns. What can you change now? What can you change in the near future?
2. Select one pattern of behavior that you want to change.
3. Fill out a Behavior Change Contract. It should include your long-term goal for change, your short-term goals, the rewards for reaching these goals, potential obstacles along the way, and strategies for overcoming these obstacles. For each goal, list the small steps and specific actions that you will take.
4. Chart your progress in a journal. At the end of a week, consider how successful you were in following your plan. What helped you be successful? What will you do differently next week?
5. Revise your plan as needed: Are the short-term goals attainable? Are the rewards satisfying?

One Student's Plan: Tranh was surprised to find he had several "yes" answers to the self-assessment section about being controlled by a drug user. He realized that his girlfriend Kim's drug use was hurting their relationship and negatively affecting his well-being. Kim smoked marijuana almost every day and took club drugs at least twice a month. Tranh often had to lie to Kim's employer if she was too incapacitated to go to work. Recently she had been in a car accident after smoking pot for several hours, which damaged Tranh's car and increased his insurance rate. And he worried whenever she went out for an evening that she was taking Ecstasy and would find herself in a compromising situation.

These worries, financial consequences, and pressure to lie all made Tranh resolve to change his responses to Kim's behavior. His first step was to plan what he wanted to say to Kim about her drug use and how it affected both of them. He also started investigating drug counseling resources at school and in the community, both for Kim and for himself to help him cope with the issues raised by Kim's drug use. Finally, he began talking to Kim's friends, who it turned out were also concerned by her behavior. They worked together to develop strategies to help Kim and provide alternatives to her drug use; Tranh also felt less alone and more supported as soon as he started reaching out to his peers.

Summary

- The six categories of drugs are prescription drugs, OTC drugs, recreational drugs, herbal preparations, illicit drugs, and commercial preparations. Routes of administration include oral ingestion, injection (intravenous, intramuscular, and subcutaneous), inhalation, inunction, and suppositories.
- People from all walks of life use illicit drugs, although college students report higher usage rates than the general population. Drug use has declined since the mid-1980s.

- Controlled substances include cocaine and its derivatives, amphetamines, newer-generation stimulants, marijuana, opiates, hallucinogens, designer drugs, inhalants, and steroids. Users tend to become addicted quickly to such drugs.
- The drug problem reaches everyone through crime and elevated health care costs. Drugs are a major problem in the workplace; workplace drug testing is one proposed solution to this problem.

Questions for Discussion and Reflection

1. What is the current theory that explains how drugs work in the body? Explain this theory.
2. Do you think there is such a thing as responsible use of illicit drugs? Would you change any of the current laws governing drugs? How would you determine what is legitimate use and illegitimate use?
3. Why do you think that many people today feel that marijuana use is not dangerous? What are the arguments in favor of legalizing marijuana? What are the arguments against legalization? How common is the use of marijuana on your campus?

4. How do you and your peers feel about illicit drug use? Has your opinion changed in recent years? If so, how and why?

5. Debate the issue of workplace drug testing. Would you apply for a job that had drug testing as an interview requirement? As a continuing requirement?

6. What could you do to help a friend who is fighting a substance abuse problem? What resources on your campus could help you?

7. Why are drugs such as Rohypnol and Ecstasy of great concern these days? If someone has "consensual" sex with another person after lacing his or her drink with one of these drugs, do you think it's a case of rape and should be prosecuted as such? Why or why not?

8. How do you think reports in the media about the use of stimulants and/or steroids by athletes affect the popularity of these drugs? Would you consider taking such a drug to improve your appearance or your athletic performance? Explain your answer.

9. What types of programs do you think would be effective in preventing drug abuse among high school and college students? How might programs for high school differ from those for college students?

Accessing Your Health on the Internet

Visit the following Internet sites to explore further topics and issues related to personal health. To visit an organization's website, go to the Companion Website for *Access to Health, Ninth Edition* at www.aw-bc.com/donatelle, click on the book image, and select "Accessing Your Health on the Internet" from the navigation menu.

1. **Club Drugs.** A website designed to disseminate science-based information about club drugs.
2. **Join Together.** An excellent site for the most current information related to substance abuse. This site also includes information on gun violence and provides advice on organizing and taking political action.
3. **National Institute on Drug Abuse.** The home page of this U.S. government agency has information on the latest statistics and findings in drug research.
4. **Substance Abuse and Mental Health Services Administration (SAMHSA).** Outstanding resource for information about national surveys, ongoing research and national drug interventions.

Further Reading

Elster, J. (ed.). *Addiction: Entries and Exits*. New York: Russell Sage Foundation, 2000.

Addresses current addiction controversies from an international perspective, with authors from the United States and Norway. Topics include whether addicts have a choice in their behavior and current addiction theories.

Goldstein, A. *Addiction: From Biology to Drug Policy*. New York: Oxford University Press, 2001.

This book discusses how drugs impact the brain, how each drug causes addiction, and how addictive drugs impact society. The author offers an explanation of what we know about drug addiction, how we know what we know, and what we can and cannot do about the drug problem.

Hales, D. and R. E. Hales. *Caring for the Mind: The Comprehensive Guide to Mental Health*. New York: Bantam, 1995.

An easy-to-understand reference that includes chapters on substance abuse problems and impulse control–related disorders, including compulsive gambling and compulsive shopping.

James, W. H. and S. L. Johnson. *Doin' Drugs: Patterns of African American Addiction*. Austin: University of Texas Press, 1997.

A concise examination of historical and current patterns of drug use in the African American community; begins with a historical overview and then proceeds to specific drugs, such as alcohol and cocaine; includes an exploration of the involvement of the church in dealing with drugs and addiction.

Reinarman, C. and H. G. Levine (eds.). *Crack in America: Demon Drugs and Social Justice*. Berkeley: University of California Press, 1997.

Examines the myths and realities of crack cocaine and how government policies toward crack may reflect racism and classism. Also explores the failure of drug prohibition.

West, J. W. *The Betty Ford Center Book of Answers: Help for Those Struggling with Substance Abuse and the People Who Love Them*. New York: Pocket Books, 1997.

Written by the former director of the Betty Ford Center, one of the leading alcohol and drug treatment centers in the United States. Provides answers to the most frequently asked questions about treatment and recovery; includes comprehensive coverage of drug abuse issues for addicts and their families.

OBJECTIVES

- Discuss the incidence, prevalence, and outcomes of cardiovascular disease in America, including its impact on society.

- Describe the anatomy and physiology of the heart and circulatory system and the importance of healthy heart function.

- Review major types of heart disease, factors that contribute to their development, diagnostic and treatment options, and the importance of fundamental lifestyle modifications aimed at prevention.

- Discuss controllable risk factors for cardiovascular disease, including smoking, cholesterol and triglycerides, certain infectious organisms, diet and obesity, exercise, hypertension, diabetes

mellitus, and stress. Examine your own risk profile, and determine those risk factors you can and cannot control.

- Discuss the issues surrounding cardiovascular disease risk and disease burden in women.

- Discuss methods of diagnosing and treating cardiovascular disease and the importance of being a wise health care consumer.

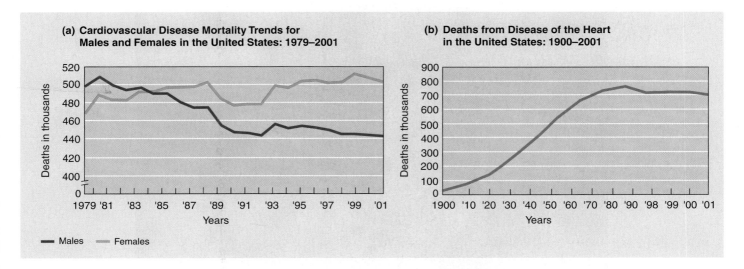

Figure 15.2

Trends in Deaths from Cardiovascular Disease

Total cardiovascular disease data are not available for much of the time period covered by this chart.

Source: (a) American Heart Association, "Statistical Fact Sheets: Women and Cardiovascular Diseases," 2004, www.americanheart.org/presenter.jhtml?identifier = 3000941 (b) American Heart Association, *Heart Disease and Stroke Statistics—2004 Update* (Dallas, TX: American Heart Association, 2004). © 2004 American Heart Association. Reproduced with permission. www.americanheart.org

- Among Hispanic Americans, 29 percent of men and 27 percent of women have CVD. They are less likely than other groups to have HBP but also are less likely to be aware of it and to be treated for it.[8]
- Along with the recent explosive increase in the prevalence of obesity and type 2 diabetes has come an increase in their related complications: hypertension, hyperlipidemia, and atherosclerotic vascular diseases.
- In terms of total deaths, in every year since 1984, CVD has claimed the lives of more women than men.

Though these statistics seem grave enough, they do not include the effects of CVD experienced by people who must live with the disease. Today, nearly 62 million Americans live with one of the major categories of CVD. Many people with CVD do not know they have a serious problem.[9] Nearly 13 million of them have a history of heart attack, angina pectoris (chest pain), or both.[10] In spite of major improvements in medication, surgery, and other health care procedures, the prognosis for many of these individuals is not good:[11]

- Twenty-five percent of men and 38 percent of women will die within one year after having an initial heart attack. In part because women have heart attacks at an older age than men do, women are more likely to die from heart attacks within just a few weeks.
- People who survive the acute stages of a heart attack have a chance of illness and death that is 1.5 to 15 times higher than that of the general population, depending on their sex and clinical outcomes. The risk of another heart attack, sudden death, angina pectoris, heart failure, and stroke—for both men and women—is substantial.
- Coronary heart disease is a major cause of death among adults at the peak of their reproductive lives.[12]
- Within six years of a recognized heart attack, 18 percent of men and 35 percent of women will have another heart attack, 7 percent of men and 6 percent of women will experience sudden death, and about 22 percent of men and 46 percent of women will be disabled with heart failure. About two-thirds of heart attack patients won't make a complete recovery, but 88 percent of those under age 65 will be able to return to their usual work.
- CHD will permanently disable 19 percent of the U.S. labor force.
- CVD death rates are highest in the southeastern regions of the United States and lowest in the Northwest and Southwest (see Figure 15.1).

Cardiovascular disease (CVD) Disease of the heart and blood vessels.

Sudden cardiac death Death that occurs as a result of sudden, abrupt loss of heart function.

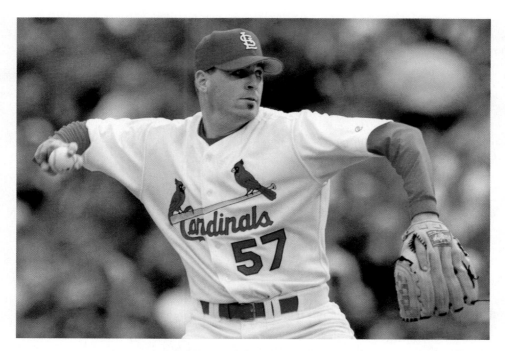

Cardiovascular disease can affect even the youngest and most fit people. Daryl Kile, a 33-year-old professional baseball player, died suddenly from atherosclerosis. It was discovered after his death that two of the main arteries in his heart were 80 to 90 percent blocked. His heart was also enlarged, weighing 20 percent more than normal.

- Although older adults are at higher risk, CVD is also one of the leading causes of death for children under the age of 15. Increasing numbers of children have congenital heart defects and strokes are a serious problem in babies under one year of age.[13] It is important to recognize that risk factors for CVD increase with age, making early prevention even more critical.

Although it is impossible to place a monetary value on human life, the economic burden of cardiovascular disease on our society is staggering—more than $368 billion is estimated for 2004.[14] This figure includes the cost of physician and nursing services, hospital and nursing home services, medications, and lost productivity resulting from disability. As Americans live longer with chronic diseases, costs will continue to increase, resulting in a tremendous burden on the health care system. The many Americans who think that CVD can be cured with a bypass or other surgical procedure, after which life simply returns to normal, are wrong. The effects of CVD can be far reaching and take a toll on quality of life. Even the best treatments exact a heavy toll on families, individuals, and society.

The best line of defense against CVD is to prevent it from developing in the first place. How can you cut your risk? Take steps now to change certain behaviors. Controlling high blood pressure and reducing intake of saturated fats and cholesterol are two examples of things you can do to lower your chances of heart attack. By maintaining your weight, exercising, decreasing your intake of sodium, not smoking, and changing your lifestyle to reduce stress, you can lower your blood pressure. You can also monitor the levels of fat and cholesterol in your blood and adjust your diet to prevent arteries from becoming blocked. Having combinations of risk factors seems to increase overall risk by a factor greater than those of the combined risks. Happily, the converse is also true: reducing several risk factors can have a dramatic effect. Answer the questions in the Assess Yourself box to determine your overall coronary risk. Understanding how your cardiovascular system works will help you understand your risk and how to reduce it.

What do you think?

Consider what happens when people who suffer a heart attack survive. ■ *What unique challenges do they face?* ■ *What difficulties might they encounter at home, at work, and in leisure time?* ■ *What might it be like to live in fear that your heart might give out or a problem could crop up at any time?* ■ *What support services are available for coping with the unique fears and anxieties faced by CVD survivors and their families?*

Understanding Your CVD Risk

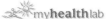

Fill out this assessment online at www.aw-bc.com/myhealthlab or www.aw-bc.com/donatelle

Each of us has a unique level of risk for various diseases. Some of these risks are things you can take action to change; others are risks that you need to consider as you plan a lifelong strategy for overall risk reduction. Complete each of the following questions and total your points in each section. If you score between 1 and 5 in any section, consider your risk. The higher the number, the greater your risk. If you answered "don't know" for any question, talk to your parents or other family members as soon as possible to find out if you have any unknown risks.

PART I: ASSESS YOUR FAMILY RISK FOR CVD

1. Do any of your primary relatives (mother, father, grandparents, siblings) have a history of heart disease or stroke? YES _____ (1 point) NO _____ (0 points) Don't Know _____

2. Do any of your primary relatives (mother, father, grandparents, siblings) have diabetes? YES _____ (1 point) NO _____ (0 points) Don't Know _____

3. Do any of your primary relatives (mother, father, grandparents, siblings) have high blood pressure? YES _____ (1 point) NO _____ (0 points) Don't Know _____

4. Do any of your primary relatives (mother, father, grandparents, siblings) have a history of high cholesterol? YES _____ (1 point) NO _____ (0 points) Don't Know _____

5. Would you say that your family consumed a high fat diet (lots of red meat, dairy, butter/margarine) during your time spent at home? YES _____ (1 point) NO _____ (0 points) Don't Know _____

Total Points _____

PART II: ASSESS YOUR LIFESTYLE RISK FOR CVD

1. Is your total cholesterol level higher than it should be? YES _____ (1 point) NO _____ (0 points) Don't Know _____

2. Do you have high blood pressure? YES _____ (1 point) NO _____ (0 points) Don't Know _____

3. Have you been diagnosed as prediabetic or diabetic? YES _____ (1 point) NO _____ (0 points) Don't Know _____

4. Do you smoke? YES _____ (1 point) NO _____ (0 points) Don't Know _____

5. Would you describe your life as being highly stressful? YES _____ (1 point) NO _____ (0 points) Don't Know _____

Total Points _____

PART III: ASSESS YOUR ADDITIONAL RISKS FOR CVD

1. How would you best describe your current weight?
   a. Lower than what it should be for my height and weight (0 points)
   b. About what it should be for my height and weight (0 points)
   c. Higher than it should be for my height and weight (1 point)

2. How would you describe the level of exercise that you get each day?
   a. Less than what I should be exercising each day (1 point)
   b. About what I should be exercising each day (0 points)
   c. More than what I should be each day (0 points)

(continues)

3. How would you describe your dietary behaviors?
   a. Eating only the recommended number of calories/day (0 points)
   b. Eating *less* than the recommended number of calories each day (0 points)
   c. Eating *more* than the recommended number of calories each day (1 point)

4. Which of the following best describes your typical dietary behavior?
   a. I eat from the major food groups, trying hard to get the recommended fruits and vegetables (0 points)
   b. I eat too much red meat and consume much saturated fat from meats and dairy products each day (1 point)
   c. Whenever possible, I try to substitute olive oil or canola oil for other forms of dietary fat. (0 points)

5. Which of the following best describes you?
   a. I watch my sodium intake and try to reduce stress in my life (0 points)
   b. I have a history of *Chlamydia* infection (1 point)
   c. I try to eat 5 to 10 milligrams of soluble fiber each day and to substitute a soy product for an animal product in my diet at least once each week. (0 points)

Total Points _____

MAKE IT HAPPEN!

Use the results of this self-assessment to begin your behavior change program. Follow the steps and use the examples on page 447 to complete your Behavior Change Contract, and use these resources to take action.

Understanding the Cardiovascular System

The **cardiovascular system** is the network of organs and elastic tubes through which blood flows as it carries oxygen and nutrients to all parts of the body and removes waste. It includes the *heart, arteries, arterioles* (small arteries), and *capillaries* (minute blood vessels). It also includes *venules* (small veins) and *veins,* the blood vessels though which blood flows as it returns to the heart and lungs.

Cardiovascular system   A complex system consisting of the heart and blood vessels that transports nutrients, oxygen, hormones, metabolic wastes, and enzymes throughout the body and regulates temperature, the water levels of cells, and the acidity levels of body components.

Atria   The two upper chambers of the heart, which receive blood.

Ventricles   The two lower chambers of the heart, which pump blood through the blood vessels.

The Heart: A Mighty Machine

The heart is a muscular, four-chambered pump, roughly the size of your fist. It is a highly efficient, extremely flexible organ that contracts 100,000 times each day, pumping the equivalent of 2,000 gallons of blood to all areas of the body. In a 70-year lifetime, an average human heart beats 2.5 billion times. This number is significantly higher for hearts that must fight to keep people moving who are out of shape and overweight.

Under normal circumstances, the human body contains approximately 6 quarts of blood. This blood transports nutrients, oxygen, waste products, hormones, and enzymes throughout the body. Blood also regulates body temperature, cellular water levels, and acidity levels of body components and aids in bodily defense against toxins and harmful microorganisms. An adequate blood supply is essential to health and well-being.

The heart's four chambers work together to recirculate blood constantly throughout the body (Figure 15.3). The two upper chambers of the heart, called **atria,** are large collecting chambers that receive blood from the rest of the body. The two lower chambers, known as **ventricles,** pump the blood out again. Small valves regulate the steady, rhythmic flow of blood between chambers and prevent inappropriate backwash. The *tricuspid valve* (located between the right

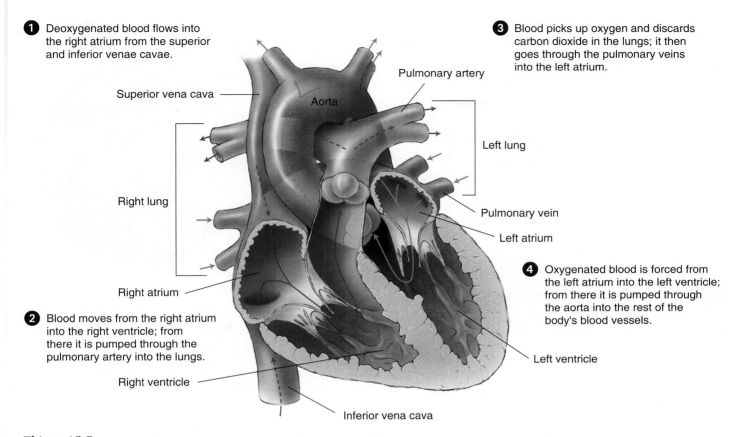

1 Deoxygenated blood flows into the right atrium from the superior and inferior venae cavae.

3 Blood picks up oxygen and discards carbon dioxide in the lungs; it then goes through the pulmonary veins into the left atrium.

Pulmonary artery

Superior vena cava

Aorta

Left lung

Right lung

Pulmonary vein

Left atrium

Right atrium

4 Oxygenated blood is forced from the left atrium into the left ventricle; from there it is pumped through the aorta into the rest of the body's blood vessels.

2 Blood moves from the right atrium into the right ventricle; from there it is pumped through the pulmonary artery into the lungs.

Right ventricle

Left ventricle

Inferior vena cava

Figure 15.3
Anatomy of the Heart

atrium and the right ventricle), the *pulmonary valve* (between the right ventricle and the pulmonary artery), the *mitral valve* (between the left atrium and left ventricle), and the *aortic valve* (between the left ventricle and the aorta) permit blood to flow in only one direction.[15]

Heart Function Heart activity depends on a complex interaction of biochemical, physical, and neurological signals. Here are the basic steps involved in heart function:

1. Deoxygenated blood enters the right atrium after having been circulated through the body.
2. From the right atrium, blood moves to the right ventricle and is pumped through the pulmonary artery to the lungs, where it receives oxygen.
3. Oxygenated blood from the lungs then returns to the left atrium of the heart.
4. Blood from the left atrium is forced into the left ventricle.
5. The left ventricle pumps blood through the aorta to all body parts.

Different types of blood vessels are required for different parts of this process. **Arteries** carry blood away from the heart; most arteries carry oxygenated blood, but the pulmonary arteries carry deoxygenated blood to the lungs, where it picks up oxygen and gives off carbon dioxide. As

the arteries branch off from the heart, they divide into smaller blood vessels called **arterioles,** and then into even smaller blood vessels called **capillaries.** Capillaries have thin walls that permit the exchange of oxygen, carbon dioxide, nutrients, and waste products with body cells. The carbon dioxide and waste products are transported to the lungs and kidneys through **veins** and **venules** (small veins).

For the heart to function properly, the four chambers must beat in an organized manner. Your heartbeat is governed by an electrical impulse that directs the heart

Arteries Vessels that carry blood away from the heart to other regions of the body.

Arterioles Branches of the arteries.

Capillaries Minute blood vessels that branch out from the arterioles; their thin walls allow for the exchange of oxygen, carbon dioxide, nutrients, and waste products among body cells.

Veins Vessels that carry blood back to the heart from other regions of the body.

Venules Branches of the veins.

muscle to move when the impulse moves across it, which results in a sequential contraction of the four chambers. This signal starts in a small bundle of highly specialized cells, the **sinoatrial node (SA node),** located in the right atrium. The SA node serves as a natural pacemaker for the heart.[16] People with a damaged SA node (either a congenital defect or one injured by disease) must often have a mechanical pacemaker implanted to ensure the smooth passage of blood through the sequential phases of the heartbeat.

The average adult heart at rest beats 70 to 80 times per minute, although a well-conditioned heart may beat only 50 to 60 times per minute to achieve the same results. When overly stressed, a heart may beat over 200 times per minute, particularly in an individual who is overweight or out of shape. A healthy heart functions more efficiently and is less likely to suffer damage from overwork.

Types of Cardiovascular Disease

There are several different types of cardiovascular disease (Figure 15.4):

- Atherosclerosis (fatty plaque buildup in arteries)
- Coronary heart disease (CHD)
- Chest pain (angina pectoris)
- Irregular heartbeat (arrhythmia)
- Congestive heart failure (CHF)
- Congenital and rheumatic heart disease
- Stroke (cerebrovascular accident)

Prevention and treatment of these diseases range from changes in diet and lifestyle to medications and surgery.

Atherosclerosis

Arteriosclerosis is a condition that underlies many cardiovascular health problems.[17] **Atherosclerosis** is actually a type of arteriosclerosis and is characterized by deposits of fatty substances, cholesterol, cellular waste products, calcium, and *fibrin* (a clotting material in the blood) in the inner lining of the artery. **Hyperlipidemia** (an abnormally high blood lipid

---

Sinoatrial node (SA node)   Cluster of electric-generating cells that serve as a form of natural pacemaker for the heart.

Arteriosclerosis   A general term for thickening and hardening of the arteries.

Atherosclerosis   Condition characterized by deposits of fatty substances, cholesterol, cellular waste products, calcium, and fibrin in the inner lining of an artery.

Hyperlipidemia   Elevated levels of lipids in the blood.

Plaque   Buildup of deposits in the arteries.

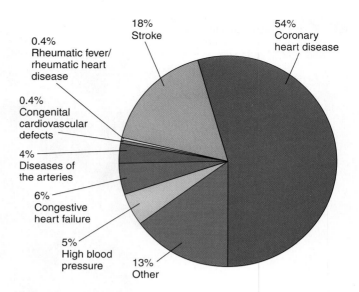

Figure 15.4

Percentage Breakdown of Deaths from Cardiovascular Disease in the United States, 2001

Source: American Heart Association. *Heart Disease and Stroke Statistics—2004 Update* (Dallas, TX: American Heart Association, 2004). © 2004 American Heart Association. Reproduced with permission. www.americanheart.org

level) is a key factor in this process, and the resulting buildup is referred to as **plaque.**[18]

Often, atherosclerosis is called *coronary artery disease (CAD)* because of the resultant damage done to coronary arteries. According to current thinking, three factors are responsible for this damage: elevated levels of cholesterol and triglycerides in the blood, high blood pressure, and tobacco smoke.[19]

Atherosclerotic plaque appears primarily in large and medium-size elastic and muscular arteries and can block blood flow to the heart, brain, or extremities. Plaque may be present throughout a person's lifetime, with the earliest formation, known as a "fatty streak," being fairly common in infants and young children.[20]

Early Theories   Initially, it was thought that plaque developed in response to injury and tended to collect at sites of injury. Many scientists believed that the process of plaque buildup begins because the protective inner lining of the artery *(endothelium)* became damaged, and fats, cholesterol, and other substances in the blood tend to aggregate in these damaged areas. High blood pressure surges, elevated cholesterol and triglyceride levels in the blood, and cigarette smoking were the main suspects in having caused this injury to artery walls. As a result of national campaigns aimed at reducing dietary fat, millions of people cut down on animal fat and dairy products. However, despite massive lifestyle changes and the use of cholesterol-lowering drugs, cardiovascular diseases continue to be the leading cause of death in the United States, Europe, and most of Asia.[21]

New Factors in CVD Risk: The Role of Homocysteine

Is it time to forget the cholesterol and fat in your diet altogether and focus on other risks? Probably not. However, researchers are investigating new factors that may contribute to CVD risk as much as that juicy steak or high-fat ice cream.

Inflammation of the walls of blood vessels may be a contributor to heart attack and stroke. Testing for C-reactive protein (CRP), a protein that increases when the body is subjected to inflammation from some form of attack, is already widely available.

Another substance that may signal increased risk for cardiovascular disease is *homocysteine*, an amino acid normally present in the blood. Some studies have indicated that high levels of homocysteine may be related to higher risk of coronary heart disease, stroke, and peripheral vascular disease. In fact, it is hypothesized that homocysteine may work in much the same way as CRP, inflaming the inner lining of arteries and promoting fat deposits on the damaged walls and development of blood clots. However, a causal link has not been established between homocysteine and CVD.

Folic acid and other B vitamins such as B_6 and B_{12} help break down homocysteine in the body, so many have jumped on the folic acid bandwagon as a preemptive action against CVD risk. Because conclusive evidence of risk reduction from folic acid is not available, authorities such as the American Heart Association do not recommend taking folic acid supplements to prevent CVD. For now, a healthy, balanced diet that includes at least five servings of fruits and vegetables a day is the best preventive action. Citrus fruit, tomatoes, vegetables, and grain products that are fortified with folic acid are good sources of the recommended 400 micrograms.

Source: American Heart Association, "Homocysteine, Folic Acid, and Cardiovascular Disease," 2004, www.americanheart.org

---

Inflammatory Risks Today, scientists are beginning to look for other factors in the formation of atherosclerotic lesions. New research has led many experts to believe that atherosclerosis is an *inflammatory* disease and that inflamed vessels are more prone to plaque formation.[22] What causes this inflammation in arterial walls? While researchers aren't sure, there is evidence that a pathogen may be at the root of it. The most likely culprits are *Chlamydia pneumoniae* (a sexually transmitted infection), *Helicobactor pylori* (which causes ulcers), *herpes simplex virus* (a virus the majority of Americans have been exposed to by the age of five), and *cytomegalovirus* (another herpes virus transmitted through body fluids and infecting most Americans before the age of 40). Clearly, if findings about these viruses holds up, there will be yet another good reason to avoid unprotected sex.

During an inflammatory reaction, C-reactive proteins (CRPs) tend to be present at high levels. Many scientists believe the presence of these proteins may signal elevated risk for angina and heart attack. Doctors could opt to test patients using a high sensitive assay (hs-CRP); if levels are high, action could be taken to prevent progression to heart attack or other coronary event. In the near future, hs-CRP tests might be given as routinely as cholesterol screening tests for heart disease.[23]

Other possible causes of inflammation include elevated low-density lipoproteins, free radicals caused by cigarette smoking, high blood pressure, diabetes mellitus, and the amino acid homocysteine (see the New Horizons in Health box).

Metabolic Syndrome According to Gerald Reaven, endocrinologist and doctor at Stanford University, when people consume too many calories, particularly carbohydrates, their bodies eventually become insulin resistant, meaning that their cells resist, or don't work properly in, handling blood glucose levels. Consequently, insulin and blood sugar levels remain high over time. These dynamics can cause a cluster of metabolic problems such as high blood pressure and glucose intolerance that raise the risk of heart disease.[24] Today, nearly 24 percent of all Americans have **metabolic syndrome,** which is defined as having three or more of the following characteristics:[25]

- Waist circumference greater than 40 inches (102 cm) in men and 35 inches (88 cm) in women
- Serum triglyceride level of 160 mg/dL or higher
- High-density lipoprotein cholesterol level less than 40 mg/dL in men and 50 mg/dL in women
- Blood pressure of 130/85 mm Hg or higher
- Fasting glucose level of 100 mg/dL or higher

Coronary Heart Disease (CHD)

Of all the major cardiovascular diseases, coronary heart disease (CHD) is the greatest killer. In fact, this year well over 1,100,000 people will suffer a heart attack, and over 40 percent

---

Metabolic syndrome A group of three or more characteristics, including waist circumference and blood pressure, that can cause metabolic problems that raise CVD risk.

What to Do in the Event of a Heart Attack

Because heart attacks are so frightening, we would prefer not to think about them. However, knowing how to act in an emergency could save your life or that of somebody else.

KNOW THE WARNING SIGNS OF A HEART ATTACK

- Uncomfortable pressure, fullness, squeezing, or pain in the center of the chest, lasting two minutes or longer
- Jaw pain and/or shortness of breath
- Pain spreading to the shoulders, neck, or arms
- Dizziness, fatigue, fainting, sweating, and/or nausea

Not all these warning signs occur in every heart attack. For instance, women's heart attacks tend to show up as shortness of breath, fatigue, and jaw pain, stretched out over hours rather than minutes. If any of these symptoms do appear, however, don't wait. Get help immediately!

KNOW WHAT TO DO IN AN EMERGENCY

- Find out which hospitals in your area have 24-hour emergency cardiac care.
- Determine (in advance) the hospital or medical facility that's nearest your home and office, and tell your family and friends to call this facility in an emergency.
- Keep a list of emergency rescue service numbers next to your telephone and in your pocket, wallet, or purse. Be aware of whether your local area has a 911 emergency service.
- If you have chest or jaw discomfort that lasts more than two minutes, call the emergency rescue service. Do not drive yourself to the hospital.

BE A HEART SAVER

- If you're with someone who is showing signs of a heart attack and the warning signs last for two minutes or longer, act immediately.
- Expect a denial. It's normal for a person with chest discomfort to deny the possibility of anything as serious as a heart attack. Don't take no for an answer, however. Insist on taking prompt action.
- Call the emergency rescue service; or
- Get to the nearest hospital emergency room that offers 24-hour emergency cardiac care.
- Give CPR (mouth-to-mouth breathing and chest compression) if it's necessary and if you're properly trained.

Source: American Heart Association, *Heart and Stroke Facts* (Dallas, TX: Author, 2004). www.americanheart.org

---

of them will die.[26] Those of you raised on a weekly dose of TV doctor programs will recognize *code blue* as the term for a **myocardial infarction (MI),** or **heart attack.** A heart attack involves an area of the heart that suffers permanent damage because its normal blood supply has been blocked. This condition is often brought on by a **coronary thrombosis,** or blood clot in the coronary artery, or through an atherosclerotic narrowing that blocks an artery. When a blood clot, or **thrombus,** becomes dislodged and moves through the circulatory system, it is called an **embolus.** When blood does not flow readily, there is a corresponding decrease in oxygen flow. If the blockage is extremely minor, an otherwise healthy heart will adapt over time by enlarging existing blood vessels and growing new ones (in a process known as *angiogenesis*) to reroute needed blood through other areas. This system, known as **collateral circulation,** is a form of self-preservation that allows an affected heart muscle to cope with the damage.

When heart blockage is more severe, however, the body is unable to adapt on its own, and outside lifesaving support is critical. The hour following a heart attack is the most crucial period—over 40 percent of heart attack victims die within this time. See the Skills for Behavior Change box to learn what to do in case of a heart attack.

Sudden death from cardiac arrest can occur within minutes, when the heart's electrical impulses become rapid (*ventricular tachycardia*) and then chaotic (*ventricular fibrillation,* or *VF*). Portable defibrillators, CPR, and other emergency techniques can save lives.

Although young adults can also succumb to cardiac arrest, abnormalities of the heart are the most likely cause. Under certain conditions, various heart medications, other prescription drugs, or illicit drugs can lead to abnormal heart

Myocardial infarction (MI)   Heart attack.

Heart attack   A blockage of normal blood supply to an area in the heart.

Coronary thrombosis   A blood clot occurring in the coronary artery.

Thrombus   Blood clot attached to the wall of a blood vessel.

Embolus   A blood clot that becomes dislodged from a blood vessel wall and moves through the circulatory system.

Collateral circulation   Adaptation of the heart to partial damage accomplished by rerouting needed blood through unused or underused blood vessels while the damaged heart muscle heals.

rhythms that cause cardiac arrest or death. Respiratory arrest caused by asthma, electrocution, high blood pressure, drowning, choking, and trauma are other potential causes.

What do you think?

What risk factors might typical college-age students have for plaque formation? ■ *What information should new CVD prevention guidelines include if the new theories discussed in this section prove true?*

Angina Pectoris

Atherosclerosis and other circulatory impairments often reduce the heart's blood and oxygen supply, a condition known as **ischemia.** People with ischemia often suffer from varying degrees of **angina pectoris,** or chest pain. In fact, an estimated 2.6 million men and 4.2 million women suffer mild to crushing forms of chest pain each day.[27] Many people experience short episodes of angina whenever they exert themselves physically. Symptoms may range from slight indigestion to a feeling that the heart is being crushed. Generally, the more serious the oxygen deprivation, the more severe the pain. Although angina pectoris is not a heart attack, it does indicate underlying heart disease.

Currently, there are several methods of treating angina. In mild cases, rest is critical. The most common treatments for more severe cases involve using drugs that affect (1) the supply of blood to the heart muscle or (2) the heart's demand for oxygen. Pain and discomfort are often relieved with *nitroglycerin,* a drug used to relax (dilate) veins, thereby reducing the amount of blood returning to the heart and thus lessening its workload. Patients whose angina is caused by spasms of the coronary arteries are often given drugs called *calcium channel blockers,* drugs that prevent calcium atoms from passing through coronary arteries and causing heart contractions. They also appear to reduce blood pressure and slow heart rate. *Beta blockers,* the other major type of drugs used to treat angina, control potential overactivity of the heart muscle.

Arrhythmias

Over 4 million Americans experience some type of **arrhythmia,** an irregularity in heart rhythm. A person who complains of a racing heart in the absence of exercise or anxiety may be experiencing *tachycardia,* the medical term for abnormally fast heartbeat. On the other end of the continuum is *bradycardia,* or abnormally slow heartbeat. When a heart goes into **fibrillation** of either the atrial or ventricular regions of the heart, it beats in a sporadic, quivering pattern resulting in extreme inefficiency in moving blood through the cardiovascular system. If untreated, fibrillation may be fatal.

Not all arrhythmias are life threatening. In many instances, excessive caffeine or nicotine consumption can trigger an arrhythmia episode. However, severe cases may require drug therapy or external electrical stimulus to prevent serious complications.

Congestive Heart Failure (CHF)

When the heart muscle is damaged or overworked and lacks the strength to keep blood circulating normally through the body, its chambers are often taxed to the limit. **Congestive heart failure (CHF)** affects over 5 million Americans and dramatically increases risk of premature death.[28] The heart muscle may be injured by a number of health conditions, including rheumatic fever, pneumonia, heart attack, or other cardiovascular problems. In some cases, the damage is due to radiation or chemotherapy treatments for cancer. These weakened muscles respond poorly, impairing blood flow out of the heart through the arteries. The return flow of blood through the veins begins to back up, causing congestion in body tissues. This pooling of blood enlarges the heart, makes it less efficient, and decreases the amount of blood that can be circulated. Fluid begins to accumulate in other body areas, such as the vessels in the legs, ankles, or lungs, causing swelling or difficulty in breathing.

Today, CHF is the single most frequent cause of hospitalization in the United States.[29] If untreated, congestive heart failure can be fatal. However, most cases respond well to treatment that includes *diuretics* (water pills) to relieve fluid accumulation; drugs, such as *digitalis,* that increase the pumping action of the heart; and drugs called *vasodilators* that expand blood vessels and decrease resistance, allowing blood to flow more easily and making the heart's work easier.

Congenital and Rheumatic Heart Disease

Approximately 1 out of every 125 children is born with some form of **congenital heart disease** (disease present at birth).[30] These forms may be relatively minor, such as slight *murmurs* (low-pitched sounds caused by turbulent blood flow through

Ischemia Reduced oxygen supply to a body organ or part.

Angina pectoris Chest pain occurring as a result of reduced oxygen flow to the heart.

Arrhythmia An irregularity in heartbeat.

Fibrillation A sporadic, quivering pattern of heartbeat resulting in extreme inefficiency in moving blood through the cardiovascular system.

Congestive heart failure (CHF) An abnormal cardiovascular condition that reflects impaired cardiac pumping and blood flow; pooling blood leads to congestion in body tissues.

Congenital heart disease Heart disease that is present at birth.

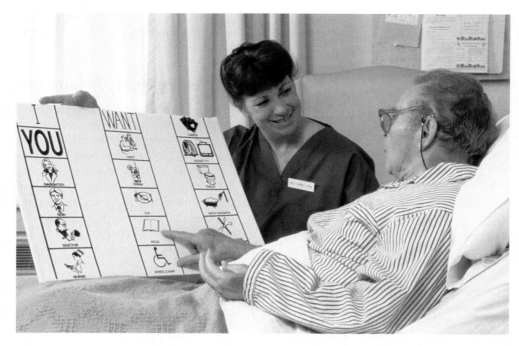

Recovery after a stroke can be a long process, often requiring therapy to improve speech and mobility.

the heart or problematic heart valve action), resulting from valve irregularities which some children outgrow. Other congenital problems involve serious complications in heart function that can be corrected only with surgery. Their underlying causes are unknown but may be related to hereditary factors; maternal diseases, such as rubella, that occurred during fetal development; or chemical intake (particularly alcohol) by the mother during pregnancy. Because of advances in pediatric cardiology, the prognosis for children with congenital heart defects is better than ever before.

Rheumatic heart disease can cause similar heart problems in children. It is attributed to rheumatic fever, an inflammatory disease that may affect many connective tissues of the body, especially those of the heart, joints, brain, or skin, and which is caused by an unresolved *streptococcal infection* of the throat (strep throat). In a small number of cases, this infection

can lead to an immune response in which antibodies attack the heart as well as the bacteria. Many of the 82,000 annual operations on heart valves in the United States (at an average cost of $85,000 each) are related to rheumatic heart disease.[31]

Stroke

Like heart muscle, brain cells must have a continuous adequate supply of oxygen in order to survive. A **stroke** (also called a *cerebrovascular accident*) occurs when the blood supply to the brain is interrupted. Strokes may be caused by a thrombus (a clot in a blood vessel), an embolus (a clot that has broken off from a blood vessel wall and is floating in the bloodstream), or an **aneurysm** (a weakening in a blood vessel that causes it to bulge and, in severe cases, burst). Figure 15.5 illustrates these blood vessel disorders. When any of these events occurs, oxygen deprivation kills brain cells, which do not have the capacity to heal or regenerate. Some strokes are mild and cause only temporary dizziness or slight weakness or numbness. More serious interruptions in blood flow may cause speech impairments, memory problems, and loss of motor control.

Other strokes affect parts of the brain that regulate heart and lung function and kill within minutes. Strokes killed 282,000 Americans in 2003 and accounted for 1 in 11.5 of our total deaths, surpassed only by CHD and cancer.[32] Each year, about 700,000 people experience a new or recurrent stroke, which averages out to one person suffering a stroke every 45 seconds and one person dying as a result every 3.3 minutes.[33]

About one in ten major strokes is preceded days, weeks, or months earlier by **transient ischemic attacks (TIAs),** brief

---

Rheumatic heart disease   A heart disease caused by untreated streptococcal infection of the throat.

Stroke   A condition occurring when the brain is damaged by disrupted blood supply.

Aneurysm   A weakened blood vessel that may bulge under pressure and, in severe cases, burst.

Transient ischemic attacks (TIAs)   Brief interruptions of the blood supply to the brain that cause only temporary impairment; often an indicator of impending major stroke.

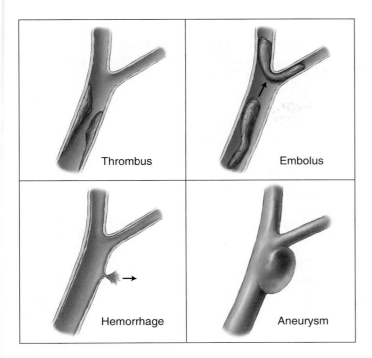

Figure 15.5
Common Blood Vessel Disorders

interruptions of the blood supply to the brain that cause only temporary impairment. Symptoms of TIAs include dizziness, particularly at first rising in the morning, weakness, temporary paralysis or numbness in the face or other regions, temporary memory loss, blurred vision, nausea, headache, slurred speech, or other unusual physiological reactions. TIAs are often indications of an impending major stroke.

The warning signs of stroke include:

- Sudden weakness or numbness of the face, arm, or leg on one side of the body
- Sudden dimness or loss of vision, particularly in only one eye
- Loss of speech or trouble talking or understanding speech
- Sudden, severe headaches with no known cause
- Unexplained dizziness, unsteadiness, or sudden falls, especially with any of the previously listed symptoms

If you experience any of these symptoms, or if you are with someone who does, seek medical help *immediately*. The earlier treatment starts, the more effective it will be.

One of the greatest medical successes in recent years has been the decline in the fatality rates from strokes, a rate that has dropped by one-third in the United States since the 1980s and continues to fall. Improved diagnostic procedures, better surgical options, clot-busting drugs injected soon after a stroke has occurred, and acute care centers specializing in stroke treatment and rehabilitation have all been factors. Increased awareness of risk factors for stroke, especially high blood pressure, knowledge of warning signals, and an emphasis on prevention also have contributed. It is estimated

that more than half of all remaining strokes could be avoided if more people followed the recommended preventive standards.

Unfortunately, those who survive a stroke do not always make a full recovery. Some 50 to 70 percent of stroke survivors regain functional independence, while 15 to 30 percent are permanently disabled and require assistance. Today, stroke is a leading cause of serious long-term disability and contributes a significant amount to Medicaid and Medicare expenses for older Americans.[34]

Reducing Your Risk for Cardiovascular Diseases

What is your own risk for heart disease? Factors that increase the risk for cardiovascular problems fall into two categories: those we can control and those we cannot. Fortunately, we can take steps to minimize many risk factors.

Risks You Can Control

Avoid Tobacco As early as 1964, the Surgeon General of the United States asserted that smoking was the greatest risk factor for heart disease. Today, one in five deaths from CVD are directly related to smoking.[35] Generally, the more a person smokes, the greater the risk for heart attack or stroke. The risk for cardiovascular disease is 70 percent greater for smokers than for nonsmokers. Smokers who have a heart attack are more likely to die suddenly (within one hour) than are nonsmokers. Evidence also indicates that chronic exposure to environmental tobacco smoke (ETS, or passive smoking) increases the risk of heart disease by as much as 30 percent.[36]

How does smoking damage the heart? There are two plausible explanations. One theory is that nicotine increases heart rate, heart output, blood pressure, and oxygen use by heart muscles. Because the carbon monoxide in cigarette smoke displaces oxygen in heart tissue, the heart is forced to work harder to obtain sufficient oxygen. The other theory states that chemicals in smoke damage the lining of the coronary arteries and cause inflammation, allowing cholesterol and plaque to accumulate more easily. This additional buildup constricts the vessels, increasing blood pressure and causing the heart to work harder.

When people stop smoking, regardless of how long or how much they've smoked, their risk of heart disease declines rapidly.[37] Three years after quitting, the risk of death from heart disease and stroke for people who smoked a pack a day or less is almost the same as for people who never smoked. Although the exact reasons are unknown, new findings from the Lung Health Study indicate that women have greater lung function improvements than their male counterparts after sustained smoking cessation.[38]

Cut Back on Saturated Fat and Cholesterol How concerned should you be about the type of fat and amount of fat and cholesterol in your diet? Very concerned. According to recent evidence, cholesterol risks may be greater than ever for Americans. When dietary experts from the National Heart, Lung, and Blood Institute met to prepare their *Third Report on Detection, Evaluation, and Treatment of Cholesterol National Guidelines,* they gave Americans a wake-up call by drastically reducing the levels of cholesterol that are considered acceptable. These guidelines not only show that cholesterol levels are out of control in the United States, but also indicate that the number of people who need cholesterol-cutting drugs may be three times what we originally thought. In fact, nearly 36 million people in the United States—one-fifth of all adults—may require medications to avoid cardiovascular problems.[39]

Why all the fuss about fats and cholesterol? Diets high in saturated fat are known to raise cholesterol levels, send the body's blood-clotting system into high gear, and make the blood more viscous in just a few hours, increasing the risk of heart attack or stroke. Studies indicate that fatty foods apparently trigger production of *factor VII,* a blood-clotting substance. Switching to a low-fat diet lowers the risk of clotting.

A fatty diet also increases the amount of cholesterol in the blood, contributing to atherosclerosis. In past years, cholesterol levels between 200 to 240 milligrams per 100 milliliters of blood (mg/dL) were considered normal. Recent research indicates that levels between 180 and 200 mg/dL are more desirable and that 150 mg/dL levels would be even better to reduce CVD risks. People with multiple risk factors for CVD are advised to follow even more stringent guidelines.[40] See Table 15.1 for recommendations.

However, it isn't just the total cholesterol level that you should be concerned about. Cholesterol comes in two main varieties: **low-density lipoprotein (LDL)** and **high-density lipoprotein (HDL).** Low-density lipoprotein, often referred to as "bad" cholesterol, is believed to build up on artery walls. In contrast, high-density lipoprotein, or "good" cholesterol, appears to remove cholesterol from artery walls, thus serving as a protector. In theory, if LDL levels get too high or HDL levels too low—largely because of too much saturated fat in the diet, a lack of physical exercise, high stress levels, or genetic predisposition—cholesterol will accumulate inside arteries

---

Table 15.1

Classification of LDL, Total, and HDL Cholesterol (mg/dL) and Recommended Levels for Adults

LDL Cholesterol

<100	Optimal
100–129	Near optimal/above optimal
130–159	Borderline high
160–189	High
=190	Very high

Total Cholesterol

<200	Desirable
200–239	Borderline high
=240	High

HDL Cholesterol

<40	Low
=60	High

Triglycerides

<150	Normal
150–199	Borderline high
200–499	High
=500	Very high

Source: National Heart, Lung, and Blood Institute, *Detection, Evaluation, and Treatment of High Blood Cholesterol in Adults* (NIH Publication No. 02-5215), 2002, www.nhlbi.nih.gov/guidelines/cholesterol/ atp3_rpt.htm

---

and lead to cardiovascular problems. Scientists now believe that there are other factors that may also increase CVD risk. A component of HDL known as Lp(a) may be the most important element of the HDL makeup. Lp(a), a lipoprotein, plays an important role in plaque accumulation and increased risk for stroke and coronary events, particularly in males. The higher the Lp(a) level, the higher the risk.[41]

The goal is to manage the ratio of HDL to total cholesterol by lowering LDL levels, raising HDL, or both. Regular exercise and a healthy diet low in saturated fat continue to be the best methods for maintaining healthy ratios. However, if dietary efforts and exercise do not reduce total cholesterol or LDL, several medications are available that may help.

Triglycerides, another type of fat in the blood, also appear to promote atherosclerosis. As people get older, heavier, or both, their triglycerides and cholesterol levels tend to rise. Although some CVD patients have elevated triglyceride levels, a causal link between high triglyceride levels and CVD has yet to be established. It may be that high triglyceride levels do not directly cause atherosclerosis but, rather, are among the abnormalities that speed its development.

Current guidelines suggest that you should reduce consumption of saturated fat (which comes mostly from animal products) to less than 7 percent of your total daily caloric intake and minimize your consumption of *trans* fats (see Chapter 8), which is found in partially hydrogenated products such as margarine, many fast foods, and many

---

Low-density lipoproteins (LDLs) Compounds that facilitate the transport of cholesterol in the blood to the body's cells.

High-density lipoproteins (HDLs) Compounds that facilitate the transport of cholesterol in the blood to the liver for metabolism and elimination from the body.

Triglycerides The most common form of fat in the body; excess calories are converted into triglycerides and stored as body fat.

---

packaged foods. (If the ingredients list includes "shortening," "partially hydrogenated vegetable oil," or "hydrogenated vegetable oil," the food contains *trans* fats.) By cutting your intake of saturated fats and *trans* fats, experts from the National Heart, Lung, and Blood Institute (NHLBI) believe that you can reduce your LDL levels by as much as 10 percent.[42] In addition, NHLBI experts indicate that you should consume fewer than 200 milligrams per day of cholesterol, which is found mainly in eggs and meat. Doing so may reduce LDL by as much as 5 percent.[43] For information on types of fat and how to reduce total fat in your diet, see "An Eating Plan for Healthy Americans: Our AHA Diet" on the American Heart Association's website (www.americanheart.org).

While it is wise to cut back on saturated fat, be aware that some fat is necessary to overall health. Ironically, the consumption of too many low-fat or fat-free foods, such as salad dressings and other products, may actually contribute to the escalating problem of obesity in America. It is better to eat foods with olive oil, canola oil, and other monounsaturated fats than to consume low-fat or no-fat products. (For a complete discussion of this topic, see Chapter 8.) Of course, all fat intake should be in moderation.

Monitor Your Cholesterol Levels To get an accurate assessment of your total cholesterol and LDL and HDL levels, consider a *lipoprotein analysis*. This analysis should be done by a reputable health provider and requires that you not eat or drink anything for 12 hours prior to the test. The LDL level is derived using a standard formula:

$$LDL = total\ cholesterol - HDL - (triglycerides \div 5)$$

For example, if the level of total cholesterol is 200, the level of HDL 45, and the level of triglycerides 150, the LDL level would be 125 (200 − 45 − 30).

In general, LDL is more closely associated with cardiovascular risk than is total cholesterol. However, most authorities agree that looking only at LDL ignores the positive effects of HDL. Perhaps the best method of evaluating risk is to examine the ratio of HDL to total cholesterol or the percentage of HDL in total cholesterol. If the level of HDL is lower than 35, the risk increases dramatically.

Change Lifestyle to Reduce Your Risk Of the more than 100 million Americans who need to worry about their cholesterol levels, almost half, particularly those at the low-to-moderate risk levels, should be able to reach their LDL and HDL goals through lifestyle changes alone. People who are at higher risk or those for whom lifestyle modifications are not effective may need to take cholesterol-lowering drugs while they continue modifying their lifestyle. Among the most commonly prescribed drugs are statins (Lipitor, Baycol, and Pravachol are examples), which are very effective in reducing LDL levels. Folic acids and niacin drugs are often prescribed for people with low HDL and high triglyceride levels.

Maintain a Healthy Weight No question about it—body weight plays a role in CVD. Researchers are not sure whether high-fat, high-sugar, high-calorie diets are a direct risk for CVD or whether they invite risk by causing obesity, which strains the heart, forcing it to push blood through the many miles of capillaries that supply each pound of fat. A heart that has to continuously move blood through an overabundance of vessels may become damaged.

Overweight people are more likely to develop heart disease and stroke even if they have no other risk factors. If you're heavy, losing even 5 to 10 pounds can make a significant difference of as much as 5 percent LDL reduction.[44] This is especially true if you're an "apple" (thicker around your upper body and waist) rather than a "pear" (thicker around your hips and thighs). Your waist measurement divided by your hip measurement should be less than 0.9 (for men) and less than 0.8 (for women).[45] (See Chapter 9 for more tips on weight management.)

Modify Other Dietary Habits The NHLBI guidelines recommend the following dietary changes to reduce CVD risk:

- Consume 5 to 10 mg per day of soluble fiber from sources such as psyllium seeds, oat bran, fruits, vegetables, and legumes (see Chapter 8). Even this small dietary modification may result in another 5 percent drop in LDL levels.
- Consume about 2 g per day of *plant sterols* or sterol derivatives from substances such as Benecol or Take Control margarine. These are the first widely available sources of sterols, but more will be on the market soon. This amount of plant sterols has the potential to reduce LDL by another 5 percent.
- Although less widely supported by rigorous research findings, many experts believe that consuming at least 25 g of soy protein from various soy foods, instead of dairy sources, could reduce LDL by 5 percent.

Exercise Regularly According to all available evidence, inactivity is a definite risk factor for CVD.[46] The good news is that you do not have to be an exercise fanatic to reduce your risk. Even modest levels of low-intensity physical activity—walking, gardening, housework, dancing—are beneficial if done regularly and over the long term. Exercise can increase HDL, lower triglycerides, and reduce coronary risks in several ways. For more information, see Chapter 10.

Making the above modifications could reduce LDL levels by as much as 35 percent—similar to taking any of the statin drugs typically prescribed.

Control Diabetes The recent NHLBI guidelines underscore the unique CVD risks for people with diabetes. Diabetics who have taken insulin for a number of years have a greater chance of developing CVD. In fact, CVD is the leading cause of death among diabetic patients. Because overweight people have a higher risk for diabetes, distinguishing between the effects of the two conditions is difficult. Diabetics also tend to have elevated blood fat levels, increased atherosclerosis, and a tendency toward deterioration of small blood vessels, particularly in the eyes and extremities. However, through a prescribed regimen of diet, exercise, and medication, diabetics can control much of their increased risk for CVD (see Chapter 18).

Control Your Blood Pressure

Hypertension refers to sustained high blood pressure. If it cannot be attributed to any specific cause, it is known as **essential hypertension.** Approximately 90 percent of all cases of hypertension fit this category. **Secondary hypertension** refers to hypertension caused by specific factors, such as kidney disease, obesity, or tumors of the adrenal glands. In general, the higher your blood pressure, the greater your risk for CVD.

Hypertension is known as the "silent killer" because it usually has no symptoms. Its prevalence has increased by over 30 percent in the last 10 years, with data indicating that there are 65 million adults in the United States with high blood pressure. This means that over one-third of all adults have blood pressure problems and may be on medication, working to reduce risk factors, or unaware that they have a problem.[47]

Blood pressure is measured in two parts and is expressed as a fraction—for example, 110/80, or 110 over 80. Both values are measured in *millimeters of mercury* (mm Hg). The first number refers to **systolic pressure,** or the pressure being applied to the walls of the arteries when the heart contracts, pumping blood to the rest of the body. The second value is **diastolic pressure,** or the pressure applied to the walls of the arteries during the heart's relaxation phase. During this phase, blood is reentering the chambers of the heart, preparing for the next heartbeat.

Normal blood pressure varies depending on weight, age, and physical condition, and for different groups of people, such as women and minorities. Systolic blood pressure tends to increase with age, while diastolic blood pressure increases until age 55 and then declines. As a rule, men have a greater risk for high blood pressure than women until age 55, when their risks become about equal. At age 75 and over, women are more likely to have high blood pressure than men.[48]

For the average person, 110 over 80 is a healthy blood pressure level. High blood pressure is usually diagnosed

Table 15.2
Blood Pressure Classifications

Classification	Systolic Reading (mm Hg)		Diastolic Reading (mm Hg)
Normal	<120	and	<80
Prehypertension	120–139	or	80–89
Hypertension			
Stage 1	140–159	or	90–99
Stage 2	≥160	or	≥100

Note: If systolic and diastolic readings fall into different categories, treatment is determined by the highest category. Readings are based on the average of 2 or more properly measured, seated readings on each of 2 or more health care provider visits.

Source: National Heart, Lung, and Blood Institute, *The Seventh Report of the Joint National Committee on Prevention, Detection, Evaluation, and Treatment of High Blood Pressure* (NIH Publication No. 03-5233) (Bethesda, MD: National Institutes of Health, May 2003).

when systolic pressure is 140 or above. Diastolic pressure does not have to be high to indicate high blood pressure. When only systolic pressure is high, the condition is known as *isolated systolic hypertension (ISH),* the most common form of high blood pressure in older Americans.[49] Causes of high blood pressure include narrowing of the arteries and the heart beating more quickly or more forcefully than it should. However, many times the underlying cause is not known. If your blood pressure exceeds 140 over 90, you need to take steps to lower it. See Table 15.2 for a summary of blood pressure values and what they mean.

Treatment of hypertension can involve dietary changes (reducing salt and calorie intake), weight loss (when appropriate), the use of diuretics and other medications (only when prescribed by a physician), regular exercise, and the practice of relaxation techniques and effective coping and communication skills.

Manage Stress

Some scientists have noted a relationship between CVD risk and a person's stress level, behavior habits, and socioeconomic status. These factors may influence established risk factors. For example, people under stress may start smoking or smoke more than they otherwise would.[50] A recent study funded by the National Heart, Lung, and Blood Institute found that impatience and hostility, two key components of the Type A behavior pattern, increase young adults' risk of developing high blood pressure. Other related factors, such as competitiveness, depression, and anxiety, did not appear to increase risk. The research was the first to study these factors as a group rather than individually and has clear implications for prevention.[51]

In other studies, researcher-physician Robert S. Eliot demonstrated that approximately one out of five people has an extreme cardiovascular reaction to stressful stimulation. These people experience alarm and resistance so strongly

Hypertension   Sustained elevated blood pressure.

Essential hypertension   Hypertension that cannot be attributed to any known cause.

Secondary hypertension   Hypertension caused by specific factors, such as kidney disease, obesity, or tumors of the adrenal glands.

Systolic pressure   The upper number in the fraction that measures blood pressure, indicating pressure on the walls of the arteries when the heart contracts.

Diastolic pressure   The lower number in the fraction that measures blood pressure, indicating pressure on the walls of the arteries during the relaxation phase of heart activity.

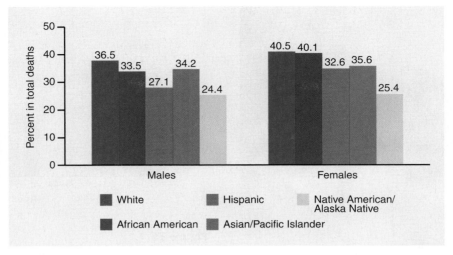

Figure 15.6

Deaths from Cardiovascular Disease in the United States by Age and Race, 2001

Source: American Heart Association, *Heart Disease and Stroke Statistics—2004 Update* (Dallas, TX: American Heart Association, 2004). © 2004 American Heart Association. Reproduced with permission. www.americanheart.org

that, when under stress, their bodies produce large amounts of stress chemicals, which in turn cause tremendous changes in the cardiovascular system, including remarkable increases in blood pressure. These people are called *hot reactors*. Although their blood pressure may be normal when they are not under stress—for example, in a doctor's office—it increases dramatically in response to even small amounts of everyday tension. *Cold reactors* are those who are able to experience stress (even to live as Type As) without showing harmful cardiovascular responses. Cold reactors may internalize stress, but their self-talk and perceptions about the stressful events lead them to a nonresponse state in which their cardiovascular system remains virtually unaffected.[52]

Since Eliot's early work, research in this area has been inconclusive, although more recent studies suggest that personality does indeed play an important role in effective coping. Some research indicates that people who have an underlying predisposition toward a toxic core personality (in other words, who are chronically hostile and hateful) may be at greatest risk for a CVD event. See Chapter 3 for tips on managing your stress, whether you are a hot or cold reactor.

What do you think?

What is your resting heart rate? You can find out by taking your pulse. Gently press the pads of your first two fingers against the inside of your wrist, just below the base of your thumb. Sit quietly, and count the number of beats that occur during a 10-second period. Multiply the number of beats by 6. Repeat the process. ■ How does your heart rate compare to that of your friends?

Risks You Cannot Control

There are, unfortunately, some risk factors for CVD that we cannot prevent or control. The most important are these:

- *Heredity.* A family history of heart disease appears to increase the risk significantly. Whether the increase is due to genetics or environment is an unresolved question.
- *Age.* Seventy-five percent of all heart attacks occur in people over age 65. The rate of CVD increases with age for both sexes.
- *Gender.* Men are at greater risk for CVD until about age 60. Women under 35 have a fairly low risk unless they have high blood pressure, kidney problems, or diabetes. Oral contraceptives and smoking also increase the risk. Hormonal factors appear to reduce risk for women, although after menopause or after estrogen levels are otherwise reduced (for example, because of hysterectomy), women's LDL levels tend to go up, increasing their chances for CVD. (For more on the gender factor, see the next section.)
- *Race.* Blacks are at 45 percent greater risk for hypertension and thus a greater risk for CVD than whites. African Americans are less likely to survive a heart attack.

Figure 15.6 reveals the impact of race on CVD risk.

What do you think?

What risk factors for heart disease do you currently have? ■ Do you know what your cholesterol level is? ■ Which of your risk factors are the most critical? ■ What actions can you start taking today to reduce your risk?

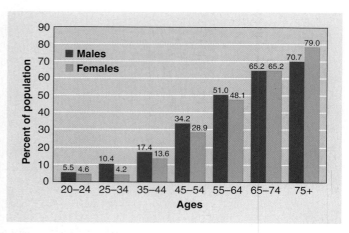

Figure 15.7
Prevalence of Cardiovascular Disease by Age and Sex

Source: American Heart Association, *Heart Disease and Stroke Statistics—2004 Update* (Dallas, TX: American Heart Association, 2004). © 2004 American Heart Association. Reproduced with permission. www.americanheart.org

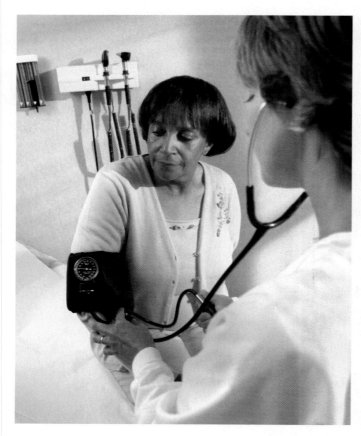

Women at risk for heart disease need to have their blood pressure and other CVD risk factors carefully monitored.

Women and Cardiovascular Disease

While men tend to have more heart attacks and to have them earlier in life than do women, some interesting trends in survivability have emerged. In 1999, CVD claimed the lives of 445,692 men and a surprising 503,927 women in the United States. Why do more men have heart attacks but more women die of them? Why do some studies say that women have about the same mortality rate after myocardial infarction and others indicate there are vast differences—and all are supported by actual numbers?

Although we understand the mechanisms that cause heart disease in men and women (or at least we think we do!), their experiences in the health care system, their reactions to life-threatening diseases, and a host of other technological and environmental factors may play a role in these statistics.

Hormone replacement therapies (HRTs) Therapies that replace estrogen in postmenopausal women.

Risk Factors for Heart Disease in Women

The Role of Estrogen Premenopausal women are unlikely candidates for heart attacks, unless they suffer from diabetes, high blood pressure, or kidney disease or have a genetic predisposition to high cholesterol levels. Family history and smoking can also increase the risk. However, once her estrogen production drops with menopause, a woman's chance of developing CVD rises rapidly. A 60-year-old woman has the same heart attack risk as a 50-year-old man. By her late 70s, a woman has the same heart attack risk as a man her age. Figure 15.7 compares CVD rates between men and women as we age. To date, much of this changing risk has been attributed to the aging process, but the role of estrogen remains unclear. Early studies of various **hormone replacement therapies (HRTs)** indicated that HRT might reduce the risk of CVD by as much as 12 to 25 percent. However, newer findings throw a huge wrench in what was previously believed to be the CVD-risk-reducing powers of HRT (see the Women's Health/Men's Health box on CVD and hormones). Even when their total blood cholesterol levels are higher than men's, however, women may be at less risk because they typically have a higher percentage of HDL.[53]

That is only part of the story. It's true that women aged 25 and over tend to have lower cholesterol levels than men of the same age—but when they reach 45, things change. Most men's cholesterol levels become more stable, while both LDL and total cholesterol levels in women start to rise. The gap widens further beyond age 55.[54]

Before age 45, women's total blood cholesterol levels average below 220 mg/dL. By the time she is 45 to 55, the average woman's blood cholesterol rises to between 223 and 246 mg/dL. Studies of men have shown that for every 1 percent drop in cholesterol, there is a 2 percent decrease in CVD

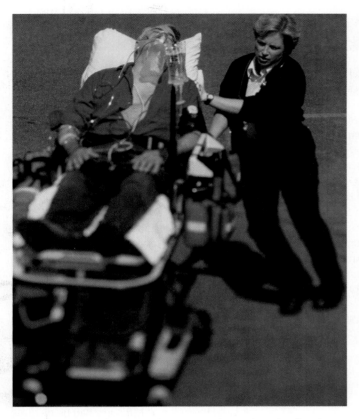

Forty percent of heart attack victims die within the first hour so immediate treatment is vital to the patient's survival.

- The fact that women's coronary arteries are often smaller than men's, making surgical or diagnostic procedures more difficult technically
- The increased incidence of postinfarction angina and heart failure in women

In addition, symptoms of heart attack often differ for women and men, making it more difficult for women to determine whether to go to the doctor (see the Women's Health/Men's Health box). While there is considerable debate over whether inequities exist in treatment of CVD in men compared to women, at least one study suggests that any disparities may reflect overtreatment of men rather than undertreatment of women.[57]

Gender Bias in CVD Research?

The traditional view that heart disease is primarily a male problem has carried over into research as well. A well-publicized example was a study suggesting that aspirin could help prevent heart attacks—based entirely on its effects in 22,000 male doctors. To address such concerns, the National Institutes of Health has launched a 15-year, $625 million study of 140,000 postmenopausal women (known as the Women's Health Initiative), focusing on the leading causes of death and disease. Researchers hope to determine how a healthy lifestyle and increased medical attention can help prevent women's heart disease, as well as cancer and osteoporosis. As discussed elsewhere, the study has already had important implications for women using HRT.

risk.[55] If this holds true for women, prevention efforts focusing on dietary intervention and exercise may significantly help postmenopausal women.

Neglect of Heart Disease Symptoms in Women

During the past decade, research has suggested three main reasons that the signs of heart disease in women may get overlooked: (1) Physicians may be gender-biased in their delivery of health care, tending to concentrate on women's reproductive organs rather than on the whole body; (2) physicians tend to view male heart disease as a more severe problem because men have traditionally had a higher incidence of the disease; and (3) women decline major procedures more often than men do. Other explanations for diagnostic and therapeutic difficulties encountered by women with heart disease include:[56]

- Delay in diagnosing a possible heart attack
- The complexity involved in interpreting chest pain in women
- Typically less aggressive treatment of female heart attack victims
- Women's older age, on average, and greater frequency of other health problems

> **What do you think?**
>
> *How do men and women differ in their experiences related to CVD?* ■ *Why do you think women's risks were largely ignored until fairly recently?* ■ *What actions do you think individuals can take to help improve the situation for both men and women?* ■ *What actions can communities and medical practitioners take?*

New Weapons Against Heart Disease

The victim of a heart attack today has many options that were not available a generation ago. Medications can strengthen heartbeat, control arrhythmias, remove fluids in case of congestive heart failure, and relieve pain. New surgical procedures are saving many lives.

Techniques of Diagnosing Heart Disease

Several techniques are used to diagnose heart disease, including electrocardiogram, angiography, and positron emission

CVD Protection or Increased Risk? The Hormone Controversy

For decades, the prevailing wisdom was that taking hormones during and after menopause would not only reduce hot flashes, it would protect against cardiovascular disease in women. The rate of CVD increases in women after menopause, leading experts to believe that keeping hormone levels high after menopause would control CVD risk. Although scientists didn't really know why this apparent relationship existed, they began to prescribe hormones to millions of women. The results of a major study in the mid-1990s, the Postmenopausal Estrogen/Progestin Intervention (PEPI) Trial, seemed to provide proof that hormone replacement therapy (HRT) lowered CVD risk by raising levels of HDL and decreasing LDL. This led to widespread promotion of HRT as a panacea for CVD risk by professional organizations, doctors, educators, and the community at large. Other studies seemed to confirm these facts, and women moved to take HRT in unprecedented numbers—some 38 percent of all post-menopausal women in the most recent data.

Women choose to take HRT for various reasons. Although reduction of CVD risk has been one of them, many women take HRT because it is the most effective treatment for menopausal symptoms such as hot flashes, night sweats, sexual dysfunction and vaginal dryness, insomnia, and hair loss. For women experiencing these problems, short term use of HRT to get them through the years when the symptoms are most disruptive may have seemed worth any small risk. Other women took HRT because it has been shown to reduce the risk of bone fractures and osteoporosis, another major threat to older women's health.

NEW FINDINGS RAISE QUESTIONS

Today, results from several new studies provide growing evidence that the advice to take HRT to prevent CVD was not only inaccurate, it may have been deadly for some of those who followed it. Consider the following:

- The 1998 Heart and Estrogen/Progestin Replacement Study (HERS), a large-scale randomized, controlled clinical trial showed that after four years on HRT, there was no difference in heart attack rates and higher rates of coronary death for those on HRT compared to those taking a placebo.
- The 2000 Estrogen Replacement and Atherosclerosis (ERA) Trial, the first

study to use angiographic images to assess the effects of HRT and Estrogen Replacement Therapy (ERT) on women with preexisting coronary disease, showed no effect on disease progression with hormone replacement.

- In 2002, investigators conducting the huge Women's Health Initiative (WHI) study stirred even more controversy. Researchers announced that women on HRT in the study were experiencing a small but unacceptable increase in heart attacks, blood clots in the lungs (pulmonary embolism) and legs (deep vein thrombosis), and stroke. Although the project was scheduled to continue until 2005, these results caused the researchers to stop it early. One version of HRT, Prempro, appeared to pose a greater risk than others.
- In 2004, a multicenter heart disease prevention study (part of WHI) found that estrogen-only therapy had no effect on coronary heart disease risk but increased the risk of stroke in postmenopausal women. The study also showed an increase in risk of deep vein thrombosis, had no effect on breast or colorectal cancer, and reduced the risk of hip and other fractures. Like its HRT counterpart, the study was stopped early and notices sent to health care providers.

Electrocardiogram (ECG)   A record of the electrical activity of the heart; may be measured during a stress test.

Angiography   A technique for examining blockages in heart arteries. A catheter is inserted into the arteries, a dye is injected, and an X ray is taken to find the blocked areas. Also called *cardiac catheterization.*

Positron emission tomography (PET scan)   Method for measuring heart activity by injecting a patient with a radioactive tracer that is scanned electronically to produce a three-dimensional image of the heart and arteries.

tomography scans. An **electrocardiogram (ECG)** is a record of the electrical activity of the heart. Patients may undergo a stress test, such as walking or running on a treadmill, while their hearts are monitored. A more accurate method of testing for heart disease is **angiography** (often referred to as *cardiac catheterization*), in which a needle-thin tube called a *catheter* is threaded through heart arteries, a dye is injected, and an X ray is taken to discover which areas are blocked. A more recent and even more effective method of measuring heart activity is **positron emission tomography (PET scan)**, which produces three-dimensional images of the heart as blood flows through it. During a PET scan, a patient receives an intravenous injection of a radioactive tracer at rest and during exercise. As the tracer decays, it emits positrons that

WHAT ARE THE IMPLICATIONS FOR CONSUMERS?

Should a woman toss out her hormones based on the WHI results? Generally, experts recommend that if you are overweight, have high cholesterol, or have a family history of heart disease, you may already be at increased risk for cardiovascular disease, and it may be prudent to look for alternatives.

How great *is* the risk? Scientists indicate that if 10,000 women took HRT for one year:

The number of women with	Would increase by	Would decrease by
Breast cancer	8[a]	
Heart attack	7	
Stroke	8	
Pulmonary embolism	8[b]	
Venous thrombosis	10[b]	
Colorectal cancer		6[c]
Hip fracture		5

a. Risk appears after four years of use
b. Risk is greatest in first two years of use
c. Benefit appears after three years of use

It should be noted that these increased risks are drawn from studies of HRT, as estrogen-alone studies are still being analyzed. They also do not apply to women who had had hysterectomies and were on HRT. The decision to use ERT or HRT is complex and should be made in consultation with knowledgeable health care providers and after reviewing the latest information from reputable sources. The most important thing to take away from the WHI findings is that HRT does not seem to prevent or improve cardiovascular risks, so no woman should take it solely to protect against heart attacks or stroke.

If you have questions about these studies or want additional information, the references below are valuable sources of information.

Sources: K. L. Brubaker et al., "Effects of Estrogen Alone Treatment in Postmenopausal Women," *Journal of the American Medical Association* 292, no. 6 (2004): 686–696; The Postmenopausal Estrogen/Progestin Intervention (PEPI) Trial, The Writing Group for the PEPI Trial, "Effects of Estrogen or Estrogen/Progestin Regimens on Heart Disease Risk Factors in Menopausal Women," *Journal of the American Medical Association* 273, no. 3 (1995):199–208; L. Mosca et al., "Hormone Replacement Therapy and Cardiovascular Disease," *Circulation* 104 (2001): 499; S. Hulley et al. "Randomized Trial of Estrogen Plus Progestin for Secondary Prevention of Coronary Heart Disease in Postmenopausal Women," Heart and Estrogen/Progestin Replacement Study (HERS) Research Group, *Journal of the American Medical Association.* 280, no. 7 (1998): 605–613; Writing Group for the Women's Health Initiative Investigators, "Risks and Benefits of Estrogen Plus Progestin in Healthy Postmenopausal Women," *Journal of the American Medical Association* 288, no. 3 (2002): 321–333; U.S. Preventive Services Task Force, "Hormone Replacement Therapy for Primary Prevention of Chronic Conditions: Recommendations and Rationale," October 2002 (Rockville, MD: Agency for Healthcare Research and Quality), http://www.ahrq.gov /clinic/3rduspstf/hrt/hrtrr.htm; C. Runowics, "A Clearer Picture of HRT," *Health News.* 8, no. 9 (September, 2002): 1–4.

---

are picked up by the scanner and transformed by a computer into color images of the heart. Newer single-photon emission computed tomography (SPECT scans) provide an even better view. Other tests include:

- *Radionuclide imaging* (includes tests such as thallium test, multinucleated gated angiography [MUGA scan], and acute infarct scintigraphy). These procedures involve injecting substances called radionuclides into the bloodstream. Computer-generated pictures can then show them in the heart. These tests can show how well the heart muscle is supplied with blood, how well the heart's chambers are functioning, and which part of the heart has been damaged by a heart attack.

- *Magnetic resonance imaging (MRI).* This test uses powerful magnets to look inside the body. Computer-generated pictures can show the heart muscle and help physicians identify damage from a heart attack, diagnose congenital heart defects, and evaluate disease of larger blood vessels such as the aorta.
- *Ultrafast computed tomography (CT).* This is an especially fast form of X ray of the heart designed to evaluate bypass grafts, diagnose ventricular function, and measure calcium deposits.
- *Digital subtraction angiography (DSA).* This modified form of computer-aided imaging records pictures of the heart and its blood vessels.

Differences Between the Sexes: Key Factors in Early Detection and Prognosis

As more research is done concerning diagnosis and treatment of CVD, it is clear that women sometimes experience different symptoms and benefit from different treatments than men do. For example, consider the following:

FEELING PAIN

Several studies have documented that women experience pain more acutely and more frequently than men, indicating that the sexes may detect and react to pain differently. In a study of dental patients, women responded more favorably than men to a class of pain relievers known as kappa opioids, including pentazocine. This finding suggests that receptors for inhibiting pain may vary by sex. Also, women appear to be less responsive than men to nonsteroidal anti-inflammatory drugs, such as ibuprofen. Women typically need slightly lower doses of aspirin and should be warned that taking 325 mg of aspirin per day may result in anticoagulation levels that exceed those of men. Surgical risks, accidents that lead to excessive bleeding, and so on, may be greater for aspirin-using women.

NOTING HEART ATTACK SYMPTOMS

Although we are taught that the classic symptom of a heart attack is chest-crushing pain, this type of pain is not that common in women. Women's heart attacks, by contrast, tend to show up as shortness of breath, fatigue, and jaw pain, stretched out over hours rather than minutes. Women tend to suffer their first heart attack ten years later than men; and, in part because they are older when they have these attacks, they are more likely to die.

TREATING CVD

Interestingly, drugs used to break up clots and stabilize erratic heartbeats are less effective in women than in men. Beta blockers, one common form of treatment for reducing blood pressure and migraines, take longer to metabolize in women than in men, meaning that women often have more difficulty regulating dosage and preventing side effects. Until recently, hormone replacement therapy had been believed to help, but recent research has shown otherwise (see the Women's Health/Men's Health box on hormone controversy, page 442). Recent studies have shown that angioplasty, a technique in which a small, flexible catheter is inserted in coronary vessels to break up plaque and clear blocked arteries, is one of the best techniques for reducing risk of heart attack.

Angioplasty versus Bypass Surgery

Coronary bypass surgery has helped many patients who suffered coronary blockages or heart attacks. In coronary bypass surgery, a blood vessel is taken from another site in the patient's body (usually the *saphenous vein* in the leg or the *internal mammary artery*) and implanted to "bypass" blocked arteries and transport blood. Bypass patients typically spend four to seven days in the hospital to recuperate. The average cost of the procedure itself is well over $50,000, and the additional intensive care treatments and follow-ups often result in total medical bills of $125,000. Death rates are generally much lower at medical centers where surgical teams and intensive care teams see large numbers of patients.[58]

Another procedure, **angioplasty** (sometimes called *balloon angioplasty*), carries fewer risks and may be more effective than bypass surgery in selected cases. As in angiography, a thin catheter is threaded through blocked heart arteries. The catheter has a balloon at the tip, which is inflated to flatten fatty deposits against the arterial walls, allowing blood to flow more freely. Angioplasty patients are generally awake but sedated during the procedure and spend only one or two days in the hospital after treatment. Most people can return to work within five days. In about 30 percent of patients, the treated arteries become clogged again within six months. Some patients may undergo the procedure as many as three times within a five-year period. Some surgeons argue that given this high rate of recurrence, bypass may be a more effective treatment.

Today, newer forms of laser angioplasty and atherectomy, a procedure that removes plaque, are being done in several clinics. These procedures are often followed by procedures in which the affected area has a small wire mesh tube (a stent) inserted to prop open the artery cleared by angioplasty.

Research suggests that in many instances, drug treatments may be just as effective in prolonging life as invasive surgical techniques, but it is critical that doctors prescribe an aggressive drug treatment program and that patients comply with it. Among the most effective are beta blockers and calcium channel blockers to reduce high blood pressure and

Coronary bypass surgery A surgical technique whereby a blood vessel is implanted to bypass a clogged coronary artery.

Angioplasty A technique in which a catheter with a balloon at the tip is inserted into a clogged artery; the balloon is inflated to flatten fatty deposits against artery walls, allowing blood to flow more freely.

Advances against Heart Disease and Stroke

Although heart disease continues to be the leading cause of death in the United States, actual rates of heart disease have declined substantially in recent decades. Every year we learn more about the functioning of the heart, and this knowledge has helped promote preventive behaviors as well as increases in longevity among those who have experienced a heart or stroke event. Health officials cite major strides in preventing and treating cardiovascular health problems:

- *High blood pressure gene.* Discovery of a gene that produces a special protein receptor that appears to serve as a "master regulator of the body's handling of salt" provides researchers with greater insight into an inherited form of high blood pressure in children. A defective gene makes the receptor stick in the "on" position, which causes the kidneys to retain salt, leading to increases in blood pressure.
- *Congenital heart defects.* A genetic defect has been identified as the cause of DiGeorge's syndrome, a condition marked by malformations of the heart and face. Identification of this missing gene, called *UFD1,* may provide clues to the prevention and treatment of congenital heart defects.

- *New diagnostic testing.* A special process called microarray analysis can detect missing or defective genes more quickly than ever before. Using this process, researchers found a genetic defect in people with Tangier disease, a blood-fat disorder caused by a shortage of HDL, the "good" cholesterol that carries fat from tissues. This knowledge may help researchers learn more about raising HDL levels for millions of individuals.
- *Reducing "stunning."* Scientists have found the cause of "stunning," a condition in which the heart's pumping action is severely weakened and that often strikes after a heart attack or heart surgery. The problem has been traced to a genetic flaw that affects a protein, troponin I, needed for normal heart contractions.
- *Tissue growth.* Remarkable advances in tissue engineering have enabled scientists to successfully grow heart valves in the laboratory. These new valves may eventually replace the mechanical valves and preserved pig valves commonly used now.
- *Diabetes link.* A link between diabetes and CVD has resulted in diabetes joining smoking, high blood pressure, high cholesterol, and lack of exercise as risk factors for heart disease and stroke. It is now believed that diabetes increases the risk of dying of heart attack, stroke, heart failure, or kidney failure by threefold.

- *New uses for an old drug.* A study of 10,000 heart and diabetes patients found that a standard high blood pressure drug, ramipril, can reduce the risk of death from a wide range of circulatory problems and may help prevent atherosclerosis.
- *New clot busters.* Experimental blood clot busters were shown to prevent brain damage and disability from stroke if given within three to six hours after the attack.
- *New imaging procedures.* New ultrafast computed tomography (CT) imaging and magnetic resonance angiography (MRA), which uses magnets and radio waves to view the inside of arteries, offer exciting new means of noninvasive diagnosis of artery blockage.
- *Robotic surgery.* Preliminary studies on the use of robotics in bypass surgery provide hope for safer options. Operating through three small holes in the chest, robotic arms mimic the actions of a surgeon working the controls. The use of robotics provides greater steadiness, eliminates human error, and increases the potential for microsurgery.

Sources: National Institutes of Health, National Heart, Lung, and Blood Institute; "Treatment Options for CVD," 2004. www.nhlbi.nih.gov; American Heart Association, "Treatment Options," 2004. www.americanheart.org.

---

treat other symptoms. Cholesterol-lowering drugs are also effective.

Aspirin for Heart Disease: Can It Help?

Research indicates that low doses of aspirin (80 mg daily or every other day) are beneficial to heart patients because of its blood-thinning properties. Higher levels do not provide significantly more protection. Aspirin has even been advised as a preventive strategy for people with no current heart disease symptoms; however, aspirin should only be taken as a preventative if under the advice of a person's own physician. Major problems associated with chronic aspirin use are gastrointestinal intolerance and a tendency for some people to

have difficulty with blood clotting, and these factors may outweigh aspirin's benefits in some cases. People taking aspirin face additional risks from emergency surgery or accidental bleeding. Although the findings concerning aspirin and heart disease are still inconclusive, the research seems promising.[59]

Thrombolysis

Whenever a heart attack occurs, prompt action is vital. When a coronary artery is blocked, the heart muscle doesn't die immediately, but time determines how much damage occurs. If a victim reaches an emergency room and is diagnosed fast enough, a form of reperfusion therapy called

thrombolysis can be performed. Thrombolysis involves injecting an agent such as TPA (tissue plasminogen activator) to dissolve the clot and restore some blood flow, thereby reducing the amount of tissue that dies from ischemia.[60] These drugs must be administered within one to three hours after a heart attack for best results.

What do you think?

With all the new diagnostic procedures, treatments, and differing philosophies about various prevention and intervention techniques, how can typical health consumers ensure that they will get the best treatment? ■ *Where can they go for information?* ■ *Why might women, members of certain minority groups, and older adults need a "health advocate" who can help them get through the system?*

Cardiac Rehabilitation

Every year, nearly 1 million people survive heart attacks. Over 7 million more have unstable angina, and about 650,000 undergo bypass surgery or angioplasty. Heart failure is the most common discharge diagnosis for hospitalized Medicare patients and the fourth most common diagnosis among all patients hospitalized in the United States. Most of these patients are eligible for cardiac rehabilitation (including exercise training and health education classes on good nutrition and CVD risk management), needing only a doctor's prescription for these services. However, many Americans do not have access to these programs. Even larger numbers are finding it difficult to afford them in light of skyrocketing costs for prescription drugs. While some patients must choose between home health care and cardiac rehabilitation, others stay away from such programs because of cost, transportation, or other factors. Perhaps the biggest deterrent is fear of having another attack due to exercise. The benefits of cardiac rehabilitation (including increased stamina and strength and faster recovery), however, far outweigh the risks when these programs are run by certified health professionals.

Personal Advocacy and Heart-Smart Behaviors

People who suspect they have cardiovascular disease are often overwhelmed and frightened. Where should they go for diagnosis? What are the best treatments? Answering these questions becomes even more difficult if they are upset, scared, or tend to listen unquestioningly to doctors' orders. If you or a loved one must face a CVD crisis, it is important to act with knowledge, strength, and assertiveness. The following suggestions will help you deal with hospitals and health care providers in the wake of a cardiac event or any major health problem (see Chapter 22 for more on being a smart consumer of health care services):

1. *Know your rights as a patient.* Ask about the risks and costs of various diagnostic tests. Some procedures, particularly angiography, may pose significant risks for people who are older, who have a history of minor strokes, or who have had chemotherapy or other treatments that could have damaged their blood vessels. Ask for test results and an explanation of any abnormalities.
2. *Find out about informed consent procedures, living wills, durable power of attorney, organ donation, and other legal issues before you become sick.* Having someone shove a clipboard in your face and ask you if life support can be terminated in case of a problem is one of the great horrors of many people's hospital experiences. Be prepared.
3. *Ask about alternative procedures.* If possible, seek a second opinion at a different health care facility (in other words, get at least two opinions from doctors who are not in the same group and who cannot read each other's diagnoses). New research indicates that doctors may not use drug treatments as aggressively as they could and that medications may be as effective as major bypass or open heart surgeries. Ask, ask, and ask again. Remember, it is your life, and there is always the possibility that another treatment will be better for you.
4. *Remain with your loved one as a "personal advocate."* If your loved one is weak and unable to ask questions, ask the questions yourself. Inquire about new medications, tests, and other potentially risky procedures that may be undertaken during the course of treatment or recovery. If you feel your loved one is being removed from intensive care or other closely monitored areas prematurely, ask if the hospital is taking this action to comply with DRGs (established limits of treatment for certain conditions) and if this action is warranted. Most hospitals have waiting areas or special rooms so family members can stay close to a patient. Exercise your right to this option.
5. *Monitor the actions of health care providers.* To control costs, some hospitals are hiring nursing aides and other personnel who may lack the training that registered nurses have in handling patients with CVD. Ask about the patient-to-nurse ratio, and make sure that people monitoring you or your loved ones have appropriate credentials.
6. *Be considerate of your care provider.* One of the most stressful jobs any person can be entrusted with is care of a critically ill person. Although questions are appropriate and your emotions are running high, be as tactful and considerate as possible. Nurses often carry a disproportionate

---

Thrombolysis Injection of an agent to dissolve clots and restore some blood flow, thereby reducing the amount of tissue that dies from ischemia.

responsibility for the care of patients during critical times and are often forced to carry a higher than optimal patient load. Try to remain out of their way, ask questions as necessary, and report any irregularities in care to the supervisor.

7. *Be patient with the patient.* The pain, suffering, and fears associated with a cardiac event often cause otherwise nice people to act in not-so-nice ways. Be patient and helpful, and allow time for the person to rest. Talk with the patient about his or her feelings, concerns, and fears. Do not ignore these concerns to ease your own anxieties.

We still have much to learn about CVD and its causes, treatments, and risk factors. Staying informed is an important part of staying healthy. Good dietary habits, regular exercise, stress management, prompt attention to suspicious symptoms, and other healthy behaviors will greatly enhance your chances of remaining CVD-free. Other factors that influence risk include how much emphasis our health care systems place on access to health care for all underserved populations, education about risk, and other community-based interventions. Action on both community and individual levels can help address the challenge of CVD.

TAKING CHARGE

MAKE IT HAPPEN!

Assessment: The Assess Yourself box on page 427 evaluates your risk of heart disease and the status of your LDL cholesterol. Based on your results and the advice of your physician, you may need to take steps to reduce your cholesterol level and risk of CVD.

Making a Change: In order to change your behavior, you need to develop a plan. Follow these steps.

1. Evaluate your behavior, and identify patterns and specific things you are doing. What can you change now? What can you change in the near future?
2. Select one pattern of behavior that you want to change.
3. Fill out a Behavior Change Contract. It should include your long-term goal for change, your short-term goals, the rewards you'll give yourself for reaching these goals, potential obstacles along the way, and strategies for overcoming these obstacles. For each goal, list the small steps and specific actions that you will take.
4. Chart your progress in a journal. At the end of a week, consider how successful you were in following your plan. What helped you be successful? What made change more difficult? What will you do differently next week?
5. Revise your plan as needed. Are the short-term goals attainable? Are the rewards satisfying?

One Student's Plan: When Nathan completed the self-assessment, he saw that his family history and eating habits were contributing to an increased risk of CVD. Nathan

couldn't do anything about his father's history of heart disease, so he knew that it was even more important to take action in the areas where he could make changes. At six feet in height, he weighed 220 pounds, which he discovered is close to obese according to body mass index calculations. He decided to manage his weight through exercise and eating better. He also expected a modified diet would help lower his cholesterol levels, which his doctor had warned him were too high.

Nathan's first step was to keep track of everything he normally ate for a week. When he analyzed his food journal, he saw that he rarely ate breakfast, which made him more likely to grab a doughnut later in the morning and a big lunch. He bought some whole wheat, high fiber cereal and skim milk and started getting up 15 minutes earlier so he had time to eat his healthy breakfast. For the days when he didn't feel like eating cold cereal, he bought some five-minute oatmeal that also contained healthy fiber and nutrients. Nathan found that he was not as tempted by doughnuts and other unhealthy snacks during the day and that he didn't overeat as much at lunch. He even had more energy during the day. As he started to lose weight, he felt more able to begin a moderate exercise program. All of these changes—losing weight, eating more fiber and less fat, and adding some exercise to his life—made Nathan confident that his next checkup would show a lower LDL level and, perhaps, lower blood pressure. When Nathan has reached a healthier range on these measures, he plans to buy himself a new DVD player.

Summary

- Cardiovascular disease incidence and prevalence rates have changed considerably in the past 50 years. Certain segments of the population have disproportionate levels of risk.

- The cardiovascular system consists of the heart and circulatory system and is a carefully regulated, integrated network of vessels that supply the body with the nutrients and oxygen necessary to perform daily functions.

- Cardiovascular diseases include atherosclerosis (hardening of the arteries), heart attack, angina pectoris, arrhythmias, congestive heart failure, congenital and rheumatic heart disease, and stroke. These combine to be the leading cause of death in the United States today.

- Many risk factors for cardiovascular disease can be controlled, such as cigarette smoking, high blood fat and cholesterol levels, hypertension, lack of exercise, high-fat diet, obesity, diabetes, and emotional stress. Some risk factors, such as age, gender, and heredity, cannot be controlled. Many of these factors have a compounded effect when combined. Dietary changes, exercise, weight reduction, and attention to lifestyle risks can greatly reduce susceptibility to cardiovascular disease.

- Women have a unique challenge in controlling their risk for CVD, particularly after menopause, when estrogen levels are no longer sufficient to be protective.

- New methods developed for treating heart blockages include coronary bypass surgery, angioplasty, and insertion of stents. Also, drugs such as beta blockers and calcium channel blockers can reduce high blood pressure and treat other symptoms. Research has provided important clues on how best to prevent or reduce risk of CVD today. Recognizing your own risks and acting now to reduce risk are important elements of lifelong cardiovascular health.

Questions for Discussion and Reflection

1. Trace the path of a drop of blood from the time it enters the heart until it reaches the extremities.
2. List the different types of CVD. Compare and contrast their symptoms, risk factors, prevention, and treatment.
3. What are the major indicators that CVD poses a particularly significant risk to people of your age? To people over 65? To people from selected minority groups?
4. Discuss the role that exercise, stress management, dietary changes, checkups, and other factors can play in reducing risk for CVD. What role might chronic infections play in CVD risk?
5. Discuss why age is such an important factor in women's risk for CVD. What can be done to decrease women's risk in later life?
6. Describe some of the diagnostic and treatment alternatives for CVD. If you had a heart attack today, which treatment would you prefer? Explain why.

Accessing Your Health on the Internet

Visit the following Internet sites to explore further topics and issues related to personal health. To visit an organization's website, go to the Companion Website for *Access to Health, Ninth Edition* at www.aw-bc.com/donatelle, click on the book image, and select "Accessing Your Health on the Internet" from the navigation menu.

1. *American Heart Association.* Homepage for the leading private organization dedicated to heart health. This site provides information, statistics, and resources regarding cardiovascular care, including an opportunity to test your own risk for CVD.
2. *Johns Hopkins Cardiac Rehabilitation Homepage.* Information about prevention of heart disease and rehabilitation from CVD from one of the best cardiac care centers in the United States, including information about programs available to help individuals stop smoking, lose weight, lower blood pressure and blood cholesterol, and reduce emotional stress.
3. *National Heart, Lung, and Blood Institute.* A valuable resource for information on all aspects of cardiovascular health and wellness.
4. *U.S. National Library of Medicine: Health Services/ Technology Assessment Text.* Access to numerous databases of health care documents outlining procedures for clinicians and patients. Choose the database for the Agency for Health Care Policy and Research (AHCPR) to review various guidelines regarding all forms of cardiac care.

Further Reading

American Heart Association. *Heart and Stroke Facts.* Dallas, TX: American Heart Association.

An annual overview providing facts and figures concerning cardiovascular disease in the United States. Supplement provides key statistics about current trends and future directions in treatment and prevention.

McCrum, Robert. *My Year Off: Recovering after a Stroke.* New York: Broadway Books, 1999.

The chronicle of a young man's recovery from a severe stroke.

Pashkow, Frederic, and Charlotte Libov. *The Women's Heart Book.* New York: Hyperion, 2001.

Gersh, Bernard and Michael Wood eds. *The Mayo Clinic Heart Book.* New York: William Morrow, 2000.

These two books provide an overview of heart disease in America, including risk factors, trends, and options for heart patients.

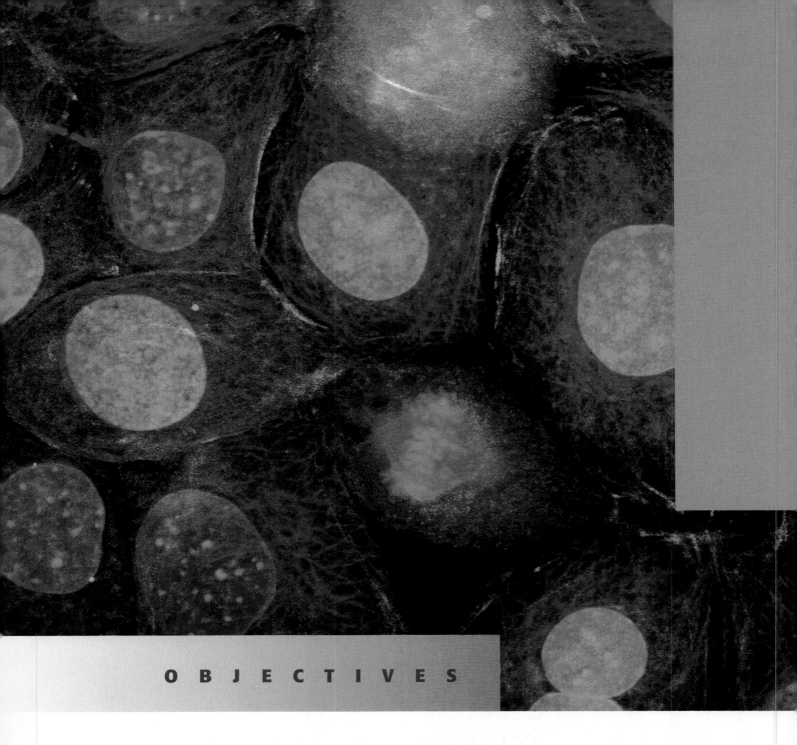

OBJECTIVES

- Define *cancer,* and discuss how it develops.

- Discuss the causes of cancer, including biological causes, occupational and environmental hazards, lifestyle, psychological factors, chemicals in foods, viruses, and medical causes.

- Describe the different types of cancer and the risks they pose to people at different ages and stages of life.

- Explain the importance of understanding and responding appropriately to self-exams, medical exams, and symptoms related to different types of cancer. Explain the importance of early detection.

- Discuss ways to prevent cancer and the implications of behavioral risks.

- Discuss cancer detection and treatment, including radiation therapy, chemotherapy, immunotherapy, and other common methods of detection and treatment.

CANCER

REDUCING YOUR RISK

IN THE NEWS

Vaccine Works to Prevent Cervical Cancer

By Denise Grady

An experimental vaccine to prevent cervical cancer, first proved effective in preliminary testing two years ago, has continued to provide protection against the disease, researchers reported yesterday.

The vaccine, which works by making people immune to a common sexually transmitted virus that causes the cancer, is not yet available. But its maker, Merck Laboratories, expects to apply for approval late next year, said Dr. Eliav Barr, a research director at the company.

Worldwide, there are 470,000 new cases of cervical cancer a year and 225,000 deaths. Most of the deaths occur in poorer countries where women do not have regular Pap tests, which can detect cancers or precancers early enough for them to be cured. In the United States, where Pap testing is widespread, 11,000 new cases are expected this year and about 4,000 deaths.

If the vaccine is approved, Dr. Barr said, it will be recommended for use in young adults and in children starting at age 9 or 10, before they become sexually active and encounter the virus. Once cancer develops, it is too late for the vaccine to help. The median age at which young people in the United States first have sex is 15.

Read the complete article online in the eThemes section of this book's website: www.aw-bc.com/donatelle.

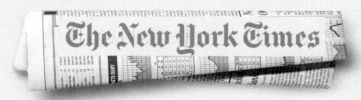

As recently as 50 years ago, a diagnosis of cancer was usually a death sentence. Health professionals could only guess at the cause, and treatments were often as deadly as the disease itself. Because we had no idea how a person "got" cancer, fears about possible infection led to ostracism and bigotry aimed at people who desperately needed support, much like people with HIV were treated in the early days of the epidemic.

Fortunately, we've come a long way since then. Today we know that there are multiple causes of cancer and few are linked to any type of infectious agent. Early detection and vast improvements in technology have dramatically improved the prognosis for most cancer patients. We also know that there are many actions we can take individually and as a society to prevent cancer. Knowing the facts about cancer, recognizing your own risk, and taking action to reduce your risk are important steps in the battle.

An Overview of Cancer

During 2004, approximately 563,700 Americans died of cancer, and nearly 1.4 million new cases were diagnosed. Cancer is the second leading cause of death, exceeded only by heart disease, in the United States.[1] Put into perspective, this means that every day more than 1,500 people die of some form of cancer. One of four deaths in the United States is from cancer. Of these, one-third of the cancers were related to poor nutrition, physical inactivity, and obesity, which means they could have been prevented.[2] Certain other cancers are related to exposure to infectious diseases such as hepatitis B virus (HBV), human papillomavirus (HPV), HIV, *Helicobacter pylori* bacterium, and others, and could be prevented through behavioral changes, vaccines, or antibiotics.[3] However, it is important to note that although more than 1.4 million people will be diagnosed with cancer in a year, over six in ten (63 percent) will be alive five years after diagnosis. Many will be considered "cured," meaning that they have no subsequent cancer in their bodies five years after diagnosis and can expect to live a long and productive life.[4]

When adjusted for normal life expectancy (factors such as dying of heart disease, accidents, etc.), a relative five-year survival of 63 percent is seen for all cancers. Some cancers that only a few decades ago presented a very poor outlook are often cured today: acute lymphocytic leukemia in children, Hodgkin's disease, Burkitt's lymphoma, Ewing's sarcoma (a form of bone cancer), Wilms' tumor (a kidney cancer in children), testicular cancer, and osteogenic (bone) sarcoma are among the most remarkable indicators of progress.

Disparities in Cancer Rates

While cancer strikes people of all ages, races, cultures, and socioeconomic levels, some Americans are at greater risk. There are many demographic and socioeconomic factors associated with health-related disparities, including income, race/ethnicity, culture, geography (urban/rural), age, sex, sexual orientation, and literacy.[5] Research into these factors includes a comprehensive review of racial and ethnic disparities in health care published in 2003 by the Institute of Medicine (IOM).[6]

Poverty is widely believed to be the most important factor affecting health and longevity.[7] People from lower socioeconomic levels tend to smoke more and are greater targets for predatory tobacco marketing,[8] are more likely to be obese and sedentary, have less access to healthy fruits and vegetables, are often under- or uninsured (and therefore can access health care only when the cancer is in its later stages of development), may not be able to afford medications or uncompensated medical charges, and have difficulty communicating with their health care providers and understanding health information. Cultural factors, including ability to speak English, beliefs about the benefits and risks of treatment, beliefs about illness, and other factors may also affect the ability to access quality health care. Culture can influence values and belief systems related to whether or not people seek care, participate in screenings, and comply with medical regimens.

How serious are the disparities? Consider the following:[9]

- Of all racial or ethnic groups in the United States, African Americans have the highest death rates from all cancer sites combined and from malignancies of the lung and bronchus, colon and rectum, female breast, prostate, and uterine cervix. Death rates for African American males are 1.4 times higher than whites, and for females, they are 1.2 times higher.
- African American, American Indian, Alaska Native, and Asian American and Pacific Island women have a lower five-year survival rate than non-Hispanic whites.
- A person living in an affluent census tract has a five-year survival rate that is 10 percent higher than a person living in a tract below the poverty level.
- The gap between socioeconomic and ethnic groups in cancer mortality rates is greater now than it was in 1975.
- Men from poorer census counties have a 22 percent higher death rate from prostate cancer than their affluent county comparison groups.
- Between 1988 and 1998, women with stage I and II breast cancer were less likely than women in more affluent counties to be treated with breast-conserving surgery and radiation if they resided in poorer counties.
- African Americans with stage I or stage II lung cancer are less likely to receive the recommended treatment of surgery than whites, a disparity that accounts for much of the difference in survival.
- African Americans with cervical cancer are more likely than whites to go unstaged (that is, not to have their cancer's progression classified) and receive no treatment.
- Whites are more likely to receive aggressive treatment for colorectal cancer.

Table 16.1
Cancer Survival Rates by Race and Year of Diagnosis (Five-Year Relative Rates)*

Site	All Races 1974–76	All Races 1983–85	All Races 1992–99	White 1974–76	White 1983–85	White 1992–99	African American 1974–76	African American 1983–85	African American 1992–99
All cancers	50	53	63†	51	54	64†	39	40	53†
Prostate	67	75	98†	68	76	98†	58	64	93†
Testis	79	91	96†	79	91	96†	76	88	87
Melanoma of the skin	80	85	90†	81	85	90†	67‡	74§	64‡
Breast (female)	75	78	87†	75	79	88†	63	64	74†
Cervix (uterine)	69	69	71†	70	71	73†	64	61	61
Colon	50	58	62†	51	58	63†	46	49	53†
Ovary	37	41	53†	37	40	52†	41	42	52†
Leukemia	34	41	46†	35	42	48†	31	34	39
Brain	22	27	33†	22	26	32†	27	32	39†
Multiple myeloma	24	28	32†	24	27	31†	28	31	33
Lung & bronchus	13	14	15†	13	14	15†	11	11	12†
Pancreas	3	3	4†	3	3	4†	3	5	4

*Survival rates are adjusted for normal life expectancy and are based on cases diagnosed from 1974–1976, 1993–1985, and 1992–1999, and followed through 2000. †The difference in rates between 1974–1976 and 1992–1999 is statistically significant (p <0.05). ‡The standard error of the survival rate is between 5 and 10 percentage points. §The standard error of the survival rate is greater than 10 percentage points.

Sources for data: NCI Surveillance, Epidemiology, and End Results Program, 1973–2000. (Bethesda, MD: National Cancer Institute, 2003): published in American Cancer Society, *Cancer Facts and Figures 2004* (Atlanta, GA: American Cancer Society, 2004). Reproduced with permission. www.cancer.org. © 2004, American Cancer Society, Inc.

While the above examples provide a disheartening look at the disparities that exist, major groups such as the IOM have called for rapid strategies to reduce disparities. Among the planned actions to be taken by the American Cancer Society are:

- *Advocacy.* Including media campaigns, information dissemination, lobbying and coalition formation and action at the federal, state, and local levels, these efforts are designed to make it easier for those who are subjected to disparities to navigate the health care system. Public policies, other legislative action, and increased funding to get the word out all help disadvantaged groups have a better chance of quality care.

- *Research.* By increasing funding for research on the mechanisms of cancer initiation and factors likely to improve treatment among the poor and disadvantaged, health outcomes for cancer patients will definitely improve.

- *Education.* By broadening the base for bilingual information and educational materials, more diverse populations will be reached with key information about signs and symptoms, risk factors, and prevention strategies. In addition, providing at-risk populations with better information about navigating in the health care system, accessing health care products and services, and other key information elements will result in earlier diagnosis and better prognosis for treatment.

For a detailed set of charts and tables that illustrate how serious this problem is for different racial and ethnic groups, visit the American Cancer Society website (www.cancer.org) and review its *Cancer Facts and Figures* document, which is updated annually. See Table 16.1 for some sample statistics from the current edition.

What do you think?

In 1991, Dr. Samual Broder, then director of the U.S. National Cancer Institute (NCI), declared that "Poverty is a carcinogen." What you believe his rationale for this statement was? Explain whether you agree or disagree with it. ▪ *Are there any specific examples that you could give with certain cancer situations that might help illustrate his point?*

What Is Cancer?

Cancer is the name given to a large group of diseases characterized by the uncontrolled growth and spread of abnormal cells.[10] Think of a healthy cell as a small computer, programmed to operate in a particular fashion. Under normal conditions, healthy cells are protected by a powerful overseer, the immune system, as they perform their daily functions of growing, replicating, and repairing body organs. When

Cancer A large group of diseases characterized by the uncontrolled growth and spread of abnormal cells.

something interrupts normal cell programming, however, uncontrolled growth and abnormal cellular development result in a new growth of tissue serving no physiological function, which is called a **neoplasm.** This neoplasmic mass often forms a clumping of cells known as a **tumor.**

Not all tumors are **malignant** (cancerous); in fact, most are **benign** (noncancerous). Benign tumors are generally harmless unless they grow in such a fashion as to obstruct or crowd out normal tissues. A benign tumor of the brain, for instance, is life threatening when it grows enough to restrict blood flow and cause a stroke. The only way to determine whether a tumor is malignant is through **biopsy,** or microscopic examination of cell development.

Benign and malignant tumors differ in several key ways. Benign tumors generally consist of ordinary-looking cells enclosed in a fibrous shell or capsule that prevents their spreading to other body areas. Malignant tumors are usually not enclosed in a protective capsule and can therefore spread to other organs. This process, known as **metastasis,** makes some forms of cancer particularly aggressive in their ability to overcome bodily defenses. By the time they are diagnosed, malignant tumors have frequently metastasized throughout the body, making treatment extremely difficult. Unlike benign tumors, which merely expand to take over a given space, malignant cells invade surrounding tissue, emitting clawlike protrusions that disturb the ribonucleic acid (RNA) and deoxyribonucleic acid (DNA) within normal cells. Disrupting these substances, which control cellular metabolism and reproduction, produces **mutant cells** that differ in form, quality, and function from normal cells. Assess your own cancer risk by completing the Assess Yourself box on page 456.

What Causes Cancer?

After decades of research, most cancer epidemiologists believe that cancers are, at least in theory, preventable, and many could be avoided by suitable choices in lifestyle and

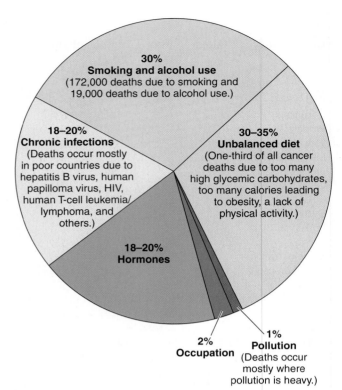

Figure 16.1
Factors Believed to Contribute to Global Causes of Cancer

Sources: S. Heacht, et al., *Public Session/Panel Discussion* (Portland, OR: Linus Pauling Institute International Conference on Diet and Optimal Health, 2001); American Cancer Society, *Cancer Facts and Figures 2004* (Atlanta, GA: American Cancer Society, 2004).

environment.[11] Many specific causes of cancer are well documented, the most important of which are smoking, obesity, and a few organic viruses. However, wide global variations in common cancers, such as those of the breast, prostate, colon, and rectum, remain unexplained (Figure 16.1).

Most research supports the idea that cancer is caused by both *external* (chemicals, radiation, viruses, and lifestyle) and *internal* (hormones, immune conditions, and inherited mutations) factors. Causal factors may act together or in sequence to promote cancer development. We do not know why some people have malignant cells in their body and never develop cancer, while others may take ten years or more to develop the disease.

Cellular Change/Mutation Theories

One theory of cancer development proposes that cancer results from spontaneous errors that occur during cell reproduction. Perhaps cells that are overworked or aged are more likely to break down, causing genetic errors that result in mutant cells.

Another theory suggests that cancer is caused by some external agent or agents that enter a normal cell and initiate the cancerous process. Numerous environmental factors,

Neoplasm A new growth of tissue that serves no physiological function and results from uncontrolled, abnormal cellular development.

Tumor A neoplasmic mass that grows more rapidly than surrounding tissue.

Malignant Very dangerous or harmful; refers to a cancerous tumor.

Benign Harmless; refers to a noncancerous tumor.

Biopsy Microscopic examination of tissue to determine if a cancer is present.

Metastasis Process by which cancer spreads from one area to different areas of the body.

Mutant cells Cells that differ in form, quality, or function from normal cells.

such as radiation, chemicals, hormonal drugs, immunosuppressant drugs (drugs that suppress the normal activity of the immune system), and other toxins, are considered possible **carcinogens** (cancer-causing agents); perhaps the most common carcinogen is the tar in cigarettes. The greater the dose or exposure to environmental hazards, the greater the risk of disease. People who are forced to work, live, and pass through areas that have high levels of environmental toxins may be at greater risk for several types of cancers.[12]

A third theory came out of research on certain viruses that are believed to cause tumors in animals. Scientists discovered **oncogenes,** suspected cancer-causing genes that are present on chromosomes. Although oncogenes are typically dormant, scientists theorize that certain conditions such as age, stress, and exposure to carcinogens, viruses, and radiation may activate them. Once activated, they grow and reproduce in an out-of-control manner.

Scientists are uncertain whether only people who develop cancer have oncogenes or whether we all have **protooncogenes,** genes that can become oncogenes under certain conditions. Many **oncologists** (physicians who specialize in the treatment of malignancies) believe that the oncogene theory may lead to a greater understanding of how individual cells function and bring us closer to developing effective treatments.

Many factors are believed to contribute to cancer, and combining risk factors can dramatically increase a person's risk of the disease.

Risks for Cancer—Lifestyle

Anyone can develop cancer; however, most cases affect adults beginning in middle age. In fact, nearly 80 percent of cancers are diagnosed at ages 55 and over.

Cancer researchers refer to one's *cancer risk* when they assess risk factors. *Lifetime risk* refers to the probability that an individual, over the course of a lifetime, will develop cancer or die from it. In the United States, men have a lifetime risk of about one in two; women have a lower risk of one in three.[13]

Relative risk is a measure of the strength of the relationship between risk factors and a particular cancer. Basically, relative risk compares your risk if you engage in certain known risk behaviors with that of someone who does not engage in such behaviors. For example, if you are a male and smoke, you have a 20-fold relative risk of developing lung cancer compared to a nonsmoker. Your chances of getting lung cancer are about 20 times greater.[14]

Over the years, researchers have found that people who engage in certain behaviors show a higher incidence of cancer. In particular, diet, sedentary lifestyle (and resultant obesity), consumption of alcohol or cigarettes, stress, and other lifestyle factors seem to play a role. Likewise, colon and rectal cancer occur more frequently among persons with a high-fat, low-fiber diet; in those who don't eat enough fruits and vegetables; and in those who are inactive. (See

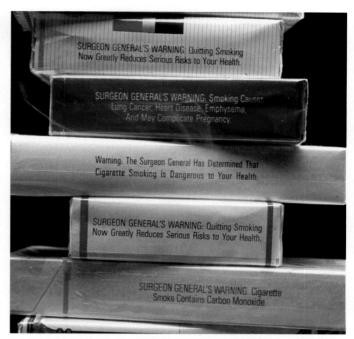

Of the several lifestyle risk factors for cancer, tobacco use is perhaps the most significant and the most preventable.

Chapter 8 on nutrition for information about certain dietary risks related to cancer and the role of supplements in prevention). More research is needed to pinpoint the mechanisms that act in the body to increase the odds of cancer. For now, there is compelling evidence that certain actions are clearly associated with a greater than average risk of the disease.

Keep in mind that a high relative risk does not guarantee cause and effect. It merely indicates the likelihood of a particular risk factor being related to a particular outcome.

Smoking and Cancer Risk Of all the potential risk factors for cancer, smoking is among the greatest. In the United States, tobacco is responsible for nearly one in five deaths annually. Tobacco use accounts for at least 30 percent of all cancer deaths and 87 percent of all lung cancer deaths.[15]

Carcinogens   Cancer-causing agents.

Oncogenes   Suspected cancer-causing genes present on chromosomes.

Protooncogenes   Genes that can become oncogenes under certain conditions.

Oncologists   Physicians who specialize in the treatment of malignancies.

Relative risk   A measure of the strength of the relationship between risk factors and the condition being studied, such as a particular cancer.

Cancer: Understanding Your Personal Risk

✨ my**health**lab

Fill out this assessment online at www.aw-bc.com/myhealthlab or www.aw-bc.com/donatelle

Although there are some types of cancer that you may be predisposed to due to genetic, biological, and/or environmental causes, there are many more that may be prevented through lifestyle changes and risk reduction strategies. If you carefully assess your risks, you can then make behavior changes that may make you less susceptible to various cancers. By answering each of the following questions, you will have an indication of your susceptibil-

ity. Of course, no single instrument can serve as a complete risk assessment or diagnostic guide. These questions merely serve as the basis for personal introspection and thoughtful planning about ways to reduce your risk.

Read each question and circle the number for your response. Be honest and accurate in order to get the most complete understanding of your cancer risks. Individual scores for specific questions should not be interpreted as a precise measure of relative risk, but the totals in each section give a general indication of your risk.

SECTION 1: BREAST CANCER

	Yes	No
1. Do you check your breasts at least monthly using breast self-exam (BSE) procedures?	1	2
2. Do you look at your breasts in the mirror regularly, checking for any irregular indentations/lumps, discharge from the nipples, or other noticeable changes?	1	2
3. Has your mother, sister, or daughter been diagnosed with breast cancer?	2	1
4. Have you ever been pregnant?	1	2
5. Have you had a history of lumps or cysts in your breasts or underarm?	2	1

Total Points _____

SECTION 2: SKIN CANCER

	Yes	No
1. Do you spend a lot of time in the sun, either at work or at play?	2	1
2. Do you use sunscreens with an SPF rating of 15 or more when you are in the sun?	1	2
3. Do you use tanning beds or sun booths regularly to maintain a tan?	2	1
4. Do you examine your skin once a month, checking any moles or other irregularities, particularly in hard-to-see areas such as your back, genitals, neck, and under your hair?	1	2
5. Do you purchase and wear sunglasses that adequately filter out harmful sun rays?	1	2

Total Points _____

SECTION 3: CANCERS OF THE REPRODUCTIVE SYSTEM

MEN

	Yes	No
1. Do you examine your penis regularly for unusual bumps or growths?	1	2
2. Do you perform regular testicular self-examinations?	1	2
3. Do you have a family history of prostate or testicular cancer?	2	1

Over the five decades since British and American epidemiologists first singled out tobacco as a culprit in lung cancer and other diseases, tar levels in British cigarettes have declined dramatically, as has the prevalence of smoking in general. As a result, the lung cancer rate for British men under age 55 has fallen by two-thirds since 1955, placing it among the lowest in the developed world. In the last 20 years, America's rates have shown a similar decline; however, lung cancer rates among men are still increasing in most developing countries and in Eastern Europe, where consumption of cigarettes remains high and is still increasing in some areas. See Chapter 13 for more on global trends in tobacco use.

	Yes	No
4. Do you practice safer sex and wear condoms with every sexual encounter?	1	2
5. Do you avoid exposure to harmful environmental hazards such as mercury, coal tars, benzene, chromate, and vinyl chloride?	1	2

Total Points _____

WOMEN

	Yes	No
1. Do you have a regularly scheduled Pap test?	1	2
2. Have you been infected with the human papilloma viruses, Epstein-Barr virus, or other viruses believed to increase cancer risk?	2	1
3. Has your mother, sister, or daughter been diagnosed with breast, cervical, endometrial, or ovarian cancer (particularly at a young age)?	2	1
4. Do you practice safer sex and use condoms with every sexual encounter?	1	2
5. Are you obese, taking estrogen, and/or consuming a diet that is very high in saturated fats?	2	1

Total Points _____

SECTION 4: CANCERS IN GENERAL

	Yes	No
1. Do you smoke cigarettes on most days of the week?	2	1
2. Do you consume a diet that is rich in fruits and vegetables?	1	2
3. Are you obese, and/or do you lead a primarily sedentary lifestyle?	2	1
4. Do you live in an area with high air pollution levels and/or work in a job where you are exposed to several chemicals on a regular basis?	2	1
5. Are you careful about the amount of animal fat in your diet, substituting olive oil or canola oil for animal fat whenever possible?	1	2
6. Do you limit your overall consumption of alcohol?	1	2
7. Do you eat foods rich in lycopene (such as tomatoes) and antioxidants?	1	2
8. Are you "body aware" and alert for changes in your body?	1	2
9. Do you have a family history of ulcers or of colorectal, stomach, or other digestive system cancers?	2	1
10. Do you avoid unnecessary exposure to radiation, cell phone emissions, and microwave emissions?	1	2

Total Points _____

ANALYZING YOUR SCORES

Take a careful look at each question for which you received a "2" score. Are there any areas in which you received mostly "2's"? Did you receive total points of 6 or higher in Sections 1 to 3? Did you receive total points of 11 or higher in Section 4? If so, you have at least one identifiable risk. The higher the score, the more risks you may have. However, rather than focusing just on your score, focus on which items you might change. Review the suggestions throughout this chapter, and list actions that you could take right now that might help you reduce your risk for these cancers.

MAKE IT HAPPEN!

Use the results of this self-assessment to begin your behavior change program. Follow the steps and use the examples on page 478 to complete your Behavior Change Contract, and then use these resources to take action.

Most authorities have believed that cigarettes cause only cancers of the lung, pancreas, bladder and kidney, and (synergistically with alcohol) the larynx, mouth, pharynx, and esophagus. However, more recent evidence indicates that several other types of cancer are also related to tobacco. Most notably, cancers of the stomach, liver, and cervix seem to be directly related to long-term smoking.

Obesity and Cancer Risk It is difficult to sort through the accumulated evidence about the role of certain nutrients, obesity, sedentary lifestyle, and related variables. Nevertheless, a body of research has emerged that points to a potential cancer link. Cancer is more common among people who are overweight, and risk increases as obesity increases. The evidence for a link is strongest for postmenopausal breast cancer and cancers of the endometrium, gallbladder, and kidney, but obesity is also implicated in other cancers. For women, the cervix and ovaries are added to this list; for men, cancers of the colon and prostate seem to be related to obesity and/or diet. The following facts provide evidence for this obesity/cancer link:[16]

- The relative risk of breast cancer in postmenopausal women is 50 percent higher for obese women than for nonobese women.
- The relative risk of colon cancer in men is 40 percent higher for obese men as compared to nonobese men.
- The relative risks of gallbladder and endometrial cancer are five times higher in obese individuals compared to individuals of "healthy" weight.
- Some studies show a positive association between obesity and cancers of the kidney, pancreas, rectum, esophagus, and liver.
- Obesity is believed to alter complex interactions among diet, metabolism, physical activity, hormones, and growth factors.

Biological Factors

Early theorists believed that we inherit a genetic predisposition toward certain forms of cancer.[17] Cancers of the breast, stomach, colon, prostate, uterus, ovaries, and lungs appear to run in families. For example, a woman runs a much higher risk of breast cancer if her mother or sisters (primary relatives) have had the disease, particularly at a young age. Hodgkin's disease and certain leukemias show similar familial patterns. Can we attribute these familial patterns to genetic susceptibility or to the fact that people in the same families experience similar environmental risks?

To date, the research in this area is inconclusive. Recent research conducted by the University of Utah indicates that genes for breast cancer exist. A rare form of eye cancer does appear to be passed genetically from mother to child. It is possible that we can inherit a tendency toward a cancer-prone, weak immune system or, conversely, that we can inherit a cancer-fighting potential. But the complex interaction of hereditary predisposition, lifestyle, and environment on the development of cancer makes it a challenge to determine a single cause. Research resulting from the Human Genome Project should help provide answers to whether there is a genetic predisposition to cancer.

Biological sex also affects the likelihood of developing certain forms of cancer. For example, breast cancer occurs primarily among females, although men do occasionally get breast cancer. Obviously, factors other than heredity and familial relationships affect which sex develops a particular cancer. In the 1950s, for example, women rarely contracted lung cancer. But with increases in the number of women who smoke and the length of time they have smoked, lung cancer rates have soared to become the leading cause of cancer death in women. However, while gender plays a role in certain cases of cancer, other variables such as lifestyle are probably more significant.

Reproductive and Hormonal Risks for Cancer The effects of reproductive factors on breast and cervical cancer have been well-documented. Late menarche, early menopause, early first childbirth, and high parity (having many children) have been shown to reduce a woman's risk of breast cancer. Pregnancy and estrogen supplementation in the form of oral contraceptives or hormone replacement therapy increase a woman's chances of breast cancer. A higher risk of endometrial cancer is also associated with hormone replacement therapy.[18]

Breast cancer is much more common in most Western countries than in developing countries. This is partly—and perhaps largely—accounted for by dietary effects (consuming a diet high in calories and fat), combined with later first childbirth, lower parity (having fewer children), shorter breast-feeding, and higher obesity rates.[19]

Occupational and Environmental Factors

Overall, workplace hazards account for only a small percentage of all cancers. However, various substances are known to cause cancer when exposure levels are high or prolonged. One of the most common occupational carcinogens is asbestos, a fibrous material once widely used in the construction, insulation, and automobile industries. Nickel, chromate, and chemicals such as benzene, arsenic, and vinyl chloride have been shown definitively to be carcinogens for humans. Also, people who routinely work with certain dyes and radioactive substances may have increased risks for cancer. Working with coal tars, as in the mining profession, or with inhalants, as in the auto-painting business, is hazardous. So is working with herbicides and pesticides, although the evidence is inconclusive for low-dose exposures. Several federal and state agencies are responsible for monitoring such exposures and ensuring that businesses comply with standards designed to protect workers.

Radiation: Ionizing and Nonionizing Ionizing radiation (IR)—radiation from X rays, radon, cosmic rays, and ultraviolet radiation (primarily ultraviolet B, or UVB radiation)—is the only form of radiation proven to cause human cancer. (See the section on skin cancer on page 468.) Incidents such as the Chernobyl accident in the 1980s focused attention on the potential risks of ionizing radiation. Evidence that high-dose IR causes cancer comes from studies of atomic bomb survivors, patients receiving radiotherapy, and certain occupational groups (for example, uranium miners). Virtually any part of the body can be affected by IR, but bone marrow and the thyroid are particularly susceptible. Radon exposures in homes can increase lung cancer risk, especially in cigarette smokers. To reduce the risk of harmful effects, diagnostic medical and dental X rays are set at the lowest dose levels possible.[20]

Table 16.2
Preventing Cancer through Diet and Lifestyle

Type	Decreases Risk	Increases Risk	Preventable by Diet
Lung	Vegetables, fruits	Smoking; some occupations	33–50%
Stomach	Vegetables, fruits; food refrigeration	Salt; salted foods	66–75%
Breast	Vegetables, fruits	Obesity; alcohol	33–50%
Colon/rectum	Vegetables; physical activity	Meat; alcohol; smoking	66–75%
Mouth/throat	Vegetables, fruits; physical activity	Salted fish; alcohol; smoking	33–50%
Liver	Vegetables	Alcohol; contaminated food	33–66%
Cervix	Vegetables, fruits	Smoking	10–20%
Esophagus	Vegetables, fruits	Deficient diet; smoking; alcohol	50–75%
Prostate	Vegetables	Meat or meat fat; dairy fat	10–20%
Bladder	Vegetables, fruits	Smoking; coffee	10–20%

Here are some tips issued by a panel of cancer researchers:

- Avoid being underweight or overweight, and limit weight gain during adulthood to less than 11 pounds.
- If you don't get much exercise at work, take a 1-hour brisk walk or similar exercise daily, and exercise vigorously for at least 1 hour a week.
- Eat 8 or more servings a day of cereals and grains (such as rice, corn, breads, and pasta), legumes (such as peas), roots (such as beets, radishes, and carrots), tubers (such as potatoes), and plantains (including bananas).
- Eat 5 or more servings a day of a variety of other vegetables and fruits.
- Limit consumption of refined sugar.
- Limit alcoholic drinks to less than 2 a day for men and 1 for women.
- Limit intake of red meat to less than 3 ounces a day, if eaten at all.
- Limit consumption of salted foods and use of cooking and table salt. Use herbs and spices to season foods.

Sources: World Cancer Research Fund; American Institute for Cancer Research.

Although nonionizing radiation produced by radio waves, cell phones, microwaves, computer screens, televisions, electric blankets, and other products has been a topic of great concern in recent years, research has not proven excess risk to date.

Social and Psychological Factors

Many researchers claim that social and psychological factors play a major role in determining whether a person gets cancer. Stress has been implicated in increased susceptibility to several types of cancers. By reducing stress levels in your daily life, you may, in fact, lower your risk for disease. A number of therapists have even established preventive treatment centers where the primary focus is on "being happy" and "thinking positive thoughts." Is it possible to laugh away cancer?

Although medical personnel are skeptical of overly simplistic solutions, we cannot rule out the possibility that negative emotional states contribute to illness. People who are under chronic, severe stress or who suffer from depression or other persistent emotional problems show higher rates of cancer than their healthy counterparts. Sleep disturbances, diet, or a combination of factors may weaken the body's immune system, increasing susceptibility to cancer. Although psychological factors may play a part in cancer development, exposure to substances such as tobacco and alcohol is far more important. Cancers of the mouth and throat pose significant risks for smokers.[21]

Chemicals in Foods

Among the food additives suspected of causing cancer is *sodium nitrate,* a chemical used to preserve and give color to red meat. The actual carcinogen is not sodium nitrate but *nitrosamines,* substances formed when the body digests the sodium nitrates. Sodium nitrate has not been banned, primarily because it kills *Clostridium botulinum,* the bacterium that causes the highly virulent foodborne disease botulism. It should also be noted that the bacteria found in the human intestinal tract may contain more nitrates than a person could ever take in from eating cured meats or other nitrate-containing food products. Nonetheless, concern about the carcinogenic properties of nitrates has led to the introduction of meats that are nitrate-free or contain reduced levels of the substance.

Much of the concern about chemicals in foods centers on the possible harm caused by pesticide and herbicide residues. While some of these chemicals cause cancer at high doses in experimental animals, the very low concentrations found in some foods are well within established government safety levels. Continued research regarding pesticide and herbicide use is essential, and scientists and consumer groups stress the importance of a balance between chemical use and the production of high-quality food products. Prevention efforts should focus on policies to protect consumers, develop low-chemical pesticides and herbicides, and reduce environmental pollution. See Table 16.2 for more information on preventing cancer through diet and lifestyle.

Viral Factors

The chances of becoming infected with a "cancer virus" are very remote. However, several forms of virus-induced cancers have been observed in laboratory animals, and there is some indication that human beings display a similar tendency toward virally transmitted cancers. For example, the *herpes-related viruses* may be involved in the development of some forms of leukemia, Hodgkin's disease, cervical cancer, and Burkitt's lymphoma. The *Epstein-Barr virus,* associated with mononucleosis, may also contribute to cancer, and cervical cancer has been linked to *human papilloma virus,* the virus that causes genital warts. The presence of *Helicobacter pylori,* a chronic gastric bacterium that causes ulcers, is a major factor in the development of stomach cancer.[22]

Many scientists believe that selected viruses help to provide an *opportunistic* environment for subsequent cancer development. It is likely that a combination of immunological bombardment by viral or chemical invaders and other risk factors substantially increases the risk of cancer.

Medical Factors

Some medical treatments increase a person's risk for cancer. One famous example is the prescription drug *diethylstilbestrol (DES),* widely used from 1940 to 1960 to control problems with bleeding during pregnancy and reduce the risk of miscarriage. Not until the 1970s did the dangers of this drug became apparent. Although DES caused few side effects in the millions of women who took it, their daughters were found to have an increased risk for cancers of the reproductive organs. Another example is the use of estrogen in treating menopausal symptoms. Estrogen use is now recognized to contribute to multiple cancer risks, and to provide fewer benefits, than originally believed. Prescriptions for estrogen therapy have declined dramatically, and many women are trying to reduce or eliminate their use of the hormone. An ironic example of another medical factor is that chemotherapy to treat one cancer may increase the risks of the patient developing other forms of cancer.

What do you think?

How do we determine whether a given factor is a risk factor for a disease? ■ Although a direct causal relationship between lung cancer and smoking has not been proved, the evidence supporting such a relationship is strong. Must a clearly established causal link exist before consumers are warned about risk? ■ Can you think of apparent dietary risks for cancer that seemed conclusive but have since been refuted? ■ How does the consumer know whom or what to believe?

Types of Cancers

As mentioned earlier, the term *cancer* refers not to a single disease, but to hundreds of different diseases. They are grouped into four broad categories based on the type of tissue from which the cancer arises.

Classifications of Cancer

- *Carcinomas.* Epithelial tissues (tissues covering body surfaces and lining most body cavities) are the most common sites for cancers. Carcinomas of the breast, lung, intestines, skin, and mouth are examples. These cancers affect the outer layer of the skin and mouth as well as the mucous membranes. They metastasize through the circulatory or lymphatic system initially and form solid tumors.
- *Sarcomas.* Sarcomas occur in the mesodermal, or middle, layers of tissue—for example, in bones, muscles, and general connective tissue. They metastasize primarily via the blood in the early stages of disease. These cancers are less common but generally more virulent than carcinomas. They also form solid tumors.
- *Lymphomas.* Lymphomas develop in the lymphatic system—the infection-fighting regions of the body—and metastasize through the lymphatic system. Hodgkin's disease is an example. Lymphomas also form solid tumors.
- *Leukemias.* Cancer of the blood-forming parts of the body, particularly the bone marrow and spleen, is called leukemia. A nonsolid tumor, leukemia is characterized by an abnormal increase in the number of white blood cells.

Trained oncologists determine the seriousness and general prognosis of a particular cancer. Once laboratory results and clinical observations have been made, cancers are rated by level and stage of development. Those diagnosed as "carcinoma in situ" are localized at the point of origin and often curable. Cancers with higher level or stage ratings have spread farther and are less likely to be cured. Figure 16.2 shows the most common sites of cancer and the number of deaths annually from each type.

Lung Cancer

Lung cancer killed an estimated 160,440 people in 2004, and it continues to be the leading cancer killer for most men and women.[23] Since 1987, more women have died each year from lung cancer than from breast cancer, which for over the previous 40 years had been the major cause of cancer deaths in women. As smoking rates have declined over the past 30 years, we have seen significant declines in male lung cancer, but these rates are not dropping as quickly among women. Another cause for concern is that although fewer adults are smoking, tobacco use among youth is again on the rise, and young women appear to be particularly vulnerable. Some 87 percent of all lung cancer deaths are caused by cigarette smoking.[24]

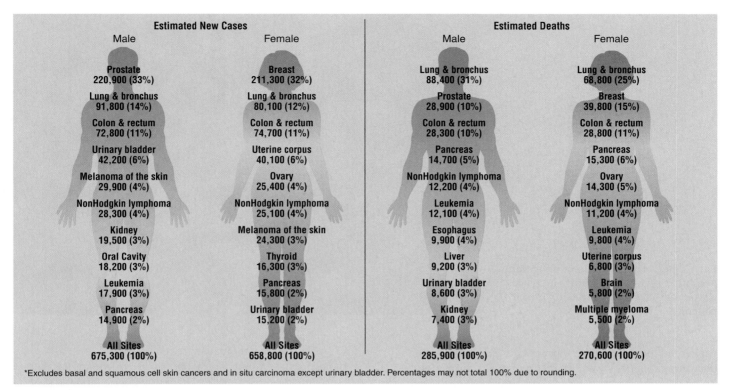

*Excludes basal and squamous cell skin cancers and in situ carcinoma except urinary bladder. Percentages may not total 100% due to rounding.

Figure 16.2
Leading Sites of New Cancer Cases and Deaths, 2003 Estimates

Source: Reprinted by permission of the American Cancer Society, *Cancer Facts and Figures 2003* (Atlanta, GA: American Cancer Society, 2003).

Symptoms of lung cancer include a persistent cough, blood-streaked sputum, chest pain, and recurrent attacks of pneumonia or bronchitis. Treatment depends on the type and stage of the cancer. Surgery, radiation therapy, and chemotherapy are all options. If the cancer is localized, surgery is usually the treatment of choice. If it has spread, surgery is combined with radiation and chemotherapy. Unfortunately, despite advances in medical technology, survival rates for lung cancer have improved only slightly over the past decade. Just 13 percent of lung cancer patients live five or more years after diagnosis. These rates improve to 47 percent with early detection, but only 15 percent of lung cancers are discovered in their early stages.[25]

Prevention Smokers, especially those who have smoked for over 20 years, and people who have been exposed to industrial substances such as arsenic and asbestos or to radiation are at the highest risk for lung cancer. The American Cancer Society estimates that in 2003, over 440,000 cancer deaths (all types) were caused by tobacco use and an additional 20,000 cancer deaths were related to alcohol use, frequently in combination with tobacco use.[26] Exposure to secondhand cigarette smoke, known as *environmental tobacco smoke* or *ETS*, increases the risk for nonsmokers. Researchers theorize that 90 percent of all lung cancers could be avoided if people did not smoke. Substantial improvements in overall

prognosis have been noted in smokers who quit at the first signs of precancerous cellular changes and allowed their bronchial linings to return to normal.

Breast Cancer

About one out of eight women will develop breast cancer at some time in her life. Although this oft-repeated ratio has frightened many women, remember that it represents lifetime risk. Thus, not until the age of 80 does a woman's risk of breast cancer rise to one in eight.[27] Here are the risks at earlier ages:

- Birth to age 39: 1 in 227
- Ages 40–59: 1 in 25
- Ages 60–79: 1 in 15
- Birth to death: 1 in 8

In 2004, approximately 215,900 women in the United States were diagnosed with invasive breast cancer for the first time. In addition, 59,390 new cases of in situ breast cancer, typically ductal carcinoma in situ (DCIS), a more localized cancer, were diagnosed. The increase in detection of DCIS is a direct result of earlier detection through mammographies.[28] In the same year, about 1,450 new cases of breast cancer were diagnosed in men. About 40,110 women (and 470 men) died, making breast cancer the second leading cause of

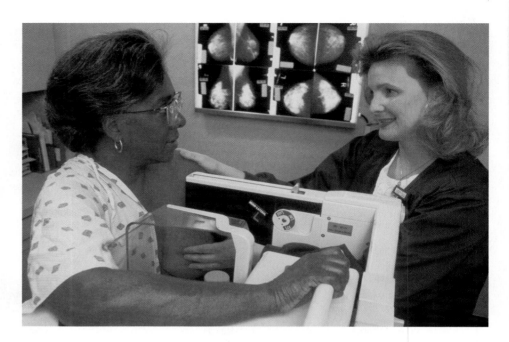

Early detection through mammography and other techniques greatly increases a woman's chance of surviving breast cancer.

cancer death for women.[29] According to the most recent data, mortality rates went down dramatically from 1990 to 2000, with the largest decrease in younger women, both white and black.[30] This decline may be due to earlier diagnosis and better treatment, as numerous studies have shown that early detection increases survival and treatment options.

The earliest signs of breast cancer are usually observable on mammograms, often before lumps can be felt. However, mammograms are not foolproof. Hence, regular breast self-examination (BSE) and careful attention to subtle body changes are important. If a mammogram detects a suspicious mass, a biopsy is performed to provide a more definitive assessment. Once breast cancer has grown to where it can be palpated, symptoms may include persistent breast changes, such as a lump in the breast or surrounding lymph nodes, thickening, dimpling, skin irritation, distortion, retraction or scaliness of the nipple, nipple discharge, or tenderness. Breast pain is commonly due to noncancerous conditions, such as fibrocystic breasts, and is not usually a first symptom. However, any time pain or tenderness persists in the breast or underarm area, it is a good idea to seek medical attention. Women who have ignored this symptom have been shocked to find out later that it was, for them, a symptom of cancer.

Risk Factors The incidence of breast cancer increases with age. Although there are many possible risk factors, those that are supported by research include:[31]

- Personal or family history of breast cancer (primary relatives such as mother, daughter, sister); the younger the relative was when diagnosed, the greater the family risk
- Biopsy-confirmed atypical hyperplasia (excessive increase in the number of cells or tissue growth)
- Long menstrual history (menstrual periods that started early and ended late in life)

- Obesity after menopause
- Recent use of oral contraceptives or postmenopausal estrogens or progestin (see the Women's Health/Men's Health box on hormones in Chapter 15)
- Never having children, or having a first child after age 30
- Consuming two or more drinks of alcohol per day
- Higher education and socioeconomic status

Risk factors that need more rigorous research before being firmly established as risks include these:[32]

- Consuming a diet high in saturated fats
- Exposure to pesticides and other chemicals
- Weight gain, particularly after menopause
- Physical inactivity
- Genetic predisposition through *BRCA1* and *BRCA2* genes (Genes appear to account for approximately 5 percent of all cases of breast cancer. Screening for these genes is recommended for women with a family history of breast cancer, when counseling is available.)

Although risk factors are useful indicators, they do not always predict individual susceptibility. However, because of increased awareness, better diagnostic techniques, and improved treatments, breast cancer patients have a better chance of surviving today. The five-year survival rate for people with localized breast cancer (which includes all people living five years after diagnosis, whether the patient is in remission, disease-free, or under treatment) has risen from 72 percent in the 1940s to 97 percent today. These statistics vary dramatically, however, based on the stage of the cancer when it is first detected. Those with early stage cancers such as DCIS appear to have the best prognosis. As with most cancers, the earlier the stage, the greater the chances of a full recovery. If the cancer has spread to surrounding tissue, the five-year survival rate is 79 percent; if it has spread to distant

How to Examine Your Breasts

The best time for a woman to examine her breasts is when the breasts are not tender or swollen. Women who are pregnant, breast-feeding, or have breast implants can also choose to examine their breasts regularly.

1. Lie down and place your right arm behind your head. The exam is done while lying down, not standing up, because when lying down the breast tissue spreads evenly over the chest wall and it is as thin as possible, making it much easier to feel all the breast tissue.

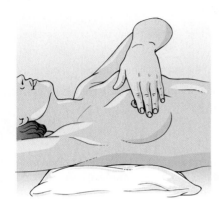

2. Use the finger pads of the three middle fingers on your left hand to feel for lumps in the right breast. Use overlapping dime-sized circular motions of the finger pads to feel the breast tissue.

3. Use three different levels of pressure to feel all the breast tissue. Light pressure is needed to feel the tissue closest to the skin; medium pressure to feel a little deeper; and firm pressure to feel the tissue closest to the chest and ribs. A firm ridge in the lower curve of each breast is normal. If you're not sure how hard to press, talk with your doctor or nurse. Use each pressure level to feel the breast tissue before moving on to the next spot.

4. Move around the breast in an up and down pattern starting at an imaginary line drawn straight down your side from the underarm and moving across the breast to the middle of the chest bone. Be sure to check the entire breast area going down until you feel only ribs and up to the neck or collar bone (clavicle).

   There is some evidence to suggest that the up and down pattern (sometimes called the vertical pattern) is the most effective pattern for covering the entire breast without missing any breast tissue.

5. Repeat the exam on your left breast, using the finger pads of the right hand.

6. While standing in front of a mirror with your hands pressing firmly down on your hips, look at your breasts for any changes of size, shape, contour, or dimpling. (The pressing down on the hips position contracts the chest wall muscles and enhances any breast changes.)

7. Examine each underarm while sitting up or standing and with your arm only slightly raised so you can easily feel in this area. (Raising your arm straight up tightens the tissue in this area and makes it difficult to examine.)

Figure 16.3
Breast Self-Examination

Note that the American Cancer Society recommends the use of mammography and clinical breast exam in addition to self-examination.

Source: American Cancer Society, "Breast Awareness and Self-Examination," 2004, www.cancer.org/docroot/CRI/content/CRI_2_4_3X_Can_breast_cancer_be_found_early_5.asp?sitearea =

parts of the body, these rates fall to 23 percent; and if the breast cancer has not spread at all, the survival rate approaches 100 percent. Survival after a diagnosis of breast cancer continues to decline beyond five years. Seventy-three percent of women diagnosed with breast cancer survive 10 years, and 59 percent survive 15 years.[33]

Patients who become actively involved in treatment decision making, who seek out the best oncologists with the most experience with their type of cancer, and who become knowledgeable about options and treatments often fare best. Of course, this takes time, access to health care providers, supportive family members, and attention to health-promoting lifestyles before, during, and after treatment.

Prevention A study of the role of exercise in reducing the risk for breast cancer generated much excitement in the scientific community. The study, involving 1,090 women who were 40 or younger (545 with breast cancer and 545 without it), analyzed subjects' exercise patterns since they began menstruating. The risk of those who averaged four hours of exercise a week since menstruation was 58 percent lower than

that of women who did no exercise at all. More good news: subjects did not have to be avid exercisers to reduce their risk. Their exercise included team sports, individual sports, dance, exercise classes, swimming, walking, and a variety of other activities. Researchers speculate that exercise may protect women by altering the production of the ovarian hormones estrogen and progesterone during menstrual cycles.

Other research has shown that vigorous athletics can delay the onset of menstruation and halt ovulation in some women. A woman's cumulative exposure to the sex hormones is associated with breast cancer risk.[34] Exercise can increase muscle mass and decrease body fat, which also lowers risk.[35]

International differences in breast cancer incidence correlate with variations in diet, especially fat intake, although a causal role for these dietary factors has not been firmly established. Sudden weight gain has also been implicated. Exciting new research about the *BRCA1* and *BRCA2* genes for breast cancer offers new hope for early detection.

Regular self-examination (Figure 16.3) and mammograms are the best ways to detect breast cancer early. The

Table 16.3
Recommendations for the Early Detection of Cancer in Asymptomatic People

Site	Recommendation
Cancer-Related Checkup	For individuals undergoing periodic health examinations, a cancer-related checkup should include health counseling and, depending on a person's age, might include examination for cancers of the thyroid, oral cavity, skin, lymph nodes, testes, and ovaries, as well as for some nonmalignant diseases.
Breast	Women 40 and older should have an annual mammogram and an annual clinical breast exam (CBE) performed by a health care professional and should perform monthly breast self-examination (BSE). Ideally, the CBE should occur before the scheduled mammogram.
	Women aged 20–39 should have a clinical breast exam performed by a health care professional every 3 years and should perform monthly breast self-examination.
Colon and Rectum	Beginning at age 50, men and women should follow one of the examination schedules below:
	• A fecal occult blood test (FOBT) every year, or a flexible sigmoidoscopy (FSIG) every five years, or annual fecal occult blood test and flexible sigmoidoscopy every 5 years*
	• A double-contrast barium enema every 5 to 10 years
	• A colonoscopy every 10 years
Prostate	The American Cancer Society recommends that both the prostate-specific antigen (PSA) blood test and the digital rectal examination be offered annually, beginning at age 50, to men who have a life expectancy of at least 10 more years.
	Men at high risk (African American men and men with a strong family history of one or more first-degree relatives diagnosed with prostate cancer at an early age) should begin testing at age 45.
	Information should be provided to patients about what is known and what is uncertain about the benefits and limitations of early detection and treatment of prostate cancer so that they can make an informed decision.
Uterus	**Cervix:** Screening should begin approximately 3 years after a woman begins having vaginal intercourse but no later than 21 years of age. Screening should be done every year with Pap tests or every 2 years using liquid-based tests. At or after age 30, women who have had 3 normal tests in a row may get screened every 2–3 years, unless they have certain risk factors, such as HIV infection or a weak immune system.
	Endometrium: The American Cancer Society recommends that all women should be informed about the risks and symptoms of endometrial cancer and strongly encouraged to report any unexpected bleeding or spotting to their physicians. Annual screening for endometrial cancer with endometrial biopsy beginning at age 35 should be offered to women with or at risk for hereditary nonpolyposis colon cancer (HNPCC).

*Combined testing is preferred over either annual FOBT or FSIG every five years alone. People who are at moderate or high risk for colorectal cancer should talk with a doctor about a different testing schedule.

Source: American Cancer Society, *Cancer Facts and Figures 2004* (Atlanta, GA: American Cancer Society, 2004). Reproduced with permission. www.cancer.org. © 2004, American Cancer Society, Inc..

American Cancer Society offers guidelines for how often women should get mammograms and checkups (Table 16.3). All women, no matter their age, should be in the habit of breast self-examination every month.

Treatment   Today, people with breast cancer (like people with nearly any type of cancer) have many treatment options to choose from. It is important to thoroughly check out a physician's track record and his or her philosophy on the best treatment. Is the physician's recommendation consistent with that of major cancer centers in the country? Check out the doctor's credentials and the experiences of patients who have seen this doctor as well as the surgeon who will perform your biopsy and other surgical techniques. If possible, seek a facility that has a significant number of breast cancer patients, does many surgeries, is regarded as a teaching facility for new oncologists, has the "latest and greatest" in terms of technology, and is highly regarded by past patients. Often, cancer support groups can provide invaluable information and advice. Treatments range from a lumpectomy to radical mastectomy to various combinations of radiation or chemotherapy. Figure 16.4 reviews these options. Among nonsurgical options, promising results have been noted among women using *selective estrogen-receptor modulators (SERMs)* such as tamoxifen and raloxifene, particularly among women whose cancers appear to grow in response to estrogen.[36] Remember that it is always a good idea to seek more than one opinion before making a decision.

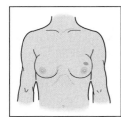

Lumpectomy
Performed when tumor is in earliest localized stages. Prognosis for recovery is better than 95%. Only tumor itself is removed. Some physicians may also remove normal tissue in surrounding area.

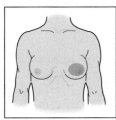

Simple mastectomy
Removal of breast and underling tissue. Prognosis for full recovery better than 80%.

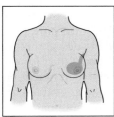

Modified radical mastectomy
Breast and lymph nodes in immediate area removed. Prognosis for full recovery dependent on level of spread.

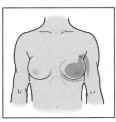

Radical mastectomy
Removal of breast, lymph nodes, pectoral muscles, all fat, and underlying tissue. Prognosis for full recovery may be as low as 60%, depending on level of spread.

Figure 16.4
Surgical Procedures for Diagnosed Breast Cancer
These surgeries are typically followed by radiation treatment and/or chemotherapy.

Colon and Rectal Cancers

Colorectal cancers (cancers of the colon and rectum) continue to be the third most common cancer in both men and women, with over 146,900 cases diagnosed in 2004.[37] Although colon cancer rates have increased steadily in recent decades, many people are unaware of their risk. In its early stages, colorectal cancer has no symptoms. Bleeding from the rectum, blood in the stool, and changes in bowel habits are the major warning signals.

Anyone can get colorectal cancer, but people who are over age 50, who are obese, who have a family history of colon and rectal cancer, a personal or family history of polyps (benign growths) in the colon or rectum, or inflammatory bowel problems such as colitis run an increased risk. Other possible risk factors include diets high in fat or low in fiber, smoking, sedentary lifestyle, high alcohol consumption, and low intake of fruits and vegetables. Indeed, approximately 90 percent of all colorectal cancers are preventable.[38] Recent studies have suggested that estrogen replacement

Table 16.4
Risk Factors for Colorectal Cancer

	Relative Risk
Family history (first-degree relative)	1.8
Physical inactivity (less than 3 hours per week)	1.7
Inflammatory bowel disease (physician-diagnosed Crohn's disease, ulcerative colitis, or pancolitis)	1.5
Obesity	1.5
Red meat consumption	1.5
Smoking	1.5
Alcohol (more than 1 drink/day)	1.4
High vegetable consumption (5 or more servings per day)	0.7
Oral contraceptive use (5 or more years of use)	0.7
Estrogen replacement (5 or more years of use)	0.8
Multivitamins containing folic acid	0.5

Modifiable factors are in **bold** text.

Source: Adapted from Kluwer Academic Publishers, Harvard Report *Cancer Causes and Control* 11 (2000), "Risk Factors for Colorectal Cancer." With the kind permission of Springer Science and Business Media.

therapy and nonsteroidal anti-inflammatories such as aspirin may reduce colorectal risk.[39] See Table 16.4 for an overview of relative risks from these and other factors.

Because colorectal cancer tends to spread slowly, the prognosis is quite good if it is caught in the early stages. Early screening can detect and remove precancerous polyps and diagnose disease at more treatable stages.[40] However, in spite of major educational campaigns, only 21 percent of all Americans over age 50 have had the most basic screening test—the fecal occult blood test—in the last five years, and 33 percent have had a colonoscopy during that same time period.[41] Colonoscopy or barium enemas are recommended screening tests for at-risk populations and everybody over age 50.

Treatment often consists of radiation or surgery. Chemotherapy, although not used extensively in the past, is today a possibility. A permanent *colostomy,* the creation of an abdominal opening to eliminate body wastes, is seldom required for people with colon cancer and even less frequently for those with rectum cancer.

As with many cancers, African Americans appear to have the highest risk of colorectal cancer, followed by whites, Asians/Pacific Islanders, American Indians/Alaska Natives, and Hispanics.[42]

Prevention and Screening Regular exercise, a diet with lots of fruits and plant-origin foods, a healthy weight, and moderation in alcohol consumption appear to be among the most promising prevention strategies. New research also suggests that aspirin-like drugs, postmenopausal hormones, folic acid, calcium supplements, selenium, and vitamin E may also contribute to prevention; however, more research must be conducted to conclusively determine if and how these substances reduce risk.[43]

The most commonly recommended screenings, particularly for those over age 50, include:[44]

- *Fecal occult blood tests (FOBT)*. Cancers and large polyps often bleed sporadically into the intestine. The FOBT detects "hidden," or "occult," blood in a stool sample. You take samples of your own stool in the privacy of your home, place them in a preservative medium, and mail them to a lab for evaluation. This is a relatively inexpensive test (less than $20 in most cases), and it has been proven to play a significant role in early detection.
- *Digital rectal exam*. In this test, a physician inserts his/her finger into the rectum to feel for irregularities. This is often part of a routine examination, but when used alone, it is not sufficient to rule out possible problems.
- *Flexible sigmoidoscopy*. In this test, a two-foot-long, slender, flexible, hollow, lighted tube is inserted into the rectum and up into the lower region of the colon. This test requires less preparation, is safer than a colonoscopy, and is a helpful early screening exam. However, it can only detect problems in the lower colon, and any polyps or other irregularities that are found will require a colonoscopy to assess the entire bowel. The cost is $150 or more.
- *Barium enema with air contrast*. For this test, the bowel must be completely clean and a white, chalky substance known as barium sulfate is introduced into the colon and allowed to spread, while air is pumped into the colon. X rays monitor irregular outcroppings and deviations that might indicate tumor invasion. The cost is $300 to $500 or more. If abnormalities are found, a colonoscopy may still need to be performed.
- *Colonoscopy*. Like the sigmoidoscopy, this test allows for direct visual examination of the colon and rectum, but it includes a much larger portion of the colon. Polyps can be removed via the colonoscope; cost is $1,000 or more.
- *Newer tests*. In the future, genetic-based fecal screening and other techniques may be widely available. It is currently possible to swallow a small camera and have a form of virtual examination of the colon as the camera passes through. However, this technique is more time-consuming and the optics are not yet as clear and reliable as the regular colonoscopic techniques. For many people—particularly older adults—the preparation for any of these tests, which may include distasteful fluids to induce bowel movements, self-enemas, long fasting, and other techniques, is an obstacle that must be reduced or overcome to ensure better participation.

Referred pain   Pain caused by a condition in one place that is felt in a different place.

Asymptomatic   Having a disease but no symptoms.

Prostate Cancer

Cancer of the prostate is the most common cancer in American males today, excluding skin cancer, and the second leading cause of cancer death in men, after lung cancer. In 2004, about 230,110 new cases of prostate cancer were diagnosed in the United States. About 1 man in 6 will be diagnosed with prostate cancer during his lifetime, but only 1 man in 33 will die of it.[45] Put into perspective, prostate cancer accounts for about 10 percent of cancer-related deaths in men each year.

Ironically, many people do not know what the prostate is or what function it serves in the body. The prostate is a muscular, walnut-sized gland that surrounds part of the urethra, the tube that transports urine and sperm out of the body. As part of the male reproductive system, its primary function is to produce seminal fluid, the fluid that transports sperm. During an orgasm, the muscles of the prostate contract to push semen through the urethra and out through the penis. Located directly below the bladder, if the prostate becomes enlarged, either through inflammation or cancerous growth, it may block the urethra, thus disrupting flow out of the bladder, or push on the bladder and cause pain or discomfort. That is why difficulty in urination and pain are often symptoms of problems with the prostate.

Symptoms   Most symptoms of prostate cancer are nonspecific, that is, they mimic signs of infection or an enlarged prostate. Symptoms may include weak or interrupted urine flow; difficulty starting or stopping urination; feeling the urge to urinate frequently; pain upon urination; blood in the urine; or **referred pain** (pain that originates in one spot but is felt elsewhere) in the low back, pelvis, or thighs. It is important to note that many men are **asymptomatic** (have no symptoms) in the early stages, which is why testing and early diagnosis are becoming more important as the risks of prostate cancer rise in the general population. Most prostate cancers grow slowly and are believed to take years to develop. Interestingly, autopsy studies indicate that some men who died of other diseases also had prostate cancer, but it never seemed to affect them and their doctors didn't know they had it.[46] New research that is particularly relevant to college-age men has found that prostate cancer may begin with a condition called *prostatic intraepithelial neoplasia (PIN)*. In this condition, there are changes in the microscopic appearance of prostate gland cells, ranging from a bit different than normal to abnormal. The important part of this is that these changes are believed to occur in men in their twenties and by the time men reach age 50, nearly 50 percent of them have these changes.[47]

Risk Factors   Although the causes of prostate cancer continue to elude health professionals, there are several factors that appear to increase risk. Among the most likely are:[48]

- *Age*. Chances of developing prostate cancer increase dramatically with age. More than 70 percent of cancers are

PSA Tests: What Do The Numbers Mean To You?

Prostate-specific antigen (PSA) tests are blood tests that detect PSA, a substance made by the prostate gland. Although PSA is found primarily in semen, a small amount is also found in the blood; hence the test involves taking a blood sample from the arm. The blood is sent to laboratory and if normal, will come back with a value of 4 nanograms per milliliter (ng/mL) of blood.

If the person has prostate cancer, these values normally go above 4. In general, the greater the value, the higher your risk of actually having cancer. If the value is between 4 and 10, you may have a 25 percent chance of having prostate cancer; if the value is greater than 10, your risk goes up proportionally. Some groups recommend that if your values are 3 or higher, you should consult with your doctor and have a more definitive test.

It is important to know that PSA tests are not perfect and many false positives (tests that show positive values but are actually negative) and false negatives (tests that show negative values when you may actually have cancer) occur. Several factors are believed to influence the reliability of these tests:

- Benign prostate hypertrophy, a non-cancerous enlargement of the prostate
- Prostatitis, inflammation of the prostate
- Ejaculation, which can cause temporary increase in blood PSA levels (you should abstain from ejaculating for two days before the test)
- Some medications, such as finasteride (Proscar or Propecia) and dutasteride (Avodart), may falsely lower PSA values

- Herbal preparations, particularly those labeled for prostate health

There are other PSA tests (such as the percent-free PSA) that are more sensitive and provide a better indicator of your risk. If you or a loved one gets a preliminary high value and none of the above factors apply, ask the doctor for a more definitive test. In addition, doctors may choose to biopsy the tissue, do digital rectal examinations, perform ultrasound tests such as a transrectal ultrasound, or employ other more sophisticated diagnostic tools. Consult the patient information websites established by the American Cancer Society and the National Cancer Institute and ask questions, particularly if you have siblings or a father who have been diagnosed previously.

Source: American Cancer Society, *Cancer Facts and Figures 2004* (Atlanta, GA: American Cancer Society, 2004). Reproduced with permission. www.cancer.org. © 2004, American Cancer Society, Inc.

diagnosed in men over the age of 65. Usually the disease has progressed to the point of displaying symptoms in these older men, or they are more likely to be seeing a doctor for other problems and get a screening test or prostate-specific antigen (PSA) test.

- *Race.* Black men are 60 percent more likely to develop prostate cancer than white men and are much more likely to be diagnosed at an advanced stage. Being diagnosed at an advanced stage means that they are also more likely to die of the disease than other races. Prostate cancer is less common among Asian men and occurs at about the same rates among Hispanic men as it does among white men.
- *Nationality.* Prostate cancer is most common in North America and northwestern Europe and less common in Asia, Africa, Central America, and South America. The reasons for these differences are not well understood but may be due to the fact that men in these countries are less likely to be diagnosed (are less likely to receive PSA testing) or that, in some countries where AIDS is a leading killer of men, men may not live long enough to develop the disease.
- *Family history.* Having a father or brother with prostate cancer more than doubles a man's risk of getting prostate cancer (interestingly, the risk is higher for men with an affected brother than it is for those with an affected father). The genes that predispose men to prostate cancer

have not been clearly identified; thus, genetic tests like those for breast cancer in women are not yet available.

- *Diet.* Although diet is widely believed to be a risk factor for prostate cancer, most studies have not yet conclusively identified specific risks. The fact that men in countries where they consume high fat diets have higher risks of prostate cancer than men in countries with lower fat diets of rice, soybean products, and vegetables provides the most compelling indicators for the role of dietary fats. Men who consume high levels of calcium also may be at greater risk, although studies have yet to confirm this. Lycopenes (found in tomatoes, pink grapefruit, and watermelon), vitamin D, vitamin E, and the mineral selenium are also being studied for their possible role in reducing prostate risk; however, studies that prove these links are not yet completed.
- *Physical activity and overweight/obesity.* Some studies have suggested that regular physical activity and maintaining a healthy weight may help reduce the risk of developing or dying from prostate cancer; however, this link is not clear.
- *Vasectomy.* Although there is concern among some groups that having a vasectomy, particularly before the age of 35, increases the risk of prostate cancer, most recent studies have not found this to be true. More research examining this issue is currently underway.

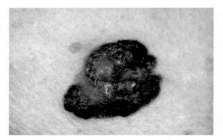 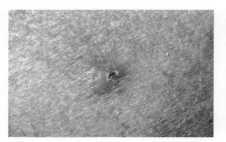 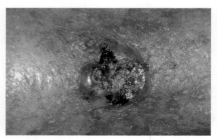

Prevention of skin cancer requires keeping a careful watch for any new pigmented growths and for changes to any moles. Melanoma symptoms, as shown in the left photo, include scalloped edges, asymmetrical shapes, discoloration, and an increase in size. Basal cell carcinoma and squamous cell carcinoma (middle and right photos, respectively) should be brought to your physician's attention but are not as deadly as melanoma.

Prevention and Treatment A quick look at the risk factors for prostate cancer tells you that many of these factors, such as age and race, are beyond your control. However, there are some things that you could do that appear promising. Eating more fruits and vegetables, particularly those containing lycopenes, may lower your risk. Some studies suggest that taking 50 milligrams (400 International Units) of vitamin E and adequate amounts of selenium in your diet may reduce risk, while consuming high levels of vitamin A may increase your risks. Until more definitive proof of nutrient effectiveness in risk reduction is available, the best advice would be to follow the Food Guide Pyramid dietary recommendations discussed in Chapter 8. Otherwise, keeping your weight levels healthy, getting regular amounts of exercise, sleeping sufficient amounts, and reducing stress levels keeps your immune system functioning effectively and may help you resist some forms of cancer development.

Another important strategy is to get diagnostic tests on the schedule recommended by the American Cancer Society and the National Cancer Institute. To date, most health organizations do not yet recommend routine testing for men under the age of 40. Every man over the age of 40 should have an annual digital rectal prostate examination. The American Cancer Society recommends that men age 50 and over have an annual **prostate-specific antigen (PSA)** test (see the Men's Health/Women's Health box on the previous page). African American men and those with brothers or fathers who have had prostate cancer need to be particularly attentive to getting PSA and other diagnostic tests and discussing their concerns with physicians.

Fortunately, even with so many generalized symptoms, 83 percent of all prostate cancers are detected while they are still in the local or regional stages and tend to progress slowly. The five-year survival rate in these early stages is 100 percent. Because most men develop the disease in their late sixties and early seventies, it is likely that they will die of other causes first. For this reason, some health care groups question the cost effectiveness and necessity of prostate surgeries and other costly procedures that may have little real effect on life expectancy. Over the past 20 years, the survival rate for all stages combined has increased from 67 percent to 96 percent, largely due to earlier diagnosis and improved treatment.

Skin Cancer: Sun Worshippers Beware

If you are one of the millions of people each year who try to get a "healthy tan," think again. In fact, that phrase isn't just an oxymoron; it stands for premature aging and wrinkling at the very least, and life-threatening illness at its worst. The damage to your skin from a single bad sunburn lasts the rest of your life! What is worse is that such damage is cumulative. Early signs of sun damage (photodamage) include sunburn, tanning, and increased freckling. Later, these "cute" freckles are followed by wrinkling, premature aging and age spots, cataracts and other forms of eye damage, sagging of the skin, and the most serious consequence: skin cancer. If you are an avid sunbather, compare areas such as your hands and face to areas that are almost always covered from the sun's rays, such as your buttocks or breasts. The differences that you see are almost always the result of sun exposure over time.[49]

The long-term effects of sun exposure can be devastating:

- Skin cancer is the most common form of cancer in the United States today, affecting over 1 million people in 2004. Most of these were *basal* or *squamous cell* skin cancers, but 55,100 were malignant melanomas.[50]
- Today, one in five adults develops skin cancer, accounting for one-third of all reported malignancies.[51]
- **Malignant melanoma,** the deadliest form of skin cancer, is beginning to occur at a much higher rate in women under age 40. In fact, while relatively few people die from

Prostate-specific antigen (PSA) An antigen found in prostate cancer patients.

Malignant melanoma A virulent cancer of the melanocytes (pigment-producing cells) of the skin.

the highly treatable basal or squamous cell skin cancers, the highly virulent malignant melanoma has become the most frequent cancer in women aged 25 to 29 and runs second only to breast cancer in women aged 30 to 34. If you think skin cancer is something that only older people get, think again![52]

- Rates of melanoma are ten times higher among whites than blacks.
- In 2004, 10,250 people died of skin cancer. Of those, 7,910 died of melanoma, and 2,340 died of other forms of skin cancer.

The sun gives off three types of harmful ultraviolet rays:[53]

1. *UVA (ultraviolet A).* These longer wavelengths penetrate deeply into the skin, damaging the skin's collagen. They result in premature aging and help prime the skin for cancers.
2. *UVB (ultraviolet B).* These are short wavelengths and are believed to be the primary rays causing sunburn and ultimately resulting in cancers.
3. *UVC (ultraviolet C).* These very short rays are deadly to plants and animals. Normally, the atmospheric ozone layer protects us by absorbing UVC rays. Interestingly, as the global ozone layer has become progressively depleted over the last decade, the incidence of skin cancer has risen dramatically, as have cases of sun-related eye damage. (See Chapter 21 for more on the effects of damage to the ozone layer.)

What happens when you expose yourself to sunlight? Biologically, the skin responds to photodamage by increasing its thickness and the number of pigment cells (melanocytes), which produce the "tan" look. An important part of the skin's immune system (the Langerhans' cells) is reduced by photodamage, lowering the normal immune protection of our skin and priming it for cancer.[54] Photodamage also causes wrinkling by impairing the elastic substances (collagens) that keep skin soft and pliable.

Although sun exposure risks have been widely reported, over 60 percent of Americans 25 years and under report that they are "working on a tan" at some point during the year. These numbers spike dramatically just prior to spring break as tanning booths fill with students and others trying to get "starter tans" before heading out to tropical climates for spring vacations. Fewer than one in three sunbathers bothers to wear UVB-thwarting sunscreen lotions. Tanning booths and other artificial tans are *not* a safe alternative to actual sun exposure (see the Reality Check box).

Who's at risk for skin cancer? Anyone who overexposes himself or herself without adequate protection. The risk is greatest for people who fit the following categories:

- Have fair skin
- Have blonde, red, or light brown hair
- Have blue, green, or gray eyes
- Always burn before tanning
- Burn easily and peel readily
- Don't tan easily, but spend lots of time outdoors

- Have previously been treated for skin cancer or have a family history of skin cancer (if you have a family history of melanoma, see your physician for regular skin exams)
- Live in or take regular vacations to high altitudes (UV exposure increases with altitude)
- Work indoors all week and try to play tanning "catch-up" on weekends
- Use no or low-SPF sunscreens

Preventing skin cancer is a matter of limiting exposure to harmful UV rays. See the Skills for Behavior Change box for strategies on safely spending time in the sun. If you do get sunburned, be careful about treating it:

- Drink more fluids than usual
- Apply cool compresses gently, without rubbing the area; when you shower or bathe, use a mild soap
- Moisturize the skin with aquaphor petroleum jelly, plain calamine lotion, or Sarna lotion. Some forms of aloe work well, but make sure you read the ingredients on the label
- Avoid "-caine" products such as benzocaine
- Take aspirin or ibuprofen to reduce inflammation
- For severe symptoms, including nausea, vomiting, chills, malaise, weakness, and blistering, stay awake and see a doctor

Many people do not know what to look for when examining themselves for skin cancer. Basal and squamous cell carcinomas can be a recurrent annoyance, showing up most commonly on the face, ears, neck, arms, hands, and legs as warty bumps, colored spots, or scaly patches. Bleeding, itchiness, pain, or oozing are other symptoms that warrant attention. Surgery may be necessary to remove them, but they are seldom life-threatening.

In striking contrast is the insidious melanoma, an invasive killer that quickly spreads to regional organs and throughout the body, accounting for over 75 percent of all skin cancer deaths. Risks increase dramatically among whites after age 20.[55] Often, melanoma starts as a normal-looking mole but quickly develops abnormal characteristics. A simple *ABCD rule* outlines the warning signs of melanoma:

- *Asymmetry.* One half of the mole does not match the other half.
- *Border irregularity.* The edges are uneven, notched, or scalloped.
- *Color.* Pigmentation is not uniform. Melanomas may vary in color from tan to deeper brown, reddish black, black, or deep bluish black.
- *Diameter.* Greater than 6 millimeters (about the size of a pea).

If you notice any of these symptoms, consult a physician promptly.

Treatment of skin cancer depends on its seriousness. Surgery is performed in 90 percent of all cases. Radiation therapy, *electrodesiccation* (tissue destruction by heat), and *cryosurgery* (tissue destruction by freezing) are also common forms of treatment. For melanoma, treatment may involve

Artificial Tans: Sacrificing Health for Beauty?

Men and women of all ages, shapes, and sizes are actively searching for an easy way to get that "summery, outdoorsy look" before or instead of spending time in the sun. Are any of the sun substitutes a safe alternative?

TANNING BOOTHS AND BEDS

On an average day, more than 1.3 million Americans visit a tanning salon, including many teenagers and young adults. Researchers using data from the *National Longitudinal Study of Adolescent Health* report that more than 25 percent of white female adolescents and 11 percent of white male adolescents used tanning booths at least three times in the last year. Factors associated with indoor tanning include being female, residence in the Midwest or South, rural school location, increased age, use of tobacco and alcohol, and increased levels of discretionary cash for personal spending. Adolescents who tanned easily were more likely to visit tanning booths, and females who reported higher levels of physical activity were less likely to use them than sedentary women.

Most tanning salon patrons incorrectly believe that tanning booths are safer than sitting in the sun. However, the truth is that there is no such thing as a safe tan from *any* source! Essentially, a tan is the skin's response to an injury, and every time you tan, you accumulate injury and increase your risk for disfiguring forms of skin cancer, premature aging, eye problems, unsightly skin spots, wrinkles and leathery skin, and possible death from melanoma. To make matters worse, the industry is difficult to monitor and regulate due to the many salons that are springing up across the country. Dermatologists cite additional factors that make tanning in a salon as bad or worse than getting a tan the old fashioned way of sitting in the sun:

✔ Tanning facilities sometimes fail to enforce regulations, such as ensuring that customers wear eye protection and that overexposure does not occur.
✔ Some tanning facilities do not calibrate the UVA output of their tanning bulbs or ensure sufficient rotation of newer and older bulbs, which can yield more or less exposure than you have paid for.
✔ Tanning facility patrons often try for a total body tan. The buttocks and genitalia are particularly sensitive to UV radiation and are prone to develop skin cancer.

Another concern is hygiene. Don't assume that those little colored water sprayers used to "clean" the inside of the beds are sufficient to kill organisms. Any time you come in contact with body secretions from others, you run the risk of getting an infectious disease. The busier the facility, the more likely you'll be to come in contact with germs that may make you sick.

SPRAY-ON TANS

During the last few years, some companies have offered a sunless option that involves spraying customers in a tanning booth with the color additive dihydroxyacetone (DHA). DHA interacts with the dead surface cells in the outermost layer of the skin to darken skin color. DHA has been approved by the FDA for use in coloring the skin since 1977 and has typically been used in lotions and creams. Its use is restricted to external application, which means that it shouldn't be sprayed in or on the mouth, eyes, or nose because the risks, if any, are unknown. If you choose to use DHA spray at home or in tanning booths, be sure to cover these areas. Remember that the spray is a dye and does not increase your protection from the damaging rays of the sun.

TANNING PILLS

Although there are no tanning pills approved by the FDA, some companies have marketed pills that contain the color additive canthaxanthin. When large amounts of canthaxanthin are ingested, the substance can turn the skin a range of colors, from orange to brown. However, canthaxanthin is only approved for use as a color additive in foods and oral medications—and then only in small amounts. Tanning pills have been associated with health problems, including an eye disorder called canthaxanthin retinopathy, which is the formation of yellow deposits on the eye's retina. Canthaxanthin has also been reported to cause liver injury and a severe itching condition called urticaria, according to the American Academy of Dermatology.

Sources: C. A. Demko, et al., "Teenagers in the UV Tanning Booth?," *Archives of Pediatric and Adolescent Medicine* 157, no. 9 (2003): 854–860; University of Alabama at Birmingham, "Dear Doctor column: Tanning Beds," 2002, www.health.uab.edu; University of Alabama at Birmingham, "Dear Doctor column: Tanning (Sunless)," 2004, www. health .uab.edu; U.S. Food and Drug Administration, "Protect the Skin You're In!," *The FDA and You* 3 (2004), www.fda.gov/cdrh/fdaandyou /issue 03.html

---

surgical removal of the regional lymph nodes, radiation, or chemotherapy.

Testicular Cancer

Testicular cancer is one of the most common types of solid tumors found in young adult males, affecting nearly 7,500 young men per year. Those between the ages of 15 and 35 are at greatest risk. There has been a steady increase in tumor frequency over the past several years in this age group.[56] Although the cause of testicular cancer is unknown, several risk factors have been identified. Males with undescended testicles appear to be at greatest risk, and some studies indicate a genetic influence.

In general, testicular tumors first appear as a painless enlargement of the testis or thickening in testicular tissue.

How to Examine your Testicles

The best time to perform a testicular self-examination is after a warm shower or bath, when the testicles descend and the scrotal skin is relaxed.

1. Use a mirror to examine the scrotum for any visible swelling.

2. Using both hands, place the index and middle fingers of each hand on the underside of the testicle and the thumbs on top. Gently roll the testicle between the thumbs and fingers.

3. Identify the epididymis, the structure behind the testicle that carries sperm, so that you don't confuse it for a lump.

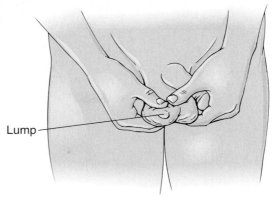

Lump

Figure 16.5
Testicular Self-Examination

Because this enlargement is often painless, it is extremely important that all young males practice regular testicular self-examination (Figure 16.5).

One of the most remarkable testicular cancer stories is the survival of Tour de France champion Lance Armstrong. Struck by an invasive form of testicular cancer that had spread to several parts of his body, including his brain, Armstrong's indomitable spirit set a wonderful example of hope for thousands of young men afflicted with the disease. He survived through a combination of superior medical care, exercise, and dietary and lifestyle changes, as well as a spiritual journey. In 2004, the Lance Armstrong Foundation received millions of dollars from sales of yellow wristbands with the words "LiveStrong" on it and now worn by millions of Americans. Figure skating Olympian Scott Hamilton has also managed to beat the disease and now devotes himself to raising awareness about risk factors and how to fight cancer.

Ovarian Cancer

Ovarian cancer is the fifth leading cause of cancer death for women, diagnosed in almost 25,580 of them in 2004 and killing over 16,090.[57] Ovarian cancer causes more deaths than any other cancer of the reproductive system because its insidious, often silent, course means women tend not to discover it until the cancer is at an advanced stage. The most common symptom is enlargement of the abdomen (or a feeling of bloating) in women over age 40. Abnormal vaginal bleeding or discharge is rarely a symptom until the disease is advanced. Other symptoms include vague digestive disturbances (stomach discomfort, gas, pressure, distention), fatigue, pain during intercourse, unexplained weight loss, unexplained changes in bowel or bladder habits, urinary frequency, and incontinence.[58] Women who have these symptoms in the absence of other problems will often be diagnosed with stomach irritability or other digestive problems. If symptoms persist, women must insist on further evaluation, including a thorough pelvic examination and other relevant tests.

Risk factors The exact causes of ovarian cancer are not known, However, studies show that the following factors may increase chances of developing the disease:[59]

- *Family history.* First-degree relatives (mother, daughter, sister) of a woman who has had ovarian cancer are at increased risk. The likelihood is especially high if two or more first-degree relatives have had it. A family history of breast or colon cancer is also associated with increased risk.
- *Age.* Chances of developing ovarian cancer increase with age. Most cases occur in women over age 50, with the highest risk in women over 60.

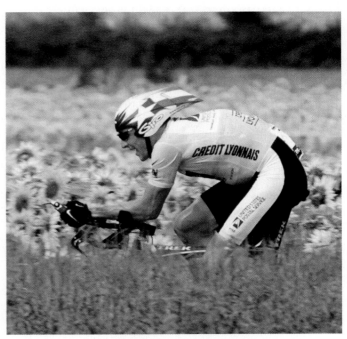

Lance Armstrong's battle with testicular cancer brought attention to a disease that strikes men who may consider themselves "too young" to be at risk for cancer.

Tips for Sun Worshippers

- Avoid the sun, or seek shade, from 10 AM to 4 PM, when the sun's rays are strongest. Even on a cloudy day, up to 80 percent of the sun's rays can get through.
- Apply an SPF 15 or higher sunscreen evenly to all uncovered skin before going outside. Check the label for the correct amount of time you should allow between applying the sunscreen and going outdoors. If the label does not specify, apply it 15 to 30 minutes before going outside. Ask a doctor before applying sunscreen to children under six months old.
- Remember to apply sunscreen to your eyelids, lips, nose, ears, neck, hands, and feet.
- If you don't have much hair, apply sunscreen to the top of your head or wear a hat.
- Reapply sunscreen often. The label will tell you how often you need to reapply it.
- Wear protective clothing and a wide-brimmed hat to protect your head and face.
- Use sunglasses with 99 to 100 percent UV protection to protect your eyes.
- Avoid artificial tanning methods such as sun lamps, tanning beds, tanning pills, and tanning makeup.
- Check your skin regularly for signs of skin cancer.

Sources: U.S. Food and Drug Administration, "Safer Sunning in Seven Steps," 2004, www.fda.gov/opacom/lowlit/sunsafty.html; Medline Plus, "Sun Exposure," 2004, www.nlm.nih. gov/medlineplus/sunexposure.html

---

- *Childbearing.* Women who have never been pregnant are more likely to develop ovarian cancer than those who have had a child, and the more children a woman has had, the less risk she faces. This may be related to exposure to the hormone estrogen. Women who use oral contraceptives that contain estrogen are also at lower risk.
- *Cancer history.* Women who have had breast or colon cancer have a greater chance of developing ovarian cancer than women who have not had either cancer.
- *Fertility drugs.* Drugs that cause a woman to ovulate may slightly increase her chance of developing ovarian cancer. Researchers are studying this possible association.
- *Talc.* Some studies suggest that women who have used talc in their genital area for many years may have increased risk.
- *Hormone replacement therapy (HRT).* Some evidence suggests that women who use HRT after menopause may have a slightly increased risk. This research is controversial and more studies are needed.
- *Genetic predisposition.* Mutation of the *BRCA1* and *BRCA2* genes (already linked to breast cancer) may also increase risk.[60] Another genetic syndrome, hereditary nonpolyposis colon cancer has also been linked to increased risk of developing ovarian cancer.[61]

Prevention   An early Yale University study indicated that diet may play a role in ovarian cancer.[62] When comparing 450 Canadian women with newly diagnosed ovarian cancer with 564 demographically similar, healthy women, the researchers found that the women without ovarian cancer had a diet lower in saturated fat. For every 10 grams of saturated fat a woman ate per day, her risk of ovarian cancer rose 20 percent. Conversely, women who lowered their saturated fat consumption by 10 grams a day experienced a 20 percent drop in risk. Every 10 grams of vegetable fiber (but not fruit or cereal fiber) added to a woman's daily menu lowered her risk by 37 percent. The study also found that each full-term pregnancy lowered risk by about 20 percent, and each year of oral contraceptive use lowered it by 5 to 10 percent. So, should you go out and get pregnant or start taking birth control pills to reduce risk? No. However, these results, particularly when combined with cardiovascular risks and other health information, provide yet another reason to eat plenty of vegetables and cut down on your fat intake. General prevention strategies focusing on diet, exercise, sleep, stress management, and weight control are good ideas for this and any of the cancers discussed in this chapter, as substantiated by recent research studying the role of lifestyle in breast and ovarian cancer.[63]

To protect yourself, thorough annual pelvic examinations are important. Pap tests, although useful in detecting cervical cancer, do not reveal ovarian cancer. Women over the age of 40 should have a cancer-related checkup every year. Transvaginal ultrasound and a tumor marker, *CA125*, may assist in diagnosis but are not recommended for routine screening.[64] If you have any symptoms of ovarian cancer and they persist, see your doctor promptly.

Cervical and Endometrial (Uterine) Cancer

In 2004, an estimated 10,520 new cases of cervical cancer and 40,320 cases of endometrial cancer were diagnosed in the United States. Most uterine cancers develop in the body of the uterus, usually in the endometrium (lining). The rest develop in the cervix, located at the base of the uterus. The overall incidence of early-stage uterine cancer—that is, cervical cancer—has increased slightly in recent years in women under the age of 50.[65] In contrast, invasive, later-stage forms of the disease appear to be decreasing. This may be due to more regular screenings of younger women using the **Pap test,** a procedure in which cells taken from the cervical region are examined for abnormal cellular activity. Although these tests are very effective for detecting early stage cervical cancer, they are less effective for detecting cancers of the uterine lining and not effective at all for detecting cancers of the fallopian tubes or ovaries.[66]

Risk factors for cervical cancer include early age at first intercourse, multiple sex partners, cigarette smoking, and certain sexually transmitted infections, including the human papilloma virus (the cause of genital warts) and the herpes virus. For endometrial cancer, risk factors include age, endometrial hyperplasia, estrogen replacement therapy, being overweight, diabetes and high blood pressure, a history of other cancers, race (white women are at higher risk), and treatment with tamoxifen for breast cancer. (Doctors emphasize that the benefits of tamoxifen far outweigh its possible risks, and close monitoring for endometrial cancer is an important part of tamoxifen treatment.) Other factors also related to estrogen include having few or no children and entering menopause late in life.[67]

Early warning signs of uterine cancer include bleeding outside the normal menstrual period or after menopause or persistent unusual vaginal discharge. These symptoms should be checked by a physician immediately.[68]

Cancer of the Pancreas

The incidence of cancer of the pancreas, known as a "silent" disease, has increased substantially during the last 25 years to 31,860 cases in 2004.[69] Chronic inflammation of the pancreas (pancreatitis), obesity, physical inactivity, diabetes, cirrhosis, and a high-fat diet may contribute to its development. Smokers have double the risk of nonsmokers.[70]

Unfortunately, pancreatic cancer is one of the worst cancers to get. Only 4 percent of patients live more than five years after diagnosis, usually because the disease is well advanced by the time there are any symptoms.

Leukemia

Leukemia is a cancer of the blood-forming tissues that leads to proliferation of millions of immature white blood cells. These abnormal cells crowd out normal white blood cells (which fight infection), platelets (which control hemorrhaging), and red blood cells (which carry oxygen to body cells). As a result, symptoms such as fatigue, paleness, weight loss, easy bruising, repeated infections, nosebleeds, and other forms of hemorrhaging occur. In children, these symptoms can appear suddenly.[71]

Leukemia can be acute or chronic in nature and can strike both sexes and all age groups. Although many people think of it as a childhood disease, leukemia struck over ten times more adults (33,440) than children (2,860) in 2004.[72] Chronic leukemia can develop over several months and have

few symptoms. The five-year survival rate for patients with chronic lymphocytic leukemia, one of the most common types, has risen to 74 percent.

Facing Cancer

While heart disease mortality rates have declined steadily over the past 50 years, cancer mortality has increased consistently in the same period. Based on current rates, about 83 million—or one in three of us now living—will eventually develop cancer. Many factors have contributed to the rise in cancer mortality, but the increased incidence of lung cancer—a largely preventable disease—is probably the most important. Despite these gloomy predictions, recent advancements in the diagnosis and treatment of many forms of cancer have reduced some of the fear and mystery that once surrounded this disease.

Detecting Cancer

The earlier cancer is diagnosed, the better the prospect for survival. Several high-tech tools to detect cancer have been developed:

- Two diagnostic imaging techniques have replaced exploratory surgery for some cancer patients. In **magnetic resonance imaging (MRI)**, a huge electromagnet detects hidden tumors by mapping the vibrations of the various atoms in the body on a computer screen. The **computerized axial tomography scan (CAT scan)** uses X rays to

Pap test A procedure in which cells taken from the cervical region are examined for abnormal cellular activity.

Magnetic resonance imaging (MRI) A device that uses magnetic fields, radio waves, and computers to generate an image of internal tissues of the body for diagnostic purposes without the use of radiation.

Computerized axial tomography (CAT scan) A machine that uses radiation to view internal organs not normally visible in X rays.

What's New in Cancer Research, Prevention, and Treatment?

THE LATEST ON FIBER

Although fiber has undergone ups and downs in popularity as a protective agent against colon and other forms of cancer, don't throw out that bran muffin just yet. A study of more than 68,000 women found that dietary fiber—particularly from breakfast cereals—can significantly decrease the risk of heart attack by improving cholesterol levels, lowering blood sugar, boosting sensitivity to insulin, and lowering the risk of blood clots. A previous study of men showed similar results. So, while some recent studies question fiber's benefits for cancer prevention, few experts believe that these findings should outweigh all the previous studies that indicate it does indeed reduce risk. In short, the scientific community is unsure of the fiber–cancer link but quite sure that the benefits in other areas more than justify a healthy high-fiber, low-fat diet.

ALCOHOL AND CANCER

Heavy drinking is associated with an increased risk for several cancers—notably, cancer of the mouth, esophagus, pharynx, larynx, liver, and pancreas. An analysis of multiple studies found that having two alcoholic drinks per day (any type of alcohol) increased a woman's chances of developing breast cancer by nearly 25 percent. The reasons for this are unclear, but researchers speculate that alcohol influences the metabolism of estrogen and that prolonged exposure to high levels of estrogen increases breast cancer risk, particularly for women on hormone replacement therapy. The effect of one drink per day is controversial, although most experts feel that one daily drink does not increase risk. But, before you toss out all of your alcohol, you should know that there is increasing evidence that a glass of red wine, with its antioxidant potential and HDL-boosting potential, seems to protect against heart disease.

NEW METHODS OF DETECTION

Several new methods of cancer detection are on the horizon:

- *Blood tests.* Researchers from the John Wayne Cancer Center in Santa Monica are developing biological markers that would identify microscopic tumors as they travel through the blood, before they are large enough to detected on conventional tests.
- *"Pap smear for the breast."* Similar to the Pap smear, which checks fluids from the cervix for abnormal cells, this newer test analyzes fluids from the breasts' milk ducts (where most tumors originate). It may be widely available soon. This test would pick up cancerous cells in their earliest, most treatable stages.
- *Better breast scans.* Researchers at the University of Chicago and elsewhere are developing better computer programs to point out questionable spots on mammograms and better, more reliable machines (such as MRIs).

Sources: American Dietetic Association, "Position Paper: Health Implications of Dietary Fiber," *Journal of the American Dietetic Association* 102 (2002): 993–1000; "Fiber and Colon Cancer . . . Again," *Nutrition Action Healthletter,* July–August 2003; U. Peters, et al., "Dietary Fibre and Colorectal Adenoma in a Colorectal Cancer Early Detection Program," *Lancet* 361, no. 9368 (2003): 1491–1495; "The Facts About Drinking and Your Health," *Johns Hopkins Medical Health Letter—Health After 50* 12, no. 5 (2000): 4–6.

examine parts of the body. In both of these painless, noninvasive procedures, cross-sectioned pictures can reveal a tumor's shape and location more accurately than can conventional X rays. (See the New Horizons in Health box.)

- *Prostatic ultrasound* (a rectal probe using ultrasonic waves to produce an image of the prostate) is being investigated as a means to increase the early detection of prostate cancer. Prostatic ultrasound has been combined with the PSA blood test.

Such medical techniques, along with regular self-examinations and checkups, play an important role in the early detection and secondary prevention of cancer. Most of the sites that pose the highest risk for cancer have screening tests available for early detection. Other common forms of cancer have readily identifiable symptoms. The key seems to be whether people have the financial resources (insurance) to seek medical diagnosis and early treatment. Health care reforms that provided coverage for regular checkups and

preventive services would help many poor and middle-class Americans seek medical care early, when the chances of a cure are best.

Regardless of insurance status, the best way to detect cancer early is to stay actively involved in your own health care. Table 16.5 lists seven warning signals of cancer. If you notice any of these signals, and they don't appear to be related to anything else, see a doctor immediately. For example, difficulty swallowing may be due to a cold or flu. However, if you are otherwise symptomless and the difficulty continues, consult your physician. Make sure you receive all appropriate diagnostic tests.

Also, make a realistic assessment of your own risk factors and avoid the ones that you can control. Do you have a family history of cancer? If so, what types? Make sure you know which symptoms to watch for, and follow the recommendations for self-exams and medical checkups in Table 16.3. Avoid known carcinogens—such as tobacco—and other environmental hazards. Eat a nutritious diet. Heeding the suggestions for primary prevention can significantly decrease your own risk for cancer.

New Hope in Cancer Treatments

Although cancer treatments have changed dramatically over the past 20 years, surgery, in which the tumor and surrounding tissue are removed, is still common. Today's surgeons tend to remove less surrounding tissue than previously and to combine surgery with either **radiotherapy** (the use of radiation) or **chemotherapy** (the use of drugs) to kill cancerous cells.

Radiation works by destroying malignant cells or stopping cell growth. It is most effective in treating localized cancer masses. Unfortunately, in the process of destroying malignant cells, radiotherapy also destroys some healthy cells. It may also increase the risk for other types of cancers. Despite these drawbacks, radiation continues to be one of the most common and effective forms of treatment.

When cancer has spread throughout the body, it is necessary to use some form of chemotherapy. Currently, over 50 different anticancer drugs are in use, some of which have excellent records of success. A chemotherapeutic regimen of four anticancer drugs combined with radiotherapy has resulted in remarkable survival rates for some cancers, including Hodgkin's disease. Ongoing research promises to result in new drugs that are less toxic to normal cells and more potent against tumor cells. Current research indicates that some tumors may actually be resistant to certain forms of chemotherapy and that the treatment drugs do not reach the core of the tumor. Scientists are working to circumvent resistance and make tumor cells more vulnerable.

Whether used alone or in combination, radiotherapy and chemotherapy have side effects, including extreme nausea, nutritional deficiencies, hair loss, and general fatigue. Long-term damage to the cardiovascular system and other body systems can be significant. It is important to discuss these matters fully with doctors when making treatment plans.

Substances found in nature, such as taxol (originally found in Pacific yew trees), are now being synthesized in laboratories and tested on a variety of cancers. Other compounds, including those derived from sea urchins, are rich in resources for anticancer drugs.

Today, researchers are targeting cancer as a genetic disease that is brought on by some form of mutation, either inherited or acquired. Promising treatments focus on stopping the cycle of these mutant cells, targeting toxins through monoclonal antibodies, and rousing the immune system to be more effective. Others include the following:[73]

- The estrogen-blocking drug *tamoxifen* is used to treat women who have breast cancer that is estrogen positive, or grows more rapidly when estrogen levels are high. This drug is often an alternative to chemotherapy.
- **Immunotherapy** enhances the body's own disease-fighting systems to help control cancer. Interferon (a naturally occurring body protein that protects healthy cells and kills cancer cells), interleukin-2 (a growth factor that stimulates cells of the immune system to find cancer), and other biological response modifiers are under study.
- One of the most exciting new approaches for spurring the immune system to ward off cancer is the use of *cancer-fighting vaccines*. Cancer vaccines are not to be confused with the vaccines for measles and other infectious diseases, which prime the body to keep bacteria and viruses from taking hold. They essentially keep people healthy, but they don't cure anything. Cancer vaccines alert the body's immune defenses; but, instead of warning of germs, they provide indicators of good cells that have gone bad. Consequently, rather than preventing disease, they help people who are already ill. Today, hundreds of studies are examining the effectiveness of possible cancer vaccines. These vaccines may be the next generation of cancer treatment.
- Research on the effectiveness of *gene therapy* has moved into early clinical trials. Scientists have found hopeful signs of a virus carrying genetic information that makes the cells it infects susceptible to an antiviral drug. Findings from human trials are expected soon. Scientists also are looking at ways to transfer genes that increase the patient's immune response to the cancerous tumor or that confer drug resistance to the bone marrow so that higher doses of chemotherapeutic drugs can be given.
- In other studies, researchers are testing compounds that may stop tumors from forming new blood vessels, a process known as *angiogenesis*. By inhibiting angiogenesis, scientists hope to inhibit the flow of nutrient- and oxygen-rich blood to the cancerous tumors and slow their growth.

Radiotherapy The use of radiation to kill cancerous cells.

Chemotherapy The use of drugs to kill cancerous cells.

Immunotherapy A process that stimulates the body's own immune system to combat cancer cells.

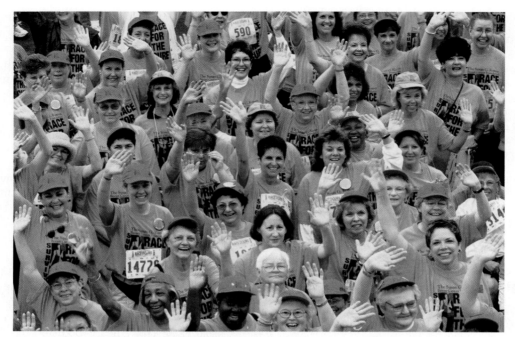

Cancer survivors can lead long and healthy lives. Some, such as these breast cancer survivors and their supporters, take part in walkathons, races, and other activities to raise money for cancer research and treatment and to increase public awareness about prevention.

- In recent years, scientists have identified various steps in what is termed the *cancer pathway*. These include onco-gene actions, hormone receptors, growth factors, metasta-sis, and angiogenesis. Preliminary studies are underway to design compounds (*rational drug design*) aimed at specific molecules along the cancer pathway with the intent of inhibiting actions at these various steps.
- Cell mutations can trigger increased production of destructive enzymes that allow them to invade surround-ing tissues and penetrate blood vessels to travel to other parts of the body. A powerful enzyme inhibitor, *TIMP-2,* shows promise for slowing the metastasis of tumor cells. A metastasis suppressor gene, *NM23,* has also been identified.
- *Neoadjuvant chemotherapy* (using chemotherapy to shrink the tumor and then removing it surgically) has been tried against various types of cancers. This is a promising new approach.
- *Stem cell research* is another promising avenue for poten-tial treatment, although controversy has stalled investiga-tion (see Chapter 19).

In addition, psychosocial and behavioral research has become increasingly important as health professionals learn more about lifestyle factors that influence risk and survivabil-ity. Health care practitioners have become more aware of the psychological needs of patients and families and have begun to tailor treatment programs to meet their diverse needs.

Talking with Your Doctor about Cancer

Any time cancer is suspected, people react with anxiety, fear, and anger. Emotional distress is sometimes so intense that they are unable to make critical health care decisions. If you find it difficult to know what to ask your doctor during a rou-tine exam, imagine how hard it would be to discuss life-or-death options for yourself or a loved one. Before you arrive at the doctor's office, prepare a list of important questions to discuss. Remember, your health care provider should be your partner and help you make the best decisions for you.

If the diagnosis is cancer, here are some suggestions for questions to ask:

- What kind of cancer do I have? What stage is it in? Based on my age and stage, what prognosis do I have?
- What are my treatment choices? Which do you recommend? Why?
- What are the benefits of each kind of treatment?
- What are the short- and long-term risks and possible side effects for each treatment?
- Would a clinical trial be appropriate for me? (Clinical trials are research studies designed to answer specific questions and to find better ways to prevent or treat cancer. Often they test new cancer-fighting treatments.)

If surgery is recommended, ask:

- What kind of operation will it be, and how long will it take? What form of anesthesia will be used? How many

Table 16.6
Five-Year Relative Survival Rates by Stage at Diagnosis*

Site	All Stages %	Local %	Regional %	Distant %
Breast (female)	86.6	97.0	78.7	23.3
Cervix (uterus)	71.3	92.2	50.9	16.5
Colon and rectum	62.3	90.1	65.5	9.2
Endometrium (uterus)	84.4	96.2	64.7	26.0
Esophagus	14.0	29.1	13.1	2.2
Kidney	62.6	89.9	60.0	9.1
Larynx	64.7	82.6	47.9	20.0
Liver	6.9	16.3	6.0	1.9
Lung	14.9	48.7	16.0	2.1
Melanoma	89.6	96.7	60.1	13.8
Oral cavity	57.2	82.1	47.9	26.1
Ovary	53.0	94.7	72.0	30.7
Pancreas	4.4	16.6	6.8	1.6
Prostate	97.5	100.0	**	34.0
Stomach	22.5	59.0	21.7	2.5
Testis	95.5	99.1	95.0	73.1
Thyroid	95.8	99.3	95.5	59.9
Urinary bladder	81.8	94.4	48.2	5.8

*Adjusted for normal life expectancy. This chart is based on cases diagnosed from 1992–1999; followed through 2000.
**Rate for local stage represents local and regional stages combined.
Source: National Cancer Institute, Surveillance, Epidemiology, and End Results Program, 1973–2000; published in American Cancer Society, *Cancer Facts and Figures 2004* (Atlanta, GA: American Cancer Society, 2004). Reproduced with permission. www.cancer.org. © 2004, American Cancer Society, Inc.

similar procedures has this surgeon done in the past month? What is his or her success rate?

- How will I feel after surgery? If I have pain, how will you help me?
- Where will the scars be? What will they look like? Will they cause disability?
- Will I have any activity limitations after surgery? What kind of physical therapy, if any, will I need? When will I get back to normal activities?

If radiation is recommended, ask:

- Why do you think this treatment is better than my other options?
- How long will I need to have treatments, and what will the side effects be in the short and long term? What body organs or systems may be damaged?
- What can I do to take care of myself during therapy? Are there services available to help me?
- What is the long-term prognosis for people of my age with my type of cancer who are using this treatment?

If chemotherapy is recommended, ask:

- Why do you think this treatment is better than my other options?
- Which drug combinations pose the fewest risks and most benefits?

- What will be the short- and long-term side effects on my body?

Before beginning any form of cancer therapy, it is imperative to be a vigilant and vocal consumer. Read and seek information from cancer support groups. Check the skills of your surgeon, your radiation therapist, and your doctor in terms of clinical experience and interpersonal interactions.

Cancer Survivors: Life after Cancer

Heightened public awareness and an improved prognosis have made the cancer experience less threatening and isolating than it once was (Table 16.6). While you may have once heard stories of recovering cancer patients experiencing job discrimination or being unable to obtain health or life insurance, these cases are decreasing. Several states have even enacted legislation to prevent insurance companies from canceling policies or instituting other forms of discrimination. Since health insurance can be obtained through large employers and large companies spread the insurance risk among many employees, insurance companies often accept new employees without underwriting.

In fact, assistance for the cancer patient is more readily available than ever before. Cancer support groups, cancer information workshops, and low-cost medical consultation are just a few of the forms of assistance now offered in many communities. Groups have successfully lobbied the U.S. Congress to increase cancer research dollars. As a result, government funding has increased substantially over the past decade. The battle for funds continues. Increasing efforts in cancer research, improvements in diagnostic equipment, and advances in treatment provide hope for the future.

TAKING CHARGE

MAKE IT HAPPEN!

Assessment: The Assess Yourself box on page 456 identifies certain behaviors that increase the risk of cancer. If you have identified particular behaviors that may be putting you at risk, consider steps you can take to change these behaviors and improve your future health.

Making a Change: In order to change your behavior, you need to develop a plan. Follow these steps.

1. Evaluate your behavior, and identify patterns and specific things you are doing. What can you change now? What can you change in the near future?
2. Select one pattern of behavior that you want to change.
3. Fill out a Behavior Change Contract. It should include your long-term goal for change, your short-term goals, the rewards you'll give yourself for reaching these goals, potential obstacles along the way, and strategies for overcoming these obstacles. For each goal, list the small steps and specific actions that you will take.
4. Chart your progress in a journal. At the end of a week, consider how successful you were in following your plan. What helped you to be successful? What made change more difficult? What will you do differently next week?

5. Revise your plan as needed. Are the short-term goals attainable? Are the rewards satisfying?

One Student's Plan: Keisha's assessment showed that, while she was taking precautions to reduce her cancer risk in most areas, she was not doing what she should about her breast cancer risk. Her score in this area was 8 because she had never been pregnant, she did not regularly examine her breasts, and her mother had been diagnosed with breast cancer two years ago. Keisha decided she needed to learn how to examine her breasts and make a plan to ensure she did it every month. After studying this textbook's illustrations, she made an appointment with her gynecologist. While she was there, she asked the doctor to confirm that she was doing the examination correctly.

Next, Keisha decided that she would spend the first ten minutes of her morning once a month to do the exam and that she would give herself a reward for each month that she examined herself on schedule. On her way to campus after doing the exam, she would treat herself to a latte and a scone. After she stuck with her schedule for six months in a row she would buy herself a new outfit. She also resolved to talk to her younger sister about the importance of the exam.

Summary

- Cancer is a group of diseases characterized by uncontrolled growth and spread of abnormal cells. These cells may create tumors. Benign (noncancerous) tumors grow in size but do not spread; malignant (cancerous) tumors spread to other parts of the body.
- Several causes of cancer have been identified. Lifestyle factors include smoking and obesity. Biological factors include inherited genes and gender. Occupational and environmental hazards are carcinogens present in people's home or work environments. Chemicals in foods

that may act as carcinogens include preservatives and pesticides. Viral diseases that may lead to cancer include herpes, mononucleosis, and human papilloma virus (which causes genital warts). Medical factors include certain drug therapies given for other conditions that may elevate the chance of cancer. Combined risk refers to a combination of the above factors, which tends to compound the risk for cancer.
- There are many different types of cancer, each of which poses different risks, depending on a number of factors.

Common forms include lung, breast, colon and rectum, prostate, skin, testicular, ovarian, uterine, and pancreatic cancers, as well as leukemia.

- Early diagnosis improves survival rate. Self-exams for breast, testicular, and skin cancer and knowledge of the seven warning signals of cancer aid early diagnosis.

- New types of cancer treatments include various combinations of radiotherapy, chemotherapy, and immunotherapy.

Questions for Discussion and Reflection

1. What is cancer? How does it spread? What is the difference between a benign and a malignant tumor?
2. List the likely causes of cancer. Do any of them put you at greater risk? What can you do to reduce this risk? What risk factors do you share with family members? Friends?
3. What are the symptoms of lung, breast, prostate, and testicular cancer? What can you do to reduce your risk of developing these cancers or increase your chances of surviving them?
4. What are the differences between carcinomas, sarcomas, lymphomas, and leukemia? Which is the most common? Least common?
5. Why are breast and testicular self-exams important for women and men? What could be the consequences of not doing these exams regularly?
6. Discuss warning signals of cancer. What could indicate that you have cancer instead of a minor illness? How soon should you seek treatment for any of the suspicious symptoms?

Accessing Your Health on the Internet

Visit the following Internet sites to explore further topics and issues related to personal health. To visit an organization's website, go to the Companion Website for *Access to Health, Ninth Edition* at www.aw-bc.com/donatelle, click on the book image, and select "Accessing Your Health on the Internet" from the navigation menu.

1. *American Cancer Society.* Resources from the leading private organization dedicated to cancer prevention. This site provides information, statistics, and resources regarding cancer.
2. *International Cancer Information Center.* Sponsored by the National Cancer Institute, this site is designed to be a comprehensive information resource on cancer for patients and health professionals.
3. *National Cancer Institute.* Check here for valuable information on clinical trials and the Physician Data Query (PDQ), a comprehensive database of cancer treatment information.
4. *National Women's Health Information Center (NWHIC).* Provides a wealth of information about cancer in women. Cosponsored by the National Cancer Institute.
5. *Oncolink.* Sponsored by the University of Pennsylvania Cancer Center, this site seeks to educate cancer patients and their families by offering information on support services, cancer causes, screening, prevention, and common questions.

Further Reading

American Cancer Institute Journal, published monthly.

Focuses on current risk factors, prevention, and treatment research in the area of cancer.

American Cancer Society. *Cancer Facts and Figures.* Atlanta, GA: American Cancer Society, published annually.

A summary of major facts relating to cancer. Provides information on incidence, prevalence, symptomology, prevention, and treatment. Available through local divisions of the American Cancer Society. Contains up-to-date information about the disease, medical options, and emotional support.

American Cancer Society. *A Breast Cancer Journey: Your Personal Guidebook,* 2nd ed. Atlanta, Georgia: American Cancer Society, 2004.

Contains up-to-date information on treatments, medicines, reconstructive surgery, and complementary and alternative options. Also includes information for caregivers, family, and friends.

Armstrong, L. *It's Not about the Bike: My Journey Back to Life.* New York: Penguin, 2000.

The incredible description by Lance Armstrong of his triumph over testicular cancer and his Tour de France victories. A book full of inspiration for young men with this disease, their families, and anyone facing cancer.

Nutrition and Cancer Journal, published monthly.

Focuses on etiological aspects of various dietary factors and research on risks for cancer development. Also includes current research on dietary factors and prevention.

- Discuss the risk factors for infectious diseases, including those you can control and those you cannot.

- Discuss the most common pathogens infecting humans today and the typical diseases caused by each.

- Explain how your immune system works to protect you and what factors may make it less effective.

- Explain the major emerging and resurgent diseases affecting humans today; discuss why they are increasing in incidence and what actions are being taken to reduce risks.

- Discuss the various sexually transmitted infections, their means of transmission, and actions that can be taken to prevent their spread.

- Discuss human immunodeficiency virus (HIV) and acquired immuno-deficiency syndrome (AIDS), trends in infection and treatment, and the impact on special populations, such as women and members of the international community.

INFECTIOUS DISEASES AND SEXUALLY TRANS-MITTED INFECTIONS

RISKS AND RESPONSIBILITIES

IN THE NEWS

Prevention: Condoms and Pelvic Inflammation

By Eric Nagourney

Women whose sexual partners regularly use condoms can reduce by half their risk of developing pelvic inflammatory disease, a painful condition that can lead to infertility, according to a new study.

Writing in the August issue of *The American Journal of Public Health,* researchers said their findings offered evidence that condoms, well established as barriers against viral infection, also help prevent the kinds of bacterial infection that can cause P.I.D., as the disease is known. The study was led by Dr. Roberta B. Ness of the University of Pittsburgh.

Each year, the researchers said, about a million American women have a serious episode of the disease. Apart from the pain it causes, it is believed to leave 100,000 women a year unable to have a baby. It can also cause pregnancy complications. A variety of bacteria can cause P.I.D., but it is usually a result of sexually transmitted diseases like gonorrhea.

For the study, the researchers asked 684 sexually active women with a history of P.I.D. to keep track of their sexual practices and recurrences of the disease over a period of almost three years. They found that the women who reported using condoms least often were the most likely to have the condition and related problems like chronic pelvic pain and infertility.

Read the complete article online in the eThemes section of this book's website: www.aw-bc.com/donatelle.

Original article published August 17, 2004. Copyright © 2004 *The New York Times.* Reprinted with permission.

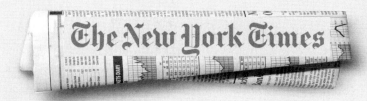

Every moment of every day, you are in contact with microscopic organisms that have the ability to make you ill or even kill you. These disease-causing agents, known as **pathogens,** are found in air and food and on nearly every object or person with whom you come in contact. Although new varieties of pathogens arise all the time, many have existed for as long as there has been life on this planet. Fossil evidence shows that infections afflicted the earliest human beings. At times, infectious diseases wiped out whole groups of people through **epidemics** such as the Black Death, or bubonic plague, that killed up to one third of the population of Europe and Asia in the 1300s. A **pandemic,** or global epidemic, of influenza killed more than 20 million people in 1918, while strains of tuberculosis and cholera continue to cause premature death among populations throughout the world.

In spite of our best efforts to eradicate them, these diseases are a continuing menace to all of us. While vaccines, pasteurization, improvements in sanitation, and other public health measures have slowed or stopped the spread of many diseases, some infections that were once held in check by antibiotics have begun to resurge, or emerge, in new and more deadly resistant forms. If we are unable to replace antibiotics as they lose their effectiveness and to limit the emergence and spread of resistance, some diseases may simply become untreatable again, much as they were in the *preantibiotic* era, when deaths from bacterial diseases were routine.

The news isn't all bad, however. Even though we are bombarded by potential pathogenic threats, our immune systems are remarkably adept at protecting us. *Endogenous microorganisms* are those that live in peaceful coexistence with their human host most of the time. For people in good health and whose immune systems are functioning properly, endogenous organisms are usually harmless. However, in sick people or those with weakened immune systems, these normally harmless pathogenic organisms can cause serious health problems.

Exogenous microorganisms are organisms that do not normally inhabit the body. When they do, however, they are apt to produce an infection and/or illness. The more easily these pathogens can gain a foothold in the body and sustain themselves, the more **virulent** (aggressive) they may be in causing disease. If your immune system is strong, you will often be able to fight off even the most virulent attacker. Just because you inhale a flu virus does not mean that you will get the flu. Just because your hands are teeming with bacteria does not mean that you will become ill. Several factors influence your susceptibility to disease.

Assessing Your Disease Risks

Most diseases are **multifactorial diseases**—that is, they are caused by the interaction of several factors from inside and outside the person. For a disease to occur, the *host* must be *susceptible,* meaning that the immune system must be in a weakened condition; an *agent* capable of *transmitting* a disease must be present; and the *environment* must be *hospitable* to the pathogen in terms of temperature, light, moisture, and other requirements. Other risk factors also apparently increase or decrease susceptibility. Figure 17.1 summarizes the body's defenses against invasion.

Risk Factors You Can't Control

Unfortunately, some risk factors are beyond our control. Here are some of the most common:

Heredity Perhaps the single greatest factor influencing longevity is the longevity of a person's parents. Being born into a family in which heart disease, cancer, or other illnesses are prevalent seems to increase a person's risk. Still other diseases are caused by direct chromosomal inheritance. For example, **sickle-cell anemia,** an inherited blood disease that primarily affects African Americans, may be transmitted to the fetus if both parents carry the sickle-cell trait. It is often unclear whether hereditary diseases occur as a result of inherited chromosomal traits or inherited insufficiencies in the immune system.

Aging After age 40, we become more vulnerable to most of the chronic diseases. Moreover, as we age, our immune systems respond less efficiently to invading organisms, increasing the risk for infection and illness. The same flu that produces an afternoon of nausea and diarrhea in a younger person may cause days of illness or even death in an older person. The very young are also at risk for many diseases, particularly if they are not vaccinated against them.

Environmental Conditions Unsanitary conditions and the presence of drugs, chemicals, and hazardous pollutants and wastes in food and water probably have a great effect on our immune systems. It is well documented that poor environmental conditions can weaken **immunological competence**—the body's ability to defend itself against pathogens.

Pathogen   A disease-causing agent.

Epidemic   Disease outbreak that affects many people in a community or region at the same time.

Pandemic   Global epidemic of a disease.

Virulent   Strong enough to overcome host resistance and cause disease.

Multifactorial disease   Disease caused by interactions of several factors.

Sickle-cell anemia   Genetic disease commonly found among African Americans; results in organ damage and premature death.

Immunological competence   Ability of the immune system to defend the body from pathogens.

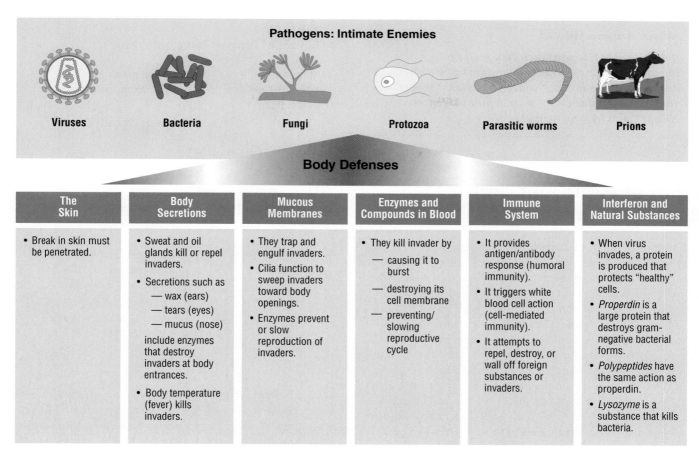

Figure 17.1
The Body's Defenses Against Disease-Causing Pathogens

Organism Resistance Some organisms, such as the food-borne organism **botulism,** are particularly virulent, and even tiny amounts may make the most hardy of us ill. Other organisms have mutated and are resistant to the body's defenses as well as other conventional treatments designed to protect against them. Still other, newer pathogens pose unique challenges for our immune systems—ones that our bodily defenses are ill-adapted to fight.

Risk Factors You Can Control

Every minute of every day, we come in contact with agents that could make us sick. Some of these agents are difficult to avoid. However, the good news is that we all have some degree of personal control over many risk factors for disease. Too much stress, inadequate nutrition, a low level of physical fitness, lack of sleep, misuse or abuse of legal and illegal substances, poor personal hygiene, high-risk behaviors, and other variables significantly increase the risk for a number of diseases. Various chapters of this text discuss these variables. Several factors influence our individual susceptibility to various diseases. Those we have the most

control over, via lifestyle decisions and behaviors, are noted on the following list with an asterisk (*):[1]

- Personal habits: smoking, alcohol use, sleep, exercise, stress levels, drug use/abuse*
- Dosage, virulence, and where the disease-causing agent enters the body
- Age at time of infection
- Preexisting level of immunity*
- Health and vigor of immune system response*
- Genetic factors controlling immune response
- Nutritional status of host*
- Comorbidities: the number of battles your immune system is fighting at the same time*
- Environmental surroundings, such as temperature, humidity, and sanitary conditions*
- Psychological factors (motivation, emotional status, and so on)*

Botulism A resistant foodborne organism that is extremely virulent.

Types of Pathogens and Routes of Transmission

Pathogens can enter the body in several ways (Table 17.1). They may be transmitted by *direct contact* between infected persons, such as during sexual relations, kissing, or touching, or by *indirect contact,* such as by touching an object the infected person has had contact with. The hands are probably the greatest source of infectious disease transmission. For example, you may touch the handle of a drinking fountain that was just touched by someone whose hands were contaminated by a recent sneeze or failure to wash after using the toilet. You may also **autoinoculate** yourself, or transmit a pathogen from one part of your body to another. For example, you may touch a sore on your lip that is teeming with viral herpes, then transmit the virus to your eye when you scratch your itchy eyelid.

Pathogens are also transmitted by *airborne contact*—you can breathe in air that carries a particular pathogen—or by *foodborne infection* if you eat something contaminated by microorganisms. Recent episodes of food poisoning from *Salmonella* bacteria in certain foods and *Escherichia coli* (*E. coli*) bacteria in undercooked beef have raised concerns about the safety of the U.S. food supply. As a direct result of these concerns, food labels caution consumers to cook meats thoroughly, wash utensils, and take other food-handling precautions.

Your best friend may be the source of *animal-borne pathogens.* Dogs, cats, livestock, and wild animals can spread numerous diseases through their bites or feces or by carrying infected insects into living areas and transmitting diseases either directly or indirectly. Although **interspecies transmission** of diseases (the passing of diseases from humans to animals and vice versa) is rare, it does occur. *Waterborne diseases* are transmitted directly from drinking water and indirectly from foods washed or sprayed with contaminated water. These pathogens can also invade your body if you wade or swim in contaminated streams, lakes, and reservoirs. Pathogens may also transmit *insectborne diseases* via mosquitoes, ticks, and other hosts that spread disease through sucking or biting. Mothers may transmit diseases *perinatally* to an infant in the womb or as the baby passes through the vagina during birth.

We can categorize pathogens into six major types: bacteria, viruses, fungi, protozoa, parasitic worms, and prions. Each has a particular route of transmission and characteristic elements that make it unique. Some are particularly virulent and can successfully invade a host and sustain themselves in a potentially hostile environment. Others are weak and die before they even penetrate the body because of the far-reaching body defense system. In the following pages we discuss each of these categories and give an overview of diseases they cause that have a significant impact on public health.

Bacteria

Bacteria are single-celled organisms that are plantlike in nature but lack chlorophyll (the pigment that gives plants their green coloring). There are three major types of bacteria: cocci, bacilli, and spirilla. Each type is distinguished by its shape, size, and other unique characteristics. Bacteria can be viewed under a standard light microscope.

Although there are several thousand species of bacteria, only approximately 100 cause diseases in humans. In many cases, it is not the bacteria themselves that cause

---

Table 17.1
Routes of Disease Transmission

Mode of Transmission	Aspects of Transmission
1. Contact	Either *direct* (e.g., skin or sexual contact) or *indirect* (e.g., infected blood or body fluid)
2. Food- or waterborne	Eating or coming in contact with contaminated food or water or products passed through them
3. Airborne	Inhalation; droplet spread as through sneezing, coughing, or talking
4. Vectorborne	Vector-transmitted via secretions, biting, egg-laying, as done by mosquitoes, ticks, snails, avians, etc; depends on how infectious the organism is
5. Perinatal	Similar to contact infection; happens in the uterus or as the baby passes through the birth canal

---

Autoinoculation Transmission of a pathogen from one part of the body to another.

Interspecies transmission Transmission of disease from humans to animals or from animals to humans.

Bacteria Single-celled organisms that may cause disease.

disease but rather the poisonous substances, called **toxins,** that they produce. The following are the most common bacterial infections.

Staphylococcal Infections   **Staphylococci** are normally present on our skin at all times and usually cause few problems; but when there is a cut or break in the **epidermis,** or outer layer of the skin, staphylococci may enter and cause a localized infection. If you have ever suffered from acne, boils, styes (infections of the eyelids), or infected wounds, you have probably had a staph infection.

At least one staph-caused disorder, **toxic shock syndrome (TSS),** is potentially fatal. Media reports in the 1980s indicated that the disorder was exclusive to menstruating women, particularly those who used high-absorbency tampons for prolonged periods of time. Although most cases of TSS have occurred in menstruating women, the disease was first reported in 1978 in a group of children and continues to appear in people recovering from wounds, surgery, or other injury.

To reduce the likelihood of TSS, take the following precautions: (1) avoid superabsorbent tampons except during the heaviest menstrual flow; (2) change tampons at least every four hours; and (3) use pads at night instead of tampons. Men and women can prevent TSS by making sure that cuts and wounds remain clean and by seeking medical attention if there are signs of skin infection such as redness, swelling, or abnormal drainage near the wound.[2] Call your doctor immediately if you experience any of the following symptoms: high fever, headache, vomiting, diarrhea and chills, stomach pains, or shocklike symptoms such as faintness, rapid pulse, pallor (which can be caused by a drop in blood pressure), or a sunburnlike rash, particularly on fingers and toes.

Streptococcal Infections   At least five types of the **streptococcus** microorganism—groups A, B, C, D, and G—are known to cause bacterial infections. Most strep infections are caused by the type A variety, including streptococcal pharyngitis ("strep throat") and scarlet fever, which is often preceded by a sore throat.[3] Most of these infections respond readily to antibiotics. However, resistant forms of streptococcal infections are emerging and pose threats for the future.

The second most common form of strep infection is the group B streptococcus (GBS), which can cause illness in newborn babies, pregnant women, the elderly, and adults with other illnesses such as diabetes or liver disease. GBS is the most common cause of life-threatening infections in newborns. In pregnant women, GBS can lead to bladder infections, womb infections, and stillbirth. Among men and nonpregnant women, it can produce blood infections and pneumonia. Approximately 20 percent of men and nonpregnant women with GBS die of the disease. This has caused increasing concern among health professionals.[4]

Pneumonia   In the early twentieth century, **pneumonia** was a leading cause of death in the United States. This disease is characterized by chronic cough, chest pain, chills, high fever,

fluid accumulation, and eventual respiratory failure. One of the most common forms of pneumonia is due to bacterial infection and responds readily to antibiotic treatment in the early stages. Other forms are caused by viruses, chemicals, or other substances in the lungs and are more difficult to treat. Although medical advances have reduced the overall incidence and severity of pneumonia, it continues to be a major threat in the United States and worldwide. Vulnerable populations include older adults and those already suffering from other illnesses such as AIDS.[5]

Legionnaire's Disease   This bacterial disorder gained widespread publicity in 1976, when several Legionnaires at an American Legion convention in Philadelphia contracted it and died before the invading organism was isolated and effective treatment devised. Although one of the lesser-known diseases, its waterborne nature has led to several recent outbreaks around the world.[6] The symptoms are similar to those for pneumonia, which sometimes makes identification difficult. In people whose resistance is lowered, particularly the elderly, delayed identification can have serious consequences.

Tuberculosis   A major killer in the United States in the early twentieth century, **tuberculosis (TB),** or "consumption" or "white death" as it was once known, was largely controlled in the United States by 1950 due to improved sanitation, isolation of infected persons, and treatment with drugs such as *rifampin* or *isoniazid*. Although many health professionals assumed that TB had been conquered, that appears not to be the case. During the past 20 years, several factors have led to an epidemic rise in the disease: deteriorating social conditions, including overcrowding and poor sanitation; failure to isolate active cases of TB; a weakening of public health infrastructure, which has led to less funding for screening; and migration of TB to the United States through international travel. In 2003, there were over 14,874 active cases of TB in the United States.[7] Over one-half of all TB cases in the United

Toxins   Poisonous substances produced by certain microorganisms that cause various diseases.

Staphylococci   Round, gram-positive bacteria, usually found in clusters.

Epidermis   The outermost layer of the skin.

Toxic shock syndrome (TSS)   A potentially life-threatening bacterial infection that is most common in menstruating women who use tampons.

Streptococcus   A round bacterium, usually found in chain formation.

Pneumonia   Bacterially caused disease of the lungs.

Tuberculosis (TB)   A disease caused by bacterial infiltration of the respiratory system.

Table 17.2
U.S. Tuberculosis Cases by Age and Race/Ethnicity, 2001

Age	Number of Cases	Percent	Rate per 100,000 Population
0–14	931	6	1.5
15–24	1,594	10	4.0
25–44	5,630	35	6.6
45–64	4,534	28	7.2
65 and over	3,295	21	9.1
Race/Ethnicity			
White, non-Hispanic	3,357	21	1.6
Black, non-Hispanic	4,796	30	13.8
Hispanic	4,001	25	11.9
American Indian/Alaskan Native	233	1	11.0
Asian/Pacific Islander	3,552	22	32.7

Source: Centers for Disease Control and Prevention, National Center for HIV, STD, and Tuberculosis Prevention, "Reported TB in the U.S.—2001," 2002, www.cdc.gov/nchstp/tb/surv/surv2001/default.htm

States in 2003 occurred in foreign-born individuals.[8] In the United States between 1998 and 2003, the top five countries of origin for foreign-born persons with TB were Mexico, the Philippines, Vietnam, India, and China.[9] Newer strains of multiple drug-resistant tuberculosis make this epidemic potentially more devastating than previous outbreaks.

People residing in overcrowded prisons and homeless shelters with poor ventilation (which means that people continuously inhale the same contaminated air) are at special risk. Early release programs for infected prisoners and the travel patterns of infected homeless people make the spread of tuberculosis difficult to control. The poor, especially children and the chronically ill, seem to be among those at greatest risk. As the HIV/AIDS epidemic has evolved, persons with compromised immune systems are also at high risk for TB infection. See Table 17.2 for a breakdown of cases by age and ethnic group.

Although tuberculosis increases in the United States are troubling, U.S. statistics pale by comparison to the staggering tuberculosis burden in the global population. The World Health Organization (WHO) ranks tuberculosis among the most serious health threats in the world. It is estimated that one-third of the world's inhabitants (over 2 billion humans) are latently infected with the TB bacterium, *Mycobacterium tuberculosis.* In addition, 7 to 8 million new cases of tuberculosis occur each year, and approximately 2 million people die of the disease. Ninety-five percent of these deaths occur in developing nations. Tuberculosis causes 25 percent of all preventable adult deaths in the developing world, and 75 percent of cases and 80 percent of deaths in these areas occur among adults aged 15 to 55.[10]

Assuming no significant improvements in prevention and control between now and 2020, WHO estimates that in the first two decades of the twenty-first century, 1 billion people will acquire a new tuberculosis infection, 200 million will develop active disease, and 35 million will die.[11] It is estimated that almost 80 percent of all cases of TB are found in 22 "high burden" countries, including China, Russia, and India, with the highest number of cases in Africa and southeast Asia.[12]

Tuberculosis is caused by bacterial infiltration of the respiratory system that results in a chronic inflammatory reaction in the lungs. Airborne transmission via the respiratory tract is the primary and most efficient mode of transmitting TB. People with active cases can transmit the disease while talking, coughing, sneezing, or singing. Fortunately, it is fairly difficult to catch, and prolonged exposure, rather than single exposure, is the typical mode of infection. Only about 20 to 30 percent of those exposed to an active case will become infected.[13] In some regions of the world, bovine tuberculosis, which is found in unpasteurized milk and dairy products from infected cattle, is more common. A rare mode of transmission is by infected urine, especially for young children using the same toilet facilities.

Many people infected with TB are contagious without actually showing any symptoms themselves. Symptoms include persistent coughing, weight loss, fever, and spitting up blood. If you or someone you know has these symptoms, check with a doctor. A simple skin test can indicate infection, to be followed by chest X rays and other confirmatory tests. Treatments are effective for most nonresistant cases. Treatment includes rest, careful infection-control procedures, and drugs to combat the infection.

Periodontal diseases Diseases of the tissue around the teeth.

Periodontal Diseases Disorders of the tissue around the teeth, called **periodontal diseases,** affect three out of four adults over age 35. Improper tooth care, including lack of flossing and poor brushing habits, and the failure to obtain professional dental care regularly lead to increased bacterial growth, caries (tooth decay), and gum infections. If left untreated, permanent tooth loss may result.

Rickettsia-Caused Diseases   Once believed to be closely related to viruses, **rickettsia** are now considered to be a small form of bacteria. They produce toxins and multiply within small blood vessels, causing vascular blockage and tissue death.

Rickettsia require an insect vector (carrier) for transmission to humans. Two common forms of human rickettsial disease are Rocky Mountain spotted fever (RMSF), carried by a tick, and typhus, carried by a louse, flea, or tick. These diseases produce similar symptoms, including high fever, weakness, rash, and coma, and both can be life threatening. You do not actually have to be bitten by a vector to contract these diseases. Because the insects harbor the developing rickettsia in their intestinal tracts, insect excrement deposited on the skin and entering the body through abrasions and scratches may be a common source of infection. Although the name *Rocky Mountain spotted fever* seems to imply a specific geographic risk, RMSF is found throughout the United States, as well as southern Canada, Mexico, Central America, and parts of South America. Between 1994 and 1998, the disease was reported in every U.S. state except Hawaii, Vermont, New Hampshire, Maine, and Alaska.[14]

What do you think?

Why do you think we are experiencing global increases in diseases such as tuberculosis today? ■ *Should we be concerned about diseases in other countries?* ■ *Do we have an obligation to help the world's population in its struggle against these diseases?* ■ *What policies, programs, and services might help?*

Viruses

Viruses are the smallest known pathogens, approximately 1/500th the size of bacteria. Because of their tiny size, they are visible only under an electron microscope and were not identified until the twentieth century.[15]

Over 150 viruses are known to cause diseases in humans, although their role in the development of various cancers and chronic diseases remains unclear. In fact, we still have much to learn about viruses, one of the most unusual microorganisms that infect humans.

Essentially, a virus consists of a protein structure that contains either *ribonucleic acid (RNA)* or *deoxyribonucleic acid (DNA)*. Incapable of carrying out the normal cell functions of respiration and metabolism, a virus cannot reproduce on its own and can exist only in a parasitic relationship with the cell it invades. In fact, some scientists question whether viruses should even be considered living organisms.

When viruses attach themselves to host cells, they inject their own RNA or DNA, causing the host cells to begin reproducing new viruses. Once they take control of a cell, these new viruses overrun it until, filled to capacity, the cell bursts, putting thousands of new viruses into circulation to begin the process of cell invasion and reproduction all over again.

Because viruses cannot reproduce outside living cells, they are especially difficult to culture in a laboratory, making their detection and study extremely time-consuming. Viral diseases can be difficult to treat because many viruses can withstand heat, formaldehyde, and large doses of radiation with little effect on their structure. In addition, some viruses may have **incubation periods** (the length of time required to develop fully and therefore cause symptoms in their hosts) that are measured in years rather than hours or days. Termed **slow-acting viruses,** these viruses infect the host and remain in a semidormant state for years, causing a slowly developing illness. HIV is the most recent deadly example of a slow-acting virus.

Drug treatment for viral infections is also limited. Drugs powerful enough to kill viruses generally kill the host cells, too, although some medications block stages in viral reproduction without damaging the host cells.

When exposed to certain viruses, the body produces a protein substance known as **interferon.** Interferon does not destroy the invading microorganisms but sets up a protective mechanism to aid healthy cells in their struggle against the invaders. Although interferon research is promising, it should be noted that not all viruses stimulate interferon production.

The Common Cold   In everyday life, perhaps no ailment is as bothersome as the common cold, with its irritating symptoms of runny nose, itchy eyes, and generally uncomfortable sensations. Colds are responsible for more days lost from work and more uncomfortable days spent at work than any other ailment.

Caused by any number of viruses (some experts claim there may be over 100 different viruses responsible), colds

---

Rickettsia   A small form of bacteria that live inside other living cells.

Viruses   Minute parasitic microbes that live inside another cell.

Incubation period   The time between exposure to a disease and the appearance of the symptoms.

Slow-acting viruses   Viruses having long incubation periods and causing slowly progressive symptoms.

Interferon   A protein substance produced by the body that aids the immune system by protecting healthy cells.

are **endemic** (always present to some degree) among people throughout the world. Current research indicates that otherwise healthy people carry cold viruses in their noses and throats most of the time. These viruses are held in check until the host's resistance is lowered. In the true sense of the word, it is possible to "catch" a cold—from the airborne droplets of another person's sneeze or from skin-to-skin or mucous membrane contact—though recent studies indicate that the hands are the greatest avenue for transmitting colds and other viruses. Obviously, then, covering your mouth with a tissue, handkerchief, or even the crook of your elbow when sneezing is better than covering it with your bare hand, particularly if you next use your hand to touch food, shake your friend's hand, or open a door.

Although numerous theories exist concerning how to "cure" the common cold, including taking megadoses of vitamin C, little hard evidence supports any of them. The best rule of thumb is to keep your resistance level high. Sound nutrition, adequate rest, stress reduction, and regular exercise appear to be the best bets in fighting off infection. Avoid people with newly developed colds (colds appear to be most contagious during the first 24 hours of onset). If you contract a cold, bed rest, plenty of fluids, and aspirin to relieve pain and discomfort are the tried-and-true remedies for adults. Children should not be given aspirin for colds or the flu because this could lead to development of *Reye's syndrome,* a potentially fatal disease. Several nonaspirin over-the-counter preparations are effective for alleviating certain symptoms.

Influenza   In otherwise healthy people, **influenza,** or flu, is usually not life-threatening. Symptoms, including aches and pains, nausea, diarrhea, fever, and coldlike ailments, generally pass quickly. (Figure 17.2 compares cold and flu symptoms.) However, in combination with other disorders, such as respiratory or heart disease, or among people over age 65 or under age 5, the flu can be very serious. Furthermore, scientists worry about the possibility of rare flu strains "jumping species" as is the case with the new avian or bird flu. If such a disease gets a foothold in the human population, there is concern that influenzal outbreaks may be similar in scope to earlier epidemics. Today, vaccines provide significant protection for vulnerable populations and these individuals receive the highest priority for annual flu shots.

Endemic   Describing a disease that is always present to some degree.

Influenza   A common viral disease of the respiratory tract.

Mononucleosis   A viral disease that causes pervasive fatigue and other long-lasting symptoms.

Hepatitis   A virally caused disease in which the liver becomes inflamed, producing symptoms such as fever, headache, and possibly jaundice.

To date, three major varieties of flu virus have been discovered, with many different strains existing within each variety. The A form of the virus is generally the most virulent, followed by the B and C varieties. If you contract one form of influenza you may develop immunity to it, but you will not necessarily be immune to other forms of the disease. Little can be done to treat flu patients once the infection has become established.

Some vaccines have proven effective against certain strains of flu virus, but they are totally ineffective against others. In spite of minor risks, it is recommended that people over age 65, pregnant women, people with heart or lung disease, and those with certain other illnesses be vaccinated. Because flu shots take two to three weeks to become effective, you should get these shots in the fall, before the flu season begins. In 2003, an inhaled vaccine called FluMist was released for use with healthy, nonpregnant adults up to age 49. Because the vaccine contains a weakened version of the live virus, people who receive the vaccine may pose a risk to anyone with a weakened immune system who is around them. More investigation into the risks are needed.[16]

In 2004, manufacturing problems caused a major shortage of flu vaccine. Even those at high risk were often unable to get vaccinated. As of this writing, the consequences of the shortage are unknown, but the crisis illustrates the importance of government oversight and regulation.

Infectious Mononucleosis   Initial symptoms of **mononucleosis,** or "mono," include sore throat, fever, headache, nausea, chills, and pervasive weakness or fatigue. As the disease progresses, lymph nodes may enlarge and jaundice, and spleen enlargement, aching joints, and body rashes may occur.

Theories on the transmission and treatment of mononucleosis are highly controversial. Caused by the *Epstein-Barr virus,* mononucleosis is readily detected through a *monospot test,* a blood test that measures the percentage of specific forms of white blood cells. Because many viruses are caused by transmission of body fluids, it was once believed that young people passed the disease on by kissing (hence its nickname, "the kissing disease"). Although this is still considered a possible cause, mononucleosis is not believed to be highly contagious. It does not appear to be easily contracted through normal, everyday personal contact. Multiple cases among family members are rare, as are cases between intimate partners.

Treatment of mononucleosis is often a lengthy process that involves bed rest, balanced nutrition, and medications. Gradually, the body develops immunity to the disease and the person returns to normal activity.

Hepatitis   One of the most highly publicized viral diseases is **hepatitis,** a virally caused inflammation of the liver. Hepatitis symptoms include fever, headache, nausea, loss of appetite, skin rashes, pain in the upper right abdomen, dark

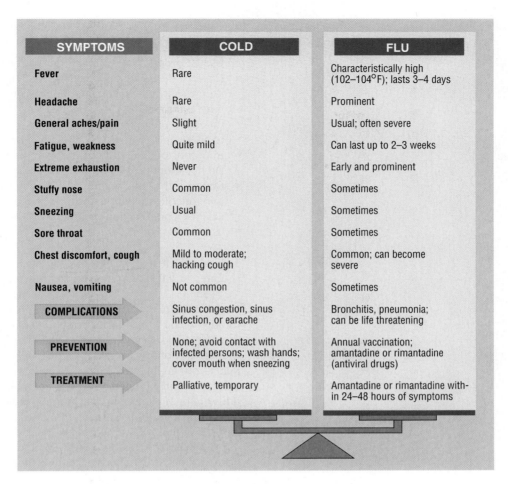

SYMPTOMS	COLD	FLU
Fever	Rare	Characteristically high (102–104°F); lasts 3–4 days
Headache	Rare	Prominent
General aches/pain	Slight	Usual; often severe
Fatigue, weakness	Quite mild	Can last up to 2–3 weeks
Extreme exhaustion	Never	Early and prominent
Stuffy nose	Common	Sometimes
Sneezing	Usual	Sometimes
Sore throat	Common	Sometimes
Chest discomfort, cough	Mild to moderate; hacking cough	Common; can become severe
Nausea, vomiting	Not common	Sometimes
COMPLICATIONS	Sinus congestion, sinus infection, or earache	Bronchitis, pneumonia; can be life threatening
PREVENTION	None; avoid contact with infected persons; wash hands; cover mouth when sneezing	Annual vaccination; amantadine or rimantadine (antiviral drugs)
TREATMENT	Palliative, temporary	Amantadine or rimantadine within 24–48 hours of symptoms

Figure 17.2
Is It a Cold or the Flu?

Source: Adapted from National Institute of Allergy and Infectious Diseases, "Is it a Cold or the Flu?" 2000.

yellow (with brownish tinge) urine, and the possibility of jaundice (yellowing of the whites of the eyes and the skin). In some regions of the United States and among certain segments of the population, hepatitis has reached epidemic proportions. Internationally, viral hepatitis is one of the most frequently reported diseases and a major contributor to acute and chronic liver disease, accounting for high morbidity and mortality. Currently, there are seven known forms of hepatitis, with hepatitis A, B, and C having the highest rate of incidence (Figure 17.3 on page 490). In the United States, hepatitis continues to be a major threat in spite of a safe blood supply and massive efforts at education about hand washing (hepatitis A) and safer sex (hepatitis B and C). Treatment of all the forms of viral hepatitis is somewhat limited. A proper diet, bed rest, and antibiotics that combat bacterial invaders, which may cause additional problems, are recommended.

Hepatitis A (HAV).   HAV is contracted from eating food or drinking water contaminated with human excrement. Today over 93,000 people in the United States are infected, typically through something in the household, sexual contact, day care attendance, or international travel.[17] Infected food handlers, people who ingest seafood from contaminated water, and those who use contaminated needles are also at risk. Fortunately, individuals infected with hepatitis A do not become chronic carriers, and vaccines for HAV are available.[18]

Hepatitis B (HBV).   This disease, one of the more virulent forms of hepatitis, is spread primarily via body fluids being shared through unprotected sex. However, it is also contracted via sharing needles when injecting drugs, through needlesticks on the job, or, in the case of a newborn baby, from an infected mother. Although 30 percent of those who are infected have no symptoms, symptoms can include jaundice, fatigue, abdominal pain, loss of appetite, nausea and vomiting, and joint pain.

One of the significant issues with HBV is that it is possible to become a chronic carrier and infect others. Approximately 90 percent of infants infected at birth, 30 percent of

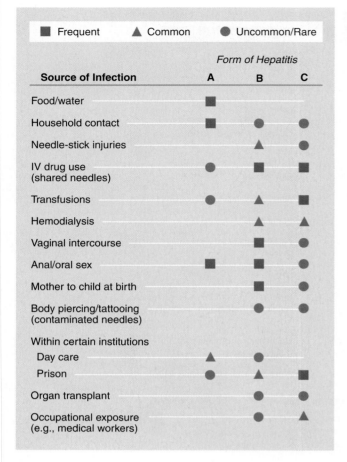

Source of Infection	Form of Hepatitis		
	A	B	C
Food/water	■		
Household contact	■	●	●
Needle-stick injuries		▲	●
IV drug use (shared needles)	●	■	■
Transfusions	●	▲	■
Hemodialysis		▲	▲
Vaginal intercourse		■	●
Anal/oral sex	■	■	●
Mother to child at birth		■	●
Body piercing/tattooing (contaminated needles)		●	●
Within certain institutions			
Day care	▲	●	
Prison	●	▲	■
Organ transplant		●	●
Occupational exposure (e.g., medical workers)		●	▲

Legend: ■ Frequent ▲ Common ● Uncommon/Rare

Figure 17.3
Ways in Which Hepatitis A, B, and C are Contracted

Source: American Liver Foundation, "Getting Hip to Hep: What You Should Know about Hepatitis A, B, and C," 2002. www .liverfoundation.org (75 Maiden Lane, Suite 603, New York, NY 10038, 1-800-GO-LIVER).

children infected between ages 1 and 5, and 6 percent of persons infected after age 5 develop chronic infections.[19] Currently more than 1.2 million people are chronic carriers.[20] Some 15 to 25 percent of all chronically infected people die from liver disease.

One of the fastest growing sexually transmitted infections in the United States, with over 300,000 new cases per year, HBV infection is more prevalent than HIV.[21] Most people recover within six months, although some become chronic carriers.

Fortunately, a vaccine for HBV has been available since 1982 and is now available on most college campuses for a modest cost. This means that HBV is one of the only vaccine-preventable sexually transmitted infections in society today. A combination series vaccine for HAV and HBV is also an option. If you work in a health care facility or plan to travel to regions of the world where HAV or HBV are prevalent, you should discuss the risk with your physician. Other ways to reduce the risk of HBV infection include:[22]

- Use latex condoms correctly every time you have sex. (*Note:* The efficacy of latex condoms in preventing infection with HBV is unknown, but their proper use may reduce transmission.)
- If you are pregnant, get a blood test for HBV; infants born to HBV-infected mothers should be given HBIG (hepatitis B immunoglobulin) and vaccine within 12 hours of birth.
- Do not shoot drugs, and never share needles.
- Consider the risks of tattoos and body piercings. Only go to reputable artists or piercers who follow established sterilization and infection control protocols.
- If you have had HBV, do not donate blood, organs, or tissues.
- If you are a health care or public safety worker, get vaccinated and follow routine barrier precautions.

Hepatitis C (HCV). This disease was spread primarily through blood transfusion or organ transplant prior to mass screenings that began in 1992. Since then, the more common means of transmission has been when blood or body fluids from an infected person follow a variety of routes to enter the body of a person who is not infected. HCV infections are on an epidemic rise in many regions of the world today. Currently, it is estimated that there are 150,000 new cases of hepatitis C in the United States each year, with over 4 million people infected.[23] Over 85 percent of those infected develop chronic infections; if the infection is left untreated, the person may develop cirrhosis of the liver, liver cancer, or liver failure. Liver failure due to chronic hepatitis C is the leading cause of liver transplants in the United States.[24] Some cases can be traced to blood transfusions or organ transplants.

Symptoms of HCV are similar to those of HBV, with jaundice, fatigue, abdominal pain, loss of appetite, and nausea occurring frequently. Dark urine is a hallmark symptom. The prognosis for a cure is bleak when compared to other forms of hepatitis. About 75 to 85 percent of those infected develop chronic HCV and 70 percent of those who become chronic carriers also develop chronic liver disease.[25]

Although there is no vaccine for HCV, one is currently being tested and may be available shortly.[26] In the absence of a vaccine, other prevention strategies include:

- Don't shoot drugs or share needles.
- Don't share personal care items that might have blood on them, such as razors or toothbrushes.
- If you are a health care worker or public safety worker, follow barrier precautions and avoid needlesticks.
- Avoid tattoos or piercings, or follow the precautions described for HBV.
- Although rare, HCV can be spread by sex. Use latex condoms.
- If you are HCV positive, don't donate blood, organs, or tissue.

Mumps Until 1968, mumps was a common viral disorder among children. That year a vaccine became available and the disease seemed to be largely under control, with reported cases declining from 80 per 100,000 people in 1968 to less than 2 per 100,000 people in 1984. Since then, mumps rates have risen steadily. Failure to vaccinate children due to public apathy, misinformation, and social and economic conditions are all responsible. Approximately one-half of all mumps infections are not apparent because they produce only minor symptoms. Many cases are never reported, so the actual incidence may be higher than indicated.

Typically, there is an incubation period of 16 to 18 days, followed by symptoms caused by the lodging of the virus in the glands of the neck. The most common symptom is the swelling of the parotid (salivary) glands; however, about one-third of all infected people never have this symptom. One of the greatest dangers associated with mumps is the potential for sterility in men who contract the disease in young adulthood. Some victims suffer hearing loss.

Chickenpox (HVZV) and Shingles Caused by the *herpes varicella zoster* virus (HVZV), chicken pox produces characteristic symptoms of fever and fatigue 13 to 17 days after exposure, followed by skin eruptions that itch, blister, and produce a clear fluid. The virus is present in these blisters for approximately one week. Symptoms are generally mild, and immunity to subsequent infection appears to be lifelong. (Some children experience more serious side effects, such as scarring, high fever, and other complications.) Although a vaccine for chicken pox is available, and all children should receive it, many parents incorrectly assume that the vaccine is not necessary. The failure to vaccinate means that many children still contract the disease.

Scientists believe that after the initial infection, the virus goes into permanent hibernation and, for most people, there are no further complications. For a small segment of the population, however, the virus may become reactivated. Blisters will develop, usually on only one side of the body and stopping abruptly at the midline. Cases in which the disease covers both sides of the body are far more serious. This disease, known as *shingles,* affects over 5 percent of the population each year. More than half the sufferers are over age 50.

Measles Technically referred to as *rubeola,* **measles** is a viral disorder that often affects young children. Symptoms, appearing about ten days after exposure, include an itchy rash and a high fever. **Rubella (German measles)** is a milder viral infection that is believed to be transmitted by inhalation, after which it multiplies in the upper respiratory tract and passes into the bloodstream. It causes a rash, especially on the upper extremities. It is not generally a serious health threat and usually runs its course in three to four days. The major exceptions to this rule are among newborns and pregnant women. Rubella can damage a fetus, particularly during the first trimester, creating a condition known as congenital rubella, in which the infant may be born blind, deaf,

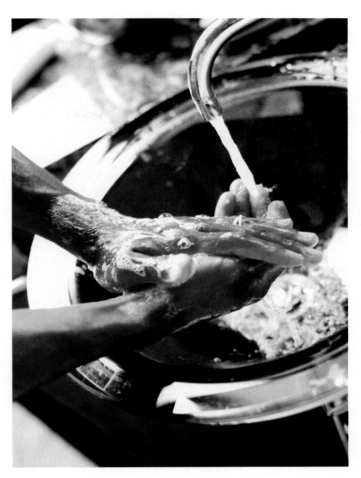

Washing your hands is a simple and effective way to stop the spread of pathogens.

retarded, or with heart defects. Immunization has reduced the incidence of both measles and rubella. Infections in children not immunized against measles can lead to fever-induced problems such as rheumatic heart disease, kidney damage, and neurological disorders.

Rabies The **rabies** virus infects many warm-blooded animals. Bats are believed to be **asymptomatic** (symptom-free) carriers. Their urine, which they spray when flying, contains the virus, and even the air of densely populated bat caves

---

Measles A viral disease that produces symptoms including an itchy rash and a high fever.

Rubella (German measles) A milder form of measles that causes a rash and mild fever in children and may cause damage to a fetus or a newborn baby.

Rabies A viral disease of the central nervous system; often transmitted through animal bites.

Asymptomatic Without symptoms, or symptom-free.

may be infectious. In most other hosts, the disease is extremely virulent and usually fatal. A characteristic behavior of rabid animals is the frenzied biting of other animals and people. Not only does this behavior cause injury, but it also spreads the virus through the infected animal's saliva. The most obvious symptoms of the disease are extreme activity in the cerebral region of the brain, rage, increased salivation, spasms in the pharynx (throat) muscles, extreme drive to find water, and the inability to swallow.

The incubation period for rabies is usually one to three months, although it may range from one week to one year. The disease may be fatal if not treated immediately with the rabies vaccine. Anyone bitten by an animal that could carry rabies should seek immediate medical attention and try to bring the animal along for testing.

Other Pathogens

Although the four other types of pathogens discussed in this section are given less attention due to space constraints, they also pose considerable risks to humans.

Fungi   Hundreds of species of **fungi,** multi- or unicellular primitive plants, inhabit our environment. Many fungi are useful, providing such foodstuffs as edible mushrooms and some cheeses. But some species of fungi can produce infections. *Candidiasis* (a vaginal yeast infection), athlete's foot, ringworm, and jock itch are examples of fungal diseases. Keeping the affected area clean and dry plus treatment with appropriate medications will generally bring prompt relief.

Protozoa   **Protozoa** are microscopic single-celled organisms that are generally associated with tropical diseases such as African sleeping sickness and malaria. Although these pathogens are prevalent in nonindustrialized countries, they are largely controlled in the United States. The most common protozoal disease in the United States is *trichomoniasis,* which we will discuss later in this chapter's section on sexually transmitted infections. A common waterborne protozoan disease in many regions of the country is *giardiasis.* Persons

who drink or are exposed to the *Giardia* pathogen may suffer intestinal pain and discomfort weeks after infection. Protection of water supplies is the key to prevention.

Parasitic Worms   **Parasitic worms** are the largest of the pathogens. Ranging in size from the relatively small pinworms typically found in children to the large tapeworms found in all warm-blooded animals, most parasitic worms are more a nuisance than a threat. Of special note today are the worm infestations associated with eating raw fish in Japanese sushi restaurants. Cooking fish and other foods to temperatures sufficient to kill the worms and their eggs can prevent this.

Prions   A **prion,** or unconventional virus, is a self-replicating, protein-based agent that can infect humans and other animals. Believed to be the underlying cause of spongiform diseases such as "mad cow disease," this agent systematically destroys brain cells. We will say more about prion-based diseases in the Emerging and Resurgent Diseases section later in this chapter.

Your Body's Defenses: Keeping You Well

Although all the pathogens just described pose a threat if they take hold in your body, the chances that they will do so are actually quite small. First, they must overcome a number of effective barriers, many of which were established in your body before you were even born.

Physical and Chemical Defenses: Your Body Responds

Perhaps our single most critical early defense system is the skin. Layered to provide an intricate web of barriers, the skin allows few pathogens to enter. **Enzymes,** complex proteins manufactured by the body that appear in body secretions such as sweat, provide additional protection, destroying microorganisms on skin surfaces by producing inhospitable pH levels. Normal body pH is 7.0, but enzymatic or biochemical changes may cause the body chemistry to become more acidic (pH of less than 7.0) or more alkaline (pH of more than 7.0). In either case, microorganisms that flourish at a selected pH will be weakened or destroyed as these changes occur. Only when cracks or breaks occur in the skin can pathogens gain easy access to the body.

The linings of the body provide yet another protection. Mucous membranes in the respiratory tract and other linings of the body trap and engulf invading organisms. *Cilia,* hairlike projections in the lungs and respiratory tract, sweep invaders toward body openings, where they are expelled. Tears, nasal secretions, ear wax, and other secretions found at body entrances contain enzymes designed to destroy or neutralize pathogens. Finally, any organism that manages to

Fungi   A group of plants that lack chlorophyll and do not produce flowers or seeds; several microscopic varieties are pathogenic.

Protozoa   Microscopic single-celled organisms.

Parasitic worms   The largest of the pathogens, most of which are more a nuisance than a threat.

Prions   A recently identified pathogen that infects humans and animals; a self-replicating protein-based agent that systematically destroys brain cells.

Enzymes   Organic substances that facilitate chemical reactions, some of which cause bodily changes and destruction of microorganisms.

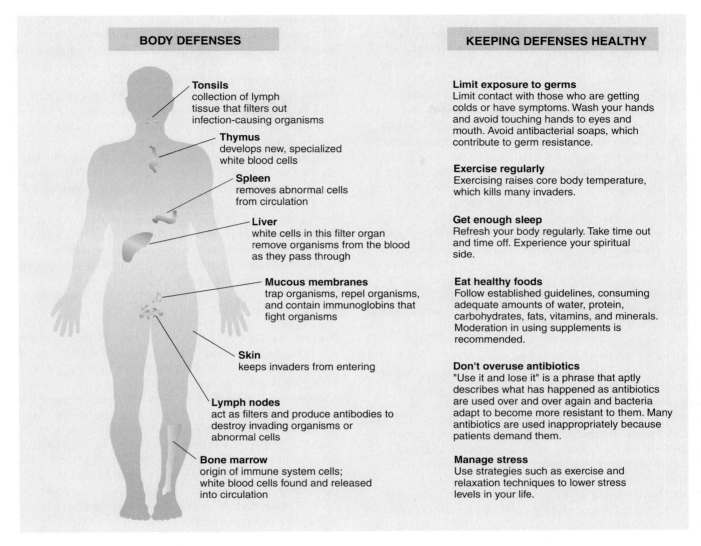

BODY DEFENSES

Tonsils
collection of lymph tissue that filters out infection-causing organisms

Thymus
develops new, specialized white blood cells

Spleen
removes abnormal cells from circulation

Liver
white cells in this filter organ remove organisms from the blood as they pass through

Mucous membranes
trap organisms, repel organisms, and contain immunoglobins that fight organisms

Skin
keeps invaders from entering

Lymph nodes
act as filters and produce antibodies to destroy invading organisms or abnormal cells

Bone marrow
origin of immune system cells; white blood cells found and released into circulation

KEEPING DEFENSES HEALTHY

Limit exposure to germs
Limit contact with those who are getting colds or have symptoms. Wash your hands and avoid touching hands to eyes and mouth. Avoid antibacterial soaps, which contribute to germ resistance.

Exercise regularly
Exercising raises core body temperature, which kills many invaders.

Get enough sleep
Refresh your body regularly. Take time out and time off. Experience your spiritual side.

Eat healthy foods
Follow established guidelines, consuming adequate amounts of water, protein, carbohydrates, fats, vitamins, and minerals. Moderation in using supplements is recommended.

Don't overuse antibiotics
"Use it and lose it" is a phrase that aptly describes what has happened as antibiotics are used over and over again and bacteria adapt to become more resistant to them. Many antibiotics are used inappropriately because patients demand them.

Manage stress
Use strategies such as exercise and relaxation techniques to lower stress levels in your life.

Figure 17.4
Bolstering Your Immune System

Source: Adapted from T. Mitchell, "Make Your Immune System Invincible," *USA Weekend,* January 7–9, 2000. Reprinted by permission of T. L. Mitchell, *USA Weekend* Health Editor.

breach these initial lines of defense faces a formidable specialized network of defenses thrown up by the immune system (Figure 17.4).

The Immune System: Your Body Fights Back

Immunity is a condition of being able to resist a particular disease by counteracting the substance that produces the disease. Any substance capable of triggering an immune response is called an **antigen.** An antigen can be a virus, a bacterium, a fungus, a parasite, or a tissue or cell from another individual. When invaded by an antigen, the body responds by forming substances called **antibodies** that are matched to that specific antigen much as a key is matched to a lock.

Antibodies belong to a mass of large molecules known as *immunoglobulins,* a group of nine chemically distinct protein substances, each of which plays a role in neutralizing, setting up for destruction, or actually destroying antigens.

Once an antigen breaches the body's initial defenses, the body begins a process of antigen analysis. It considers the size and shape of the invader, verifies that the antigen is not part of the body itself, and then produces a specific

Antigen Substance capable of triggering an immune response.

Antibodies Substances produced by the body that are individually matched to specific antigens.

antibody to destroy or weaken the antigen. This process, which is much more complex than described here, is part of a system called the *humoral immune response.* Humoral immunity is the body's major defense against many bacteria and bacterial toxins.

Cell-mediated immunity is characterized by the formation of a population of lymphocytes that can attack and destroy the foreign invader. These lymphocytes constitute the body's main defense against viruses, fungi, parasites, and some bacteria. Key players in this immune response are specialized groups of white blood cells known as *macrophages* (a type of phagocytic, or cell-eating, cell) and *lymphocytes,* other white blood cells found in the blood, lymph nodes, bone marrow, and certain glands.

Two forms of lymphocytes in particular, the *B lymphocytes* (B cells) and *T lymphocytes* (T cells), are involved in the immune response. B cells are named according to the area of the body in which they develop: most are manufactured in the soft tissue of the hollow shafts of the long bones. T cells, in contrast, develop and multiply in the thymus, a multilobed organ that lies behind the breastbone.

T cells assist the immune system in several ways. *Regulatory T cells* help direct the activities of the immune system and assist other cells, particularly B cells, to produce antibodies. Dubbed "helper T's," these cells are essential for activating B cells, other T cells, and macrophages. Another form of T cell, known as the "killer T's" or "cytotoxic T's," directly attacks infected or malignant cells. Killer T's enable the body to rid itself of cells that have been infected by viruses or transformed by cancer; they are also responsible for the rejection of tissue and organ grafts. The third type of T cells, "suppressor T's," turns off or suppresses the activity of B cells, killer T's, and macrophages. Suppressor T cells circulate in the bloodstream and lymphatic system, neutralizing or destroying antigens, enhancing the effects of the immune response, and helping to return the activated immune system to normal levels.

After a successful attack on a pathogen, some of the attacker T and B cells are preserved as *memory T and B cells,* enabling the body to quickly recognize and respond to subsequent attacks by the same kind of organism at a later time. Thus macrophages, T and B cells, and antibodies are the key factors in mounting an immune response.

Once people have survived certain infectious diseases, they become immune to those diseases, meaning that in all probability they will not develop them again. Upon subsequent attack by the disease-causing microorganisms, their memory T and B cells are quickly activated to come to their defense.

Referred pain   Pain that is present at one point, although the source of pain is elsewhere.

Vaccination   Inoculation with killed or weakened pathogens or similar, less dangerous antigens in order to prevent or lessen the effects of some disease.

Autoimmune Diseases   Although white blood cells and the antigen–antibody response generally work in our favor by neutralizing or destroying harmful antigens, the body sometimes makes a mistake and targets its own tissue as the enemy, builds up antibodies against that tissue, and attempts to destroy it. This is known as *autoimmune* disease (*auto* means "self"). Common autoimmune disorders are rheumatoid arthritis, lupus erythematosus, and myasthenia gravis, and are discussed further in Chapter 18.

In some cases, the antigen–antibody response completely fails to function. The result is a form of *immunodeficiency syndrome.* Perhaps the most dramatic case of this syndrome was the "bubble boy," a youngster who died in 1984 after living his short life inside a sealed-off environment designed to protect him from all antigens. A much more common immune system disorder is *acquired immunodeficiency syndrome (AIDS),* which we will discuss later in this chapter (page 511).

Fever

If an infection is localized, pus formation, redness, swelling, and irritation often occur. These symptoms indicate that the invading organisms are being fought systematically. Another indication is the development of a *fever,* or a rise in body temperature above the norm of 98.6°F. Fever frequently results from toxins secreted by pathogens that interfere with the control of body temperature. Although extremely elevated temperature is often harmful to the body, fever is believed to act as a form of protection. Raising body temperature by even one or two degrees provides an environment that destroys some disease-causing organisms. A fever also stimulates the body to produce more white blood cells, which destroy more invaders.

Pain

Although we do not usually think of pain as a defense mechanism, it is a response to injury, and it plays a valuable role in the body's response to invasion. Pain may be either direct, caused by the stimulation of nerve endings in an affected area, or referred, meaning it is present in one place although the source is elsewhere. An example of **referred pain** is the pain in the arm or jaw often experienced by someone having a heart attack. Most pain responses are accompanied by inflammation. Pain tends to be the earliest sign that an injury has occurred and often causes the person to slow down or stop the activity that was aggravating the injury, thereby protecting against further damage. Because it is often one of the first warnings of disease, persistent pain should not be overlooked or masked with short-term pain relievers.

Vaccines: Bolstering Your Immunity

Recall that once people have been exposed to a specific pathogen, subsequent attacks will activate their memory T and B cells, giving them immunity. This is the principle on which **vaccination** is based.

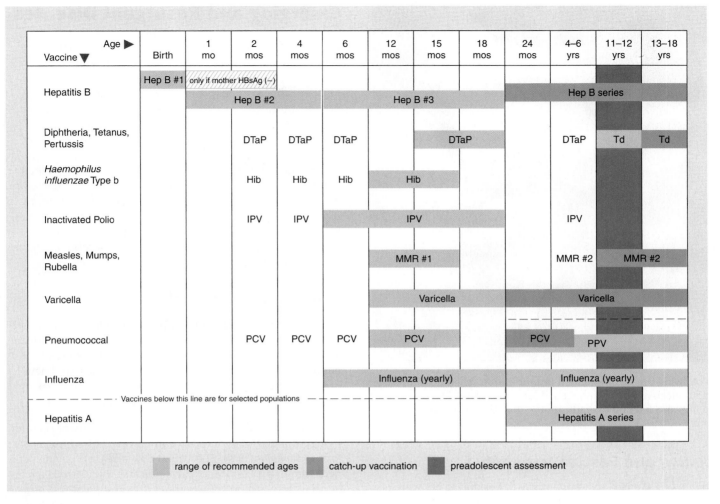

Age ▶ Vaccine ▼	Birth	1 mo	2 mos	4 mos	6 mos	12 mos	15 mos	18 mos	24 mos	4–6 yrs	11–12 yrs	13–18 yrs
Hepatitis B	Hep B #1	only if mother HBsAg (–)									Hep B series	
		Hep B #2			Hep B #3							
Diphtheria, Tetanus, Pertussis		DTaP	DTaP	DTaP		DTaP			DTaP	Td	Td	
Haemophilus influenzae Type b		Hib	Hib	Hib	Hib							
Inactivated Polio		IPV	IPV		IPV				IPV			
Measles, Mumps, Rubella					MMR #1				MMR #2	MMR #2		
Varicella					Varicella				Varicella			
Pneumococcal		PCV	PCV	PCV	PCV			PCV	PPV			
Influenza					Influenza (yearly)				Influenza (yearly)			
— — — — Vaccines below this line are for selected populations — — — —												
Hepatitis A									Hepatitis A series			

▨ range of recommended ages   ▨ catch-up vaccination   ▨ preadolescent assessment

Figure 17.5

Recommended Childhood and Adolescent Immunization Schedule, 2004

Note that there are important explanations and additions to these recommendations that should be consulted by checking the latest schedule (available on the Centers for Disease Control and Prevention website).

Source: Centers for Disease Control and Prevention, "Recommended Childhood and Adolescent Immunization Schedule, July–December 2004," 2004, www.cdc.gov/nip/recs/child-schedule.htm

A vaccine consists of killed or attenuated (weakened) versions of a disease-causing microorganism or an antigen that is similar to but less dangerous than the disease antigen. It is administered to stimulate the person's immune system to produce antibodies against future attacks—without actually causing the disease (or by causing a very minor case of the disease). Vaccines are given orally or by injection, and this form of artificial immunity is termed **acquired immunity,** in contrast to **natural immunity,** which a mother passes to her fetus via their shared blood supply.

Depending on the virulence of the organism, vaccines containing live, attenuated, or dead organisms are given for a variety of diseases. In some instances, if a person is already weakened by other health problems, vaccination may provoke an actual mild case of the disease so the decision as to whether an ill person should receive the vaccine should be discussed with that person's physician. Figure 17.5 shows the recommended schedule for childhood vaccinations.

Acquired immunity Immunity developed after birth in response to disease, vaccination, or exposure.

Natural immunity Immunity passed to a fetus by its mother.

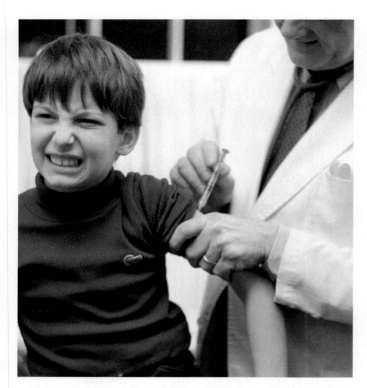

Following the recommended immunization schedule is an easy and effective way to protect a child from serious illnesses, while also helping to eradicate life-threatening disease.

Active and Passive Immunity

If you are exposed to an organism, either during daily life or through vaccination, you will eventually develop an active acquired immunity to that organism. Your body will produce its own antibodies, and, in most cases, you will not have to worry about subsequent exposures to that disease.

In some cases, however, the risks associated with contracting a disease are so severe that a person may not be able to wait the days or weeks that the body needs to produce antibodies. Also, in the event that resistance is terribly weakened as a result of cancer chemotherapy or other reasons, the body may be unable to produce its own antibodies. In this case, antibodies formed in another person or animal (called the donor) are often given. Termed **passive immunity,** this type of immunity is often short-lived but provides the necessary boost to get a person through a potentially critical period. Antibodies utilized for passive immunity are taken from *gamma globulins,* proteins synthesized from a donor's blood. A mother also confers passive immunity on her newborn baby through breastfeeding.

Passive immunity Antibodies formed in another person or animal, and then given to someone with a weakened immune system.

Emerging and Resurgent Diseases

Although our immune systems are remarkably adept at responding to challenges, they are threatened by an army of microbes that is so diverse, virulent, and insidious that the invaders appear to be gaining ground. Within the past decade, rates for infectious diseases have rapidly increased, particularly for reemerging diseases such as tuberculosis. This can be attributed to a combination of overpopulation, inadequate health care systems, increasing poverty, extreme environmental degradation, and drug resistance.[27] As international travel increases (over 1 million people per day cross international boundaries), with germs transported from remote regions to huge urban centers within hours, the likelihood of infection by microbes previously unknown on U.S. soil increases. Table 17.3 identifies major contributors to the emergence and resurgence of infectious diseases.

Tiny Microbes: Lethal Threats

Today's arsenal of antibiotics appears to be increasingly ineffective, with penicillin-resistant strains of diseases on the rise as microbes are able to outlast and outsmart even the best of our antibiotic weapons.[28] Old scourges are back, and new ones are emerging. See the New Horizons in Health box on page 498 that discusses increases in antibiotic resistance.

"Mad Cow Disease"   The American cattle industry is under new scrutiny, with the first confirmed case of *bovine spongiform encephalopthy* (BSE, or "mad cow disease") having been detected in late 2003. Evidence indicates that there is a relationship between ongoing outbreaks in Europe of BSE and a disease in humans known as *new variant Creutzfeldt-Jakob disease* (NvCJD).[29] Both disorders are invariably fatal brain diseases with unusually long incubation periods measured in years, and both are caused by unconventional transmittable agents known as *prions.*

BSE is thought to have been transmitted when cows were fed a protein-based substance (slaughterhouse leftovers from scrapie-infected sheep and BSE-infected cows) to help them put on weight and grow faster. (*Scrapie* is another prion-derived disease found in sheep.) Failure to treat this protein by-product sufficiently to kill the BSE organism allowed it to infect the cows. The disease is believed to be transmitted to humans through the meat of these slaughtered cows. The resultant variant of BSE in humans, NvCJD, is characterized by progressively worsening neurological damage and death.

As scientists continue to investigate this possible link, it should be noted that such a link has not yet been scientifically verified, and it is extremely unlikely that BSE would be a foodborne hazard in the United States.[30] People living in the United States who have developed the disease are believed to have been infected during international travel.

A related prion-caused disease similar to BSE, *chronic wasting disease*, has been found in deer. Studies are underway to investigate the implications of this disease for human health.

Table 17.3
Factors Contributing to Emergent/Resurgent Disease Spread and Possible Solutions

Contributing Factors	Possible Solutions
Hardier bugs: tiny size, adaptability, resistant strains, misuse of antibiotics	Increased pharmaceutical efforts, new drug development, selective use of new drugs; improved vaccination rates; funding of new research
Failure to prioritize public health initiatives on national level	Increased government funding; improved efforts aimed at prevention and intervention (Less than 1 percent of the federal budget goes to prevention programs.)
Explosive population growth: resource degradation, overcrowding, land use atrocities, increased urbanization	Population control, wise use of natural resources, environmental controls, reduced deforestation, and increased pollution prevention efforts
International travel	Education or risk reduction; restrictions related to unvaccinated populations; improved air quality and venting on commercial airlines
Human behaviors, particularly intravenous (IV) drug use and risky sexual behavior	Education about risky behaviors; incentives for improved behaviors; increased personal motivation
Vector management failures: widespread overuse/misuse of pesticides and antimicrobial agents that hasten resistance	Management of pesticide use; focus on pollution prevention; regulation; enforcement of laws
Food and water contamination; globalization of food supply and centralized processing	Control of population growth; animal controls; food controls; improved environmental legislation; food safety; pollution prevention
Complacency and apathy	Education—develop "we" mentality rather than "me" mentality
Poverty	Government support; international aid for vaccination programs, early diagnosis, and treatment; care for disadvantaged
War and mass refugee migration, famine, disasters	Government intervention; international aid
Aging of population	Support for prevention/intervention against controllable age-related health problems
Irrigation, deforestation, and reforestation projects that alter habitats of disease-carrying insects and animals	Improved techniques for conservation; responsible use of resources; policies and programs that protect environment
Increased human contact with tropical rainforests and other wilderness habitats that are reservoirs for insects and animals that harbor unknown infectious agents	Increased regulation to reduce human impact; more research to improve interactions between humans and environment

Sources: Author; information from Centers for Disease Control and Prevention, "Emerging Infectious Diseases: A Strategy for the 21st Century," 2001, www.cdc.gov/ncidod/emergplan

Dengue and Dengue Hemorrhagic Fever   Transmitted by mosquitoes, **dengue** viruses are the most widespread insect-borne viruses in the world. Today, dengue is found on most continents, and over one-half of all United Nations member states are threatened.[31] Dengue symptoms include flulike nausea, aches, and chronic fatigue and weakness. As urban areas become increasingly infected with mosquitoes, nearly 1.5 billion people worldwide, including about 600 million children, are at risk. Each year, it is estimated that more than 100 million people are infected, and over 8,000 die.[32] A more serious form of the disease, **dengue hemorrhagic fever,** can kill children in 6 to 12 hours, as the virus causes capillaries to leak and spill fluid and blood into surrounding tissue. Dengue is on the rise in the United States, largely due to increased international travel.

Ebola Hemorrhagic Fever (Ebola HF)   Another emerging disease, Ebola HF is a severe, often fatal disease in humans and nonhuman primates (monkeys, gorillas, and chimpanzees). Although much about Ebola is unknown, researchers believe that the virus is zoonotic (animal-borne) and normally occurs in animal hosts that are native to the African continent.[33] The

Dengue   A disease transmitted by mosquitoes; causes flulike symptoms.

Dengue hemorrhagic fever   A more serious form of dengue.

Antibiotic Resistance: What Doesn't Kill Them Makes Them Stronger

Imagine a world where people die from common colds, diarrhea, ear infections, and superficial cuts and infections. If this sounds like the stuff of science fiction or bioterrorism run amok, the facts indicate that such a scenario is not that outrageous. In fact, according to the World Health Organization, "People of the world may only have a decade or two to make use of many of the medicines presently available to stop infectious diseases before antimicrobial resistance begins to be a major threat to health." Either we develop entirely new classes of antibiotics at a previously unheard-of rate, or we face the inevitable truth about the dwindling effectiveness of penicillin and other antibiotics. Our health care system has become increasingly dependent on the availability and efficacy of antibiotics as a part of a $24.5 million industry designed to quickly treat bacterial infections.

RESISTANT INFECTIONS

Drug-resistant infectious agents—those that are not killed or inhibited by antimicrobial compounds—are an increasingly important public health concern. Tuberculosis, gonorrhea, malaria, and childhood ear infections are just a few of the diseases that have become difficult, if not impossible, to treat due to the emergence of drug-resistant pathogens. The Institute of Medicine, part of the National Academy of Sciences, has estimated that the annual cost of treating antibiotic-resistant infections in the United States may be as high as $30 billion. How serious is the problem? Consider the following facts:

- Strains of *Staphylococcus aureus* resistant to most antibiotics are endemic in many hospitals today. In some cities 31 percent of staph infections are resistant, and in nursing homes as many as 71 percent of staph infections defy traditional antibiotic regimens.
- *Streptococcus pneumoniae* causes thousands of cases of meningitis and pneumonia and 7 million cases of ear infections in the United States each year. Currently, about 30 percent of these cases are resistant to penicillin, the primary drug for treatment. Many penicillin-resistant strains are also resistant to other antibiotics.
- An estimated 300 to 500 million people worldwide are infected with parasites that cause malaria, and an estimated 700,000 to 2.7 million people die each year from the disease. Resistance to chloroquine, once a widely used and highly effective treatment, is now found in most regions of the world, with other treatments losing their effectiveness at alarming rates.
- Strains of multidrug-resistant tuberculosis have emerged over the last decade and pose a particular threat to HIV-positive individuals.
- Diarrheal diseases cause almost 3 million deaths per year—mostly in developing countries where resistant forms of *Campylobacter, Shigella, Escherichia coli, Vibrio cholerae,* and *Salmonella* food poisoning have emerged. In some areas, as much as 50 percent of the *Campylobacter* cases are resistant to Cipro, the most effective treatment. A potentially deadly "superbug" known as *Salmonella enterica* Typhimurium, resistant to most antibiotics, has appeared in Europe, Canada, and the United States.
- Resistant fungal diseases such as *Pneumocystis carinii* pneumonia are on the rise internationally.
- Viral resistance to HIV treatment has meant that many drugs quickly lose their effectiveness in treating HIV.

In the battle between drugs and bugs, the bugs are clearly scoring some big wins.

WHY IS ANTIMICROBIAL RESISTANCE GROWING?

Although the actual mechanisms are complex, antibiotics typically wipe out certain bacteria that are susceptible to them.

---

virus is spread via direct contact with blood and/or secretions and may be aerosol disseminated (airborne). With an incubation period of 2 to 21 days, the course of the disease is quick and characterized by fever, headache, joint and muscle aches, sore throat, and weakness, followed by diarrhea, vomiting, and stomach pain. A rash, red eyes, hiccups, and internal and external bleeding often occur in later phases.[34] Although there have been no known cases of human transmission in the United States, several outbreaks have occurred in various regions of Africa. One outbreak in 1995 in Zaire killed 245 of the 316 people infected, forcing strict government-enforced quarantine of the entire region. Subsequent infections in other regions of the world have caused increasing concern in the global community. Fortunately, Ebola is not as prevalent worldwide as dengue fever. See the New Horizons in Health box on page 500 for information on another virus originating in Africa: West Nile virus.

Cryptosporidium In 1993, the intestinal parasite *Cryptosporidium* infected the municipal water supply of Milwaukee, Wisconsin. The result was the largest waterborne coccidian protozoan disease outbreak ever recognized in this country, causing many deaths and sickening hundreds of thousands of people. Exactly how the water supply became infected remains in question; since humans, birds, and other animals can carry the infective agent, there are many possible routes.

However, when used improperly, the antibiotics kill the weak bacteria and leave the strongest versions to thrive and replicate. Because bacteria can swap genes with one another under the right conditions, drug-resistant, hardy germs can share their resistance mechanisms with other germs. Eventually, an entire colony of resistant bugs grows and passes on its resistance traits to new generations of bacteria.

In developing countries, resistance commonly stems from underuse of drugs. For example, some patients may begin an antibiotic regimen, start to feel better, and stop taking the drug to save money by using the drug another time. The surviving bacteria then build immunity to the drugs used to treat them. In the United States, patients have historically failed to comply with their antibiotic regimens, leaving pills in the bottle that should have been used to kill all remnants of the bacteria. Also, doctors have overused antibiotics; the CDC estimates that one-third of the 150 million prescriptions written each year are unnecessary, resulting in bacterial strains that are tougher than the drugs used to fight them.

While patient noncompliance and doctor overuse are believed to be the most significant contributors to our epidemic of resistant bacteria, other factors are also contributors.

- Overuse of antibiotics in food production has contributed to increased drug resistance. About 50 percent of antibiotic production today is used to treat sick animals and encourage growth in livestock and poultry. Although research is only in its infancy, many believe that ingesting meats and animal products that are rich in antibiotics may actually contribute to antibiotic-resistance in humans.
- Another area of concern is the American obsession with cleanliness. One need only look at the antibacterial soaps, cleaning products, and other products on the shelves to know that personal and home cleaning products are the rage. Just how much these soaps and other products contribute to overall resistance is also in question; as with antibiotics, the germs these products do not kill may become stronger than before.

REDUCING THE RISK OF ANTIMICROBIAL RESISTANCE

What can be done to slow the growth of resistant organisms? Individual and community actions include the following:

- Enact policies that severely restrict the use of antibiotics, growth hormones, and other products in our food supply
- Buy foods and products that are antibiotic-free
- Motivate people to take medications as prescribed and to finish all medications: killing the bugs the first time, all the time
- Encourage doctors to prescribe antibiotics only when absolutely necessary and to educate patients about their use
- Encourage consumers not to pressure doctors to give them antibiotics for their ailments
- Educate consumers about the fact that germs are not inherently bad and that exposure to many of them helps our immune systems develop arsenals capable of fighting pathogens
- Educate people that washing their hands with a good flow of water and regular soap for a bit longer time than normal is better than using antibacterial soaps
- Encourage pharmaceutical companies to develop, test, and market newer classes of antibiotics to keep up with growing resistance

Sources: National Institute of Allergy and Infectious Diseases, "Fact Sheet: Antimicrobial Resistance," 2004, www.niaid.nih.gov /factsheets/antimicro.htm; National Center for Infectious Diseases, "Malaria Fact Sheet," 2004, www.cdc.gov/malaria/facts.htm; S. B. Levy, *The Antibiotic Paradox: How the Misuse of Antibiotics Destroys Their Curative Powers* (Cambridge, MA: Perseus Publishing, 2002); Harvard Health Letter, "Overdoing Antibiotics," 2002, www.health.harvard.edu; L. Bren, "Battle of the Bugs: Fighting Antibiotic Resistance," *FDA Consumer* 36, no. 4 (October 31, 2002), 28–36.

Escherichia coli O157:H7 *E. coli* O157:H7, as it is commonly referred to, is one of over 170 types of *E. coli* bacteria that can infect humans. While most *E. coli* organisms are harmless and live in the intestines of healthy animals and humans, *E. coli* O157:H7 produces a lethal toxin and can cause severe illness or death.

E. coli O157:H7 can live in the intestines of healthy cattle and then contaminate food products at slaughterhouses. Eating ground beef that is rare or undercooked is a common way of becoming infected (see Chapter 8 for more information on safe food handling practices). Drinking unpasteurized milk or juice and drinking or swimming in sewage-contaminated water or public pools can also cause infection via ingestion of feces that contain *E. coli*. Several children were infected at a fair in Oregon when they petted infected farm animals and did not wash their hands.

A symptom of infection is nonbloody diarrhea, usually two to eight days after exposure; however, asymptomatic cases have been noted. Children and older adults are particularly vulnerable to such serious side effects as kidney failure, as are persons whose immune systems have been weakened by other diseases.

While *E. coli* organisms continue to pose threats to public health, strengthened regulations on the cooking of meat and regulation of chlorine levels in pools have helped. Recent findings indicate that eliminating grains from the diet of cattle in the days prior to slaughter may reduce the growth of *E. coli* in their stomachs.

New Scourge on the Land: West Nile Virus and Its Cousins

Until 1999, few Americans had heard of *West Nile virus (WNV)*, a disease that was endemic in many other regions of the world. However, when thousands of birds (primarily crows) began to drop from the skies in the eastern United States, scientists from the Centers for Disease Control and Prevention (CDC) were quick to note that it looked a lot like WNV was to blame. They weren't sure that it really was this disease; hence, the original designation of West Nile-*like* virus. Subsequent testing confirmed that the virus actually was the authentic disease and today the "look-alike" designation has been dropped. Attention to the disease intensified as horses, dogs, cats, and other birds throughout the eastern and central United States were stricken by the disease and peaked when the first human cases were confirmed. In 1999, 62 cases of severe disease were confirmed; 7 deaths resulted from this infection in New York state. Today, the disease has crossed the Mississippi and only a few states remain disease-free (see map).

TRANSMISSION

West Nile virus is spread by the bite of an infected mosquito of the *Culex* species. The basic transmission cycle starts with the mosquitoes, which feed on infected birds. (Over 110 species of birds are known to be infected.) Although birds, particularly crows and jays, can die when infected, most survive, and the virus then circulates freely between the birds and mosquitoes in an ongoing cycle of infection. When a virus-free mosquito feeds on the bird, it contracts the virus. The virus is located in the mosquito's salivary glands, so when the insect bites a human or animal for a blood meal, it injects the virus into its victim, where the virus multiplies and causes illness.

As of this date, there is no evidence to suggest that West Nile virus can be spread from person to person. However, the CDC has reported a suspected case of a baby contracting the disease from breast-feeding. Cases where people may have become infected from organ donation or blood transfusion are currently under investigation.

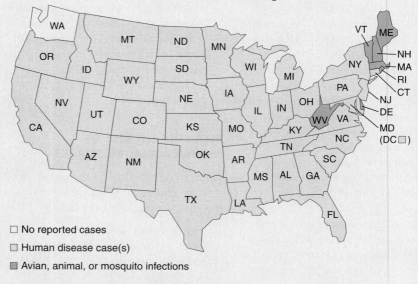

□ No reported cases

□ Human disease case(s)

▨ Avian, animal, or mosquito infections

West Nile Virus in the United States, 2004

Source: Centers for Disease Control and Prevention, "West Nile Virus—Statistics, Surveillance, and Control," 2004, www.cdc.gov/ncidod/dvbid/westnile

---

Cholera   Cholera, an infectious disease transmitted through fecal contamination of food or water supplies, has been rare in the United States for most of this century. Recent epidemic outbreaks in the Western hemisphere (over 900,000 cases), however, have started to affect the United States. One theory of how cholera is introduced into distant regions of the world is that ships from endemic areas release contaminated bilge water into port towns, contaminating local shellfish.[35] Efforts to control cholera may be increasingly difficult as international travel and trade increase.

Hantavirus   Transmitted via rodent feces, this virus was responsible for many deaths in the desert southwestern United States in 1994 before experts were able to identify the culprit.

Victims were believed to have come into contact with this organism through breathing the virus-laden dust in rodent-infested homes. Within hours, victims' lungs filled with fluid and they experienced respiratory collapse and died. Today, cases of hantavirus have been noted in over 20 states, and vaccines are being developed to counteract it.

Listeriosis   Caused by a potent bacterium found in plants and animals, listeriosis has proved fatal in many cases in recent years. Early symptoms begin with mild or low fever and progress to headache and inflammation of the brain. Those who are immunocompromised and pregnant women are at greatest risk. Foods that are improperly cooked or that don't require cooking (such as luncheon meats) are particularly

SYMPTOMS AND TREATMENT

Most people who become infected with West Nile virus will have either mild symptoms or none at all. However, on rare occasions, West Nile virus infection can result in severe and sometimes fatal illness. When symptoms appear, they include fever, headache, and body aches, often with skin rash and swollen lymph glands. More severe symptoms include a form of encephalitis, or inflammation of the brain, that can cause high fever, neck stiffness, stupor, disorientation, coma, tremors, convulsions, muscle weakness, paralysis, and death.

Unfortunately, there is no vaccine on the horizon for WNV and no specific antiviral medication. For severe symptoms, hospitalization with IV fluids, breathing management and respiratory support, and prevention of secondary infections are necessary.

If you think you have the disease, see your doctor as soon as possible.

PREVENTION

Avoiding WNV infection means avoiding mosquito bites. Follow these strategies:

- Apply mosquito repellents containing DEET (diethyl toluamide) when you're outdoors. Note that supersprays with high percentages of DEET are generally not any more effective than milder forms and may cause side effects.

- When possible, wear long-sleeved clothing and long pants treated with repellents. Do not apply repellents containing permethrin directly to exposed skin.
- Consider staying indoors at dawn, dusk, and in the early evening, which are peak mosquito feeding times.
- Limit mosquito egg laying areas by getting rid of any standing water sources around the home. One flower pot with water standing in it may be home to thousands of mosquitoes.
- Work with your local government to institute some form of mosquito control program in your neighborhood.

OTHER VIRUSES

Although West Nile virus has captured the media's attention for now, it is important to note that we are just in the early stages of being infected with several marauding viruses that may hop the world's oceans and infect America. Whether they arrive by bird, plane, ship, or food source, three noteworthy diseases are likely invaders and have public health officials worried:

Japanese Encephalitis (JE)

Related to St. Louis encephalitis, JE is the leading cause of viral encephalitis in Asia, infecting 35,000 to 60,000 people each year and killing about 4,000. It is far more severe than West Nile virus. Symptoms include fever, headache, neck stiffness, and disorientation, with progression to convulsions and coma. Mosquitoes transmit it after feeding on infected birds or pigs, and then biting humans or other animals. So far the mosquito that spreads this disease has not been found in the United States, but experts fear that other mosquitoes can adapt and carry the virus if it does arrive. There is a preventive vaccine available.

Rift Valley Fever (RVF)

Like West Nile virus, Rift Valley fever was first found in Africa. Mosquitoes help spread it both by biting people and animals and by laying infected eggs that are ingested by livestock. It has many varying symptoms, including severe headaches and eye pain. About 10 percent of victims have lasting eye damage, and about 1 percent die. There is no vaccine.

Ross River Fever (RRF)

A relatively mild mosquito-borne virus that causes fever and joint pains, RRF has infected thousands in Australia and can cause lethargy that often lasts more than three months and sometimes more than two years. No vaccine is available.

Source: Centers for Disease Control and Prevention, "West Nile Virus," 2004, www.cdc.gov /ncidod/dvbid/westnile/index.htm

---

susceptible. New regulations that require strict monitoring of food processing plants should help reduce the risk of listeria infection.

Malaria In the 1960s, after massive international efforts, malaria, a vectorborne disease transmitted by the *Anopheles* mosquito, seemed to be on the decline. However, today there has been a major resurgence of malaria outbreaks, particularly in Africa, Asia, and Latin America. Currently, the malaria prevention effort is focused on personal protection against bites rather than elimination of mosquitoes.

Bioterrorism: The New Global Threat The idea of using infectious microorganisms as weapons is not new. In fact, during the English wars with American Indians, blankets impregnated with scabs from smallpox patients were traded to Native Americans in hopes of causing disease.[36] In the 1980s, a large community outbreak of salmonellosis in Oregon was believed to originate from intentional contamination of salad bars in multiple restaurants, carried out by followers of an extremist religious group.[37]

The threat of delivering a lethal load of anthrax or other deadly microorganisms in the warheads of missiles or by a single person is a topic of much discussion among today's world leaders, particularly after the cases of anthrax delivered via the mail following the September 11, 2001, terrorist attacks. For a complete listing of biological threats considered to pose the greatest risk, see the New Horizons in Health box on bioterrorism in Chapter 4.

Table 17.4
Common Sexually Transmitted Infections

STI	Incidence (Estimated Number of New Cases per Year)	Prevalence (Estimated Number of People Currently Infected)
Chlamydia	3 million	2 million
Gonorrhea	650,000	Not available*
Syphilis	70,000	Not available*
Herpes	1 million	45 million
Human papillomavirus (HPV)	5.5 million	20 million
Hepatitis B	120,000	417,000
Trichomoniasis	5 million	Not available*

*No recent surveys on national prevalence for gonorrhea, syphilis, or trichomoniasis have been conducted.

Source: Centers for Disease Control and Prevention, "Tracking the Hidden Epidemics: Trends in STDs in the United States—2002," www.cdcnpin.org/std.start.htm

Necrotizing Fasciitis ("Flesh-Eating Strep") The stuff of science fiction, this organism caused hysteria in the United States in 1994 as hospital patients fell prey to an illness that slowly invaded and killed tissue in healing wounds. The culprit? An otherwise treatable form of streptococcus that had suddenly become the victor in the delicate war between antibiotics and microbes. In this case, our then-current arsenal of drugs was too weak to fight the microbe, until a newer antibiotic was found to stop it. There are 500 to 1,500 cases of necrotizing fasciitis in the United States each year. They range in severity in their effects. [38]

Sexually Transmitted Infections

Sexually transmitted infections (STIs) have been with us since our earliest recorded days on earth. Today, there are more than 20 known types of STIs. Once referred to as "venereal diseases" and then "sexually transmitted diseases," the most current terminology is more reflective of the number and types of these communicable diseases. More virulent strains and more antibiotic-resistant forms spell trouble for at-risk populations in the days ahead.

STIs affect men and women of all backgrounds and socioeconomic levels. The most recent report issued by the Centers for Disease Control and Prevention (CDC) indicated that annual new occurrences of STIs increased by over 3.5 million from 1988 to 1999.[39] Although exact numbers are not available for each STI, the number of cases did increase for several in 2001 after years of decline. Syphilis was among those showing the greatest increase.[40]

In the United States alone, an estimated 15.3 million new cases of STIs are reported each year. Table 17.4 gives an overview of the reported cases of selected STIs. Additional facts to note include the following:

- More than 65 million people are currently living with an incurable STI.[41]
- Two-thirds of all STIs occur in people 25 years of age or younger.[42]
- One in four new STI infections occurs in teenagers.[43]
- One in five Americans has genital herpes, with 500,000 new cases each year[44]

STIs disproportionately affect women, minorities, and infants. In addition, STIs are most prevalent in teens and young adults.[45] In 2003, approximately 47 percent of high school students had never engaged in sexual intercourse, and 14 percent had had four or more sex partners. Some 37 percent did not use a condom in their most recent sexual encounter.[46]

Early symptoms of an STI are often mild and unrecognizable (Figure 17.6). Left untreated, some of these infections can have grave consequences, such as sterility, blindness, central nervous system destruction, disfigurement, and even death. Infants born to mothers carrying the organisms for these infections are at risk for a variety of health problems.

As with many communicable diseases, much of the pain, suffering, and anguish associated with STIs can be eliminated through education, responsible action, simple preventive strategies, and prompt treatment. STIs can happen to anyone, but they won't if you take appropriate precautions when you decide to engage in a sexual relationship.

Possible Causes: Why Me?

Several reasons have been proposed to explain the present high rates of STIs. The first relates to the moral and social stigma associated with these infections. Shame and embarrassment often keep infected people from seeking treatment. Unfortunately, these people usually continue to be sexually active, thereby infecting unsuspecting partners. People who

---

Sexually transmitted infections (STIs) Infectious diseases transmitted via some form of intimate, usually sexual, contact.

are uncomfortable discussing sexual issues may also be less likely to use and ask their partners to use condoms to protect against STIs and pregnancy.

Another reason proposed for the STI epidemic is our casual attitude about sex. Bombarded by media hype that glamorizes easy sex, many people take sexual partners without considering the consequences. Others are pressured into sexual relationships they don't really want. Generally, the more sexual partners a person has, the greater the risk for contracting an STI. Evaluate your own attitude about STIs by completing the Assess Yourself box.

Ignorance—about the infections, their symptoms, and the fact that someone can be asymptomatic but still be infected—is also a factor. A person who is infected but symptom-free can unknowingly spread an STI to an unsuspecting partner, who may in turn ignore or misinterpret any symptoms. By the time either partner seeks medical help, he or she may have infected several others.

Modes of Transmission

Sexually transmitted infections are generally spread through some form of intimate sexual contact. Sexual intercourse, oral–genital contact, hand–genital contact, and anal intercourse are the most common modes of transmission. More rarely, pathogens for STIs are transmitted mouth to mouth or through contact with fluids from body sores. Although each STI is a different infection caused by a different pathogen, all STI pathogens prefer dark, moist places, especially the mucous membranes lining the reproductive organs. Most of them are susceptible to light, excess heat, cold, and dryness, and many die quickly on exposure to air. (The toilet seat is not a likely breeding ground for most STIs!) Although most STIs are passed on by sexual contact, other kinds of close contact, such as sleeping on sheets used by someone who has pubic lice, may also infect you.

Like other communicable infections, STIs have both pathogen-specific incubation periods and periods of time during which transmission is most likely, called periods of communicability.

Chlamydia

Chlamydia, a disease that often presents no symptoms, tops the list of the most commonly reported infections in the United States. Chlamydia infects about 2.8 million people annually in the United States, the majority of them women.[47] Public health officials believe that the actual number of cases is probably higher because these figures represent only those cases reported. College students account for over 10 percent of infections, and these numbers seem to be increasing yearly.

The name of the disease is derived from the Greek verb *chlamys,* meaning "to cloak," because, unlike most bacteria, chlamydia can live and grow only inside other cells. Although many people classify chlamydia as either

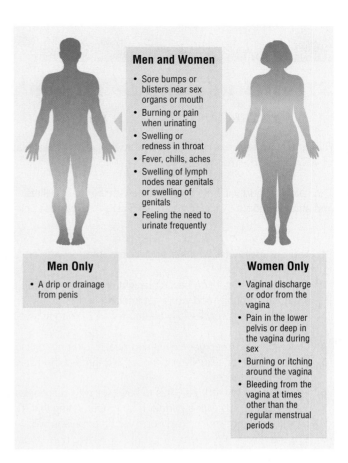

Figure 17.6
Signs or Symptoms of Sexually Transmitted Infections (STIs)
In their early stages, many STIs may be asymptomatic or have such mild symptoms that they are easy to overlook.

nonspecific or *nongonococcal urethritis (NGU),* a person may have NGU without having the organism for chlamydia.

In males, early symptoms may include painful and difficult urination, frequent urination, and a watery, puslike discharge from the penis. Symptoms in females may include a yellowish discharge, spotting between periods, and occasional spotting after intercourse. However, many chlamydia victims display no symptoms and therefore do not seek help until the disease has done secondary damage. Females are especially likely to be asymptomatic; over 70 percent do not realize they have the disease until secondary damage occurs.

The secondary damage resulting from chlamydia is serious in both genders. Men can suffer injury to the prostate gland, seminal vesicles, and bulbourethral glands, as well as arthritis-like symptoms and damage to the blood vessels and

Chlamydia   Bacterially caused STI of the urogenital tract.

STI Attitude and Belief Scale

myhealthlab

Fill out this assessment online at www.aw-bc.com/myhealthlab or www.aw-bc.com/donatelle

The following quiz will help you evaluate whether your beliefs and attitudes about STIs lead you to take risks that increase your risk of infection. Indicate that you believe the following items are true or false by marking the appropriate column. Then consult the answer key that follows.

	True	False
1. You can usually tell whether someone is infected with an STI, especially HIV infection.	❑	❑
2. Chances are that if you haven't caught an STI by now, you probably have a natural immunity and won't get infected in the future.	❑	❑
3. A person who is successfully treated for an STI needn't worry about getting it again.	❑	❑
4. So long as you keep yourself fit and healthy, you needn't worry about STIs.	❑	❑
5. The best way for sexually active people to protect themselves from STIs is to practice safer sex.	❑	❑
6. The only way to catch an STI is to have sex with someone who has one.	❑	❑
7. Talking about STIs with a partner is so embarrassing that it's better not to raise the subject and instead hope the other person will.	❑	❑
8. STIs are mostly a problem for people who have numerous sex partners.	❑	❑
9. You don't need to worry about contracting an STI so long as you wash yourself thoroughly with soap and hot water immediately after sex.	❑	❑
10. You don't need to worry about AIDS if no one you know has ever come down with it.	❑	❑
11. When it comes to STIs, it's all in the cards. Either you're lucky or you're not.	❑	❑
12. The time to worry about STIs is when you come down with one.	❑	❑
13. As long as you avoid risky sexual practices, such as anal intercourse, you're pretty safe from STIs.	❑	❑
14. The time to talk about safer sex is before any sexual contact occurs.	❑	❑
15. A person needn't be concerned about an STI if the symptoms clear up on their own in a few weeks.	❑	❑

SCORING KEY

1. *False.* While some STIs have telltale signs, such as the appearance of sores or blisters on the genitals or disagreeable genital odors, others do not. Several STIs, such as chlamydia, gonorrhea (especially in women), internal genital warts, and even HIV infection in its early stages, cause few if any obvious signs or symptoms. You often cannot tell whether your partner is infected with an STI. Many of the nicest-looking and well-groomed people carry STIs, often unknowingly. The only way to know whether a person is infected with HIV is by means of an HIV-antibody test.

2. *False.* If you practice unprotected sex and have not contracted an STI to this point, count your blessings. The thing about good luck is that it eventually runs out.

3. *False.* Sorry. Successful treatment does not render immunity against reinfection. You still need to take precautions to avoid reinfection, even if you have had an STI in the past and were successfully treated. If you answered true to this item, you're not alone. About one in five college students polled in a recent survey of more than 5,500 college students across Canada believed that a person who gets an STI cannot get it again.

4. *False.* Even people in prime physical condition can be felled by the tiniest of microbes that cause STIs. Physical fitness is no protection against these microscopic invaders.

5. *True.* If you are sexually active, practicing safer sex is the best protection against contracting an STI.

6. *False.* STIs can also be transmitted through nonsexual means, such as by sharing contaminated needles or, in some cases, through contact with disease-causing organisms on towels and bedsheets.

7. *False.* Because of the social stigma attached to STIs, it's understandable that you may feel embarrassed about raising the subject with your partner—but don't let embarrassment prevent you from taking steps to protect your own and your partner's welfare.

8. *False.* While it stands to reason that people who are sexually active with numerous partners stand a greater chance that one of their sexual partners will carry an STI, all it takes is one infected partner to pass along an STI to you, even if he or she is the only partner you've had or even if the two of you had sex only once. STIs are a potential problem for anyone who is sexually active.

9. *False.* While washing your genitals immediately after sex may have some limited protective value, it is no substitute for practicing safer sex.

10. *False.* You can never know whether you may be the first among your friends and acquaintances to become infected. Moreover, symptoms of HIV infection may not appear for years after initial infection with the virus, so you may have sexual contacts with people who are infected but don't know it and who are capable of passing along the virus to you. You in turn may then pass it along to others, whether or not you are aware of any symptoms.

11. *False.* Nonsense. While luck may play a part in determining whether you have sexual contact with an infected partner, you can significantly reduce your risk of contracting an STI.

12. *False.* The time to start thinking about STIs (thinking helps, but worrying only makes you more anxious than you need be) is now, not after you have contracted an infection. Some STIs, like herpes and AIDS, cannot be cured. The only real protection you have against them is prevention.

13. *False.* Any sexual contact between the genitals, between the genitals and the anus, or between the mouth and genitals, is risky if one of the partners is infected with an STI.

14. *True.* Unfortunately, too many couples wait until they have commenced sexual relations to have "a talk." By then it may already be too late to prevent the transmission of an STI. The time to talk is before *any* intimate sexual contact occurs.

15. *False.* Several STIs, notably syphilis, HIV infection, and herpes, may produce initial symptoms that clear up in a few weeks. But while the early symptoms may subside, the infection is still at work within the body and requires medical attention. Also, as noted previously, the infected person is capable of passing along the infection to others, regardless of whether noticeable symptoms were ever present.

INTERPRETING YOUR SCORE

Add up the number of items you got right. The higher your score, the lower your risk. The lower your score, the greater your risk. A score of 13 correct or better may indicate that your attitudes toward STIs would probably decrease your risk of contracting them. Yet even one wrong response on this test may increase your risk of contracting an STI. You should also recognize that attitudes have little effect on behavior unless they are carried into action. Knowledge alone isn't sufficient to protect yourself from STIs. You need to ask yourself how you are going to put knowledge into action by changing your behavior to reduce your chances of contracting an STI.

MAKE IT HAPPEN!

Use the results of this self-assessment to begin your behavior change program. Follow the steps and use the examples on page 519 to complete your Behavior Change Contract, and use these resources to take action.

Source: From Jeffrey S. Nevid, *Choices: Sex in the Age of STDs*, 2nd ed. (Boston: Allyn & Bacon, 1998). © Pearson Education. Reprinted by permission.

---

heart. In women, chlamydia-related inflammation can injure the cervix or uterine tubes, causing sterility, and damage the inner pelvic structure, leading to pelvic inflammatory disease (PID). If an infected woman becomes pregnant, she has a high risk for miscarriage and stillbirth. Chlamydia may also be responsible for one type of **conjunctivitis**, an eye infection that affects not only adults but also infants, who can contract the disease from an infected mother during delivery. Untreated conjunctivitis can cause blindness.

If detected early, chlamydia is easily treatable with antibiotics such as tetracycline, doxycycline, or erythromycin.

In most cases, treatment is successfully completed in two to three weeks. Unfortunately, chlamydia tests are not a routine part of many health clinics' testing procedures. Usually a person must specifically request a chlamydia check.

> **Conjunctivitis** Serious inflammation of the eye caused by any number of pathogens or irritants; can be caused by STDs such as chlamydia.

Pelvic Inflammatory Disease (PID)

Pelvic inflammatory disease (PID) is a term used to describe a number of infections of the uterus, uterine tubes, and ovaries. Although PID often results from an untreated sexually transmitted infection, especially chlamydia or gonorrhea, it is not actually an STI. Several nonsexual factors increase the risk of PID, particularly excessive vaginal douching, cigarette smoking, and substance abuse.

Approximately one million women develop PID each year and approximately 100,000 become infertile as a result. A large number of ectopic pregnancies occur each year due to PID, and 150 women die from PID or its complications.[48] Symptoms of PID vary but generally include lower abdominal pain, fever, unusual vaginal discharge, painful intercourse, painful urination, and irregular menstrual bleeding.[49] Major consequences of untreated PID are infertility, ectopic pregnancy, chronic pelvic pain, and recurrent upper genital infections. Risk factors include young age at first sexual intercourse, multiple sex partners, high frequency of sexual intercourse, and change of sexual partners within the past 30 days. Regular gynecological examinations and early treatment for STI symptoms reduce risk.

Gonorrhea

Gonorrhea is one of the most common STIs in the United States, surpassed only by chlamydia in number of cases. The CDC estimates that there are over 700,000 cases per year, plus numbers that go unreported.[50] Health economists estimate that the annual cost of gonorrhea and its complications is over $1.1 billion.[51] Caused by the bacterial pathogen *Neisseria gonorrhoeae,* this infection primarily infects the linings of the urethra, genital tract, pharynx, and rectum. It

Pelvic inflammatory disease (PID) Term used to describe various infections of the female reproductive tract.

Gonorrhea Second most common STD in the United States; if untreated, may cause sterility.

Syphilis One of the most widespread STDs; characterized by distinct phases and potentially serious results.

Chancre Sore often found at the site of syphilis infection.

may spread to the eyes or other body regions via the hands or body fluids, typically during vaginal, oral, or anal sex. Most victims are males between the ages of 20 and 24, with sexually active females between the ages of 15 and 19 also at high risk.[52]

In males, a typical symptom is a white, milky discharge from the penis accompanied by painful, burning urination two to nine days after contact. This is usually enough to send most men to the physician for treatment. However, about 20 percent of all males with gonorrhea are asymptomatic.

In females, the situation is just the opposite: only 20 percent experience any discharge, and few develop a burning sensation upon urinating until much later in the course of the infection (if ever). The organism can remain in the woman's vagina, cervix, uterus, or uterine tubes for long periods with no apparent symptoms other than an occasional slight fever. Thus a woman can be unaware that she has been infected and that she is infecting her sexual partners.

If the infection is detected early, an antibiotic regimen using penicillin, tetracycline, spectinomycin, ceftriaxone, or other drugs is generally effective within a short period of time. If the infection goes undetected in a woman, it can spread throughout the urogenital tract to the uterine tubes and ovaries, causing sterility, or at the very least, severe inflammation and PID. The bacteria can also spread up the reproductive tract, or more rarely, through the blood and infect the joints, heart valves, or brain. If an infected woman becomes pregnant, the infection can cause conjunctivitis in her infant. To prevent this, physicians routinely administer silver nitrate or penicillin preparations to the eyes of newborn babies.

In a man, untreated gonorrhea may spread to the prostate, testicles, urinary tract, kidney, and bladder. Blockage of the ductus deferentia due to scar tissue formation may cause sterility. In some cases, the penis develops a painful curvature during erection.

Syphilis

Syphilis is also caused by a bacterial organism, the *spirochete* known as *Treponema pallidum.* Because it is extremely delicate and dies readily upon exposure to air, dryness, or cold, the organism is generally transferred only through direct sexual contact. Typically, this means contact between sexual organs during intercourse; but, in rare instances, the organism enters the body through a break in the skin, through deep kissing in which body fluids are exchanged, or through some other transmission of body fluids.

Syphilis is called the "great imitator" because its symptoms resemble those of several other infections. Left untreated, syphilis generally progresses through several distinct stages. It should be noted, however, that some people experience no symptoms at all.

Primary Syphilis The first stage of syphilis, particularly for males, is often characterized by the development of a **chancre** (pronounced "shank-er"), a sore located most

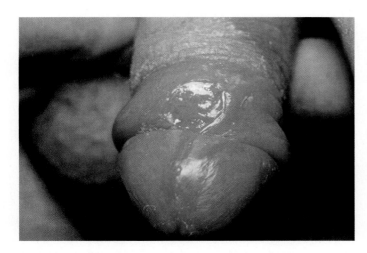

A chancre on the site of the initial infection is a symptom of primary syphilis.

frequently at the site of initial infection. Although painless, the dime-sized chancre is oozing with bacteria, ready to infect an unsuspecting partner. Usually it appears three to four weeks after contact.

In males, the site of the chancre tends to be the penis or scrotum because this is where the organism first enters the body. But, if the infection was contracted through oral sex, the sore can appear in the mouth, throat, or other first contact area. In females, the site of infection is often internal, on the vaginal wall or high on the cervix. Because the chancre is not readily apparent in females, the likelihood of detection is not great. In both males and females, the chancre will completely disappear in three to six weeks.

Secondary Syphilis   A month to a year after the chancre disappears, secondary symptoms may appear, including a rash or white patches on the skin or on the mucous membranes of the mouth, throat, or genitals. Hair loss may occur, lymph nodes may enlarge, and the victim may develop a slight fever or headache. In rare cases, sores develop around the mouth or genitals. As during the active chancre phase, these sores contain infectious bacteria, and contact with them can spread the infection. In a few cases, there may be arthritic pain in the joints. Because symptoms vary so much and appear so much later than the sexual contact that caused them, the victim seldom connects the two. The infection thus often goes undetected even at this second stage. Symptoms may persist for a few weeks or months and then disappear, leaving the person thinking that all is well.

Latent Syphilis   After the secondary stage, the syphilis spirochetes begin to invade body organs. Symptoms, including infectious lesions, may reappear periodically for two to four years after the secondary period. After this period, the infection is rarely transmitted to others, except during

pregnancy, when it can be passed to the fetus. The child will then be born with *congenital syphilis*, which can cause death or severe birth defects such as blindness, deafness, or disfigurement. Because in most cases the fetus does not become infected until after the first trimester, treatment of the mother during this period will usually prevent infection of the fetus.

In some instances, a child born to an infected mother will show no signs of the infection at birth but, within several weeks, will develop body rashes, a runny nose, and symptoms of paralysis. Congenital syphilis is usually detected before it progresses much further. But sometimes the child's immune system will ward off the invading organism, and further symptoms may not surface until the teenage years. One way that some states protect against congenital syphilis is by requiring prospective marriage partners to be tested for syphilis prior to obtaining a marriage license.

In addition to causing congenital syphilis, latent syphilis, if untreated, will progress and infect more and more organs.

Late Syphilis   Years after syphilis has entered the body, its effects become all too evident. Late-stage syphilis indications include heart damage, central nervous system damage, blindness, deafness, paralysis, premature senility, and, ultimately, dementia.

Treatment for Syphilis   Because the organism is bacterial, it is treated with antibiotics, usually penicillin, benzathine penicillin G, or doxycycline. The major obstacle to treatment is misdiagnosis of this "imitator" infection.

Pubic Lice

Pubic lice, often called "crabs," are small parasites that are usually transmitted during sexual contact. More annoying than dangerous, they move easily from partner to partner during sex. They have an affinity for pubic hair, attaching themselves to the base of these hairs, where they deposit their eggs (nits). One to two weeks later, these nits develop into adults that lay eggs and migrate to other body parts, thus perpetuating the cycle.

Treatment includes washing clothing, furniture, and linens that may harbor the eggs. It usually takes two to three weeks to kill all larval forms. Although sexual contact is the most common mode of transmission, you can "catch" pubic lice from lying on sheets that an infected person has slept on. Sleeping in hotel and dormitory rooms in which sheets are not washed regularly or sitting on toilet seats where the nits or larvae have been dropped and lie in wait for a new carrier increases your risk.

> **Pubic lice (crabs)**   Parasites that can inhabit various body areas, especially the genitals.

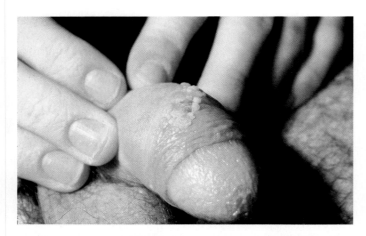

Genital warts are caused by the human papillomavirus and can be either full-blown or flat.

Genital HPV

Genital warts (also known as venereal warts or condylomas) are caused by a small group of viruses known as **human papillomaviruses (HPVs).** A person becomes infected when HPV penetrates the skin and mucous membranes of the genitals or anus through sexual contact. HPV is among the most common forms of STI, infecting over 5.5 million Americans each year. The virus appears to be relatively easy to catch. The typical incubation period is from six to eight weeks after contact. Many people have no symptoms, particularly if the warts are located inside the reproductive tract. Others may develop a series of itchy bumps on the genitals, ranging in size from small pinheads to large cauliflower-like growths. On dry skin (such as the shaft of the penis), the warts are commonly small, hard, and yellowish gray, resembling warts that appear on other parts of the body.

Genital warts are of two different types: (1) *full-blown genital warts* that are noticeable as tiny bumps or growths, and (2) the much more prevalent *flat warts* that are not usually visible to the naked eye. In females, these flat warts are often first detected by a doctor during a routine Pap test. Abnormal Pap results may prompt the physician to perform a procedure in which a vinegar-like solution is applied to the insides of the vaginal walls and cervix to bleach potential warts. The area is then viewed through a special magnifying instrument known as a colposcope. A relatively new photographic procedure known as a cerviscope can also detect genital warts. During a cerviscope, vinegar is applied to the vaginal and cervical areas, and an image of the area is projected onto a screen for a specialist to diagnose. This

technique is relatively inexpensive and is believed to be five times more sensitive than standard colposcopy. An even newer method is the *DNA probe,* a technique that identifies the genetic makeup of possible warts.

Whereas women must see a physician for a diagnosis, a male can check for suspicious lesions by wrapping his penis in vinegar-soaked gauze or cloth, waiting for five minutes, and then checking for white bleached areas indicative of flat warts. However, genital warts of the rectum must be diagnosed by a physician.

Risks of Genital Warts Many genital warts eventually disappear on their own. Others grow and generate unsightly flaps of irregular flesh on the external genitalia. If they grow large enough to obstruct urinary flow or become irritated by clothing or sexual intercourse, they can cause significant problems.

The greatest threat from genital warts may lie in the apparent relationship between them and a tendency for *dysplasia,* or changes in cells that may lead to a precancerous condition. Exactly how HPV infection leads to cervical cancer is uncertain. It is known that within five years after infection, 30 percent of all HPV cases will progress to the precancerous stage. Of those cases that become precancerous and are left untreated, 70 percent will eventually result in actual cancer. In addition, genital warts may pose a threat to a pregnant woman's unborn fetus if the fetus is exposed to the virus during birth. Cesarean deliveries may be considered in serious cases.

New research has also implicated HPV as a possible risk factor for coronary artery disease. It is hypothesized that HPV causes an inflammatory response in the artery walls, which makes cholesterol and plaque build up. (See Chapter 14.)

Treatment for Genital Warts Treatment for genital warts may take several forms:

1. Warts may be painted with a medication called *podophyllin* during a visit to the doctor's office. The podophyllin is washed off after about four hours, and a few days later the warts begin to dry up and fall off. Sometimes more than one trip to the doctor is necessary. This procedure is relatively painless, but there are potential side effects. Because podophyllin may be absorbed through the skin, pregnant women should not use it. Some patients may experience skin reactions.
2. Warts may be removed by *cryosurgery,* a procedure in which an instrument treated with liquid nitrogen is held to the affected area, freezing the tissue. Within a few days, the warts fall off.
3. Depending on size and location, some warts are removed by *simple excision.*
4. For larger warts, *laser surgery* is often used. This is a major procedure that usually requires general anesthesia. The frequency of laser use for wart removal is currently being questioned by many health experts. (Precautions

---

Genital warts Warts that appear in the genital area or the anus; caused by the human papillomaviruses (HPVs).

Human papilloma viruses (HPVs) A small group of viruses that cause genital warts.

must also be taken during this procedure to shield medical staff from infection by viral spray.)

5. Creams containing *5-fluorouracil* (an anticancer drug) are being used to prevent further precancerous cell development.

6. For external warts, injections of *interferon* are sometimes given to keep the virus from spreading to healthy tissue. This treatment shows promise, but it is expensive and, in large doses, may cause flulike symptoms.

Prevention is clearly the best approach. The same strategies that help protect you against AIDS can also protect you from genital warts and other STIs (see the section on AIDS prevention later in this chapter).

Candidiasis (Moniliasis)

Unlike many STIs, which are caused by pathogens that come from outside the body, the yeastlike fungus caused by the *Candida albicans* organism normally inhabits the vaginal tract in most women. Only under certain conditions, in which the normal chemical balance of the vagina is disturbed, will these organisms multiply to abnormal quantities and begin to cause problems. Factors affecting this balance include:

- Antibiotics
- Changes in hormone levels brought on by pregnancy, breast-feeding, or menopause
- Douches or spermicides
- Sexual intercourse
- Other sexually transmitted infections

The likelihood of **candidiasis** (also known as moniliasis or a *yeast infection*) increases if a woman has diabetes, if her immune system is overtaxed or malfunctioning, if she is taking birth control pills or other hormones, or if she is taking broad-spectrum antibiotics. All of these factors decrease the acidity of the vagina and create favorable conditions for a yeastlike infection.

Symptoms of candidiasis include severe vaginal itching and burning of the vagina and vulva. A white, cheesy discharge and swelling of the vulva may also occur. These symptoms are often collectively called **vaginitis,** which means an inflammation of the vagina. When this microbe infects the mouth, whitish patches form, and the condition is referred to as *thrush.* This monilial infection also occurs in males and is easily transmitted between sexual partners.

Candidiasis strikes at least half a million American women a year. Antifungal drugs applied on the surface or by suppository usually cure it in just a few days. For approximately one out of ten women, however, nothing seems to work, and the infection returns again and again. Symptoms can be aggravated by contact of the vagina with scented soaps, douches, perfumed toilet paper, chlorinated water, and spermicides. Tight-fitting jeans and pantyhose can provide the combination of moisture and irritant the organism thrives on.

Trichomoniasis

Unlike many STIs, **trichomoniasis** is caused by a protozoan. Although as many as half of the men and women in the United States may carry this organism, most remain free of symptoms until their bodily defenses are weakened. Both men and women may transmit the infection, but women are the more likely candidates for infection. Symptoms include a foamy, yellowish, unpleasant-smelling discharge accompanied by a burning sensation, itching, and painful urination. These symptoms are most likely to occur during or shortly after menstruation, but they can appear at any time or be absent altogether.

Although usually transmitted by sexual contact, the "trich" organism can also be spread by toilet seats, wet towels, or other items that have discharged fluids on them. You can also contract trichomoniasis by sitting naked on the locker-room bench at your local health spa or gym. Treatment includes oral metronidazole, usually given to both sexual partners to avoid the possible "ping-pong" effect of repeated cross-infection so typical of STIs.

General Urinary Tract Infections (UTIs)

Although *general urinary tract infections (UTIs)* can be caused by various factors, particularly the insertion of catheters and other devices during hospitalization, some forms are sexually transmitted. Any time invading organisms enter the genital area, they can travel up the urethra and enter the bladder. Similarly, organisms normally living in the rectum, urethra, or bladder may travel to the sexual organs and eventually be transmitted to another person.

You can also get a UTI through autoinoculation, often during the simple task of wiping yourself after defecating. Wiping from the anus forward can transmit organisms found in feces to the vaginal opening or the urethra. Contact between the hands and the urethra and between the urethra and other objects are also common means of autoinoculation. Women, with their shorter urethras, are more likely to contract UTIs. Handwashing with soap and water prior to sexual intimacy, foreplay, and so on, is recommended.

Treatment depends on the nature and type of pathogen. For minor infections of the urinary tract proper, some practitioners recommend drinking eight to ten glasses of fluids per day, particularly acidic liquids such as cranberry juice, to alter the acidity of the urine and kill the pathogen. If the infection has spread to a woman's vagina, this treatment

Candidiasis (yeast infection, moniliasis) Yeastlike fungal disease often transmitted sexually.

Vaginitis Set of symptoms characterized by vaginal itching, swelling, and burning.

Trichomoniasis Protozoan infection characterized by foamy, yellowish discharge and unpleasant odor.

is generally considered worthless, however, since it has been estimated that a person would have to drink over four quarts of cranberry juice a day for several days to even begin to alter vaginal acidity. Considering the caloric intake, cost of the juice, and minimal effectiveness of this home treatment, you may be better off visiting a doctor and obtaining proven medications from a pharmacy.

Herpes

Herpes is a general term for a family of infections characterized by sores or eruptions on the skin. Caused by herpesviruses, the herpes family of diseases is not transmitted exclusively sexually. Kissing or sharing eating utensils can also exchange saliva and transmit the infection. Herpes infections range from mildly uncomfortable to extremely serious. **Genital herpes** is an infection caused by the herpes simplex virus (HSV).

There are two types of herpes simplex virus (HSV). Historically, the herpes simplex type 2 virus was considered the primary culprit in genital herpes, and herpes simplex type 1 was thought to affect the area of the lips and other body areas.[53] We now know that both type 1 and type 2 can infect any area of the body, producing lesions (sores) in and around the vaginal area, on the penis, around the anal opening, and on the buttocks or thighs. For example, you may have a type 1 infection on your lip and transmit the HSV-1 organism to your partner's genitals during oral sex. Practically speaking, the resulting symptoms would be virtually the same as if you had transmitted the type 2 virus. Occasionally, sores appear on other parts of the body. HSV remains in certain nerve cells for life and can flare up, or cause symptoms, when the body's ability to maintain itself is weakened.

The *prodromal* (precursor) phase of the infection is characterized by a burning sensation and redness at the site of infection. During this time prescription medicines such as acyclovir and over-the-counter medications such as Abreva will often keep the disease from spreading. However, this phase of the disease is quickly followed by the second phase, in which a blister filled with a clear fluid containing the virus forms. If you pick at this blister or otherwise touch the site and spread this fluid with fingers, lipstick, lip balm, or other products, you can autoinoculate other body parts. Particularly dangerous is the possibility of spreading the infection to your eyes, for a herpes lesion on the eye can cause blindness.

Over a period of days, the unsightly blister will crust over, dry up, and disappear, and the virus will travel to the base of an affected nerve supplying the area and become dormant. Only when the victim becomes overly stressed, when diet and sleep are inadequate, when the immune

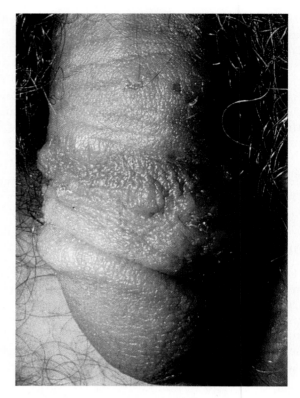

Genital herpes is a highly contagious and incurable STI. It is characterized by recurring cycles of painful blisters on the genitalia.

system is overworked, or when excessive exposure to sunlight or other stressors occurs will the virus become reactivated (at the same site every time) and begin the blistering cycle all over again. These sores cast off (shed) viruses that can be highly infectious. However, it is important to note that a herpes site can shed the virus even when no overt sore is present, particularly during the interval between the earliest symptoms and blistering. People may get genital herpes by having sexual contact with others who don't know they are infected or who are having outbreaks of herpes without any sores. A person with genital herpes can also infect a sexual partner during oral sex. The virus is spread only rarely, if at all, by touching objects such as a toilet seat or hot tub seat.[54] In fact, if you are seated on a toilet seat properly, the only thing in contact with your genitals should be air, and thus, the likelihood of contact exposure would be exceedingly rare!

Genital herpes is especially serious in pregnant women because the baby can be infected as it passes through the vagina during birth. Many physicians recommend cesarean deliveries for infected women. Additionally, women with a history of genital herpes appear to have a greater risk of developing cervical cancer.

Although there is no cure for herpes at present, certain drugs can reduce symptoms. Unfortunately, they seem to work only if the infection is confirmed during the first few hours after contact. As you may guess, this is rather rare. The

Genital herpes   STI caused by the herpes simplex virus.

effectiveness of other treatments, such as L-lysine, is largely unsubstantiated. Newer over-the-counter medications seem to be moderately effective in reducing the severity of symptoms. Although lip balms and cold-sore medications may provide temporary anesthetic relief, remember that rubbing anything on a herpes blister can spread herpes-laden fluids to other body parts.

Preventing Herpes You can take precautions to reduce your risk of herpes:

- Avoid any form of kissing if you notice a sore or blister on your partner's mouth. Kiss no one, not even a peck on the cheek, if you know that you have a herpes lesion or if you see one on a person you want to kiss. Although there is no set time period for safe kissing, the longer you refrain from deep kissing after a herpes sore has been present, the better. (Sores typically take two to four weeks to heal, depending on the health of your immune system.[55]) Keeping your lips healthy, moist, and crack-free will also reduce risk of infection.
- Be extremely cautious if you have casual sexual affairs. Not every partner will feel obligated to tell you that he or she has a problem. It's up to you to protect yourself.
- Wash your hands immediately with soap and water after any form of sexual contact.
- If you have questionable sores or lesions, seek medical help at once. Do not be afraid to name your contacts.
- If you have herpes, be responsible in your sexual contacts with others. If you have any suspicious lesions that might put your partner at risk, say so. Find an appropriate time and place, and hold a candid discussion.
- Reduce your risk of herpes outbreaks by avoiding excessive stress, sunlight, or whatever else appears to trigger an episode.
- Do not share lip balms or lipstick.

HIV/AIDS

Acquired immunodeficiency syndrome (AIDS) is a significant global health threat. Since 1981, when AIDS was first recognized, over 60 million people in the world have become infected with **human immunodeficiency virus (HIV),** the virus that causes AIDS. Today, over 37.8 million people are estimated to be living with HIV or AIDS and an estimated 4.8 million new cases were diagnosed worldwide in 2003.[56] Women are becoming increasingly affected by the virus, accounting for approximately 50 percent of cases.[57] In the United States, as of 2002, over 886,575 men, women, and children with AIDS have been reported to the Centers for Disease Control and Prevention (CDC), and at least 501,669 have died.[58] The CDC estimates that at least 40,000 new infections occur each year in the United States. See the Health in a Diverse World box for more on the global impact of HIV/AIDS.

The Onset of AIDS

Researchers believe that the AIDS virus may actually have been present in the United States since the early 1950s, although medical and government officials did not note problems related to the disease until the spring of 1981. Suddenly, federal officials began to receive an increasing number of requests for an experimental drug used to treat a rare disease called *Pneumocystis carinii pneumonia (PCP)*. Caused by a protozoan, PCP appeared to be affecting significant numbers of previously healthy young men in New York and California.

At about the same time, increasing numbers of men in California were being diagnosed with a rare form of cancer known as *Kaposi's sarcoma*. These two groups of patients—those with PCP and those with Kaposi's sarcoma—tended to share many characteristics. They were typically white and homosexual, came from similar geographical regions, used specific types of drugs, and had generalized lymphadenopathy (chronic swelling of the lymph nodes) and general malfunctioning of the immune system. Because of the last problem, many of these people developed several diseases at the same time, making diagnosis of one underlying cause extremely difficult.

For many months, epidemiologists investigated possible causes of this disease, including the types of drugs used by many gay men and the water supplies in their communities. In 1984, two researchers, Robert C. Gallo at the National Cancer Institute in the United States and Luc Montagnier at the Pasteur Institute in Paris, independently isolated the retrovirus (a type of slow-acting virus) that causes AIDS. Initially called the human T cell lymphotropic virus type III (HTLV-III) by most American researchers, this pathogen is today generally referred to as the human immunodeficiency virus (HIV).

Although during the early days of the epidemic it appeared that HIV infected only homosexuals, it quickly became apparent that the disease was not confined to groups of people, but rather was related to high-risk behaviors such as unprotected sexual intercourse and sharing needles.

A Shifting Epidemic

Initially, people with HIV were diagnosed as having AIDS only when they developed blood infections, the cancer known as Kaposi's sarcoma, or any of 21 other indicator diseases, most of which were common in male AIDS patients.

Acquired immunodeficiency syndrome (AIDS) Extremely virulent sexually transmitted disease that renders the immune system inoperative.

Human immunodeficiency virus (HIV) The slow-acting virus that causes AIDS.

The Staggering Toll of HIV/AIDS in the Global Community

Although the rates of HIV/AIDS may be slowing in the United States, the disease has had an increasingly devastating impact on other regions of the world. By the year 2004, an estimated 39.4 million people from all regions of the world were infected with HIV, translating to nearly 11 out of every 1,000 men, women, and children. For many years, women, children, and teenagers seemed to be on the periphery of the HIV/AIDS pandemic, but this is no longer true. Every day in 2004, an estimated 13,500 people were newly infected with HIV. Here are some facts about this global epidemic.

AFRICA

- In southern Africa, one in every five people is now infected. Almost 35 percent of the population in Botswana and Swaziland is living with HIV.

- Two-thirds of all people living with HIV live in sub-Saharan Africa, an area that is home to just 10 percent of the world's population.

LATIN AMERICA AND THE CARIBBEAN

- In 2004, over 2 million people were living with HIV. The epidemic was mainly spread through heterosexual intercourse, injecting drug use, and men who have sex with men.
- Haiti was worst hit, with 280,000 adults infected as of 2004.

EASTERN EUROPE AND CENTRAL ASIA

- In eastern Europe and central Asia combined, an estimated 1.4 million people were living with the AIDS virus at the end of 2004.
- Rates of infection are increasing among drug users sharing needles in Estonia, Latvia, the Russian Federation, and Ukraine.

ASIA

- An estimated 8.2 million people in the region were living with the AIDS virus in 2004.
- Thailand and Cambodia seem to have controlled the once-rampant spread of HIV by promoting condom use, especially among sex workers.
- An estimated 5.1 million people in India live with the virus, the second highest national total behind South Africa, with an infection rate of 0.7 percent.

Source: Joint United Nations Programme on HIV/AIDS (UNAIDS), "AIDS Epidemic Update," December 2004, www.unaids.org /wad2004/report.html

---

The CDC has expanded the indicator list to include pulmonary tuberculosis, recurrent pneumonia, and invasive cervical cancer. Perhaps the most significant new indicator is a drop in the level of the body's master immune cells, called CD4s, to 200 per cubic millimeter (one-fifth the level in a healthy person).

AIDS cases have been reported state by state throughout the United States since the early 1980s as a means of tracking the disease. While the numbers of actual reported cases have always been suspect, improved reporting and surveillance methods have helped increase accuracy. Today, the CDC recommends that all states report HIV infections as well as AIDS. Because of medical advances in treatment and increasing numbers of HIV-infected persons who do not progress to AIDS, it is believed that AIDS incidence statistics may not provide a true picture of the epidemic, the long-term costs of treating HIV-infected individuals, and other key information. HIV incidence data also provide a better picture of infection trends. Currently, most states mandate that those

who test positive for the HIV antibody be reported. Although there is significant pressure to mandate reporting in all states, there is controversy over implementing such a mandate. Many believe that if we require reporting of HIV-positive tests, many people will refuse to be tested even if they suspect they are infected.

What do you think?

Do you favor mandatory reporting of HIV and AIDS cases? ■ *If you knew that your name and vital statistics would be "on file" if you tested positive for HIV, would you be less likely to take the HIV test to begin with?* ■ *On the other hand, do people who carry this contagious fatal disease have a responsibility to inform the general public and the health professionals who will provide their care?* ■ *Explain your answer.*

Women and AIDS

HIV is an equal-opportunity pathogen that can attack anyone who engages in high-risk behaviors. This is true regardless of race, gender, sexual orientation, or socioeconomic status. Consider the following facts:[59]

- In new HIV infections, 60 percent of males and 75 percent of females contracted the virus through heterosexual contact.[60]
- By 2002, women accounted for over 50 percent of all AIDS cases in the United States.[61]
- HIV/AIDS due to heterosexual sexual transmission is increasing faster in rural America than in any other part of the country. Women most at risk are ethnic minorities and the economically disadvantaged. Among sexually active heterosexual teenagers, college students, and health care workers, nearly 60 percent of HIV cases are women.
- Most women with AIDS were infected through heterosexual exposure to HIV, followed by injection drug use (sharing needles).
- Women of color are disproportionately affected by HIV. Although African American and Hispanic females comprise less than 25 percent of all U.S. women, together they account for 76 percent of AIDS cases among women in the United States.
- Of all AIDS cases among women, 61 percent were reported from five states: New York (26 percent), Florida (13 percent), New Jersey (10 percent), California (7 percent), and Texas (5 percent).
- AIDS is the leading cause of death among African American women aged 25 to 44, and the fourth leading cause of death among all American women in this age group.
- AIDS is one of the top ten causes of death for people age 15 to 64 in the United States.

Compounding the problems of women with HIV are serious deficiencies in our health and social service systems, including inadequate treatment for female addicts and lack of access to child care, health care, and social services for families headed by single women. Women with HIV/AIDS are also the major source of infection in infants. Virtually all new HIV infections among children in the United States are attributable to perinatal transmission of HIV.[62]

Special Concerns of Women with HIV/AIDS   Although contracting HIV is a serious problem for both males and females, women often have an even more difficult time protecting themselves from infection and taking care of themselves if they become ill. Irrefutable evidence indicates that HIV/AIDS disproportionately affects women, who, as mentioned earlier, are four to ten times more likely than men to contract HIV through unprotected sexual intercourse with an infected partner. This discrepancy can be traced to both biological and socioeconomic factors.

Biological factors include:

- HIV can enter through mucous membrane surfaces of the genital tract; the vagina has a greater exposed mucous membrane area than does the urethra of the penis.
- The vaginal area is more likely to incur microtears during sexual intercourse, which facilitates entry of HIV.
- During intercourse, a woman is exposed to more semen than is the male to vaginal fluids.
- Semen is more likely to enter the vagina with force, whereas vaginal fluids do not enter the penis with force.
- Women who have STIs are more likely to be asymptomatic and therefore unaware they have a disease; STIs increase the risk of HIV transmission.

Socioeconomic factors include:

- Currently there are more HIV-infected men than HIV-infected women in the United States; thus, it is more likely for a woman to have an HIV-infected male partner than for a man to have an HIV-infected female partner.
- Women have been underrepresented in clinical trials for HIV treatment and prevention.
- Many cultural norms place women in subordination to men, especially in developing nations. This reduces women's decision-making power and ability to negotiate safer sex.
- Women are more vulnerable to sexual abuse from their male partners and are more likely to be involved in nonconsensual sex or sex without condoms.
- Women are more likely to be economically dependent on men.
- Women may be less likely to seek medical treatment because of caregiving burdens, transportation problems, and lack of money.
- In the United States, HIV-positive women are likely to be younger and less educated than HIV-positive men.
- Traditionally, women have played a relatively passive role in taking responsibility for protection during sexual intercourse and in general sexual decision making, particularly in third world countries.

Efforts must be initiated to help women take control of their sexual health and participate actively in sexual decisions made with their partners. In addition, women often carry the responsibility for caring for their children or for others who may be infected with HIV or suffering from AIDS. If the mother's role as caretaker must be abandoned due to illness, family members often suffer. As more and more women become infected with HIV, national efforts aimed at prevention, intervention, and treatment will undoubtedly increase. ■

What do you think?

Why do you think HIV/AIDS is increasing among women and minority groups in America? ■ Why are some women particularly vulnerable to diseases such as AIDS? ■ What actions can we take as a nation to reduce the spread of HIV/AIDS among women and minority groups? ■ Should Americans be concerned about the global HIV/AIDS epidemic? Why or why not?

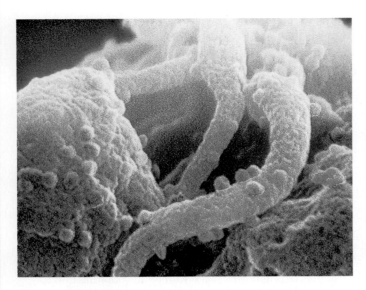

Viruses attach themselves to host cells and inject their own DNA or RNA in order to reproduce new cells. Some viruses run their course and expire. Others, such as HIV, shown here in green, are destructive over the long term.

How HIV Is Transmitted

HIV typically enters one person's body when another person's infected body fluids (semen, vaginal secretions, blood, etc.) gain entry through a breach in body defenses. Mucous membranes of the genital organs and the anus provide the easiest route of entry. If there is a break in the mucous membranes (as can occur during sexual intercourse, particularly anal intercourse), the virus enters and begins to multiply.

After initial infection, HIV multiplies rapidly, invading the bloodstream and cerebrospinal fluid. It progressively destroys helper T cells, weakening the body's resistance to disease. The virus also changes the genetic structure of the cells it attacks. In response to this invasion, the body quickly begins to produce antibodies.

Despite some myths, HIV is not a highly contagious virus. Studies of people living in households with an AIDS patient have turned up no documented cases of HIV infection due to casual contact.[63] Other investigations provide overwhelming evidence that insect bites do not transmit HIV.

Engaging in High-Risk Behaviors AIDS is not a disease of gay people or minority groups. If you engage in high-risk behaviors, you increase your risk for the disease. If you do not practice these behaviors, your risk is minimal. It is as simple as that.

Unfortunately, the message has not gotten through to many Americans. They assume that because they are heterosexual, do not inject illegal drugs, and do not have sex with sex workers, they are not at risk. They couldn't be more wrong. Anyone who engages in unprotected sex is at risk, especially sex with a partner who has engaged in other high-risk behaviors. Sex with multiple partners is the greatest threat.

You can't determine the presence of HIV by looking at a person; you can't tell by questioning unless the person has been tested recently, is HIV negative, *and* is giving an honest answer. So what should you do?

Of course, the simplest answer is abstinence. If you don't exchange body fluids, you won't get the disease. As a second line of defense, if you decide to be intimate, the next best option is to use a condom. However, in spite of all the educational campaigns, surveys consistently indicate that most college students throw caution to the wind if they think they "know" someone—they have unprotected sex. Even when they do not know the individual involved well, most of them have unprotected sex.

Why do so many of us act so irresponsibly when the outcome is so deadly? The answer is probably a combination of ignorance, denial that it could be *you* who is HIV positive, a certain degree of apathy, and a bit of very real fear. People who are afraid often avoid testing. If they have symptoms, they may still avoid testing out of fear that they may be diagnosed positive and not have any real options for a cure.

Recognize the risk factors, and remember, if you do not engage in activities that are known to spread the virus, your chances of becoming infected are extremely small. The following activities are high-risk behaviors.

Exchange of Body Fluids The greatest risk factor is the exchange of HIV-infected body fluids during vaginal or anal intercourse. Substantial research indicates that blood, semen, and vaginal secretions are the major fluids of concern. However, even though these risks are well documented, millions of Americans report inconsistent safer sex practices, particularly when drugs or alcohol affect rational thinking.

Although the virus was found in one person's saliva (out of 71 people in a study population), most health officials state that saliva is not a high-risk body fluid unless blood is present; saliva is a less significant risk than other shared body fluids (see the Reality Check box on tattooing and piercing for additional risks). The fact that the virus has been found in saliva does provide a good rationale for caution when engaging in deep, wet kissing.

Initially, public health officials also included breast milk in the list of high-risk fluids because a few infants apparently contracted HIV while breast-feeding. Subsequent research has indicated that HIV could have been transmitted by bleeding nipples as well as by actual consumption of breast milk and other fluids. Infection through contact with feces and urine is believed to be highly unlikely though technically possible.

Receiving a Blood Transfusion Prior to 1985 A small group of people have become infected after receiving blood transfusions or infected organ transplants. In 1985, the Red Cross and other blood donation programs implemented a

Body Piercing and Tattooing: Risks to Health

A look around almost any college campus reveals many examples of the widespread trend of body piercing and tattooing, also referred to as "body art." In record numbers, people are getting their eyebrows, tongues, lips, noses, navels, nipples, and genitals pierced. Many view the trend as a fulfillment of a desire for self-expression, as this University of Wisconsin–Madison student points out: "The nipple [ring] was one of those things that I did as a kind of empowerment, claiming my body as my own and refuting the stereotypes that people have about me. . . .The tattoo was kind of a lark and came along the same lines and I like it too. . . .[T]hey both give me a secret smile." Whatever the reason, there is a booming business in both tattooing and the "art" of body piercing.

However, health professionals cite several concerns over health risks. The most common health-related problems associated with tattoos and body piercing include skin reactions, infections, and scarring. The average healing times for piercings depend on the size of the insert, location, and the person's overall health. Tongue piercings are especially prone to infection because the mouth has so much bacteria. Because the hands are great germ transmitters, "fingering" pierced areas poses a significant risk for infection.

Of even greater concern is the potential transmission of dangerous pathogens that any puncture of the human body exacerbates. The use of unsterile needles—which can cause serious infections and can transmit HIV, hepatitis B and C, tetanus, and a host of other diseases—poses a very real risk. (Consider actress Pamela Anderson, who claims to have contracted hepatitis C from sharing a tattoo needle with her ex-husband Tommy Lee.) Body piercing and tattooing are often performed by unlicensed "professionals" who generally have learned their trade from other body artists. Laws and policies regulating body piercing and tattooing vary greatly by state. While some states don't allow tattoo and body-piercing parlors, others may regulate them carefully, and still others provide few regulations and standards by which parlors have to abide. Standards for safety usually include minimum age of use, standards of sanitation, use of aseptic techniques, sterilization of equipment, informed risks, instructions for skin care, record keeping, and recommendations for dealing with adverse reactions. Because of the lack of standards regulating this business and the potential for transmission of dangerous pathogens, anyone who receives a tattoo, body piercing, or permanent makeup tattoo cannot donate blood for one year.

If you opt for tattooing or body piercing, remember the following points:

✔ Look for clean, well-lit work areas, and ask about sterilization procedures.

✔ Before having the work done, watch the artist at work. Tattoo removal is expensive and often impossible. Make sure the tattoo is one you can live with for years.

✔ Immediately before piercing or tattooing, the body area should be carefully sterilized. The artist should put on new latex gloves and touch nothing else while working.

✔ Packaged, sterilized needles should be used only once and then discarded. A piercing gun should not be used because it cannot be sterilized properly.

✔ Only jewelry made of noncorrosive metal, such as surgical stainless steel, niobium, or solid 14-karat gold, is safe for new piercing.

✔ Leftover tattoo ink should be discarded after each procedure. Do not allow the artist to reuse ink that has been used for other customers.

✔ If any signs of pus, swelling, redness, or discoloration persist, remove the piercing object and contact a physician.

Sources: Center for Food Safety and Applied Nutrition, Office of Cosmetics Fact Sheet: "Tattoos and Permanent Makeup," 2004, www.cfsan.fda.gov/~dms/cos-204.html; M. L. Armstrong and K. P. Murphy, "Adolescent Tattooing and Body Piercing," *The Prevention Researcher* (Integrated Research Services, Eugene, OR) 5, no. 3 (1998): 5.

---

stringent testing program for all donated blood. Today, because of these massive screening efforts, the risk of receiving HIV-infected blood is almost nonexistent.

Injecting Drugs A significant percentage of AIDS cases in the United States result from sharing or using HIV-contaminated needles and syringes. Though users of illegal drugs are commonly considered the only members of this category, others may also share needles—for example, people with

diabetes who inject insulin or athletes who inject steroids. People who share needles and also engage in sexual activities with members of high-risk groups, such as those who exchange sex for drugs, increase their risks dramatically.

Mother-to-Infant (Perinatal) Transmission Approximately one in three of the children who has contracted AIDS received the virus from their infected mothers while in the womb or while passing through the vaginal tract during delivery.

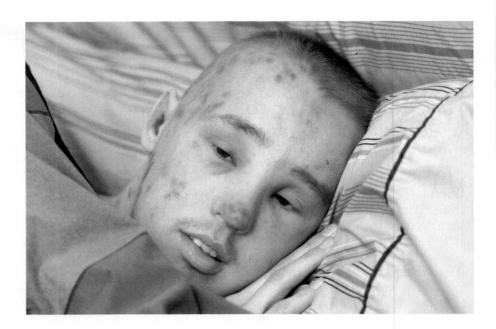

The effects of HIV/AIDS can be seen here in the form of Kaposi's sarcoma and AIDS-wasting syndrome.

Symptoms of HIV Disease

A person may go for months or years after infection by HIV before any significant symptoms appear. The incubation time varies greatly from person to person. Children have shorter incubation periods than adults. Newborns and infants are particularly vulnerable to AIDS because human beings do not become fully immunocompetent (that is, their immune system is not fully developed) until they are 6 to 15 months old. New information suggests that some very young children show the adult progression of AIDS.[64]

For adults who receive no medical treatment, it takes an average of eight to ten years for the virus to cause the slow, degenerative changes in the immune system that are characteristic of AIDS. During this time, the person may experience a large number of opportunistic infections (infections that gain a foothold when the immune system is not functioning effectively). Colds, sore throats, fever, tiredness, nausea, night sweats, and other generally nonlife-threatening conditions commonly appear and are described as pre-AIDS symptoms.

ELISA Blood test that detects presence of antibodies to the HIV virus.

Western blot A test more accurate than the ELISA to confirm presence of HIV antibodies.

Testing for HIV Antibodies

Once antibodies have formed in reaction to HIV, a blood test known as the **ELISA** test may detect their presence. If sufficient antibodies are present, the ELISA results will be positive. When a person who previously tested *negative* (no HIV antibodies present) has a subsequent test that is *positive*, seroconversion is said to have occurred. In such a situation, the person would typically take another ELISA test, followed by a more expensive, precise test known as the **Western blot** to confirm the presence of HIV antibodies.

Although the ELISA is viewed as quite accurate, it is a conservative test in that it errs on the side of caution, meaning it produces a large number of *false-positive results*. It was deliberately designed to do this because it was intended as a test for screening the nation's blood supply. There have also been instances of *false-negative results*. Some health professionals believe that there are chronic carriers of HIV who, for unknown reasons, continually show false-negative results on both the ELISA and Western blot tests. This, of course, raises serious concerns about risks for these people's sexual partners.

It should be noted that these tests are not AIDS tests per se. Rather, they detect antibodies for the disease, indicating the presence of HIV in the person's system. Whether the person will develop AIDS depends to some extent on the strength of the immune system. Although we have made remarkable progress in prolonging the relatively symptom-free period between infection, HIV-positive status, and progression to symptomatic AIDS, it is important to note that a cure does not yet exist. The vast majority of all infected people eventually develop some form of the disease.

As testing for HIV antibodies has improved, scientists have explored various ways of making it easier for individuals to be tested. Health officials distinguish between *reported* and *actual* cases of HIV infection because it is believed that many HIV-positive people avoid being tested. One reason is fear of knowing the truth. Another is the fear of recrimination from employers, insurance companies, and medical staff if a positive test result becomes known to others. (Although it is illegal to discriminate against a person who is HIV positive or has AIDS, discrimination is not always an overt act that is easily punished. Subtle acts of discrimination and harassment continue to be reported.) Early detection and reporting are important, because immediate treatment for someone in the early stages of HIV disease is critical.

New Hope and Treatments

New drugs and new drug combinations have slowed the progression from HIV to AIDS and have prolonged life expectancies for most AIDS patients. While these new therapies offer the promise of extended life for many, they may have inadvertently led to a recent increase in risky behaviors and a rise in cases of infection. Although AIDS fell from the top ten to the fourteenth leading cause of death in 1997 and has held steady at that ranking, many experts fear that we are taking steps backward. Advocates for AIDS patients believe the medications still cost too much money and cause too many side effects. The cost of multidrug treatment for one person now exceeds $20,000 per year. Medical costs for people with AIDS, from the time of diagnosis until death, typically exceed $102,000.[65] A new study, conducted by the Agency for Healthcare Research and Quality (AHRQ), will provide an up-to-date estimate of HIV/AIDS costs soon. Until then, the cost implications of improved treatments remain unclear.

Current treatments combine selected drugs, especially protease inhibitors and reverse transcriptase inhibitors. Protease inhibitors (for example, amprenavir, ritonavir, and saquinavir) resemble pieces of the protein chain that the HIV protease normally cuts. They block the HIV protease enzyme from cutting the protein chains needed to produce new viruses. Other drugs, including the nucleoside analogs (such as AZT, ddI, ddC, d4T, and 3TC), inhibit the HIV enzyme reverse transcriptase before the virus has invaded the cell. Protease inhibitors act to prevent the production of the virus in chronically infected cells that HIV has already invaded. In effect, the older drugs work by preventing the virus from infecting new cells, and the protease inhibitors work by preventing infected cells from reproducing new HIVs.

While protease inhibitors show promise, they have proved difficult to manufacture, and some have failed while others are successful. Side effects vary from person to person, and getting the right dose is critical for effectiveness. All of the protease drugs seem to work best in combination with other therapies. These combination treatments are still quite experimental, and no combination has proved to be absolute for all people as yet. Also, as with other antiviral treatments, resistance to the drugs can develop. Individuals who already show resistance to AZT may not be able to use a protease-AZT combination. This can pose a problem for many people who have been taking the common drugs and then find their options for combination therapy limited.

Although these drugs provide new hope and longer survival rates for people living with HIV, it is important to maintain caution. We are still a long way from a cure. Apathy and carelessness may abound if too much confidence is placed in these treatments. Newer drugs that held much promise are becoming less effective as HIV develops resistance to them. Costs of taking multiple drugs are becoming prohibitive and side effects common. There is no cure. Furthermore, the number of people becoming HIV-infected each year has stabilized and even increased in some communities, meaning that we are still a long way from beating this disease. In fact, while AIDS death rates in America dropped nearly 66 percent during the 1995–1998 period, we are now seeing modest increases in the rate, as drug regimens lose effectiveness and rates of infection rise.[66]

Preventing HIV Infection

Although scientists have been working on a variety of HIV vaccine trials none are currently available.[67] The only way to prevent HIV infection is to avoid risky behaviors. HIV infection and AIDS are not uncontrollable conditions. You can reduce your risk by the choices you make in sexual behaviors and by taking responsibility for your own health and the health of your loved ones. The Skills for Behavior Change box presents ways to reduce your risk for contracting HIV and other STIs.

Because the status of your immune system is an important factor in your susceptibility to any of the STIs, it is important that you do everything possible to protect yourself. Adequate nutrition, sleep, stress management, vaccinations, and other preventive maintenance strategies can do a great deal to ensure your long-term health.

Where to Go for Help If you are concerned about your own risk or the risk of a close friend, arrange a confidential meeting with the health educator or other health professional at your college health service. He or she will provide you with the information that you need to decide whether you should be tested for HIV antibodies. If the student health service is not an option for you, seek assistance through your local public health department or community STI clinic. Local physicians, counselors, professors, and other responsible people can help you discover the answers you are looking for.

Staying Safe in an Unsafe Sexual World

HIV transmission depends on behavior; this is true of other STIs as well. To protect yourself and reduce your risk:

- Avoid casual sexual partners. Ideally, have sex only if you are in a long-term, mutually monogamous relationship with someone who is equally committed to the relationship and whose HIV status is negative.
- Avoid unprotected sexual activity involving the exchange of blood, semen, or vaginal secretions with people whose present or past behaviors put them at risk for infection. Do not be afraid to ask intimate questions about your partner's sexual past. Remember, whenever you choose to have sexual relations, you expose yourself to your partner's history. Postpone sexual involvement until you are assured that he or she is not infected.
- All sexually active adults who are not in a lifelong monogamous relationship should practice safer sex by using latex condoms. Remember, however, that condoms are not 100 percent safe.
- Never share injecting needles with anyone for any reason.
- Never share any devices through which the exchange of blood could occur, including needles, razors, tattoo instruments, body-piercing instruments, and any other sharp objects.
- Avoid injury to body tissue during sexual activity. HIV can enter the bloodstream through microscopic tears in anal or vaginal tissues.
- Avoid unprotected oral sex or any sexual activity in which semen, blood, or vaginal secretions could penetrate mucous membranes through breaks in the membrane. Always use a condom or a dental dam during oral sex.
- Avoid using drugs or alcohol that may dull your senses and affect your ability to make decisions about responsible

precautions with potential sex partners.
- Wash your hands before and after sexual encounters. Urinate after sexual relations and, if possible, wash your genitals.
- Although total abstinence is the only absolute means of preventing the sexual transmission of HIV, abstinence can be a difficult choice to make. If you have any doubt about the potential risks of having sex, consider other means of intimacy, at least until you can assure your safety. Try massage, dry kissing, hugging, holding and touching, and masturbation (alone or with a partner).
- Be sure medical professionals take appropriate precautions to prevent potential transmission, including washing their hands and wearing gloves and masks. All equipment used for treatment should be properly sterilized.
- If you are worried about your own HIV status, have yourself tested. Don't risk infecting others.
- If you are a woman and HIV positive, you should take the steps necessary to ensure that you do not become pregnant.
- If you suspect that you may be infected or if you test positive for HIV antibodies, do not donate blood, semen, or body organs.

At no time in your life is it more important to communicate openly than when you are considering an intimate relationship. Ask questions so you can make an informed decision about whether to get involved. Remember that you can't tell if someone has a sexually transmitted infection just by looking. Anyone who has ever had sex with anyone else or has injected drugs is at risk, and they may not even know it. To communicate about potential risks:

- Remember that you have a responsibility to your partner to disclose your own status. You also have a responsibility to yourself to stay healthy. Ask about your partner's HIV status. Suggest going through the testing together as a means of sharing something important.

- Be direct, honest, and determined in talking about sex before you become involved. Do not act silly or evasive. Get to the point, ask clear questions, and do not be put off in receiving a response. A person who does not care enough to talk about sex probably does not care enough to take responsibility for his or her actions.
- Discuss the issues without sounding defensive or accusatory. Develop a personal comfort level with the subject prior to raising the issue with your partner. Be prepared with complete information, and articulate your feelings clearly. Reassure your partner that your reasons for desiring abstinence or safer sex arise from respect and not distrust. Sharing feelings is easier in a calm, suspicion-free environment in which both people feel comfortable.
- Encourage your partner to be honest and share feelings. This will not happen overnight. If you have never had a serious conversation with this person before you get into an intimate situation, you cannot expect honesty and openness when the lights go out.
- Analyze your own beliefs and values ahead of time. Know where you will draw the line on certain actions, and be very clear with your partner about what you expect. If you believe that using a condom is necessary, make sure you communicate this.
- Decide what you will do if your partner does not agree with you. Anticipate potential objections or excuses, and prepare your responses accordingly.
- Ask about your partner's history. Although it may seem as though you are prying into another person's business, your own future depends upon knowing basic information about your partner's past sexual practices and use of injectable drugs.
- Discuss the significance of monogamy in your partner's relationships. Ask, "How important is a committed relationship to you?" Decide early how important this relationship is to you and how much you are willing to work on an acceptable compromise in lifestyle.

MAKE IT HAPPEN!

Assessment: The Assess Yourself box on page 504 gave you the chance to consider your beliefs and attitudes about STIs and the possible risks you may be facing. Now that you have considered these results, you can begin to take steps toward changing certain behaviors that may be putting you at risk.

Making a Change: In order to change your behavior, you need to develop a plan. Follow these steps.

1. Evaluate your behavior, and identify patterns and specific things you are doing. What can you change now? What can you change in the near future?
2. Select one pattern of behavior that you want to change.
3. Fill out a Behavior Change Contract. It should include your long-term goal for change, your short-term goals, the rewards you'll give yourself for reaching these goals, potential obstacles along the way, and strategies for overcoming these obstacles. For each goal, list the small steps and specific actions that you will take.
4. Chart your progress in a journal. At the end of a week, consider how successful you were in following your plan. What helped you to be successful? What made change more difficult? What will you do differently next week?
5. Revise your plan as needed. Are the short-term goals attainable? Are the rewards satisfying?

One Student's Plan: Carlos had never thought that he was at risk for an STI. He only dated one woman at a time, and he had never had an STI himself. After he reviewed his answers to the self-assessment, however, he saw that there were several ways in which he was putting himself at risk.

He had thought that he would be able to tell whether someone was infected with an STI, but the answer to question #1 described how, especially among women, there are few if any obvious signs or symptoms of some STIs. Carlos also believed that he was not at risk because he dated only one woman at a time, but the answer to question #8 pointed out that a person can pass on an STI that he or she contracted from a previous sex partner. Carlos decided it was time to take responsibility for his sexual activity. He had been on three dates with Sherry and felt things were progressing to a more intimate stage soon. He wanted to be sure that they took the time to discuss STIs before they put themselves at risk.

Carlos was nervous when he thought about talking to Sherry about STIs so he wrote out a few ideas of ways to bring up the subject. This made him more confident that he would be able to talk honestly with Sherry before they became more intimate. He also made sure that he had a supply of condoms, so there wouldn't be any reason not to practice safe sex. At the end of their next date, Carlos asked Sherry if they could have a serious conversation about the next step. When he told her that he wanted to talk about STIs, she told him that she was relieved that he had brought up the subject. She knew that she was healthy and hadn't been sure how to find out his status. Carlos was relieved that Sherry was as concerned about the issue as he was, and they were both glad that embarrassment had not prevented them from having this conversation.

Summary

- The major uncontrollable risk factors for contracting infectious diseases are heredity, age, environmental conditions, and organism resistance. Major controllable risk factors include stress, nutrition, fitness level, sleep, hygiene, avoidance of high-risk behaviors, and drug use.
- The major pathogens are bacteria, viruses, fungi, protozoa, prions, and parasitic worms. Bacterial infections include staphylococcal infections, streptococcal infections, pneumonia, Legionnaire's disease, tuberculosis, periodontal diseases, and rickettsia. Major viral infections include the common cold, influenza, infectious mononucleosis, hepatitis, mumps, chickenpox and shingles, measles, and rabies.
- Your body uses a number of defense systems to keep pathogens from invading. The skin is our major protection, helped by enzymes. The immune system creates antibodies to destroy antigens. In addition, fever and pain play a role in defending the body. Vaccines bolster the body's immune system against specific diseases.

- Emerging and resurgent diseases pose significant threats for future generations. Many factors contribute to these risks. Possible solutions focus on a public health approach to prevention.
- Sexually transmitted infections are spread through intercourse, oral sex, anal sex, hand–genital contact, and sometimes mouth-to-mouth contact. Major STIs include chlamydia, pelvic inflammatory disease, gonorrhea, syphilis, pubic lice, genital warts, candidiasis, trichomoniasis, and herpes.
- Acquired immunodeficiency syndrome (AIDS) is caused by the human immunodeficiency virus (HIV). HIV is not confined to certain high-risk groups. Globally, HIV/AIDS has become a major threat to the world's population. Anyone can get HIV by engaging in high-risk sexual activities that include exchange of body fluids, by having received a blood transfusion or organ transplant before 1985, by injecting drugs, or by having sex with anyone who engages in any of these high-risk activities. Women appear to be particularly susceptible to infection. You can cut your risk for AIDS significantly by deciding not to engage in risky sexual activities.

Questions for Discussion and Reflection

1. What are the major controllable risk factors for contracting infectious diseases? Using this knowledge, how would you change your current lifestyle to prevent such infection?
2. What is a pathogen? What are the similarities and differences between pathogens and antigens? Discuss uncontrollable and controllable risk factors that can threaten your health. What can you do to limit the effects of either type of risk factor?
3. What are the six types of pathogens? What are the various means by which they can be transmitted? How have social conditions among the poor and homeless increased the risks for certain diseases, such as tuberculosis, influenza, and hepatitis? Why are these conditions a challenge to the efforts of public health officials?

4. What is the difference between active and passive immunity? How do they compare to natural and acquired immunity? Explain why it is important to wash your hands often when you have a cold.
5. Identify possible reasons for the spread of emerging and resurgent diseases. Indicate public policies and programs that might reduce this trend.
6. Identify five sexually transmitted infections. What are their symptoms? How do they develop? What are their potential long-term effects?
7. Why are women more susceptible to HIV infection than men? What implication does this have for prevention, treatment, and research?
8. Should Americans be concerned about soaring HIV/AIDS rates elsewhere in the world? Explain your answer.

Accessing Your Health on the Internet

Visit the following Internet sites to explore further topics and issues related to personal health. To visit an organization's website, go to the Companion Website for *Access to Health, Ninth Edition* at www.aw-bc.com/donatelle, click on the book image, and select "Accessing Your Health on the Internet" from the navigation menu.

1. *Centers for Disease Control and Prevention (CDC).* Homepage for the government agency dedicated to disease intervention and prevention, with links to all the latest data and publications put out by the CDC, including the *Morbidity and Mortality Weekly Report (MMWR), HIV/AIDS Surveillance Report,* and the *Journal of Emerging Infectious Diseases,* and access to the CDC research database, Wonder.

2. *National Center for Infectious Disease.* Up-to-date perspectives on infectious diseases of significance to the global community.
3. *The New England Journal of Medicine Online.* Online version of a weekly journal reporting the results of important medical research worldwide; includes articles from current and past publications.
4. *World Health Organization.* Access to the latest information on world health issues; direct access to publications and fact sheets; with keywords to find topics of interest.

Further Reading

Addressing Emerging Infectious Disease Threats: A Prevention Strategy for the U.S. Atlanta: Centers for Disease Control, 1998.

Useful slides and narrative addressing risks and threats of emerging diseases as well as a national strategy for prevention and control.

Champeau, D. and R. Donatelle. *AIDS and STIs: A Global Perspective.* Englewood Cliffs, NJ: Prentice Hall, 2002.

An overview of issues, trends, and ethics surrounding the global pandemic of HIV/AIDS and sexually transmitted infections.

Chin, J., ed. *Control of Communicable Diseases Manual,* 17th ed. Washington, DC: American Public Health Association, 2003.

Outstanding pocket reference for information on infectious diseases. Updated every three to five years to cover emerging diseases.

Levy, S. B. *The Antibiotic Paradox: How the Misuse of Antibiotics Destroys Their Curative Powers.* Cambridge, MA: Perseus Publishing, 2002.

A discussion of microbial resistance, history, progression, and implications for public health.

■ Discuss chronic lung diseases, including allergies, hay fever, asthma, emphysema, chronic bronchitis, and other problems.

■ Describe common gender-related disorders, risk factors for these conditions, their symptoms, and methods to control or prevent them.

■ Discuss the varied musculoskeletal diseases, including arthritis and other bone and joint problems, and their effects on the body.

■ Explain common neurological disorders, including headaches and seizure disorders.

■ Discuss diabetes and other digestion-related disorders, including their symptoms, prevention, and control.

■ Describe chronic fatigue syndrome and job-related disorders.

18

NONINFECTIOUS CONDITIONS

THE MODERN MALADIES

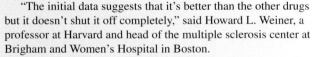

F.D.A. Approves a Multiple Sclerosis Drug

By Andrew Pollack

The Food and Drug Administration yesterday approved a drug for multiple sclerosis that has shown early evidence of being more effective than existing drugs.

The drug, Tysabri, was developed by Biogen Idec and Elan and was called Antegren until the F.D.A. requested a name change to avoid confusion with other drugs. Some analysts predict annual sales will eventually surpass $2 billion.

Doctors and analysts say the drug represents an advance but is far from a cure. Long-term data on safety and efficacy are still lacking.

"The initial data suggests that it's better than the other drugs but it doesn't shut it off completely," said Howard L. Weiner, a professor at Harvard and head of the multiple sclerosis center at Brigham and Women's Hospital in Boston.

The F.D.A. approved the drug based on only one year's worth of data from clinical trials, rather than the two customarily required, because of positive results. In one trial, Tysabri reduced the rate of relapses—the flaring up of symptoms—by two-thirds, to 25 per 100 patients per year compared with 74 per 100 patients per year for a placebo.

Read the complete article online in the eThemes section of this book's website: www.aw-bc.com/donatelle.

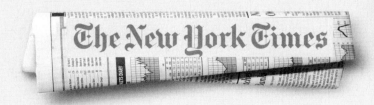

Typically, when we think of the major ailments and diseases affecting Americans today, we think of "killer" diseases such as cancer and heart disease. Clearly, these diseases make up the major portion of life-threatening diseases, accounting for nearly two-thirds of all deaths. Yet although they do not capture much media attention, other forms of chronic disease can also cause substantial pain, suffering, and disability. Fortunately, most of them can be prevented or their symptoms relieved.

Generally, noninfectious conditions are not transmitted by a pathogen or by any form of personal contact. They often develop over a long period of time and cause progressive damage to human tissues. Although these conditions normally do not result in death, they do lead to illness and suffering for many people. Lifestyle and personal health habits are often implicated as underlying causes; however, a number of "newer" maladies seem to defy conventional wisdom about causation. For those known maladies and **idiopathic** (of unknown cause) disorders, education, reasonable changes in lifestyle, pharmacological agents, and public health efforts aimed at research, prevention, and control can minimize their effects. In this chapter, we will discuss common noninfectious conditions and the factors that contribute to them.

Chronic Lung Diseases

Chronic obstructive pulmonary diseases (COPDs) are slowly progressive diseases of the airways that are characterized by a gradual loss of lung function.[1] Many victims suffer with a condition known as chronic **dyspnea,** a form of uncomfortable breathlessness. Others have a chronic cough and lots of sputum production, leading to a distinctive gurgling cough sound. People with these lung diseases are particularly susceptible to problems when they get colds or infections or live in areas where air quality is poor.

Typically in the United States, the term COPD includes *bronchitis, chronic obstructive bronchitis, emphysema,* or

combinations of these conditions. The conditions are often distinguished from one another according to whether it is the upper or lower region of the respiratory system that is affected.

Regardless of the specific lung disease, any time a person's breathing is impaired, the heart must work harder to supply oxygen-rich blood to the body. Prolonged strain on the heart can eventually lead to heart failure and death. Breathing difficulty can also make it hard for individuals to perform activities of daily living (ADLs) such as walking, performing household tasks, or dressing themselves. As the lungs become more impaired, they begin to fill with fluid or mucus and lose their ability to move air in and out of the body. In severe cases, oxygen tanks and mechanical breathing devices become necessary.

As these diseases progress, death is often the end result. How serious is COPD? It is the fourth leading cause of death in the United States, causing over 119,000 deaths annually.[2] By the year 2020, it is projected to be the third leading cause of death. Fortunately, COPDs are largely preventable. One of the leading causes is cigarette smoking. Other causes include smoking pipes and cigars, passive exposure to tobacco smoke, and exposure to occupational dusts and chemicals.

Allergy-Induced Respiratory Problems

An **allergy** occurs as a part of the body's attempt to defend itself against a specific *antigen* or *allergen* by producing specific *antibodies.* When foreign pathogens such as bacteria or viruses invade the body, it responds by producing antibodies to destroy these invading antigens. Under normal conditions, the production of antibodies is a positive element in the body's defense system. However, for unknown reasons, in some people the body overreacts by developing an overly elaborate protective mechanism against relatively harmless substances. The resultant *hypersensitivity reaction* to specific allergens or antigens in the environment is fairly common, as anyone who has awakened with a runny nose or itchy eyes will testify. Most commonly, these hypersensitivity, or allergic, responses occur as a reaction to environmental antigens such as molds, animal dander (hair and dead skin), pollen, ragweed, or dust. Once excessive antibodies to these antigens are produced, they trigger the release of **histamines**, chemical substances that dilate blood vessels, increase mucous secretions, cause tissues to swell, and produce other allergy-like symptoms, particularly in the respiratory system (Figure 18.1).

Over 60 million Americans have asthma or allergies.[3] Although many people think of allergies as childhood diseases, in reality allergies tend to become progressively worse with time and with increased exposure to allergens. In these circumstances, allergic responses become chronic in nature, and treatment becomes difficult. Many people take allergy shots to reduce the severity of their symptoms, with some success. In most cases, once the offending antigen has disappeared, allergy-prone people suffer few symptoms.

Idiopathic   Of unknown cause.

Chronic obstructive pulmonary diseases (COPDs) A collection of chronic lung diseases including asthma, emphysema, and chronic bronchitis.

Dyspnea   Shortness of breath, usually associated with disease of the heart or lungs.

Allergy   Hypersensitive reaction to a specific antigen or allergen in the environment in which the body produces excessive antibodies to that antigen or allergen.

Histamines   Chemical substances that dilate blood vessels, increase mucous secretions, and produce other symptoms of allergies.

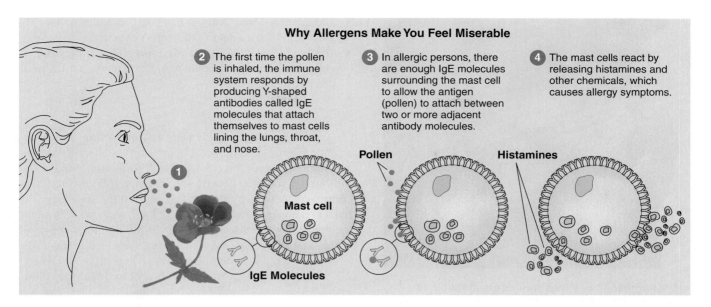

Why Allergens Make You Feel Miserable

2 The first time the pollen is inhaled, the immune system responds by producing Y-shaped antibodies called IgE molecules that attach themselves to mast cells lining the lungs, throat, and nose.

3 In allergic persons, there are enough IgE molecules surrounding the mast cell to allow the antigen (pollen) to attach between two or more adjacent antibody molecules.

4 The mast cells react by releasing histamines and other chemicals, which causes allergy symptoms.

Pollen

Histamines

Mast cell

IgE Molecules

Figure 18.1
Steps of an Allergic Response

Hay Fever Perhaps the best example of a chronic respiratory disease is **hay fever.** Usually considered a seasonally related disease (most prevalent when ragweed and flowers are blooming), hay fever is common throughout the world. Hay fever attacks, which are characterized by sneezing and itchy, watery eyes and nose, make countless people miserable. The disorder appears to run in families, and research indicates that lifestyle is not as great a factor in developing hay fever as it is in other chronic diseases. Instead, an overzealous immune system and exposure to environmental allergens including pet dander, dust, pollen from various plants, and other substances appear to be the critical factors that determine vulnerability. For those people who are unable to get away from the cause of their hay fever response, medical assistance in the form of injections or antihistamines may provide the only relief. Over 18 million adults and 7.5 million children have a diagnosis of hay fever.[4]

Asthma

Unfortunately, for many people who suffer from allergies such as hay fever, their condition often becomes complicated by the development of one of the major COPDs: asthma, emphysema, or bronchitis. **Asthma** is a long-term, chronic inflammatory disorder that blocks air flow in and out of the lungs. Asthma causes tiny airways in the lung to overreact with spasms in response to certain triggers. Although most asthma attacks are mild and nonlife-threatening, they can trigger bronchospasms (contractions of the bronchial tubes in the lungs) that are so severe that without rapid treatment, death may occur.

The good news is that asthma is a treatable condition, and flare-ups can be prevented. All asthma attacks give a warning. Learning to recognize the warning signs and treat-

ing the symptoms early can help prevent attacks or keep them from getting worse.[5] Warning signs and symptoms can include increased shortness of breath or wheezing, disturbed sleep caused by shortness of breath, cough or wheezing, chest tightness or pain, increased need to use bronchodilators (medications that open up airways by relaxing the surrounding muscles), and a fall in peak flow rates (as measured by a simple device that allows monitoring of lung function).

A number of factors can trigger an asthma attack or increase your risk of having one. These include living in a large urban area, exposure to secondhand smoke, exposure to occupational chemicals, having one or both parents with asthma, respiratory infections in childhood, low birth weight, obesity, and gastroesophageal reflux disease. Exposure to indoor air pollutants (see Chapter 21) and exposure to allergens such as dust mites, cockroach saliva, and pet dander can cause reactions. In some individuals, stress, exercise, certain medications, cold air, and sulfites are also potential triggers.

Asthma can occur at any age but is most likely to appear in children between infancy and age 5 and in adults before age 40. In childhood, asthma strikes more boys than girls; in adulthood, it afflicts more women than men. Also, the asthma rate is 50 percent higher among African Americans than whites, and four times as many African Americans

---

Hay fever A chronic respiratory disorder that is most prevalent when ragweed and flowers bloom.

Asthma A chronic respiratory disease characterized by attacks of wheezing, shortness of breath, and coughing spasms.

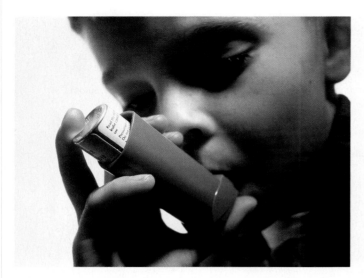

Although a number of new medications are available to relieve the symptoms of asthma, the marked increase of this respiratory problem among young children worries health officials.

die of asthma than do whites.[6] Midwesterners and Southeasterners appear to be more prone to asthma than people from other areas of the country. If you are younger than 30, your asthma is probably triggered by some type of allergy. Over age 30, attacks are often triggered by environmental irritants.

In the last decade, asthma rates have risen dramatically, particularly among children in the inner city. Consider these points regarding its spread:[7]

- Asthma is the only chronic disease, besides AIDS and tuberculosis, with an increasing death rate. Each day 14 Americans die from asthma.
- Asthma has become the most common chronic disease of childhood, accounting for one-fourth of all school absences and affecting more than one child in 20.
- Asthma affects over 17 million Americans, including 5 million children; 13 percent of all students aged 5 to 19 have it.
- The annual direct costs of asthma are over $15 billion. Among adults, asthma is the fourth leading cause of work absence, resulting in over 9 million lost workdays per year.
- The number of asthma sufferers has increased by more than 65 percent since the 1980s; one in ten new cases is diagnosed in people over age 65.

Emphysema A respiratory disease in which the alveoli become distended or ruptured and are no longer functional.

Alveoli Tiny air sacs of the lungs where gas exchange occurs (oxygen enters the body and carbon dioxide is removed).

- The death toll from asthma has nearly doubled since 1980, to more than 5,000 persons per year.
- The World Health Organization estimates that between 100 and 150 million people worldwide have asthma, and this number is rising.
- Worldwide rates of asthma are rising, on average, by 50 percent every decade.

Ask a hundred experts what causes asthma, and you might get a hundred different answers. Clearly, many factors contribute to increased risk. Although some studies have indicated a potential genetic link, much of this research is controversial, with critics pointing out that the gene pool hasn't changed much in the past few decades, yet asthma incidence has increased substantially. Most experts point to a potential allergenic cause, whereas others look to environmental, infectious, and familial links to explain the increase.

People with asthma fall into one of two distinctly different types. *Intrinsic asthma* may have allergic triggers, but any unpleasant event or stimulant may trigger an attack. In contrast, the most common form of asthma, known as *extrinsic* (or *slow onset*) *asthma*, is associated with allergic triggers. This type tends to run in families and develop in childhood. Often, by adulthood, a person has few episodes, or the disorder completely goes away. A common form of extrinsic asthma is *exercise-induced asthma (EIA)*, which may or may not have an allergic connection. Some athletes have no allergies, yet live with asthma. Cold, dry air is believed to exacerbate EIA; thus, keeping the lungs moist and warming up prior to working out may help. The warm, moist air around a swimming pool is one of the best environments for people with asthma.

Relaxation techniques appear to help some asthma sufferers. Drugs may be necessary for serious cases. Determining whether a specific allergen provokes asthma attacks, taking steps to reduce exposure, avoiding triggers such as certain types of exercise or stress, and finding the most effective medications are big steps in asthma prevention and control. Numerous new drugs are available that cause fewer side effects than older medications. Finding a doctor who specializes in asthma treatment and stays up-to-date on possible options is critical. Today the focus is on disease management and controlling triggers. The Skills for Behavior Change box identifies important preventive measures.

Emphysema

If you have ever heard someone gasping for air for no apparent reason or watched someone hooked up to an oxygen tank and struggling to breathe while climbing a flight of stairs, you have probably witnessed an emphysemic episode. **Emphysema** involves the gradual destruction of the **alveoli** (tiny air sacs through which gas exchange occurs) of the lungs. As the alveoli are destroyed, the affected person finds it more and more difficult to exhale. The victim struggles to take in a fresh supply of air before the air held in the lungs

Keys to Asthma Prevention

Although asthma rates continue to increase around the world, there is much that individuals and communities can do to reduce risk:

- Work with local leaders to reduce air pollution in your community. Investigate regulations on the burning of household and yard trash, field burning, wood-burning stoves, and second-hand smoke from cigarettes—all known triggers for asthma attacks—and work to revise them as necessary.
- Purchase a good air filter for your home, and clean furnace filters regularly. Clean house often, using a high-suction vacuum rather than a broom to reduce dust particles in suspended air.
- Wash pillows regularly to avoid pesty mites and other debris inside the pillows. Use pillow protectors and mattress protectors, which keep dust mites and other critters out of your face and trapped inside the pillow or mattress. Don't purchase used mattresses, which may be teeming with mites.
- Avoid having cats or dogs that are known for high dander production in the home. If you're a pet lover but animal dander bothers you, try a non-shedding breed such as a poodle. Keep all pets off your bed, and wash them and their bedding weekly. Vacuum their hair regularly.
- Have asthma medications handy, and know where they are kept in case of an emergency.
- Keep your home clean and pest free; cockroaches and other vermin have enzymes in their saliva or particles on their bodies that may trigger allergic reactions.
- Keep mold concentrations low by using antimold cleaners or by running a dehumidifier to keep moisture levels down.
- Avoid mowing the lawn or excessive outdoor exposure to pollen during high-pollen times. Local news stations often provide pollen warnings. If you must be outdoors, wear a pollen mask.
- Exercise regularly to keep your lungs functioning well.
- Avoid cigarette, cigar, and pipe smoke.
- If you have a fireplace or wood-burning stove, check it regularly to make sure that it is not spewing smoke and particulate matter.
- Let people close to you know that you are asthmatic, and educate them about what to do if you have an asthmatic attack. Understanding and knowledge are powerful tools for health consumers. Make sure your loved ones have access to information.

---

has been expended. Over time the chest cavity gradually expands, producing the barrel-shaped chest characteristic of the chronic emphysema patient.

The cause of emphysema is uncertain. There is, however, a strong relationship between emphysema and long-term cigarette smoking and exposure to air pollution. Victims of emphysema often suffer discomfort for many years. In fact, studies show that lung function decline may begin well before age 50, and the early morning "smoker's cough" may signal that the damage has already begun.[8] What most of us take for granted—the easy, rhythmic flow of air in and out of the lungs—becomes a continuous struggle for people with emphysema. Inadequate oxygen supply, combined with the stress of overexertion on the heart, eventually takes its toll on the cardiovascular system and leads to premature death.

Bronchitis

Bronchitis refers to an inflammation of the lining of the bronchial tubes. These tubes, the bronchi, connect the windpipe (trachea) with the lungs. When the bronchi become inflamed or infected, less air is able to flow from the lungs, and heavy mucus begins to form. **Acute bronchitis** is the most common of the bronchial diseases, resulting in millions of visits to the doctor every year.[9] Over 95 percent of these acute cases are caused by viruses; however, they are often misdiagnosed and treated with antibiotics, even though little evidence supports this treatment. Typically, misdiagnosis occurs when a cluster of symptoms is labeled as bronchitis, despite the fact that there is no true laboratory diagnosis.

Chronic bronchitis, on the other hand, is defined by the presence of a productive (mucus-laden) cough most days of the month, over three months of a year for two successive years without underlying disease to explain the cough. Other symptoms may include soreness and feeling of chest constriction, dyspnea, wheezing, chills, malaise, and slight fever. Typically, cigarette smoking causes chronic bronchitis; once bronchitis begins, secondary bacterial or viral infections often make the condition worse. Air pollution and industrial dusts and fumes are also risk factors.

Bronchitis An inflammation of the lining of the bronchial tubes.

Acute bronchitis A form of bronchitis most often caused by viruses.

Chronic bronchitis A serious respiratory disorder in which the bronchial tubes become so inflamed and swollen that respiratory function is impaired.

If you have either type of bronchitis, the following recommendations can help you reduce your risk of complications and lung damage:

- See your doctor or follow your doctor's instructions at the beginning of a cold or respiratory infection.
- Get a flu shot if you are at risk for COPDs.
- Don't smoke. If you do, quit.
- Follow a nutritious, well-balanced diet, get enough sleep, and maintain your ideal body weight.
- Exercise regularly.
- Do breathing exercises regularly to keep lungs healthy.
- Avoid exposure to colds and flu and to respiratory irritants such as secondhand smoke, dust, and air pollutants.

Sleep Apnea

Annoyed by your parent's, partner's, or roommate's snoring? Have you ever heard someone sleeping in your room stop breathing? What you have witnessed may be the warning signs of a problem known as **sleep apnea,** a problem that may be as pervasive as diabetes in the United States and believed to affect more than 18 million adults, particularly those with weight problems. What is it? The word *apnea* means "without breath," and, in this case, it refers to a serious, potentially life-threatening condition that involves brief interruptions in breathing. There are two major types of sleep apnea: central and obstructive. *Central sleep apnea* occurs when the brain fails to tell the breathing muscles to initiate breathing. Abuse of alcohol and other medications can help cause this condition. The more common form, *obstructive sleep apnea,* occurs when air cannot move in and out of a person's nose or mouth, even though the body tries to breathe.

It is a common misperception that breathing always stops entirely during the apnea phases of sleep. Often, breathing continues and the chest rises and falls, but the level of air that is exchanged is minimal. Some people may have 20 to 60 episodes of virtually no air exchange or low air exchange in an hour. Their breathing pauses or low breathing patterns usually are accompanied by snoring. When the body doesn't get enough oxygen, the heart races, blood pressure goes up, body chemistry may change, and a host of other subtle and not so subtle events occur. Most importantly, as oxygen saturation levels in the blood fall, the body's autonomic nervous system moves to protect you and signals your body to breathe, which often explains the sudden gasp of breath that may occur. Essentially, your body tries to wake you up and often knocks you out of deep, restorative sleep. If this happens over and over again in the night, people may think that they have slept; but, in fact, they rarely reached deep sleep, and they may wake up tired

and not feeling well. This is often one of the first symptoms of a person with sleep apnea.

What causes sleep apnea? Typically, obstructive apnea occurs when a person's throat muscles and tongue relax during sleep and block the airways. When the muscles of the soft palate at the base of the tongue and uvula (small fleshy tissue hanging from the center at the back of the throat) relax and sag, airways become blocked, making breathing labored and noisy and occasionally stopping breathing.[10] People who are overweight or obese often have more tissue to flap or sag, making their risk of apnea greater; however, not all people with sleep apnea are obese.

Why should we be concerned? Other than the annoyance of having a snorer in the room, there are real threats to the person affected. Chronic high blood pressure, irregular heart beats, heart attack, and stroke are among the more serious risks. Chronic fatigue, inattentiveness when driving, and general feelings of tiredness and depression may also be of concern. Some people have early morning headaches. People with untreated sleep apnea are three times more likely to have automobile accidents than people who do not suffer from it.[11]

Because sleep apnea is increasing in recognition and prevalence, more and more clinics specializing in diagnosis and treatment are available. Usually, patients are required to stay overnight in a sleep lab, which measures vital functions, sleep and arousal patterns, oxygen levels during sleep, REM (rapid eye movement) sleep, and other factors. If diagnosed, there are several options available for treatment, the most common of which is a *continuous positive airway pressure* (CPAP) device, which consists of an air flow device, long tube, and mask. Persons with sleep apnea wear this mask during sleep, and air is forced into the nose to keep the airway open. Snoring and sleep disturbances generally stop with the use of this machine. There are also surgical, laser, and other techniques for treating sleep apnea, but the results of these treatments are mixed. In people who have weight problems, losing weight often reduces the number and severity of apnea events; however, since many apnea patients have a hereditary predisposition to loose skin in the throat area without being obese, weight loss does not always solve the problem.

Sleep apnea Disorder in which a person has numerous episodes of breathing stoppage during a night's sleep.

What do you think?

Which of the respiratory diseases described in this section do you or your family have problems with? ■ *How many of your college friends have these COPDs?* ■ *What difficulties do they have in controlling their diseases?* ■ *Why do you think the incidence of COPDs, as a group, is increasing?* ■ *What actions can you or the people in your community take to reduce risks and problems from these diseases?*

Disparities in Disease Trends

In a review of the leading causes of death in the United States, clear gender, racial, and ethnic differences exist. African Americans, Hispanic Americans, Asian Americans, and white Americans display vastly different risk profiles. These differences are found not only among life-threatening diseases such as cardiovascular disease and cancer, but in many chronic conditions as well. Consider the following:

- Prevalence rates of asthma are consistently higher for blacks than for whites by approximately 50 percent. Among Hispanic Americans, death rates due to asthma are approximately 50 percent higher than among non-Hispanics.

- Females report approximately 50 percent more chronic bronchitis than males, and whites are 50 percent more likely to develop the condition than are blacks.
- Osteoarthritis is more common among males under age 45 than among their female counterparts. However, over the age of 54, osteoarthritis is more common among women than men.
- No significant racial differences in morbidity for rheumatoid arthritis are apparent; however, several American Indian tribes show a high prevalence of the disease, including the Yakima of Central Washington and the Mille-Lac Band of Chippewa in Minnesota.
- Older Americans and minority populations suffer disproportionately high rates of diabetes and diabetes-related complications.

- The prevalence of type 1 diabetes is higher among whites than among people of other races (relative risk of 1.4). In contrast, type 2 diabetes is more common among races other than whites, including blacks (1.3), Hispanic Americans (3.1), and American Indians (10.1).
- Parkinson's disease rates are higher among men than among women and more common in whites than in blacks.

Sources: R. C. Brownson, P. L. Remington, and J. Davis (eds.), *Chronic Disease Epidemiology and Control* (Washington, DC: American Public Health Association, 1998); National Center for Health Statistics, *Health: United States, 2003,* 2004, www.cdc .gov/nchs

Neurological Disorders

Headaches

If you think you are alone when you get a headache, think again. Over 50 million people see their doctors for headaches each year, and many more just silently put up with the pain or pop pain relievers to blunt the symptoms. Over 80 percent of women and 65 percent of men experience them on a regular basis.[12]

It is small comfort to know that headaches are usually not the sign of a serious disease or underlying condition and will go away fairly quickly. Over 90 percent of all headaches are of three major types: *tension headaches, migraines,* and *cluster headaches.*

Tension Headaches   These are the most common type of headache and produce what is usually a mild to moderate level of diffuse pain in the head. The name implies that stress and muscular tension in the jaw, neck, or other body areas cause this type of headache; however, newer thinking is that this headache is due to chemical and neuronal imbalances in the brain or other, as yet unknown, causes. Possible triggers for this imbalance include red wine, lack of sleep, fasting or extreme dieting (such as in the early stages of the Atkins diet), menstruation, or certain food additives or preservatives. If you suffer from this type of headache, the best thing to do might be to take over-the-counter pain medications such as aspirin, get more sleep, and record when you seem to have

symptoms. If stress is a trigger, try to relax with a hot bath, relaxing music, hot compresses, massage, or other relaxation technique. If you seem to get these headaches after eating certain foods or with other triggers, avoid them. The good news is that these types of headaches are often short lived. If they occur frequently or in combination with migraine symptoms, consult your doctor.

Migraine Headaches   More than 28 million Americans— three times more women than men—suffer from **migraines,** a type of headache that often has severe, debilitating symptoms. One of four households has a migraine sufferer.[13] While all headaches can be painful, migraines can be disabling. Symptoms vary greatly by individual, and attacks can last anywhere from 4 to 72 hours, with distinct phases of symptoms. Usually migraine incidence peaks in young adulthood, the prime years for college students, aged 20 to 45.[14] Migraines are often hereditary. If both parents have them, there is a 75 percent chance their children will have them; if only one parent has them, there is a 50 percent chance their children will have them. If any of your relatives have them, there is a 20 percent risk for you.[15] In about 15 percent of cases, migraines are preceded by a sensory warning sign

Migraine   A condition characterized by localized headaches that possibly result from alternating dilation and constriction of blood vessels.

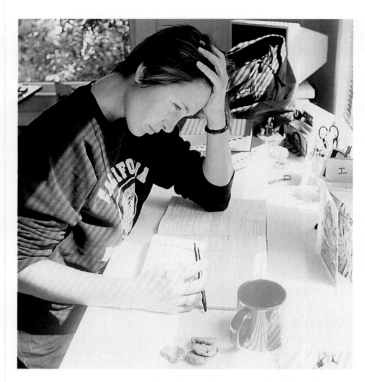

Tension headaches are triggered by many factors, including lack of sleep, stress, and strain on head and neck muscles.

known as an *aura*, such as flashes of light, flickering vision, blind spots, tingling in arms or legs, or sensation of odor or taste. Sometimes, nausea, vomiting, and extreme sensitivity to light and sound are present.[16] Symptoms of migraines include pain behind or around one eye and usually on the same side of the head. Pain may be excruciating and can last for hours or days. In some people, there is sinus pain, neck pain, or an aura without headache.

Patients report that migraines can be triggered by emotional stress, weather, certain foods, lack of sleep, and a litany of other causes. When tested under laboratory settings, however, much of this evidence is inconclusive. What is known is that migraines occur when blood vessels dilate in the membrane that surrounds the brain. Historically, treatments have centered on reversing or preventing this dilation, with the most common treatment derived from the rye fungus *ergot*. Today, fast-acting ergot compounds are available by nasal spray, vastly increasing the speed of relief. However, ergot drugs have many side effects, the least of which may be that they are habit forming, causing users to wake up with "rebound" headaches each morning after use.[17]

Critics of the blood vessel dilation theory question why only blood vessels of the head dilate in these situations.

Epilepsy   A neurological disorder caused by abnormal electrical brain activity; can be accompanied by altered consciousness or convulsions.

Furthermore, why aren't people who take hot baths or those who exercise more prone to migraine attacks? They suggest that migraines originate in the cortex of the brain, where certain pain sensors are stimulated.

According to pioneering work by Harvard University neurology professor Michael Moskowitz, triggers, such as caffeine or wine, set off an electrical ripple on the surface of the cortex. Waves of nerve cells fire and then go quiet, creating an aura. This spurs a reaction in the meninges, the membranes above the cortex. The meninges contain endings of one of the brain's major nerves, the *trigeminus,* which release chemicals that inflame nearby tissues. The result is pain.[18]

Other doctors believe that pain signals begin deep in the brain in areas normally rich in the painkilling chemical serotonin. Migraines are started by disturbances that keep the pain-regulating chemicals from doing their job. Susceptibility to these disturbances may be hereditary. This theory would explain why drugs that interact with serotonin reduce headaches. (It must be said that there is no proof that serotonin irregularities cause headaches—only that serotonin drugs work.)[19]

When true migraines occur, relaxation is only minimally effective as a treatment. Often, strong pain-relieving drugs prescribed by a physician are necessary. Imitrex, a drug tailor-made for migraines, works for about 80 percent of those who try it. However, Imitrex is expensive and its side effects make it inappropriate for anyone with uncontrolled high blood pressure or heart disease. Recently, treatment with lidocaine has shown promising results, and newer drugs called triptans, such as Zomig, Amerge, and Maxalt, are now available. All triptans, however, are cleared from the body in a few hours, and the migraine sometimes returns.[20]

Cluster Headaches   Fortunately, cluster headaches are among the more rare forms of headache, affecting less than 1 percent of people, usually men.[21] Although cluster headaches are less common than migraines, the pain can be worse. Usually these headaches cause stabbing pain on one side of the head, behind the eye, or in one defined spot. They can last for weeks and disappear quickly but, most commonly, last for 30 to 45 minutes.[22] Oxygen therapy, drugs, and even surgery have been used to treat severe cases.

Secondary Headaches   Secondary headaches arise as a result of some other underlying, usually organic, condition. Hypertension, blocked sinuses, allergies, low blood sugar, diseases of the spine, the common cold, poorly fitted dentures, problems with eyesight, and other types of pain or injury can trigger this condition. Relaxation and pain relievers such as aspirin are of little help in treating secondary headaches. Rather, medications or other therapies to relieve the underlying organic cause of the headache must be included in the treatment regimen.

Seizure Disorders

The word *epilepsy* derives from the Greek *epilepsia,* meaning "seizure." Reports of epilepsy appeared in Greek medical records as early as 300 BC. Ancient peoples interpreted seizures as invasions of the body by evil spirits or as punishments by the gods. Although much of the mystery surrounding epileptic seizures has been solved in recent years, the stigma and lack of understanding remain. Approximately 2 million people in the United States suffer from some form of seizure-related disorder, and between 5 and 10 percent of the population will experience at least one seizure in their lives.[23]

These disorders are generally caused by abnormal electrical activity in the brain and are characterized by loss of control of muscular activity and unconsciousness. Symptoms vary widely from person to person and can range from temporary confusion to major motor seizing.

Epilepsy is most common in childhood and after age 65 but can occur at any time. Typically seizures fall into one of two categories. When they seem related to abnormal activity in just one region of the brain, they are classified as partial. When they involve all or most parts of the brain, they are generalized. Common seizure disorders include:[24]

- *Narcolepsy.* A condition in which the individual falls asleep at unpredictable times
- *Grand mal, or major motor seizure.* These seizures are often preceded by a shrill cry or a seizure aura (body sensations such as ringing in the ears or a specific smell or taste). Convulsions and loss of consciousness generally occur and may last from 30 seconds to several minutes or more. Keeping track of the length of time elapsed is one aspect of first aid.
- *Petit mal, or minor, seizure.* These seizures involve no convulsions. Rather, a minor loss of consciousness occurs, which may even go unnoticed. Minor twitching of muscles may take place, usually for a shorter time than grand mal convulsions.
- *Psychomotor seizure.* These seizures involve both mental processes and muscular activity. Symptoms include mental confusion and a listless state characterized by activities such as lip smacking, chewing, and repetitive movements.
- *Jacksonian, or focal, seizure.* This is a progressive seizure that often begins in one part of the body, such as the fingers, and moves to other parts, such as the hand or arm. Usually only one side of the body is affected.

About half of all cases of seizure disorder are of unknown origin. Stroke and head injury or trauma are possible causes; other causes include congenital abnormalities, injury or illness resulting in inflammation of the brain or spinal column, drug or chemical poisoning, tumors, nutritional deficiency, and heredity.

In most cases, people afflicted with seizure disorders can lead normal, seizure-free lives when under medical supervision. Public ignorance about these disorders is one of the most serious obstacles confronting them. Improvements in medication and surgical interventions to reduce some causes of seizures are among the most promising treatments today.

Providing First Aid for Seizures   There are several things you can do to help people during and after seizures.

1. *Note the length of the attack.* Seizures in which a person remains unconscious for long periods of time should be monitored closely. If medical help arrives, be sure to tell the medical personnel how long it has been since the person became unconscious.
2. *Remove obstacles that could harm the victim.* Because seizure victims may lose motor control during a convulsion, they inadvertently thrash around. To reduce the chances of serious injury, clear away any objects that could pose a threat.
3. *Loosen clothing, and turn the victim's head to the side.* This procedure will ensure adequate ventilation and allow fluids or vomit to drain from the mouth.
4. *Do not force objects into the victim's mouth.* Although seizure victims may bite their tongues, causing possible damage, they will not swallow them. If the victim's mouth is clamped shut, forcing objects into the mouth may break teeth or cause more harm than doing nothing.
5. *Get help.* After you have completed steps 1 through 4, get help or send someone for help. This is particularly important if the victim does not regain consciousness within a few minutes.
6. *Reassure the victim.* In too many instances, the seizure victim regains consciousness only to face a crowd of staring people. When administering first aid, try to dissuade curious bystanders from hanging around. Calmly reassure the victim that everything is okay.
7. *Allow the person to rest.* After a seizure, many people will be exhausted. Allow them to sleep if possible.

What do you think?

Do you suffer from recurrent headaches or other neurological problems? ■ *What might cause your problems?* ■ *What actions could you take to reduce your risks and symptoms?*

Parkinson's Disease

Until recently, most people thought of Parkinson's disease as something that afflicted only older people. Many were surprised when one of the younger generation, actor Michael J. Fox, announced that he suffers from the disease. Over 1.5 million Americans are believed to have **Parkinson's disease**, a chronic, slowly progressive neurological condition that typically strikes after age 50. Rates of Parkinson's have

Parkinson's disease   A chronic, progressive neurological condition that causes tremors and other symptoms.

quadrupled in the past 30 years and may increase even more dramatically as growing numbers of baby boomers pass age 60. Nearly 60,000 new cases are diagnosed each year. Fifteen percent of the people diagnosed are under age 50.[25]

The hallmark of Parkinson's disease, and the symptom most commonly associated with it, is a tremor or "shaking palsy." Tremors can become so severe that the simplest tasks, such as eating or brushing one's teeth, become difficult or impossible. Additional symptoms may include:

- Tremor of the hand when in a relaxed position or when under stress
- Rigid or stiff muscles
- Slowness in movement and a delay in initiating movements
- Poor balance
- Difficulty in walking, shuffling steps, and inability to take next steps
- Slurred speech, slowness in thought, and small, cramped handwriting

Although many theories exist concerning the causes of this disease, most are only speculative. The most common factors being studied include:[26]

- Familial predisposition, particularly for younger patients (about 15 to 20 percent of those who have Parkinson's have a close relative with it). However, newer research indicates that heredity is probably not as great a factor as previously believed.
- Acceleration of age-related changes
- Exposure to environmental toxins such as pesticides
- Past illnesses/disorders
- Trauma

Parkinson's is progressive and incurable. However, new drug therapies, including levodopa, dopamine antagonists, and MAOIs, work to keep symptoms under control, possibly for years. Surgical options such as brain tissue transplants and the use of fetal tissue or genetically engineered cell transplants have also provided promising results.

Multiple Sclerosis (MS)

Multiple sclerosis (MS) is a degenerative neurological disease in which the myelin, a fatty material that serves as an insulator that facilitates transmission of nerve impulses,

breaks down and causes nerve malfunction, or short-circuiting. As the myelin degenerates, it scars; hence the sclerotic (scar) terminology. Typically, MS appears between ages 15 and 50 and is characterized by periods of relapse (when symptoms flare up) and remissions (when symptoms are not present).

Symptoms of MS vary considerably from one person to the next. Some experience mild problems of episodic numbness, dizziness, fatigue, changes in gait, and temporary vision loss. Others face more severe symptoms, including loss of bladder control and severe muscle weakness, necessitating a wheelchair for mobility. Most MS patients lead fairly normal lives and have few disease flare-ups.

Though several hypotheses address possible causes of MS, none has been proved conclusively. Allergies, viral exposure to an unknown pathogen, and environmental factors all have been considered as possible causes.

Those who have been diagnosed with MS should practice commonsense strategies for preventing flare-ups. As with most neurological problems, risk reduction includes practicing a healthy lifestyle—particularly getting adequate sleep, eating a well-balanced diet, and controlling stress.[27] Temperature extremes, including exposure to cold, damp weather or to excessive heat and humidity can make symptoms flare.

Gender-Related Disorders

Fibrocystic Breast Condition

A common, noncancerous problem among women in the United States is **fibrocystic breast condition.** Symptoms range in severity from one small, palpable lump to large masses of irregular tissue found in both breasts. The underlying causes of the condition are unknown. Although some experts relate it to hormonal changes that occur during the normal menstrual cycle, many women report that their conditions neither worsen nor improve during their cycles. In fact, in most cases, the condition appears to run in families and to become progressively worse with age, irrespective of pregnancy or other hormonal disruptions. Although most cyst formations consist of fibrous tissue, some are filled with fluid. Treatment often involves removing fluid from the affected area or surgically removing the cyst itself.

Does fibrocystic breast condition predispose a woman to breast cancer? Experts believe that the risks for breast cancer among women with certain types of fibrocystic disease may be slightly higher than among the general populace, but it is likely that other factors, discussed in detail in Chapter 16, present much greater risks.

Endometriosis

Endometriosis is characterized by the abnormal growth and development of endometrial tissue (the tissue lining the uterus) in regions of the body other than the uterus. It is

---

Multiple sclerosis (MS) A degenerative neurological disease in which myelin, an insulator of nerves, breaks down.

Fibrocystic breast condition A common, noncancerous condition in which a woman's breasts contain fibrous or fluid-filled cysts.

Endometriosis Abnormal development of endometrial tissue outside the uterus, resulting in serious side effects.

Uterine Fibroids

Severe abdominal cramps. Incontinence. Infertility. Excessive bleeding during the menstrual cycle. Back pain. If you are one of the many women who suffer from these symptoms but can't figure out what might be wrong, a trip to your gynecologist should be on your schedule. For the majority of women who have these symptoms, it isn't cancer that is stalking you; it is more likely to be the fairly common problem of uterine fibroids.

Uterine fibroids are benign (noncancerous) growths that can develop in a woman's uterine tissue. They may range in size from pea-sized growths to the size of a football or larger, weighing in at over 20 pounds. It is not uncommon for a woman to have several at a time. Many fibroids grow in the thick inner walls (endometrium) of the uterus; others may develop from the outer walls of the uterus on stalks or as large masses.

Who is susceptible to fibroids? Although they are typically found in women between the ages of 35 to 50, fibroids can occur at any age. African American women are two to three times more likely to have fibroids and typically develop them at younger ages than other groups of women. Asian women have the lowest incidence.

Risk factors associated with fibroids include obesity and the consumption of red meat, pork, and ham. Green leafy vegetables, fruit, and fish seem to bestow some type of protective effect resulting in a reduced incidence of fibroids.

Fibroid symptoms include obvious changes in menstruation (excessive bleeding and cramps, longer periods, bleeding between periods, anemia) and pain in the lower back or abdomen. Other symptoms include a feeling of pressure, abdominal cramping, the need to urinate more frequently, constipation, and/or pain during sex. However, some women have none of these symptoms. Fibroids may grow and obstruct the uterine tubes, leading to infertility, or they may obstruct the bowel or other body parts, leading to dysfunction.

If symptoms become severe or persist, a woman must choose the treatment that's best for her situation. Because most fibroids grow in the presence of estrogen, if a woman is near menopause, the fibroids may shrink on their own as a part of natural hormone depletion. Thus, if the pain or problems are tolerable, a woman can "wait them out," and the fibroids may shrivel and never cause further problems.

Other women may opt for surgical removal of the fibroids. Women of childbearing age may choose to have a *myomectomy* (removal of the fibroids only, preserving the uterus), a *hysterectomy* (removal of the uterus and/or one or both ovaries), a *fibroid embolization* (a catheter is placed in an artery and guided to the uterus, where small particles are injected to block the blood supply feeding the fibroids, eventually killing them), or other techniques designed to destroy the fibroids' ability to grow.

It is estimated that 30 to 80 percent of all women may have fibroids of varying size during their lives. Many never know they have them. Fibroids can be detected during an annual pelvic examination and verified by ultrasound, laparoscopy, magnetic resonance imaging (MRI), or computerized tomography (CT) scans. While little can be done to prevent fibroids, paying attention to changes or unusual events with the menstrual cycle and to general body health may help detect them early. Regular checkups are important for early detection and monitoring before the fibroids develop into more serious problems.

Source: National Uterine Fibroids Foundation, "About Uterine Fibroids," 2004, www.nuff .org/health.htm

---

most likely to appear between the ages of 20 and 40. It is difficult to determine whether the incidence of endometriosis is on the rise in the United States or whether the disorder is simply attracting more attention.

Symptoms of endometriosis include severe cramping during and between menstrual cycles, irregular periods, unusually heavy or light menstrual flow, abdominal bloating, fatigue, painful bowel movements with periods, painful intercourse, constipation, diarrhea, menstrual pain, infertility, and low back pain. Among the most widely accepted theories concerning the causes of endometriosis are the transmission of endometrial tissue to other regions of the body during surgery or through the birthing process; the movement of menstrual fluid backward through the uterine tubes during menstruation; and abnormal cell migration through body-fluid movement. Women with cycles shorter than 27 days or flows lasting over a week are at increased risk. The more aerobic exercise a woman engages in and the earlier she starts it, the less likely she is to develop endometriosis.

Treatment ranges from bed rest and stress reduction to **hysterectomy** (the removal of the uterus) and/or the removal of one or both ovaries and the uterine tubes. Physicians have been criticized for being too quick to select hysterectomy as the treatment of choice. More conservative treatments that involve dilation and curettage, surgically scraping endometrial tissue off the uterine tubes and other reproductive organs, and combinations of hormone therapy have become more acceptable. Hormonal treatments include gonadotropin-releasing hormone (GnRH) analogs, various synthetic progesterone-like drugs (Provera), and oral contraceptives. (See the Reality Check box for information about another problem of the female reproductive system: uterine fibroids.)

Hysterectomy   Surgical removal of the uterus.

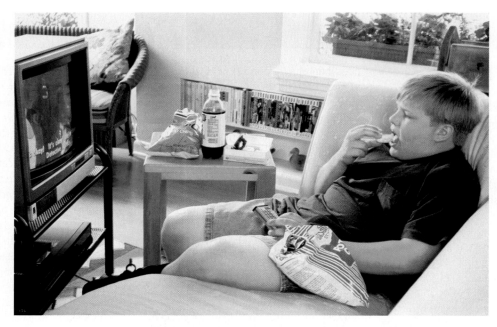

Unhealthy eating habits and a sedentary lifestyle can lead to type 2 diabetes even among children.

What do you think?

Which of the preceding health problems do you think causes the most problems for women in the United States? ■ *For college-age women?* ■ *Why might certain groups of women have more difficulties than others?* ■ *What actions could be taken to increase awareness and understanding of these conditions?*

Digestion-Related Disorders

Diabetes: Disabling, Deadly, and on the Rise

Diabetes is a serious, widespread, and costly chronic disease, affecting not just the 18 million Americans who must live with it, but their families and communities. Between 1980 and 2002, diagnosed diabetes increased over 50 percent among U.S. adults, giving it the dubious distinction of being the fastest growing chronic disease in American history.[28] (Figure 18.2 shows the rapid spread of diabetes since 1990.) A recent study by the Centers for Disease Control indicated that diabetes seems to be increasing even more dramatically among younger adults—it is up by almost 70 percent among those in their thirties.[29]

Over 2,200 people are diagnosed with diabetes each day in America and over 200,000 die each year of related complications, making diabetes the sixth leading cause of death in America today.[30] Diabetes has its greatest impact on the elderly and certain racial and ethnic groups. One in five adults over age 65 has diabetes. Among adults aged 20 and older, African Americans are twice as likely as whites to have diabetes, and American Indians and Alaska Natives are 2.6 times more likely to develop it.[31] Overall diabetes rates are projected to double by 2050.

What causes this serious disease? In healthy people, the *pancreas,* a powerful enzyme-producing organ, produces the hormone **insulin** in sufficient quantities to allow the body to use or store glucose (blood sugar). When the pancreas fails to produce enough insulin to regulate sugar metabolism or when the body fails to use insulin effectively, a disease known as **diabetes mellitus** occurs (Figure 18.3). Diabetics exhibit **hyperglycemia,** or elevated blood sugar levels, and high glucose levels in their urine. Other symptoms include excessive thirst, frequent urination, hunger, tendency to tire easily, wounds that heal slowly, numbness or tingling in the extremities, changes in vision, skin eruptions, and, in women, a tendency toward vaginal yeast infections. Of the 17 million people in the United States today who have diabetes, nearly 6 million are unaware of their condition.

Insulin   A hormone produced by the pancreas; required by the body for the metabolism of carbohydrates.

Diabetes mellitus   A disease in which the pancreas fails to produce enough insulin or the body fails to use insulin effectively.

Hyperglycemia   Elevated blood sugar levels.

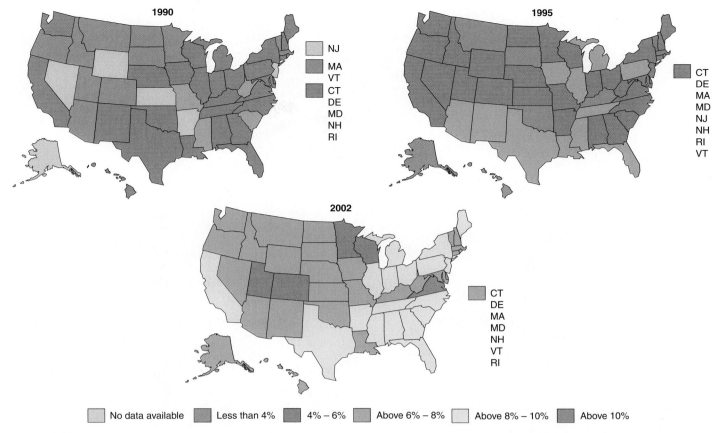

Figure 18.2

Percentage of Adults with Diagnosed Diabetes*

*includes women with gestational diabetes

Source: Centers for Disease Control and Prevention, "Diabetes: Disabling, Deadly and on the Rise, At A Glance 2004," 2004, www.cdc.gov/nccdphp/aag/aag/ddt.htm

How does a person become diabetic? The more serious form, known as *type 1 diabetes* (formerly known as insulin-dependent, or juvenile, diabetes), is an autoimmune disease in which the immune system destroys the insulin-making beta cells and most often appears during childhood or adolescence.[32] Type 1 diabetics typically must depend on insulin injections or oral medications for the rest of their lives because insulin is not present in their bodies.

In *type 2 diabetes* (formerly known as noninsulin-dependent, or adult-onset, diabetes), insulin production is deficient or the body is unable to utilize available insulin. Type 2 diabetes accounts for 90 to 95 percent of all diabetes cases and most often appears after age 40.[33] However, type 2 diabetes is now being diagnosed at younger ages, even among children and teens. This form of diabetes is typically linked to obesity and physical inactivity, both of which can be modified to control diabetes and improve health. If people with type 2 diabetes change their lifestyle, they may be able to avoid oral medications or insulin indefinitely.

A third type of diabetes, called *gestational diabetes,* can develop in a woman during pregnancy and affects 2 to 5 percent of all pregnant women. The condition usually disappears after childbirth, but it does leave the woman at greater risk of developing type 2 diabetes at some point. Other, less common, forms of diabetes can result from genetic syndromes, surgery, drugs, malnutrition, infections, and other illnesses.[34]

Understanding Risk Factors   Diabetes tends to run in families. Being overweight, coupled with inactivity, dramatically increases the risk of type 2 diabetes. Older persons and mothers of babies weighing over 9 pounds also run an increased risk. Approximately 80 percent of all type 2 patients are overweight at the time of diagnosis. Weight loss, better nutrition, control of blood glucose levels, and regular exercise are important factors in lowering blood sugar and improving the efficiency of cellular use of insulin. These improvements can help to prevent overwork of the pancreas and the development of diabetes. In fact, recent findings show that modest, consistent physical activity and a healthy diet can cut a person's risk of type 2 diabetes by nearly 60 percent.[35] African Americans, Hispanics, and American Indians have the highest

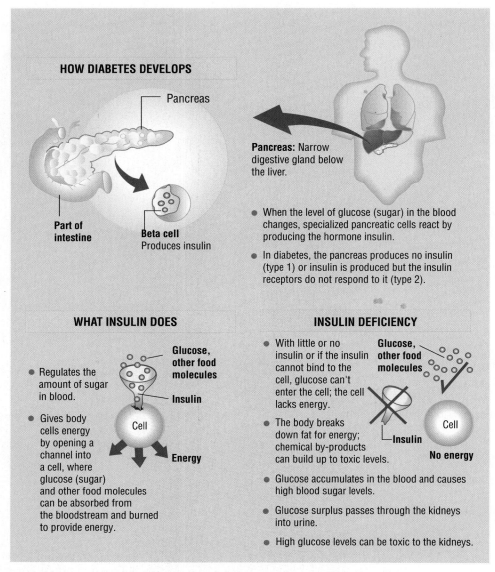

HOW DIABETES DEVELOPS

Pancreas

Part of intestine

Beta cell
Produces insulin

Pancreas: Narrow digestive gland below the liver.

- When the level of glucose (sugar) in the blood changes, specialized pancreatic cells react by producing the hormone insulin.

- In diabetes, the pancreas produces no insulin (type 1) or insulin is produced but the insulin receptors do not respond to it (type 2).

WHAT INSULIN DOES

Glucose, other food molecules

Insulin

Cell

Energy

- Regulates the amount of sugar in blood.

- Gives body cells energy by opening a channel into a cell, where glucose (sugar) and other food molecules can be absorbed from the bloodstream and burned to provide energy.

INSULIN DEFICIENCY

Glucose, other food molecules

Insulin

Cell
No energy

- With little or no insulin or if the insulin cannot bind to the cell, glucose can't enter the cell; the cell lacks energy.

- The body breaks down fat for energy; chemical by-products can build up to toxic levels.

- Glucose accumulates in the blood and causes high blood sugar levels.

- Glucose surplus passes through the kidneys into urine.

- High glucose levels can be toxic to the kidneys.

Figure 18.3
Diabetes

Sources: Adaptation based on *Oregonian,* September 5, 2000, A6; *FDA Consumer* magazine; J. Mordis and W. Manis, *The Healing Handbook for Persons with Diabetes,* 3rd ed., 2000. www.umassmed.edu/diabeteshandbook; L. Urdang, ed., *The Bantam Medical Dictionary,* 3rd ed. (New York: Bantam, 2000); American Medical Association, *American Medical Association Family Medical Guide,* 4th ed. (New York: Wiley, 2004); research by Jutta Scheibe.

rates of type 2 diabetes in the world—much higher than that of whites. The reasons for this increased risk are not clear.[36] (See Figure 18.4 for a comparison of rates.)

People who develop diabetes today have a much better prognosis than just 20 years ago. Recognize your own risk for this disease and take steps to reduce it. The Assess Yourself box will help you determine if you are at risk for diabetes.

Controlling Diabetes Most physicians attempt to control type 1 and later stages of type 2 diabetes with a variety of

insulin-related drugs. Most of these drugs are taken orally, although self-administered hypodermic injections are prescribed when other treatments are inadequate. Recent breakthroughs in individual monitoring and implantable insulin monitors and insulin infusion pumps that regulate insulin intake "on demand" have provided many people with diabetes the opportunity to lead normal lives.

Newer forms of insulin that last longer in the body and have fewer side effects are now available. As we go to press, an insulin inhaler is being tested for possible widespread use.

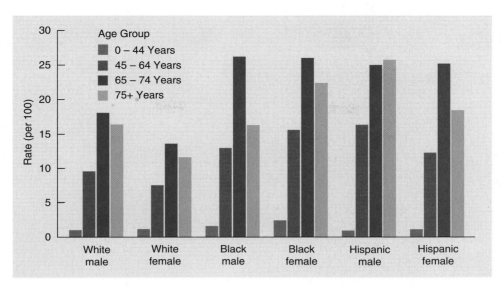

Figure 18.4
Age-Specific Prevalence of Diagnosed Diabetes, by Race/Ethnicity and Sex, 2002

Source: Centers for Disease Control and Prevention, "Diabetes Surveillance System," 2004, www.cdc.gov/diabetes/statistics/prev/national/fig2002.htm

All of these treatments come at a price. On average, health care costs for diabetics are $10,000 to $20,000 higher per year than for healthy patients. The direct and indirect costs of treating diabetes in the United States total $132 billion per year.[37] However, the full burden of diabetes is hard to measure: death records often do not reflect the role of diabetes in a person's death, and the costs related to undiagnosed diabetes are unknown.

Some people find that they can manage their diabetes effectively by eating foods that are rich in complex carbohydrates, low in sodium, and high in fiber; by losing weight; and by getting regular exercise. Developing a routine for monitoring and controlling this disease can be stressful, particularly in the beginning. Some reports even suggest that people with diabetes may be at a greater-than-average risk for clinical depression.[38] Attention to psychosocial needs is often an important aspect of diabetic health.

Preventing Complications   Depending on the type and severity of the disease, diabetes can cause many complications and increase the severity of other existing conditions. If diabetes rates can be reduced, the real impact may be seen in reductions in diabetes complications and prevention of diabetes-related diseases. Consider the following problems that diabetes causes or contributes to and actions that may help reduce their burden:[39]

- *Eye disease and blindness.* Each year, 12,000–24,000 people become blind because of diabetic eye disease. In fact, it is the leading cause of new blindness in America today. Screenings and care could prevent up to 90 percent of diabetes-related blindness, but only 64.2 percent of people with diabetes received annual dilated eye exams in 2002.
- *Kidney disease.* In 2002, 42,813 people with diabetes developed kidney failure; each year over 100,000 are in treatment for this condition. Better control of blood pressure and blood glucose levels could reduce diabetes-related kidney failure by about 50 percent.
- *Amputations.* About 82,000 people have diabetes-related leg and foot amputations each year. Foot care programs that include regular examinations and patient education could prevent up to 85 percent of these amputations.
- *Cardiovascular disease.* Heart disease and stroke cause about 65 percent of deaths among people with diabetes. These deaths could be reduced by 30 percent with improved care to control blood pressure and blood glucose and lipid levels.
- *Pregnancy complications.* About 18,000 women with preexisting diabetes deliver babies each year, and an estimated 135,000 expectant mothers are diagnosed with gestational diabetes. These women and their babies have an increased risk for serious complications. Screenings and diabetes care before and after pregnancy can reduce the risk for complications such as stillbirths, congenital malformations, and the need for cesarean sections.
- *Flu- and pneumonia-related deaths.* Each year, 10,000 to 30,000 people with diabetes die of complications from flu or pneumonia. They are roughly three times more likely to die of these complications than people without diabetes, yet only 55 percent of people with diabetes get an annual flu shot. In the 2004–2005 flu season, vaccine shortages may increase the risk for diabetics.

Are You at Risk for Diabetes?

myhealthlab

Fill out this assessment online at www.aw-bc.com/myhealthlab or www.aw-bc.com/donatelle

Certain characteristics place people at greater risk for diabetes. Nevertheless, many people remain unaware of the symptoms of diabetes until after the disease has begun to progress. If you answer yes to three or more of the following questions, you should consider seeking medical advice. Talk to health professionals at your student health center, or make an appointment with your family physician.

		Yes	No
1.	Do you have a history of diabetes in your family?	❏	❏
2.	Do any of your primary relatives (mother, father, sister, brother, grandparents) have diabetes?	❏	❏
3.	Are you overweight or obese?	❏	❏
4.	Are you typically sedentary (seldom, if ever, engage in vigorous aerobic exercise)?	❏	❏
5.	Have you noticed an increase in your craving for water or other beverages?	❏	❏
6.	Have you noticed that you have to urinate more frequently than you used to during a typical day?	❏	❏
7.	Have you noticed any tingling or numbness in your hands and feet, which might indicate circulatory problems?	❏	❏
8.	Do you often feel a gnawing hunger during the day, even though you usually eat regular meals?	❏	❏
9.	Have you noticed that you are losing weight but don't seem to be doing anything in particular to make this happen?	❏	❏
10.	Are you often so tired that you find it difficult to stay awake to study, watch television, or engage in other activities?	❏	❏
11.	Have you noticed that you have skin irritations more frequently and that minor infections don't heal as quickly as they used to?	❏	❏
12.	Have you noticed any unusual changes in your vision (blurring, difficulty in focusing, etc.)?	❏	❏
13.	Have you noticed unusual pain or swelling in your joints?	❏	❏
14.	Do you often feel weak or nauseated if you wait too long to eat a meal?	❏	❏
15.	If you are a woman, have you had several vaginal (yeast) infections during the past year?	❏	❏

MAKE IT HAPPEN!

Use the results of this self-assessment to begin your behavior change program. Follow the steps and use the examples on page 545 to complete your Behavior Change Contract, and use these resources to take action.

Lactose Intolerance

As many as 50 million Americans are unable to eat dairy products such as milk, cheese, or ice cream. They suffer from **lactose intolerance,** meaning that they have lost the ability to produce the digestive enzyme lactase, which is necessary for the body to convert milk sugar (lactose) into glucose. That cold glass of milk becomes a source of stomach cramping, diarrhea, nausea, gas, and related symptoms. (See Chapter 8 for a discussion of other things we eat that may cause intolerance.) Lactose intolerance, however, may not require avoiding all dairy products. Once diagnosed, it can be treated by introducing low-lactose or lactose-free foods into the diet. Through trial and error, individuals usually find that they can tolerate one type of low-lactose food better than others. As an alternative to consuming foods without lactose, some people purchase special products that supply the missing lactase and thus eat dairy foods without serious side effects. Most large grocery chains, food cooperatives, and drug stores have these products available in liquid or tablet form. It should be noted, however, that these products do not work for everyone; someone who is lactose intolerant may need to experiment before settling into a diet that works. Furthermore, many people who think they are lactose intolerant actually are not. If you suspect that you are lactose intolerant, diagnostic tests can provide conclusive evidence.

> **Lactose intolerance** The inability to produce lactase, an enzyme needed to convert milk sugar into glucose.

Colitis and Irritable Bowel Syndrome

Ulcerative colitis is a disease of the large intestine in which the mucous membranes of the intestinal walls become inflamed. Victims with severe cases may have as many as 20 bouts of bloody diarrhea a day. Colitis can also produce severe stomach cramps, weight loss, nausea, sweating, and fever. Although some experts believe that colitis occurs more frequently in people with high stress levels, this theory is controversial. Hypersensitivity reactions, particularly to milk and certain foods, have also been considered as a possible cause. It is difficult to determine the cause of colitis because the disease goes into unexplained remission and then recurs without apparent reason. This pattern often continues over periods of years and may be related to the later development of colorectal cancer. Because the cause of colitis remains unknown, treatment focuses on relieving the symptoms. Increasing fiber intake and taking anti-inflammatory drugs, steroids, and other medications to reduce inflammation and soothe irritated intestinal walls can relieve symptoms.

Many people with colitis develop a related condition known as **irritable bowel syndrome (IBS),** characterized by nausea, pain, gas, diarrhea attacks, or cramps occurring after eating certain foods or during unusual stress. IBS symptoms commonly begin in early adulthood. Symptoms may vary from week to week and can fade for long periods of time, only to return.

The cause is unknown, but researchers suspect that people with IBS have digestive systems that are overly sensitive to what they eat and drink, to stress, and to certain hormonal changes. They may also be more sensitive to pain signals from the stomach. Stress management, relaxation techniques, regular activity, and diet can control IBS in the vast majority of cases. Problems with diarrhea can be reduced by cutting down on fat and avoiding caffeine and excessive amounts of sorbitol, a sweetener found in dietetic foods and chewing gum. Many IBS patients are lactose intolerant. Constipation can be relieved by a gradual increase in fiber. Some sufferers benefit from anticholinergic drugs, which relax the intestinal muscle, or from antidepressant drugs and psychological counseling. Medical advice should be sought whenever such conditions persist.

Diverticulosis

Diverticulosis occurs when the walls of the intestine weaken for undetermined reasons and small pea-sized bulges develop. These bulges often fill with feces and, over time, become irritated and infected, causing pain and discomfort. If this irritation persists, bleeding and chronic obstruction may occur, either of which can be life threatening.

Although diverticulosis may appear in any part of the intestinal wall, it most commonly occurs in the small intestine. Often the person affected may be unaware that the problem exists. However, in some cases, a person may actually have an attack similar to the pain of appendicitis except that the pain is on the left side of the body instead of the right, where the appendix is located. Although diverticulosis most frequently occurs during and after middle age, it can appear at any age. If you have persistent discomfort in the lower abdominal region, seek medical attention at once.

Peptic Ulcers

An ulcer is a lesion or wound that forms in body tissue as a result of some form of irritant. A **peptic ulcer** is a chronic ulcer that occurs in the lining of the stomach or the section of the small intestine known as the *duodenum.* It has been thought to be caused by the erosive effect of digestive juices on these tissues. The lining of these organs becomes irritated, the protective covering of mucus is reduced, and the gastric acid begins to digest the dying tissue, just as it would a piece of food. Typically, this irritation causes pain that disappears when the person eats but returns about an hour later.

For many years, doctors believed that peptic ulcers were caused by eating spicy foods and acid-reducing drugs were the accepted treatment. However, research now indicates that a common bacterium, *Helicobacter pylori,* causes most ulcers. This means that antibiotics can effectively treat this disorder, which affects over 4 million Americans every year, and significantly reduce the risk of recurrence. In addition to antibiotic treatment, people with ulcers should also avoid high-fat foods, alcohol, and substances such as aspirin that may irritate organ linings or cause increased secretion of stomach acids and thereby exacerbate this condition. In extreme cases, surgery is necessary to relieve persistent symptoms.

Gallbladder Disease

Also known as *cholecystitis,* **gallbladder disease** occurs when the gallbladder has been repeatedly irritated by chemicals, infection, or overuse, thus reducing its ability to release bile used for the digestion of fats. Usually, gallstones, consisting of calcium, cholesterol, and other minerals, form in the gallbladder itself. When the patient eats foods that are high in fat, the gallbladder contracts to release bile and presses on

---

Ulcerative colitis An inflammatory disorder that affects the mucous membranes of the large intestine, producing bloody diarrhea.

Irritable bowel syndrome (IBS) Nausea, pain, gas, or diarrhea caused by certain foods or stress.

Diverticulosis A condition in which bulges form in the walls of the intestine; results in irritation and infection of the intestine.

Peptic ulcer Damage to the stomach or intestinal lining, usually caused by digestive juices.

Gallbladder disease A disease caused by repeated irritation of the gallbladder, which leads to the formation of gallstones.

the gallstones. One of the characteristic symptoms of gall-bladder disease is acute pain in the upper right portion of the abdomen after eating fatty foods. This pain, which can last for several hours, may feel like a heart attack or an ulcer and is often accompanied by nausea.

Who gets gallbladder disease? The old adage about the "five f's" of risk factors frequently holds true. Anyone who is "female, fat, fair, forty, and flatulent" (prone to passing gas) appears to be at increased risk. However, people who don't fit this picture also get the disease.

Current treatment of gallbladder disease usually involves medication to reduce irritation, restriction of fat consumption, and surgery to remove the gallstones. New medications designed to dissolve small gallstones may help some patients. Another option is a procedure called *lithotripsy*, in which a series of noninvasive shock waves breaks up small stones. Surgery may be performed with lasers and various forms of laparoscopy to eliminate the risks associated with large surgical incisions.

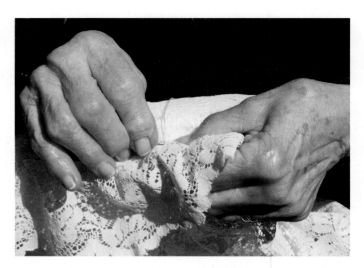

Arthritis can make simple tasks both painful and difficult to accomplish.

What do you think?

What role can a healthy diet play in reducing risks for and symptoms of the diseases discussed here? ■ *Are you or any of your family members at risk for these problems?* ■ *What actions can you take today that will cut your risk?*

Musculoskeletal Diseases

Most of us will encounter chronic musculoskeletal disease during our lifetime. Some form of arthritis will afflict half of those over 65; low back pain hits 80 percent of us at some point. Arthritis and musculoskeletal diseases are the most common causes of physical disability in the United States.[40]

Arthritis: Many Types, Many Problems

Called "the nation's primary crippler," **arthritis** strikes one in seven Americans, or over 38 million people. Symptoms range from the occasional tendinitis of the weekend athlete to the horrific pain of rheumatoid arthritis. There are over 100 types of arthritis diagnosed today, accounting for over 30 million lost workdays annually. The cost to the U.S. economy is over

$65 billion per year in lost wages and productivity and untold amounts in hospital and nursing home services, prescriptions, and over-the-counter pain relief.[41]

Osteoarthritis (OA), also known as degenerative joint disease, is a progressive deterioration of bones and joints that has been associated with the "wear and tear" theory of aging. More recent research indicates that as joints are used, they release enzymes that digest cartilage, while other cells in the cartilage try to repair the damage. When the enzymatic breakdown overpowers cellular repair, the cartilage is destroyed. Bones rub directly against each other, causing the pain, swelling, and limited movement characteristic of arthritis. Weather extremes, excessive strain, and injury often lead to osteoarthritis flare-ups, but a specific precipitating event does not seem to be necessary. Obesity, joint trauma, and repetitive joint usage all increase the risk and thus are important targets for prevention.

Although age and injury are undoubtedly factors in osteoarthritis, heredity, abnormal use of the joint, diet, abnormalities in joint structure, and impaired blood supply to the joint may also contribute. Osteoarthritis of the hands seems to have a particularly strong genetic component. Over 80 percent of those with OA report an activity limitation; OA of the knee can be as disabling as any cardiovascular disease short of stroke.[42] When joints become so distorted that they impair activity, surgical intervention is often necessary. Joint replacement and bone fusion are common surgical repair techniques. For most people, anti-inflammatory drugs and pain relievers such as aspirin and cortisone-related agents ease discomfort. In some sufferers, applications of heat, mild exercise, and massage may also relieve the pain. Today 20.7 million Americans have osteoarthritis, the majority of them women.[43]

Rheumatoid arthritis is an autoimmune disease involving chronic inflammation that can appear at any age, but it most commonly appears between ages 20 and 45 and affects over 2.1 million Americans. It is three times more common among women than among men during early

---

Arthritis   Painful inflammatory disease of the joints.

Osteoarthritis (OA)   A progressive deterioration of bones and joints that has been associated with the "wear and tear" theory of aging.

Rheumatoid arthritis   A serious inflammatory joint disease.

---

adulthood but equally common among men and women in the over-70 age group. Symptoms include stiffness, pain, redness, and swelling of multiple joints, often including the hands and wrists, and can be gradually progressive or sporadic, with occasional unexplained remissions. Other symptoms include loss of appetite, fever, loss of energy, anemia, and generalized aches.[44]

Rheumatoid arthritis typically attacks the synovial membrane, which produces the lubricating fluids for the joints. Advanced rheumatoid arthritis often involves destruction of the bony ends of joints. The remedy for this condition is typically bone fusion, which leaves the joint immobile. In some instances, joint replacement may be a viable alternative.

Although the cause of rheumatoid arthritis is unknown, some theorists believe it is caused by some form of invading microorganism that takes over the joint. Toxic chemicals and stress have also been mentioned as possible causes. Genetic predisposition is a strong predictor of risk, and a genetic marker called *HLA-DR4* has been identified.[45]

Regardless of the cause, treatment of rheumatoid arthritis is similar to that for osteoarthritis treatments, emphasizing pain relief and improved functional mobility of the patient. In some instances, immunosuppressant drugs can reduce the inflammatory response.

Fibromyalgia

Fibromyalgia is a chronic, painful, rheumatoid-like disorder that affects 5 to 6 percent of the general population with bouts of muscle pain and extreme fatigue. Persons with fibromyalgia experience an array of other symptoms including headaches, dizziness, numbness and tingling, itching, fluid retention, chronic joint pain, abdominal or pelvic pain, and even occasional diarrhea. Suspected causes have ranged from sleep disturbances, stress, emotional distress, and viruses to autoimmune disorders; however, none has been proved in clinical trials. Because of fibromyalgia's multiple symptoms, it is usually diagnosed only after myriad tests have ruled out other disorders. The American College of Rheumatology identifies these major diagnostic criteria:[46]

- History of widespread pain of at least three months' duration in the axial skeleton as well as in all four quadrants of the body.
- Pain in at least 11 of 18 paired tender points on digital palpation of about 4 kilograms of pressure.

Fibromyalgia is primarily diagnosed in women in their thirties and forties, and it can be extremely debilitating due to unrelieved pain, feelings of bloating or swelling, and fatigue. Many people with fibromyalgia also become depressed and report chronic fatigue–like symptoms.

Treatments vary based on the severity of symptoms. Typically, adequate rest, stress management, relaxation techniques, dietary supplements and selected herbal remedies, and pain medications are prescribed. Patients are advised to avoid extreme temperatures, which can exacerbate symptoms.

Systemic Lupus Erythematosus (SLE)

Systemic lupus erythematosus (SLE, or lupus) is an autoimmune disease in which antibodies destroy or injure organs such as the kidneys, brain, and heart. The symptoms include sensitivity to sunlight, arthritis, kidney problems, anemia, and multiple infections; they range from mild to severe and may disappear for periods of time. A butterfly-shaped rash covering the bridge of the nose and both cheeks is common. Nearly all SLE sufferers have aching joints and muscles, and 60 percent of them develop redness and swelling that move from joint to joint. The disease affects 1 in 700 Caucasians but 1 in 250 African Americans; 90 percent of all victims are females who show initial symptoms between the ages of 18 and 45. Extensive research has not yet found a cure for this sometimes fatal disease, although new studies suggest that there may be a genetic predisposition to it.

Scleroderma

Scleroderma (hardening of the skin) is a disease characterized by an increasing fibrous growth of connective tissue underlying the skin and body organs. These areas may form hard skin patches or a more generalized "ever-tightening case of steel," making movement difficult. Some cases of scleroderma are related to certain occupations, such as working with vibrating machines and exposure to chemicals in plastics or in mining. Others have an abrupt, unknown etiology. Scleroderma may cause swelling of the hands, face, or feet. Symptoms range from minor discomfort to severe pain. In some instances, scleroderma is life-threatening.

Raynaud's Syndrome

For most of us, a few minutes in the cold causes only minor discomfort. For people suffering from **Raynaud's syndrome,** fingers and toes go numb, then turn white, then deep purple; as fingers and toes warm, they throb. Raynaud's is caused by exaggerated constriction of small arteries in the extremities that shunts blood away from them and toward the vital

---

Fibromyalgia A chronic, rheumatoid-like disorder that can be highly painful and difficult to diagnose.

Systemic lupus erythematosus (SLE, or lupus) A disease in which the immune system attacks the body, producing antibodies that destroy or injure organs such as the kidneys, brain, and heart.

Scleroderma A disease in which fibrous growth of connective tissue underlying the skin and body organs hardens and makes movement difficult.

Raynaud's syndrome A disease in which exposure to cold temperatures produces exaggerated constriction of the small arteries in the extremities, causing fingers and toes to go numb, turn white, and then turn deep purple.

Funding Allocations: What's Fair?

It seems logical that we should allocate research dollars to health problems based on the number of people affected and the risk for death and disability associated with a particular disease. However, that is not necessarily how money is distributed. Disability rankings are based on complex formulas and calculations in which numbers of persons affected, age, degree of functional capacity lost, and death are factored together to assess the level of disability that a condition represents in a population. For example, if many people die or are disabled at a very young age from a particular condition, it would be ranked as more severe than if it killed only older people, due to accounting for years of potential life lost.

Consider the expenditures and disability rankings for the conditions shown below. Although heart disease exacts the greatest human toll, its funding for research, prevention, and intervention does not fully reflect the significance of its impact.

Do you notice any other large discrepancies between societal impact and

Disease Areas	NIH Funding in 2005: Millions of Dollars for Research (Estimates)	Disability ranking
HIV/AIDS	2,930	15
Heart disease	2,125	1
Diabetes	1,024	8
Breast cancer	768	14
Prostate cancer	417	19
Schizophrenia	354	10
Stroke	352	4
Lung cancer	321	6
Asthma	279	17
Parkinson's disease	243	21
Multiple sclerosis	103	25

level of federal funding for battling a disease? Do the ranking or funding for any disease surprise you? If so, why? What factors might influence the amount of funding allocated for fighting a given disease or disability? What factors should influence funding priorities? Does the guideline of providing major research funding mainly for conditions that afflict

numerous individuals disadvantage any groups of people? Explain your answer.

Source: National Institutes of Health, "Estimates of Funding for Various Diseases, Conditions, Research Areas," 2004, www.nih .gov/news/fundingresearchareas.htm

organs. Why this disease occurs in people whose lives are not threatened by the cold (in which case vasoconstriction serves a vital function by sending blood to the body core) is unknown. It is believed that Raynaud's affects 5 to 10 percent of the population, with women accounting for the majority of sufferers. In women, onset is usually between the ages of 15 and 40; men tend to develop Raynaud's later in life. Treatment for Raynaud's consists of controlling body temperature by wearing warm gloves and boots, avoiding drugs that may alter blood flow (for example, nicotine), taking drugs to regulate blood flow, and surgery to improve circulation or repair damaged areas.

Low Back Pain

Approximately 80 percent of all Americans will experience low back pain (LBP) at some point. Some of these episodes result from muscular damage and are short-lived and acute; others may involve dislocations, fractures, or other problems with spinal vertebrae or discs, resulting in chronic pain or

requiring surgery. Low back pain is epidemic throughout the world and the major cause of disability for people aged 20 to 45 in the United States, who suffer more frequently and severely from this problem than older people do.[47]

LBP causes more lost work time in the United States than any other illness except upper respiratory infections. In fact, costs associated with back injury exceed those associated with all other industrial injuries combined. Back injuries are the most frequently mentioned complaints in injury-related lawsuits and result in high medical and rehabilitation bills, costing businesses and industries in the United States over $50 billion annually in direct and indirect costs.[48] As a result, employers throughout the country have become increasingly interested in preventing these injuries. These figures do not include the costs of human suffering, damaged self-worth, and other emotional problems that occur when a person becomes disabled. Interestingly, funding for research into LBP is much lower than its impact would lead you to expect; see the Health Ethics box for more information on spending priorities.

Table 18.1
Other Modern Afflictions

Disease	Description	Treatment
Cystic fibrosis	Inherited disease occurring in 1 out of every 1,600 births. Characterized by pooling of large amounts of mucus in lungs, digestive disturbances, and excessive sodium excretion. Results in premature death.	Most treatments are geared toward relief of symptoms. Antibiotics are administered for infection. Recent strides in genetic research suggest better treatments and potential cure in the near future.
Sickle-cell anemia	Inherited disease affecting 8–10% of all African Americans. Disease affects hemoglobin, forming sickle-shaped red blood cells that interfere with oxygenation. Results in severe pain, anemia, and premature death.	Reduce stress, and attend to minor infections immediately. Seek genetic counseling.
Cerebral palsy	Disorder characterized by the loss of voluntary control over motor functioning. Believed to be caused by a lack of oxygen to the brain at birth, brain disorders, an accident before or after birth, poisoning, or brain infections.	Follow preventive actions to reduce accident risks; improved neonatal and birthing techniques show promise.
Graves' disease	A thyroid disorder characterized by swelling of the eyes, staring gaze, and retraction of the eyelid. Can result in loss of sight. The cause is unknown, and the disease can occur at any age.	Medication may help control symptoms. Radioactive iodine supplements may also be administered.

Risk Factors for Low Back Pain   Health experts believe that the following factors contribute to LBP:

- *Age.* People between the ages of 20 and 45 run the greatest risk of LBP. At age 50, the condition becomes less common. After age 65, the incidence again rises, apparently because of bone and joint deterioration.
- *Body type.* Many studies have indicated that people who are very tall, are overweight, or have lanky body types run an increased risk of LBP. However, much of this research is controversial.
- *Posture.* Poor posture may be one of the greatest contributors to LBP. If you routinely slouch, particularly during daily tasks, you run an increased risk.
- *Strength and fitness.* People with LBP tend to have less overall trunk strength than do other people. Weak abdominal muscles and back muscles also increase risk. In addition, total level of fitness and conditioning is a factor. The more fit you are, the better.
- *Psychological factors.* Numerous psychological factors appear to increase risk for LBP. Depression, apathy, inattentiveness, boredom, emotional upsets, drug abuse, and family and financial problems all heighten risk.
- *Occupational risk.* Evidence indicates that employees who are new to a particular job run the greatest risk of LBP problems. Type of work and work conditions greatly affect risk. For example, truck drivers, who must endure the bumps and jolts of the road while in a sitting position, frequently suffer from back pain.

Preventing Back Pain and Injury   What can you do to protect yourself from possible back injury? Almost 90 percent of all back problems occur in the lumbar region of the spine (lower back). You can avoid many problems by consciously maintaining good posture. Other preventive hints include the following.

- Purchase a supportive mattress, and avoid sleeping on your stomach.
- Avoid high-heeled shoes, which tilt the pelvis forward.
- Control your weight.
- Lift objects with your legs, not your back.
- Buy a good chair for doing your work, preferably one with lumbar support.
- Move your car seat forward so your knees are elevated slightly.
- Warm up before exercising.
- Exercise regularly—in particular do exercises that strengthen the abdominal muscles and stretch the back muscles.

Other Maladies

During the past 20 years, several afflictions have surfaced that seem to be products of our times. Some of these health problems relate to specific groups of people, some are due to technological advances, and others have not been explained (Table 18.1).

Chronic Fatigue Syndrome

Fatigue is a subjective condition in which people feel tired before they begin activities, lack the energy to accomplish tasks that require sustained effort and attention, or become

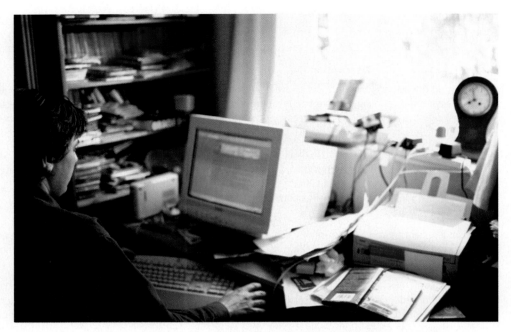

Poorly designed or crowded workspaces, long hours at a computer, and repetitive procedures are all potential causes of repetitive stress injuries.

abnormally exhausted after normal activities. All of us experience fatigue occasionally. Since the late 1980s, several U.S. clinics have noted a characteristic set of symptoms including chronic fatigue, headaches, fever, sore throat, enlarged lymph nodes, depression, poor memory, general weakness, nausea, and symptoms remarkably similar to those of mononucleosis. Researchers initially believed these symptoms were caused by the same virus as mononucleosis, the Epstein-Barr virus. At first the disease was called *chronic Epstein-Barr disease,* or the "yuppie flu," because the pattern of symptoms appeared most commonly in baby boomers in their early thirties. Some cases were so severe that patients required hospitalization. Since those initial studies, however, researchers have all but ruled out the Epstein-Barr virus. Despite extensive testing, no viral cause has been found to date.[49]

Today, in the absence of a known pathogen, many researchers believe that the illness, now commonly referred to as **chronic fatigue syndrome (CFS),** may have strong psychosocial roots. Our heightened awareness of health makes some of us scrutinize our bodies so carefully that the slightest deviation becomes amplified. The more we focus on the body and on our perception of health, the worse we feel. In addition, the growing number of people who suffer from depression seem to be good candidates for chronic fatigue syndrome. Experts worry, however, that too many people approach CFS as something that is "in the person's head" and that such an attitude may prevent scientists from doing the serious research needed to find a cure.

The diagnosis of chronic fatigue syndrome depends on two major criteria and eight or more minor criteria. The major criteria are debilitating fatigue that persists for at least six months and the absence of other illnesses that could cause the symptoms. Minor criteria include headaches, fever, sore throat, painful lymph nodes, weakness, fatigue after exercise, sleep problems, and rapid onset of these symptoms. Because the cause is not apparent, treatment of CFS focuses on improved nutrition, rest, counseling for depression, judicious exercise, and development of a strong support network.

Repetitive Stress Injuries

It's the end of the term, and you have finished the last of several papers. After hours of nonstop typing, your hands are numb and you feel an intense, burning pain that makes the thought of typing one more word almost unbearable. If you are like one of the thousands of students and workers who every year must quit a particular task due to pain, you may be suffering from a **repetitive stress injury (RSI).** These are injuries to nerves, soft tissue, or joints that result from the physical stress of repeated motions.

Chronic fatigue syndrome (CFS) A condition of unknown cause characterized by extreme fatigue that is not caused by other illness.

Repetitive stress injury (RSI) An injury to nerves, soft tissue, or joints due to the physical stress of repeated motions.

While no good mechanism of reporting exists for students suffering from RSIs, the U.S. Bureau of Labor Statistics estimates that 25 percent of all injuries in the labor force that result in lost work time are due to repetitive motion or stress injuries. RSIs cost employers over $22 billion a year in workers' compensation and an additional $85 billion in related costs, such as absenteeism.

One of the most common RSIs is **carpal tunnel syndrome,** a product of both the information age and the age of technology in general. Hours spent typing at the computer, flipping groceries through computerized scanners, or other jobs "made simpler" by technology can irritate the median nerve in the wrist, causing numbness, tingling, and pain in the fingers and hands. Although carpal tunnel syndrome risk can be reduced by proper placement of the keyboard, mouse, wrist pads, and other techniques, RSIs are often overlooked until significant damage has been done. Better education and ergonomic workplace designs can eliminate many injuries of this nature.

> **Carpal tunnel syndrome** A common occupational injury in which the median nerve in the wrist becomes irritated, causing numbness, tingling, and pain in the fingers and hands.

TAKING CHARGE

MAKE IT HAPPEN!

Assessment: The Assess Yourself box on page 538 asks you to evaluate whether you are at risk for diabetes. Now that you have considered your results, you may need to take steps to further understand and address your risks.

Making a Change: In order to change your behavior, you need to develop a plan. Follow these steps.

1. Evaluate your behavior, and identify patterns and specific things you are doing. What can you change now? What can you change in the near future?
2. Select one pattern of behavior that you want to change.
3. Fill out a Behavior Change Contract. It should include your long-term goal for change, your short-term goals, the rewards you'll give yourself for reaching these goals, potential obstacles along the way, and strategies for overcoming these obstacles. For each goal, list the small steps and specific actions that you will take.
4. Chart your progress in a journal. At the end of a week, consider how successful you were in following your plan. What helped you to be successful? What made change more difficult? What will you do differently next week?
5. Revise your plan as needed. Are the short-term goals attainable? Are the rewards satisfying?

One Student's Plan: When Jamie answered the questions in the self-assessment, he found that he had three "yes" answers. He was overweight (which he knew from calculating his body mass index), he was typically sedentary, since he didn't have a regular exercise program, and he felt like he was always hungry, even though he had regular meals. He

decided to check into his family's medical history to further consider his risk for diabetes.

When Jamie spoke to his mother, he was surprised to find out that both his father and his grandmother had diabetes. Even more surprising, his 12-year-old brother had recently been diagnosed as being at risk.

Jamie immediately made an appointment at his student health center and soon was tested. His results were borderline normal, but he was advised to make changes to prevent developing diabetes. Among the changes were reducing his weight, eating more fiber, and starting a regular exercise program. Jamie talked to his roommates about his results, and they helped him come up with some ideas to make these changes. His first step was to ride his bicycle to campus every day, instead of driving. This gave him some physical activity that didn't take too much extra time from his day. Jamie also knew that he needed to improve his diet, by cutting down on junk food and looking for ways to include more fiber in his meals. He decided to start bringing snacks of carrots or apples with him to school. This would help him eat a balanced diet and keep him from buying candy from the vending machines. He also made sure to pay attention to his various options when he ate at the dining hall and to try to steer clear of the high fat entrees and desserts.

Jamie's blood sugar will be retested in two months. If the level has come down to closer to the normal range, he will reward himself with tickets to see his favorite baseball team play their cross-town rivals.

Summary

- Chronic lung diseases include allergies, hay fever, asthma, emphysema, and chronic bronchitis. Allergies are part of the body's natural defense system. Chronic obstructive pulmonary diseases are the fourth leading cause of death in the United States. Sleep apnea is another breathing-related malady increasing in prevalence.

- Neurological conditions include headaches and seizure disorders. Headaches may be caused by a variety of factors, the most common of which are tension, dilation and/or contraction of blood vessels in the brain, chemical influences on muscles and vessels that cause inflammation and pain, and underlying physiological and psychological disorders. The most common types of headache are tension, migraine, and cluster. Other disorders include Parkinson's disease and multiple sclerosis.

- Several modern maladies affect only women. Fibrocystic breast condition is a common, noncancerous buildup of irregular tissue. Endometriosis is the buildup of endometrial tissue in regions of the body other than the uterus.

- Diabetes occurs when the pancreas fails to produce enough insulin to regulate sugar metabolism. Its increase in prevalence is related to increases in obesity and other factors. Other conditions, such as colitis, irritable bowel syndrome, gallbladder disease, and peptic ulcers, are the direct result of functional problems in various digestion-related organs or systems. Pathogens, problems in enzyme or hormone production, anxiety or stress, functional abnormalities, and other problems are possible causes.

- Musculoskeletal diseases such as arthritis, lower back pain, repetitive stress injuries, and other problems cause significant pain and disability in millions of people. Age, occupation, gender, posture, abdominal strength, and psychological factors contribute to the development of lower back problems.

- Chronic fatigue syndrome (CFS) and repetitive stress injuries (such as carpal tunnel syndrome) have emerged as major chronic maladies. CFS is associated with depression. Repetitive stress injuries are preventable by proper equipment placement and usage.

Questions for Discussion and Reflection

1. What are some of the major noninfectious chronic diseases affecting Americans today? Do you think there is a pattern in the types of diseases that we get? What are the common risk factors?

2. List the common respiratory diseases affecting Americans. Which of these diseases has a genetic basis? An environmental basis? An individual basis? What, if anything, is being done to prevent, treat, or control each of these conditions?

3. Compare and contrast the different types of headaches, including their symptoms and treatments.

4. What are the medical risks of fibrocystic breast condition and endometriosis? How can they be treated?

5. Describe the risk factors for diabetes and its symptoms and treatment. What is the difference between type 1 diabetes and type 2 diabetes?

6. Compare the symptoms of colitis, diverticulosis, peptic ulcers, and gallbladder disease. How can you tell whether your stomach is reacting to final exams or telling you that you have a serious medical condition?

7. What are the major disorders of the musculoskeletal system? Why do you think there aren't any cures? Describe the difference between osteoarthritis and rheumatoid arthritis.

8. Chronic fatigue syndrome (CFS) is often associated with depression. Experts argue about whether depression precedes CFS or CFS causes depression. What do you think?

Accessing Your Health on the Internet

Visit the following Internet sites to explore further topics and issues related to personal health. To visit an organization's website, go to the Companion Website for *Access to Health, Ninth Edition* at www.aw-bc.com/donatelle, click on the book image, and select "Accessing Your Health on the Internet" from the navigation menu.

1. ***American Academy of Allergy, Asthma, and Immunology.*** Provides an overview of asthma information, particularly as it applies to children with allergies. Offers interactive quizzes to test your knowledge as well as an "ask the expert" section.

2. ***American Diabetes Association.*** Excellent resource for diabetes information.

3. ***American Lung Association.*** Includes the latest in asthma news, including a free monthly newsletter, *The Breathe Easy/Asthma Digest.*

4. ***ChronicIllnet.*** A multimedia information source dedicated to chronic illnesses, including AIDS, cancer, Gulf War syndrome, autoimmune diseases, chronic fatigue syndrome, heart disease, and neurological diseases.

5. ***National Center for Chronic Disease Prevention and Health Promotion (NCCDPHP).*** Access to a wide range of information from this CDC-linked organization dedicated to chronic diseases and health promotion.

6. ***National Institute of Neurological Disorders and Stroke.*** Many of the modern maladies result in chronic pain. This site provides up-to-date information to help you cope with pain-related difficulties.

Further Reading

Brownson, R., P. Remington, and J. Davis. *Chronic Disease Epidemiology and Control,* 2nd ed. Washington, DC: American Public Health Association, 1998.

An excellent book covering the epidemiology of major human illnesses. Provides historical, pathological, and epidemiological perspectives on illness and infirmity.

National Center for Health Statistics. *Monthly Vital Statistics Report* and *Advance Data from Vital and Health Statistics.* Hyattsville, MD: Public Health Service.

Detailed government reports, usually published monthly, concerning mortality and morbidity data for the United States, including changes occurring in the rates of particular diseases and in health practices so patterns and trends can be analyzed.

Public Health Services, Centers for Disease Control. *Chronic Disease News and Notes.* Washington, DC: U.S. Department of Health and Human Services.

Quarterly publication focusing on relevant chronic disease topics and issues.

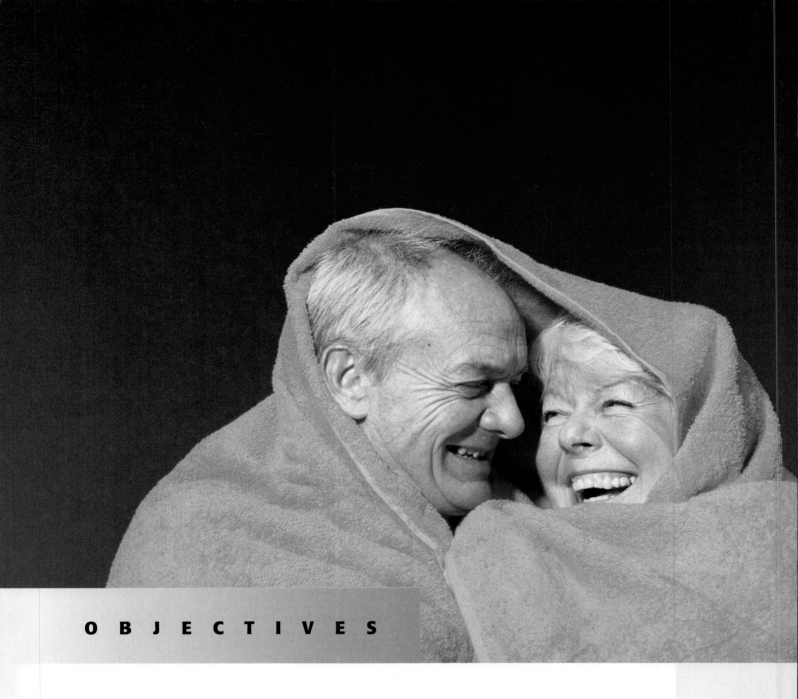

OBJECTIVES

■ Define *aging,* and explain the related concepts of biological, psychological, social, legal, and functional age.

■ Explain how the growing population of older adults will impact society, including considerations of economics, health care, living arrangements, and ethical and moral issues.

■ Discuss the biological and psychosocial theories of aging, and examine how knowledge of these theories may have an impact on your own aging process.

■ Summarize major physiological changes that occur as a result of the aging process.

■ Discuss unique health challenges faced by older adults, such as alcohol abuse, use of prescription medication and over-the-counter drugs, osteoporosis, urinary incontinence, depression, and Alzheimer's disease.

■ Discuss strategies for healthy aging that can begin during young adulthood.

HEALTHY AGING

A LIFELONG PROCESS

IN THE NEWS

Aging: Sharper Minds With Bustling Feet

By Eric Nagourney

Just going out regularly for an easy walk appears to help elderly people ward off a decline in their mental abilities, two new studies have found.

One of the studies, which tracked the health and exercise habits of more than 18,000 women over a period of about 12 years, found that those who walked regularly had the mental acuity usually associated with people several years younger.

"We're looking at two or three hours of walking at an easy pace," said the lead author, Dr. Jennifer Weuve, an epidemiologist at the Harvard School of Public Health. The second study, led by Dr. Robert D. Abbott of the University of

Virginia School of Medicine, followed the health of almost 2,300 men, ages 71 to 93, and found that those who walked the least had twice the risk of developing dementia as those who walked two or more miles a day. Both studies were published in the Sept. 22 issue of *The Journal of the American Medical Association*.

Read the complete article online in the eThemes section of this book's website: www.aw-bc.com/donatelle.

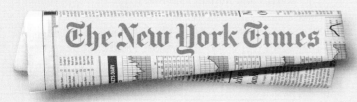

Grow old along with me!
The best is yet to be,
The last of life, for which the first was made . . .
        —Robert Browning, *Rabbi Ben Ezra*

In a society that seems to worship youth, researchers have begun to offer good—even revolutionary—news about the aging process: growing old doesn't have to mean a slow slide to disability, loneliness, and declining physical and mental health. Health promotion, disease prevention, and wellness-oriented activities can prolong vigor and productivity, even among those who haven't always led model lifestyles or made healthful habits a priority. In fact, getting older can mean getting better in many ways—particularly socially, psychologically, and intellectually.

Growing Old: Life Passages

Every moment of every day, we are involved in a steady aging process. Everything in the universe—animals, plants, mountains, rivers, planets, even atoms—changes over time. This process is commonly referred to as *aging*. Aging is something that we cannot avoid, despite the perennial human quest for a fountain of youth. Since you can't stop the clock, why not resolve to have a positive aging experience by improving your understanding of this process, taking steps to maximize your potential, and developing strengths you can draw upon over a lifetime?

The manner in which you view aging (either as a natural part of living or an inevitable decline toward disease and death) is a crucial factor in how successfully you will adapt to life's transitions. If you view these transitions as periods of growth, as changes that will lead to improved mental, emotional, spiritual, and physical phases in your development as a human being, your journey through even the most difficult times will be easier. No doubt you have encountered vigorous 80-year-olds who wake up every morning looking forward to whatever challenges the day may bring. Such persons are socially active, have a zest for life, and seem much younger than their chronological ages. In contrast, you have probably met 50-year-olds who lack energy and enthusiasm, who seem resigned to tread water for the rest of their lives. These people often appear much older than their chronological age. In short, people experience the aging process in different ways. Explore your own notions about aging with the Assess Yourself box.

Aging The patterns of life changes that occur in members of all species as they grow older.

Ageism Discrimination based on age.

Gerontology The study of individual and collective aging processes.

Aging has traditionally been described as the patterns of life changes that occur in members of all species as they grow older. Some believe that it begins at the moment of conception. Others contend that it starts at birth. Still others believe that true aging does not begin until we reach our forties.

Typically, experts and laypersons alike have used chronological age to assign a person to a particular life-cycle stage. However, people of different chronological ages view age very differently. To the 4-year-old, a college freshman seems quite old. To the 20-year-old, parents in their forties are over the hill. Have you ever heard your 65-year-old grandparents talking about "those old people down the street"? Views of aging are also colored by occupation. Most professional athletes are considering other careers by the time they reach 40. Airline pilots and police officers often retire in their fifties, while actors, writers, musicians, and even college professors may work well into their seventies and eighties. Perhaps we need to reexamine our traditional definitions of aging.

Redefining Aging

Discrimination against people based on age is known as **ageism.** This type of discrimination carries with it social ostracism and negative portrayals of older people. A developmental task approach to life-span changes tends to reduce the potential for ageist or negatively biased perceptions about what occurs as a person ages chronologically.

The study of individual and collective aging processes, known as **gerontology,** explores the reasons for aging and the ways in which people cope with and adapt to this process. Gerontologists have identified several age-related characteristics that define where a person is in terms of biological, psychological, social, legal, and functional life-stage development:[1]

- *Biological age* refers to the relative age or condition of the person's organs and body systems. There are 70-year-old runners who have the cardiovascular system of a 40-year-old, and 40-year-olds who have less energy than their parents. Smoking, obesity, and chronic health conditions such as arthritis can accelerate the aging process.[2]
- *Psychological age* refers to a person's adaptive capacities, such as coping abilities and intelligence, and to the person's awareness of his or her individual capabilities, self-efficacy, and general ability to adapt to new situations. Research documents that people who maintain a positive attitude and stay mentally active are more likely to age well and be happy.[3] Even if chronic illness renders someone physically handicapped, the person may have tremendous psychological reserves and remain alert and fully capable of making decisions.
- *Social age* refers to a person's habits and roles relative to society's expectations. People in a particular life stage often share similar tastes in music and television shows, for example.

Where Do You Want to Be?

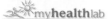

Fill out this assessment online at www.aw-bc.com/myhealthlab or www.aw-bc.com/donatelle

When we are young, aging most likely is the furthest thing from our minds. However, thinking about aging and what we expect from life are important elements of a satisfying adult development process. Take a few minutes to answer the following questions. Your answers may tell you a great deal about yourself.

1. At this point in your life, what do you value most?
2. What do you think will be most important to you when you reach your forties? Fifties? Sixties? What similarities and differences do you notice, and what causes these similarities and differences?
3. Do you think your parents are happy and content with the way their lives have turned out? If they could change anything, what do you think they might do differently?
4. What about your own direction thus far in life? Is it similar to that of your parents? What have you done differently? Are the similarities and differences good? Why or why not?

5. What do you think are the keys to a happy and satisfying life?
6. What do you want to accomplish by the time you are 40? 50? 60?
7. Have you ever thought of retirement? Describe your retirement.
8. Describe the "you" that you would like to be at age 70. How is that person similar to or different from the "you" of today? What actions will you need to take to be that "you" in the future?

MAKE IT HAPPEN!

Use the results of this self-assessment to begin your behavior change program. Follow the steps and use the examples on page 565 to complete your Behavior Change Contract, and use these resources to take action.

- *Legal age* is probably the most common definition of age in the United States. Based on chronological years, legal age is used as a factor in determining voting rights, driving privileges, drinking age, eligibility for Social Security payments, and a host of other rights and obligations.
- *Functional age* refers to the ways—heart rate, hearing, etc.—in which people compare to others of a similar age. It is difficult to separate functional aging from many of the other types of aging, particularly chronological and biological aging.

What Is Successful Aging?

As people pass through critical periods in their lives, gerontologists discuss whether they are aging "successfully." Those who are successful usually develop positive coping skills that carry over into other areas of their lives. They have realistic, achievable goals that bring them pleasure and tend to think confidently and independently. In short, successful agers are more prepared to "experience" life. Those who are less successful in these rites of passage either develop a sense of learned helplessness and lose confidence in their ability to succeed or learn to compensate for their failures in other ways.

Today, it is easier to find positive examples of aging than at any other time in our history. Many of today's "elderly" individuals lead active, productive lives. For instance, 49,000 Americans aged 65 and older are currently enrolled in college, and 14 percent are employed. Seventy-two percent of U.S. citizens aged 65 to 74 voted in the 2000 presidential election—a higher percentage than any other age group.[4]

Typically, people who have aged successfully have the following characteristics:

- In general, they have managed to avoid serious, debilitating diseases and disability.
- They function well physically, live independently, and engage in most normal activities of daily living.
- They have maintained cognitive function and are actively engaged in mentally challenging and stimulating activities.
- They are actively engaged in social and productive pursuits.
- They are resilient and able to cope reasonably well with physical, social, and emotional changes.

Although the process of aging has often been viewed with dread due to physical changes that inevitably occur, only in the past decade have we begun to fully appreciate the gains and positive aspects of normal adult development

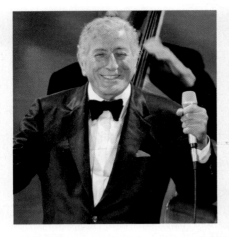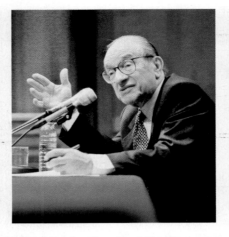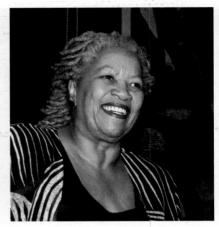

Singer Tony Bennett, economist Alan Greenspan, and author Toni Morrison are examples of people who stay active and vigorous in their professions well into their seventies and eighties.

throughout the life span. According to gerontologist Dr. Karen Hooker, older adults as a population display much more differentiation in personalities, coping styles, and "possible selves" than any other age group. She states that "successful aging and development as individuals can be viewed as dynamic processes of adaptation between the self and the environment. Throughout our lives we make choices and respond to changes in vastly different ways. Each person is born with certain traits that stay reasonably stable throughout life, but character is deeply affected by personal action constructs that change with time and life history."[5] Thus, aging is not a static process, but one in which each of us changes and becomes someone uniquely fashioned by our life's story.

Gerontologists have devised several categories for specific age-related characteristics. People aged 65 to 74 are viewed as the **young-old;** those aged 75 to 84 are the **middle-old** group; those 85 and over are classified as the **old-old.**

However, chronological age is not the only issue to be considered. The question is not how many years someone has lived, but how much life the person has packed into those years. This *quality-of-life index,* combined with the chronological process, appears to be the best indicator of the phenomenon of "aging gracefully." Most experts agree that the best way to experience a productive, full, and satisfying old age is to lead a productive, full, and satisfying life prior to old age. Essentially, older people are the product of their lifelong experiences and behaviors.

Young-old People aged 65 to 74.

Middle-old People aged 75 to 84.

Old-old People aged 85 and over.

What do you think?

What factors influence the aging process? ■ *Which of these factors do you have the power to change through the behaviors that you engage in right now?*

Older Adults: A Growing Population

There are more than 35 million people aged 65 or older in the United States, nearly 13 percent of the total population. The number of older Americans has increased more than tenfold since 1900, when there were 3 million people aged 65 or older (4 percent of the total population), and the number of those 65 and over is projected to double between 2000 and 2030[6] (Figure 19.1). Other nations report a similar trend. The World Health Organization predicts that, worldwide by 2025, there will be 1.2 billion people over the age of 60.[7] (See the Health in a Diverse World box.) In the United States, according to researchers at the Administration on Aging, the growth of the 65-plus population will accelerate between 2010 and 2030 as the 77-million-strong "baby boom generation" reaches age 65. Some researchers predict that this will have as big an impact on our society as immigration did at the turn of the last century.[8]

What will this growth of the over-65 population mean to the American economy, health care system, and social structure? Leaders must take a proactive stance in developing programs and services to promote health and prevent premature disease and disability. In Utah, state officials are targeting 40-year-olds through their Healthy Aging program, encouraging regular checkups, exercise, healthy eating habits, and overall improved health behaviors. More health plans are considering ways to motivate clients to take more initiative, to work harder at health improvements that will

Aging: The World's Oldest Countries

The growth of older populations around the world results from major achievements—reliable birth control that has decreased fertility rates, improvements in medical care and sanitation that have reduced infant and maternal mortality and infectious and parasitic diseases, and improvements in nutrition and education. Every month, the net increase in the world's population aged 60 and over is more than 1 million; 70 percent of this increase occurs in developing countries and 30 percent in industrialized countries. Between 1991 and 2020, the world population over age 60 is projected to increase by 59 percent in industrialized nations and 159 percent in less developed countries. The world's older population—defined here as persons aged 60 and over—numbers 495 million today and is expected to exceed 1 billion by the year 2020. Almost half of today's older adults live in just four nations: the People's Republic of China, India, Russia, and the United States. (The chart shows countries with the highest percentages of people over 60.) There is intense debate over issues—social security costs, health care, educational investments, and so on—that are directly linked to this changing age structure of societies.

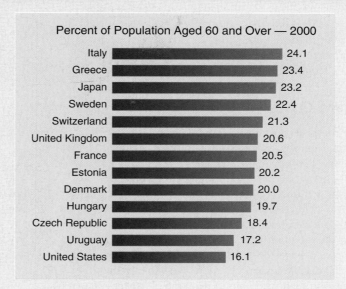

Percent of Population Aged 60 and Over — 2000

Country	Percent
Italy	24.1
Greece	23.4
Japan	23.2
Sweden	22.4
Switzerland	21.3
United Kingdom	20.6
France	20.5
Estonia	20.2
Denmark	20.0
Hungary	19.7
Czech Republic	18.4
Uruguay	17.2
United States	16.1

Source: United Nations Population Division, "World Population Prospects Population Database," 2002, http://esa.un.org/unpp

Sources: United Nations, "International Plan of Action on Aging: Demographic Background," updated January 15, 2003, www.un.org/esa/socdev/ageing/ageipaa.htm; U.S. Bureau of the Census, *Global Aging: Comparative Indicators and Future Trends* (Washington, DC: Government Printing Office, 1991); U.S. Bureau of the Census, International Programs Center, International Data Base, 1998.

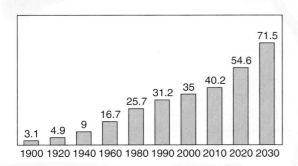

Figure 19.1
Number of Americans Aged 65 and Older (in Millions)

Source: Department of Health and Human Services, Administration on Aging, *A Profile of Older Americans: 2003*, 2003, www.aoa.gov/prof/Statistics/profile/2003/4_pf.asp

save insurers money in the long run. Instead of focusing on negative aspects of aging, more health and social service leaders are focusing on "successful aging—what it means and what it will take to ensure that each of us can achieve it." By enhancing collective understanding of the aging process and the role of current behaviors in developing lifetime habits to inoculate us against the stresses and strains of living, we will improve our chances of achieving our "possible selves."

Health Issues for an Aging Society

The concerns of government officials over the impending growth in the older population center around meeting their financial and medical needs. No doubt you have heard discussions on the potential bankruptcy of the Social Security system and the large increases in out-of-pocket costs for people on Medicare. According to the latest statistics, life expectancy for a person born in 2001 is 77.2 years, about 30 years longer than for a child born in 1900.[9]

With fewer people contributing to the system and greater numbers drawing on it, the likelihood of problems arising is great. Where will these older people live? How will they pay for their medical costs, and how long will they need to work to support themselves? These and other questions pose many challenges for all of us.

Health Care Costs

Today, older Americans average $3,586 per year in out-of-pocket medical expenses, an increase of 45 percent since 1992.[10] As people live longer, the chances of developing a costly chronic disease increase, and as technology improves, chronic illnesses that once were quickly fatal may now be treated successfully for years. Projected future costs are staggering. Health care expenditures rise with age, and 77 million baby boomers are now in middle age. Compared with people ages 18 to 44, people ages 45 to 64 are nearly three times more likely to be disabled, six times more likely to have high blood pressure, and 15 times more likely to die of cancer. Meeting the nation's long-term care needs will become even more challenging as the population ages and more people require assistance with living. At least 4 million Americans are 85 or older, the segment most in need of long-term care. By 2040, that number is projected to triple to more than 14 million.[11]

If Social Security goes bankrupt, large numbers of Americans will no longer have Medicare coverage. Even if they could afford to buy their own health insurance, most older individuals would face high out-of-pocket expenses and limited choices in treatments. Today, persons on Medicare already pay over $3,000 each in out-of-pocket health care expenses. These numbers are certain to increase.

Another large group of Americans falls into the category of "uninsured" or "underinsured"—those having only small levels of insurance, usually insufficient for their needs. It is important to note here that the highest rate of uninsured Americans today (22 percent) occurs in the 15- to 44-year-old age group; another 13 percent are in the 45- to 64-year-old age group. If insurance is too expensive or unavailable during the years when people are employed, is it likely that they will be able to afford insurance when they are retired or on a fixed income? Recent stock market downturns and company failures that wiped out retirement savings may make it even more difficult for older Americans to afford health insurance in the next decade.

Major questions loom: Will working Americans be willing to pay an increased share of the health care costs for people on fixed incomes who cannot pay for themselves? If not, what will become of older Americans? Perhaps most important, who will ultimately pay?

Housing and Living Arrangements

Contrary to popular opinion, most older people (over 95 percent) never live in a nursing home. Many continue to live

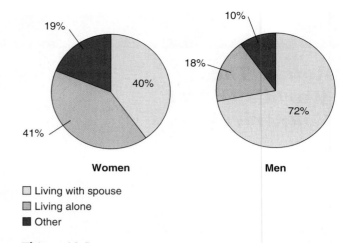

Figure 19.2
Living Arrangements of Americans Aged 65 and Older

Source: Department of Health and Human Services, Administration on Aging, *A Profile of Older Americans: 2003.* 2003, www.aoa.gov/prof/Statistics/profile/2003/4_pf.asp

with a spouse; others live alone or make other arrangements such as living with relatives or friends (Figure 19.2). Community living, assisted living, skilled nursing care, and other options are new possibilities for those who have financial means or who have purchased some form of long-term care insurance. However, housing problems for the low-income elderly remain. Who will provide the necessary social services, and who will pay the bill? Will the family of the future be forced to coexist with several generations under one roof?

Ethical and Moral Considerations

Difficult ethical questions arise when we consider the implications of an increasing population of older adults for an already overburdened health care system. Given the shortage of donor organs, will we be forced to decide whether a 50-year-old should receive a heart transplant instead of a 75-year-old? The debate over stem cell research asks us to balance scientific achievements with questions of morality (see the Health Ethics box). Is the prolongation of life at all costs a moral imperative, or will future generations be forced to devise a set of criteria for deciding who will be helped and who will not? Understanding the process of aging and knowing what actions you can take to prolong your own healthy years are part of our collective responsibility.

What do you think?

What do you think people over 65 would do if they suddenly didn't have Medicare? ■ *Why are the aging of the population and the impending difficulties with health care costs and access important to all of us?*

The Debate Over Stem Cells

Stem cells are unique—and controversial. Stem cells are body cells with two important characteristics: (1) they are unspecialized and capable of renewing themselves by dividing repeatedly, and (2) they can be induced to become specialized cells that perform specific functions, such as muscle cells that make the heart beat or nerve cells that enable the brain to function.

These qualities have led many scientists to feel that stem cells have the potential to cure debilitating health problems such as Alzheimer's, heart disease, diabetes, Parkinson's, and glaucoma. These conditions all involve the destruction of certain crucial cells; for example, in the case of Type 1 diabetes, it is the pancreatic cells that secrete insulin, the hormone that regulates blood glucose. In the laboratory, researchers are working to coax stem cells to develop into these pancreatic cells. The plan is to transplant the new cells into diabetic patients, where they could replace the patients' damaged cells and produce insulin. If successful, this approach could prevent the destructive complications of the disease and free diabetics from the painful burden of injecting insulin for the rest of their lives. Other therapies under investigation involve growing new cells to replace those ravaged by spinal injuries, heart attacks, muscular dystrophy, and vision and hearing loss.

The controversy over stem cells arises from their origins. Generally stem cells are derived from eggs that were fertilized in vitro. Typically these are "extra" embryos created during fertility treatments at clinics but not used for implantation. Only four to five days old, embryonic stem cells are *pluripotent* (capable of developing into many different cell types).

Embryonic stem cell research has provoked fierce debate. Opponents believe that an embryo is a human being and that we have no right to create life and then destroy it, even for humanitarian purposes. Advocates counter that the eggs from which these embryos developed were given freely by donors and would otherwise be discarded.

Are adult stem cells a solution to this ethical dilemma? An adult stem cell is an undifferentiated cell, found in body tissues, that can specialize to replace certain types of cells. For example, human bone marrow contains at least two kinds of adult stem cells. One kind gives rise to the various types of blood cells, while the other can differentiate into bone, cartilage, fat, or fibrous connective tissue. Other tissues that may contain adult stem cells include the brain, liver, skeletal muscles, and blood vessels. While research indicates that adult stem cells may be more versatile than previously thought, many scientists believe that embryonic stem cells, with their unlimited potential, are far more promising medically.

In the United States, embryonic stem cell research is limited by law. Federal funding—a major source of support for universities and labs—is restricted to experiments on only 71 stem cell lines (a stem cell line refers to a set of pluripotent, embryonic stem cells that have grown in the laboratory for at least six months), all of which were established prior to the legislation taking effect. Some scientists worry that this pool is too small to develop valid medical therapies. Opponents believe that even this compromise allows unethical research practices to continue. In 2004, the state of California voted to fund stem-cell research itself, in order to avoid federal restrictions.

As the debate continues, embryonic stem cell research is moving forward in a few countries. For example, South Korean scientists claim to have successfully cloned a human embryo and extracted stem cells, and the United Kingdom has licensed a British university to clone stem cells for diabetes research.

Do you feel that embryonic stem cell research is ethical? Explain your answer. Would you feel differently if you or a loved one suffered from a disease that might respond to stem cell therapy?

Sources: National Institutes of Health, Stem Cell Information, "Stem Cell Basics," revised June 10, 2004, http://stemcells.nih.gov /info/basics/; M. Waldholz and A. Regalado, "Biggest Struggles in Stem-Cell Fight May Be in the Lab," *The Wall Street Journal,* August 12, 2004, pp. A1, A6; International Society for Stem Cell Research, "The Ethics of Embryonic Stem Cell Research," updated June 10, 2004, http://www.isscr.org/public /ethics.htm; Associated Press, "U.K. Grants First Cloning License to Develop Research Stem Cells," *The Wall Street Journal,* August 12, 2004, p. D3.

Theories on Aging

Biological Theories

Explanations for the biological causes of aging include the following:

- *The wear-and-tear theory* states that, like everything else in the universe, the human body wears out. Inherent in this theory is the idea that the more you abuse your body, the faster it will wear out. Fortunately, today's older adults can achieve high levels of fitness without having to be marathoners. Strength training, walking, gardening, yoga, tai chi, and other activities allow even the most out of shape to improve. You don't have to feel pain to realize healthy gains.

- *The cellular theory* states that at birth we have only a certain number of usable cells, which are genetically programmed to divide or reproduce a limited number of times. Once these cells reach the end of their reproductive cycle, they die, and the organs they make up begin to deteriorate. The rate of deterioration varies from person to person, and its impact depends on the system involved.

- *The autoimmune theory* attributes aging to the decline of the body's immunological system. Studies indicate that as we age, our immune systems become less effective in fighting disease. Eventually, bodies that are subjected to too much stress, lack of sleep, and so on, show signs of disease and infirmity, especially if these factors are coupled with poor nutrition. In some instances, the immune system appears to lose control and turn its protective mechanisms inward, actually attacking the person's own body. Although autoimmune disorders occur in all age groups, some gerontologists believe that they increase in frequency and severity with age.

- *The genetic mutation theory* proposes that the number of cells exhibiting unusual or different characteristics increases with age. Proponents of this theory believe that aging is related to the amount of mutational damage within the genes. The greater the mutation, the greater the chance that cells will not function properly, leading to eventual dysfunction of body organs and systems.

Psychosocial Impacts on Aging

Numerous psychological and sociological factors also influence the manner in which people age. Psychologists Erik Erikson and Robert Peck have formulated theories of personality development that emphasize adaptation and adjustment. In his developmental model, Erikson states that people must progress through eight critical stages during a lifetime. If a person does not receive the proper stimulus or develop effective methods of coping with life's turmoil from infancy onward, problems are likely to develop later in life. According to this theory, maladjustments in old age are often a result of problems encountered in earlier stages of a person's life.

Peck argues that during middle and old age, people face a series of increasingly stressful tasks. Those who are poorly adjusted psychologically or who have not developed appropriate coping skills are likely to undergo a painful aging process.

Both Erikson and Peck suggest that a combination of psychosocial and biological factors and environmental "trigger mechanisms" causes each of us to age in a unique manner. But what is normal and what is unique in aging? How much change is inevitable, and how much can we avoid?

Rosacea Skin disorder that causes facial redness, puffiness, and other symptoms.

Osteoporosis A degenerative bone disorder characterized by increasingly porous bones.

Changes in the Body and Mind

Typical Physical Changes

Although the physiological consequences of aging can differ in severity and timing, certain standard changes occur as a result of the aging process.

The Skin As a normal consequence of aging, the skin becomes thinner and loses elasticity, particularly in the outer surfaces. Fat deposits, which add to the soft lines and shape of the skin, diminish. Starting at about age 30, lines develop on the forehead as a result of sun exposure and facial expressions such as smiling and squinting. These lines become more pronounced, with added "crow's-feet" around the eyes, during the forties. During a person's fifties and sixties, the skin begins to sag and lose color, leading to pallor in the seventies. Body fat in underlying layers of skin continues to be redistributed away from the limbs and extremities into the trunk region of the body. Age spots become more numerous because of excessive pigment accumulation under the skin, particularly in those with heavy sun exposure.

A common skin disorder that affects millions of Americans is **rosacea** (pronounced roh-ZAY-sha). One symptom is redness on the cheeks, nose, chin, or forehead, particularly after exercise or drinking alcohol. This redness looks like a blush or sunburn in the early stages and fades fairly quickly. However, as the condition worsens, the blush may deepen in color and last longer. Other symptoms include small visible blood vessels on the nose or cheeks, small bumps and/or pimples on the skin surface, watery or itchy eyes along with a tendency for red eyes and stye development, enlargement of the nose after recurrent swelling of nasal tissue, and a puffy, red appearance of the face. While the cause of rosacea is unknown and there is no cure, prescription medications can treat and control the symptoms. People who suspect that they have rosacea should visit a dermatologist, who will treat the symptoms and help avoid more serious damage to facial tissue.

Bones and Joints Throughout the life span, bones are continually changing because of the accumulation and loss of minerals. By the third or fourth decade of life, mineral loss from bones becomes more prevalent than mineral accumulation, resulting in a weakening and porosity (diminishing density) of bony tissue. This loss of minerals (particularly calcium) occurs in both sexes, although it is much more common in females. Loss of calcium can contribute to **osteoporosis,** a disease characterized by low bone density and structural deterioration of bone tissue. These porous, fragile bones are susceptible to fracture.[12] (See the Reality Check box.)

The Head With age, features of the head enlarge and become more noticeable. Increased cartilage and fatty tissue cause the nose to grow a half inch wider and another half

Osteoporosis: Preventing an Age-Old Problem

When you hear that someone has osteoporosis, the image that may come to mind is a slumped-over woman with a characteristic "dowager's hump" in the upper back; however, this is a relatively rare, extreme version of the disease. Although many people consider osteoporosis to be a disease only of older women, osteoporosis can occur at any age, and it can pose a problem for men, too. Osteoporosis is progressive and occurs over many years. Without proper prevention in the form of diet, weight-bearing exercise, and overall fitness (see Chapter 10), each of us risks developing this condition. As awareness increases, millions of Americans are requesting bone density tests to determine just how far gone their bones and joints really may be. Health care providers, responding to the estimated $14 billion in direct and indirect costs that osteoporosis patients incur, are also motivated to focus on controlling risks.

EPIDEMIOLOGY

Prevalence data indicate the following:

✔ The hips, wrists, and spine are most vulnerable to the ravages of osteoporosis.
✔ In the United States, osteoporosis affects over 44 million Americans, 68 percent of whom are women.
✔ Each year osteoporosis causes 1.5 million fractures: 300,000 at the hip, 700,000 in the vertebrae, 250,000 in the wrists, and more than 300,000 at other sites.
✔ One out of every two women and one in four men over age 50 will have an osteoporosis-related fracture sometime in life.
✔ More than 2 million American men have osteoporosis and millions more are at risk. Each year, 80,000 men suffer a hip fracture, and one-third of them die within a year.

RISK FACTORS

A number of factors may predispose a person to developing osteoporosis. Risk factors that we cannot control include:

✔ *Gender.* Chances of developing osteoporosis are greater if you are a woman. Women have less bone tissue and lose bone more rapidly than men because of the hormonal changes resulting from menopause.
✔ *Age.* The older you are, the greater your risk of osteoporosis. Your bones become less dense and weaker as you age.
✔ *Body size.* Small, thin-boned women are at greatest risk.
✔ *Ethnicity.* Caucasian and Asian women are at highest risk; African American and Latino women have a lower but still significant risk.
✔ *Family history.* Susceptibility to fracture may be, in part, hereditary. People whose parents have a history of fractures also seem to have reduced bone mass.

The following risk factors can be modified by our choices in lifestyle behaviors, medication, and diet:

✔ Levels of sex hormones—abnormal absence of menstrual periods (amenorrhea), low estrogen levels (menopause), and low testosterone levels in men may signal potential problems.
✔ Anorexia or being very thin—women who are underweight produce less estrogen. Patients with severe anorexia can develop osteoporosis as early as their twenties.
✔ A lifetime diet low in calcium and vitamin D.
✔ Use of certain medications, such as glucocorticoids or some anticonvulsants.
✔ An inactive lifestyle or extended bed rest.
✔ Cigarette smoking.
✔ Excessive consumption of alcohol.

PREVENTION

Increased calcium and vitamin D intake and consistent weight-bearing exercise can help everyone reduce their risk of osteoporosis.

Many studies have indicated that if you don't consume enough calcium, you will be at increased risk for osteoporosis. Calcium requirements change over the course of a lifetime, with greater needs during childhood and adolescence when the skeleton is growing and during pregnancy and breast-feeding. Postmenopausal women and older men also need more, and medications may deplete calcium reserves as well. Be sure to take vitamin D, which helps the body absorb and utilize calcium more efficiently.

Like muscle, bone is living tissue that responds to exercise by becoming stronger. The best exercise for the bones is weight-bearing exercise that forces you to work against gravity. Examples include walking, hiking, jogging, weight training, tennis, and dancing.

Research conducted by Dr. Christine M. Snow, director of Oregon State University's bone research lab and internationally known exercise scientist, has shed interesting light on the importance of exercise for residents of nursing homes. Residents were given modest exercises to do while wearing weighted vests. They improved not only bone density, but also balance and strength, which together can reduce the risk of falling and fracturing bones. In addition, residents were able to walk faster, which made them less likely to fall if they lost balance. In studies of young gymnasts, Snow has found that bone density can be increased through various types of exercise. She emphasizes that it is vitally important to begin exercising early in life to ensure bone health in later years.

Sources: National Institutes of Health, Osteoporosis and Related Bone Diseases National Resource Center, "What People with Anorexia Nervosa Need to Know About Osteoporosis," revised October 2002. www.osteo.org/newfile.asp?doc=r803i &doctitle=What+People+with+Anorexia +Nervosa+Need+to+Know+About +Osteoporosis&doctype=HTML+Fact+Sheet; National Institutes of Health, Osteoporosis and Related Bone Diseases National Resource Center, "Fast Facts," December 2002, www.osteo.org/osteo.html

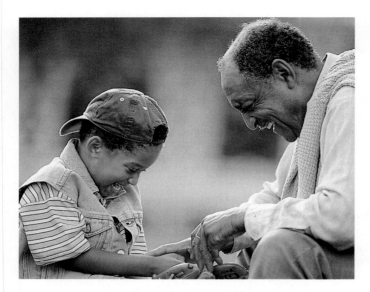

Learning to cope with challenges and changes early in life develops attitudes and skills that contribute to a full and satisfying old age.

inch longer. Earlobes get fatter and longer, while overall head circumference increases one quarter of an inch per decade, even though the brain itself shrinks, because the skull becomes thicker with age.

The Urinary Tract   At age 70, the kidneys can filter waste from the blood only half as fast as they could at age 30. The need to urinate more frequently occurs because the bladder's capacity declines from 2 cups of urine at age 30 to 1 cup at age 70.

One problem sometimes associated with aging is **urinary incontinence,** which ranges from passing a few drops of urine while laughing or sneezing to having no control over urination. Approximately 35 percent of older women and 22 percent of older men have some degree of urinary incontinence.[13] Incontinence can pose major social, physical, and emotional problems. Embarrassment and fear of wetting oneself may cause an older person to become isolated and avoid social functions. Caregivers may become frustrated with incontinent patients. Prolonged wetness and the inability to properly care for oneself can lead to irritation, infections, and other problems.

Urinary incontinence   The inability to control urination.

Cataracts   Clouding of the lens that interrupts the focusing of light on the retina, resulting in blurred vision or eventual blindness.

Glaucoma   Elevation of pressure within the eyeball, leading to hardening of the eyeball, impaired vision, and possible blindness.

However, incontinence is not an inevitable part of aging. Most cases are caused by medications, highly treatable neurological problems that affect the central nervous system, infections of the pelvic muscles, weakness in the pelvic wall, or other problems. When the problem is treated, the incontinence usually vanishes.[14] Drug therapy can slow bladder contractions, increase bladder capacity, contract or relax the bladder sphincter, and increase fluid output. In addition, women can learn Kegel exercises to strengthen the pelvic floor and reduce their susceptibility to this problem later in life. Biofeedback to control urine flow and improve mind/body responses is another approach to prevention. Surgery to repair the pelvic floor is often successful in stress incontinence. Improved access to toilet facilities, artificial devices that slow urine flow, and other treatments have also shown promise.

The Heart and Lungs   Resting heart rate stays about the same over the course of a person's life, but the stroke volume (the amount of blood the muscle pushes out per beat) diminishes as heart muscles deteriorate. Vital capacity, or the amount of air that moves when you inhale and exhale at maximum effort, also declines with age. Exercise can do a great deal to preserve heart and lung function.

Eyesight   By age 30, the lens of the eye begins to harden, causing problems by the early forties. The lens begins to yellow and loses transparency, while the pupil of the eye shrinks, allowing less light to penetrate. Activities such as reading become more difficult, particularly in dim light. By age 60, depth perception declines and farsightedness often develops. A need for reading glasses usually develops in the forties, and this evolves into a need for bifocals or trifocals. Eventually a tendency toward color blindness may develop, especially for shades of blue and green. In addition to these normal changes, some elderly people develop an eye disease such as cataracts, glaucoma, or macular degeneration.

Approximately 20.5 million adult Americans suffer from **cataracts** (clouding of the lens).[15] Normally, the lens is a transparent structure inside the eye that focuses incoming light and images. Over time, the lens can darken or become clouded by clumps of protein, blurring images and impairing night vision. Smoking, diabetes, and extensive exposure to sunlight increase the risk of developing cataracts. Fortunately, most cataracts can be removed surgically with a high success rate; 90 percent of people who undergo cataract surgery enjoy better vision afterward.[16]

Glaucoma (elevated pressure within the eyeball) affects about 2.2 million adult Americans.[17] Inside the front of the eye, there is a space called the anterior chamber. Normally, a clear fluid flows freely in and out of this chamber to nourish nearby tissues. If for some reason the fluid cannot drain from the anterior chamber, pressure can build up inside the eyeball and eventually damage the optic nerve that carries visual information to the brain. Glaucoma is usually painless, and many people don't realize they have it until they have already lost some vision permanently. Risk factors include nearsightedness, age (most cases develop after age 60), and a family history of the disease. For unknown reasons, Mexican Americans and African Americans have a higher risk. There is no cure for glaucoma, but medicated eyedrops can lower the pressure and control the disease. Surgery may also help.[18]

Approximately 1.8 million Americans over age 40 have advanced **macular degeneration**, and another 7.3 million are at high risk for vision loss from it.[19] This condition breaks down the macula, the part of the retina responsible for the sharp, direct vision needed to read, watch television, or drive. Macular degeneration can cause permanent blindness in the central vision plane. The exact causes of age-related macular degeneration are unknown; however, smoking, high blood pressure, farsightedness, obesity, and a family history of the condition tend to increase the risk. Although many researchers and eye specialists believe that certain nutrients such as zinc, antioxidants such as vitamins A, C, and E, and lutein may reduce risks, these theories have not been proven in clinical trials. Efforts to treat macular degeneration are underway, but progress to date has been slow.

Hearing The ability to hear high-frequency consonants (for example, *s, t,* and *z*) diminishes with age. Much of the actual hearing loss lies in the ability to distinguish extreme ranges of sound rather than normal conversational tones.

Sexual Changes As men age, they experience notable alterations in sexual function. Whereas the degree and rate of change vary greatly from person to person, changes that generally occur in men include:

- slowed ability to obtain an erection
- diminished ability to maintain an erection
- increased length of the refractory period between orgasms
- a decline in angle of the erection
- shortened duration of orgasm

Women also experience several changes:

- Menopause usually occurs between the ages of 45 and 55. Women may experience hot flashes, mood swings, weight gain, development of facial hair, or other hormone-related symptoms.
- The walls of the vagina become less elastic and the epithelium thins, possibly making intercourse painful.
- Vaginal secretions, particularly during sexual activity, diminish.
- The breasts become less firm. Loss of fat in various areas leads to fewer curves, with a decrease in the soft lines of body contours.

While these physiological changes may sound somewhat discouraging, the fact is that many people remain sexually active throughout their entire adult lives.[20] Indeed, a landmark study by the National Council on Aging refuted long-held beliefs that sexual desire decreases as we age. Results indicated that nearly half of Americans over age 60

engage in sexual activity at least once a month, and 4 out of 10 would like to have sex more frequently than they currently do.[21] With the advent of drugs designed to treat sexual dysfunction, such as Viagra, many older adults may get their wish.

Body Comfort Because of the loss of body fat, thinning epithelium, and diminished glandular activity, older adults experience greater difficulty regulating body temperature. This limits their ability to withstand extreme cold or heat, increasing the risks of hypothermia, heatstroke, and heat exhaustion. Thinning skin also makes older adults more vulnerable to bed sores and other skin ulcers.

What do you think?

Of the health conditions discussed in this section, which ones can you prevent? ■ *Which ones can you delay?* ■ *What actions can you take now to protect yourself from these problems?*

Mental Changes

Intelligence Recent research demonstrates that many of our previous beliefs about the intelligence of older adults were based on inappropriate testing procedures. Given an appropriate length of time, older people learn and develop skills in a similar manner to younger people. Researchers have also determined that what many older adults lack in speed of learning they make up for in practical knowledge—that is, the "wisdom of age."

Memory Have you ever wondered why your grandfather seems unable to remember what he did last weekend but can vividly describe an event that occurred 40 years ago? This phenomenon is not unusual. Research indicates that although short-term memory may fluctuate on a daily basis, the ability to remember events from past decades seems to remain largely unchanged.

Flexibility versus Rigidity Although it is widely believed that people become more like one another as they age, nothing could be further from the truth. Having lived through a multitude of experiences and faced diverse joys, sorrows, and obstacles, the typical older person has developed unique methods of coping with life. These unique adaptive variations make for interesting differences in how they confront

---

Macular degeneration Disease that breaks down the macula, the light-sensitive part of the retina responsible for sharp, direct vision.

the many changes brought on by the aging process. As a group, the elderly are extremely heterogeneous. They flex and adapt and "make do" in ways that younger adults may not be able to duplicate. Labeling this highly flexible and resilient group as rigid or unmovable is inaccurate and misleading.

Depression   Most adults continue to lead healthy, fulfilling lives. However, some older people do suffer from mental and emotional disturbances. Some research indicates that depression may be the most common psychological problem facing older adults. However, the rate of major depression is actually lower among older people than among younger adults.

Regardless of age, people who have a poor perception of their health, have multiple chronic illnesses, take a lot of medications, abuse alcohol and other drugs, lack social support, and do not exercise face more challenges that require many emotional strengths to get through them. Strong coping skills and support systems will often lessen the duration and severity of the depression. However, those who are ill-equipped to deal with life's changes or who lack close ties may consider suicide as a means of solving their problems.

Senility: Getting Rid of Ageist Attitudes   Over the years, older adults have often suffered from ageist attitudes. People who were chronologically old were often labeled "senile" whenever they displayed memory failure, errors in judgment, disorientation, or erratic behavior. Today scientists recognize that these same symptoms can occur at any age and for various reasons, including disease (such as vitamin B deficiency) or the use of over-the-counter and prescription drugs. When the underlying problems are corrected, the memory loss and disorientation also improve. Currently, the term *senility* is seldom used except to describe a very small group of organic disorders.

Alzheimer's Disease   **Dementias** are progressive brain impairments that interfere with memory and normal intellectual functioning. Although there are many types of dementia, one of the most common forms is **Alzheimer's disease,** also known as **AD.** Attacking over 4 million Americans and killing over 100,000 of them every year, this disease is one of the most painful and devastating conditions that families can

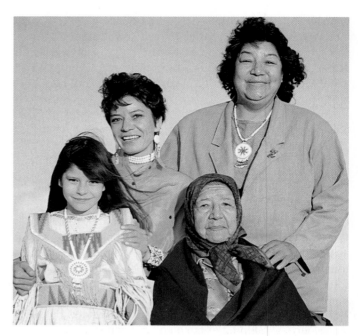

In most cases, you need look no further than your family tree to get an idea of the effects that aging will have on you.

endure. It kills its victims twice: first through a slow loss of personhood (memory loss, disorientation, personality changes, and eventual loss of the ability to function independently), and then through the deterioration of bodily systems as they gradually succumb to the powerful impact of neurological problems.

Currently, Alzheimer's afflicts an estimated one in ten people over the age of 65 and nearly half of people over age 85, including actor Charlton Heston and the late president Ronald Reagan, and costs society over $100 billion a year. With the U.S. population gradually aging, the number of people afflicted and the economic burden are certain to increase.[22] Patients with Alzheimer's live for an average of 8 years after diagnosis, though the disease can last for up to 20 years.[23] While most people associate the disease with the aged, Alzheimer's has been diagnosed in people in their late forties. In fact, about 5 percent of all cases occur before age 65.

Contrary to what many people think, Alzheimer's is not a new disease. Named after Alois Alzheimer, a German neuropathologist who recorded it as early as 1906, Alzheimer's refers to a degenerative disease of the brain in which nerve cells stop communicating with one another. Ordinarily, brain cells communicate by releasing chemicals that allow the cells to receive and transmit messages for various types of behavior. In Alzheimer's patients, the brain doesn't produce enough of these chemicals, cells can't communicate, and eventually the cells die.

This degeneration occurs in the sections of the brain that affect memory, speech, and personality, leaving the parts that control other bodily functions, such as heartbeat

---

Senility   A term associated with judgment and orientation problems and the loss of memory occurring in a small percentage of the elderly.

Dementias   Progressive brain impairments that interfere with memory and normal intellectual functioning.

Alzheimer's disease (AD)   A chronic condition involving changes in nerve fibers of the brain that results in mental deterioration.

and breathing, functioning at near normal levels. Thus, the mind begins to go while the body lives on. It all happens in a slow, progressive manner, and it may take 20 years before symptoms are noticed.

Alzheimer's is generally detected first by families, who note changes, particularly memory lapses and personality changes, in their loved ones. Medical tests rule out underlying causes, and certain neurological tests help confirm the diagnosis.

Alzheimer's disease characteristically progresses in three stages. During the *first stage*, symptoms include forgetfulness, memory loss, impaired judgment, increasing inability to handle routine tasks, disorientation, lack of interest in one's surroundings, and depression. These symptoms accelerate in the *second stage*, which also includes agitation and restlessness (especially at night), loss of sensory perceptions, muscle twitching, and repetitive actions. Many patients become depressed, combative, and aggressive. In the *final stage*, disorientation is often complete. The person becomes completely dependent on others for eating, dressing, and other activities. Identity loss and speech problems are common. Eventually, control of bodily functions may be lost.

Researchers are investigating a number of possible causes of the disease, including genetic predisposition, malfunction of the immune system, a slow-acting virus, chromosomal or genetic defects, chronic inflammation, and neurotransmitter imbalance. Preliminary research indicates that a defect in the chromosomes may be the most likely cause, partly because virtually everyone with Down syndrome eventually develops Alzheimer's. A recent study indicates that being overweight or obese may predispose individuals to Alzheimer's.[24] While the link is not clear, obesity increases the incidence of high blood pressure, high cholesterol, and high blood sugar, all of which have been implicated as risk factors. However, more research with greater numbers of participants and sufficient controls will be needed to validate these initial findings.

Treatment for Alzheimer's focuses on several drugs that have been approved by the U.S. Food and Drug Administration. Cognex, the first drug to be approved, is used only rarely because of side effects, including possible liver damage. Aricept, Exelon, and Reminyl are all cholinesterase inhibitors. They seem to slow the loss of memory by preventing the destruction of neurotransmitters. Although the drugs were associated with better results for users in memory and thinking tests than for patients taking a placebo, the differences were modest, and more than half of the patients showed no improvement at all.[25] In 2003 the FDA approved another type of drug, Memantine, that regulates levels of brain chemicals involved in information storage and memory.[26] Some physicians prescribe vitamin E supplements for Alzheimer's patients, since the vitamin may help protect brain cells against damage from free radicals.

Some researchers are looking at anti-inflammatory drugs, theorizing that Alzheimer's may develop in response to an inflammatory ailment. Others are focusing on stimulating the brains of Alzheimer's-prone individuals, believing that as people learn, more connections between cells are formed that may offset those that are lost.

Much attention has also focused on the family, as the family is often another victim when Alzheimer's occurs. Having to decide between tending to a loved one at home or seeking the assistance of a long-term care facility can be heartbreaking. Caring for Alzheimer's patients is a challenge for even the most dedicated family members. And even the best preparation for the final days of a loved one with this disease does not make the process easy. Knowing what the options are and being able to recognize the differences between normal physiological aging and the ravages of certain diseases can make it easier to cope with age-related problems, for both older patients and their families.

Table 19.1 Percentage of Older Americans Reporting Selected Chronic Health Conditions	
Hypertension	49.2 %
Arthritis	36.1 %
Heart disease	31.1 %
Cancer	20.0 %
Sinusitis	15.1 %
Diabetes	15.0 %

Source: U.S. Department of Health and Human Services, Administration on Aging, *A Profile of Older Americans 2003: Health and Health Care*, updated March 8, 2004, www.aoa.gov/prof/Statistics/profile/2003/14.asp

Health Challenges of Older Adults

Some health problems common in older adults are brought on by failing health (Table 19.1), others by society or a perceived loss of control over life's events—watching loved ones die, facing health problems, and confronting an uncertain economy on a fixed income. Developing life skills and a network of social support during earlier years can significantly reduce problems in old age.

Alcohol Use and Abuse

Early studies reported that 2 to 10 percent of older Americans were alcoholics, but the exact percentages are controversial today. However, a person who is prone to alcoholism during the younger and middle years is more likely to continue during later years. The older alcoholic is probably no more common in American society than the young alcoholic, despite the stereotype of the old, lost soul, hiding his or her sorrows in a bottle. Often, when people think they see a drunken older person, they are really seeing a confused individual who has taken too many different prescription medications and is experiencing a form of drug interaction.

Men tend to have a higher risk for alcoholism at all ages. Alcohol abuse is five times more common among older men than among older women. Yet as many as half of all older men and an even higher proportion of older women don't drink at all. Those who do drink do so less than younger persons, consuming only five to six drinks weekly.

If the more recent studies are accurate, the reason there aren't many heavy drinkers among older adults may be that very heavy drinkers tend either to die of alcoholic complications before they reach old age or to reform their drinking habits. Some older people reduce their consumption because they find they cannot process alcohol as readily as they did when they were younger or because they are afraid of combining it with the prescription drugs they must take. If the older reports are accurate, alcoholism among the elderly may be disguised by a tendency among health professionals and family members to associate forgetfulness, incontinence, poor grooming, dementia-like reactions, injuries, and so on with old age rather than with an alcohol problem. It is important to note that most older adults who consume alcohol are neither alcoholics nor people who drink to cope with their losses. Most drinking among older people is social and may, in fact, be much less of a problem than previously thought.

Prescription Drug Use

It is extremely rare for older people to use illicit drugs, but some do overuse and grow dependent on prescription drugs. Some take four to six prescription drugs a day. Reported numbers of drugs taken are substantially higher for residents of health care institutions, but this may be because drugs that many of us purchase over the counter, such as aspirin, are counted in the total numbers.

Anyone who combines different drugs runs the risk of dangerous drug interactions. The risks of adverse effects are even greater for people with impaired circulation and declining kidney and liver function. Older people displaying symptoms of these drug-induced effects, which may include bizarre behavior patterns or disorientation, are all too often misdiagnosed as senile rather than examined for underlying causes and treated.

Currently there is no one system that tracks all of a patient's prescriptions. Pharmacists may not know about other drugs, vitamins, or herbal supplements that a patient is taking and thus may not warn of possible drug interactions. Illness or physiological abnormalities may affect the way drugs are metabolized, contributing to dose irregularities and other problems. To avoid drug interactions and other problems, older adults should use the same pharmacy consistently, ask questions about medicines and dosages, and read the directions carefully.

Sarcopenia   Age-related loss of muscle mass.

Over-the-Counter Remedies

A substantial segment of the over-60 population avoids professional medical treatment, viewing it as only a last resort. This is becoming increasingly true as Medicare coverage becomes less adequate and older adults are forced to pay larger medical bills out of their own resources. The poor are particularly prone to turn to folk medicine and over-the-counter (OTC) preparations as cheaper, less intimidating alternatives. Aspirin and laxatives head the list of commonly used OTC medications.

Strategies for Healthy Aging

As you know from reading this book, you can do many things to prolong your life and improve the quality of your life. To provide for healthy older years, make each of the following part of your younger years.

Develop and Maintain Healthy Relationships

Social bonds lend vigor and energy to life. Be willing to give to others, and seek variety in your relationships rather than befriending only people who agree with you. By experiencing diverse people and interacting with different points of view, we gain a new perspective on life.

Enrich the Spiritual Side of Life

Although we often take this for granted, cultivating a relationship with nature, the environment, a higher being, and yourself is a key factor in personal growth and development. Take time for thought and quiet contemplation, and enjoy the sunsets, sounds, and energy of life. These moments spent in time prioritized for "you" will leave you invigorated and fresh—better able to cope with the ups and downs of life. If you don't take time for yourself now, it just may be that you won't have time in the later years.

Improve Fitness

If you're basically sedentary, just about any moderate-intensity exercise that gets your heart beating faster and increases strength and/or flexibility will maximize your physical health and functional years. The research presented in Chapter 10 shows that there is hope even for the most die-hard couch potato.

One of the inevitable physical changes that the body undergoes is **sarcopenia,** age-associated loss of muscle mass. The less muscle you have, the less energy you will burn even while resting. The lower your metabolic rate, the more likely you will gain weight. With regular strength training, you can increase your muscle mass, boost your metabolism, strengthen your bones, lower the risk of osteoporosis, and, in general, feel better and function more efficiently. The Skills for Behavior Change box provides tips for exercise.

Aging and Exercise

Whether you're 20, 50, or 80 years old, you can exercise and improve your health. Exercising has even helped 90-year-olds living in nursing homes to grow stronger and more independent.

Staying physically active is a key to good health well into later years. Yet only about one in four older adults exercises regularly. Many think they are too old or too frail, but nothing could be further from the truth. Physical activity of any kind—from heavy-duty exercises such as jogging or bicycling to easier efforts like walking—is good for you. Vigorous exercise can help strengthen your heart and lungs. Taking a brisk walk regularly will lower your risk of health problems like heart disease and depression. Climbing stairs, calisthenics, and housework will increase strength, stamina, and self-confidence. Weight lifting or strength training is a good way to slow down muscle and bone loss. Your daily activities will become easier as you feel better.

You can exercise at home alone, with a buddy, or as part of a group. Talk to your doctor before you begin, especially if you are over 40 or have a medical problem. Move at your own speed, and don't take on too much at first. A class can be a good idea if you haven't exercised for a long time or are just beginning. A qualified teacher will make sure you are doing the exercise in the right way.

Set a goal of 30 minutes of moderate activity every day. You don't have to exercise for 30 minutes all at once. Short bursts of activity, like taking the stairs instead of the elevator or walking instead of driving, can add up to 30 minutes of exercise a day. Raking leaves, playing actively with children, gardening, and even doing household chores can count toward your daily total.

Include a mix of stretching, strength training, and aerobic or endurance exercise in your exercise plan. People who are weak or frail should start slowly. Begin with stretching and strength training; add aerobic exercises later. Aerobic exercises are safer and easier once you feel balanced and your muscles are stronger.

Stretching improves flexibility, eases movement, and lowers the risk of injury and muscle strain. It also increases blood flow and gets your body ready for exercise. A warm-up and cool-down period of 5 to 15 minutes should be done slowly and carefully, before and after all types of exercise. In addition to being relaxing, stretching can loosen muscles in the arms, shoulders, back, chest, stomach, buttocks, thighs, and calves.

Strength training (also called resistance training or weight lifting) builds muscle and bone, both of which decline with age. Lifting weights or working out with machines or an elastic band will strengthen the upper and lower body. It is very important to have an expert teach you how to work with weights; otherwise you could get hurt. With help, older adults can work their way up to many of the same weight-lifting routines as younger adults. Once you know what to do, you can do simple strength training exercises at home. Try using household items, such as soup cans or milk jugs filled with water or sand, as weights. Strength training does not have to take a lot of time; 30 to 40 minutes at least two or three times each week are all that's needed. Try not to exercise the same muscles two days in a row.

Aerobic exercises (also called endurance exercises) strengthen the heart and improve overall fitness by increasing the body's ability to use oxygen. Swimming, walking, and dancing are "low-impact" aerobic activities. They avoid the muscle and joint pounding of more "high-impact" exercises like jogging and jumping rope. Aerobic exercises raise the number of heartbeats each minute (heart rate). Try to get your heart rate to a certain level and keep it there for 20 minutes or more. If you have not exercised in a while, start slowly. As you get stronger, try to increase your heart rate. Aerobics should be done for 20 to 40 minutes at least three times each week.

Before starting any aerobics program, check with your doctor and ask about your target heart rate. Some blood pressure medicines, for example, can affect how you calculate target heart rate.

Not sure where to start? Local gyms, universities, or hospitals can help you find a teacher or program that works for you. You can also check with local churches or synagogues, senior and civic centers, parks, recreation associations, YMCAs, YWCAs, and even local shopping malls for exercise and wellness programs. Many community centers also offer programs for older people who are worried about special health problems like heart disease or falling. Look for books and tapes at your local library.

Source: Adapted from U.S. Department of Health and Human Services, National Institute on Aging, "Don't Take It Easy—Exercise!" (Gaithersburg, MD: National Institute on Aging, n.d.), www.medaccess.com /seniors/agepg/ap41.htm

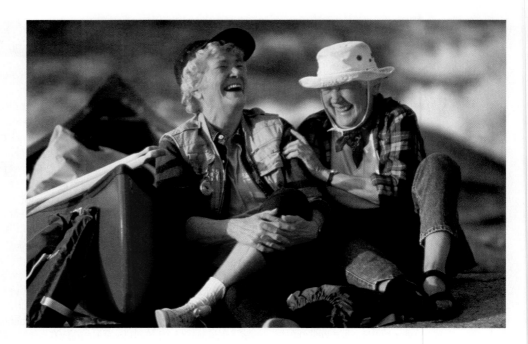

For many, the secret to aging well is to stay active and enjoy the company of good friends.

So, get moving and keep moving, no matter what the activity is. And remember, it is never too late to start. Even if you're in your sixties or seventies, exercise can increase life expectancy by improving circulation, reducing blood pressure, and reducing overall health risks. A lifetime of exercise and movement will pay dividends in later years.

Eat for Health

Although other chapters in this text provide detailed information about nutrition and weight control, certain nutrients are especially essential to healthy aging:

- *Calcium.* Bone loss tends to increase in women, particularly in the hip region, shortly before menopause. During perimenopause and menopause, this bone loss accelerates rapidly, with an average of about 3 percent skeletal mass lost per year over a five-year period. The result is an increased risk for fracture and disability. Few women actually consume the 1,000 milligrams of calcium recommended during the younger years or the 1,500 milligrams recommended during and after menopause.
- *Vitamin D.* Vitamin D is necessary for adequate calcium absorption, yet as people age, particularly in their fifties and sixties, they do not absorb vitamin D from foods as readily as they did in their younger years. If vitamin D is unavailable, calcium levels are also likely to be lower.

Comorbidity   The presence of a number of diseases at the same time.

- *Protein.* As older adults become more concerned about cholesterol and fatty foods, and as their budgets shrink, one nutrient that often takes the "hit" is protein. It costs more, takes longer to cook, and often has that "fat" stigma associated with animal products. Many older people cut back on protein to a point that is below the recommended daily amount. Large numbers of women in particular cut back so far that they get less than half of the daily amount necessary. Because protein is necessary for muscle mass, protein insufficiencies can spell trouble.

Other nutrients, including vitamin E, folic acid (folate), iron, potassium, and vitamin B_{12} (cobalamin), are important to the aging process, and most of these are readily available in any diet that follows food pyramid recommendations.

In summary, aging is not just a static state that you suddenly achieve. You can feel old at a very young age or feel young at a very old age. You can have an engaging and active life full of challenges, friends, and fulfillment, or you can become socially isolated, bored, and unhappy. Many of these end products in life have to do with the path you choose to follow now.

Caring for Older Adults

Older women far outnumber older men in American society, and the discrepancy increases with age. Because women live seven years longer than men on average, older women are more likely to be living alone. Further, they are more likely to experience poverty and multiple chronic health problems, a situation referred to as **comorbidity.** Consequently, more older women than men are likely to need assistance from children, other relatives, friends, and neighbors.

Women have usually been the primary caregivers for older Americans, often for their ailing husbands. Research also indicates that women spend more hours than men (38 hours versus 27 hours per week) in caregiving activities and perform a wider range of activities. Regardless of the time spent, caregiving is a difficult and stressful experience for both women and men. **Respite care,** or care that is given by someone who relieves the primary caregiver, should be available to ease the burden. As the population ages and more older adults require care, it will become even more important to support caregivers' health and well-being.

What do you think?

Why are women often the primary caregivers for aging spouses and other family members? ▪ *What problems can such caregiving cause?* ▪ *How can caregivers learn to cope with the stresses and strains of their situation?*

Respite care   The care provided by substitute caregivers to relieve the principal caregiver from his or her continuous responsibility.

TAKING CHARGE

MAKE IT HAPPEN!

Assessment: The Assess Yourself box earlier in this chapter (page 551) encouraged you to consider some of the deepest questions in life: What are your values? How do you want your life to compare with that of your parents? How would you like to be described at age 70? Now that you have considered your answers, perhaps there are actions you can take that will help you create the life you want.

Making a Change: In order to change your behavior, you need to develop a plan. Follow these steps:

1. Evaluate your behavior, and identify patterns and specific things you are doing. What can you change now? What can you change in the near future?
2. Select one pattern of behavior that you want to change.
3. Fill out a Behavior Change Contract. It should include your long-term goal for change, your short-term goals, the rewards you'll give yourself for reaching these goals, potential obstacles along the way, and strategies for overcoming these obstacles. For each goal, list the small steps and specific actions that you will take.
4. Chart your progress in a journal. At the end of a week, consider how successful you were in following your plan.

What helped you be successful? What made change more difficult? What will you do differently next week?
5. Revise your plan as needed: Are the short-term goals attainable? Are the rewards satisfying?

One Student's Plan: When Eric answered the Assess Yourself questions, he realized he had not thought deeply about where he wanted to be at various stages in his life. In particular, he wanted to take more time to look at his parents' lives and careers, as well as those of older adults around him in the community. He set a goal of asking his parents and grandparents some of these same questions about their goals and lives to see where he might agree and disagree with them and how he might develop his own values and priorities. As he began thinking more seriously about the types of careers that he thought might be fulfilling, he arranged to meet with adults who had gone into professions that he was considering. He also decided to take a philosophy class as one of his electives in the next year, in which he could actually get school credit for thinking about these big questions.

Summary

- Aging can be defined in terms of biological age, referring to a person's physical condition; psychological age, referring to a person's coping abilities and intelligence; social age, referring to a person's habits and roles relative to society's expectations; legal age, based on chronological years; or functional age, relative to how other people function at varied ages.

- The growing numbers of older adults (people age 65 and older) will have an important impact on society in terms of the economy, health care, housing, and ethical considerations.

- Two broad groups of theories—biological and psychosocial—purport to explain the physiological and psychological changes that occur with aging. The biological theories include the wear-and-tear theory, the cellular theory, the autoimmune theory, and the genetic mutation theory. Psychosocial theories center on adaptation and adjustments related to self-development.

- Aging changes the body and mind in many ways. Physical changes occur in the skin, bones and joints, head, urinary tract, heart and lungs, senses, sexual functioning, and temperature regulation. Major physical concerns are osteoporosis, urinary incontinence, and changes in eyesight and hearing. Most older people maintain a high level of intelligence and memory. Potential mental problems include depression and Alzheimer's disease.

- Special challenges for older adults include alcohol abuse, prescription drug and OTC interactions, questions about vitamin and mineral supplementation, and issues regarding caregiving.

- Lifestyle choices we make today will affect health status later in life. Choosing to exercise, eat a healthy diet, and foster lasting relationships will contribute to healthy aging. Decisions about caring for older adults and stresses related to caregiving are ongoing concerns as the U.S. population ages.

Questions for Discussion and Reflection

1. Discuss the various definitions of aging. At what age would you place your parents for each category?
2. As the older population grows, how will it affect your life? Would you be willing to pay higher taxes to support government social programs for older adults? For example, do you believe that Social Security should continue its yearly increases in payments, which are pegged to inflation? Why or why not?
3. Which of the biological theories of aging do you think is most correct? Why?
4. List the major physiological changes that occur with aging. Which of these, if any, can you change?
5. Explain the major health challenges that older people may face. What advice would you give to your grandparents before they took a prescription or OTC drug?
6. Discuss actions you can start taking now to help ensure a healthier aging process.

Accessing Your Health on the Internet

Visit the following Internet sites to explore further topics and issues related to personal health. To visit an organization's website, go to the Companion Website for *Access to Health, Ninth Edition* at www.aw-bc.com/donatelle, click on the book image, and select "Accessing Your Health on the Internet" from the navigation menu.

1. **Administration on Aging.** A link to the U.S. Department of Health and Human Services agency dedicated to addressing the health needs of older Americans.
2. **Alzheimer's Association.** Archives of media releases and position statements, fact sheets on Alzheimer's disease, medical and research updates, and a brochure on how to recognize the ten warning signs of Alzheimer's.
3. **SeniorCom.** Home page to a link to numerous resources for senior citizens, including chat rooms, databases, and services dedicated to assisting the aging.
4. **Social Security Online.** Provides information about Social Security benefits and entitlements. Also offers links to related sites.

Further Reading

Gaby, A. R. *Preventing and Reversing Osteoporosis: Every Woman's Essential Guide.* Roseville, CA: Prima Publishing, 1995.

Excellent reference text focusing on osteoporosis risk factors and what you can do to reduce risks.

The Johns Hopkins Medical Letter—Health After 50. www.hopkinsafter50.com

Monthly newsletter providing comprehensive, accurate overviews of health topics relevant to older adults.

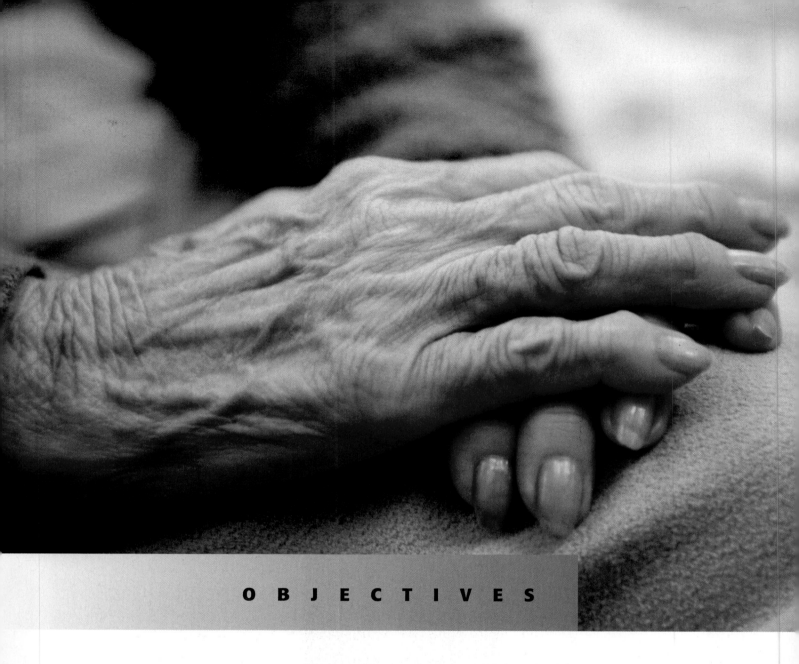

OBJECTIVES

- Define *death,* and analyze why people deny death in Western culture.

- Discuss the stages of the grieving process and strategies for coping more effectively with death.

- Explain the ethical concerns that arise from the concepts of the right to die and rational suicide.

- Review the decisions that need to be made when someone is dying or has died, including hospice care, funeral arrangements, wills, and organ donations.

DYING AND DEATH

THE FINAL TRANSITION

IN THE NEWS

Ruling Upholds Oregon Law Authorizing Assisted Suicide

By Adam Liptak

A federal appeals court yesterday upheld the only law in the nation authorizing doctors to help their terminally ill patients commit suicide. The decision, by a divided three-judge panel of the United States Court of Appeals for the Ninth Circuit, in San Francisco, said the Justice Department did not have the power to punish the doctors involved.

The majority used unusually pointed language to rebuke Attorney General John Ashcroft, saying he had overstepped his authority in trying to block enforcement of the state law, Oregon's Death With Dignity Act.

"The attorney general's unilateral attempt to regulate general medical practices historically entrusted to state lawmakers," Judge Richard C. Tallman wrote for the majority, "interferes with the democratic debate about physician-assisted suicide and far exceeds the scope of his authority under federal law."

Charles Miller, a Justice Department spokesman, said lawyers there were reviewing the decision and had not decided on their next move. The government could ask an 11-member panel of the Ninth Circuit to rehear the case or try to appeal to the United States Supreme Court.

Read the complete article online in the eThemes section of this book's website: www.aw-bc.com/donatelle.

Original article published May 27, 2004. Copyright © 2004 *The New York Times*. Reprinted with permission.

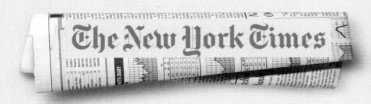

Death eventually comes to everyone, but if you live life to the fullest and learn as much about end-of-life issues as you can, you will be better able to accept the inevitable. Distractions and denial may postpone the reality of death, but they cannot eliminate it. The acceptance of death helps shape attitudes about the importance of life.

Throughout history, humans have attempted to determine the nature and meaning of death. This quest continues today. Although we will touch on moral and philosophical questions about death in this chapter, we will not explore such issues in depth. Rather, our primary focus is to present dying and death as normal components of life and to discuss how we can cope with these events.

Confrontations with death elicit different feelings depending on many factors, including age, religious beliefs, family orientation, health, personal experience with death, and the circumstances of the death itself. To cope effectively with dying, we must address the individual needs of those involved. We will identify some of these needs and offer information and suggestions that have been helpful to many people as they face this final transition. See the Assess Yourself box to evaluate your personal level of anxiety about death.

Understanding Death

Large-scale and impersonal death seems to surround us. Often sensationalized by the news media, it is regularly woven into our entertainment. In the context of this routine exposure, it seems paradoxical that Western society in the twenty-first century has been characterized as "death-denying." Why is it that we wish to deny, or even postpone, death? Let's begin by investigating what death means, at least in medical terms.

Defining Death

Dying is the process of decline in body functions resulting in the death of an organism. **Death** can be defined as the "final cessation of the vital functions" and also refers to a state in which these functions are "incapable of being restored."[1] This definition has become more significant as medical and scientific advances make it increasingly possible to postpone death.

Legal and ethical issues related to death and dying led to the Uniform Determination of Death Act in 1981, which was endorsed by the American Medical Association, the

American Bar Association, and the National Conference for Commissioners on Uniform State Laws. This act, which has been adopted by several states, reads as follows: "An individual who has sustained either (1) irreversible cessation of circulatory and respiratory functions, or (2) irreversible cessation of all functions of the entire brain, including the brainstem, is dead. A determination of death must be made in accordance with accepted medical standards."[2]

The concept of **brain death,** defined as the irreversible cessation of all functions of the entire brainstem, has gained increasing credence. (The brainstem is a relay site for sensory and motor pathways and contains structures responsible for mediating such critical body functions as respiration, heart rate, and general levels of alertness.) As defined by the Ad Hoc Committee of the Harvard Medical School, brain death occurs when the following criteria are met:[3]

- Unreceptivity and unresponsiveness—that is, no response even to painful stimuli.
- No movement for a continuous hour after observation by a physician, and no breathing after three minutes off a respirator.
- No reflexes, including brainstem reflexes; fixed and dilated pupils.
- A "flat" electroencephalogram (EEG, which measures electrical activity of the brain) for at least 10 minutes.
- All of these tests repeated at least 24 hours later with no change.
- Certainty that hypothermia (extreme loss of body heat) and depression of the central nervous system caused by use of drugs such as barbiturates are not responsible for these conditions.

The Harvard report provides useful guidelines; however, the definition of *death* and all its ramifications continue to concern us.

What do you think?

Why is there so much concern over the definition of death? ■ *How does modern technology complicate the understanding of when death occurs?*

Denying Death

Attitudes toward death tend to fall on a continuum. At one end of the continuum, death is viewed as the mortal enemy of humankind. Both medical science and religion have promoted this idea of death. At the other end of the continuum, death is accepted and even welcomed.[4] For people whose attitudes fall at this end, death is a passage to a better state of being. Most of us, however, perceive ourselves to be in the middle of this continuum. From this perspective, death is a bewildering mystery that elicits fear and apprehension while

---

Dying   The process of decline in body functions, resulting in the death of an organism.

Death   The permanent ending of all vital functions.

Brain death   The irreversible cessation of all functions of the entire brainstem.

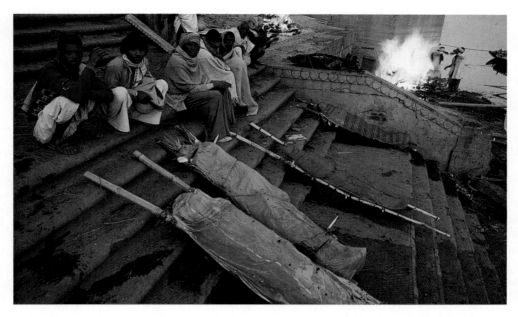

There is no single way to mourn. Each culture has its own unique ways of saying goodbye to the deceased.

profoundly influencing attitudes, beliefs, and actions throughout life.

In the United States, a high level of discomfort is associated with death and dying. As a result, we may avoid speaking about death in an effort to limit our own discomfort. Those who deny death tend to:

- Avoid people who are grieving after the death of a loved one so they won't have to talk about it.
- Fail to validate a dying person's frightening situation by talking to the person as if nothing were wrong.
- Substitute euphemisms for the word *death* (for example, "passing away," "no longer with us," or "going to a better place").
- Give false reassurances to people who are dying by saying things like "everything is going to be okay."
- Shut off conversation about death by silencing people who are trying to talk about it.
- Avoid touching people who are dying.

Death denial has long been a predominant characteristic of our society, but we must keep in mind that social attitudes change over time. It is therefore important to understand the climate in which these perceptions developed and took hold.

Major changes in attitudes toward death accompanied the Industrial Revolution. An emphasis on autonomy and rejection of magic meant that, as a culture, Americans had to be independent and autonomous. Yet American rituals centered on connections to other people. Recent years have shown a greater effort on the part of the American public to mourn openly, as indicated by roadside crosses and memorials placed at the sites of violent or unexpected deaths.

Although these are fairly new additions to the American landscape, these memorials have long been popular in other parts of the world, particularly in predominantly Catholic countries.[5]

The attitudes we develop about death are influenced by many factors, including modern technology, personal experience and beliefs, the environment, age, access to health care, and many other factors. The complex social environment we live in has added new experiences and sometimes confusion to the complexity of our own personal beliefs about death.

What do you think?

"The art of living well and the art of dying well are one." What do you think this quote from the Greek philosopher Epicurus means? ■ Do you agree?

The Process of Dying

Dying is a complex process that includes physical, intellectual, social, spiritual, and emotional dimensions. Now that we have examined the physical indicators of death, we must consider the emotional aspects of dying and "social death."

Coping Emotionally with Death

Science and medicine have enabled us to understand changes associated with growth, development, aging, and social roles throughout the life span, but they have not fully

Death-Related Anxiety Scale

✳myhealthlab

Fill out this assessment online at www.aw-bc.com/myhealthlab or www.aw-bc.com/donatelle

How anxious or accepting are you about the prospect of your death? Indicate how well each statement describes your attitude.

Not true at all 0   Mainly not true 1   Not sure 2   Somewhat true 3   Very true 4

1. I tend not to be very brave in crisis situations. _____
2. I am an unusually anxious person. _____
3. I am something of a hypochondriac and am perhaps obsessively worried about infections. _____
4. I have never had a semimystical, spiritual, out-of-the-body, near-death, or "peak" experience. _____
5. I tend to be unusually frightened in planes at takeoff and landing. _____
6. I do not have a particular religion or philosophy that helps me to face dying. _____
7. I do not believe in any form of survival of the soul after death. _____
8. Personally, I would give a lot to be immortal in this body. _____
9. I am very much a city person and not really close to nature. _____
10. Anxiety about death spoils the quality of my life. _____
11. I am superstitious that preparing for dying might hasten my death. _____
12. I don't like the way some of my relatives died and fear that my death could be like theirs. _____
13. My actual experience of friends dying has been undilutedly negative. _____
14. I would feel easier being with a dying relative if he or she had not been told he or she was dying. _____
15. I have fears of dying alone without friends around me. _____
16. I have fears of dying slowly. _____
17. I have fears of dying suddenly. _____
18. I have fears of dying before my time or while my children are still young. _____
19. I have fears of dying before fulfilling my potential and fully using my talents. _____
20. I have fears of dying without adequately having expressed my love to those I am close to. _____
21. I have fears of dying before having really experienced much *joie de vivre*. _____
22. I have fears of what may or may not happen after death. _____
23. I have fears of what could happen to my family after my death. _____
24. I have fears of dying in a hospital or an institution. _____
25. I have fears of those caring for me feeling overwhelmed by the strain of it. _____
26. I have fears of not getting help with euthanasia when the time comes. _____
27. I have fears of being given unofficial and unwanted euthanasia. _____
28. I have fears of getting insufficient pain control while dying. _____
29. I have fears of being overmedicated and unconscious while dying. _____
30. I have fears of being declared dead when not really dead or being buried alive. _____
31. I have fears of getting confused at death or not being able to follow my spiritual practices. _____
32. I have fears of what may happen to my body after death. _____
33. I have fears of an Alzheimer's-type mental degeneration near death. _____
34. Overall I would say that I am unusually anxious about death and dying. _____

Total Points _____

Add up your scores. If you are extremely anxious (scoring 65 or more), you might consider counseling or therapy; if you are unusually anxious (scoring between 40 and 64), you might want to find a method of meditation, philosophy, or spiritual practice to help experience, explore, and accept your feelings about death. Average anxiety is a score under 40. Continue to have a thoughtful and open ability to consider your own death in time.

MAKE IT HAPPEN!

Use the results of this self-assessment to begin your behavior change program. Follow the steps and use the examples on page 587 to complete your Behavior Change Contract, and then use these resources to take action.

Source: The New Natural Death Handbook, 3rd ed. (2000). Copyright © 2000 The Natural Death Centre. Reprinted with permission.

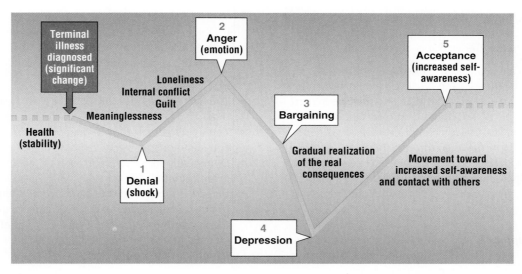

Figure 20.1
Kübler-Ross's Stages of Dying

explained the nature of death. This may partially explain why the transition from life to death evokes so much mystery and emotion. Although emotional reactions to dying vary, many people share similar experiences during this process.

Tasks, stages, and phases are all terms that have been used in models that have been developed to understand the process of dying. The late Elisabeth Kübler-Ross is perhaps the most well known of writers on the topic, but researchers such as Charles Corr have continued to expand on her great work. Research leading to a better understanding of the process of dying will continue as new psychological perspectives are explored.

Kübler-Ross and the Stages of Dying   Much of our knowledge about reactions to dying stems from the work of Elisabeth Kübler-Ross, a pioneer in **thanatology,** the study of death and dying. In 1969, Kübler-Ross published *On Death and Dying,* a sensitive analysis of the reactions of terminally ill patients. This pioneering work encouraged the development of death education as a discipline and prompted efforts to improve the care of dying patients. Kübler-Ross identified five psychological stages (Figure 20.1) that terminally ill patients often experience as they approach death:

1. *Denial.* ("Not me, there must be a mistake.") This is usually the first stage, experienced as a sensation of shock and disbelief. A person intellectually accepts the impending death but rejects it emotionally. The patient is too confused and stunned to comprehend "not being" and thus rejects the idea.
2. *Anger.* ("Why me?") Anger is another common reaction to the realization of imminent death. The person becomes angry at having to face death when others are healthy.

The dying person perceives the situation as "unfair" or "senseless" and may be hostile to friends, family, physicians, or the world in general.

3. *Bargaining.* ("If I'm allowed to live, I promise . . .") This stage generally occurs at about the middle of the progression. The dying person may resolve to be a better person in return for an extension of life or may secretly pray for a short reprieve from death in order to experience a special event, such as a family wedding or birth.
4. *Depression.* ("It's really going to happen to me, and I can't do anything about it.") Depression eventually sets in as vitality diminishes and the person begins to experience symptoms with increasing frequency. The person's deteriorating condition becomes impossible for him or her to deny, and feelings of doom and tremendous loss may become unbearably pervasive. Feelings of worthlessness and guilt are also common because the dying person may feel responsible for the emotional suffering of loved ones and the arduous efforts of caregivers.
5. *Acceptance.* ("I'm ready.") This is often the final stage. The patient stops battling with emotions and becomes tired and weak. The need to sleep increases, and wakeful periods become shorter and less frequent. With acceptance, the person does not "give up" and become sullen or resentfully resigned to death, but rather becomes passive. According to one dying person, the acceptance stage is "almost void of feelings . . . as if the pain had gone, the struggle is over, and there comes a time for the final rest before the long journey."[6] As he or she lets go, the dying

Thanatology   The study of death and dying.

person may no longer welcome visitors and may not wish to engage in conversation. Death usually occurs quietly and painlessly while the victim is unconscious.

The health care profession immediately embraced Kübler-Ross's "stage theory" and applied it in clinical settings. However, subsequent research has indicated that the experiences of dying people do not fit easily into specific stages. Although it is normal to grieve when a severe loss has been sustained, some people never go through this process; others may pass back and forth between the stages. Even if it is not accurate in all its particulars, however, Kübler-Ross's theory offers valuable insights for those dealing with the process of dying.

Corr's Coping Approach   Since Kübler-Ross's work, others have developed alternative models for understanding the ways in which we cope with death and other significant losses. Charles Corr believes that there are unique challenges and responses for the dying person and those who love them.[7] He suggests four dimensions of coping with loss: *physical*—doing everything possible to make ourselves comfortable and minimize pain; *psychological*—living to the fullest, focusing on life accomplishments, and seeking satisfaction in daily activities; *social*—nurturing relationships, keeping loved ones involved, and sharing emotions; and *spiritual*—identifying what matters in life and reaffirming meaningful experiences.

What do you think?

Do you agree with Elisabeth Kübler-Ross's stages of dying, or do you think the stages should be expanded to include Corr's model? ■ *Do you think it is important to help a person get through all the stages that Kübler-Ross has identified?* ■ *Why or why not?*

Social Death

The need for recognition and appreciation within a social group is nearly universal. Denying a person normal social interaction is **social death,** a seemingly irreversible situation in which a person is not treated like an active member of society. Dramatic examples of social death include the exile of nonconformists from their native countries or the

excommunication of dissident members of religious groups. Numerous studies indicate that people who are dying are treated differently too. The following common behaviors contribute to the social death that often isolates people who are terminally ill:[8]

- The dying person is referred to as if he or she were already dead.
- The dying person may be inadvertently excluded from conversations.
- Dying patients are often moved to terminal wards and given minimal care.
- Bereaved family members are avoided, often for extended periods, because friends and neighbors are afraid of feeling uncomfortable in the presence of grief.
- Medical personnel may make degrading comments about patients in their presence.

This decrease in meaningful social interaction often strips dying and bereaved people of their identity as valued members of society at a time when belonging is critical. Some dying people choose not to speak of their inevitable fate in an attempt to make others feel more comfortable and thus preserve vital relationships.

Coping with Loss

The losses resulting from the death of a loved one are extremely difficult to cope with. The dying person, as well as close family and friends, frequently suffers emotionally and physically from the impending loss of critical relationships and roles. Words used to describe feelings and behavior related to losses resulting from death include *bereavement, grief, grief work,* and *mourning.* These terms are related but not identical in meaning. Understanding them will help in comprehending the emotional processes associated with loss and the cultural constraints that often inhibit normal coping behavior (Figure 20.2).

Bereavement is generally defined as the loss or deprivation experienced by a survivor when a loved one dies. Because relationships vary in type and intensity, reactions to losses also vary. The death of a parent, spouse, sibling, child, friend, or pet will result in different kinds of feelings. In the lives of the bereaved or of close survivors, the loss of loved ones leaves "holes." We can think of bereavement as the awareness of these holes. Time and courage are necessary to fill these spaces.

A special case of bereavement occurs in old age. Loss is an intrinsic part of growing old. The longer we live, the more losses we are likely to experience. These losses include physical, social, and emotional losses as our bodies deteriorate and more and more of our loved ones die. The theory of *bereavement overload* has been proposed to explain the effects of multiple losses and the accumulation of sorrow in the lives of some older adults. This theory suggests that the gloomy outlook, disturbing behavior patterns, and apparent apathy that characterize some people may be related more to bereavement overload than to intrinsic physiological degeneration in old age.[9]

Social death   A seemingly irreversible situation in which a person is not treated like an active member of society.

Bereavement   The loss or deprivation experienced by a survivor when a loved one dies.

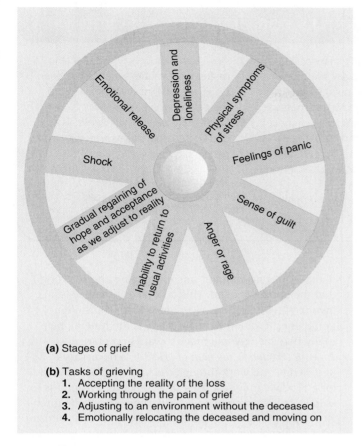

(a) Stages of grief

(b) Tasks of grieving
1. Accepting the reality of the loss
2. Working through the pain of grief
3. Adjusting to an environment without the deceased
4. Emotionally relocating the deceased and moving on

Figure 20.2

The Stages and Tasks of Grief
(a) People react differently to losses, but most eventually adapt. Generally, the stronger the social support system, the smoother the progression through the stages of grief. (b) Worden's developmental tasks associated with grief are another way to understand the grieving process.

Grief is a state of mental distress that occurs in reaction to significant loss, including one's own impending death, the death of a loved one, or a quasi-death experience (to be discussed later in this chapter). Grief reactions include any adjustments needed for one to "make it through the day" and may include changes in patterns of eating, sleeping, working, and even thinking.

When a person experiences a loss that cannot be openly acknowledged, publicly mourned, or socially supported, coping may be much more difficult. This type of grief is referred to as **disenfranchised grief**.[10] It may occur among those who miscarry during pregnancy, are developmentally disabled, or are close friends rather than relatives of the deceased. It may also include relationships that are not socially approved, such as those between extramarital lovers or gay and lesbian couples. When society does not assign significance to a high-grief death, grieving becomes even more difficult for the bereaved.

The term *mourning* is often incorrectly equated with the term *grief*. As we have noted, *grief* refers to a wide variety of feelings and actions that occur in response to bereavement. **Mourning,** in contrast, refers to culturally prescribed and accepted time periods and behavior patterns for the expression of grief. In Judaism, for example, "sitting *shiva*" is a designated mourning period of seven days that involves prescribed rituals and prayers. Depending on a person's relationship with the deceased, various other rituals may continue for up to a year.

In some cases, people are so overwhelmed by grief that they do not return to normal daily living. Support and counseling should be sought when this occurs. Doctors, nurses, psychologists, psychiatrists, and clergy can be helpful in solving problems associated with the loss of a loved one.

Symptoms of grief vary in severity and duration, depending on the situation and the individual. However, the bereaved person can benefit from emotional and social support from family, friends, clergy, employers, and traditional support organizations, including the medical community and the funeral industry. The larger and stronger the support system, the easier readjustment is likely to be. See the Skills for Behavior Change box to learn about how you can best help a grieving friend.

Religion provides comfort to many dying and grieving people. Although some people question the existence of an afterlife, others gain support from religious beliefs that provide a purpose and meaning to life. By accepting dying as a part of the continuum of life, many people are able to make necessary readjustments after the death of a loved one. This holistic concept, which accepts dying as a part of the total life experience, is shared by both believers and nonbelievers.

What Is "Normal" Grief?

This is a difficult question to answer. Grief responses vary widely from person to person, but a classic acute grief syndrome often includes the following symptoms:

- Periodic waves of physical distress lasting 20 minutes to an hour.
- A feeling of tightness in the throat.
- Choking and shortness of breath.
- A frequent need to sigh.
- A feeling of emptiness in the abdomen.
- A sensation of muscular weakness.
- Intense anxiety that is described as actually painful.

Grief   The state of mental distress that occurs in reaction to significant loss, including one's own impending death, the death of a loved one, or a quasi-death experience.

Disenfranchised grief   Grief concerning a loss that cannot be openly acknowledged, publicly mourned, or socially supported.

Mourning   The culturally prescribed behavior patterns for the expression of grief.

Talking to Friends When Someone Dies

It's always hard to know just what to say and how to say it when talking with a grieving friend or relative. Sometimes, even though we mean well, our actions can hurt more than help. Here are some do's and don'ts.

1. Be honest. If you don't know what to say, don't be afraid to say so.
2. Respect your friend's need for privacy.
3. Send a card with a handwritten message, note, or letter expressing your sorrow.
4. Share your fond memories of the person who died.
5. Don't judge the way in which a person grieves.
6. Don't assume that the person thinks the death was "for the best."
7. Don't say "I know how you feel"—no matter what your experience has been.
8. Don't ask for things that belonged to the person who passed away.
9. Don't make parallels with animals—don't compare a dog's death with a person's.

Source: L. Kelly, *Don't Ask for the Dead Man's Golf Clubs: What to Do and Say (And What Not To) When a Friend Loses a Loved One* (New York: Workman, 2000).

Other common symptoms of grief include insomnia, memory lapses, loss of appetite, difficulty concentrating, a tendency to engage in repetitive or purposeless behavior, an "observer" sensation or feeling of unreality, difficulty in making decisions, lack of organization, excessive speech, social withdrawal or hostility, guilt feelings, and preoccupation with the image of the deceased. Susceptibility to disease increases with grief and may even be life-threatening in severe and enduring cases.

A bereaved person may suffer emotional pain and may exhibit a variety of grief responses for many months after the death. The rate of the healing process depends on the amount and quality of grief work that a person does. **Grief work** is the process of integrating the reality of the loss into everyday life and learning to feel better. Often, the bereaved person must deliberately and systematically work at reducing denial and coping with the pain that results from memories of the deceased. This process takes time and requires emotional effort.

Not everyone grieves in the same way. For differences between how women and men grieve, see the Women's Health/Men's Health box.

Worden's Model of Grieving Tasks

William Worden, a researcher into the death process, developed a more active grieving model that defined four tasks necessary for the individual to complete (Figure 20.2).[11] He explained that each person reacts differently to loss but, in general, the work of bereavement entails the following developmental tasks:

1. *To accept the reality of the loss.* At first, people may react to the death of their loved one with numbness, shock, and denial. This task requires acknowledging and realizing that the person is dead. This task takes time because it involves an intellectual acceptance as well as an emotional one. Traditional rituals, such as the funeral, help many bereaved people move toward acceptance.

2. *To work through to the pain of grief.* It is necessary to acknowledge and work through the pain associated with loss, or it will manifest itself through other symptoms or behaviors. Not everyone will experience the same intensity of pain or feel it in the same way. One of the aims of grief counseling is to help facilitate people through this difficult second task so they don't carry the intense pain with them throughout their life.

3. *To adjust to an environment in which the deceased is missing.* Adjusting to a new environment means different things to different people depending on what the relationship was with the deceased. The bereaved may feel lonely and uncertain about a new identity without the person who has died. This loss confronts them with the challenge of adjusting to their own sense of self.

4. *To emotionally relocate the deceased and move on with life.* Individuals never lose memories of a significant relationship, yet eventually grieving individuals need to look forward and continue with their lives. They may need help in letting go of the emotional energy that used to be invested in the person who has died, and they may need help in finding an appropriate place for the deceased in their emotional lives. Completing the necessary grief work enables them to focus less on the loss and to connect with other people by investing new energy in ongoing relationships.

In summary, models of the grief process can be viewed as "generalized maps," in that each theory is an attempt by an investigator to understand and guide the grieving individual through their pain. However, humans are unique and cannot be forced into particular patterns of behavior. Each individual will travel through grief at his/her own speed using an appropriate route.

Grief work The process of accepting the reality of a person's death and coping with memories of the deceased.

Gender Differences in the Bereavement Experience

Although men and women suffer through similar stages of bereavement, a Harvard study pointed out interesting differences in how men and women interpret their feelings of loss immediately after the death of a spouse.

WOMEN

- Women emphasized a sense of abandonment and spoke of being alone. They felt deprived of a comforting person.

- Women tended to regard the funeral director and staff as supportive and caring people, rather than business people.
- The funeral process was important for women in reaching the realization that their spouses were gone forever.
- Widows showed more emotions to other people.
- Women most often provided help to others.

MEN

- Men reported feeling a sort of dismemberment, as if both arms and legs were being cut off.
- Men expressed less gratitude toward the funeral directors and usually expressed concern over cost.

- Men felt that the funeral was just something to get through.
- Widowers showed fewer emotions to other people. Those offering help to the widower were more likely to offer practical help rather than emotional support.
- Widowers began dating and remarrying sooner than did widows, but this did not mean they had worked through their emotional attachment to their late spouse.

Source: Adapted from R. J. Kastenbaum, *Death, Society, and Human Experience,* 7th ed. (Boston: Allyn & Bacon, 2001). Copyright © 2001 by Pearson Education.

What do you think?

If you have experienced a death among your family or friends, how did you grieve? ■ *Did you accomplish Worden's tasks?* ■ *Does the model match your experience?*

When an Infant or Child Dies

At the beginning of the twentieth century, children under the age of 15 made up 34 percent of the U.S. population but accounted for 53 percent of total deaths. Today, children continue to benefit from advances in medicine and social policy that have reduced mortality rates by more than 90 percent since 1900.[12] Children are highly valued in our society, and their deaths are considered major tragedies. No matter what the cause of death—miscarriage, fatal birth defects, childhood illness, accident, suicide, homicide, natural disaster, neglect, or war injuries—the grief experienced when a child dies may be overwhelming.

The death of a child is terribly painful for the whole family. However, for several reasons, the siblings of the deceased child have a particularly hard time with grief work. Bereaved children usually have limited experience with death and therefore have not yet learned how to deal with major loss. Children may feel uncomfortable talking about death, and they may also receive less social support and sympathy than their parents. Because so much attention

and energy are devoted to the deceased child, the surviving children may feel emotionally abandoned by their parents.

A Child's Response to Death

In the past, children were thought to be miniature adults and were expected to behave as adults. It is now understood that children and adults react to death quite differently. Often, when children suffer a loss, they will react in ways that seem "normal" to the adult observer. However, children often do not show their feelings as openly as adults do. Although their actions may not reveal what they are truly feeling, children tend to experience more prolonged mourning periods. They typically grapple with these questions: (1) Did I cause the death to happen? (2) Is it going to happen to me? (3) Who is going to take care of me?[13] A child's grieving period may be less stressful when adults are open and honest and include the child in the funeral process as much as possible.

Quasi-Death Experiences

Many cultures provide social and emotional support for the bereaved in the aftermath of death. Typically, however, little support is offered when people face many other significant losses in life. Losses that in many ways resemble death and that may involve a heavy burden of grief include a child running away from home, an abduction or kidnapping, a divorce, a move to a distant place, a move to a nursing home, the loss of a romance

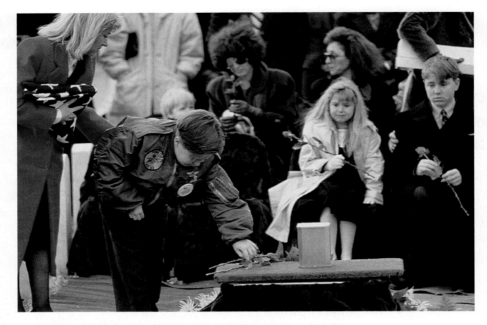

A significant loss can be particularly difficult for children.

or intimate friendship, retirement, job termination, finishing a "terminal" academic degree, or ending an athletic career.

These **quasi-death experiences**[14] resemble death in that they involve separation, termination, loss, and a change in identity or self-perception. If grief results from these losses, the pattern of the grief response will probably follow the same course as responses to death. Factors that may complicate the grieving process associated with quasi-death include uncomfortable contact with the object of loss (for example, an ex-spouse) and a lack of adequate social and institutional support.

Living with Death and Loss

The reality of death and loss touches everyone. Although the accompanying grief causes painful emotions, it can also bring strength. C. M. Parkes, a British researcher in the psychiatric aspects of bereavement, observed that:

> The experience of grieving can strengthen and bring maturity to those who have previously been protected from misfortune. The pain of grief is just as much a part of life as the joy of love; it is, perhaps, the price we pay for love, the cost of commitment. To ignore this fact, or to pretend that it is not so [would] leave us unprepared for the losses that will inevitably occur in our lives and unprepared to help others cope with the losses in theirs.[15]

Quasi-death experience A loss or experience that resembles death, in that it involves separation, termination, significant loss, a change of personal identity, and grief.

Life-and-Death Decision Making

Many complex—and often expensive—life-and-death decisions must be made during a highly distressing period in people's lives. These emotion-laden decisions are compounded by the stresses of dying and bereavement. We will not attempt to present definitive answers to moral and philosophical questions about death; instead, we offer these topics for your consideration. We hope that this discussion of the needs of the dying person and the bereaved will help you negotiate these difficult decisions in the future.

The Right to Die

Few people would object to a proposal for the right to a dignified death. Going beyond that concept, however, many people today believe that they should be allowed to die if their condition is terminal and their existence depends on mechanical life-support devices or artificial feeding or hydration systems. Artificial life-support techniques that may be legally refused by competent patients in some states include:

- Electrical or mechanical heart resuscitation
- Mechanical respiration by machine
- Nasogastric tube feedings
- Intravenous nutrition
- Gastrostomy (tube feeding directly into the stomach)
- Medications to treat life-threatening infections

As long as a person is conscious and competent, he or she has the legal right to refuse treatment, even if this decision will hasten death. However, when a person is in a coma

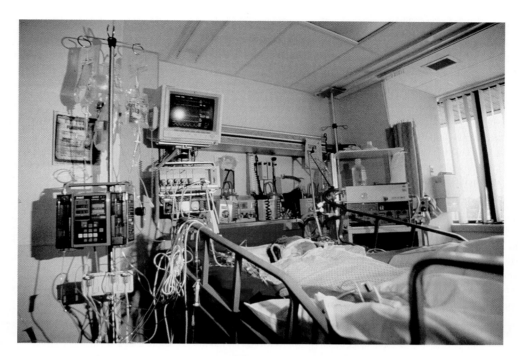

Sophisticated life-support technology allows a patient's life to be prolonged even in cases of terminal illness or mortal injury. It has also raised legal and moral questions for patients, their families, and health care professionals.

or otherwise incapable of speaking on his or her own behalf, medical personnel and administrative policy will dictate treatment. This issue has evolved into a battle involving personal freedom, legal rulings, health care administration policy, and physician responsibility. The living will and other advance directives were developed to assist in solving conflicts among these people and agencies.

Cases have been reported in which the wishes of people who had signed a living will (or other directive) indicating their desire not to receive artificial life support were not honored by their physician or medical institution. This problem can be avoided by choosing both a physician and a hospital that will carry out the directives of the living will. Taking this precaution and discussing your personal philosophy and wishes with your family should eliminate anxiety about how you will be treated at the end of your life (Figure 20.3).

Many legal experts suggest that you take the following steps to ensure that your wishes are carried out:

1. *Be specific.* Rather than signing an advance directive (that only speaks in generalities), complete a directive that permits you to make specific choices about a variety of procedures, including cardiopulmonary resuscitation (CPR); dialysis; being placed on a ventilator; being given food, water, or medication through tubes; being given pain medication; and organ donation. It is also essential to attach that document to a completed copy of the standard advance directive for your state.

2. *Get an agent.* Even the most detailed directive cannot possibly anticipate every situation that may arise. You may want to also appoint a family member or friend to act as your agent, or *proxy,* by making out a form known as either a *durable power of attorney for health care* or a *health care proxy.*

3. *Discuss your wishes.* Discuss your preferences in detail with your proxy and your doctor. Your doctor or proxy may misinterpret or ignore your wishes. Going over the situations described in the form will give them a clear idea of just how much you are willing to endure to preserve your life.

4. *Deliver the directive.* Distribute several copies, not only to your doctor and your agent, but also to your lawyer and to immediate family members or a close friend. Make sure *someone* knows to bring a copy to the hospital in the event you are hospitalized.[16]

Rational Suicide

We have discussed suicide in earlier chapters as a consequence of depression or other factors. The concept of **rational suicide** as an alternative to an extended dying

Rational suicide The decision to kill oneself rather than endure constant pain and slow decay.

This directive is made this _____ day of _____ (month) _____ (year).
I, _____ being of sound mind, willfully and voluntarily make known my desire

(a) ☐ **That my life shall not be artificially prolonged** and

(b) ☐ **That my life shall be ended with the aid of a physician under circumstances set forth below, and do hereby declare:**
(You must initial (a) or (b), or both.)

_____

1. If at any time I should have a terminal condition or illness certified to be terminal by two physicians, and they determine that my death will occur within six months,

   (a) ☐ **I direct that life-sustaining procedures be withheld or withdrawn** and

   (b) ☐ **I direct that my physician administer aid-in-dying in a humane and dignified manner.** (You must initial (a) or (b), or both.)

   (c) ☐ **I have attached Special Instructions on a separate page to the directive.** (Initial if you have attached a separate page.)

   The action taken under this paragraph shall be at the time of my own choosing if I am competent.

2. In the absence of my ability to give directions regarding the termination of my life, it is my intention that this directive shall be honored by my family, agent (described in paragraph 4), and physician(s) as the final expression of my legal right to

   (a) ☐ **Refuse medical or surgical treatment,** and

   (b) ☐ **To choose to die in a humane and dignified manner.** (You must initial (a) or (b), or both and you must initial one box below.)

   ☐ If I am unable to give directions, I *do not* want my attorney-in-fact to request aid-in-dying.

   ☐ If I am unable to give directions, I *do* want my attorney-in-fact to ask my physician for aid-in-dying.

3. I understand that a terminal condition is one in which I am not likely to live for more than six months.

4. a. I, _____
   do hereby designate and appoint _____
   as my attorney-in-fact (agent) to make health-care decisions for me if I am in a coma or otherwise unable to decide for myself as authorized in this document. For the purpose of this document, "health-care decision" means consent, refusal of consent, or withdrawal of consent to any care, treatment, service, or procedure to maintain, diagnose, or treat an individual's physical or mental condition, or to administer aid-in-dying.

   b. By this document I intend to create a Durable Power of Attorney for Health Care under The Oregon Death With Dignity Act and ORS Section 126.407. This power of attorney shall not be affected by my subsequent incapacity, except by revocation.

   c. Subject to any limitations in this document, I hereby grant to my agent full power and authority to make health-care decisions for me to the same extent that I could make these decisions for myself if I had the capacity to do so. In exercising this authority, my agent shall make health-care decisions that are consistent with my desires as stated in this document or otherwise made known to my agent, including, but not limited to, my desires concerning obtaining, refusing, or withdrawing life-prolonging care, treatment, services, and procedures, and administration of aid-in-dying.

5. This directive shall have no force or effect seven years from the date filled in above, unless I am competent to act on my own behalf and then it shall remain valid until my competency is restored.

6. I recognize that a physician's judgment is not always certain, and that medical science continues to make progress in extending life, but in spite of these facts, I nevertheless wish aid-in-dying rather than letting my terminal condition take its natural course.

7. My family has been informed of my request to die, their opinions have been taken into consideration, but the final decision remains mine, so long as I am competent.

8. The exact time of my death will be determined by me and my physician with my desire or my attorney-in-fact's instructions paramount.

I have given full consideration and understand the full import of this directive, and I am emotionally and mentally competent to make this directive. I accept the moral and legal responsibility for receiving aid-in-dying.

This directive will not be valid unless it is signed by two qualified witnesses who are present when you sign or acknowledge your signature. The witnesses must not be related to you by blood, marriage, or adoption; they must not be entitled to any part of your estate; and they must not include a physician or other person responsible for, or employed by anyone responsible for, your health care. If you have attached any additional pages to this form, you must date and sign each of the additional pages at the same time you date and sign this power of attorney.

Signed: _____

_____
City, County, and State of Residence

This document must be witnessed by two qualified adult witnesses. None of the following may be used as witnesses: (1) a health-care provider who is involved in any way with the treatment of the declarant, (2) an employee of a health-care provider who is involved in any way with the treatment of the declarant, (3) the operator of a community care facility where the declarant resides, (4) an employee of an operator of a community care facility who is involved in any way with the treatment of the declarant.

Figure 20.3

Directive to Physicians

An example of a directive that can be used to specify end-of-life treatments.

Source: The Oregon Death with Dignity Act, Oregon Revised Statute, Chapter 97 (1990).

Is Physician-Assisted Suicide Ethical?

Physician-assisted suicide (PAS) has caused a furor in the media and debate within the medical and legal professions. Consider the reasoning that follows as you develop your own position on this issue.

ARGUMENTS IN FAVOR OF PAS

Those who believe that PAS is ethically justified offer the following reasons:

1. *Respect for autonomy.* Decisions about time and circumstances of death are very personal. Competent persons should have the right to choose death.
2. *Justice.* Justice requires that we "treat like cases alike." Competent terminally ill patients are allowed to hasten death by refusing treatment; but for some patients, cutting off treatment will not suffice to hasten death—their only real option is suicide. Justice requires that we should allow assisted death for these patients.
3. *Compassion.* Suffering means more than pain; other physical and psychological burdens also accompany some forms of terminal illness. It is not always possible to relieve suffering. Thus PAS may be a compassionate response to unbearable suffering.
4. *Individual liberty versus state interest.* Though society has a strong interest in preserving life, that interest lessens when a person is terminally ill and has a strong desire to end life. A complete prohibition on assisted death excessively limits personal liberty. Therefore PAS should be allowed in certain cases.
5. *Openness of discussion.* Some would argue that assisted death already occurs, albeit in secret. For example, morphine drips ostensibly for pain relief may be a covert form of assisted death or euthanasia. The fact that PAS is illegal prevents open discussion of the issue and fosters secrecy in administration of PAS. Legalization would promote open discussion.

ARGUMENTS AGAINST PAS

Those who believe that PAS should remain illegal present these arguments:

1. *Sanctity of life.* There are strong religious and secular traditions against taking human life. Assisted suicide is morally wrong because it contradicts these beliefs.
2. *Passive versus active distinction.* There is an important difference between passively "letting die" and actively "killing." Refusing treatment or withholding treatment is equivalent to letting die (a passive measure) and therefore justifiable, whereas PAS is equivalent to killing (an active measure) and is not justifiable.
3. *Potential for abuse.* Certain groups of people, lacking access to care and support, may be pushed into assisted death. Furthermore, assisted death may become a cost-containment strat-

egy. Burdened family members and health care providers may unscrupulously encourage the option of assisted death in certain cases. To protect against these abuses, PAS should remain illegal.
4. *Professional integrity.* The historical ethical traditions of medicine, which promote strongly opposition to taking life. For instance, the Hippocratic oath states, "I will not administer poison to anyone where asked" and "Be of benefit, or at least do no harm." Furthermore, major professional groups (such as the American Medical Association and the American Geriatrics Society) oppose assisted death because linking PAS to the practice of medicine could harm the public's image of the profession.
5. *Fallibility of the profession.* Physicians will make mistakes. For instance, there may be uncertainty in diagnosis and prognosis, errors in diagnosis and treatment of depression, or inadequate treatment of pain. Thus the state has an obligation to protect lives from these inevitable mistakes.

What are your feelings about PAS? Under what circumstances might you consider it an acceptable option? Under what circumstances should it not be an option? Where should the line be drawn?

Source: Excerpted from C. H. Braddock and M. R. Tonelli, "Physician-Assisted Suicide," *Ethics in Medicine,* February 22, 1999, http://eduserv.hscer.washington.edu /bioethics/topics/pas.html

---

process, however, deserves mention here. Rational suicide is a result of a reasoned, coherent process in which a person chooses death as a preferable alternative to unbearable pain.

Although exact numbers are not known, medical ethicists, experts in rational suicide, and specialists in forensic medicine (the study of legal issues in medicine) estimate that thousands of terminally ill people every year decide to kill themselves rather than endure constant pain and slow decay. To these people, the prospect of an undignified death is unac-

ceptable. This issue has been complicated by advances in death prevention techniques that allow terminally ill patients to exist in an irreversible disease state for extended periods of time. Medical personnel, clergy, lawyers, and patients all must struggle with this ethical dilemma.

Still, questions remain. Do we have a right to die? If so, is this an unlimited right, or does it apply only to certain conditions? If terminally ill patients are allowed to commit suicide legally, what other groups will demand this option?

Should the courts be involved in private decisions? Should any organization be allowed to distribute information that may encourage suicide? Should loved ones or medical care-givers be allowed to assist the person who wants to die by providing the means?

Euthanasia is often referred to as "mercy killing." The term *active euthanasia* has been given to ending the life of a person (or animal) that is suffering greatly and has no chance of recovery. An example might be a physician-prescribed lethal injection. **Passive euthanasia** refers to the intentional withholding of treatment that would prolong life. Deciding not to place a person with massive brain trauma on life support is an example of passive euthanasia.

Dr. Jack Kevorkian, a physician in Michigan, has started a one-person campaign to force the medical profession to change its position regarding physician-assisted death. Kevorkian has assisted many terminally ill patients in dying and, until recently, had escaped conviction despite being taken into court several times for his actions. Kevorkian has argued that the Hippocratic oath, an ancient ethical pledge still taken by medical students, is not binding. He believes that the present situations in our society demand a shift in the thinking and practices that medicine has had throughout most of human history. He believes that acceptance of eu-thanasia, specifically physician-assisted death, is one of those changes. In 1998, Kevorkian took his argument to prime time, as the CBS News program *60 Minutes* broadcast his latest case of assisting a terminally ill patient with ending his life. This time, however, the courts determined that Kevorkian's meth-ods had gone too far; he was convicted of murder and sen-tenced to prison, where he remains.

Kevorkian's actions have focused attention on the issue, causing many to discuss the merits of physician-assisted suicide. According to public opinion polls, most Americans believe that suicide is morally wrong but are di-vided on whether physician-assisted suicide is morally ac-ceptable. Roughly six in ten Americans say they think people have a right to end their own life only if they have an incur-able disease.[17]

Legalization of assisted suicide has been debated in many states across the nation. Currently, 38 states have en-acted statues explicitly prohibiting assisted suicide, 4 states are undecided (meaning there are no statutes or case law specifically prohibiting assisted suicide), and Oregon is the only state that allows physician-assisted suicide under certain circumstances. According to Oregon's right-to-die law, a pa-tient must: be at least 18 years old, be an Oregon resident, have a terminal illness with less than six months to live, and make three requests for a prescription (one written and two verbal) with at least 15 days between each request. In addi-tion, the prescribing doctor and a consulting physician are required to confirm the terminal diagnosis and prognosis, determine that the patient is capable and acting voluntarily, and refer the patient for counseling if either believes the pa-tient's judgment is impaired by a psychiatric or psychological disorder. The doctor must also inform the patient of alterna-tives such as hospice care.[18]

What do you think?

Are there any end-of-life situations in which you would ask a physician to help you die? Explain your answer. ■ *Do you believe people should have the right to ask a physician to help them die? Why or why not?* ■ *See the Health Ethics box for more debate on physician-assisted suicide.*

Making Final Arrangements

Caring for dying people and dealing with the practical and legal questions surrounding death can be difficult and painful. The problems of the dying person and the bereaved loved ones involve a wide variety of psychological, legal, so-cial, spiritual, economic, and interpersonal issues.

Hospice Care: Positive Alternatives

Since the mid-1970s, **hospice** programs have grown from a mere handful to more than 2,500, available in nearly every community. Improving the quality of care at the end of life is a top priority of the American Medical Association.

The primary goals of the hospice program are to re-lieve the dying person's pain, offer emotional support to the dying person and loved ones, and restore a sense of control to the dying person, family, and friends. Although home care with maximum involvement by loved ones is emphasized, hospice programs are directed by cooperat-ing physicians, coordinated by specially trained nurses, and fortified with the services of counselors, clergy, and trained volunteers. Hospital inpatient beds are available if necessary. Hospice programs usually include the following characteristics:

1. The patient and family constitute the unit of care because the physical, psychological, social, and spiritual problems of dying confront the family as well as the patient.

Active euthanasia "Mercy killing," in which a person or organization knowingly acts to hasten the death of a terminally ill person.

Passive euthanasia The intentional withholding of treatment that would prolong life.

Hospice A concept of care for terminally ill patients de-signed to maximize quality of life.

Preparing to Support a Dying Person

Whether we have months to prepare for death or it comes suddenly, most people have difficulty knowing what to do. We push death from our consciousness in ways that may lead to problems as the moment of death comes for loved ones and after that moment passes. Although you can never be fully prepared for the loss of a loved one, you can learn skills that will help you through the trauma of loss. The following things to think about may help, particularly in situations such as hospice care where you have time to prepare yourself.

1. *Follow the wishes of the patient.* Make sure that a copy of his or her advance directive is available and is accepted as the wishes of the patient. Most people, particularly in hospice, want a natural death. Think in terms of "comfort," not "cure." Whenever possible, talk to the patient and allow choices to be made about the dying process. For example, if the person wants to stay in her own bed but a hospital bed would be easier for those providing care at home, talk it out with her.

2. *Help with comfort and rest.* Don't be afraid to ask for medications to help the patient with pain, sleeping, or anxiety.

3. *Prepare a list of people to call near the time of death, including family, friends, and religious support.* Talk about who the patient wants present, if anyone. Make a list of people to notify once death occurs. Keep a list of home health nurses, hospice staff, and physicians nearby, so that they can be contacted without delay.

4. *Call for professional help if any of the following occur:*
   - Extreme pain or discomfort.
   - Difficulty breathing. Oxygen can help calm the patient and make the last hours more comfortable.
   - Trouble urinating or passing stool. Usually the urine will be dark and in small quantity. Medications can help ease discomfort.
   - Emotions getting the best of you. Thoughts of impending loss can prevent you from being supportive to the dying person.

5. *Touch is often comforting for the dying person.* Give back, hand, or foot rubs. Do not stand back and avoid contact. Help the patient adjust his or her position in bed if at all possible. Usually an extra sheet under the patient and the aid of a second person will make this easier.

6. *Make the person as physically comfortable as possible.* Moisten the eyes and lips with warm, damp cloths and apply skin lotion to ensure comfort. Apply warm or cool compresses if the person wants them.

7. *Know what to expect.* Be ready to say goodbye. Talk to the person. In some cases soft, relaxing music may be comforting. During the last moments of life, the body begins to slow down, breathing rates slow, sometimes there are long pauses between breaths. Sometimes the person will appear to wake up and may or may not be able to speak or recognize you. Usually this means patients are in or near coma state, and they may progress to longer and longer periods of sleep. The skin may be cool, especially around the feet and hands, and may become blue- or gray-tinged. In the last stages, as death nears, the person may become incontinent or lose bowel control. Finally, the chest will stop rising, the eyes may appear glassy, and there will be no more pulse.

8. *Prepare for the activities that will occur after death.* You may choose to assist with preparing the body for transport to the funeral home or other facility, or you may choose to let others take over. Try to think about this in advance and make decisions based on your own preferences and needs.

---

2. Emphasis is placed on controlling symptoms, primarily the alleviation of pain. Curative treatments are curtailed as requested by the patient, but sound judgment must be applied to avoid a feeling of abandonment.

3. There is overall medical direction of the program, with all health care being provided under the direction of a qualified physician.

4. Services are provided by an interdisciplinary team because no one person can provide all the needed care.

5. Coverage is provided 24 hours a day, seven days a week, with emphasis on the availability of medical and nursing skills.

6. Carefully selected and extensively trained volunteers are an integral part of the health care team, augmenting staff service but not replacing it.

7. Care of the family extends through the bereavement period.

8. Patients are accepted on the basis of their health needs, not their ability to pay.

Despite the growing number of people considering the hospice option, many people prefer to go to a hospital to die. Others choose to die at home, without the intervention of medical staff or life-prolonging equipment. Each dying person and his or her family should decide as early as possible what type of terminal care is most desirable and feasible. This will allow time for necessary emotional, physical, and financial preparations. Hospice care may also help the survivors cope better with the death experience. See the Skills for Behavior Change box for information on how to prepare yourself if you expect to be with a dying person.

Funeral and Mourning Customs around the World

Traditions associated with death vary around the world, reflecting differing cultures and religious practices. However, every culture recognizes death as a significant rite of passage. Here is a global sampling of funeral customs:

BUDDHISM

In several Japanese Buddhist traditions, a funeral ceremony resembles a Christian ceremony, with a eulogy and prayers at a funeral home. Cambodian, Thai, and Sri Lankan traditions may have up to three ceremonies. In the first, which is held two days after the death, monks conduct a ceremony at the home of the bereaved. In the second, two to five days after the death, monks hold a service at a funeral home, and the third, seven days after burial or cremation, is a monk-led ceremony at a temple or the home of the bereaved. This last ceremony, called a "merit transference," seeks to generate good energy for the deceased in his or her new incarnation. There is always an open casket, with the sight of the body reminding guests of the impermanence of life.

GREEK ORTHODOX CHURCH

Mourners bow in front of the open casket and kiss an icon or cross placed on the chest of the deceased. The traditional words said to the bereaved are "May you have an abundant life" and "May their memory be eternal." At the graveside, there is a five-minute prayer ceremony and each person present places one flower on the casket. A memorial service is held on the Sunday closest to the fortieth day after the death.

HINDUISM

The body remains at the home until it is taken to the place of cremation, usually 24 hours after death. It is customary to wear white at the funeral. The major officiants at the service are Hindu priests or senior male members of the family. Special books containing mantras for funeral services are used but only by the priests. At the cremation, a last food offering is symbolically made to the deceased and then the body is cremated. An additional ceremony at home, performed 10 days after death for the Brahmin caste and 30 days after death for other castes, liberates the soul of the deceased for its ascent to heaven.

ISLAM

Mourners wash the body of the deceased, perfume it, and wrap it in white cloth. Mourners face Mecca and recite prayers, and then a silent procession carries the body to its burial place. All the mourners participate in filling the grave with soil.

JUDAISM

A Jewish funeral is a time of intense mourning and public grieving. Traditional Jewish law forbids cremation, but it is allowed among Reform Jews. Flowers are never appropriate for Orthodox or Conservative funerals but are sometimes appropriate for Reform funerals. There is never an open casket, and the officiants are a rabbi (who delivers a eulogy), a cantor (who sings), and family members or friends (who may also deliver a eulogy or memorial). At the simplest graveside service, the rabbi recites prayers and leads the family in the mourner's *kaddish*, the prayer for the deceased. At a traditional service, there is a slow procession to the grave itself with several pauses along the way. After prayers and *kaddish* have been recited, each person puts one spade of earth into the grave.

The family sits in mourning for seven days after the funeral, called the *shiva* period. To symbolize the mourners' lack of interest in their comfort or how they appear to others, family members may cover mirrors in the home, wear a black ribbon that has been cut and slippers or socks rather than shoes, and, for men, refrain from shaving. A special memorial candle may be burned for seven days.

NATIVE AMERICAN RELIGIONS

Funeral and mourning rituals are linked to the belief that this is the beginning of a journey into the next world. Strict rules govern the behavior of the living relatives so as to ensure the deceased a good start on their journey. Some Potawatomi, for instance, set a place for the deceased at a funeral feast so the spirit can partake of the food. Among the Yuchi, personal items such as a hunting rifle, blanket, and tobacco may be placed in an adult male's coffin, reflecting the belief that needs in the next life are not significantly different from needs in this one.

While Native beliefs assert that death is not necessarily the termination of life, the bereaved still mourn the absence of the one who has died. Many tribes restrict what bereaved relatives can eat or the activities they can engage in. This represents a sacrifice by the living for those who have moved on.

SOCIETY OF FRIENDS (QUAKERS)

There are two types of Quaker funerals. An unprogrammed meeting is held in the traditional manner of Friends on the basis of silence. Worshippers sit and wait for divine guidance; if so moved, they speak to the group. Programmed meetings are planned in advance and usually include singing, prayers, Bible reading, silent worship, and a sermon.

Source: Excerpt is from *How to Be a Perfect Stranger: The Essential Religious Etiquette Handbook* © 2003 SkyLight Paths Publishing. Edited by Stuart M. Matlins and Arthur J. Magida. Permission granted by SkyLight Paths Publishing. P.O. Box 237, Woodstock, VT 05091, www.skylightpaths.com

Making Funeral Arrangements

Anthropological evidence indicates that all cultures throughout history have developed some sort of funeral ritual. For this reason, social scientists agree that funerals assist survivors of the deceased in coping with their loss.

In the United States, with its diversity of religious, regional, and ethnic customs, funeral patterns vary. (See the Health in a Diverse World box for information on the practices of several religious traditions.) In some faiths, prior to body disposal, the deceased may be displayed to formalize last respects and increase social support of the bereaved. This part of the funeral ritual is referred to as a **wake** or **viewing.** The body of the deceased is usually embalmed prior to viewing to retard decomposition and minimize offensive odors. The funeral service may be held in a church, in a funeral chapel, or at the burial site. Some people choose to replace the funeral service with a simple memorial service held within a few days of the burial. Social interaction associated with funeral and memorial services is valuable in helping survivors cope with their losses.

Common methods of body disposal include burial in the ground, entombment above ground in a mausoleum, cremation, and anatomical donation. Expenses involved in body disposal vary according to the method chosen and the available options. It should be noted that if burial is selected, an additional charge may be assessed for a burial vault. Burial vaults—concrete or metal containers that hold the casket—are required by most cemeteries to limit settling of the gravesite as the casket disintegrates and collapses. Choosing the actual container for the remains is only one of many tasks that must be dealt with when a person dies. There are many other decisions concerning the funeral ritual that can also be difficult for survivors.

Pressures on Survivors

Funeral practices in the United States today are extremely varied. A great number of decisions have to be made, usually within 24 hours. These decisions relate to the method and details of body disposal, the type of memorial service, display of the body, the site of burial or body disposition, the cost of funeral options, organ donation decisions, ordering floral displays, contacting friends and relatives, planning for the arrival of guests, choosing markers, gathering and submitting obituary information to newspapers, printing memorial folders, and many other details. Even though funeral directors are available to facilitate decision making, the bereaved may experience undue stress, especially in the event of a sudden death.

In our society, people who make their own funeral arrangements can save their loved ones from having to deal with unnecessary problems. Even making the decision regarding the method of body disposal can greatly reduce the stress on survivors.

Wills

The issue of inheritance is controversial in some families and should be resolved before the person dies to reduce both conflict and needless expense. Unfortunately, many people are so intimidated by the thought of making a will that they never do so and die **intestate** (without a will). This is tragic, especially because the procedure for establishing a legal will is relatively simple and inexpensive. In addition, if you don't make a will before you die, the courts (as directed by state laws) will make a will for you. Legal issues, rather than your wishes, will preside. Settling an estate also takes longer when a person dies without a will.

For example, let's explore what happens if you die in Massachusetts without a will. If you have a minor child or children, a guardian may have to be appointed to manage their property under the supervision of the Probate Court, a very costly legal procedure. If you die with a spouse and children, the property is passed to both the spouse and children. If you die with a spouse and no children, all of your property goes to your spouse, but part of your estate goes to your parents. Think about the problems this poses for those who choose to cohabitate or are homosexual: without a will, their partners get *nothing*. Or think of the problems posed when stepchildren who choose not to support the surviving spouse are involved. Clearly, we all need wills and to update them regularly.

In some cases, other types of wills may substitute for the traditional legal will. One alternative is the **holographic will,** written in the handwriting of the **testator** (person who leaves a will) and unwitnessed. Be very cautious concerning alternatives to legally written and witnessed wills because they are not honored in all states. For example, holographic wills are contestable in court. Think of the parents who never approved of the fact that their child lived with someone outside marriage: they could successfully challenge a holographic will in court.

Organ Donation

Another decision concerns organ donation. Organ transplant techniques have become so refined, and the demand for transplant tissues and organs has become so great, that

---

Wake or **viewing** Displaying of the deceased to formalize last respects and increase social support of the bereaved.

Intestate Not having made a will.

Holographic will A will written in the testator's own handwriting and unwitnessed.

Testator A person who leaves a will or testament at death.

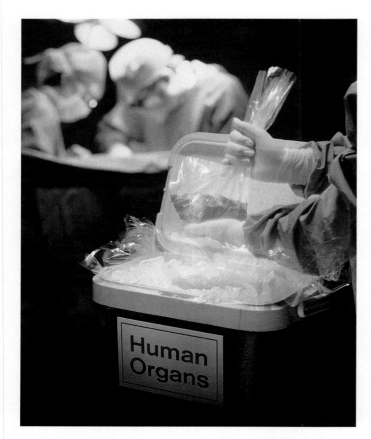

Organ donor programs provide registered donors with the satisfaction of knowing that they may save another person's life. Taking time to register with such a program also expedites the transfer of viable organs when the donor dies.

National Kidney Foundation
Please detach and give this portion
of the card to my family

This is to inform you that, should the occasion ever arise, I would like to be an organ and tissue donor. Please see that my wishes are carried out by informing the attending medical personnel that I have indicated my wishes to become a donor.
Thank you.

_____
Signature   Date

For further information write or call:
National Kidney Foundation
30 East 33rd Street, New York, NY 10016
(800) 622-9010

- -

Uniform Donor Card

Of _____
(print or type name of donor)

In the hope that I may help others, I hereby make this anatomical gift, if medically acceptable, to take effect upon my death. The words and marks below indicate my wishes.

I give: ☐ any needed organs or parts
☐ only the following organs or parts

_____
(specify the organ(s), tissue(s) or part(s))

for the purposes of transplantation, therapy, medical research or education;
☐ my body for anatomical study if needed.

Limitations or special wishes, if any: _____

Figure 20.4
Organ Donor Card

Source: Reprinted with permission from "Uniform Donor Card."
© National Kidney Foundation.

many people are being encouraged to donate these "gifts of life" upon death. Uniform donor cards are available through the National Kidney Foundation, donor information is printed on the backs of drivers' licenses, and many hospitals include the opportunity for organ donor registration in their admis-

sion procedures (Figure 20.4). Although some people are opposed to organ transplants and tissue donation, many others experience personal fulfillment from knowing that their organs may extend and improve someone else's life after their own deaths.

TAKING CHARGE

MAKE IT HAPPEN!

Assessment: The Assess Yourself box earlier in this chapter (page 572) encouraged you to assess your anxiety related to death. How anxious are you? Do you want to reduce your fears and increase your acceptance of this inevitable process?

Making a Change: In order to change your behavior, you need to develop a plan. Follow these steps:

1. Evaluate your behavior and identify patterns. What can you change now? What can you change in the near future?
2. Select one pattern of behavior that you want to change.
3. Fill out a Behavior Change Contract. It should include your long-term goal for change, your short-term goals, the rewards for reaching these goals, potential obstacles along the way, and strategies for overcoming these obstacles. For each goal, list the small steps and specific actions that you will take.
4. Chart your progress in a journal. At the end of a week, consider how successful you were in following your plan. What helped you to be successful? What will you do differently next week?
5. Revise your plan as needed: Are the short-term goals attainable? Are the rewards satisfying?

One Student's Plan: Peter's score of 60 points on the self-assessment indicated that he was unusually anxious about death. The experience of his grandmother's death had been a very difficult one. He was only six years old at the time of her death, and no one in his family discussed it with him. He visited her once in the hospital and witnessed an argument between his parents and her doctors over the steps that should be taken to prolong her life.

Peter decided that one way to feel more in control and less anxious about death would be to learn about advance directives. He went to a low-cost legal clinic near campus and asked for information. There, he was given a sample directive to discuss with his parents and his physician. It listed various medical procedures for him to indicate which he did and did not want taken.

Peter also decided to fill out an organ donation card. He wanted to be sure his parents knew what he wanted done after his death, and he believed that donating any needed body parts was a worthy and fulfilling decision.

Summary

- *Death* can be defined biologically in terms of brain death and/or the final cessation of vital functions. Denial of death results in limited communication about death, which can lead to further denial.
- Death is a multifaceted process, and individuals may experience emotional stages of dying including denial, anger, bargaining, depression, and acceptance, as noted by Kübler-Ross. Social death results when a person is no longer treated as living. Grief is the state of distress felt after loss. Worden proposes developmental tasks associated with grieving. Men and women differ in their responses to grief. Children, too, need to be helped through the process of grieving.

- The right to die by rational suicide involves ethical, moral, and legal issues.
- Practical and legal issues surround dying and death. Choices of care for the terminally ill include hospice care. After death, funeral arrangements must be made almost immediately, adding to pressures on survivors. As many decisions as possible should be made in advance of death through wills and organ donation cards.

Questions for Discussion and Reflection

1. Discuss why so many of us deny death. How could death become a more acceptable topic to discuss?
2. What are the stages that Kübler-Ross believed that terminally ill patients experience? Do you agree with the five-stage theory? Explain why or why not.
3. Define *social death* and *quasi-death experiences*.
4. Discuss coping with grief, the different grief experiences of men and women, and how to help children deal with death.
5. Identify at least one development—legal, medical, or social—that has occurred in the past five years and that has affected the way we view death.
6. Debate whether rational suicide should be legalized for the terminally ill. What restrictions would you include in such a law?
7. Compare and contrast the hospital experience with hospice care. What must one consider before arranging for hospice care?
8. Discuss the legal matters surrounding death, including wills, physician directives, organ donations, and funeral arrangements.

Accessing Your Health on the Internet

Visit the following Internet sites to explore further topics and issues related to personal health. To visit an organization's website, go to the Companion Website for *Access to Health, Ninth Edition* at www.aw-bc.com/donatelle, click on the book image, and select "Accessing Your Health on the Internet" from the navigation menu.

1. ***Beyond Indigo.*** This site addresses all aspects of grief and loss, including terminal illness, legal issues, and funeral planning.
2. ***Doctor-Assisted Suicide—a Guide to Web Sites and the Literature.*** A comprehensive look at the current status of physician-assisted suicide. Sources presented are very informative and up-to-date.
3. ***Funerals: A Consumer Guide.*** This site guides the consumer through the thinking process of planning for a funeral, including preplanning, types of funerals, costs, choosing a casket, burial, and many other aspects of funeral preparation.
4. ***GriefNet.org.*** Resources to help people deal with the loss of loved ones, including memorial pages and e-mail support groups.
5. ***Hospice Web.*** Information and links about hospice, including frequently asked questions.
6. ***Loss, Grief, and Bereavement.*** This site from the National Cancer Institute covers a variety of topics related to loss, grief, and bereavement. Among the contents is a summary written by cancer experts.
7. ***Terminal Illness and Hospice.*** This site addresses all aspects of dealing with terminal illness, including loss, ALS (Lou Gehrig's disease), Alzheimer's disease, legal issues, and funeral planning.

Further Reading

Humphrey, D. and M. Clement. *Freedom to Die: People, Politics, and the Right-to-Die Movement.* Torrance, CA: Griffin, 2000.

Describes the history of the right-to-die movement and all sides of the debate.

Jacobs Altman, L. *Death: An Introduction to Medical–Ethical Dilemmas.* Berkeley Heights, NJ: Enslow, 2000.

A multifaceted exploration of death that gives the reader much to consider.

Mims, C. A. *When We Die: The Science, Culture, and Rituals of Death.* Torrance, CA: Griffin, 2000.

A look at how society views and portrays death in science and culture.

Muth, A. S. (ed.). *Death and Dying Sourcebook: Basic Consumer Health Information for the Layperson About End-of-Life Care and Related Ethical and Legal Issues.* Detroit, MI: Omnigraphics, 2000.

Provides up-to-date information on the issues of nursing care, living wills, pain management, and counseling.

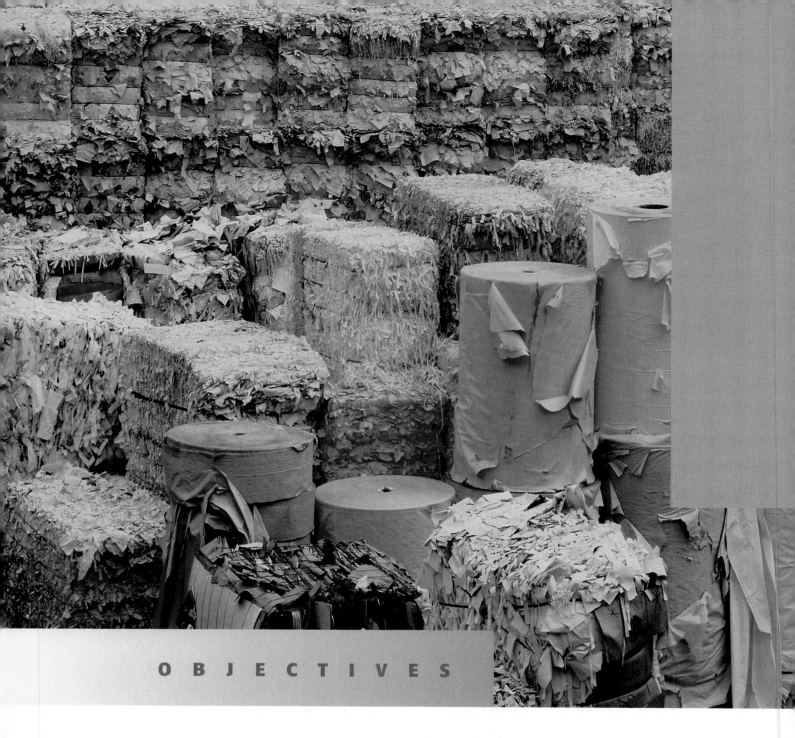

OBJECTIVES

- Explain problems and ethical issues associated with current levels of global population growth.

- Discuss major causes of air pollution, including photochemical smog and acid rain, and the global consequences of the accumulation of greenhouse gases and ozone depletion.

- Identify sources of water pollution and chemical contaminants often found in water.

- Describe the physiological consequences of noise pollution.

- Distinguish between municipal solid waste and hazardous waste.

- Discuss the health concerns associated with ionizing and nonionizing radiation.

ENVIRONMENTAL HEALTH

THINKING GLOBALLY, ACTING LOCALLY

IN THE NEWS

E.P.A. Says Mercury Taints Fish Across U.S.

By Michael Janofsky

The head of the Environmental Protection Agency said on Tuesday that fish in virtually all of the nation's lakes and rivers were contaminated with mercury, a highly toxic metal that poses health risks for pregnant women and young children.

Michael O. Leavitt, the E.P.A. administrator, drew his conclusion from the agency's latest annual survey of fish advisories, which showed that 48 states—all but Wyoming and Alaska—issued warnings about mercury last year. That compared with 44 states in 1993, when the surveys were first conducted.

The latest survey also shows that 19 states, including New York, have now put all their lakes and rivers under a statewide advisory for fish consumption. But Mr. Leavitt said that the widespread presence of mercury reflected a surge in monitoring—not an increase in emissions—as part of growing state efforts to warn local anglers about the fish they are catching. Last year, states issued 3,094 advisories for toxic substances, compared with 1,233 in 1993.

"Mercury is everywhere," Mr. Leavitt said at a news conference in his office. "The more waters we monitor, the more we find mercury. Monitoring is up and will continue to go up. But emissions are down and will continue to go down."

Read the complete article online in the eThemes section of this book's website: www.aw-bc.com/donatelle.

Original article published August 25, 2004. Copyright © 2004 *The New York Times*. Reprinted with permission.

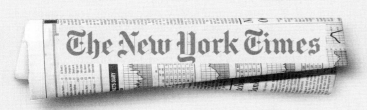

Human health, well-being, and the survival of all living things depend on the health and integrity of the planet on which we live. Today the natural world is under siege from the pressures of a burgeoning population that uses massive amounts of natural resources to survive. Consequently, many citizens are interested in the health effects of environmental concerns such as global warming; depletion of the ozone layer; air, water, and solid waste pollution; deforestation; human population control; and the impact of too many people on dwindling natural resources.

In response to public and political concerns, there has been a surge in federal and state regulations along with a multibillion-dollar national infrastructure—but doubt remains as to the effectiveness of that infrastructure in reducing environmental health risks.[1] In addition, during the recent economic downturn, politicians dismantled some environmental gains by reducing regulations, easing compliance deadlines, weakening protections for endangered species, and undermining other environmental programs labeled by some in Congress as "antibusiness."[2] Today, while the federal government has decided not to participate in several international policy and planning groups designed to protect the global environment, environmental problems continue to escalate. National and international groups continue to promote an agenda based on sustainable development, or efforts to ensure that the level of productivity and activity that are undertaken in one generation do not compromise the environmental integrity or needed resources of the next generation.[3] In such a period of environmental pressures, an informed citizenry with a strong commitment to be responsible for the planet is essential to the survival of Earth and all living things. This chapter reviews major global environmental issues that affect us today and will continue to affect generations to come.

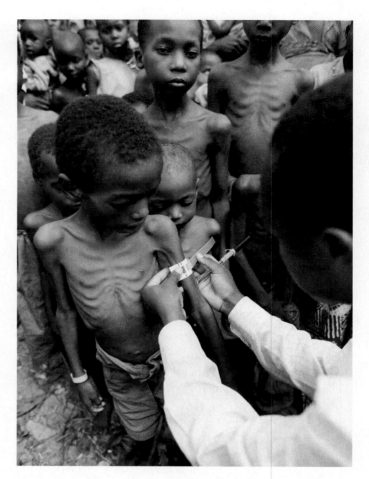

As populations increase, countries' resources become overloaded. In many parts of the world, governments cannot meet the needs of their most vulnerable citizens, and outside organizations must get involved.

Overpopulation

Anthropologist Margaret Mead wrote, "Every human society is faced with not one population problem but two: how to beget and rear enough children and how not to beget and rear too many."[4] The United Nations projects that the world population will grow from its present total of 6.4 billion to 9.4 billion by 2050 and to 11.5 billion by 2150.[5] Though our population is expanding, the earth's resources are not. Population experts believe that many areas of the world are already struggling with "demographic fatigue" and the most critical environmental challenge today is to slow the population growth of the world.[6] See the Health Ethics box for ethical concerns related to overpopulation.

The global population explosion is not distributed equally, with vast differences in growth rates between most developing and industrialized nations. Nearly 99 percent of all population increases take place in poor countries, while population size is static or declining in wealthy countries. Nations that can least afford a high birth rate in terms of economic, social, health, and nutritional needs are the ones with the most rapidly expanding populations. Overpopulation threats are most evident in Latin America, Africa, and parts of Asia—areas where poverty, devastating infectious diseases such as HIV, and problems with food and water are already prevalent.

The country projected to have the largest increase in population is India, which could add another 600 million people by the year 2050 and surpass China as the most populous country in the world. Put into perspective, the U.S. population had not yet reached 300 million by the end of 2004.[7]

Why should we be concerned? Whether you live in an area of heavy population growth or zero population growth, the drain on the environment that will result with exponential population growth is expected to be staggering. Many argue that at the current rate, we are already exceeding our capacity to provide food, provide clean water, and dispose of human waste. Every week, the population of the world's urban centers grows by more than 1 million.[8] In 1800, London was the only city in the world with a 1 million people; today, 14 cities have megacity status with populations

Population Control

The world's population tops 6.4 billion. Ninety-nine percent of each year's population growth occurs in the poorest parts of the world. Consider the following statistics:

- An estimated 300 million women desire family planning but lack the information or the means to obtain it.
- Over 1 billion people have no access to health care.
- Roughly 1.3 billion people live in poverty.
- An estimated 840 million people are malnourished.
- Eighty-five countries lack the ability to grow or purchase enough food to feed their own citizens.
- Over 1 billion people lack access to safe drinking water.
- Approximately 2.6 billion live without adequate sanitation.

The United Nations projects that world population will increase to 9.4 billion by 2050. The statistics listed above are sure to rise as the population increases.

Overpopulation has contributed to environmental degradation, resulting in the loss of immense tracts of forest and tons of arable topsoil. Many scientists suggest that increased industrialization and consumption threaten the atmosphere and world climate. Unrestricted population growth could lead to worldwide shortages of food and energy.

Already women, particularly in the developing world, suffer the ill health effects of having too many children too close together. Often these children live in poverty and are malnourished. Particularly in regions where HIV and poverty are rampant, many women neglect their own health to care for sick partners and children.

For the past half century, those concerned about overpopulation have called for population control. A number of organizations, such as the International Planned Parenthood Federation, advocate women's access to family planning information and contraception. Unfortunately, even if many of these women had access to family planning services, cultural mores or religious beliefs could prevent their use of these resources. Recently, U.S. funding for such programs has been sharply curtailed.

Another solution some have offered is government regulation of population growth. In the 1970s, China instituted a strictly enforced one child–one family policy that allowed each family to have only a single child. While the policy has been effective in cities, where people tend to be more educated and space is already extremely limited, it has not been successful in rural areas, where families whose survival depends on having enough labor continue to have multiple children. One unintended consequence of this policy has been female infanticide, in order for the family to make sure that its one child will be a boy.

Other recommendations are under consideration. One of these gives each woman born the right to have two babies. If the woman chooses not to exercise this right, she can sell her rights on the open market. If people want a large family, they must have enough resources to buy the baby rights and therefore, in all likelihood, the ability to support these children financially. Another option might be to pay a woman not to reproduce: for each year of her childbearing years that she does not have a child, she is rewarded financially.

Finally, some people suggest that the problem is not overpopulation but the unequal consumption of resources by a minority of the world's population. They believe that poverty results not from overpopulation, but from the inequitable distribution of wealth.

Do you think overpopulation is a problem? Do you think population control is the answer? How do you think population control should be effected? Do you think inequality is a greater problem than overpopulation? If so, what do you think should be done to bring about greater equality worldwide?

over 10 million, and by 2015, at current rates, there will be 26 megacities on earth.[9]

As the global population expands, so does competition for the earth's resources. There is already heavy pressure on the capacity of natural resources to support human life and world health.[10] Experts speculate that as nations of "haves" and "have-nots" fight over scarce life necessities such as water and food, wars may escalate and international instability may become pervasive.

Recognizing that population control will be essential in the decades ahead, many countries have already enacted strict population control measures or have encouraged their citizens to limit the size of their families. By 2000, Italy, Spain, Portugal, Greece, and Sweden were among the first to achieve zero-population growth.[11] Germany, Russia, Ukraine, Hungary, and Bulgaria had actually achieved negative population growth.[12] Ironically, while other nations, many of which consume far fewer natural resources and contribute far less to environmental decline, have worked hard to achieve zero or negative population growth, the United States is the only major industrialized nation to continue to have significant population growth. In 2004, the rate of U.S. growth is estimated to be nearly 1 percent, far greater than that of Canada, England, or other world leaders.[13] Why do Americans continue to grow their population at a time when other nations are downsizing? There are many reasons for this growth, including religious beliefs, government programs that promote family growth by giving tax breaks and other incentives for families, American values that revere the family unit, and economics that support a family consumer

Table 21.1
Oil Consumption (Thousands of Barrels per Day) in Selected Countries

Country	1992	2003	Percentage of World Consumption
United States	17,033	20,071	25.1
Japan	5,521	5,451	6.8
China	2,662	5,982	7.6
India	1,296	2,426	3.1
Canada	1,708	2,149	2.6
Brazil	1,328	1,817	2.3
Saudi Arabia	1,095	1,437	1.8
Iran	1,017	1,132	1.5
Australia	679	845	1.0
Egypt	457	550	0.7
South Africa	369	513	0.7

Source: British Petroleum, "BP Statistical Review of World Energy, 2004," 2004, www.bp.com

system. Unless the United States plays a leadership role and takes action to further reduce population growth at home and diminish our heavy consumption patterns, we will continue to be part of the problem instead of part of the solution.

We can also do our part by recognizing that the United States consumes far more energy and raw materials per person than any other nation on Earth. Many of these resources come from other countries, and our consumption is depleting the resource balance of those countries. (See Table 21.1 for a comparison of U.S. oil consumption with that of selected other countries.)

Perhaps the simplest course of action is to control our own reproductivity, as mentioned earlier. The concept of *zero population growth (ZPG)* was introduced in the 1960s. Proponents of this idea believed that each couple should produce only two offspring. When the parents die, these two children are their replacements, allowing the population to stabilize. Globally, certain nations have made great strides toward achieving this rate. For example, in 1970, the worldwide total fertility rate peaked at an estimated 5 births per woman; at present it is 2.7 births. However, while that may sound good, even as rates go down in many regions of the world, the sheer magnitude of the population means that the actual number of births continues to rise at an unprecedented rate.

Sulfur dioxide A yellowish brown gaseous by-product of the burning of fossil fuels.

We have a long way to go before the population of the world levels out or begins to decline.

The continued preference for large families in many developing nations is related to several factors: high infant mortality rates; the traditional view of children as "social security" (working from a young age to assist families in daily survival and supporting parents when they grow too old to work); the low educational and economic status of women that often leaves women in positions of powerlessness with respect to reproductive choices; and the traditional desire for sons, which keeps parents of several daughters reproducing until they have male offspring.

Education may be the single biggest contributor to zero population growth. As education levels of women increase and women achieve equality in pay and job status, fertility rates decline. However, U.S. funding for this kind of education and family planning has declined dramatically in the last four years as highly controversial "abstinence only" messages have been promoted as the only allowable interventions in many regions of the world. Most public health professionals, particularly those in the field of research and prevention, support a much more ecological approach to population planning. They believe that a vast array of social, cultural, biological, psychological, economic, and other factors contribute to population growth and unwanted pregnancies and that simple solutions such as abstinence programs are destined to fail.

Policies that encourage low birth rates in society and educate citizens about the consequences of unchecked population growth may be effective. In countries such as the United States, policies that encourage zero population rates or provide incentives to young parents through tax breaks for reduced family size may be a viable option.

Air Pollution

Although we often assume that the air we breathe is safe, the daily impact of a growing population makes clean air more difficult to find. Concern about air quality prompted Congress to pass the Clean Air Act in 1970 and to amend it in 1977 and again in 1990. The goal was to develop standards for six of the most widespread air pollutants that seriously affect health: sulfur dioxide, particulates, carbon monoxide, ozone, nitrogen dioxide, and lead. The Air Quality Index is the best way for the public to assess the daily quality of the air we breathe (see the Reality Check box).

Sources of Air Pollution

Sulfur Dioxide A yellowish brown gas, **sulfur dioxide** is a by-product of burning fossil fuels. Electricity-generating stations, smelters, refineries, and industrial boilers are the main sources. In humans, sulfur dioxide aggravates symptoms of heart and lung disease, obstructs breathing passages, and increases the incidence of respiratory diseases such as colds,

What Is the AQI?

Air quality affects how we live and breathe. Like the weather, it can change from day to day or even hour to hour. The U.S. Environmental Protection Agency (EPA) and other groups are working to make information about outdoor air quality as available to the public as a weather report. A key tool in this effort is the Air Quality Index, or AQI.

A measure of daily air quality, the AQI tells you how clean or polluted your air is and what associated health concerns you should be aware of. The AQI focuses on health effects that can happen within a few hours or days after breathing polluted air. It reflects national air quality standards for five major air pollutants regulated by the Clean Air Act: ground-level ozone, particulate matter, carbon monoxide, sulfur dioxide, and nitrogen dioxide.

HOW DOES THE AQI WORK?

Think of the AQI as a yardstick that runs from 0 to 500. The higher the AQI value, the greater the level of air pollution and associated health risks. An AQI value of 100 generally corresponds to the national air quality standard for the pollutant, which is the level the EPA has set to protect public health. AQI values below 100 are generally considered satisfactory. When AQI values rise above 100, air quality is considered to be unhealthy—at first, for certain groups of people, then for everyone.

UNDERSTANDING THE AQI

The EPA has divided the AQI scale into six categories and color codes as follows:

AQI Range	Air Quality Condition / Level of Health Concern	Color
0–50	Good	Green
51–100	Moderate	Yellow
101–150	Unhealthy for sensitive groups	Orange
151–200	Unhealthy	Red
201–300	Very unhealthy	Purple
301–500	Hazardous	Maroon

✔ *Good.* Air quality is satisfactory for all groups.
✔ *Moderate.* Air quality is acceptable except for a very small group of individuals. For example, people who are unusually sensitive to ozone may experience respiratory symptoms.
✔ *Unhealthy for sensitive groups.* The general public is not likely to be affected, but certain individuals may experience health effects. For example, children and adults who are active outdoors and people with respiratory disease are at greater risk from exposure to ozone, while people with heart disease are at greater risk from carbon monoxide.
✔ *Unhealthy.* At this point the general public may begin to notice symptoms.
✔ *Very unhealthy.* This may trigger a health alert, meaning everyone may experience serious health effects.
✔ *Hazardous.* The entire population is likely to be affected, and a warning of emergency conditions will be triggered.

Source: U.S. Environmental Protection Agency, "Air Quality Index (AQI)," 2004, www.epa.gov/airnow/aqi.html

asthma, bronchitis, and emphysema. It is toxic to plants, destroys some paint pigments, corrodes metals, impairs visibility, and is a precursor to acid deposition (acid rain), which we discuss later in this chapter.

Particulates **Particulates** are tiny solid particles or liquid droplets that are suspended in the air. Cigarette smoke releases particulates. They are also by-products of industrial processes and the internal combustion engine. Particulates irritate the lungs and can carry heavy metals and carcinogenic agents deep into the lungs. When combined with sulfur dioxide, they exacerbate respiratory diseases. Particulates can also corrode metals and obscure visibility. Numerous scientific studies have found significant links between exposure to air particulate concentrations at or below current standards and adverse health effects, including premature death.[14] A recent study of workplace smoking bans in Montana showed significant improvement in worker health after bans were implemented.[15]

Carbon Monoxide An odorless, colorless gas, **carbon monoxide** originates primarily from motor vehicle emissions. Carbon monoxide interferes with the blood's ability

Particulates Nongaseous air pollutants.

Carbon monoxide An odorless, colorless gas that originates primarily from motor vehicle emissions.

What Can I Do to Preserve the Environment?

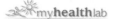 my**health**lab

Fill out this assessment online at www.aw-bc.com/myhealthlab or www.aw-bc.com/donatelle

Environmental problems often seem too big for an individual to make a difference. Each day, though, there are things you can do that contribute to the health of the planet.

MAKING A DIFFERENCE

For each statement, indicate how commonly you follow the described behavior:

	Always	Usually	Sometimes	Never
1. Whenever I can, I walk or ride my bicycle rather than take a car.	1	2	3	4
2. I carpool to school or work with others.	1	2	3	4
3. I have my car tuned up and inspected every year.	1	2	3	4
4. When I have the oil in my car changed, I make sure the oil goes into a recycling bin, not on the ground or into a floor drain.	1	2	3	4
5. I save fuel by not using the air conditioner except in extreme conditions.	1	2	3	4
6. I turn off the lights when a room is not being used.	1	2	3	4
7. I take a shower rather than a bath most of the time.	1	2	3	4
8. I have water-saving devices installed on my shower and sinks.	1	2	3	4
9. I make sure faucets and toilets do not leak.	1	2	3	4
10. I use my bath towels more than once before putting them in the wash.	1	2	3	4
11. I wear my clothes more than once between washings.	1	2	3	4
12. I make sure that the washing machine is full before I wash a load of clothes.	1	2	3	4
13. I purchase biodegradable soaps and detergents.	1	2	3	4
14. I use biodegradable trash bags.	1	2	3	4

to absorb and carry oxygen and can impair thinking, slow reflexes, and cause drowsiness, unconsciousness, and death. Home monitors are available to test for carbon monoxide.

Ozone Ground-level **ozone** is a form of oxygen that is produced when nitrogen dioxide reacts with hydrogen chloride. These gases release oxygen, which is altered by sunlight to produce ozone. In the lower atmosphere, ozone irritates the mucous membranes of the respiratory system, causing

coughing and choking. It can impair lung function, reduce resistance to colds and pneumonia, and aggravate heart disease, asthma, bronchitis, and pneumonia. One of the irritants found in smog, this ozone corrodes rubber and paint and can kill vegetation. The natural ozone found in the upper atmosphere (sometimes called "good" ozone), however, serves as a protective shield against heat and radiation from the sun. We will discuss this atmospheric ozone layer later in the chapter.

Nitrogen Dioxide Coal-powered electrical utility boilers and motor vehicles emit **nitrogen dioxide.** High concentrations of the gas can be fatal, while lower concentrations increase susceptibility to colds and flu, bronchitis, and pneumonia. Nitrogen dioxide is also toxic to plant life and causes a brown discoloration of the atmosphere. It is a precursor of ozone and, along with sulfur dioxide, of acid rain.

Ozone A gas formed when nitrogen dioxide interacts with hydrogen chloride.

Nitrogen dioxide An amber-colored gas found in smog; can cause eye and respiratory irritations.

		Always	Usually	Sometimes	Never
15.	At home, I use dishes and silverware rather than Styrofoam or other single-use dishes or utensils.	1	2	3	4
16.	When I buy prepackaged foods, I choose the ones with the least packaging.	1	2	3	4
17.	I try not to subscribe to newspapers and magazines when I can view them online.	1	2	3	4
18.	I try not to use a hair dryer.	1	2	3	4
19.	I recycle plastic shopping bags.	1	2	3	4
20.	I don't run water continuously when washing the dishes, shaving, or brushing my teeth.	1	2	3	4
21.	I prefer to use unbleached or recycled paper.	1	2	3	4
22.	I use both sides of printer paper and other paper when possible.	1	2	3	4
23.	If I have items I do not want to use anymore, I donate them to charity so someone else can use them.	1	2	3	4
24.	I try not to buy drinks in cans with plastic rings attached to them.	1	2	3	4
25.	I try not to buy bottled water in small plastic containers.	1	2	3	4
26.	I clean up after myself while enjoying the outdoors (picnicking, camping, etc.).	1	2	3	4
27.	I volunteer for clean-up days in the community in which I live.	1	2	3	4
28.	I consider candidates' positions on environmental issues before casting my vote.	1	2	3	4

FOR FURTHER THOUGHT

Review your scores. Are your responses mostly 1s and 2s? If not, what actions can you take to become more environmentally responsible? Does the list suggest ways to help the environment that you had not considered? Are there behaviors not on the list that you are already doing?

MAKE IT HAPPEN!

Use the results of this self-assessment to begin your behavior change program. Follow the steps and use the examples on page 614 to complete your Behavior Change Contract and use these resources to take action.

Lead Lead is a metal pollutant found in paint, batteries, drinking water, pipes, dishes with lead-glazed bases, dirt, soldered cans, and some candies made in Mexico. It affects the circulatory, reproductive, urinary, and nervous systems and can accumulate in bone and other tissues. Lead is particularly detrimental to children and fetuses. It can cause birth defects, behavioral abnormalities, and decreased learning abilities.[16]

The elimination of lead from gasoline and auto exhaust in the 1970s was one of the great public health accomplishments of all time. However, although stricter standards prevail, an estimated 300,000 children in the United States still have unsafe blood lead levels.

Hydrocarbons Although not listed as one of the six major air pollutants in the Clean Air Act, hydrocarbons encompass a wide variety of chemical pollutants in the air. Sometimes known as *volatile organic compounds (VOCs),* **hydrocarbons** are chemical compounds containing different combinations of carbon and hydrogen. The principal source is the internal combustion engine. Most automobile engines emit hundreds of different hydrocarbon compounds. By themselves, hydrocarbons seem to cause few problems, but when they combine with sunlight and other pollutants, they form such poisons as formaldehyde, ketones, and peroxyacetylnitrate (PAN), all of which are respiratory irritants. Hydrocarbon combinations such as benzene and benzo[a]pyrene are carcinogenic. In addition, hydrocarbons play a major part in the formation of smog.

Lead A metal found in the exhaust of motor vehicles powered by fuel containing lead and in emissions from lead smelters and processing plants.

Hydrocarbons Chemical compounds that contain carbon and hydrogen.

Photochemical Smog

Photochemical smog is a brown, hazy mix of particulates and gases that forms when oxygen-containing compounds of nitrogen and hydrocarbons react in the presence of sunlight. It is sometimes called *ozone pollution* because ozone is created when vehicle exhaust reacts with sunlight. In most cases, smog forms in areas that experience a **temperature inversion,** a weather condition in which a cool layer of air is trapped under a layer of warmer air, preventing the air from circulating. When gases such as hydrocarbons and nitrogen oxides are released into the cool air layer, they remain suspended until winds remove the warmer air layer. Sunlight filtering through the air causes chemical changes in the hydrocarbons and nitrogen oxides, which results in smog. (*Smog* is a combined term derived from "smoke" and "fog.") Smog is more likely to be produced in valley regions blocked by hills or mountains—for example, Los Angeles, Denver, and Tokyo.

The most noticeable adverse effects of smog are difficulty in breathing, burning eyes, headaches, and nausea. Long-term exposure poses serious health risks, particularly for children, older adults, pregnant women, and people with chronic respiratory disorders such as asthma and emphysema.

What do you think?

Should automakers be responsible for developing cars with low emissions? ■ *As a motorist, how can you help eliminate carbon monoxide emissions?*

Acid Deposition and Acid Rain

Acid deposition is a broad term that encompasses the acidification process that occurs when rain, sleet, snow, clouds, and fog hold acid particles. In most scientific circles, it is replacing the term *acid rain*. Acid deposition refers to precipitation that has fallen through acidic air pollutants, particularly

---

Photochemical smog   The brownish yellow haze resulting from the combination of hydrocarbons and nitrogen oxides.

Temperature inversion   A weather condition occurring when a layer of cool air is trapped under a layer of warmer air.

Acid deposition   The acidification process that occurs when pollutants are deposited in precipitation, directly on the land, or by clouds.

Leach   To dissolve and filter through soil.

---

those containing sulfur dioxides and nitrogen dioxides. When introduced into lakes and ponds, this precipitation gradually acidifies the water. When the acid content of the water reaches a certain level, plant and animal life cannot survive. Ironically, acidified lakes and ponds become a crystal-clear deep blue, giving the illusion of beauty and health.

Acidic pollutants can be deposited in three ways:[17]

- Wet deposition. Pollutants are deposited in rain and snow (what is commonly termed acid rain or acid precipitation). This is the major acid deposition found in most of the Northern Hemisphere.
- Dry deposition. Gases and particles are deposited directly onto the land. This is the most common form of acid deposition in much of Europe.
- Cloud deposition. Clouds can provide a significant input of acidic pollutants over high ground.

Sources of Acid Deposition   More than 95 percent of acid deposition originates in human actions, chiefly the burning of fossil fuels. The greatest sources of acid deposition in the United States are coal-fired power plants, ore smelters, oil refineries, and steel mills.

When these and other industries burn fuels, the sulfur and nitrogen in the emissions combine with oxygen and sunlight in the air to become sulfur dioxide and nitrogen oxides (precursors of sulfuric acid and nitric acids, respectively). Small acid particles are then carried by the wind and combine with moisture to produce acidic rain or snow. Rain is more acidic in the summertime because of higher concentrations of sunlight. The ability of a lake to cleanse itself and neutralize its acidity depends on several factors, the most critical of which is the buffering ability of the underlying bedrock.

Effects of Acid Deposition   In addition to damaging lakes and ponds, every year acid deposition destroys millions of trees in Europe and North America. Scientists have concluded that much of Europe's forestlands are now experiencing damaging levels of sulfur deposition. Forests in every country on the continent are affected.[18] Emissions of sulfur dioxide in the United States rose 4 percent in 2003, while other pollutants—carbon monoxide, lead, and nitrous oxide—have decreased since 2001.[19]

Doctors believe that acid deposition aggravates and may even cause bronchitis, asthma, and other respiratory problems. People with emphysema and those with a history of heart disease may also suffer from exposure. It may also be hazardous to a pregnant woman's unborn child.

Acidic deposition can cause metals such as aluminum, cadmium, lead, and mercury to **leach** (dissolve and filter) out of the soil. If these metals make their way into water or food supplies (particularly fish), they can cause cancer in humans who consume them. Acid deposition also damages crops; laboratory experiments show that it can reduce seed yield by up to 23 percent. Actual crop losses are being reported with

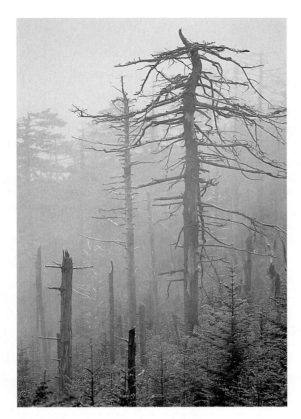

Acid deposition has many harmful effects on the environment. Because its toxins seep into groundwater and enter the food chain, it also poses health hazards to humans.

increasing frequency. A final consequence is the destruction of public monuments and structures, with billions of dollars in projected building damage each year.

Indoor Air Pollution

In the last several years, a growing body of scientific evidence has indicated that the air within homes and other buildings can be more polluted than the outdoor air in even the most industrialized cities. Research also indicates that some of the most vulnerable people, particularly the young, older adults, and those who are sick, often spend over 90 percent of their time indoors.[20]

Most indoor air pollution comes from sources that release gases or particles into the air. Inadequate ventilation, particularly in heavily insulated buildings with airtight windows, may increase pollution by not allowing in outside air.

Table 21.2 describes major sources of indoor air pollution and possible health effects from these pollutants. However, the relative dose of any given chemical and the degree of its toxicity are key variables in determining risk. Some sources, such as building materials, furnishings, and household products such as air fresheners, release pollutants continuously. Others release pollutants intermittently. Health

effects may develop over years of exposure or occur in response to toxic levels of pollutants. Several factors affect risk, including age, preexisting medical conditions, individual sensitivity, room temperature and humidity, and functioning of the liver, immune, and respiratory systems.[21]

Prevention of indoor air pollution should focus on three main areas: source control (eliminating or reducing individual contaminants), ventilation improvements (increasing the amount of outdoor air coming indoors), and air cleaners (removing particulates from the air).[22]

How serious is the problem? Indoor air can be 10 to 40 times more hazardous than outdoor air. There are 20 to 100 potentially dangerous chemical compounds in the average American home. Indoor air pollution comes primarily from these sources: woodstoves, furnaces, passive cigarette exposure (see Chapter 13), asbestos, formaldehyde, radon, and household chemicals. An emerging source of indoor air pollution is mold (see the New Horizons in Health box). It is not yet clear how widespread the effects of mold are.

Home Heating   Woodstoves emit significant levels of particulates and carbon monoxide in addition to other pollutants, such as sulfur dioxide. If you rely on wood for heating, make sure that your stove is properly installed, vented, and maintained. Burning properly seasoned wood reduces particulates.

People who rely on oil- or gas-fired furnaces also need to make sure that these appliances are properly installed, ventilated, and maintained. Inadequate cleaning and maintenance can allow deadly carbon monoxide to build up in the home.

Asbestos   Asbestos is a mineral that was commonly used in insulating materials in buildings constructed before 1970. When bonded to other materials, asbestos is relatively harmless, but if its tiny fibers become loosened and airborne, they can embed themselves in the lungs. Their presence leads to cancer of the lungs, stomach, and chest lining, and a fatal lung disease called mesothelioma.

Formaldehyde   Formaldehyde is a colorless, strong-smelling gas present in some carpets, draperies, furniture, particleboard, plywood, wood paneling, countertops, and many adhesives. It is released into the air in a process called *outgassing*. Outgassing is highest in new products, but the process can continue for many years.

Exposure to formaldehyde can cause respiratory problems, dizziness, fatigue, nausea, and rashes. Long-term exposure can lead to central nervous system disorders and cancer.

Asbestos   A substance that separates into stringy fibers and lodges in the lungs, where it can cause various diseases.

Formaldehyde   A colorless, strong-smelling gas released through outgassing; causes respiratory and other health problems.

Table 21.2
Health Effects of Indoor Air Pollution

Type of Pollutant	Sources	Health Effects
Radon	Uranium in the soil or rock on which homes are built; well water also can be a source	Lung cancer from exposure in air, other health risks from swallowing in water
Environmental tobacco smoke	Smoke that comes from burning end of cigarette, pipe, or cigar	Complex mixture of more than 4,000 compounds, over 40 of which cause cancer
Biological contaminants (molds, mildew, viruses, animal dander and cat saliva, dust mites, cockroaches, and pollen)	Improper ventilation and moisture buildup, lack of cleanliness/sanitation, contaminated heating systems, household pets, rodents, insects, damp carpets, etc.	Allergic reactions, including hypersensitivity, rhinitis, asthma, infectious illnesses, sneezing, watering eyes, coughing, shortness of breath, dizziness, lethargy, fever, digestive problems
Combustion products	Unvented kerosene heaters, woodstoves, fireplaces, gas stoves	Carbon monoxide causes headaches, dizziness, weakness, nausea, confusion and disorientation, chest pain, death. Nitrogen dioxide causes irritation of nose, eyes, respiratory distress. Particles cause lung damage and irritation.
Household chemicals (see partial list below)	Paints, varnishes, cleaning products, solvents, degreasers, hobby products, etc.	Variable symptoms dependent on exposure level, including eye and respiratory tract problems, headaches, dizziness, visual disorders, and memory impairment
• Benzene	Paint, new carpet, new drapes, upholstery, fast-drying glues, caulks	Headaches, eye/skin irritation, fatigue, cancer
• Formaldehyde	Tobacco smoke, plywood, cabinets, furniture, particle board, new carpet and drapes, wallpaper, ceiling tile, paneling	Headaches, eye/skin irritation, drowsiness, fatigue, respiratory problems, memory loss, depression, gynecological problems, cancer
• Chloroform	Paint, new drapes, new carpet, upholstery	Headaches, asthma attacks, dizziness, eye/skin irritations
• Toluene	All paper products, most finished wood products	Headaches, eye/skin irritation, sinus problems, dizziness, cancer
• Hydrocarbons	Tobacco smoke, gas burners and furnaces	Headaches, fatigue, nausea, dizziness, breathing difficulty
• Ammonia	Tobacco smoke, cleaning supplies, animal urine	Eye/skin irritation, headaches, nosebleeds, sinus problems
• Trichloroethylene	Paints, glues, caulking, vinyl coatings, wallpaper	Headaches, eye/skin irritation, upper respiratory irritation

Source: U.S. Environmental Protection Agency, "The Inside Story: A Guide to Indoor Air Quality" (EPA Document #402-K-93-007), 1995, http://epa.gov/iaq/pubs/insidest.html

Ask about the formaldehyde content of products you purchase, and avoid those that contain this gas. Some houseplants, such as philodendrons and spider plants, help clean formaldehyde from the air. If you experience symptoms of formaldehyde exposure, have your home tested by a city, county, or state health agency.

Radon A naturally occurring radioactive gas resulting from the decay of certain radioactive elements.

Radon Radon, an odorless, colorless gas, is the natural by-product of the decay of uranium and radium in the soil. Radon penetrates homes through cracks, pipes, sump pits, and other openings in the foundation. An estimated 15,000 to 22,000 lung cancer deaths per year have been attributed to radon, making it second only to smoking as a cause of lung cancer.[23]

The EPA estimates that 1 in 15 American homes has an elevated radon level.[24] A home-testing kit from a hardware store will enable you to test your home yourself. "Alpha track" detectors are commonly used for this type of short-term testing. They must remain in your home for 2 to 90 days, depending on the device.

Are Environmental Molds Making You Sick?

If you've heard tales of people getting sick from living in homes or working in buildings with molds growing in the walls or attics, you are not alone. Molds seem to have captured the public interest in recent years, particularly in states such as Oregon where rain, fog, and dampness permeate just about everything for several months of the year.

What are molds, and why all the concern? Molds are actually fungi that can be found both indoors and outdoors in most regions of the country. There are literally thousands of different mold types; and, for the most part, we live with them in peaceful coexistence. Molds produce tiny spores to reproduce, and the spores waft through the indoor and outdoor air continually. When they land on a damp spot indoors, they may begin growing and digesting whatever they are growing on, including wood, paper, carpet, and food.

However, some people are sensitive to molds, and exposure may lead to nasal stuffiness, running nose and eyes, itchy skin, or much more serious consequences. For those who are really sensitive, living in a home where mold is in the walls or under the carpets may lead to fever, headache, shortness of breath, nausea, light-headedness, or severe respiratory problems. Some people have experienced extreme autoimmune-like symptoms.

In general, the best way to prevent problems is to avoid areas that are likely to have molds, such as compost piles, cut grass, and wooded areas. Antique shops, greenhouses, saunas, flower shops, lake or beach houses, attics, and basements are all likely mold growth areas.

If you have mold in your home, you should clean it up and fix sources of dampness that may be contributing to them. Mold growth can be stopped by using a solution of bleach and water or by purchasing antimold products designed to kill growth in showers and other areas of the home. If you suspect mold-related problems in your work or school and to find out how to arrange for an inspection, contact your local health department.

Specific recommendations for reducing mold exposure include:

- Keep the humidity level in the house between 40 and 60 percent.
- Use an air conditioner or a dehumidifier during humid months.
- Be sure your home has adequate ventilation, including exhaust fans in the kitchen or bath. If there are no fans, open windows.
- Add mold inhibitors to paints before application.
- Clean bathrooms with mold-killing products
- Do not carpet bathrooms and basements.
- Wash rugs in entryways and other areas where moisture can accumulate.
- Get rid of mattresses and other furniture that may have been exposed to moisture during moving or through bed-wetting or other situations where slow drying may occur.
- Dry clothing thoroughly before folding and putting in drawers or hanging in dark closets.

Source: National Center for Environmental Health, "Molds in the Environment," 2004, www.cdc.gov/nceh/airpollution/mold /moldfacts.htm

---

Household Chemicals   Use cleansers and other cleaning products in a well-ventilated room, and be conservative in their use. Those caustic chemicals that zap mildew and grease also pose a major risk to water and the environment. Avoid buildup. Regular cleanings will reduce the need to use potentially harmful substances. Cut down on dry cleaning, as the chemicals used by many cleaners can cause cancer. If your newly cleaned clothes smell of dry-cleaning chemicals, return them to the cleaner or hang them in the open air until the smell is gone. Avoid household air freshener products containing the carcinogenic agent *dichlorobenzene*.

Indoor air pollution is also a concern in the classroom and workplace. Studies show that one in five U.S. schools has indoor air quality problems, and one in four had ventilation problems.[25] Poor air quality in classrooms may lead to drowsiness, headaches, and lack of concentration. It may also affect physical growth and development. Children with asthma are particularly at risk. Many people who work indoors complain of maladies that lessen or vanish when they leave the building. **Sick building syndrome (SBS)** is said to exist when 80 percent of a building's occupants report problems. Poor ventilation is a primary cause of sick building syndrome. Other causes include faulty furnaces that emit carbon monoxide, nitrogen dioxide, and sulfur dioxide; biological air pollutants such as dander, molds, and dust; VOCs from products including hairspray, cleaners, and adhesives; and heavy metals such as lead, particularly in older buildings. Symptoms include eye irritation, sore throat, queasiness, and worsened asthma.[26]

> **Sick building syndrome (SBS)**   Problem that exists when 80 percent of a building's occupants report maladies that tend to lessen or vanish when they leave the building.

Ozone Layer Depletion

As mentioned earlier, the *ozone* layer forms a protective layer in the earth's stratosphere—the highest level of the earth's atmosphere, located 12 to 30 miles above the earth's surface. The ozone layer in the stratosphere protects our planet and its inhabitants from ultraviolet B (UVB) radiation, a primary cause of skin cancer. UVB radiation may also damage DNA and weaken immune systems in both humans and animals. Thus, the ozone layer is crucial to life on the planet's surface.

In the 1970s, scientists began to warn of a breakdown in the earth's ozone layer. Instruments developed to test atmospheric contents indicated that chemicals used on earth, **chlorofluorocarbons (CFCs)**, were contributing to its rapid depletion.

At first believed to be miracle chemicals, chlorofluorocarbons were used as refrigerants (Freon), as aerosol propellants in hairsprays and deodorants, as cleaning solvents, and in medical sterilizers, rigid foam insulation, and Styrofoam. But, along with halons (found in many fire extinguishers), methyl chloroform, and carbon tetrachloride (cleaning solvents), CFCs were eventually found to be a major cause of ozone depletion. When released into the air through spraying or outgassing, CFCs migrate upward toward the ozone layer, where they decompose and release chlorine atoms. These atoms cause ozone molecules to break apart (Figure 21.1).

The U.S. government banned the use of aerosol sprays containing CFCs in the 1970s. The discovery of an "ozone hole" over Antarctica led to the 1987 Montreal Protocol, a treaty whereby the United States and other nations agreed to further reduce the use of CFCs and other ozone-depleting chemicals. The treaty was amended in 1995 to ban CFC production in developed countries. Today, over 160 countries have signed the treaty, as the international community strives to preserve the ozone layer.[27]

Although the ban on CFCs is believed to be responsible for slowing the depletion of the ozone layer, CFC replacements (including the greenhouse gases termed hydrofluorocarbons and perfluorocarbons) appear to be equally damaging. A United Nations treaty signed in Kyoto in 1997 attempted to control these newer greenhouse gases. Unfortunately, the United States refused to sign the treaty in 2001, amid much controversy. As the greatest producer of greenhouse gases, the United States would have been required to reduce emissions by 33 percent.

Global Warming

More than 100 years ago, scientists theorized that carbon dioxide emissions from fossil-fuel burning would create a buildup of *greenhouse gases* in the Earth's atmosphere that

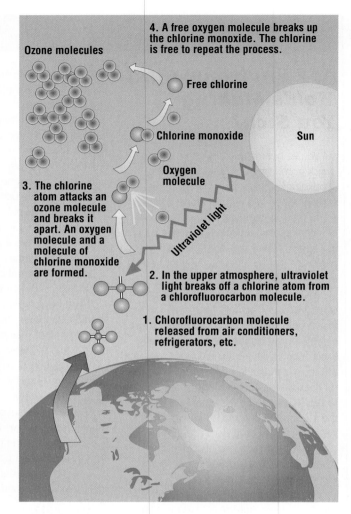

Figure 21.1
How the Ozone Layer Is Being Depleted

could have a warming effect on the planet's surface. The century-old predictions now seem to be coming true, with alarming results. According to the National Academy of Sciences, the Earth's surface temperature has risen 1 degree Fahrenheit in the past century, with accelerated warming in the past two decades,[28] and there is new and strong evidence that most of the warming over the last 50 years is due to human activities.[29]

With average global temperatures higher today than at any time since global temperatures were first recorded, the change in atmospheric temperature may be taking a heavy toll on human beings and crops. Climate researchers predicted in 1975 that the buildup of greenhouse gases would produce life-threatening natural phenomena, including drought in the midwestern United States, more frequent and severe forest fires, flooding in India and Bangladesh, extended heat waves over large areas of the Earth, and killer hurricanes. Recently, the planet has experienced all of these phenomena, although whether they are connected to global warming remains a matter of debate.

Chlorofluorocarbons (CFCs)   Chemicals that contribute to the depletion of the ozone layer.

Greenhouse gases include carbon dioxide, CFCs, ground-level ozone, nitrous oxide, and methane. They become part of a gaseous layer that encircles the Earth, allowing solar heat to pass through and then trapping it close to the Earth's surface. The most predominant is carbon dioxide, which accounts for 49 percent of all greenhouse gases, and Eastern Europe and North America are responsible for approximately half of all carbon dioxide emissions. Since the late nineteenth century, carbon dioxide concentrations in the atmosphere have increased by 30 percent, with half of this increase occurring since the 1950s. Carbon emissions from the burning of fossil fuels, oil, coal, and gas continue to climb. The United States is the greatest producer of greenhouse gases, responsible for over 20 percent of all output.

Rapid deforestation of the tropical rain forests of Central and South America, Africa, and Southeast Asia also contributes to the rapid rise in greenhouse gases. Trees take in carbon dioxide, transform it, store the carbon for food, and then release oxygen into the air. As we lose forests at the rate of hundreds of acres per hour, we lose the capacity to dissipate carbon dioxide.

Reducing Air Pollution

Air pollution problems are rooted in our energy, transportation, and industrial practices. We must develop comprehensive national strategies to address the problem of air pollution in order to clean the air for the future. We must support policies that encourage the use of renewable resources such as solar, wind, and water power as the providers of most of the world's energy. Table 21.3 indicates global trends in sources of energy consumption.

Most experts agree that shifting away from automobiles as the primary source of transportation is the only way to reduce air pollution significantly. Many cities have taken steps in this direction by setting high parking fees, imposing bans on city driving, and establishing high road-usage tolls. Community governments should be encouraged to provide convenient, inexpensive, and easily accessible public transportation.

Table 21.3
Global Trends in Energy Use, by Source, 1990–1997

Energy Source	Annual Rate of Growth (%)
Wind power	25.7
Solar power	16.8
Geothermal power	3.0
Natural gas	21.1
Hydroelectric power	1.6
Oil	1.4
Nuclear power	0.6

Source: C. Flavin and S. Dunn, *Vital Signs Brief 98-6: Merger Signals Beginning of Geriatric Era for Oil Industry* (Washington, DC: Worldwatch Institute, 1998).

Table 21.4
Daily per Capita Water Use (in Gallons) in Single-Family Homes

Type of Use	With Water-Conserving Devices	Without Water-Conserving Devices
Showers	10.0	12.6
Washing machines	10.6	15.1
Toilets	9.3	20.1
Dishwashers	1.0	1.0
Baths	1.2	1.2
Leaks	5.0	10.0
Faucets	10.8	11.1
Other domestic use	1.5	1.5
Total	**49.4**	**72.6**

Total savings: 23.3 gallons per day

Source: Adapted from "1999 Residential Water Use Summary," by permission. Copyright © 2002, American Water Works Association.

Although stricter laws on carbon emissions from cars and trucks and new hybrid cars that operate on electricity and gas are promising, we have a long way to go to reduce fossil fuel consumption. One promising initiative is "bicycle power," with bicycles gaining popularity worldwide. Currently, China leads the world in bicycle use, followed by India. In Germany, bicycle use has increased by 50 percent, and England has a plan to quadruple bicycle use by the year 2012.[30] Hybrid cars, capable of significantly lower emissions and less reliance on fossil fuels, have gained popularity in the United States and abroad. Improved technology, tax incentives, and other initiatives have made these a more real-istic alternative to traditional cars.

Water Pollution

Seventy-five percent of the Earth is covered with water in the form of oceans, seas, lakes, rivers, streams, and wetlands. Beneath the landmass are reservoirs of groundwater. We draw our drinking water from either this underground source or from surface freshwater. However, just 1 percent of our entire water supply is available for human use—the rest is too salty or locked away in polar ice caps.[31] Considering that this water must meet the world's agricultural, manufacturing, community, personal, and sanitation needs, it is no wonder that clean water is a precious commodity. Table 21.4 shows how much water might be saved daily through simple conservation actions.

Greenhouse gases Gases that contribute to global warming by trapping heat near the Earth's surface.

We cannot take the safety of our water supply for granted. Local and state governments, public water systems, and the EPA spend billions of dollars per year to protect and maintain water quality.[32] The status of our water supply reflects the pollution level of our communities and, ultimately, of the whole Earth.

How serious is our shortage of safe water for global populations? According to a 2004 World Health Organization/ UNICEF report, the world faces a silent emergency of a shortage of clean water for almost half the world's population. More than 2.6 billion people, about 40 percent of those on the planet, have no access to basic sanitation or adequate toilet facilities. More than a billion have no access to clean water, and over 4,000 children die every day from illnesses caused by contaminated water and lack of sanitation. By 2015, over 800 million people will have no safe water.[33]

Water Contamination

Many factors can contribute to water contamination. Microorganisms can flourish if water temperature and oxygen levels become hospitable to their growth, and these microbes can cause disease. In 1993, an outbreak of cryptosporidiosis caused over 400,000 people to become sick from contaminated city water in Milwaukee, Wisconsin. Waterborne diseases such as hepatitis A, cholera, and amoebic dysentery can cause severe illness and death.

In addition to microbial contamination, water can become polluted by toxic chemicals such as pesticides, herbicides, fertilizers, and a host of other chemicals. You need only go to your local hardware store and note the aisles of chemicals that we can spray on our lawns to keep them green, to kill weeds, kill insects, and remove paint and stains to fully appreciate the magnitude of toxic load that we wash down with water every day of our lives. These substances end up in our sewers, our water supplies, and our general environment. The potential health hazards of mixing these thousands of chemicals together can barely be imagined.[34]

Any substance that gets into the soil can potentially enter the water supply. Industrial pollutants, acid deposition, and pesticides eventually work their way into the soil, then into groundwater. Underground storage tanks for gasoline may leak. Oil spills contaminate coastal waterways and spill into local rivers, along with hazardous farming and industrial wastes.

The U.S. Congress has coined two terms, *point source* and *nonpoint source,* to describe the two general sources of

water pollution. **Point source pollutants** enter a waterway at a specific point through a pipe, ditch, culvert, or other conduit. The two major sources of this type of pollution are sewage treatment plants and industrial facilities.

Nonpoint source pollutants—commonly known as *runoff* and *sedimentation*—run off or seep into waterways from broad areas of land rather than through a discrete conduit. It is estimated that 99 percent of the sediment in our waterways, 98 percent of the bacterial contaminants, 84 percent of the phosphorus, and 82 percent of the nitrogen come from nonpoint sources.[35] Nonpoint pollution results from a variety of human land use practices. It includes soil erosion and sedimentation, construction wastes, pesticide and fertilizer runoff, urban street runoff, wastes from engineering projects, acid mine drainage, leakage from septic tanks, and sewage sludge.[36] (See Figure 21.2.)

Septic Systems Bacteria from human waste can leach into the water supply from improperly installed septic systems. Toxic chemicals that are dumped into septic systems can also enter groundwater.

Landfills Landfills and dumps generate a liquid called **leachate**, a mixture of soluble chemicals from household garbage, office waste, biological waste, and industrial waste. If a landfill has not been properly lined, leachate trickles through its layers of garbage and eventually into the water supply as acid and into the atmosphere as methane gas.

Gasoline and Petroleum Products In the United States, there are more than 2 million underground storage tanks for gasoline and petroleum products, most of which are located at gasoline filling stations. One-quarter of them are thought to be leaking.[37]

Most of these tanks were installed 25 to 30 years ago. They were made of fabricated steel that was unprotected from corrosion. Over time, pinpoint holes develop in the steel, and the petroleum products leak into groundwater. The most common way to detect the presence of petroleum products in water is to test for benzene, a component of oil and gasoline. Benzene is highly toxic and associated with the development of cancer.

Chemical Contaminants *Organic solvents* are chemicals designed to dissolve grease and oil. These extremely toxic substances, such as carbon tetrachloride, tetrachloroethylene, and trichloroethylene (TCE), are used to clean clothing, painting equipment, plastics, and metal parts. Many household products, such as stain and spot removers, degreasers, drain cleaners, septic system cleaners, and paint removers, also contain these toxic chemicals.

Organic solvents work their way into the water supply in different ways. Consumers often dump leftover products into the toilet or into street drains. Industries pour leftovers into large barrels, which are then buried. After a while, the chemicals eat their way out of the barrels and leach into groundwater.

Point source pollutants Pollutants that enter waterways at a specific point.

Nonpoint source pollutants Pollutants that run off or seep into waterways from broad areas of land.

Leachate A liquid consisting of soluble chemicals that come from garbage and industrial waste that seeps into the water supply from landfills and dumps.

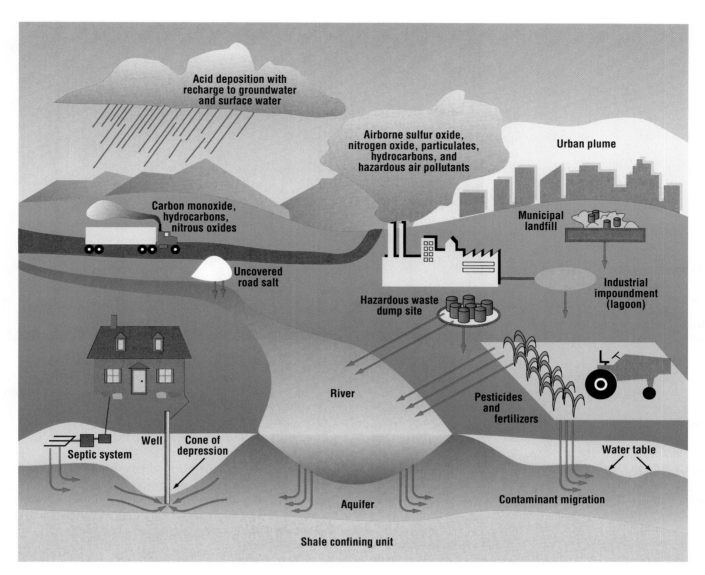

Figure 21.2
Sources of Groundwater Contamination

One related group of toxic substances contains chlorinated hydrocarbons. The most notorious of these substances are the **polychlorinated biphenyls (PCBs),** their cousins the *polybromated biphenyls (PBBs),* and the *dioxins.*

PCBs Fire resistant and stable at high temperatures, PCBs were used for many years as insulating materials in high-voltage electrical equipment such as transformers. PCBs bioaccumulate, meaning that the body does not excrete them but rather stores them in fatty tissues and the liver. PCBs are associated with birth defects, and exposure to them is known to cause cancer. The manufacture of PCBs was discontinued in the United States in 1977, but approximately 500 million pounds of them have been dumped into landfills and waterways, where they continue to pose an environmental threat.[38] Western European countries phased out the use of many of these chemicals in the 1970s; however, elevated

levels can still be detected at the mouths of major rivers, and some countries continue to produce them. PCBs bind to dust particles in the air, are deposited on plants, and end up in the food supply.[39]

Dioxins **Dioxins** are chlorinated hydrocarbons found in herbicides (chemicals that are used to kill vegetation) and pro-

> **Polychlorinated biphenyls (PCBs)** Toxic chemicals that were once used as insulating materials in high-voltage electrical equipment.
>
> **Dioxins** Highly toxic chlorinated hydrocarbons contained in herbicides and produced during certain industrial processes.

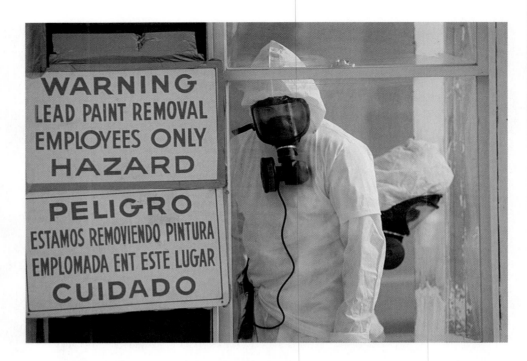

Although an expensive and cumbersome project, deleading a house is now one of the most important considerations of prospective homeowners, especially those with children.

duced during certain industrial processes. Dioxins have the ability to bioaccumulate and are much more toxic than PCBs.

The long-term effects of bioaccumulation of these toxic substances include possible damage to the immune system and increased risk of infections and cancer. Exposure to high concentrations of PCBs or dioxins for a short period of time can also have severe consequences, including nausea, vomiting, diarrhea, painful rashes and sores, and chloracne, an ailment in which the skin develops hard, black, painful pimples that may never go away.

Pesticides   **Pesticides** are chemicals that are designed to kill insects, rodents, plants, and fungi. Americans use more than 1.2 billion pounds of pesticides each year, but only 10 percent actually reach the targeted organisms. The remaining 1.1 billion pounds of pesticides settle on the land and in our air and water. Many pesticides, such as DDT, that are banned in the United States are shipped abroad. Mexico, a major crop producer for the American market, continues to use DDT.[40]

Pesticides are volatile and evaporate readily, often being dispersed by winds over a large area or carried to the sea. This is particularly true in tropical regions, where many farmers use pesticides heavily and the climate promotes their rapid release into the atmosphere. In Nigeria, for example, 98 percent of the DDT applied to a cowpea crop evaporated within four years.[41]

Pesticide residues cling to fresh fruits and vegetables and can accumulate in the body when people eat these items. One study found a correlation between breast cancer and dieldrin, a popular pesticide used until the 1970s.[42]

Women who had the highest traces of dieldrin in their blood were twice as likely to develop breast cancer as were women with the lowest levels. Other potential hazards associated with exposure to pesticides include birth defects, liver and kidney damage, and nervous system disorders.

Lead   The EPA has issued new standards to reduce dramatically the levels of lead in U.S. drinking water. These standards are already in place in many municipalities and will eventually reduce lead exposure for approximately 130 million people. The new rules stipulate that tap water lead values must not exceed 15 parts per billion (the previous standard allowed an average lead level of 50 parts per billion). When water suppliers identify problem areas, they will have to lower the water's acidity with chemical treatment (because acidity increases water's ability to leach lead from the pipes through which it passes), or they will have to replace old lead plumbing in the service lines.

If lead does exist in your home's water, you can reduce your risk by running tap water for several minutes before taking a drink or cooking with it. This flushes out water that has been standing overnight in lead-contaminated lines. Although leaded paints and ceramic glazes used to pose health risks, particularly for small children who put painted toys in their mouths, the use of lead in such products has been effectively reduced in recent years.

Pesticides   Chemicals that kill pests.

What do you think?

Who should bear the financial responsibility for cleaning up hazardous waste leaks? ■ *What can you do to avoid contributing to water contamination?*

Taking Action for the Environment

Protecting the environment involves much more than recycling your paper and plastic and using environmentally friendly household products. It means making a commitment to being an activist and working to change national, state, and local policies so that sustainable development becomes the rule, not the exception. It also means working to elect public officials who represent your views on the environment. There are several things that you can do to help win the battle to preserve and protect the environment for future generations:

- Listen carefully to what political candidates are saying about the environment. Environmental issues have received a low priority in recent national debates and political platforms. Concern for the environment, for all forms of life, and for future generations who must live in the environment we create should be part of the debate in America over moral responsibility. Whether your spiritual self relates to organized religion or to a love of nature and the environment, a part of spiritual health centers on respect and caring for the world we live in and an unselfish consideration, respect, and love for the natural environment. Vote for politicians who prioritize environmental issues and actively promote preservation, protection, and sustainable development.
- Carefully consider state and federal initiatives on issues such as logging, preservation of parks, oil and natural gas drilling, protection of the food supply, restrictions on industrial polluters, solid waste disposal, and water quality. Take the time to read both sides of the issues, consider who is making the

arguments and their motivation for arguing in a particular way. Write to your legislators and let them know your opinions. Talk to others and encourage them to think about the implications of proposed changes.
- Consider "species-ism" in your decision making about endangered species acts, commercial agribusiness, fishing and drift net practices, and other practices that we engage in for the sake of profit and mass production of foods, products, and services. Who decides which living creatures should be treated in a particular way? Who should protect them? What are the ramifications of animal protection? Should humans have the sole right to decide the fate of entire species because of our own interests or needs? What policies, philosophies, or values should guide our decisions about care and protection of other forms of life?
- Become an active environmental-oriented consumer. Buy products with less packaging, foods that are produced with minimal energy, and foods that have fewer chemicals and pesticides. Buy organic whenever possible.
- Do not use caustic cleansers, chemicals that remove film in your shower, or dyes and fragrances in your laundry products. Use soap and water to clean surfaces, not disposable cleaning cloths and spray-on shower cleaners. All these chemicals are flushed down the drain and into the local water supply.
- Let your congressional representative and senators know how you feel about environmental issues and that you will vote according to their record on the issues. When writing to any public official, remember to keep the letter simple and to the point; avoid inflammatory statements or attacks; state the facts, cite reputable sources, and indicate what you want changed; and try

to say what you have to say in one page or less. Proofread the letter to ensure accuracy.
- If you buy a product with excessive packaging, call the toll-free number on the package, and let the manufacturer know about your concerns.
- Educate yourself and others. Organize a discussion group of friends to read books or articles or discuss speakers focused on environmental issues. Test your ideas by engaging others who you think would disagree with you in the discussion. Journal clubs, book clubs, and other forums are excellent opportunities to share ideas, discuss issues, and reach consensus.
- Request environmental speakers in your class or at campus events. Help organize events such as Earth Week and other environmental-oriented projects. Participate in cleanup days and recycling drives. Try to increase others' exposure to people and issues focused on environmental topics.
- Stop buying plastic bottles of water and other beverages. Plastics are among the fastest growing sources of pollution in America. Purchase a hard plastic, wide-mouth water bottle and fill it from a filtered source. Reuse the bottle, and wash it frequently.
- Get active in community groups that deal with environmental issues. Volunteer for commissions, boards, and other groups involved in decision making. Parks, land use, animal control, zoning, public transit, street cleanup, and trash collection are a few of the many issues that have environmental components.
- Run for student government. Help your school become more involved in environmental issues. Seek practicum or internship credits working for environmental causes. Take coursework in environmental health or science.

Table 21.5
Noise Levels of Various Activities (in Decibels)

Decibels (db) measure the volume of sounds. Here are the decibel levels of some common sounds.

Type of Sound	Noise Level (db)
Carrier deck jet operation	150
Jet takeoff from 200 feet	140
Rock concert	120 (painful)
Auto horn (3 feet)	110 (extremely loud)
Motorcycle	100
Garbage truck	100
Pneumatic drill	90
Lawnmower	90
Heavy traffic	80
Alarm clock	80
Shouting, arguing	80 (very loud)
Vacuum cleaner	75 (loud)
Freight train from 50 feet	70
Freeway traffic	65
Normal conversation	60
Light auto traffic	50 (moderate)
Library	40
Soft whisper	30 (faint)

the duration of allowable daily exposure to different decibel levels is exceeded, hearing loss will result.

Unfortunately, despite increasing awareness that noise pollution is more than just a nuisance, noise control programs at federal, state, and local levels have received low budgetary priority in the United States. The European Union has been more active in combating certain forms of noise pollution, such as aircraft noise.[43] Still, the European Environment Agency estimates that over 120 million people in the European Union are exposed daily to noise levels greater than 55 decibels on the front facade of their homes.[44]

Clearly, to protect your hearing, you must take it upon yourself to avoid exposure to excessive noise. Playing stereos in your car and home at reasonable levels, wearing ear plugs when you use power equipment, and establishing barriers such as closed windows between you and noise will help keep your hearing intact.

What do you think?

What do you currently do that places your hearing at risk? ■ *What changes can you make in your lifestyle to protect your hearing?*

Noise Pollution

Loud noise has become commonplace. We are often painfully aware of construction crews in our streets, jet airplanes roaring overhead, stereos blaring next door, and trucks rumbling down nearby freeways. Our bodies show definite physiological responses to noise, and it can become a source of physical and mental distress. Short-term exposure to loud noise reduces productivity, concentration levels, and attention spans and may affect mental and emotional health. Symptoms of noise-related distress include disturbed sleep patterns, headaches, and tension. Physically, our bodies respond to noise in a variety of ways. Blood pressure increases, blood vessels in the brain dilate, and vessels in other parts of the body constrict. The pupils of the eye dilate. Cholesterol levels in the blood rise, and some endocrine glands secrete additional stimulating hormones, such as adrenaline, into the bloodstream.

Hearing can be damaged by varying lengths of exposure to sound, which is measured in decibels (Table 21.5). If

Municipal solid waste Solid wastes such as durable goods, nondurable goods, containers and packaging, food wastes, yard wastes, and miscellaneous wastes from residential, commercial, institutional, and industrial sources.

Land Pollution

Solid Waste

Each day, every person in the United States generates about 4 pounds of **municipal solid waste**—containers and packaging, discarded food, yard debris, and refuse from residential, commercial, institutional, and industrial sources. Approximately 73 percent of this waste is buried in landfills. Cities

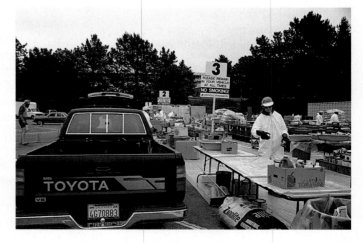

Many communities now provide special programs where their residents can drop off any kind of hazardous waste for safe disposal.

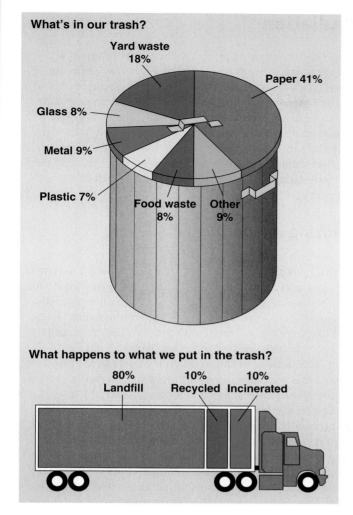

What's in our trash?

Yard waste 18%

Paper 41%

Glass 8%

Metal 9%

Plastic 7%

Food waste 8%

Other 9%

What happens to what we put in the trash?

80% Landfill   10% Recycled   10% Incinerated

Figure 21.3
The Composition and Disposal of Trash

throughout the country are in danger of exhausting their landfill space.

As communities run out of landfill space, it is becoming more common to haul garbage out to sea to dump it or ship it to landfills in developing countries. Figure 21.3 shows the composition of our trash and what happens to our garbage after disposal. Although experts believe that up to 90 percent of our trash is recyclable, only 26 percent of it is currently recycled. In today's throwaway society, we need to become aware of the amount of waste we generate every day and to look for ways to recycle, reuse, and—most desirable of all—reduce what we use.

Hazardous Waste

The community of Love Canal, New York, has come to symbolize **hazardous waste** dump sites. The Hooker Chemical Company used Love Canal as a chemical dump site from 1947 to 1952. The area was later filled in by land developers and built up with homes and schools. In 1976, homeowners began noticing strange seepage in their basements and strong chemical odors. Babies were born with abnormal hearts and kidneys, two sets of teeth, mental handicaps, epilepsy, liver disease, and abnormal rectal bleeding. The rate of cancer and miscarriages was far above normal. The New York State Department of Health investigated and found high concentrations of PCBs in the storm sewers near the old canal, but it took the department another two years to order the evacuation of Love Canal homes. Over 900 families were evacuated, and the state purchased their homes. Finally, in 1978, the expensive process of cleaning up the waste dump began and continued for several years.

In 1980, the Comprehensive Environmental Response Compensation and Liability Act **(Superfund)** was enacted to provide funds for cleaning up chemical dump sites that endanger public health and land. This fund is financed through taxes on the chemical and petroleum industries (87 percent) and through general federal tax revenues (13 percent). Cleanup cost estimates made in the late 1990s for cleanup covering the years 1990 through 2020 ranged from $106 billion to as high as $500 billion. Billions continue to be spent annually.[45]

To date, 32,500 potentially hazardous waste sites have been identified across the nation. After investigation, 17,800 of these sites were determined to require no further action. However, 1,498 sites were listed on the National Priorities List (NPL), and 46 percent of the sites assessed from 1992 through 1996 were considered a hazard to human health.[46] As of the end of 2004, cleanup work had been completed at 926 of the sites. Funding for several projects was scaled back or "deobligated" and overall efforts have slowed as competing economic priorities made these projects more difficult to complete.

The large number of hazardous waste dump sites in the United States indicates the severity of our toxic chemical problem. American manufacturers generate more than 1 ton of chemical waste per person per year (approximately 275 million tons). The Agency for Toxic Substances and Disease Registry (ATSDR) and the EPA evaluate and rank the chemicals that are considered hazardous substances (Table 21.6 on page 610).

The EPA and the states have undertaken an aggressive program to manage hazardous wastes by monitoring their generation, transportation, storage, treatment, and final disposal. To ensure that hazardous wastes being generated

Hazardous waste   Solid waste that, due to its toxic properties, poses a hazard to humans or to the environment.

Superfund   Fund established under the Comprehensive Environmental Response Compensation and Liability Act to be used for cleaning up toxic waste dumps.

today do not become complex and expensive cleanup problems tomorrow, the following steps are being taken:[47]

- Many wastes are now banned from land disposal or are being treated to reduce their toxicity before they become part of land disposal sites.
- The EPA has developed protective requirements for land disposal facilities, such as double liners, detection systems for substances that may leach into groundwater, and groundwater monitoring systems.
- Hazardous waste handlers must now clean up contamination resulting from past waste management practices as well as from current activities.
- The EPA is exploring economic incentives to encourage ingenuity in waste minimization practices and recycling.

See the Health in a Diverse World box for a description of the devastating effects of hazardous waste, oil contamination, and other environmental problems on minority communities.

What do you think?

What items do you currently recycle? ■ *What are some of the reasons you do not recycle?* ■ *What might encourage you to recycle more than you do?* ■ *What concerns would you have about living near a landfill or hazardous waste disposal site?*

Ionizing radiation Radiation produced by photons having high enough energy to ionize atoms

Radiation absorbed doses (rads) Units that measure exposure to radioactivity.

Radiation

A substance is said to be radioactive when it emits high-energy particles from the nuclei of its atoms. There are three types of radiation: alpha particles, beta particles, and gamma rays. *Alpha particles* are relatively massive and are not capable of penetrating human skin. They pose health hazards only when inhaled or ingested. *Beta particles* can penetrate the skin slightly and are harmful if ingested or inhaled. *Gamma rays* are the most dangerous because they can pass straight through the skin, causing serious damage to organs and other vital structures.

Ionizing Radiation

Exposure to ionizing radiation is an inescapable part of life on this planet. **Ionizing radiation** is caused by the release of particles and electromagnetic rays from atomic nuclei during the normal process of disintegration. Some naturally occurring elements, such as uranium, emit radiation. Radiation can wreak havoc on human cells, leading to mutations, cancer, miscarriages, and other problems.

Reactions to radiation differ from person to person. Exposure is measured in **radiation absorbed doses,** or **rads** (also called *roentgens*). Recommended maximum "safe" dosages range from 0.5 to 5 rads per year. Approximately 50 percent of the radiation to which we are exposed comes from natural sources, such as building materials. Another 45 percent comes from medical and dental X rays. The remaining 5 percent comes from computer display screens, microwave ovens, television sets, luminous watch dials, and radar screens and waves. Most of us are exposed to far less radiation than the "safe" maximum dosage per year.

Radiation can cause damage at dosages as low as 100 to 200 rads. At this level, signs of radiation sickness include nausea, diarrhea, fatigue, anemia, sore throat, and hair loss, but death is unlikely. At 350 to 500 rads, these symptoms become more severe, and death may result because the radiation hinders bone marrow production of the white blood cells we need to protect us from disease. Dosages above 600 to 700 rads are invariably fatal. The effects of long-term exposure to relatively low levels of radiation are unknown. Some scientists believe that such exposure can cause lung cancer, leukemia, skin cancer, bone cancer, and skeletal deformities.

Researchers are now investigating links between the radio frequency waves generated by cell phones and cancer, but results are inconclusive (see the New Horizons in Health box).

EMFs: Emerging Risks?

If you believe what you hear on TV or read in the papers, electromagnetic fields (EMFs) generated by electric power delivery systems are responsible for risks for cancer

Environmental Racism

Environmental racism has meant, among other things, that toxic waste dumps, landfills, and industrial plants are much more likely to be placed in communities of color and in the developing world than in predominantly white communities. The adverse health effects of environmental racism have been devastating in the United States and throughout the world.

A clear example comes from the Amazon rain forest of Ecuador. Over a 21-year period, an American oil company systematically dumped more than 16 million gallons of oil and toxic wastewater into the Amazon River. Three indigenous groups lived in the area where the oil company operated—the Cofan, the Secoya, and the Siona. The Cofan, who numbered approximately 15,000 when the oil company built its first well in 1971, now number only a few hundred. The Secoya and Siona populations have also declined. Each of these three groups was a fishing culture when the oil company first came to the Amazon. Now, because of oil contamination, they can no longer fish in the rivers and so face starvation. Often young people migrate to the cities and take low-wage jobs. The result of the contamination of the environment has effectively been the decimation of these three cultures.

After a decade of legal maneuvering, the surviving indigenous people filed suit against the oil company, claiming that it had violated their right to a healthy environment. The case is now underway in Ecuador, but attorneys say that the decision will be binding on an American corporation. The tribes allege that the company's decision to dump millions of gallons of toxins in the rain forest led to the cultural genocide of the three tribes, amounting to racial and ethnic discrimination. One of the tribes' attorneys commented, "The fact is when [the oil company] drills for oil where white people live, they do it safely and according to industry standards. When they drilled in the headwaters of the Amazon River, however, they blatantly ignored these standards while knowingly wreaking havoc on the local people, almost all of whom are people of color." The oil company continues to fight the lawsuit and refuses to clean up the Amazon, while indigenous leaders have launched a national media campaign in the United States, charging the oil company with racism. The company denies that race played any role in its actions.

Scientific literature clearly demonstrates that crude oil and toxic wastewater produced by oil drilling are highly carcinogenic. A public health study of San Carlos, an Ecuadorian town containing more than 30 oil wells, found cancer rates 30 times greater than normal, despite the fact that local inhabitants do not smoke, eat a healthy diet, and are not exposed to urban contamination. Additionally, no other industries in the area release cancer-causing toxins. The water in San Carlos contained nearly 150 times the amount of hydrocarbons considered safe by internationally recognized limits.

Examples of environmental racism can also be found throughout the United States:

- In Los Angeles, recycling plants are located in low-income, primarily Latino neighborhoods. Local residents consistently complain of dustlike glass particles in the air.
- In Augusta, Georgia, a wood preservant factory leaked creosote into the ground, and a scrap metal company leaked arsenic. This ethnic minority community now reports high rates of cancer and skin disease. The plants are also located near an elementary school, and students there experience high rates of learning disabilities, allergies, and asthma.
- The predominantly African American area of Chester, Pennsylvania, contains four hazardous and municipal waste facilities. That area has the highest percentage of low-weight births in the state, as well as mortality and lung cancer rates 60 percent higher than in the rest of the county.

Many health, civil rights, and environmental activists have become proponents of environmental justice. They argue that everyone has the right to be protected from hazardous substances and that environmental policy should be based on mutual respect and justice for all people.

(particularly among children), reproductive dysfunction, birth defects, neurological disorders, Alzheimer's disease, and other ailments. Does research support these claims about EMFs? Though many believe that the threat is legitimate, others point to major discrepancies and inconsistencies in the research. In spite of many questions, fears have increased, and there is probably more potential for exploitation of consumers than real hazard to health from this nonionizing form of exposure.

A six-year study by the National Institute of Environmental Health Sciences (NIEHS) found that the evidence for a link between cancer and EMFs is "weak," although the director of NIEHS warned that efforts to reduce exposure should continue. The study did find a slight increase in risk for childhood leukemia, as well as chronic lymphocytic leukemia in occupationally exposed adults such as utility workers, machinists, and welders. Since then, numerous studies in the United States, Canada, Sweden, Taiwan, New Zealand, and other regions have found only a small association or none at all between cancer and EMFs. Although rates of brain tumors and other cancers are on the increase, a clear link to EMFs has not been established. NIEHS suggests that the lack of consistent, positive findings weakens the contention that EMFs cause cancer.[48]

Wireless Worries: Cell Phones and Risks to Health

In less than a decade, cell phones have become a household staple, with the number of subscribers skyrocketing from 16 million in 1994 to over 110 million today and still rising by 1 million per month.

Although cell phones have become commonplace, their use continues to spur controversy, particularly regarding questions of potential health risk. While the cell phone industry assures consumers that phones are completely safe, a former industry research director, Dr. George Carlo, argues that past studies have not provided conclusive evidence of safety and we do not know the effects of cell phone usage on future generations. He observed, "This is the first generation that has put relatively high-powered transmitters against the head, hour after hour, day after day." Depending on how close the cell phone antenna is to the head, as much as 60 percent of microwave radiation may be absorbed by and actually penetrate the area around the head, some reaching an inch to an inch-and-a-half into the brain.

Are increases in the incidence and prevalence of brain tumors and other neurological conditions in the last decade related to cell phone use? At high power levels, radiofrequency energy, which is the energy used in cell phones, can rapidly heat biological tissue and cause damage, such as burns. However, cell phones operate at power levels well below the level at which such heating effects occur. Many countries, including the United States and most of Europe, use standards set by the Federal Communications Commission (FCC) for radiofrequency energy based on research by several scientific groups.

These groups identified a whole-body *specific absorption rate (SAR)* value for exposure to radiofrequency energy. Four watts per kilogram was identified as a threshold level of exposure at which harmful biological effects may occur. The FCC requires wireless phones to comply with a safety limit of 1.6 watts per kilogram. To find the SAR for your phone, see this website: www.fda.gov/cellphones/qa.html.

The U.S. Food and Drug Administration (FDA), the World Health Organization, and other major health agencies agree that the research to date has not shown radiofrequency energy emitted from cell phones to be harmful. However, they also point to the need for more research and caution that because cell phones have only been widely used for less than a decade and no long-term studies have been done, there is not enough information to say they are risk-free. Three large case-control studies and one large cohort study have compared cell phone use among brain cancer patients and individuals free of brain cancer. Key findings from these studies indicate that:

- Brain cancer patients did not report more cellular phone use overall than did the control group. In fact, most of the studies showed a lower risk of brain cancer among cell phone users, for unclear reasons.
- None of the studies showed a clear link between the side of the head on which the cancer occurred and the side on which the phone was used.
- There was no correlation between brain tumor risk and dose of exposure, as assessed by duration of use, date since first subscription, age at first subscription, or type of cellular phone used.

However, these studies are not conclusive, and preliminary results from smaller, well-designed studies have continued to raise questions. A recent Swedish study found higher risk of a benign brain tumor among adults who had used analog cell phones (which produce higher exposure levels than their digital counterparts) for at least ten years. At the moment, the biggest risk from cell phones appears to come from using them while driving, with a corresponding increase in vehicle crashes. However, if you prefer to err on the side of caution, follow these hints to lower your risk:

- Use lighter- or dash-mounted phones or headphones/ear buds when driving. This not only keeps your hands free, helping to avoid accidents, but, if subsequent studies indicate potential health risk, you will have minimized your exposure to radiofrequency energy. Exposure levels drop dramatically with distance.
- Limit cell phone usage. Use land-based phones whenever possible.
- Check the SAR level of your phone. Purchase one with a lower level if yours is near the FCC limit.
- Digital phones have lower radiofrequencies than analog phones. An upgrade might be in order.

Sources: S. Grund, "Cell Phones: Do They Cause Cancer?" Medline Plus, 2004 update, www.nlm.nih.gov/medlineplus/ency/article/007151.htm; S. Lönn et al., "Mobile Phone Use and the Risk of Acoustic Neuroma," *Epidemiology* 15, no. 6 (2004): 653–659. H. Frumkin and M. Thun, "Environmental Carcinogens—Cellular Phones and Risk of Brain Tumors," *California Cancer Journal for Clinicians* 51 (2001): 137–141; R. Westerman and B. Hocking, "Diseases of Modern Living: Neurological Changes Associated with Mobile Phones and Radiofrequency Radiation in Humans," *Neuroscience Letter* 361, no. 1–3 (2004): 13–16; U.S. Food and Drug Administration, "Cell Phone Facts: Consumer Information on Wireless Phones," 2004, www.fda.gov/cellphones/qa.html.

Nuclear Power Plants

Nuclear power plants account for less than 1 percent of the total radiation to which we are exposed. Other producers of radioactive waste include medical facilities that use radioactive materials as treatment and diagnostic tools and nuclear weapons production facilities.

Proponents of nuclear energy believe that it is a safe and efficient way to generate electricity. Initial costs of building nuclear power plants are high, but actual power generation is relatively inexpensive. A 1,000-megawatt reactor produces enough energy for 650,000 homes and saves 420 million gallons of fossil fuels each year. In some areas where nuclear power plants were decommissioned, electricity bills tripled when power companies turned to hydroelectric or fossil fuel sources to generate electricity.

Nuclear reactors also discharge fewer carbon oxides into the air than fossil fuel–powered generators. Advocates believe that conversion to nuclear power could help slow the global warming trend. Over the past 15 years, carbon emissions were reduced by 298 million tons, or 5 percent.

All these advantages of nuclear energy must be weighed against the disadvantages. First, disposal of nuclear wastes is extremely problematic. Additionally, a reactor core meltdown could pose serious threats to a plant's immediate environment and to the world in general.

A **meltdown** occurs when the temperature in the core of a nuclear reactor increases enough to melt both the nuclear fuel and the containment vessel that holds it. Most modern facilities seal their reactors and containment vessels in concrete buildings with pools of cold water on the bottom. If a meltdown occurs, the building and the pool are supposed to prevent the escape of radioactivity.

Two serious nuclear accidents within seven years of each other caused a steep decline in public support for nuclear energy. The first occurred in 1979 at Three Mile Island near Harrisburg, Pennsylvania, when a mechanical failure caused a partial meltdown of one reactor core and small amounts of radioactive steam were released into the atmosphere. No loss of human life was reported, although residents in the area were evacuated. Miscarriages, birth defects, and cancer rates in the area are reported to have increased, but no public health statistics have been released.

Human error and mechanical failure were the reported causes of the 1986 reactor core fire and explosion at the Chernobyl nuclear power plant in Russia. In just 4.5 seconds, the temperature in the reactor rose to 120 times normal, causing the explosion. Eighteen people were killed immediately, 30 workers died later from radiation sickness, and 200 other workers were hospitalized for severe radiation sickness. Officials evacuated towns and villages near the plant. Some medical workers estimate that the eventual death toll from radiation-induced cancers related to the Chernobyl incident topped 100,000.

Radioactive fallout from the Chernobyl disaster spread over most of the Northern Hemisphere. Milk, meat, and vegetables in Scandinavian countries were contaminated with radioactive iodine and cesium and were declared unfit for human consumption. Thousands of reindeer in Lapland were contaminated and had to be destroyed. In Great Britain, thousands of sheep had to be destroyed, and three years later sheep in the northern regions of the country were still found to be contaminated. Direct costs of the disaster totaled more than $13 billion, including lost agricultural output and the cost of replacing the power plant. Nuclear accidents continue to pose risks to human health, even in well-controlled settings.

What do you think?

How much exposure do you have to ionizing and nonionizing radiation in a year? ■ *What measures could you take to reduce your exposure?* ■ *Do you feel the advantages outweigh the disadvantages of nuclear power? Explain why or why not.*

Meltdown An accident that results when the temperature in the core of a nuclear reactor increases enough to melt the nuclear fuel and the containment vessel housing it.

TAKING CHARGE

MAKE IT HAPPEN!

Assessment: The Assess Yourself box earlier in this chapter (page 596) gave you the chance to look at your behavior and consider ways of saving water, reducing waste, and other ways to protect the planet. Now that you have considered these results, you can begin to take steps toward taking action to become more environmentally responsible.

Making a Change: In order to change your behavior, you need to develop a plan. Follow these steps:

1. Evaluate your behavior, and identify patterns. What can you change now? What can you change in the near future?
2. Select one pattern of behavior that you want to change.
3. Fill out a Behavior Change Contract. It should include your long-term goal for change, your short-term goals, the rewards for reaching these goals, potential obstacles along the way, and strategies for overcoming these obstacles. For each goal, list the small steps and specific actions that you will take.
4. Chart your progress in a journal. At the end of a week, consider how successful you were in following your plan. What helped you be successful? What will you do differently next week?

5. Revise your plan as needed: Are the short-term goals attainable? Are the rewards satisfying?

One Student's Plan: Marta saw that she was already doing several of the items recommended in the self-assessment. However, she had not considered several of the ideas regarding excess packaging of her food, drinks, and so on, although she knew that extra plastic wraps and other excess packaging contribute to the need for more landfills and other environmental problems. She decided that for a week she would try to pay more attention to the packaging of her favorite foods and to buy large sizes of the food whenever possible instead of individually packed products. This meant spending more time in the grocery store to be sure she found items with the least packaging (although she also didn't have to make as many trips to the store that week). The next week, Marta looked at how many plastic bottles she used for her water each day. She bought a durable plastic bottle and started washing it and filling it with water each day before she left the house. After a week she discovered that her garbage was no longer full of plastic water bottles, and she had actually saved herself some money.

Summary

- Population growth is the single largest factor affecting the demands made on the environment. Demand for more food, products, and energy—as well as sites to dispose of waste, particularly in the industrialized world—places great strain on the Earth's resources.
- The primary constituents of air pollution are sulfur dioxide, particulate matter, carbon monoxide, nitrogen dioxide, ozone, lead, and hydrocarbons. Air pollution takes the forms of photochemical smog and acid deposition, among others. Indoor air pollution is caused primarily by woodstove smoke, furnace emissions, asbestos, passive smoke, formaldehyde, radon, and household chemicals. Pollution is depleting the Earth's protective ozone layer, contributing to global warming.
- Water pollution can be caused by either point (direct entry through a pipeline, ditch, etc.) or nonpoint (runoff or seepage from a broad area of land) sources. Major contributors to water pollution include dioxins, pesticides, and lead.

- Noise pollution affects our hearing and produces other symptoms such as reduced productivity, reduced concentration, headaches, and tension.
- Solid waste pollution includes household trash, plastics, glass, metal products, and paper; limited landfill space creates problems. Hazardous waste is toxic; its improper disposal creates health hazards for those in surrounding communities.
- Ionizing radiation results from the natural erosion of atomic nuclei. Nonionizing radiation is caused by the electromagnetic fields around power lines and household appliances, among other sources. The disposal and storage of radioactive wastes from nuclear power plants and weapons production pose serious potential problems for public health.

Questions for Discussion and Reflection

1. How are the rapidly increasing global population and consumption of resources related? Is population control the best solution? Why or why not?
2. What are the primary sources of air pollution? What can be done to reduce air pollution?
3. What causes poor indoor air quality? How does indoor air pollution affect schoolchildren?
4. What are the causes and consequences of global warming?
5. What are point and nonpoint sources of water pollution? What can be done to reduce or prevent water pollution?
6. What are the physiological consequences of noise pollution? What can you do to lessen your exposure to noise pollution?
7. Why do you think so little recycling occurs in the United States?
8. Would you feel comfortable living near a nuclear power plant? Do you think nuclear power will be an important source of energy in the future? Why or why not?

Accessing Your Health on the Internet

Visit the following Internet sites to explore further topics and issues related to personal health. To visit an organization's website, go to the Companion Website for *Access to Health, Ninth Edition* at www.aw-bc.com/donatelle, click on the book image, and select "Accessing Your Health on the Internet" from the navigation menu.

1. *American Cancer Society Environmental Cancer Risks.* Provides a searchable database of information about specific cancers and environmental risks, as well as a risk assessment and information about carcinogens.
2. *Data Online for Population, Health, and Nutrition (DOLPHN) Database.* DOLPHN provides demographic and health trend data relevant to the U.S. Agency for International Development. Subjects include child survival, family planning, access to clean water, and many other subjects.
3. *Environmental Protection Agency.* A source for up-to-date statistics and background information about major risks to health from environmental hazards.
4. *GeoHive.* A resource for general statistics on human population and health-related factors.
5. *National Center for Environmental Health.* A section of the Centers for Disease Control and Prevention, with information on a wide variety of environmental health issues, including a series of helpful fact sheets.
6. *National Environmental Health Association (NEHA).* This organization provides educational resources and opportunities for environmental health professionals. The NEHA website lists conferences, training, and publications and offers informational position papers.

Further Reading

Cayne, B. and J. Tesar. *Food and Water: Threats, Shortages, and Solutions.* New York: Facts on File, 2002.

A basic introduction that discusses the vital importance of having an adequate supply of food and water and the need for alternative water storage and agricultural strategies.

Kennedy, R. F. *Crimes Against Nature: How George W. Bush and His Corporate Pals Are Plundering the Country and Hijacking Our Democracy.* New York: HarperCollins, 2004.

Michaels, P. *Meltdown: The Predictable Distortion of Global Warming by Scientists, Politicians, and the Media.* Washington, DC: Cato Institute, 2004.

These two books offer sharply contrasting perspectives on the environment and public policy and will provoke debate and discussion. The factual basis of the assertions made in both books should be compared to commentary and statistics available from objective sources in the scientific community.

Speth, J. G. *Red Sky at Morning: America and the Crisis of the Global Environment.* New Haven, CT: Yale University Press, 2004.

Overview of major environmental threats to health and projections for the future.

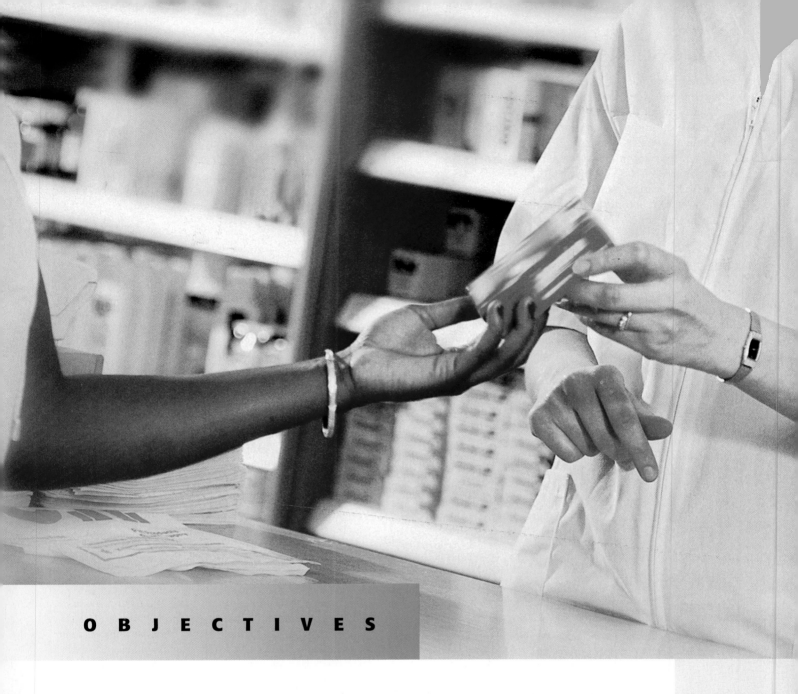

- Explain why responsible consumerism is important to Americans today and how to encourage consumers to take action.

- Explain why self-diagnosis, self-help, and self-care are becoming increasingly important in our quest for health and well-being.

- Compare choices in prescription and over-the-counter drugs and actions that will maximize the benefit received from such drugs.

- Discuss the choices available to Americans who seek health care through allopathic avenues, as well as factors that should be considered in making decisions about health care.

- Describe the U.S. health care system in terms of types of medical practice, provider groups, and the changing structures of managed care and other options.

- Discuss key issues in American health care services in terms of cost, quality, and access to services.

- Discuss the different types of health insurance available in the United States and the role that they play in providing health care.

CONSUMERISM

SELECTING HEALTH CARE PRODUCTS AND SERVICES

IN THE NEWS

At F.D.A., Strong Drug Ties and Less Monitoring

By Gardiner Harris

When federal drug officials suspected in 1992 that a popular allergy pill might cause heart problems, they turned to their own scientists. Their trial confirmed the danger, and the drug was pulled from the market.

Eight years later, similar worries surrounded the arthritis pill Vioxx. But by then, the Food and Drug Administration had shifted gears, slashing its laboratories and network of independent drug safety experts in favor of hiring more people to approve drugs—changes that arose under an unusual agreement that has left the agency increasingly reliant on and bound by drug

company money. Discovering Vioxx's dangers would take four more years.

That delay has led to a firestorm of criticism. Members of Congress, an internal F.D.A. whistleblower and prominent medical journals have said that the agency is incapable of uncovering the perils of drugs that have been approved and are in wide distribution. Some have accused it of being cozy with drug makers.

Dozens of former and current F.D.A. officials, outside scientists and advocates for patients say that the agency's efforts to monitor the ill effects of drugs that are on the market are a shadow of what they should be because the White House and Congress forced a marriage between the agency and industry years ago for the rich dowry that industry offered.

Read the complete article online in the eThemes section of this book's website: www.aw-bc.com/donatelle.

Original article published December 6, 2004. Copyright © 2004 *The New York Times.* Reprinted with permission.

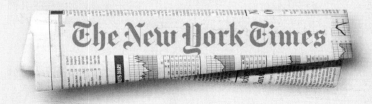

There are many reasons to be an informed health care consumer. Most important, you have only one body—if you don't treat it with care, you will pay a major price in terms of financial costs and health consequences. Doing everything you can to prevent illness, stay healthy, and recover rapidly when you do get sick will enhance every other part of your life.

Here is yet another reason to be an active health consumer: as a citizen or resident of the United States, you have no constitutional right to health care. Our society generally treats health care as a private-consumption good or service to be bought and sold rather than as a social good to which everyone is entitled.

Therefore, to obtain high-quality health care at an affordable cost, you need to be both informed and assertive. However, as you may already know, medical and health care services are much harder to evaluate for need, availability, cost, and quality than are, say, clothes or vegetables. In addition, you may seek health care services in circumstances of physical or emotional distress when your decision-making powers are compromised and you find yourself very vulnerable.

This chapter will help you make better decisions about your health and health care. Our health care system is a maze of health care providers, payers (insurance, government, and individuals), and products, and many of us find it hard to thread our way through it. Health care is the fifth largest industry in our country, accounting for over 10 percent of our workforce, and many different companies aggressively market health products and services to the public. Increasingly, health care organizations are "for-profit" businesses, sold and traded on the stock market, and making a profit is the goal. Both medical professionals and consumers report that they feel overwhelmed, confused, and frustrated by the multitude of choices, seemingly divergent interests, and lack of coordination in our system.

Responsible Consumerism: Choices and Challenges

Perhaps the single greatest difficulty that we face as health consumers is the sheer magnitude of choices. If you try to select a general practitioner from the telephone book, you have to thumb through dozens of pages of specialists. When you want to purchase cough syrup, you are confronted with hundreds of options, each claiming to do more for you than the brand next to it. Even trained pharmacists find it impossible to keep up with the explosion of new drugs and health-related products.

Because there are so many profit-seekers competing for a share of the lucrative health market and because misinformation is so common, wise health consumers use every means at their disposal to ensure that they are acting responsibly and economically. Answer the questions in the Assess

Yourself box to see how you might become a better health care consumer.

Attracting Consumers' Dollars

Today's marketing specialists identify a target audience for a given product and go after it with an arsenal of gimmicks, subtle persuaders, and sophisticated strategies. Different techniques are used to attract new customers, maintain existing customers, and encourage former consumers of the product to come back. Advertisements may present a product as a status symbol or play on inner fears and insecurities, causing you to wonder whether your deodorant is working, your breath is bad, or your skin is greasy.

Whatever your desires or fears, countless products and services are available to meet them. Although some marketing tactics are obvious, others are subtle and difficult to discern. Perfume advertisements that depict passionate embraces and automobile ads that feature expensive sports cars with beautiful young men and women are common. The implied message is that if you purchase a given perfume, your love life will improve, and if you buy that flashy car, attractive people will flock to you.

Many other marketing strategies revolve around "trendy" news items. A good example is the current fascination with the use of herbs to treat the common cold and wearable magnets to treat arthritis and painful joints. Increasingly, these advertising techniques are used for medical products as aggressively as they are for other items.

Putting *Cure* into Perspective

People often fall victim to false health claims because they mistakenly believe that a product or provider has helped them. Frequently this belief arises from two conditions: spontaneous remission and the placebo effect.

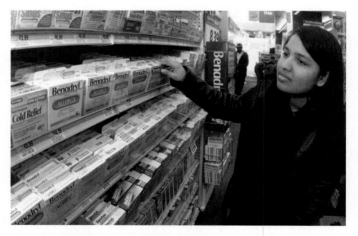

Deciding when to contact a physician can be difficult. Most people first try to diagnose and treat their condition themselves.

Being a Better Health Consumer

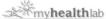

Fill out this assessment online at www.aw-bc.com/myhealthlab or www.aw-bc.com/donatelle

Answer the following questions, and determine what you might do to become a better health consumer.

1. Do you have a physician?
2. Do you have health insurance?
3. Have you determined which services are available free or at a reduced cost in your area? If so, what are they?
4. When you receive a prescription, do you ask the pharmacist if a generic brand could be substituted?
5. Do you ask the pharmacist for potential side-effects before or after the prescription is filled?
6. Do you take medication as directed?
7. Do you report any unusual side effects to your doctor?
8. When you receive a diagnosis, do you seek more information about the diagnosis and treatment?
9. If surgery or an invasive type of treatment is indicated by your doctor, do you seek a second opinion?
10. Where do you find most health information?
11. How do you know this source of information is a reliable and credible source?
12. When you purchase an over-the-counter (OTC) medication, do you read the label?
13. What attracts you most to a new product? (Check all that apply.)
    _____ price
    _____ promises of a new lifestyle
    _____ appears to meet a need
    _____ positive testimonials
    _____ savings or coupons
    _____ spokesperson
    _____ testing for product safety
14. How big a role do you think advertising plays in your decision to purchase a new product?

MAKE IT HAPPEN!

Use the results of this self-assessment to begin your behavior change program. Follow the steps and use the examples on page 641 to complete your Behavior Change Contract, and use these resources to take action.

Spontaneous Remission It is said that if you treat a cold, it will disappear in a week, but if you leave it alone, it will last seven days. A **spontaneous remission** from an ailment refers to the disappearance of symptoms without any apparent cause or treatment. Many illnesses, like the common cold and even back strain, are self-limiting and will improve in time, with or without treatment. Other illnesses, such as multiple sclerosis and some cancers, are characterized by alternating periods of severe symptoms and sudden remissions. People experiencing spontaneous remissions can easily attribute their "cure" to a treatment that in fact had no real effect.

Placebo Effect The **placebo effect** is an apparent cure or improved state of health brought about by a substance, product, or procedure that has no generally recognized therapeutic value. It is not uncommon for patients to report improvements based on what they expect, desire, or were told

would happen after taking simple sugar pills that they believed were powerful drugs. About 10 percent of the population is thought to be exceptionally susceptible to the power of suggestion and may be easy targets for aggressive marketing of products that are really placebos. Although the placebo effect is generally harmless, it does account for the expenditure of millions of dollars on health products and services every year. Megadoses of vitamin C have never been proven to treat cancer, nor do mud baths smooth wrinkled skin.

> **Spontaneous remission** The disappearance of symptoms without any apparent cause or treatment.
>
> **Placebo effect** An apparent cure or improved state of health brought about by a substance or product that has no medicinal value.

People who use placebos when medical treatment is needed increase their risk for health problems. However, those who use low-cost, no-risk placebos and find relief, even for just a short time, should not be criticized.

Taking Responsibility for Your Health Care

As the health care industry has become more sophisticated about seeking your business, so must you become more sophisticated about purchasing its products and services. Learn how, when, and where to enter the massive technological maze that is our health care system without incurring unnecessary risk and expense. Acting responsibly in times of illness can be difficult, but the person best able to act on your behalf is you.

If you are not feeling well, you must first decide whether you really need to seek medical advice. A decade ago, as many as 70 percent of all trips to the doctor and nearly half of all hospital stays were believed to be unnecessary and potentially harmful.[1] These figures have been reduced considerably, however, with the advent of managed care, which carries with it a degree of out-of-pocket shared costs. Theoretically, patients who have to pay for a portion of their care will not seek care unnecessarily. As we will discuss later in this chapter, managed care involves a number of measures designed to keep people out of hospitals and emergency rooms, which are typically the most expensive form of nonemergency health care.[2]

Yet critics of managed care point to cost savings as a part of the problem with quality and access. Not seeking treatment, whether due to high costs or limited coverage, or trying to medicate yourself when more rigorous methods of treatment are needed, is dangerous. Being knowledgeable about the benefits and limits of self-care is critical for responsible consumerism.

Self-Help or Self-Care

A recent concept in health consumerism proposes that the patient is the primary health care provider or first line of defense in health. We can practice behaviors that promote health, prevent disease, and minimize reliance on the formal medical system. We can also interpret basic changes in our own physical and emotional health and treat minor afflictions without seeking professional help. Self-care consists of knowing your body, paying attention to its signals, and taking appropriate action to improve your health and stop the progression of illness or injury.

Common forms of self-care include the following:

- Diagnosing symptoms or conditions that occur frequently but may not need physician visits (for example, colds, minor abrasions)
- Performing breast and testicular self-examinations (monthly)

- Learning first aid for common, uncomplicated injuries and conditions
- Checking blood pressure, pulse, and temperature
- Using home pregnancy and ovulation kits and HIV test kits
- Monitoring cervical mucus for natural family planning
- Doing periodic checks for blood cholesterol
- Using home stool test kits for blood and early colon cancer detection
- Learning from reliable self-help books, tapes, software, websites, and videos
- Benefiting from relaxation techniques, including meditation, nutrition, rest, and exercise

When to Seek Help

Effective self-care also means understanding when to seek professional medical attention rather than treating a condition yourself. Deciding which conditions warrant professional advice is not always easy. Generally, you should consult a physician if you experience *any* of the following:

- A serious accident or injury
- Sudden or severe chest pains causing breathing difficulties
- Trauma to the head or spine accompanied by persistent headache, blurred vision, loss of consciousness, vomiting, convulsions, or paralysis
- Sudden high fever or recurring high temperature (over 102°F for children and 103°F for adults) and/or sweats
- Tingling sensation in the arm accompanied by slurred speech or impaired thought processes
- Adverse reactions to a drug or insect bite (shortness of breath, severe swelling, dizziness)
- Unexplained bleeding or loss of body fluid from any body opening
- Unexplained sudden weight loss
- Persistent or recurrent diarrhea or vomiting
- Blue-colored lips, eyelids, or nail beds
- Any lump, swelling, thickness, or sore that does not subside or that grows for over a month
- Any marked change or pain in bowel or bladder habits
- Yellowing of the skin or the whites of the eyes
- Any symptom that is unusual and recurs over time
- Pregnancy

With the vast array of home diagnostic devices currently available, it seems relatively easy for most people to take care of themselves. But some caution is in order here: although many of these devices are valuable for making an initial diagnosis, home health tests are no substitute for regular, complete examinations by a trained practitioner. The Skills for Behavior Change box offers valuable information about taking an active role in your own health care.

Assessing Health Professionals

Suppose you decide that you do need medical help. You must then identify what type of help you need and where to

Being Proactive in Your Own Health Care

Throughout this book, we have emphasized the importance of healthy preventive behaviors. Sometimes, however, regardless of the steps you take to care for yourself, you still get sick. At such times, it is important that you continue to be actively involved in your care. The more you know about your own body and the factors that can affect your health, the better you will be at communicating with your doctor. It also helps you make informed decisions and recognize when a certain treatment may not be right for you. The following points can help:

- Know your own and your family's medical history.
- Be knowledgeable about your condition—causes, physiological effects, possible treatments, prognosis. Don't rely on the doctor for this information. Do some research.
- Bring a friend or relative along for medical visits to help you review what the doctor says. If you go alone, take notes.
- Ask the practitioner to explain the problem and possible treatments, tests, and drugs in a clear and understandable way. If you don't understand something, ask for clarification.
- If the doctor prescribes any medications, ask whether you can take generic equivalents that cost less.
- Ask for a written summary of the results of your visit and of any lab tests.
- If you have any doubt about the doctor's recommended treatment, seek a second opinion.

- If you will need to take a prescription medication for an extended time, ask for the maximum number of doses allowed by your plan if you have a small pharmacy copayment.

After seeing a health care professional, consider these ideas:

- Write down an accurate account of what happened and what was said. Be sure to include the names of the doctor and all other people involved in your care, the date, and the place.
- Shop around drugstores for the best prices in the same way that you would when shopping for clothes. Be aware that some insurance companies will only pay for part (or even none) of the cost of prescriptions if you do not use pharmacies they recommend.
- When filling prescriptions, ask to see the pharmacist's package inserts that list medical considerations concerning the medicines. Request detailed information about potential drug and food interactions. Make sure the pharmacist is aware of all prescription and nonprescription medications *and* all supplements you are currently using (including dosages).
- Write clear instructions on the label to avoid risk to others who may take the drug in error.

Just like you, doctors are human. Their decisions are based on the best information they have available to them and may be influenced by a number of factors—workload, limited information, personal views. Therefore, in addition to following the practical steps listed above, being proactively involved in your health care also means that you should be aware of

your rights as a patient. Your rights include the following:

- The right of informed consent means that, *before* receiving any care, you should be fully informed of what is being planned, the risks and potential benefits, and possible alternative forms of treatment, including the option of no treatment. Your consent must be voluntary and without any form of coercion. It is critical that you read any consent forms carefully and amend them as necessary before signing.
- You are entitled to know whether the treatment you are receiving is standard or experimental. In experimental conditions, you have the legal and ethical right to know if the study is one in which some people receive treatment while others do not in order to compare the results, and if any drug is being used in the research project for a purpose not approved by the U.S. Food and Drug Administration (FDA).
- You have the right to privacy, which includes the source of payment for treatment and care. It also includes protecting your right to make personal decisions concerning all reproductive matters.
- You have the right to receive care. You also have the legal right to refuse treatment at any time and to cease treatment at any time.
- You are entitled to access all your medical records and to have those records remain confidential.
- You have the right to seek the opinions of other health care professionals regarding your condition.

obtain it. Selecting a professional may seem simple, yet many people have no idea how to assess the qualifications of a health care provider.

Knowledge of both traditional medical specialties and alternative, or complementary, medical treatment is critical to making an intelligent selection. In addition, numerous studies document the importance of good communication skills: the most satisfied patients are those who feel their

physician explains diagnosis and treatment options thoroughly and involves them in decisions regarding their own care.[3]

When selecting from a network of providers, make sure you understand your coverage options and consider the following factors about prospective health care providers:

- What professional educational training have they had? What license or board certification do they hold? Note that there is a difference between "board eligible" and "board certified." *Board certified* indicates that they have passed the national board examination for their specialty (such as pediatrics) and have been certified as competent in that specialty. In contrast, *board eligible* merely means that they are eligible to take the specialty board's exam but have not necessarily passed it.

- Are they affiliated with an accredited medical facility or institution? The Joint Commission on Accreditation of Healthcare Organizations (JCAHO) requires these institutions to verify all education, licensing, and training claims of their affiliated practitioners. What other doctors are in their group, and who will assist in your treatment?
- Are they open to complementary or alternative strategies? Would they refer you for different treatment modalities if appropriate?
- Do they indicate clearly how long a given treatment may last, what side effects you might expect, and what problems you should watch for?
- Are their diagnoses, treatments, and general statements consistent with established scientific theory and practice?
- Who will be responsible for your care when the doctor is on vacation or off call?
- Do they listen to you, respect you as an individual, and give you time to ask questions? Do they return your calls, and are they available to answer questions?

When a doctor orders a test, treatment, or medication, you might ask questions like these:

- How often has the doctor performed this test, surgery, or procedure and with what proportion of successful outcome?
- What are the side effects, and can these side effects be treated or reduced?
- Does this procedure require an overnight stay at a hospital, or can it be performed in a doctor's office?
- Why has this test been ordered? What is the doctor trying to find or exclude?

Asking the right questions at the right time may save you personal suffering and expense. Many patients find that writing their questions down before an appointment helps them get answers to all their questions. You should not accept a defensive or hostile response; asking questions is your right as a patient.

A recent survey found that nearly two-thirds of Americans are confident that the medical information given to them by their doctor is accurate, while the remaining third

opt for a second opinion on important issues or do independent research.[4]

Choices in Health Products: Prescription and Over-the-Counter Drugs

Recall from Chapter 14 that prescription drugs can be obtained only with a written prescription from a physician, while over-the-counter drugs can be purchased without a prescription. Just as making wise decisions about providers is an important aspect of responsible health care, so is making wise decisions about medications. Consider the benefits, risks, and possible interactions related to a given drug.

Prescription Drugs

In about two-thirds of doctor visits, the physician administers or prescribes at least one medication. In fact, prescription drug use has risen by 25 percent over the past decade.[5] Even though these drugs are administered under medical supervision, the wise consumer still takes precautions. Hazards and complications arising from the use of prescription drugs are common. Responsible decision making requires the consumer to acquire basic drug knowledge.

Types of Prescription Drugs Prescription drugs can be divided into dozens of categories. We discuss some of the most common here. Others are explored in the chapters on birth control, infectious and sexually transmitted diseases, cancer, and cardiovascular disease.

Antibiotics are drugs used to fight bacterial infection. Bacterial infections continue to be the most common serious diseases in the United States and throughout the world. The vast majority of these can be cured with antibiotic treatment. There are currently close to 100 different antibiotic drugs used to kill or stop bacterial growth. They may be dispensed by intramuscular injection or in tablet or capsule form. Some, called broad-spectrum antibiotics, are designed to control disease caused by a number of bacterial species. However, these medications may also kill helpful bacteria in the body, thus triggering secondary infections. For example, some vaginal infections are related to long-term use of antibiotics. Other hazards of antibiotic overuse are discussed in Chapter 17.

Sedatives are central nervous system depressants that induce sleep and relieve anxiety. Because of the high incidence of anxiety and sleep disorders in the United States, drugs that encourage relaxation and drowsiness are frequently prescribed. The potential for addiction is high. Detoxification can be life-threatening and must be medically supervised. Because doctors do not prescribe sedatives as frequently as they did in past decades, users often purchase them illegally.

Antibiotics   Prescription drugs designed to fight bacterial infection.

Sedatives   Central nervous system depressants that induce sleep and relieve anxiety.

Tranquilizers, another form of central nervous system depressant, are classified as major and minor tranquilizers. The most powerful tranquilizers are used to treat major psychiatric illnesses. When used appropriately, these strong sedatives can reduce aggressive and self-destructive impulses.

The so-called minor tranquilizers gained much notoriety in the 1970s when consumer groups discovered that these drugs—known by their trade names Valium, Librium, and Miltown—were the most commonly prescribed medications in the United States. They were often prescribed for women who suffered from anxiety. These drugs have a high potential for addiction, and many people became physically and psychologically dependent on them. When the media reported on the widespread and casual prescribing of these drugs, physicians were forced to reevaluate the practice. Today a doctor is more likely to suggest psychotherapy or counseling for patients suffering from anxiety.

Antidepressants are medications typically used to treat major depression, although occasionally they are used to treat other forms of depression that may be resistant to conventional therapy. There are several groups of antidepressant medications approved for use in the United States (Table 22.1). The first to be used to treat depression were monoamine oxidase inhibitors (MAOIs), which were discovered in the 1960s. The most commonly used antidepressants are the tricyclic medications, but perhaps the best known are the selective serotonin reuptake inhibitors or SSRIs, which include the drugs Prozac and Zoloft. Antidepressants are among the three most commonly prescribed classes of drugs. Over the past decade, the use of antidepressant drugs in the United States has increased by 48 percent overall and by 124 percent in children.[6] **Amphetamines** are stimulants that are prescribed less commonly now than in the past. Like many psychoactive drugs, they are purchased both legally and illegally. Amphetamines suppress appetite and elevate respiration, blood pressure, and pulse rate. Ritalin and Cylert are prescription amphetamines that are used to treat attention deficit hyperactivity disorder in children, and Pondimin is used to treat obesity.

Tolerance to these powerful stimulants develops rapidly, and the user trying to cut down or quit may experience unpleasant **rebound effects.** These severe withdrawal symptoms, peculiar to stimulants, include depression, irritability, violent behavior, headaches, nausea, and deep fatigue.

Generic Drugs   Generic drugs, medications sold under a chemical name rather than a brand name, have gained popularity in recent years. They contain the same active ingredients as brand-name drugs, but their price is often less than half that of the brand-name medications. If your doctor prescribes a drug, always ask if a generic equivalent exists and if it would be safe and effective for you to try.

Be aware, though, that there is some controversy about the effectiveness of generic drugs because substitutions are often made in minor ingredients that can affect the way the drug is absorbed, causing discomfort or even an allergic

Table 22.1 Antidepressants	
Type/Generic Name	**Trade Name**
Monoamine Oxidase Inhibitors (MAOIs)	
Phenelzine	Nardil
Tranylcypromine	Parnate
Tricyclic Medications	
Amitriptyline	Elavil, Endep, Tryptanol
Amoxapine	Asendin
Clomipramine	Anafranil
Desipramine	Norpramin, Pertofrane
Doxepin	Adapin, Sinequan
Imipramine	Janimine, Tofranil
Maprotiline	Ludiomil
Nortriptyline	Aventyl, Pamelor
Protriptyline	Concordin, Triptil, Vivactil
Trazodone	Desyrel, Molipaxin
Trimipramine	Surmontil
Selective Serotonin Reuptake Inhibitors (SSRIs)	
Citalopram	Cipramil
Fluoxetine	Prozac
Fluvoxamine	Luvox
Paroxetine	Paxil
Sertraline	Lustral, Zoloft
Other Antidepressants	
Bupropion	Wellbutrin
Nefazodone	Serzone
Venlafaxine	Effexor

reaction in some users. Always note any reactions you have to medications and tell your doctor. Also, not all drugs are available as generics.

Over-the-Counter Drugs

Over-the-counter (OTC) drugs are nonprescription substances we use in the course of self-diagnosis and self-medication. More than one-third of the time people treat their own health

Tranquilizers   Central nervous system depressants that relax the body and calm anxiety.

Antidepressants   Prescription drugs used to treat clinically diagnosed depression.

Amphetamines   Prescription stimulants not commonly used today because of the dangers associated with them.

Rebound effects   Severe withdrawal effects experienced by users of stimulants, including depression, nausea, and violent behavior.

Generic drugs   Drugs marketed by chemical name rather than brand name.

The Debate over Rapid Drug Approval

In 1993, the Food and Drug Administration (FDA) changed its policies to speed the approval process of new drugs. These changes were made for humanitarian reasons, in response to activists seeking rapid approval of experimental drugs that offered at least a ray of hope to AIDS patients who otherwise faced certain death. The "accelerated development/review" process can be used for drugs that appear to offer significant improvement over existing treatments or that could benefit life-threatening illnesses for which no treatment currently exists.

Hundreds of new drugs have been approved for OTC status since then. Of that number, seven have been withdrawn after reports of deaths and severe side effects. Examples of drugs that have been placed on the pharmacy shelves as a result of the FDA's more lenient approach—but have yielded fatal results—include Redux and Lotronex. The diet pill Redux, approved despite an advisory committee's vote against it, was taken off the shelves after one year when several patients taking it developed heart-valve damage. Lotronex, a drug for treating irritable bowel syndrome, was approved despite warnings. It has now been linked to five deaths, the removal of one patient's colon, and other bowel surgeries. Lotronex was pulled from the market after only ten months.

Reports of adverse drug reactions made to the FDA are considered by public health officials to be the most reliable early warning that a product may be dangerous. The reports are filed to the FDA by health professionals, consumers, and drug manufacturers. These reports become part of the "Adverse Event Reporting System" database, which is monitored by clinical reviewers for early signs of safety problems. This information is also made available 24 hours a day to health care professionals. More than 250,000 side effects linked to prescription drugs, including injuries and deaths, are reported each year. However, since these adverse-event reports are voluntary, experts, including Dr. Brian L. Strom, chair of epidemiology at the University of Pennsylvania, believe they represent only 1 to 10 percent of all such events. "There is no incentive at all for a physician to report [an adverse drug reaction]," said Strom, who has documented the process. "The underreporting is vast."

To be sure, many events—some of them outside FDA control—can affect the safe use of a prescription drug. A lapse at any of the following steps could prove dangerous:

- The companies' conduct of clinical studies
- The FDA's regulatory actions
- The doctor's decision to prescribe
- The pharmacist's filling of a handwritten prescription
- The patient's ability and willingness to take the drug as directed

Even if all these steps proceed normally, there is still the potential for interactions with foods or other medicines. The patient's state of health is also a factor, since underlying health problems could make almost any drug more risky.

When serious side effects emerge, FDA officials have championed using package labeling to warn of potential risks. Yet the agency typically has no way to know if the labels—dense, lengthy, and in tiny print—are read or followed by doctors and their patients. The FDA often addresses unresolved safety questions by asking companies to conduct studies after the product is approved. However, this research frequently has not been performed.

To address this lack of follow-through, the inspector general of the Department of Health and Human Services issued the following statement: "The FDA can move to withdraw drugs from the market if the post-marketing studies are not completed with due diligence." However, since that time the FDA has not withdrawn any drug because of a company's failure to complete a postapproval safety study.

What standards should the FDA use in deciding whether a drug can be sold over the counter? Are current standards too strict or too lenient? Explain your answer. How might consumers benefit from a rapid drug approval process? What assumptions has the FDA made about the way consumers use drug labels?

Sources: Center for Drug Evaluation and Research, "Adverse Event Reporting System (AERS)," August 7, 2002, www.fda.gov/cder /aers/default.htm; U.S. Food and Drug Administration, "Accelerated Development /Review," www.fda.gov/cder/handbook /accel.htm; "How a New Policy Led to Seven Deadly Drugs," David Willman, *Los Angeles Times,* December 20, 2000. Reprinted by permission of Tribune Media Services International.

problems with OTC medications. Self-care for many of us results from eagerness to save money and time on an office visit to the physician. We therefore diagnose our own illnesses and go to the nearest discount pharmacy to stock up on the latest and best-advertised cure for what we think ails us.

In fact, American consumers spend billions of dollars yearly on OTC preparations for relief of everything from runny noses to ingrown toenails. There are 40,000 OTC drugs and more than 300,000 brand names for those drugs. Most of these products are manufactured from a basic group of 1,000 chemicals. The many different OTC drugs available to us are produced by combining as few as two and as many as ten substances.

How Prescription Drugs Become OTC Drugs The U.S. Food and Drug Administration (FDA) regularly reviews prescription drugs to evaluate how suitable they would be as OTC products. (See the Health Ethics box.) Typically, these are drugs for conditions that consumers can diagnose readily and manage themselves and for which clear, understandable directions can be included. For a drug to be switched from prescription to OTC status, it must meet the following criteria:

1. The drug has been marketed as a prescription medication for at least three years.
2. The use of the drug has been relatively high during the time it was available as a prescription drug.
3. Adverse drug reactions are not alarming, potential adverse effects are printed on the drug label, and the frequency of side effects has not increased during the time it was available to the public.

Since this policy has been in effect, the FDA has switched hundreds of drugs from prescription to OTC status. Some examples are the analgesic/anti-inflammatory medicines ibuprofen (Advil, Nuprin) and naproxen sodium (Aleve), the antihistamine Benadryl, the vaginal antifungal Gyne-Lotrimin, the bronchodilator Bronkaid Mist, the hydrocortisone Cortaid, and the allergy reliever Claritin. Many more prescription drugs are currently being considered for OTC status.

Types of OTC Drugs The FDA has categorized 26 types of OTC preparations. Those most commonly used are analgesics, cold/cough/allergy and asthma relievers, stimulants, sleeping aids and relaxants, and dieting aids.

Analgesics We spend more than $2 billion annually on **analgesics** (pain relievers), the largest sales category of OTC drugs in the United States. Although these pain relievers come in several forms, aspirin, acetaminophen (Tylenol, Pamprin, Panadol), and ibuprofen-like drugs such as naproxen (Aleve) and ketoprofen (Orudis) are the most common.

Most pain relievers work at receptor sites by interrupting pain signals. Some are categorized as NSAIDs (nonsteroidal anti-inflammatory drugs), also called **prostaglandin inhibitors.** Prostaglandins are chemicals that resemble hormones and are released by the body in response to pain. (Scientists believe that the additional pain caused by the release of prostaglandins signals the body to begin the healing process.) Prostaglandin inhibitors restrain the release of prostaglandins, thereby reducing the pain. Common NSAIDs include ibuprofen (including Motrin), naproxen sodium (such as Anaprox), and aspirin.

In addition to relieving pain, aspirin lowers fever by increasing the flow of blood to the skin surface, which causes sweating, thereby cooling the body. Aspirin has also long been used to reduce the inflammation and swelling associated with arthritis. Recently it has been discovered that aspirin's anticoagulant (interference with blood clotting) effects make it useful for reducing the risk of heart attack and stroke.

Although aspirin has been popular for nearly a century, it is not as harmless as many people think. Possible side effects—for it and many other NSAIDS—include allergic reactions, ringing in the ears, stomach bleeding, and ulcers. Combining aspirin with alcohol can compound aspirin's gastric irritant properties. As with all drugs, read the labels. Some analgesic labels caution against driving or operating heavy machinery when using the drug, and most warn that analgesics should not be taken with alcohol.

In addition, research has linked aspirin to a potentially fatal condition called Reye's syndrome. Children, teenagers, and young adults (up to age 19) who are treated with aspirin while recovering from the flu or chicken pox are at risk for developing the syndrome. Aspirin substitutes are recommended for people in these age groups.

Acetaminophen is an aspirin substitute found in Tylenol and related medications. Like aspirin, acetaminophen is an effective analgesic and antipyretic (fever-reducing drug). It does not, however, relieve inflamed or swollen joints. The side effects associated with acetaminophen are generally minimal, though overdose can cause liver damage.

Several analgesics are available as prescription or OTC drugs. Generally, the OTC drugs (for example, Nuprin, Advil, and Aleve) are milder versions of the prescription varieties. Aleve's main distinction is its lasting effect: while other analgesics must be taken every 4 to 6 hours, once every 8 to 12 hours is sufficient for Aleve.

Cold, Cough, Allergy, and Asthma Relievers **The operative word** in this category is *reliever*. Most of these medications are designed to alleviate the uncomfortable symptoms associated with maladies of the upper respiratory tract, but no drugs exist to cure the actual diseases. The drugs available provide only temporary relief until the sufferer's immune system prevails over the disease. Aspirin or acetaminophen is used in some cold preparations, as are several other ingredients. Both aspirin and acetaminophen are on the government's lists of medications that are Generally Recognized as Safe **(GRAS)** and Generally Recognized as Effective **(GRAE).**

Basic types of OTC cold, cough, and allergy relievers include the following:

- *Expectorants.* These drugs are formulated to loosen phlegm, allowing the user to cough it up and clear congested respiratory passages. GRAS and GRAE reviewers question the effectiveness of many expectorants. In addition, when combined with other medications, particularly among frail or very ill individuals, safety issues may arise.

Analgesics Pain relievers.

Prostaglandin inhibitors Drugs that inhibit the production and release of prostaglandins associated with arthritis or menstrual pain.

GRAS list A list of drugs generally recognized as safe, which seldom cause side effects when used properly.

GRAE list A list of drugs generally recognized as effective, which work for their intended purpose when used properly.

- *Antitussives.* These OTC drugs calm or curtail the cough reflex. They are most effective when the cough is "dry," or does not produce phlegm. Oral codeine, dextromethorphan, and diphenhydramine are the most common antitussives that are on both the GRAE and GRAS lists.
- *Antihistamines.* These central nervous system depressants dry runny noses, clear postnasal drip, clear sinus congestion, and reduce tears.
- *Decongestants.* These remedies reduce nasal stuffiness due to colds.
- *Anticholinergics.* These substances are often added to cold preparations to reduce nasal secretions and tears. None of the preparations tested was found to be GRAE/GRAS. Some cold compounds can make users extremely drowsy, and some contain alcohol in concentrations that may exceed 40 percent.

Stimulants   College students who have neglected assignments and other obligations until the last minute sometimes use OTC stimulants. The active ingredient in these stimulants is caffeine, which heightens wakefulness, increases alertness, and relieves fatigue. None of the OTC stimulants has been judged GRAS or GRAE.

Sleeping Aids and Relaxants   A study by the World Health Organization, conducted in 15 health centers around the globe, found that 27 percent of patients reported difficulties with sleeping. A U.S. survey found that 10 percent of American adults experienced chronic insomnia.[7] Many people routinely treat their insomnia with OTC sleep aids (such as Nytol, Sleep-Eze, and Sominex) that are advertised as providing a "safe and restful" sleep. These drugs are used to induce the drowsy feelings that precede sleep. The principal ingredient in OTC sleeping aids is an antihistamine called pyrilamine maleate. Chronic reliance on sleeping aids may lead to addiction; people accustomed to using these products may eventually find it impossible to sleep without them.

Dieting Aids   In the United States, there is a $200 million market for dieting aids. Some of these drugs (such as Acutrim and Dexatrim) are advertised as "appetite suppressants." The FDA has pulled several appetite suppressants off the market because their active ingredient was phenylpropanolamine (PPA), which is a **sympathomimetic** (affecting the sympathetic nervous system). This causes reactions similar to those experienced when angry or excited, such as dry mouth and lack of appetite. PPA has been linked to increased risk of stroke.[8]

Estimates show that, when taken as recommended, even the best OTC dieting aids significantly reduce appetite in less than 30 percent of users, and tolerance occurs in only one to three days of use. Manufacturers of appetite suppressants often include a written 1,200-calorie diet to complement their drug. However, most people who limit themselves to 1,200 calories per day will lose weight—without any help from appetite suppressants. Clearly, these products have no value in treating obesity.

Some people rely on **laxatives** and **diuretics** ("water pills") to lose weight. Frequent use of laxatives disrupts the body's natural elimination patterns and may cause constipation or even *obstipation* (inability to have a bowel movement). The use of laxatives to produce weight loss has generally unspectacular results and robs the body of needed fluids, salts, and minerals. Abuse of laxatives is associated with eating disorders (Chapter 9).

Taking diuretics to lose weight is also dangerous. Not only will the user gain the weight back upon drinking fluids, but diuretic use may contribute to dangerous chemical imbalances. The potassium and sodium eliminated by diuretics play important roles in maintaining electrolyte balance. Depletion of these vital minerals may cause weakness, dizziness, fatigue, and sometimes death. (See Table 22.2 for side effects of other OTC drugs.)

Rules for Proper OTC Drug Use   Despite a common belief that OTC products are safe and effective, indiscriminate use and abuse can occur with these drugs as with all others. For example, people who frequently drop medication into their eyes to "get the red out" or pop antacids after every meal are likely to become dependent. Many people also experience adverse side effects because they ignore warning labels or simply do not read them. The FDA has developed a standard label that appears on most OTC products (Figure 22.1 on page 628). It provides directions for use, warnings, and other useful information. (Diet supplements, which are regulated as food products, have their own type of label that includes a Supplements Facts panel.)

OTC medications are far more powerful than ever before, and the science behind them is stronger as well. Most of us are self-medicators at one time or another. We find it easier to function, for example, if the headache and stuffiness of the common cold do not interfere with our studies or work. Most of us can use OTC products safely with adequate precautions, but for some people, OTCs can be as toxic as the most dangerous chemicals. Therefore, before you use any type of medication, do your homework. Observe the following rules when taking nonprescription drugs:

1. Always know what you are taking. Identify the active ingredients in the product.
2. Know the effects. Be sure you know both the desired and potentially undesired effects of each active ingredient.
3. Read the warnings and cautions.
4. Don't use anything for longer than one or two weeks. If your symptoms persist, consult a doctor.

Sympathomimetics   Drugs found in appetite suppressants that affect the sympathetic nervous system.

Laxatives   Medications used to soften stool and relieve constipation.

Diuretics   Drugs that increase the excretion of urine from the body.

Table 22.2
Some Side Effects of OTC Drugs

Drug	Possible Hazards
Acetaminophen	• Bloody urine, painful urination, skin rash, bleeding and bruising, yellowing of the eyes or skin (even for normal doses) • Difficulty in diagnosing overdose because reaction may be delayed up to a week • Liver damage from chronic low-level use
Antacids	• Reduced mineral absorption from food • Possible concealment of ulcer • Reduction of effectiveness for anticlotting medications • Prevention of certain antibiotics' functioning (for antacids that contain aluminum) • Worsening of high blood pressure (for antacids that contain sodium) • Aggravation of kidney problems
Aspirin	• Stomach upset and vomiting, stomach bleeding, worsening of ulcers • Enhancement of the action of anticlotting medications • Potentiation of hearing damage from loud noise • Severe allergic reaction • Association with Reye's syndrome in children and teenagers • Prolonged bleeding time (when combined with alcohol)
Cold medications	• Loss of consciousness (if taken with prescription tranquilizers)
Diet pills, caffeine, decongestants	• Organ damage or death from cerebral hemorrhage
Ibuprofen	• Allergic reaction in some people with aspirin allergy • Fluid retention or edema • Liver damage similar to that from acetaminophen • Enhancement of action of anticlotting medications • Digestive disturbances (half as often as with aspirin)
Laxatives	• Reduced absorption of minerals from food • Creation of dependency
Naproxen sodium	• Potential digestive tract bleeding • Possible stomach cramps or ulcers
Toothache medications	• Destruction of the still-healthy part of a damaged tooth (for medications that contain clove oil)

5. Be particularly cautious if you are also taking prescription drugs.
6. If you have questions, ask your pharmacist.
7. *If you don't need it, don't take it!*

Drug Interactions   Sharing medications, using outdated prescriptions, taking higher doses than recommended, or using medications as a substitute for dealing with personal problems may result in serious health consequences. But so may **polydrug use:** taking several medications or illegal drugs simultaneously may result in very dangerous problems associated with drug interactions. The most hazardous interactions are synergism, antagonism, inhibition, and intolerance. Hazardous interactions may also occur between drugs and foods and beverages (see Table 22.3 for common drug–nutrient interactions).

Synergism, also known as potentiation, is an interaction of two or more drugs in which the effects of the individual drugs are multiplied beyond what would normally be expected if they were taken alone—rather like saying 1 + 1 = 6. A synergistic interaction is most likely to occur when *central nervous system depressants* are combined. Included in this category are alcohol, opiates (morphine, heroin), antihistamines (cold remedies), sedative hypnotics (Quaalude), minor tranquilizers (Valium, Librium, and Xanax), and barbiturates. The worst possible combination is alcohol and barbiturates (sleeping preparations such as Seconal and phenobarbital) because combining these depressants slows down the brain centers that normally control vital functions. Respiration, heart rate, and blood pressure can drop to the point of inducing coma and even death.

Polydrug use   The use of multiple medications or illicit drugs simultaneously.

Synergism   An interaction of two or more drugs that produces more profound effects than would be expected if the drugs were taken separately.

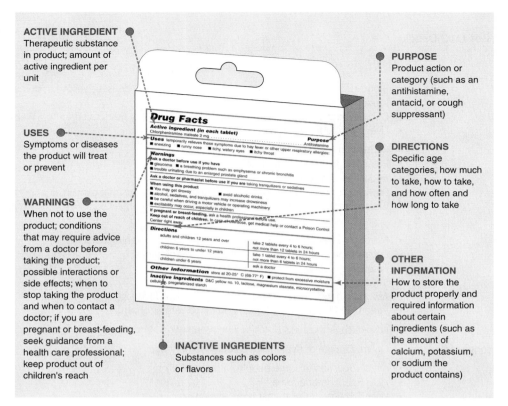

ACTIVE INGREDIENT
Therapeutic substance in product; amount of active ingredient per unit

USES
Symptoms or diseases the product will treat or prevent

WARNINGS
When not to use the product; conditions that may require advice from a doctor before taking the product; possible interactions or side effects; when to stop taking the product and when to contact a doctor; if you are pregnant or breast-feeding, seek guidance from a health care professional; keep product out of children's reach

INACTIVE INGREDIENTS
Substances such as colors or flavors

PURPOSE
Product action or category (such as an antihistamine, antacid, or cough suppressant)

DIRECTIONS
Specific age categories, how much to take, how to take, and how often and how long to take

OTHER INFORMATION
How to store the product properly and required information about certain ingredients (such as the amount of calcium, potassium, or sodium the product contains)

Drug Facts

Active ingredient (in each tablet)
Chlorpheniramine maleate 2 mg .... **Purpose** Antihistamine

Uses temporarily relieves those symptoms due to hay fever or other upper respiratory allergies:
■ sneezing ■ runny nose ■ itchy, watery eyes ■ itchy throat

Warnings
Ask a doctor before use if you have
■ glaucoma ■ a breathing problem such as emphysema or chronic bronchitis
■ trouble urinating due to an enlarged prostate gland
Ask a doctor or pharmacist before use if you are taking tranquilizers or sedatives
When using this product
■ You may get drowsy   ■ avoid alcoholic drinks
■ alcohol, sedatives, and tranquilizers may increase drowsiness
■ be careful when driving a motor vehicle or operating machinery
■ excitability may occur, especially in children
If pregnant or breast-feeding, ask a health professional before use.
Keep out of reach of children. In case of overdose, get medical help or contact a Poison Control Center right away.

Directions
adults and children 12 years and over	take 2 tablets every 4 to 6 hours; not more than 12 tablets in 24 hours
children 6 years to under 12 years	take 1 tablet every 4 to 6 hours; not more than 6 tablets in 24 hours
children under 6 years	ask a doctor

Other information store at 20-25° C (68-77° F) ■ protect from excessive moisture
Inactive ingredients D&C yellow no. 10, lactose, magnesium stearate, microcrystalline cellulose, pregelatinized starch

Figure 22.1
The New Over-the-Counter Medicine Label

Source: Consumer Healthcare Products Association, "The New Over-the-Counter Medicine Label," 2002. Reprinted by permission.

Prescription and OTC drugs carry labels warning the user not to combine the drug with certain other drugs or with alcohol. Because the dangers associated with synergism are so great, you should always verify any possible drug interactions before using a prescribed or OTC drug. Pharmacists, physicians, drug information centers, or community drug education centers can answer your questions. Even if one of the drugs in question is an illegal substance, you should still attempt to determine the dangers involved in combining it with other drugs. Health care professionals are legally bound to maintain confidentiality even when they know that a client is using illegal substances.

Antagonism A type of interaction in which two or more drugs work at the same receptor site.

Inhibition A type of interaction in which the effects of one drug are eliminated or reduced by the presence of another drug at the receptor site.

Intolerance A type of interaction in which two or more drugs produce extremely uncomfortable symptoms.

Cross-tolerance The development of a tolerance to one drug that reduces the effects of another, similar drug.

Antagonism, although not usually as serious as synergism, can produce unwanted and unpleasant effects. In an antagonistic reaction, drugs work at the same receptor site so that one drug blocks the action of the other. The "blocking" drug occupies the receptor site and prevents the other drug from attaching, thus altering its absorption and action.

With **inhibition,** the effects of one drug are eliminated or reduced by the presence of another drug at the receptor site. One common inhibitory reaction occurs between antacid tablets and aspirin. The antacid inhibits the absorption of aspirin, making it less effective as a pain reliever. Other inhibitory reactions occur between alcohol and contraceptive pills and between antibiotics and contraceptive pills. Both alcohol and antibiotics may make birth control pills less effective.

Intolerance occurs when drugs combine in the body to produce extremely uncomfortable reactions. The drug Antabuse, used to help alcoholics give up alcohol, works by producing this type of interaction. It binds liver enzymes (the chemicals the liver produces to break down alcohol), making it impossible for the body to metabolize alcohol. As a result, an Antabuse user who drinks alcohol experiences nausea, vomiting, and, occasionally, fever.

Cross-tolerance occurs when a person develops a physiological tolerance to one drug and shows a similar tolerance to selected other drugs as a result. Taking one medication

Table 22.3
Foods and Drugs That Don't Mix

Drugs	Common Brands	Effects and Precautions
Allergy and Cold Medications		
Antihistamines	Benadryl, Allegra, Claritin, Zyrtec, Chlor-trimeton, Tavist, Dimetane	Antihistamines should be taken on an empty stomach to increase their effectiveness. Avoid alcohol; some antihistamines may increase drowsiness and slow mental function and motor performance when taken with alcohol.
Antibiotics		
Erythromycin	ERYC, Erythrocot, Erythrocin	Best taken with water. Fruit juice, vegetable juice, and soda may interfere with drug absorption.
Sulfonamides	Bactrin, Septra	Long-term therapy may cause a deficiency in folic acid; talk with your doctor about adding a multivitamin or folate-rich foods to your diet. Take on empty stomach 1 hour before or 2 hours after meal.
Tetracycline	Vibramycin, Minocin, Achromycin, Sumycin	Dairy products and other foods rich in calcium may interfere with drug absorption. Take on empty stomach 1 hour before or 2 hours after meal.
Analgesics		
Acetaminophen	Tylenol	Avoid or limit the use of alcohol because chronic alcohol use can increase the risk of liver damage or stomach bleeding.
Nonsteroidal Anti-Inflammatory Drugs (NSAIDs)		
Aspirin, ibuprofen, naproxen, celecoxib, nabumetone	Bayer, Motrin, Advil, Aleve, Ecotrin, Relafen, Anaprox, Naprosyn	Because these medications can irritate the stomach, it is best to take them with food or milk. Avoid or limit the use of alcohol; chronic alcohol use can increase the risk of liver damage or stomach bleeding.
Antidepressants		
Paroxetine, sertraline, fluoxetine, citalopram	Paxil, Zoloft, Prozac, Celexa	Individuals taking these drugs should avoid the use of alcohol.
Monoamine Oxidase Inhibitors (MAOIs)		
Phenelzine, tranylcypromine	Nardil, Parnate	Foods high in tyramine should be avoided. Check with physician for complete list; examples include Parmesan cheese, cured meats, avocados, caffeine-containing products, alcoholic beverages, and nonalcoholic beer and wine.
Hormone Preparations		
Oral contraceptives	Demulen, Loestrin, Triphasil	Salty foods increase fluid retention. Increase intake of foods high in calcium, vitamin K, potassium, and protein to avoid deficiencies.
Steroids	Cortef, Deltasone, Prednisone, Sterapred	Salty foods increase fluid retention. Increase intake of foods high in calcium, vitamin K, potassium, and protein to avoid deficiencies.
Thyroid drugs	Tapazole	Avoid taking with iodine-rich foods, which can reduce the drug's efficacy.
Laxatives		
Mineral Oil	Lansoyl, Liqui-Doss, Magnolax	Frequent use can lead to deficiency in vitamins A, D, E, and K.

Source: Adapted in part from "Food and Drug Interactions," National Consumers League, 2000.

may actually increase the body's tolerance to another. For example, cross-tolerance can develop between alcohol and barbiturates, two depressant drugs.

What do you think?

What are some situations in which students misuse drugs? ■ *Other than alcohol, which drugs (prescription or OTC) do students tend to abuse while they are at college?*

Women and Medications

Women menstruate, can become pregnant, and go through menopause. These normal conditions all affect how women's bodies react to medication. On average, women take more prescription and nonprescription medications than do men. For these reasons, women should be especially concerned about which substances they take and about how and when they take them.

Many women use oral contraceptives, commonly known as "the pill." Failure to take the pill each day can

Table 22.4
Allopathic/Traditional Medical Professionals

Allergist	A specialist who diagnoses and treats allergies
Anesthesiologist	A specialist who administers drugs during surgical procedures to reduce pain or induce unconsciousness
Cardiologist	A specialist in the diagnosis and treatment of heart and blood vessel disorders
Dermatologist	A specialist in the diagnosis and treatment of skin disorders
Dietitian	A specialist in the field of diet and human nutrition
Endocrinologist	A specialist in the diagnosis and treatment of glandular disorders
Family practitioner	A physician who offers routine medical service for a variety of ailments
Gastroenterologist	A specialist who diagnoses and treats disorders of the stomach and intestinal tract
Hematologist	A specialist who diagnoses and treats blood-related disorders
Internist	A specialist who diagnoses and treats disorders of the internal organs
Neurologist	A specialist who diagnoses and treats diseases of the brain, nervous system, and spinal cord
Nurse practitioner	Nurse specialist with additional training in a specific area, such as OB-Gyn
Obstetrician-gynecologist (OB-Gyn)	A specialist who diagnoses and treats problems of the female reproductive system
Oncologist	A specialist who diagnoses and treats cancerous growths and tumors
Orthopedist and orthopedic surgeon	Specialists who diagnose, treat, and/or provide surgical care for bone and joint injuries and problems
Otolaryngologist	A specialist who treats ear, nose, and throat disorders
Pediatrician	A physician who treats childhood diseases
Physical therapist	A specialist who rehabilitates people after impairment due to injury or disease
Plastic surgeon	A specialist who provides corrective surgery for irregularities of body or facial contours
Podiatrist	A specialist who diagnoses and treats disorders of the feet
Pulmonary specialist	A specialist who diagnoses and treats disorders of the respiratory system
Radiologist	A specialist in the diagnosis of disease by using x rays and other imaging techniques
Rheumatologist	A specialist who diagnoses and treats medical conditions of joints and surrounding tissues
Urologist	A specialist who diagnoses and treats disorders of the urinary tract

result in pregnancy, yet 25 percent of women on the pill miss or skip days. Women may also become pregnant accidentally because some medicines—such as penicillin, some sleeping pills, tuberculosis drugs, and anxiety medicines—can keep oral contraceptives from working. When a woman is prescribed a new medication, she should inform her health care provider that she is on the pill.

A woman should also inform her physician if she is taking any medication while pregnant or breastfeeding. Medications taken during these times may be passed to her fetus or baby, and some can severely affect the developmental process, resulting in physical or mental impairments or even death. The physician may be able to prescribe a different drug or a different way to take the medication that will not affect the fetus or baby.

Choices in Medical Care

How can you choose the best health care provider for your needs? Familiarize yourself with the various health professions and subspecialties (see the list in Table 22.4). These professionals all subscribe to allopathic medical procedures. Most people believe that **allopathic medicine,** or traditional Western medical practice, is based on scientifically validated methods, but be aware that not all allopathic treatments have undergone the extensive clinical trials and long-term studies of outcomes that

are necessary to conclusively prove effectiveness in different populations. Even when studies appear to support the health benefits of a particular treatment or product, other studies with equal or better scientific validity often refute these claims. Also, what is recommended treatment today may change dramatically in the future as new technology and medical advances replace older practices. Like other professionals, medical doctors are only as good as their training, continuing knowledge acquisition, and resources allow them to be. A "consumer beware" attitude is always prudent, especially when making critical health care decisions.

Traditional Western (Allopathic) Medicine

Selecting a **primary care practitioner**—a medical practitioner whom you can visit for routine ailments, preventive care, general medical advice, and appropriate referrals—is not an easy task. The primary care practitioner for most people is a family practitioner, an internist, a pediatrician, or an obstetrician-gynecologist. Many people routinely see nurse practitioners or physician assistants who work for an individual doctor or a medical group, and others use nontraditional providers as their primary source of care.

Active participation in your own treatment is the only sensible course in a health care environment that encourages "defensive medicine." In a recent survey, 91 percent of U.S.

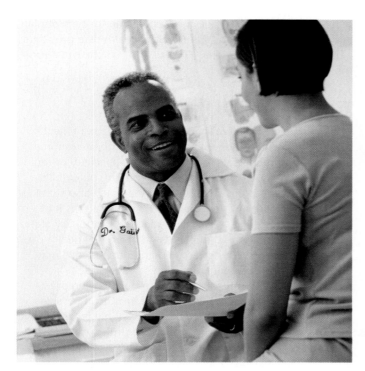

It is important to have an open and honest relationship with your health care provider. Asking questions and providing accurate information will help you make the best decisions about your medical treatment.

physicians admitted they sometimes order unnecessary medical tests because they are concerned about being sued for malpractice. Approximately 50 percent of physicians have ordered unnecessary invasive procedures such as tissue biopsies, and 41 percent have prescribed unneeded drugs such as antibiotics.[9] Unnecessary drugs and procedures do not improve health outcomes, and in some cases they may even create new health problems.

Informed consent refers to your right to have explained to you—in nontechnical language you can understand—all possible side effects, benefits, and consequences of a procedure, as well as available alternatives to it. It also means that you have the right to refuse a treatment and to seek a second or even third opinion from unbiased, noninvolved providers.[10]

What do you think?

Have you ever opted for a treatment other than what was recommended by your allopathic medical provider? ■ *What was the response?* ■ *Did your health insurer cooperate fully and pay the bill?*

Other Allopathic Specialties

Although Table 22.4 provides an overview of common sources of health care, it is by no means all-inclusive. Other specialists include **osteopaths,** general practitioners who

receive training similar to a medical doctor's but who place special emphasis on the skeletal and muscular systems. Their treatments may involve manipulation of the muscles and joints. Osteopaths receive the degree of doctor of osteopathy (DO) rather than doctor of medicine (MD).

Much confusion exists about the roles of ophthalmologists and optometrists. An **ophthalmologist** holds a medical degree and can perform surgery and prescribe medications. An **optometrist** typically evaluates visual problems and fits glasses but is not a trained physician. If you have an eye infection, glaucoma, or other eye condition needing diagnosis and treatment, you need to see an ophthalmologist.

Dentists are specialists who diagnose and treat diseases of the teeth, gums, and oral cavity. They attend dental school for four years and receive the title of doctor of dental surgery (DDS) or doctor of medical dentistry (DMD). They must also pass both state and national board examinations before receiving their licenses to practice. The field of dentistry includes many specialties. For example, **orthodontists** are specialists in the alignment of teeth. **Oral surgeons** perform surgical procedures to correct problems of the mouth, face, and jaw.

Nurses are highly trained and strictly regulated health practitioners who provide a wide range of services for patients and their families, including patient education, counseling, community health and disease prevention information, and

Allopathic medicine   Traditional, Western medical practice; in theory, based on scientifically validated methods and procedures.

Primary care practitioner   A medical practitioner who treats routine ailments, advises on preventive care, gives general medical advice, and makes appropriate referrals when necessary.

Osteopath   General practitioner who receives training similar to a medical doctor's but with an emphasis on the skeletal and muscular systems, often using spinal manipulation as part of treatment.

Ophthalmologist   Physician who specializes in the medical and surgical care of the eyes, including prescriptions for glasses.

Optometrist   Eye specialist whose practice is limited to prescribing and fitting lenses.

Dentist   Specialist who diagnoses and treats diseases of the teeth, gums, and oral cavity.

Orthodontist   Dentist who specializes in the alignment of teeth.

Oral surgeon   Dentist who performs surgical procedures to correct problems of the mouth, jaw, and face.

Nurse   Health practitioner who provides many services for patients and who may work in a variety of settings.

administration of medications. They may choose from several training options. There are over 2.4 million licensed registered nurses (RN) in the United States who have completed either a four-year program leading to a bachelor of science in nursing (BSN) degree or a two-year associate degree program. More than half a million lower-level licensed practical or vocational nurses (LPN or LVN) have completed a one- to two-year training program, which may be community college–based or hospital-based.

Nurse practitioners (NP) are professional nurses having advanced training obtained through either a master's degree program or a specialized nurse practitioner program. Nurse practitioners have the training and authority to conduct diagnostic tests and prescribe medications (in some states). They work in a variety of settings, particularly in HMOs (health maintenance organizations), clinics, and student health centers. Nurses may also earn the clinical doctor of nursing degree (ND) or doctor of nursing science (DNS and DNSc), or a research-based PhD in nursing.

More than 30,000 **physician assistants** (PA) currently practice in the United States. Most of these are in office-based practices, including school health centers, but approximately 40 percent practice in areas where physicians are in short supply. Studies have shown that this relatively new class of midlevel practitioners may competently care for the majority of patients seeking primary care. All physician assistants must work under the supervision of a licensed physician, and they are legally permitted to prescribe drugs in 47 states.[11]

Health Care Organizations, Programs, and Facilities

Today, managed care is the dominant health payer system in the United States. Because of this, many people are restricted in their choice of a health care provider. Selective contracting between insurers or employers and health providers has limited the freedom of choice that some Americans previously enjoyed under a fee-for-service system. Two critical decisions

---

Physician assistant   A midlevel practitioner trained to handle most standard cases of care.

Group practice   A group of physicians who combine resources, sharing offices, equipment, and staff costs, to render care to patients.

Solo practitioner   Physician who renders care to patients independently of other practitioners.

Nonprofit (voluntary) hospitals   Hospitals run by religious or other humanitarian groups that reinvest their earnings in the hospital to improve health care.

For-profit (proprietary) hospitals   Hospitals that provide a return on earnings to the investors who own them.

---

to make are (1) choosing an insurance carrier or type of plan, and then (2) choosing from among the health care providers who participate in that plan. This section lists the most common choices.

Types of Medical Practices

In the highly competitive market for patients, many health care providers have found it essential to combine resources into a **group practice,** which can be single-specialty or multi-specialty. Physicians share offices, equipment, utility bills, and staff costs. Besides sharing costs, they may also share profits. Proponents of group practice maintain that it provides better coordination of care, reduces unnecessary duplication of equipment, and improves the quality of health care through peer review. Critics argue that group practice may limit competition and patients' access to services.

Solo practitioners are medical providers who practice independently of other practitioners. It is difficult for solo practitioners to survive in today's high-cost, high-technology health care market. They often have little time away from their offices and have to trade on-call hours with other doctors. For these reasons, there are far fewer solo practices today than in the past. Most solo practitioners are doctors who established their practices years ago, have a specialty that's in high demand, or work in a rural or underserved area.

Integrated Health Care Organizations

Both hospitals and clinics provide a range of health care services, including emergency treatment, diagnostic tests, and inpatient and outpatient (ambulatory) care. Your selection of a hospital or clinic will depend on your particular needs, income, and insurance coverage, plus the availability of services in your community. As the number of hospitals has decreased in recent years due to an oversupply of hospital beds, a decreasing reliance on inpatient care, and an increase in competition, the number of hospital-based outpatient clinics has grown. These integrated health care organizations range from groups of loosely affiliated health service organizations and hospitals to HMOs that control their own very tightly joined hospitals, clinics, pharmacies, and even home health agencies.

There are several ways to classify hospitals: by profit status (nonprofit or for-profit); ownership (private, city, county, state, federal); specialty (children's, maternity, chronic care, psychiatric, general acute); teaching status (teaching-affiliated or not); size; and whether they are part of a chain of hospitals.

Nonprofit (voluntary) hospitals have traditionally been run by religious or other humanitarian groups. Earnings have generally been reinvested in the hospital to improve health care. These hospitals have often cared for patients whether they could pay or not.

The number of **for-profit (proprietary) hospitals** has multiplied over the past two decades. Today they constitute

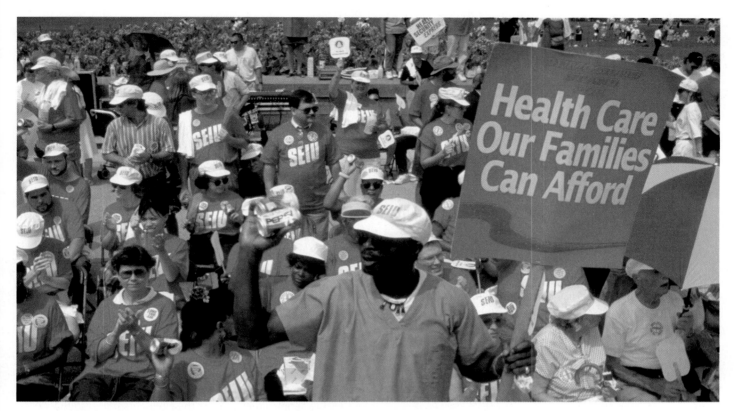

Increasing health care costs have mobilized people to take political action. Debate continues over the proper role of government, the insurance industry, and other parties.

over 20 percent of nongovernmental acute-care hospitals. For-profit hospitals, which do not receive tax breaks, are not compelled to operate as a charity and typically provide fewer free services to the community than do nonprofit hospitals. Historically, some for-profit hospitals quickly transferred indigent (poor) or uninsured patients to public hospitals (those that are not heavily supported by taxes) or to nonprofit hospitals. This practice, known as *patient dumping,* was prohibited by federal law in 1986. Today, all hospital emergency rooms are required to perform a screening exam on all patients, regardless of their ability to pay. Legally, patients must be determined to be "medically stable" before they can be discharged from the emergency room or transferred to another facility, although consumer groups allege that some hospitals continue to dump less-profitable patients.[12]

More treatments and services, including surgery, are delivered on an **outpatient (ambulatory) care** basis (care that does not involve an overnight stay) by hospitals, traditional clinics, student health clinics, and nontraditional clinical centers. One type of ambulatory facility that is becoming common is the *surgicenter*—a place where minor, low-risk procedures such as vasectomies, tubal ligations, tissue biopsies, cosmetic surgery, abortions, and minor eye operations are performed. In 1980, the U.S. hospitalization rate was 168 per 1,000 people; since then it has fallen by more than 30 percent.[13]

To reduce the distance patients have to travel, many hospitals locate satellite clinics in cities' outlying areas, sometimes in shopping centers. A few hospitals have designated their satellites as freestanding emergency centers, or surgicenters, that function like hospital emergency rooms for uncomplicated immediate-care cases but have lower operating costs. Some consumers refer to these as "doc-in-the-box" centers.

Many hospitals and group practices are affiliated with freestanding imaging and diagnostic laboratory centers through direct ownership or other profit-sharing arrangements. Significant debate surrounds this practice. Critics argue that when doctors own the diagnostic and laboratory services to which they refer patients, they may order an excessive number of tests. Today, such practices amount to "conflict of interest situations" and are largely prohibited by antikickback legislation.

Once located within hospitals, most health clinics today are likely to be independent facilities run by medical practitioners. Other health clinics are run by county health

---

Outpatient (ambulatory) care   Treatment that does not involve an overnight stay in a hospital.

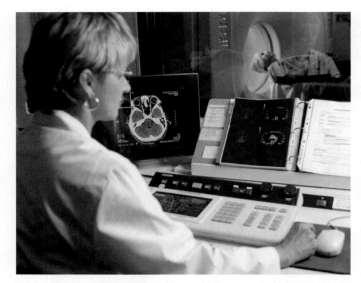

Modern technology has vastly improved treatment for many illnesses, but it has also played a major role in the escalating costs of medical care.

departments; these offer low-cost diagnosis and treatment for financially needy patients. Some 1,500 college campuses also have student health centers that, along with county, city, or community clinics, supply low-cost family planning, tests, and services related to vaccinations, sexually transmitted infections, and gynecological services.

Consumers who consider using a hospital or clinic should scrutinize the facility's accreditation. Accredited hospitals have met rigorous standards set by the Joint Commission on Accreditation of Healthcare Organizations (JCAHO). If you choose an institution that has this accreditation, you have a greater likelihood of quality care.

People can also obtain information regarding prior provider malpractice insurance or sanctions from state licensure boards and the National Practitioner Data Bank. It is the responsibility of all health care consumers to report concerns about health care providers to local or state medical societies or licensing agencies for investigation. Report concerns about billing-related fraud or abuse directly to the Health Care Finance Administration (HCFA).

For more tips on how to evaluate hospitals and health care providers, see the Reality Check box.

What do you think?

Do you assume that your physicians and health care centers are licensed, certified, and accredited? ■ *Have you ever checked on a doctor's or health care facility's credentials?* ■ *If so, what did you decide?*

Issues Facing Today's Health Care System

Many Americans believe that our health care system needs fundamental reform. What are the problems that have brought us to this point? Cost, access, malpractice, restricted choices in providers and treatments, unnecessary procedures, complicated and cumbersome insurance rules, and dramatic ranges in quality are among the issues of concern. One of the most frequently voiced criticisms concerns lack of access to adequate health insurance, as many Americans have had increasing difficulty obtaining comprehensive coverage from their employers. Until recently, insurance benefits were often lost when employees changed jobs, causing many to remain in undesirable positions in order to avoid losing health benefits. This phenomenon, known as *job lock,* led the federal government to pass legislation mandating the "portability" of health insurance benefits from one job to the next, thereby guaranteeing coverage during the transition. Today, individuals who leave their jobs have the option of continuing their group health insurance benefits under the Consolidated Omnibus Budget Reconciliation Act (COBRA). COBRA gives former employees, retirees, spouses, and dependents the right to continue their insurance temporarily at group rates. COBRA beneficiaries pay for their benefits but usually have better coverage than they could receive as individuals.

Over 90 million people in the United States suffer from chronic health conditions that should be at least monitored by medical practitioners.[14] Their access to care is largely determined by whether they have health insurance. Catastrophic or chronic illness among only 10 percent of the population accounts for 75 percent of all health expenditures.[15] Since we cannot perfectly predict who will fall into that 10 percent, every American is potentially vulnerable to the high cost and devastating effects of such illnesses.

Cost

Both per capita and as a percentage of gross domestic product (GDP), we spend more on health care than any other nation. Yet, unlike the rest of the industrialized world, we do not provide access for our entire population. Already, we spend over $1.4 trillion annually on health care, over $5,035 for every man, woman, and child. This translates into 14.1 percent of our GDP. Does this sound like a lot? Consider that health care expenditures are projected to grow by 7.3 percent each year until they reach $3.1 trillion annually by 2012—nearly 18 percent of our GDP.[16]

Why do health care costs continue to spiral upward? There are many factors involved: excess administrative costs; duplication of services; an aging population; growing rates of obesity, inactivity, and related health problems; demand for new diagnostic and treatment technologies; an emphasis on crisis-oriented care instead of prevention; inappropriate utilization of services by consumers; and related factors.

Evaluating Hospitals and Health Care Providers

Suppose that you decide to buy a car. No doubt you would do some research first and compare information on various models and dealers to obtain the best vehicle for your needs.

Now suppose that you are told you need surgery. Wouldn't you like to be able to do the same kind of research on hospitals and surgeons, so you could identify the best health care providers for your case?

Until recently, it has been much easier to obtain ratings on cars than hospitals. This situation is slowly changing, as consumer groups, health insurance plans, and a few states start making data available online to help consumers compare health care facilities and providers. Below are some of the most helpful sources.

THE LEAPFROG GROUP

www.leapfroggroup.org

A nationwide coalition of more than 150 public and private organizations, the Leapfrog Group focuses on identifying problems in the U.S. hospital system that can lead to medical errors and devising solutions. For example, more than 1 million medication errors occur each year in United States hospitals. These errors include administering the wrong drug, administering the right drug but the wrong dose, or overlooking drug allergies and interactions. A report by the Institute of Medicine estimates that serious medication errors account for 7,000 deaths annually in the U.S. The causes of these errors can be as tragically simple as misreading a doctor's handwritten prescription or misplacing a decimal point. Leapfrog advocates that all hospitals adopt a Computer Physician Order Entry (CPOE) system that lets doctors enter prescriptions into a computer rather than on paper. The computer then verifies the prescription and checks for potential problems such as interactions, dosage, and allergies. In follow-up studies, the CPOE reduced medication errors by 55 to 88 percent.

Leapfrog issues hospitals a quality rating based on CPOE implementation and other safety practices. Its website posts the results of its hospital safety survey and ranks hospitals around the country. Note that hospital participation in the program is voluntary, and many hospitals do not participate at present.

HEALTHGRADES

www.healthgrades.com

This company provides quality reports on physicians as well as hospitals, nursing homes, and other health care facilities. In its hospital ratings, the website incorporates data from nearly 5,000 hospitals on surgery volume (how many procedures of this type are performed at that particular hospital) and patient outcomes (complication and mortality rates). Ratings of physicians detail the doctor's specialty, training, board certification, and whether there have been any governmental disciplinary actions taken against him or her.

HEALTHSCOPE

www.healthscope.org

Operated by the nonprofit coalition Pacific Business Group on Health, this website rates hospitals, medical groups, and health plans in California. Hospital ratings are based on patient questionnaires, mortality reports, patient discharge records, and quality assessments from the Leapfrog Group. Hospital participation is voluntary.

HEALTHFINDER

www.myhealthfinder.com

Sponsored by the Niagara Health Quality Coalition, this site provides quality assessments of hospitals, health insurance plans, and long-term care facilities in New York State. Hospital ratings are based on information from patients, the Joint Commission on Accreditation of Health Care Organizations, HealthGrades, and various reports. Ratings include data on surgery volume and mortality rates for coronary bypass surgery.

PENNSYLVANIA HEALTH CARE COST CONTAINMENT COUNCIL

www.phc4.org

This independent state agency seeks to lower health care costs by stimulating competition in the health care market. It collects, analyzes, and makes available to the public information on the cost and quality of health care in Pennsylvania. Hospital ratings include data such as patients' length of stay in the hospital, readmission for any reason, readmission for complications or infections, rate of transfer to acute care, mortality rates, and average hospital charges.

Our system has more than 2,000 health insurance companies, each with different coverage structures and administrative requirements. This lack of uniformity prevents our system from achieving the *economies of scale* (bulk purchasing at a reduced cost) and administrative efficiency realized in countries where there is a single-payer delivery system. According to the Health Insurance Association of America (HIAA), commercial insurance companies commonly experience administrative costs greater than 10 percent of the total health care insurance premium, whereas the administrative cost of the government's Medicare program is less than 4 percent. Administrative expenses in the private sector contribute to the high cost of health care and force companies to require employees to share more of the costs, cut back on benefits, and drop some benefits altogether. These costs are largely passed on to consumers in the form of higher prices for goods and services. See Figure 22.2 for a breakdown of how health care dollars are spent.

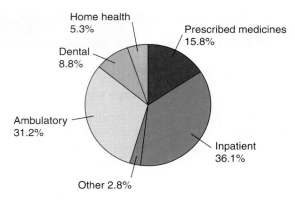

Figure 22.2

Where Do We Spend Our Health-Care Dollars?

Source: G. L. Olin and S. R. Machlin, "Health Care Expenses in the Community Population, 1999," *Medical Expenditure Panel Survey* (MEPS Chartbook No. 11) (Rockville, MD: Agency for Healthcare Research and Quality, 2003).

The declining availability of health insurance coverage means more Americans are uninsured or underinsured. These people are unable to access preventive care and seek care only in the event of an emergency or crisis. Since emergency care is extraordinarily expensive, they often are unable to pay, and the cost is absorbed by those who *can* pay—the insured or taxpayers. This process is known as *cost shifting*.

Access

Access to health care is determined by numerous factors, including the supply of providers and facilities, proximity to care, ability to maneuver in the system, health status, and insurance coverage. Although there are approximately 700,000 physicians in the United States, many Americans lack adequate access to health services because of insurance barriers or maldistribution of providers. There is an oversupply of higher-paid specialists and a shortage of lower-paid primary care physicians (family practitioners, pediatricians, internists, OB-Gyns, geriatricians). Inner cities and some rural areas face constant shortages of physicians.

Managed care health plans determine access on the basis of participating providers, health plan benefits, and administrative rules. Often this means that consumers do not have the freedom to choose specialists, facilities, or treatment options beyond those contracted with the health plan and recommended by their primary care provider (also known as *gatekeeper*). In the United States, consumer demand has led to an expansion of benefits to include such nonallopathic therapies as chiropractic and acupuncture (see Chapter 23). However, many nonallopathic treatments remain unavailable, even to a limited degree, through current health plans.

Quality and Malpractice

The U.S. health care system employs several mechanisms for ensuring quality services: education, licensure, certification/ registration, accreditation, peer review, and, as a last resort, the legal system of malpractice litigation. Some of these mechanisms are mandatory before a professional or organization may provide care, whereas others are purely voluntary. (Be aware that licensure, although state mandated for some practitioners and facilities, is only a minimum guarantee of quality.) Insurance companies and government payers may also require a higher level of quality by linking payment to whether a practitioner is board certified or a facility is accredited by the appropriate agency. In addition, most insurance plans now require prior authorization and/or second opinions not only to reduce costs, but also to improve quality of care.

Consumer, provider, and advocacy groups focus on the great variation in quality as a major problem in our health care system. A newer form of quality measurement uses "outcome" as the primary indicator for measuring health care quality at the individual level. With outcome measurements, we don't look just at what is done to the patient but at what subsequently happens to the patient's health status. Thus, mortality rates and complication rates (such as infections) become very important statistics in assessing individual practitioners and facilities.

Medical errors and mistakes do happen. An Institute of Medicine report indicates that as many as 44,000 to 98,000 people die in U.S. hospitals each year as the result of medical errors—more than the number who die from motor vehicle accidents, breast cancer, or AIDS.[17] The Reality Check box discusses what "actionable" malpractice really is. Clearly, we must be as proactive as possible in our health care.

What do you think?

Do you believe prospective patients should have access to information about practitioners' and facilities' malpractice records? ■ How about their success and failure rates or outcomes of various procedures?

Third-Party Payers

The fundamental principle of insurance underwriting is that the cost of health care can be predicted for large populations. This is how health care premiums (payments) are determined. Policyholders pay premiums into a pool, which fills as reserves until needed. When you are sick or injured, the insurance company pays out of the pool, regardless of your total amount of contribution. Depending on circumstances, you may never pay for what your medical care costs or you

"Actionable" Medical Malpractice: What Is It, and When Should You Consider It?

Actionable medical malpractice or medical negligence occurs when a physician fails to properly treat a medical condition and the negligent act or omission causes a new or aggravated injury to the patient. Obviously, the physician cannot be held responsible for the original underlying health problem. The negligence in medical malpractice cases can occur in a variety of situations including, but not limited to, the following:

✔ Delay or failure in diagnosing a disease
✔ Surgical or anesthesia-related mishap during an operative procedure
✔ Failure to gain the informed consent of the patient for an operation or surgical procedure
✔ Failure to properly treat the disease process after making the correct diagnosis
✔ Misuse of prescription drugs or a medical device or implant

Typically, patients must secure an attorney who is well versed in medical law and who can quickly determine whether there is an actionable case. Usually, a medical expert who is qualified to give a medical opinion and board certified in the relevant field of medicine is also necessary. The attorney agrees up front to advance costs and to be repaid in the event the case is won, with a percentage of the gross recovery as the established fee for service.

Medical malpractice lawsuits are costly and complex and may take years to win. Careful record keeping of procedures and actions is an important part of the entire case. Having a health advocate who has witnessed the events is another key element in determining success or failure.

Source: "Actionable Medical Malpractice Civil Rights and the Law," January 2002, www.civilrights.com/medical.html

---

may pay much more for insurance than your medical bills ever total. The idea is that you pay in affordable premiums so that you never have to face catastrophic bills. In today's profit-oriented system, insurers prefer to have healthy people in their plans who put money into risk pools without taking money out.

Unfortunately, not everyone has health insurance. Forty-seven million Americans (18.8 percent of the non-elderly population) are uninsured—that is, they have no private health insurance and are not eligible for Medicare, Medicaid, or other health programs.[18] The number of uninsured has grown since the late 1970s. Lack of health insurance has been associated with delayed health care and increased mortality. *Underinsurance* (that is, the inability to pay out-of-pocket expenses despite having insurance) also may result in adverse health consequences. Another 41 million Americans are estimated to be underinsured (at risk for spending more than 10 percent of their income on medical care because their insurance is inadequate).[19]

Contrary to the common belief that the uninsured are unemployed, 75 percent of them are either workers or the dependents of workers. One-quarter of all the uninsured are children under age 16. College students are one of the largest groups of the uninsured not in the labor force. This presents a difficult dilemma for both universities and students when they must seek care because most university insurance plans are designed as short-term, noncatastrophic plans having low upper limits of benefits. As a full-time student, you should consider purchasing a higher level catastrophic plan to protect yourself in the event of a rare, but very costly, illness or accident.

For the uninsured and many of the underinsured, health care may not be available through any source because of their inability to pay. Many either will not or cannot seek care from charitable providers, so they fail to receive the medical care they need. People without health care coverage are less likely than other Americans to have their children immunized, seek early prenatal care, obtain annual blood pressure checks, and seek attention for serious symptoms of illness. Many experts believe that this ultimately leads to higher system costs because their conditions deteriorate to a more debilitating and costly stage before they are forced to seek help.

Private Health Insurance

Our current health system began in the past century and its growth accelerated in the post–World War II era to its current massive, complex web. Hospitals became the engines of medicine in the midtwentieth century. Doctors became the drivers or conductors of this rapidly moving system. The system was fueled by a variety of funding sources but, chiefly, first by the growth of tax-exempt, nonprofit private insurance companies established in the 1940s and later by the growth of for-profit insurance companies.

Originally, health insurance originally consisted solely of coverage for hospital costs (it was called *major medical*) but gradually was extended to routine physicians' treatment and other areas such as dental services and pharmaceuticals. Payment mechanisms used until recently laid the groundwork for today's steadily-rising health care costs. Hospitals were reimbursed on a cost-plus basis after services were rendered. That is, they billed for the costs of providing care plus an amount for profit. This system provided no incentive to contain costs, limit the number of procedures, or curtail capital investment in redundant equipment and facilities. Physicians were reimbursed on a fee-for-service (indemnity) basis determined by "usual, customary, and reasonable" fees. These were calculated by comparing what a doctor charged for a service with what that same doctor charged last year for the service and with what other doctors in the area charged. This system encouraged physicians to charge high fees, raise them often, and perform as many procedures as possible. At the same time, because most insurance did not cover routine or preventive services, consumers were encouraged to use hospitals whenever possible (the coverage was better) and to wait until illness developed to seek help instead of seeking preventive care. Consumers were also free to choose any provider or service they wished, including even inappropriate—and often very expensive—levels of care.

Private insurance companies have increasingly employed several mechanisms to limit potential losses and control consumers' use of insurance. These mechanisms include cost sharing (in the form of deductibles, copayments, and coinsurance), exclusions, "preexisting condition" clauses, waiting periods, and upper limits on payments. *Deductibles* are front-end payments (commonly $250 to $1,000) that you must make to your provider before your insurance company will start paying for any services you use. *Copayments* are set amounts that you pay per service received regardless of the cost of the services (for example, $20 per doctor visit or per prescription). *Coinsurance* is the percentage of the bill that you must pay throughout the course of treatment (for example, 20 percent of whatever the total is). *Preexisting condition clauses* limit the insurance company's liability for medical conditions that a consumer had before obtaining insurance coverage (for example, if a woman takes out coverage while she is pregnant, the insurance company may cover pregnancy complications and infant care but not charges related to "normal pregnancy"). Because many insurance companies use a combination of these mechanisms, keeping track of the costs you are responsible for can become very difficult.

Group plans of large employers (government agencies, school districts, or corporations, for example) generally do not have preexisting condition clauses in their plans. But smaller group plans (a group may be as small as two) often do. Some plans never cover services for preexisting conditions, while others specify a waiting period (such as six months) before they will provide coverage. All insurers set some limits on the types of services they will cover (for example, most exclude cosmetic surgery, private rooms, and experimental procedures). Some insurance plans may also include an upper or lifetime limit, after which coverage will end. Although $250,000 may seem like an enormous sum, medical bills for a sick child or chronic disease can easily run this high within a few years.

Medicare and Medicaid

After years of debate about whether we should have a national health program like those of most industrialized countries, the U.S. government directed the system toward a mixed private and public approach in the 1960s. Most Americans obtained their health insurance through their employers, but this left out two groups—the nonworking poor and the aged. In 1965, amendments to the 1935 Social Security Act established Medicare and Medicaid. Although enacted simultaneously, these programs are vastly different.

Medicare, basically federal social insurance covering 99 percent of the elderly over 65 years of age, all totally and permanently disabled people (after a waiting period), and all people with end-stage kidney failure, is a universal program that covers a broad range of services except long-term care and pharmaceuticals. It currently covers over 39 million people.[20] Medicare is widely accepted by physicians and hospitals and has relatively low administrative costs.

On the other hand, **Medicaid,** covering approximately 40 million people, is a federal-state matching funds welfare program for people who are defined as poor (blind, disabled, aged, or those receiving Aid to Families with Dependent Children) and relies on matching funds provided by federal and state sources.[21] Because each state determines income eligibility levels and payments to providers, there are vast differences in the way Medicaid operates from state to state.

To control hospital costs, in 1983 the federal government set up a prospective payment system based on **diagnosis-related groups (DRGs)** for Medicare. Using a complicated formula, nearly 500 groupings of diagnoses were created to establish how much a hospital would be reimbursed for a particular patient. If a hospital can treat the patient for less than that amount, it can keep the difference. However, if a patient's care costs more than the set amount, the hospital must absorb the difference (with a few exceptions that must be reviewed by a panel). This system gives hospitals the incentive to discharge patients quickly after doing as little as possible for them, provide more ambulatory care, and admit only patients with favorable (profitable) DRGs. Many private health insurance companies have followed the federal government in adopting this type of reimbursement. In 1998, the federal HCFA expanded the

---

Medicare Federal health insurance program for the elderly and the permanently disabled.

Medicaid Federal-state health insurance program for the poor.

Diagnosis-related groups (DRGs) Diagnostic categories established by the federal government to determine in advance how much hospitals will be reimbursed for the care of a particular Medicare patient.

---

prospective payment system to include payments for outpatient surgery and skilled nursing care.

In its continuing effort to control rising costs, HCFA has encouraged the growth of prepaid HMO senior plans for Medicare-eligible persons. Under this system, commercial managed care insurance plans receive a fixed per capita premium from HCFA and then offer more preventive services with lower out-of-pocket copayments. These managed care plans encourage providers and patients to utilize health care resources under administrative rules similar to commercial HMO plans. Similarly, states have encouraged the growth of managed Medicaid programs.

Managed Care

Managed care describes a health care delivery system comprised of the following elements:

1. A budget based on an estimate of the annual cost of delivering health care for a given population
2. A network of physicians, hospitals, and other providers and facilities linked contractually to deliver comprehensive health benefits within that predetermined budget, sharing economic risk for any budget deficit or surplus
3. An established set of administrative rules requiring patients to follow the advice of participating health care providers in order to have their health care paid for under the terms of the health plan

Many such plans pay their contracted health care providers through **capitation,** that is, prepayment of a fixed monthly amount for each patient without regard for the type or number of health services provided. Some plans pay health care providers a salary, and some are still fee-for-service plans. As with other insurance plans, enrollees are members of a risk pool, and it is expected that some persons will use no services, some will use a modest amount, and others will have high-cost utilization over a given year. Doctors have the incentive to keep their patient pool healthy and avoid catastrophic ailments that are preventable; usually such incentives come back in terms of increased salaries, bonuses, and other benefits. As such, prevention and health education to reduce risk and intervene early to avoid major problems should be capstone components of such plans.

Managed care plans have grown steadily over the past decade with a proportionate decline of enrollment in traditional indemnity insurance plans. The reason for this shift is that indemnity insurance, which pays providers and hospitals on a fee-for-service basis with no built-in incentives to control costs, has become unaffordable or unavailable for most Americans.

With the growth of managed care organizations, concerns have arisen about the quality of care offered under this type of payment system. These concerns compelled consumer groups and public health organizations to require managed care insurers to compile quality care "report cards," known as HEDIS (Health Employer Data Information Set)

Reports, so that health outcomes could be compared across different plans. The quality measures include preventive services (childhood immunizations, Pap smears, mammograms), disease indicators (eye exams and glucose control tests for diabetics), and screening exams (routine physical exams, including gynecological exams). These reports are available from most managed care health plans on request. Still, such information is difficult for the consumer to evaluate due to inconsistent data collection and reporting techniques. This problem has given rise to skepticism and controversy over the validity of these reports.

Types of managed care plans include health maintenance organizations (HMOs), preferred provider organizations (PPOs), and point of service (POS). Approximately 166 million Americans are enrolled in HMOs, the most common type.[22]

Health Maintenance Organization (HMO) HMOs provide a wide range of covered health benefits (such as checkups, surgery, doctor visits, lab tests) for a fixed amount prepaid by you, the employer, Medicaid, or Medicare. Usually, HMO premiums are the least expensive form of managed care (saving between 10 and 40 percent more than other plans) but also are the most restrictive (offering little or no choice in doctors and certain services). These premiums are 8 to 10 percent lower than for traditional plans, there are low or no deductibles or coinsurance payments, and copayments are $10 to $20 per office visit. HMOs contract with providers to supply health services for enrollees through various systems, such as these:[23]

- *The staff model.* You receive care from salaried staff doctors at the HMO's facility.
- *The group network model.* The HMO contracts with one or several groups of doctors, who provide care for a fixed amount per plan member. Groups often practice in one facility.
- *The independent practice association (IPA).* Doctors in private practice form an association that contracts with HMOs. The physicians generally work in their own offices.

The downside of HMOs is that patients are typically required to use the plan's doctors and hospitals and to get approval from a "gatekeeper" or primary care physician for treatment and referrals.[24] As more and more people enroll in HMOs, criticisms of the plans are mounting. Currently, a class action suit is pending against a major HMO over "denial of service" that plaintiffs claim endangered their lives. If

---

Managed care   Cost-control procedures used by health insurers to coordinate treatment.

Capitation   Prepayment of a fixed monthly amount for each patient without regard to the type or number of services provided.

such cases succeed, HMOs may need to change their business practices or face significant financial risk. Other concerns about HMOs include questions such as:

- Do highly paid administrators and stockholders ration care, allocating more care to those who are better able to pay and enjoy better health?
- Does the huge administrative structure imposed by the HMO make it virtually impossible for patients to sue in the event of clear violations?
- Are patients denied costly diagnostic tests because such tests cut into bottom-line profits? Are some tests given too late because of cost concerns?
- Do HMOs really focus on prevention or intervention? Critics charge that the fee structure of many HMOs actually discourages basic preventive services, such as immunizations.
- Are doctors allowed to treat patients using their best judgment and skills, or do policies and profit-motivated concerns interfere with their roles as advocates for patients?
- Are the obstacles imposed by HMOs too daunting for patients in need of urgent care?
- Do HMO cost-saving policies force patients out of hospitals and treatment centers too early?

Preferred Provider Organization (PPO) PPOs are networks of independent doctors and hospitals that contract to provide care at discounted rates. Although they offer greater choices in doctors than HMOs do, they are less likely to coordinate a patient's care. In addition, while members have a choice of seeing doctors who are not on the preferred list, this choice may come at considerable cost (such as having to pay 30 percent of the charges out of pocket, rather than 10 to 20 percent for PPO doctors and services).[25]

Point of Service (POS) This option—a hybrid of the HMO and PPO types—provides a more acceptable form of managed care for those used to the traditional indemnity plan of insurance, which probably explains why it is among the fastest growing of the managed care plans. Under POS, patients can go to providers outside their HMO for care but must pay for the extra cost. Usually this is a reasonable alternative for middle-class or wealthy Americans who are willing to pay extra for choices in care.[26]

What do you think?

Why is it important that private insurance cover preventive or lower-level care as well as hospitalization and high-technology interventions? ■ *What kinds of incentives would cause you to seek help early rather than delay care?*

What Are Your Options?

The United States and South Africa are currently the only industrialized nations that do not have a national health program that guarantees all citizens access to at least a basic set of health benefits. The United States has seen four major political movements supporting national health insurance during the past century, but none has succeeded. Whether universal coverage will—or should—be achieved and through what mechanism remain hotly debated topics. Many analysts believe that health care reform has failed due to a combination of circumstances and influences: lobbying efforts by the insurance industry and the medical community, proposed plans that were too complicated, and interest groups who felt that the plans either went "too far" or "not far enough." Some people also believe that our current system serves people well.

One critical point must be made, though: we are paying for the most expensive system in the world without obtaining full coverage. We pay for people who don't have insurance through cost shifting that increases premiums and taxes, and we spend more than necessary because prevention and early treatment are not emphasized. We also pay for much duplication of services and technologies, for practitioners who practice defensive medicine and who refer patients to their own diagnostic labs for profit reasons, and for the vast bureaucracy made inevitable by over 2,000 private health insurance companies.

One proposal for reform involves the federalization and incremental expansion of Medicaid. The idea is to eliminate state disparities and improve coverage gradually through progressive general tax financing. First would come federalization of Medicaid eligibility, benefits, and reimbursement to improve access for those determined eligible. Next would come a step-by-step expansion raising the age limits for children, then covering all pregnant women, then allowing "intact" poor families to obtain coverage, then increasing the income limit to incorporate the uninsured near-poor, and finally allowing the middle class to buy into the program. This type of plan could work well if reimbursements were set high enough to encourage provider participation. However, it would take a long time to provide universal coverage, and it is not a likely option at this time.

The Institute of Medicine, a nonpartisan organization that advises the federal government on health issues, recommends a single-payer, tax-financed scheme that severs insurance ties from employment.[27] Similar to the Canadian model, it would cover everyone—regardless of income or other factors such as health status. It would offer many different ways to tailor a plan to the needs of U.S. citizens. A single federal plan or a privately administered plan paid for by general tax funds or earmarked taxes could be created. Thus, all (or most) private insurers would be eliminated or would see their role limited to that of fiscal administrators. Benefits would be comprehensive and provide incentives for cost-effective care. Benefits would be "portable": they would remain in effect when individuals changed jobs or moved to a different area of the country. Freedom of choice in terms of providers might actually improve in a single-payer system, given how restrictive our current private health insurance system has become. Such a plan would allow far greater control over resource and personnel planning and improve access to preventive services, and it could eliminate duplicate services and technology. Such a single-payer system would be expensive, but researchers estimate that it could save upward of $130 billion annually in administrative costs—enough to provide coverage to all uninsured Americans.[28] Claims that the Canadian system has long waiting lists have either proved entirely untrue or exaggerated: modest waits do not appear to result in any reduction of health status.

Given the delay in realizing national health care reform, several states have sought ways to contain costs and improve access for their populations. At the federal level, Congress continues to debate strategies for bolstering Social Security and Medicare.

What do you think?

Do you believe that the time is right for another national discussion on health care reform?
■ *Do you think we are moving to a more profit-oriented health care system or a single-payer system?* ■ *Which would you prefer?* ■ *Is health care a right or a privilege?*

TAKING CHARGE

MAKE IT HAPPEN!

Assessment: The Assess Yourself box on page 619 asks you to look at your behavior as a health care consumer. Once you have considered your responses, you may want to change certain behaviors in order to get the best treatment from your health care provider and the health care system.

Making a Change: In order to change your behavior, you need to develop a plan. Follow these steps.

1. Evaluate your behavior, and identify patterns and specific things you are doing. What can you change now? What can you change in the near future?
2. Select one pattern of behavior that you want to change.
3. Fill out a Behavior Change Contract. It should include your long-term goal for change, your short-term goals, the rewards you'll give yourself for reaching these goals, potential obstacles along the way, and strategies for overcoming these obstacles. For each goal, list the small steps and specific actions that you will take.
4. Chart your progress in a journal. At the end of a week, consider how successful you were in following your plan. What helped you to be successful? What made change more difficult? What will you do differently next week?
5. Revise your plan as needed. Are the short-term goals attainable? Are the rewards satisfying?

One Student's Plan: When Theo reviewed his answers in the self-assessment, he realized that he needed to pay more attention to the medication he took for his asthma. Although he was supposed to take the same dose every day, when he was feeling good he would take only half of the prescribed dosage in order to save money. Theo also wasn't sure what side effects were considered normal with his medication and had not mentioned any of them to his physician, Dr. Hanako. He also had recently started taking an herbal supplement that his roommate had recommended to help his weightlifting, but he hadn't mentioned the supplement to his doctor either.

Theo's first step was to make an appointment with Dr. Hanako to discuss his questions and concerns. He made a list ahead of time of what he wanted to talk about to be sure he didn't forget any questions. He also started keeping track of the side effects he was experiencing so he could give the doctor a clear picture of his health. Finally, he made a note of the name and ingredients of the supplement and decided to stop taking it until he could ask about potential interactions with his asthma medication.

Theo's meeting with Dr. Hanako went well. When Theo explained that he was trying to save money by using less of the medication than prescribed, Dr. Hanako found a generic equivalent that cost much less. He reminded Theo about the importance of taking the correct dose and explained that some of the side effects that he reported were caused by the variation in the amount of medication he was taking. He also told Theo that the herbal supplement would make the asthma medication much less effective, an interaction not disclosed on the supplement's label. Theo agreed that now he could afford to take the medication exactly as prescribed, and he scheduled a follow-up appointment in six months to discuss any further concerns that might arise.

Summary

- Advertisers of health care products and services use sophisticated tactics to attract attention and get business. Advertising claims sometimes appear to be supported by spontaneous remission (symptoms disappearing without any apparent cause) or the placebo effect (symptoms disappearing because people think they should), rather than the efficacy of the product or service.

- Self-care and individual responsibility are key factors in reducing rising health care costs and improving health status. Advance planning can help a person navigate health care treatment in unfamiliar situations or emergencies. Assess health professionals by considering their qualifications, their record of treating problems like yours, and their ability to work with you.

- In theory, allopathic (traditional Western) medicine is based on scientifically validated methods and procedures. Medical doctors, specialists of various kinds, nurses, physician assistants, and other health professionals practice allopathic medicine.

- Prescription drugs are administered under medical supervision. Categories include antibiotics, sedatives, tranquilizers, antidepressants, and amphetamines. Generic drugs can often be substituted for more expensive brand-name drugs. Over-the-counter drug categories include analgesics; cold, cough, allergy, and asthma relievers; stimulants; sleeping aids and relaxants; and dieting aids. Exercise personal responsibility by reading directions for OTC drugs and asking your pharmacist or doctor if any special precautions are advised when taking these substances.

- Health care providers may provide services as solo practitioners or in group practices (which share overhead costs). Hospitals and clinics are classified by profit status, ownership, specialty, teaching status, size, and whether they are part of a chain.

- Concerns about the U.S. health care system include cost, access, choice of treatment modality, quality and malpractice, and fraud and abuse.

- Health insurance is based on the concept of spreading risk. Insurance is provided by private insurance companies (who charge premiums) and the government Medicare and Medicaid programs (funded by taxes). Managed care (in the form of HMOs, POS plans, and PPOs) attempts to control costs by streamlining administrative procedures and stressing preventive care (among other initiatives).

Questions for Discussion and Reflection

1. What claims do marketers use to get people to try health-related products? Why are consumers susceptible to such ploys? What could be done to increase the accuracy of messages related to health care?

2. List several conditions (resulting from illness or accident) for which you don't need to seek medical help. When would you consider each condition to be bad enough to require medical attention? How would you decide to whom and where to go for treatment?

3. Explain the terms *synergism, antagonism,* and *inhibition.*

4. What are the advantages and disadvantages associated with generic drugs?

5. What are the pros and cons of group practices? Of non-profit and for-profit hospitals? If you had health insurance, where do you believe you would get the best care? On what do you base your answer?

6. What are the inherent benefits and risks of managed care organizations?

7. Discuss the problems of the U.S. health care system. If you were president, what would you propose as a solution? Which groups might oppose your plan? Which groups might support it?

8. Explain the differences between traditional indemnity insurance and managed health care. Which would you feel more comfortable with? Should insurance companies set rates for various medical tests and procedures in an attempt to keep prices down?

Accessing Your Health on the Internet

Visit the following Internet sites to explore further topics and issues related to personal health. To visit an organization's website, go to the Companion Website for *Access to Health, Ninth Edition* at www.aw-bc.com/donatelle, click on the book image, and select "Accessing Your Health on the Internet" from the navigation menu.

1. ***Agency for Health Care Research and Quality.*** A gateway to consumer health information, providing links to sites that can address health care concerns and provide information on questions to ask, what to look for, and what you should know when making critical decisions about personal care.

2. ***Food and Drug Administration.*** News on the latest government-approved generic drugs and investigations.

3. ***Health Touch.*** Search for prescription and over-the-counter drug uses and side effects, plus other health-related resources.

4. ***National Committee for Quality Assurance.*** The NCQA assesses and reports on the quality of managed care plans, including health maintenance organizations.

5. ***National Library of Medicine—General Information Center for Health-Related Research.*** Supports Medline/Pubmed information retrieval systems in addition to providing public health information for consumers.

Further Reading

Birenbaum, A. *Wounded Profession: American Medicine Enters the Age of Managed Care.* Westport, CT: Praeger Publishers, 2002.

Birenbaum describes the rise of HMOs in the nineties and the increasing backlash, and he presents ideas for reform of the health care system.

Geyman, J. *Health Care in America: Can Our Ailing System Be Healed?* London: Butterworth-Heinemann, 2001.

Written from the perspective of a physician, this book focuses on the challenges—escalating costs, limitations of access, and a wide range of quality—facing the health care system.

Greenburg, S. *2002 Physician's Desk Reference for Nonprescription Drugs and Dietary Supplements,* 21st ed. Oradell, NJ: Medical Economics Data, 2002.

Outlines proper uses, possible dangers, and effective ingredients of nonprescription medications.

Griffith, W. H. *A Complete Guide to Prescription and Nonprescription Drugs, 2001.* San Francisco, CA: Berkeley Publishing Group, 2001.

This essential guide answers every conceivable question about prescription and nonprescription drugs and contains information about dosages, side effects, precautions, interactions, and more. More than 5,000 brand name and 700 generic drugs are profiled in an easy-to-use format.

Lee, P. and C. Estes. *The Nation's Health,* 7th ed. Sudbury, MA: Jones and Bartlett, 2003.

Overview of factors affecting the health of Americans and the roles of public health, medical care, and the community in ensuring the nation's health. Special emphasis on health determinants, women's health, long-term care, and the uncertainties of tomorrow's health care system.

- Describe complementary and alternative medicine (CAM), and identify its typical domains. Explain why it is growing in popularity in the United States and throughout the world and who is most likely to use it.

- Discuss major types of complementary and alternative medicine providers and common treatments that they offer.

- Discuss the various types of complementary and alternative medicines being used in America today, their patterns of use, and their potential benefits and risks.

- Explain how to evaluate testimonials and claims related to complementary and alternative products and services and how to ensure that you are getting accurate information and sound treatment.

- Discuss the challenges and opportunities related to complementary and alternative medicine in ensuring our health and wellness.

COMPLEMENTARY AND ALTERNATIVE MEDICINE

NEW CHOICES AND RESPONSIBILITIES FOR HEALTHWISE CONSUMERS

IN THE NEWS

Acupuncture Moves Toward the Mainstream

By Anahad O'Connor

Three years ago, Alfred Szymanski could not seem to get his blood pressure under control. He ran 10 miles a week, stuck to a healthy diet and was on a hypertension medication, all to no avail. His doctor suggested switching medications, but Mr. Szymanski, wary of side effects, decided to try something he had always wondered about: acupuncture.

After three 20-minute sessions, each covered by his medical plan, his blood pressure plunged 20 points.

"Every time I left I was so relaxed; it was like euphoria," said Mr. Szymanski, 61, who lives in New York. "My blood pressure stayed down for quite a while."

Acupuncture, long shunned by mainstream medicine but for centuries considered the crown jewel of alternative therapy, is slowly gaining ground in doctors' offices around the country. While some experts still question its effectiveness, studies in recent years—including one at Duke last week—have thrown scientific weight behind its benefits, supporting its usefulness in alleviating conditions from morning sickness to carpal tunnel syndrome.

Read the complete article online in the eThemes section of this book's website: www.aw-bc.com/donatelle.

Original article published September 28, 2004. Copyright © 2004 *The New York Times.* Reprinted with permission.

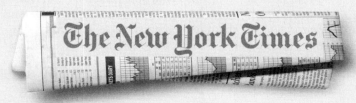

Consumers today face an amazing array of choices when they consider taking action to improve their health or seek care for a health problem. In increasing numbers they are looking beyond conventional Western medicine for at least some of their health care. One of the newest movements toward self-care and health promotion focuses on **complementary and alternative medicine (CAM).** Whether taking herbs to lift their mood or reduce pain, doing yoga or Pilates to reduce stress and increase strength, receiving acupuncture for low back pain, or following naturopathic tenets for cancer treatment, over half of all Americans go outside the traditional health care system to prevent disease, enhance health, or treat symptoms. A new survey by the National Center for Complementary and Alternative Medicine (NCCAM) and the National Center for Health Statistics provides a clear picture of CAM's popularity in the United States (Figure 23.1).

After dismissing CAM therapies as quackery for the better part of a century, the medical establishment now finds itself racing to evaluate them. Many of the country's leading hospitals and research institutions are studying the effects of herbs, acupuncture, tai chi, and biofeedback as rigorously as they would a new antibiotic.[1] The short-term goal of this investigation is to identify CAM practices with the greatest benefits and the fewest hazards and to make these part of clinical practice; the long-term goal is to foster a new kind of medicine—an *integrative* medicine that employs the rigor of modern science without being constrained by it.[2] If these CAM remedies prove effective, a merger of traditional medicine and CAM will change the face of modern medicine in ways that few would have imagined only a decade ago.

Be aware that few CAM therapies have been thoroughly evaluated in controlled studies, so their effectiveness is still widely debated. While there has been much progress in research and testing since the National Institutes of Health opened NCCAM as a full-strength federal agency in 1998, the science of CAM is still in its infancy.

The challenge for consumers is to keep informed of current research, to know how and where to find information about the effectiveness and risks of particular therapies, and to examine any therapy (traditional or alternative) thoroughly. Although the excitement and enthusiasm for CAM are unmistakable, wise consumers will apply the same caution to CAM therapies they would employ in any health decision making. Many of us use the Internet to research CAM therapies, so the NCCAM has developed guidelines for evaluating health-related websites (see the Reality Check box).

Complementary and alternative medicine (CAM)
Forms of treatment distinct from traditional allopathic medicine that until recently were neither taught widely in U.S. medical schools nor generally available in U.S. hospitals.

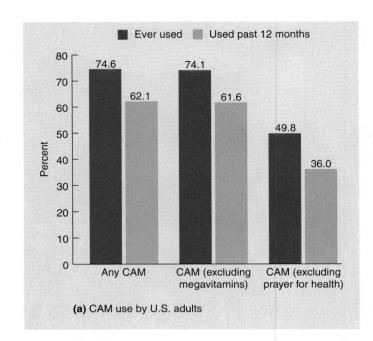

(a) CAM use by U.S. adults

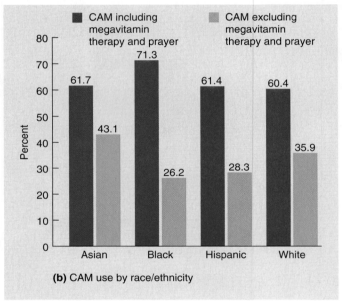

(b) CAM use by race/ethnicity

Figure 23.1
Use of Complementary and Alternative Medicine in the United States

Source: P. Barnes et al., "CDC Advance Data Report #343: Complementary and Alternative Medicine among Adults: United States, 2002," 2004, http://nccam.nih.gov/news/camsurvey.htm

How does the average consumer know what to believe? How do we separate genuinely helpful CAM therapies from those that might be risky? This chapter attempts to present a research-based and unbiased perspective on modern CAM treatments. As you read, look for answers to your own questions, and think about how this information relates to your interests and lifestyle.

Evaluating Medical Resources on the Web

Planning to research health information online? The National Center for Complementary and Alternative Medicine recommends that you ask these questions about any website you visit.

1. *Who runs this site?* Any good health-related website should be clear about who is responsible for the site and its information, with the name of the site's sponsor and a link to its homepage on every major page of the site.

2. *Who pays for the site?* It costs money to run a website, so how does the site pay for its existence? The source of its funding should be clearly stated or readily apparent. For example, Web addresses ending in ".gov" denote a federal government–sponsored site. Does the site sell advertising? Is it sponsored by a drug company? The source of funding can affect what content is presented, how the content is presented, and what the site owners want to accomplish.

3. *What is the purpose of the site?* This question is related to who owns and pays for the site. An "About This Site" link appears on many sites; if it's there, use it. The purpose of the site should be clearly stated and should help you evaluate the trustworthiness of the information.

4. *Where does the information come from?* Many health and medical sites post information collected from other websites or sources. If the person or organization in charge of the site did not create the information, the original source should be clearly identified.

5. *What is the basis of the information?* In addition to identifying who wrote the material you are reading, the site should describe the evidence that the material is based on. Medical facts and figures should have references (such as to articles in medical journals). Also, opinions or advice should be clearly set apart from information that is evidence-based (that is, information based on research results).

6. *How is the information selected?* Is there an editorial board listed for the site? Do people with excellent professional and scientific qualifications review the material before it is posted?

7. *How current is the information?* Websites should be reviewed and updated on a regular basis. It is particularly important that medical information be current. The most recent update or review date should be clearly posted. Even if the information has not changed, you want to know whether the site owners have reviewed it recently to ensure that it is still valid.

8. *How does the site choose links to other sites?* Websites usually have a policy about how they establish links to other sites. Some medical sites take a conservative approach and don't link to any other sites. Some link to any site that asks, or pays, for a link. Others link only to sites that have met certain criteria.

9. *What information about you does the site collect, and why?* Websites routinely track the paths visitors take through their sites to determine which pages are being used. However, many health websites ask for you to "subscribe" or "become a member." In some cases, this may be so that they can collect a user fee or select information for you that is relevant to your concerns. In all cases, this will give the site personal information about you. Any credible health site asking for this kind of information should tell you exactly what will and will not be done with it. Many commercial sites sell "aggregate" (collected) data about their users to other companies—information such as what percentage of their users are women with breast cancer, for example. In some cases they may collect and reuse information that is "personally identifiable," such as your Zip code, gender, and birth date. Be certain that you read and understand any privacy policy or similar language on the site, and don't sign up for anything that you do not fully understand.

10. *How does the site manage interactions with visitors?* There should always be a way for you to contact the site owner if you run across problems or have questions or feedback. If the site hosts chatrooms or other online discussion areas, it should tell visitors what the terms of using this service are. Is it moderated? If so, by whom, and why? It is always a good idea to spend time reading the discussion without joining in, so that you feel comfortable with the environment before becoming a participant.

Source: National Center for Complementary and Alternative Medicine, "Ten Things to Know about Evaluating Medical Resources on the Web," 2002, http://nccam.nih.gov /health/webresources

Evaluating Complementary and Alternative Medicine

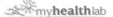

Fill out this assessment online at www.aw-bc.com/myhealthlab or www.aw-bc.com/donatelle

You may have a range of opinions about CAM, depending on the therapies described. Use the questions below to explore your assumptions about CAM.

1. What types of medical professionals do you think should call themselves *holistic health practitioners*?

2. What is meant by the term *mind–body medicine?*

3. What type of person do you think is most likely to seek alternative or complementary medical treatment?

4. Would you tell your doctor if you were taking herbal supplements?

5. Would you tell your doctor if you were consulting an alternative medicine practitioner?

6. Would you try hypnosis to quit smoking or lose weight? Why or why not?

7. Do you consider yoga or tai chi forms of alternative medicine?

8. If a person with severe pain claimed that wearing a magnetic bracelet worked, would you try it? Would you recommend it to someone else?

9. Should health insurance cover complementary and alternative medical treatments?

10. Should herbal supplements be tested and regulated by the federal government?

MAKE IT HAPPEN!

Use the results of this self-assessment to begin your behavior change program. Follow the steps and use the examples on page 667 to complete your Behavior Change Contract, and use these resources to take action.

CAM: What Is It and Who Uses It?

If you think that alternative medicine is just a fad, you are in for a surprise. Today, Americans and people from most other cultures of the world are much more likely to try therapies once considered exotic and strange. This is particularly true as America becomes a composite of people from different regions and cultures of the world. Many of these cultures are contributing their unique beliefs about remedies to restore health and treat afflictions. Referred to as *complementary and alternative medicine,* these therapies are generically defined as "neither being taught widely in U.S. medical schools nor generally available in U.S. hospitals during the previous year."[3] Although often used interchangeably, there is a distinction between the terms *complementary* and *alternative*. **Complementary medicine** is used *together with* conventional medicine, as part of the modern integrative medicine approach. An aromatherapist might work with an oncologist to reduce a patient's nausea during chemotherapy, for example. **Alternative medicine** is used *in place of* conventional medi-cine. An example of this would be using a special diet or herbal remedy to treat cancer instead of using radiation, surgery, or other traditional treatments.[4]

Complementary and alternative therapies vary widely in terms of nature of treatment, extent of therapy, and types of problems for which they offer help. Typically, CAM therapies are compared with the conventional medicine. Conventional medicine is practiced by holders of M.D. (medical doctor) or DO (doctor of osteopathy) degrees and by allied health professionals, such as physical therapists, psychologists, and registered nurses. Other terms for conventional medicine include *allopathy, Western, mainstream, orthodox,* and *biomedicine.*[5] In general, practitioners of conventional medicine have graduated from U.S.–sanctioned schools of medicine or are licensed medical practitioners recognized by the American Medical Association (AMA). Some conventional medical practitioners are also CAM practitioners.

The list of practices that are considered CAM changes continually as CAM therapies are proven safe and effective and become accepted as "mainstream."[6] CAM therapies, in general, serve as alternatives to an allopathic system that some people regard as too invasive, too high tech, and too toxic in terms of laboratory-produced medications. CAM users are often people who seek what they perceive as a more natural, gentle approach to healing. Other CAM patients distrust the traditional medical approach and believe that alternative practices will give them greater control over their own health care. Explore your own attitudes toward CAM in the Assess Yourself box.

> **Complementary medicine** Treatment used in conjunction with conventional medicine.
>
> **Alternative medicine** Treatment used in place of conventional medicine.

Who Seeks Alternative Medical Treatment?

People who decide to use complementary and alternative medicine tend not to make this decision on a whim. In many cases, they are more educated than people who rely solely on traditional health care. They are also more likely to be middle-aged and have a middle-class socioeconomic status. A randomized study of several thousand patients seeking care for low back pain through traditional allopathic providers versus chiropractic providers found that those opting for chiropractic help were more likely to question their providers about the nature and extent of recommended treatments. People who seek alternative care usually do so for one of three reasons:

1. *Dissatisfaction.* Patients may be unhappy with ineffective treatment or treatment that has resulted in adverse effects, may find traditional allopathic medicine too impersonal and techno-logically oriented, or may find it too costly. Managed care may have pushed some people out of the allopathic system, after they or family members have experienced problems.

2. *Need for personal control.* Patients view CAM therapies as less authoritarian and more empowering.

3. *Philosophical congruence.* For some people, CAM is just a better fit. Referred to as *cultural creatives,* these CAM users tend to be committed to the environment; to feminism; to involvement with esoteric forms of spirituality and personal growth psychology, including self-actualization and self-expression; and to exploring anything foreign and exotic. They also identify with cultural change and innovation and are among those most likely to adopt alternative treatments.

Research has also revealed the following:

✔ CAM users didn't have a particularly negative attitude toward traditional medicine.
✔ Racial or ethnic status didn't predict CAM usage.
✔ Men and women were equally likely to use CAM.
✔ Those with poorer health were more likely to use CAM.
✔ Some conditions, particularly low back pain and other chronic pain conditions, predict higher CAM usage.
✔ Those who had gone through a transformational experience that had changed their world view were more likely to use CAM.

Sources: P. Barnes et al., "CDC Advance Data Report #343: Complementary and Alternative Medicine among Adults: United States, 2002," 2004, http://nccam.nih.gov/news/camsurvey.htm; J. Astin, "Why Patients Use Alternative Medicine: Results of a National Study," *Journal of the American Medical Association* 279 (1998): 1548–1552; D. M. Eisenberg, R. Davis, and S. Ettner, "Trends in Alternative Medicine Use in the United States, 1990–1997: Results of a Follow-Up National Study," *Journal of the American Medical Association* 280 (1998): 1569–1579; R. Donatelle, J. Nyiendo, and M. Haas, "Health Care Decision-Making Among Those Seeking Care for Low Back Pain from Traditional Medical and Chiropractic Physicians" (paper presented at the American Public Health Association's annual meeting, 1998); R. H. Ray, "The Emerging Culture," *American Demographics*, February 1997.

In short, people choose alternative therapies for a variety of practical and deeply personal reasons (see the Reality Check box). Others continue to consult traditional medical providers, believing that there is safety in government-controlled licensing, regulation of procedures, and drug testing and approval.

A Historical Perspective

America's zeal for the healing power of herbs and plant medicines marks a return to a simpler life. In fact, it takes us back thousands of years. For example, poppy extract was used to quiet crying children in the time of the pharaohs, eons before the medical use of opiates. Although the United States has been somewhat slow to accept plant remedies as standard treatment, an estimated 25 percent of all modern pharmaceutical drugs are derived from herbs, including aspirin (white willow bark), the heart medication digitalis (foxglove), and the cancer treatment Taxol (Pacific yew tree).

Although plant-based medicines were used widely in the United States until World War II, a new generation of FDA-tested pharmaceuticals took over in the later years of the twentieth century. Nontraditional treatments fell out of favor among all but a few segments of the U.S. population and were associated with the undeveloped and impoverished parts of the world. After decades of languishing, however, and with a growing dissatisfaction of the populace with the technowizardry of late twentieth- and early twenty-first-century U.S. medicine, many nontraditional treatments reemerged in treatment arsenals.

To better understand why Americans behave as they do when confronted with an illness or disorder, it is necessary to understand fears, concerns, and sources of hope for a positive outcome. Many of us have a powerful distrust of traditional medical practice. Through either direct experience or media portrayals of problems with today's health care system, many people believe that when sick, the worst place to be is in a hospital or health care setting.

The shift to alternatives is not surprising, considering what has happened in other regions of the world. Reports of miracle cures from ancient remedies, more gentle and holistic means of treatment, and positive outcomes from alternative treatments have led many to seek answers from other cultures. In fact, a number of our recent pharmacological advances have their roots in the herbal remedies used in cultures throughout the world. Eastern medicine, in particular, has been very influential in today's alternative therapies. Chinese medicine and other ancient healing practices, such as Ayurvedic medicine, provide reasonable alternatives to traditional Western treatment.

The Emergence of CAM in the United States

Prior to the early 1990s, we knew little about who was using CAM therapies and their reasons for choosing them. In 1993, a landmark study showed that one in three Americans sought some form of alternative care.[7] Not only did this shock health care providers and public health professionals alike, but it essentially indicated that CAM was here to stay and that we had better take a long, hard look at the implications of CAM use for American consumers. A follow-up study in 1997 showed that an unprecedented increase in CAM use had occurred; almost half of all Americans (47 percent) were using some form of CAM.[8] Although the exact amount spent on CAM therapies was difficult to determine, estimates of spending in excess of $300 billion per year stunned the health care marketplace—this figure was comparable to the total out-of-pocket spending for all U.S. physician services.

As a direct result of these early studies, the U.S. government not only sanctioned the concept of CAM in prevention and treatment, but also created a new National Institutes of Health center, the National Center for Complementary and Alternative Medicine, in 1998. NCCAM is a clearinghouse for CAM information and a focal point for research initiatives, policy development, and general recommendations.

Biologically-based practices   Treatments using substances found in nature, such as herbs, special diets, or vitamin megadoses.

Energy medicine   Therapies using energy fields, such as magnetic fields or biofields.

Manipulative and body-based practices   Treatments involving manipulation or movement of one or more body parts.

Mind–body medicine   Techniques designed to enhance the mind's ability to affect bodily function and symptoms.

Whole medical systems   Complete systems of theory and practice that involve several CAM domains.

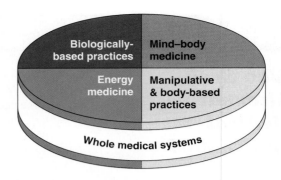

Figure 23.2
The Domains of Complementary and Alternative Medicine

Source: P. Barnes, et al., "CDC Advance Data Report #343: Complementary and Alternative Medicine among Adults: United States, 2002," 2004, http://nccam.nih.gov/news/camsurvey.htm

Major Domains of CAM

The many varieties of CAM have been grouped by the NCCAM into four domains of practice (Figure 23.2), recognizing that the domains may overlap. The domains are as follows:[9]

- **Biologically-based practices** use substances found in nature, such as herbs, special diets, or vitamins (in doses outside those used in conventional medicine)
- **Energy medicine** involves the use of energy fields, such as magnetic fields or biofields (energy fields that some believe surround and penetrate the body)
- **Manipulative and body-based practices** are based on manipulation or movement of one or more body parts
- **Mind–body medicine** uses a variety of techniques designed to enhance the mind's ability to affect bodily function and symptoms

An additional area of study is **whole medical systems,** which cut across all domains and are built upon complete systems of theory and practice. Often these systems evolved apart from and earlier than the conventional medical approach.

CAM Use: Who, What, and Why?

Although previous studies indicated widespread CAM use and prompted government recognition and research, it wasn't until 2004 that comprehensive and reliable data was available on not only the CAM therapies that Americans were using, but who was using them and why. The survey was completed by over 31,000 Americans and revealed that 36 percent of adults are using some form of CAM.[10] While this number is lower than the 1997 survey results, it is important to note that the new survey did not include prayer or the use of megavitamins as forms of CAM. If these two modalities are included, the use of CAM would be over 62 percent. In general, when prayer is not included as a CAM therapy, biologically-based therapies are most commonly used (22 percent of adults), with mind–body medicine being second (17 percent).[11]

Who actually uses CAM? There are distinct patterns of use that emerged from the 2004 survey:

- More women than men
- People with higher educational levels
- People who had been hospitalized in the past year
- Former smokers (compared with current smokers or those who have never smoked)
- People with back, neck, head, or joint aches or other painful conditions
- People with gastrointestinal disorders or sleeping problems

Interesting information about *why* people use CAM also surfaced from the survey. Some 55 percent of people believed that CAM would improve health when used in combination with conventional therapy, while 28 percent used it because they believed that conventional medicine could not help. Fifty percent thought that CAM would be interesting to try, while 26 percent had a recommendation from a medical professional to try a CAM therapy. Finally, 13 percent tried CAM because conventional medical treatment was too expensive.

Alternative Medical System Options

Alternative medical systems involve complete systems of theory and practice that have evolved independently of, and often prior to, the conventional biomedical approach that we tend to consider "traditional." In the United States, the terms *traditional* and *allopathic* have historically referred to a system that is directed by the AMA guidelines for licensing and that most insurance plans cover as fairly standard and acceptable procedure. In contrast, *nonallopathic* medicine has been dubbed "alternative." This situation is changing. In the past decade, some specialists in nonallopathic medicine have been accepted by professional groups, and their inclusion in mainstream medicine is growing daily. Many traditional medical schools are now offering coursework in CAM, and many traditional doctors refer patients to alternative providers, who are in turn reimbursed by the patients' health insurance plans. Modalities that have received the greatest degree of acceptance include chiropractic medicine, acupuncture, herbal and homeopathic medicine, and naturopathy. However, it is important to realize that there are many other traditional systems of medicine that have been practiced by various cultures throughout the world. Many come from venerable Asian approaches.

Traditional Chinese Medicine and Ayurveda

Two major systems that are at the root of much of our CAM thinking today are traditional Chinese medicine and Ayurveda, which is India's traditional system of medicine. **Traditional Chinese medicine (TCM)** emphasizes the proper balance or disturbances of *qi* (pronounced "chee"), or vital energy in health and disease, respectively. In TCM, diagnosis is based on history, on observation of the body (especially the tongue), on palpation, and on pulse diagnosis, an elaborate procedure requiring considerable skill and experience by the practitioner. Techniques such as acupuncture, herbal medicine, massage, and *qi gong* (a form of energy therapy described in more detail later in this chapter) are among the TCM approaches to health and healing.

Ayurveda (or **Ayurvedic medicine**) relates to the "science of life," which places equal emphasis on body, mind, and spirit and strives to restore the innate harmony of the individual. Ayurvedic practitioners diagnose mainly by observation and touch and assign patients to one of three major body types and a variety of subtypes. Once classified, patients are treated mostly through dietary modifications and herbal remedies that have been drawn from the vast botanical wealth of the Indian subcontinent. Treatments may also include animal and mineral ingredients, even powdered gemstones. Massage, steam baths, exposure to sunlight, and controlled breathing are among the more common Ayurvedic treatments.[12]

Homeopathy and Naturopathy

Other alternative systems of medicine include *homeopathy* and *naturopathy*. **Homeopathic medicine** is an unconventional Western system based on the principle that "like cures like." In other words, the same substance that in large doses produces the symptoms of an illness will, in very small

---

Traditional Chinese medicine (TCM) Comprehensive system of diagnosis and treatment in which dietary change, touch, massage, medicinal teas, and other herbal medicines are used extensively.

Qi Element of traditional Oriental medicine that refers to the vital energy force that courses through the body. When qi is in balance, health is restored.

Ayurveda (Ayurvedic medicine) A method of treatment derived largely from ancient India, in which practitioners diagnose by observation and touch, and then assign a largely dietary treatment laced with herbal medicines.

Homeopathic medicine Unconventional Western system of medicine based on the principle that "like cures like."

Table 23.1
Popular Complementary Treatments

Aromatherapy	Aromatherapists use scented materials to evoke sensations through the smell centers of the body. Treatment focuses on odors regarded as pleasurable.
Food therapy	Treatment is based on the belief that many disorders are based on allergies and toxic synergism among food combinations. Naturopaths test for and treat food allergies and assign special diets designed to produce nutritional balance.
Hypnosis	Diseases are treated by suggestion while the patient is in a hypnotic trance.
Massage	Massage involves rubbing, stroking, kneading, or lightly pounding the body with the hands or other instruments.
Megavitamins	Treatment with megavitamins promotes the consumption of large doses of common essential vitamins and minerals to prevent disease and heal illness.
Relaxation techniques	The goal is to remove stress and promote healing. Techniques include yoga, meditation, breathing and posture exercises, and visualization.

doses, cure the illness.[13] Essentially, homeopathic physicians use herbal medicine, minerals, and chemicals in extremely diluted forms as natural agents to kill infectious agents or ward off illnesses that are caused by more potent forms or doses of those agents.

Naturopathic medicine views disease as a manifestation of an alteration in the processes by which the body naturally heals itself. Disease results from the body's effort to ward off impurities and harmful substances from the environment. Naturopathic physicians emphasize restoring health rather than curing disease. They employ an array of healing practices, including diet and clinical nutrition; homeopathy; acupuncture; herbal medicine; hydrotherapy (the use of water in a range of temperatures and methods of application); spinal and soft-tissue manipulation; physical therapies involving electric currents, ultrasound, and light therapy; therapeutic counseling; and pharmacology. Several major naturopathic schools in the United States and Canada provide training, conferring the *naturopathic doctor (ND)* degree on students who have completed a four-year graduate program that emphasizes humanistically oriented family medicine.

While these medical philosophies and patterns of treatment have exerted great influence on populations worldwide, other, more regionally limited, medical traditions are also noteworthy. American Indian, Aboriginal, African, Middle Eastern, Tibetan, and South American cultures also have their own unique alternative systems. International surveys of CAM outside the United States suggest that alternative therapies are popular throughout most of the world. Public opinion polls and consumer surveys in Europe and the United Kingdom suggest high CAM use in Italy, France, Denmark, Finland, and Australia, in addition to most Asian cultures.[14]

As the number of alternative therapists grows and systems become intertwined, so do the number of health care options available to consumers (see Table 23.1 for examples). Before considering any medical systems, wise consumers will consult the most reliable resources to thoroughly evaluate risks, the scientific basis of claimed benefits, and any contraindications to using the CAM product or service. Avoid practitioners who promote their treatments as a cure-all for every health problem or who seem to promise remedies that have thus far defied the best scientific efforts of mainstream medicine. Wise consumers apply the same strategies to researching CAM as they do to choosing allopathic care (see Chapter 22).

Manipulative and Body-Based Methods

Another category of CAM includes methods that are based on manipulation and/or movement of the body. For example, chiropractors focus on the relationship between the body's structures (primarily the spine) and functions and on how that relationship affects the preservation and restoration of health. Chiropractors employ manipulation as a key therapy.

Chiropractic Medicine

Chiropractic medicine has been practiced for over 100 years. Allopathic medicine and chiropractic medicine were in direct competition over a century ago.[15] Today, however, many managed care organizations work closely with chiropractors, and many insurance companies will pay for chiropractic

---

Naturopathic medicine System of medicine that attempts to restore natural processes of the body and promote healing through natural means.

Chiropractic medicine Manipulation of the spine to allow proper energy flow.

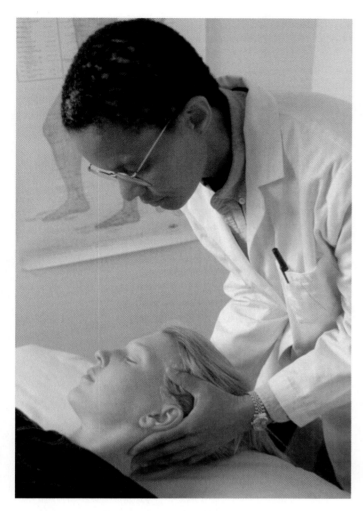

A chiropractor treats a patient using a variety of techniques to manipulate the spine into proper alignment.

treatment, particularly if it is recommended by a medical doctor. More than 20 million Americans now visit chiropractors each year.

Chiropractic medicine is based on the idea that a life-giving energy flows through the spine via the nervous system. If the spine is subluxated (partly misaligned or dislocated), that force is disrupted. Chiropractors use a variety of techniques to manipulate the spine back into proper alignment so the life-giving energy can flow unimpeded through the nervous system. It has been established that their treatment can be effective for back pain, neck pain, and headaches.

The average chiropractic training program requires four years of intensive courses in biochemistry, anatomy, physiology, diagnostics, pathology, nutrition, and related topics, combined with hands-on clinical training. Many chiropractors continue their training to obtain specialized certification, for instance, in women's health, gerontology, or pediatrics. There are currently 16 chiropractic colleges in the United States, with a combined enrollment of over 14,000 students.

Six states require a bachelor's degree in addition to the doctor of chiropractic degree for licensure. The practice of chiropractic is licensed and regulated in all 50 states.[16]

You should investigate and question a chiropractor as carefully as you would any licensed medical doctor. As with many health professionals, you may note vast differences in technique among specialists. It is recommended that you choose a chiropractor who follows standard chiropractic regimens for treating musculoskeletal conditions. Avoid those who promote adjustment as a cure-all for all disorders or whose treatments are not based on manipulation of the spine.

Other Manipulation Therapies

There are other specialties that involve manipulation of the body. Recall from Chapter 22 that *DOs,* or *doctors of osteopathy,* place particular emphasis on the musculoskeletal system. Osteopathic practitioners believe that all of the body's systems work together and that disturbances in one system may have an impact upon function elsewhere in the body.[17] As such, they specialize in body manipulation yet also have a more traditional form of medical school training.

Energy Medicine

Energy medicine, also called energy therapies, focuses either on energy fields thought to originate with the body (biofields) or on fields from other sources (electromagnetic fields). Biofield therapies are intended to affect energy fields said to surround and penetrate the human body. The existence of these fields has not been experimentally proven. Some forms of energy therapy manipulate biofields by applying pressure and/or manipulating the body by placing the hands in, or through, these fields.[18]

Popular examples of biofield therapy include *qi gong, reiki,* and *therapeutic touch. Qi gong,* a component of traditional Chinese medicine, combines movement, meditation, and regulation of breathing to enhance the flow of vital energy (qi), improve blood circulation, and enhance immune function.[19] *Reiki,* whose name derives from the Japanese word representing "universal life energy," is based on the belief that by channeling spiritual energy through the practitioner the spirit is healed, and it in turn heals the physical body.[20] *Therapeutic touch* derives from the ancient technique of "laying on of hands" and is based on the premise that the healing force of the therapist brings about the patient's recovery and that healing is promoted when the body's energies are in balance. By passing the hands over the body, the healers identify bodily imbalances.[21]

Bioelectromagnetic-based therapies involve the unconventional use of electromagnetic fields, such as pulsed fields, magnetic fields, or alternating current or direct current fields, to treat asthma, cancer, pain, migraines, and other conditions.

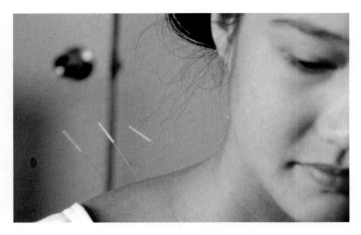

Acupuncture has been found to be effective in treating many problems but should always be performed by a licensed practitioner.

There is little scientific documentation to support claims for energy fields techniques at this point. However, two derivatives of energy therapy have gained much wider acceptance in recent years: acupuncture and acupressure.

Acupuncture and Acupressure

Chinese medical treatments are growing in popularity and offer an important complement to Western biomedical care. **Acupuncture,** one of the more popular forms of Chinese medicine among Americans, is sought for a wide variety of health conditions, including musculoskeletal dysfunction, mood enhancement, and wellness promotion. Following acupuncture, most respondents report high satisfaction with the treatment, improved quality of life, improvement in or cure of the condition, and reduced reliance on prescription drugs and surgery.[22]

Acupuncturists in the United States are state-licensed, and each state has specific requirements regarding training programs. Most acupuncturists have either completed a two-to-three-year postgraduate program to obtain a master of traditional Oriental medicine (MTOM) degree or attended a shorter certification program in North America or Asia. They may be licensed in multiple areas—for example, the MTOM is also trained in the use of herbs and moxibustion (the application of a heated herbal moxa stick). Some licensed MDs and chiropractors have trained in acupuncture and obtained certification to use this treatment.

Acupuncture The insertion of long, thin needles to affect the energy flow within the body.

Acupressure Application of pressure to selected body points to balance energy.

Acupressure is similar to acupuncture but does not use needles. Instead, the practitioner applies pressure to points critical to balancing yin and yang, the two Chinese principles that interact to influence overall harmony (health) of the body. Practitioners must have the same basic understanding of energy pathways as do acupuncturists. Acupressure should not be applied by an untrained person to pregnant women or to anyone with a chronic health condition.

What do you think?

Why do you think more and more people are opting for complementary and alternative treatments? ■ What are the potential benefits of these treatments? ■ What are the potential risks? ■ What types of controls are reasonable to regulate the quality and consistency of foreign-trained health care providers?

Mind–Body Medicine

Mind–body interventions employ a variety of techniques to facilitate the mind's capacity to affect bodily functions and symptoms. Many therapies might fall under this category; but some areas, such as biofeedback, patient education, and cognitive-behavior techniques, have been so well investigated that they are no longer considered alternative. However, meditation, yoga, tai chi, certain uses of hypnosis, dance, music and art therapy, prayer and mental healing, and several others are still categorized as complementary and alternative.

Body Work

Body work actually consists of several different forms of exercise. *Feldenkrais* therapy work is a system of the movements, floor exercises, and body work designed to retrain the central nervous system to help it find new pathways around areas of blockage or damage. It is gentle and effective in rehabilitating trauma victims. *Rolfing* is a more invasive form of body work, aimed at restructuring the musculoskeletal system by working on patterns of tension held in deep tissue. The therapist applies firm—sometimes painful—pressure to different areas of the body. Rolfing can release repressed emotions as well as dissipate muscle tension. *Shiatsu* is a traditional healing art from Japan that makes use of firm finger pressure applied to specified points on the body and is intended to increase the circulation of vital energy. The client lies on the floor, with the therapist seated alongside. *Trager therapy,* one of the least invasive forms of body work, employs gentle rocking and bouncing motions to induce states of deep, pleasant relaxation.[23]

Psychoneuroimmunology

As briefly discussed in Chapter 3, **psychoneuroimmunology (PNI)** is a relatively new field of study. Seaward defines it as the "interaction of consciousness (psycho), brain and central nervous system (neuro), and the body's defense against external infection and internal aberrant cell division (immunology)."[24] A number of researchers have postulated over the years that excessive stress and maladaptive coping will ultimately serve to create dysfunction of the immune system and increase risk for a variety of infectious and chronic diseases. To counteract the negative impact on health, scientists are exploring ways in which relaxation, biofeedback, meditation, yoga, laughter, exercise, and activities that involve either conscious or unconscious mind "quieting" and harnessing of negative energy may interact to counteract negative stressors. As such, several of the above mind–body activities designed to slow heartbeat and breathing and to bring about homeostasis in the body are being studied. A classic study of PNI and mind–body health attempted to assess the effects of relaxation and coping techniques on the immune system by studying nursing home patients. Participants were divided into three groups: those who were taught relaxation techniques, those who were provided with abundant social contact, and those who received no special techniques or contact. After a one-month period, immune system function was greatly improved in those people who received stress management therapy as compared to the control group.[25] Several other studies have attempted to show similar positive effects of mind–body techniques that encourage relaxation and other stress-reduction strategies.

> ### What do you think?
>
> *Have you ever tried any of these CAM therapies?* ■ *Which of them are offered on your campus or in your community?* ■ *What role do CAM exercises have in your personal quest for physical fitness? Spiritual fitness?*

Biologically-based Practices

Biologically-based therapy is perhaps one of the most controversial domains of CAM practice, largely because of the sheer numbers of options that are available and the myriad claims that are made about their supposedly magical effects. To date, many of these claims have not been thoroughly investigated, and regulation of this aspect of CAM has been relatively slow in coming.

Biologically-based therapies include natural and biologically-based practices, interventions, and products, many of which overlap with conventional medicine's use of dietary supplements. Included are *herbal, special dietary, orthomolec-*

ular, and *individual* biological therapies. Practitioners who base their therapies primarily on the medicinal qualities of plants and herbs are referred to as *herbalists.*

Herbal remedies are not to be taken lightly. Just because something is natural does not necessarily mean that it is safe. For example, a recent FDA Consumer Advisory warned that kava products may be associated with severe liver damage.[26] Other reports remind consumers that even rigorously tested products can be risky. Many plants are poisonous, and some can be toxic if ingested in high doses. Others may be dangerous when combined with prescription or over-the-counter drugs, or they could disrupt the normal action of the drugs.

Properly trained herbalists and homeopaths have received graduate-level training in special programs such as herbal nutrition or traditional Chinese medicine. These practitioners have been trained in diagnosis; in mixing herbs, titrations, and dosages; and in the follow-up care of patients.

Checking on the education and training of anyone who recommends or sells herbal medications is a part of intelligent consumerism as well as just plain good sense. Also, it is important to look at the research surrounding individual substances and remedies. The NCCAM website is a good place to start, because it includes summaries of recent research. It is a good resource for information on the effectiveness and risks of any CAM therapy discussed in this chapter.

Herbal Remedies

Largely derived from Ayurvedic or traditional Chinese medicine, herbal medications are widely available in the United States. Fueled by mass advertising and promoted as part of multiple vitamin and mineral regimens by major drug manufacturers, herbal supplements represent the hottest trend in the health market.

Herbal remedies come in several different forms. **Tinctures** (extracts of fresh or dried plants) usually contain a high percentage of grain alcohol to prevent spoilage and are among the best herbal options. Freeze-dried extracts are very stable and offer good value for your money. Standardized extracts are also among the more reliable forms of herbal preparations.

In general, herbal medicines tend to be milder than chemical drugs and produce their effects more slowly; they also are much less likely to cause toxicity because they are diluted rather than concentrated forms of drugs.[27] But diluted or not, herbals are still drugs. They should not be taken

> **Psychoneuroimmunology (PNI)** Use of stress-management and other techniques to enhance the function of the immune system.
>
> **Tinctures** Herbal extracts usually combined with grain alcohol to prevent spoilage.

casually, any more than you would take over-the-counter or prescription drugs without really needing them or knowing their side effects. No matter how natural they are, herbs still contain many of the same chemicals as synthetic prescription drugs. Too much of any herb can cause problems, particularly one from nonstandardized extracts. Some herbs and specific dietary supplements can pose risks to consumers by interacting with prescription drugs or causing unusual side effects.

The following discussion gives an overview of some of the most common herbal supplements on the market.

Ginkgo Biloba Ginkgo biloba is an extract from the leaves of a deciduous tree that lives up to 1,000 years. It is one of the world's oldest living tree species, one that can be traced back more than 200 million years. The ginkgo was almost destroyed during the last ice age in all regions of the world except China, where it is considered a sacred tree with medicinal properties.[28] Today, ginkgo leaf extracts are widely prescribed in many countries and gaining in popularity.

Gingko biloba is said to have many benefits and is used to treat depression, impotence, premenstrual syndrome, diseases of the eye (such as retinopathy and macular degeneration), and general vascular disease. In particular, it has been shown to improve short-term memory and concentration for individuals with impaired blood flow to the brain due to narrowing of vessels or clogging of key arteries. Reports of improvements in circulation and anti-aging properties are interesting but, as yet, unsubstantiated. An early Harvard-based study of 202 men and women with mild to moderately severe dementia caused by stroke or Alzheimer's disease was among the first to promote ginkgo in the United States. After one year, the group receiving ginkgo experienced significant improvement in cognitive performance (memory, learning, reading) and social functioning (carrying on conversations, recognizing familiar faces) compared to those in the placebo (nonginkgo) group.[29] Much of this improvement was believed to be due to the antioxidant properties of the herb and its blood-thinning properties, which seem to improve blood and oxygen flow to clogged blood vessels. Whether this herb will improve memory in people with normal blood flow remains largely unexplored to date. Claims that ginkgo will improve short- and long-term memory in the typical person are not scientifically based.

Most nutritional experts and physicians recommend that people who are considering using ginkgo take a 40-milligram tablet three times a day for a month or so to determine whether there is any improvement. If there is none, continuing to take this supplement is largely unwarranted. It has been shown to cause gastric irritation. Also, remember that disturbing memory loss or difficulty thinking, regardless of age, should be checked by a doctor to determine underlying causes.

Because the main action of ginkgo appears to be as a blood thinner, it should not be taken with other blood-thinning agents, such as aspirin, vitamin E, garlic, ginger, the

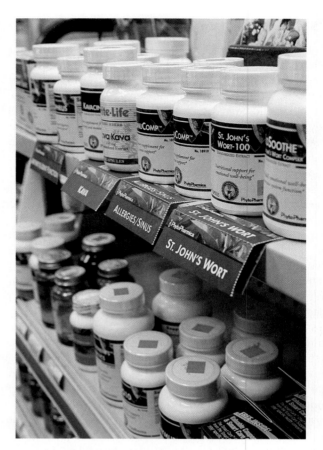

Buying herbal supplements can be confusing, since so many brands exist and their manufacture is not strictly regulated for potency or quality.

prescription drug warfarin (trade name: Coumadin), or any other medications that list thinning of the blood as a potential side effect.[30] Doing so could increase the risk of hemorrhage.

Today, much of what we know about ginkgo biloba remains controversial, even though extensive research on its effects has been conducted. Today, trials are in progress to test its effectiveness in treating asthma, cardiovascular disease (CVD), sexual function, memory, digestive problems, diabetes, and several other areas. Until the results of these tests are available, consumers should use caution in any use of ginkgo.[31]

St. John's Wort The bright yellow, star-shaped flowers of St. John's wort (SJW) have a rich and varied history in Europe, Asia, and Africa. The name for this herb dates back to early Christian times and relates to the red oil that glands in the flowers secrete when they are pinched or cut. Christians believed that the flowers secreted this blood-red oil on August 29, the anniversary of the beheading of St. John the Baptist, and that they bloomed on June 24, St. John's birthday. *Wort* is Old English for "root" or "plant."[32] Colonists who came to the United States brought SJW with them, only to find that

Native Americans were already using it for everything from snake bite to general health enhancement. In the United States, SJW grows in abundance in northern California and southern Oregon and is also referred to as *klammath weed*.[33]

Today, SJW enjoys global popularity. It is the favored therapy for depression in a number of countries, including Germany, actually surpassing most standard antidepressants as the first mode of treatment for clinical depression. Research into the herb has yielded mixed results: some studies have indicated it is more effective than a placebo and has fewer side effects than prescription antidepressants, while others have found no effect on depression at all.

A review of 23 well-designed clinical trials published in the *British Medical Journal* concluded that extracts of SJW "are more effective than placebo for the treatment of mild to moderately severe depressive disorders." This review also found evidence from eight other studies that SJW may work as well as some other drugs in countering mild depression. The research team called for more rigorously controlled, larger sample–sized studies comparing this herb with prescription doses of Prozac and other antidepressant drugs.[34] However, the results of one such study, a randomized, double-blind trial conducted at multiple sites and reported in the *Journal of the American Medical Association*, found that SJW was no more effective for treating major depression of moderate severity than was a placebo.[35] Since this study refutes the results of several less rigorously controlled trials, reports on it were front-page news. Other studies have provided a conflicting array of results about potential benefits.[36] As other well-designed studies are published, consumers will have more information on which to base their decision.

Proponents believe SJW has the following effects:[37]

- Acts as a positive mood enhancer by helping maintain serotonin levels and as natural neurotransmitters that help brain function and calm the body[38]
- Helps as a sleep enhancer for those having difficulty sleeping[39]
- Supports immune function by suppressing the release of interleukin-6, a protein that controls certain aspects of the immune response.[40]

Like other plants, SJW contains a number of different chemicals, many of which are not clearly understood. We do know that there seems to be more to SJW than myth and the simplistic explanations that many health food stores give their customers, and researchers are beginning to view the herb in a less favorable light.

The herb also has several side effects. Most are more bothersome than severe and range from slight gastrointestinal upset to fatigue, dry mouth, dizziness, skin rashes, and itching. Some people develop extreme sensitivity to sunlight. Most of these side effects are minor, however, when compared with those of prescription antidepressant medicines.

Due to conflicting news about SJW, consumers should proceed with caution. Since the herb is sold in the United States as a dietary supplement, not a drug, it is not regulated by the FDA and rigorous testing has not been done. Anyone suffering from clinical depression should be under a physician's and psychologist's care.

In addition, SJW should never be taken in combination with prescription antidepressants. When combined with other serotonin-enhancing drugs, such as Prozac, SJW may result in serotonin overload, leading to tremors, agitation, or convulsions. SJW also should not be used by pregnant women or women who are nursing, by young children, or by the frail elderly, because the safety margins have not been established.

Echinacea Echinacea, or the *purple coneflower*, is found primarily in the Midwest and prairie regions of the United States. Two of the nine species of echinacea in the United States are now on the federal endangered species list, a cause of growing concern for many environmentalists as the herb's popularity has grown. Believed to be used extensively by Native Americans for centuries, echinacea eventually gained widespread acceptance in the United States before being shipped to Europe, where its use grew gradually over the eighteenth and nineteenth centuries.

Today, echinacea is the best-selling herb in health and natural food stores in the United States and is widely used throughout most of the world. It is said to stimulate the immune system and increase the effectiveness of the white blood cells that attack bacteria and viruses. Many people believe it to be helpful in preventing and treating the symptoms of a cold or flu.

However, echinacea remains controversial. While many studies in Europe have provided preliminary evidence of its effectiveness, recent controlled trials in the United States indicate that echinacea is no more effective than a placebo in preventing a cold.[41]

As with many herbal treatments, little valid research has been conducted on the benefits and risks of echinacea. Because it can affect the immune system, people with autoimmune diseases such as arthritis should not take it. Other people who should avoid echinacea include pregnant women, people with diabetes or multiple sclerosis, anyone allergic to the daisy family of plants, and anyone undergoing chemotherapy.[42] Recent studies have also raised concerns about increased risks for people who take echinacea before surgery.[43]

Green Tea Several studies have shown promising links between green and white tea consumption and cancer prevention, although investigation continues. Now, new research from Japan suggests that drinking one or two cups of green tea per day may keep the heart attack doctors away.[44] Findings indicate that tea drinkers had lower rates of heart attack, indicating a possible protective effect. Some scientists suspect that green tea may boost heart health because it contains high levels of flavonoids. These plant compounds, which are also found in fruits, vegetables, and red wine, are

Table 23.2
Herbal Remedies for Common Conditions

Condition	Herbal Product	Dose	Side Effects
Constipation	Aloe	20–30 mg hydroxyanthracene derivatives/day	Electrolyte and fluid imbalance
	Buckthorn	20–30 mg glycofrangulin per day	None known
	Cascara	20–30 mg cascaroside/day	None known
	Flaxseed	1 tbs. whole flaxseed with 8 oz. water 2–3 times/day	None if taken as directed
	Manna	20–30 g/day	Nausea, flatulence
	Psyllium	12–40 g (seed) or 4–20 g (husk) daily with 8 oz. water for every 5 g drug	Allergic reaction (rare)
	Senna leaf	20–30 mg sennoside per day	Electrolyte and fluid imbalance; can produce rebound constipation if used longer than 1–2 weeks
Dysmenorrhea (menstrual cramps)	Black cohosh	40–60% extract with alcohol	Occasionally, gastric discomfort
	Potentilla	4–6 g powdered herb	Aggravates any gastric discomforts
Leg cramps and swelling	Butcher's broom	7–11 mg ruscogenin in extract	Gastric disturbance, nausea in rare cases
	Horse chestnut	250–312.5 mg extract 2 times/day	Itching, nausea in rare cases
	Sweet clover	3–30 mg coumarin/day	May cause headache
Menopausal symptoms	Black cohosh	40–60% extract with alcohol	Occasionally, gastric discomfort
	Chaste tree fruit	30–40 mg in aqueous-alcohol extracts	May cause itching, rash
Premenstrual syndrome	Black cohosh	40–60% extract with alcohol	Occasionally, gastric discomfort
	Chaste tree fruit	30–40 mg in aqueous-alcohol extracts	May cause itching, rash
	Yarrow	4.5 g powder for infusion	None known
Sleep disturbances	Hops flower	0.5 g powder for infusion	None known
	Valerian root	2–3 g powder for infusion	None known

Source: From "New Guides to Herbal Remedies: Examples of Herbs Approved by German Commission E," *Harvard Women's Health Watch,* February 1999, © 1999, President and Fellows of Harvard College. Reprinted by permission.

thought to boost health by combating oxidation, a process in which cell-damaging free radicals accumulate. Oxidative damage can be caused by outside factors, such as cigarette smoking, or by factors on the cellular level. Oxidation is suspected of increasing the risk of heart disease, stroke, and several other diseases. Although promising, more research on the role of green tea in CVD risk must be conducted to determine whether the effect is actually due to the tea or to some other characteristic that tea drinkers have in common.

Ephedra (Ma Huang)   An herbal ingredient formerly found in many weight loss and fitness supplements, ephedra's active ingredient is ephedrine, which is similar to amphetamine. After years of controversy, a comprehensive study conducted by the RAND Corporation for the U.S. Food and Drug Administration (FDA) indicated that there was limited evidence of an effect of ephedra on short-term weight loss and minimal evidence of an effect on performance enhancement in physical

activity. Furthermore, the study reviewed over 16,000 reported adverse effects from ephedra and noted that heart attack, stroke, and death had occurred in the absence of other contributing factors. Other side effects such as heart palpitations, psychiatric problems, upper gastrointestinal effects, tremor, insomnia and other problems had also occurred at rates much greater than expected.[45] In 2004, the FDA banned the sale of all supplements containing ephedra. These products are no longer legally available for sale.

See Table 23.2 for other herbal remedies that are popular for treating common health conditions.

Special Supplements

The FDA defines dietary supplements as "products (other than tobacco) that are intended to supplement or add to the diet and contain one or more of the following ingredients: vitamins, minerals, amino acids, herbs, or other substance that increases total dietary intake, and that is intended for ingestion in the form of a capsule, powder, soft gel, or gel-cap, and is not represented as a conventional food or as a sole item." Typically, people take these supplements to improve health, prevent disease, or enhance mood. In recent years, we've heard increasing reports on the health benefits of a number of vitamins and minerals.

When taken to increase work output or the potential for it, dietary supplements are labeled as **ergogenic aids.** Examples include bee pollen, caffeine, glycine, carnitine, lecithin, brewer's yeast, and gelatin. In recent years, a new generation of performance-enhancing ergogenic aids has hit the market. Many of these claim to increase muscular strength and performance, boost energy, and enhance resistance to disease.

Muscle Enhancers As described in Chapter 14, baseball player Mark McGwire made headline news in 1998 not only for his home run record, but also for admitting that he took the diet supplement androstenedione. "Andro," a substance that is found naturally in meat and some plants and is also produced in the human body by the adrenal glands and gonads, is a precursor to the human hormone testosterone. In other words, the body converts andro directly into testosterone, which enables an athlete to train harder and recover more quickly. Ironically, although major league baseball, the NCAA, the NFL, and the International Olympic Committee have banned andro, it is readily available over the counter.

Research indicates that andro has a chemical structure very similar to that of anabolic steroids. When taken over time and in sufficient quantities, andro may increase the risk of serious medical conditions. Alarmed by a 2004 *Monitoring the Future* survey that showed that one in 40 high school seniors had used andro in the past year, the U.S. Department of Health and Human Services has called for prompt action to regulate andro as a controlled substance. As of this writing, action to restrict use and sanction offenders is still pending.

Creatine is a naturally occurring compound found primarily in skeletal muscle that helps to optimize the muscles' energy levels. In recent years, the use of creatine supplements has increased dramatically because of claims that it increases muscle energy and allows a person to work harder with less muscle fatigue and build muscle mass with less effort. Reports of creatine's benefits, however, appear exaggerated. Over one-third of those taking creatine are unable to absorb it in the muscles and thus achieve no benefit. Side effects include muscle cramping, muscle strains, and possible liver and kidney damage.[46]

Ginseng Grown commercially throughout many regions of North America, ginseng is much prized for its reported sexual restorative value. It is believed that ginseng affects the pituitary gland, increasing resistance to stress, affecting metabolism, aiding skin and muscle tone, and providing the hormonal balance necessary for a healthy sex life. Other purported benefits include improved endurance, muscle strength, recovery from exercise, oxygen metabolism during exercise, auditory and visual reaction time, and mental concentration.[47]

Studies of the effectiveness of ginseng, however, have raised questions about the appropriate dosages and how long it should be taken to realize benefits. Because the potency of plants varies considerably, dosage is difficult to control and side effects are fairly common. Noteworthy side effects of high doses include nervousness, insomnia, high blood pressure, headaches, skin eruptions, chest pain, depression, and abnormal vaginal bleeding.[48]

Glucosamine Glucosamine is a substance produced by the body that plays a key role in the growth and development of cartilage. When present in sufficient amounts, it stimulates the manufacture of substances necessary for proper joint function and joint repair. It is manufactured commercially and sold under a variety of different names, usually glucosamine sulfate.

Glucosamine has been shown to be effective for treating osteoarthritis and related degenerative joint diseases and appears to relieve swelling and decrease pain. Unlike many other herbal supplements, glucosamine sulfate has a good safety record with few noteworthy side effects. However, questions have arisen as to its effectiveness in recent years. While results of meta-analysis reviews and industry-sponsored research have shown it to be moderately effective, smaller independent studies have shown no significant benefits. Currently the Glucosamine Arthritis Intervention Trial is being conducted by the NIH and NCCAM to examine possible benefits. Results should be available in 2005.[49]

Chromium Picolinate A few years ago, chromium picolinate was believed to be the new miracle for anyone interested in weight loss. Since then, at least two major studies at the U.S. Department of Agriculture Human Nutrition Research Center have shown no benefit.[50]

SAMe SAMe (pronounced "Sammy") is the nickname for S-adenosyl-L-methionine, a compound produced biochemically in all humans to help perform some 40 functions in the body, ranging from bone preservation (hence its purported osteoarthritis benefits) to DNA replication.

SAMe has been reported to have a significant effect on mild-to-moderate depression without many of the typical side effects of prescription medications, such as sexual dysfunction, weight gain, and sleep disturbance. Scientists speculate that SAMe somehow affects brain levels of the neurotransmitters noradrenaline, serotonin, and, possibly,

> **Ergogenic aids** Special dietary supplements taken to increase strength, energy, and the ability to work.

dopamine, all of which are related to the human stress response and the origins of depression in the body.[51]

While there has been much ado about the wonders of this natural antidepressant, much of the hype has not been substantiated in large, randomized clinical trials, the type of research necessary to validate drug claims. Also, the research has been of short duration, meaning that little is known about potential long-term side effects such as toxicity to the liver or carcinogenic properties. Questions still remain over how much SAMe a person should take and in what form it should be administered.

Anyone considering SAMe use should consider these factors:[52]

- While one large, randomized trial showed modest pain relief in osteoarthritis patients using SAMe, results were not significantly better than results obtained using standard treatments.
- Many question the high cost of SAMe (between $15 and $35 or higher for 20 pills).
- Clinical depression requires more than self-treatment. Any depressed person should consult a physician to explore all options, including counseling as well as pharmaceutical and natural remedies.
- People with a family history of cardiovascular disease should not take SAMe, due to preliminary indications that it may trigger heart problems.
- Side effects such as restlessness, anxiety, insomnia, and mania occasionally occur with use and are more common in people with bipolar disorder.

Under no circumstances should SAMe be taken by anyone on prescription antidepressants. The time lag between taking the prescription and beginning SAMe, and vice versa, should be carefully considered.[53]

Antioxidants   Although covered in depth in Chapter 8, it should be noted here that antioxidants are among the most sought-after supplements on the market. Primary antioxidants include beta-carotene, selenium, vitamin C, and vitamin E.

Foods as Healing Agents

Many Americans rely on *functional foods*—foods or supplements designed to improve some aspect of physical or mental functioning. Sometimes referred to as **nutraceuticals,** for their combined nutritional and pharmaceutical benefit, several are believed to actually work in much the same way as pharmaceutical drugs in making a person well or bolstering the immune system.

Foods contain many nonnutrient active ingredients that can affect us in different ways. For example, chili peppers contain ingredients that make your eyes water and clear your sinuses. Many of these active ingredients, or constituents, can promote good health. A number of foods, such as sweet potatoes, tangerines, and red peppers, are recognized as excellent sources of antioxidants. Onion and garlic contain allium compounds that reduce blood clotting. Other foods have natural anti-inflammatory properties or aid digestion. Some are known by the term *probiotics,* foods that promote good bacteria in the body that may help fight off infection.[54]

Some of the most common healthful foods and their purported benefits include the following:

- *Plant stanol.* Can lower "bad" (LDL) cholesterol.
- *Oat fiber.* Can lower "bad" (LDL) cholesterol; serves as a natural soother of nerves; stabilizes blood sugar levels.
- *Sunflower.* Can lower risk of heart disease; may prevent angina.
- *Soy protein.* May lower heart disease risk; provides protective estrogen-like effect; may reduce risk from certain cancers.
- *Red meats and dark green, leafy vegetables.* Contain B vitamins (B_6, B_{12}, folate), which can lower levels of homocysteine, an amino acid associated with heart disease.
- *Garlic.* Lowers cholesterol and reduces clotting tendency of blood; lowers blood pressure; may serve as form of antibiotic.
- *Green tea.* Lowers cholesterol; may have a role in fighting certain cancers (see earlier section).
- *Ginger.* Fights motion sickness, stomach pain and upset; discourages blood clots; may relieve rheumatism.
- *Yogurt.* Yogurt that is labeled "Live Active Culture" contains active, friendly bacteria that can fight off infections.

Table 23.3 lists other foods and supplements with their risks and benefits.

Many people purchase foods labeled *organic* because they expect these products to contain only health-promoting substances. See Chapter 8 for a complete discussion of what it means for a food to be labeled organic.

Protecting Consumers and Regulating Claims

While many CAM products appear promising, be aware that most of them are not regulated in the United States as strictly as are foods and drugs. This is in sharp contrast to nations such as Germany, where the government holds companies to strict standards for ingredients and manufacturing. In the United States, nutritional supplements have had a long history

---

Nutraceuticals   Term often used interchangeably with *functional foods*; refers to the combined nutritional and pharmaceutical benefit derived through use of foods or food supplements.

Table 23.3
Common Herbal, Vitamin, and Mineral Supplements: Benefits versus Risks

Supplement	Use	Claims of Benefits	Risks
Chaparral	Sold as teas and pills	Fights cancer and purifies blood	Linked to serious liver damage
Comfrey	Originated as a poultice to reduce swelling, but later used internally	Wound healing, infection control	Contains alkaloids toxic to the liver, and animal studies suggest it is carcinogenic
Melatonin	"Clock hormone"	Role in regulating circadian rhythms and sleep patterns	Anti-aging claims unfounded
DHEA (dehydroepiandrosterone)	Hormone that turns into estrogen and testosterone in the body	Fights aging, boosts immunity, strengthens bones, and improves brain functioning	No anti-aging benefits proven; could increase cancer risk and lead to liver damage, even when taken briefly
Dieter's teas	Herbal blends containing senna, aloe, rhubarb root, buckthorn, cascara, and castor oil	Act as laxatives	Can disrupt potassium levels and cause heart arrhythmias; linked to diarrhea, vomiting, chronic constipation, fainting, and death
Pennyroyal (member of the mint family)	—	Soothing effect in teas	Pregnancy-related complications, heart arrhythmias, coma, convulsions, death
Sassafras	Once a flavoring in root beer, used in tonics and teas	No real claims	Shown to cause liver cancer in animals
Flaxseeds	Produce linseed oil	Omega-3 fatty acid benefits	Delay absorption of medicine
Kava	—	—	Increases the effects of alcohol and other drugs
High-dose vitamin E	Antioxidants	Reduces risk of heart disease; better survivability after heart attack	Causes bleeding when taking blood thinners
Vitamin C	Antioxidant, manufactures collagen, wound repair, nerve transmission	Improves blood vessel relaxation in people with CVD, diabetes, hypertension, and other problems; can relieve pain of angina pectoris	None known
L-Carnitine	Amino acid	Improves metabolism in heart muscle, purported to increase fat-burning enzymes	Heart palpitations, arrhythmias, sudden death; claims largely unsubstantiated
Licorice root	Sweetener, used in cough drops	None proven	Speeds potassium loss
Niacin (vitamin B$_3$)	Reduces serum lipids, vasodilation, and increases blood flow	—	Skin flushing, gastrointestinal distress, stomach pain, nausea and vomiting
Chondroitin (shark cartilage or sea cucumber)	—	Improves osteoporosis and arthritis by improving cartilage function	Fewer benefits than glucosamine; benefits still unproven

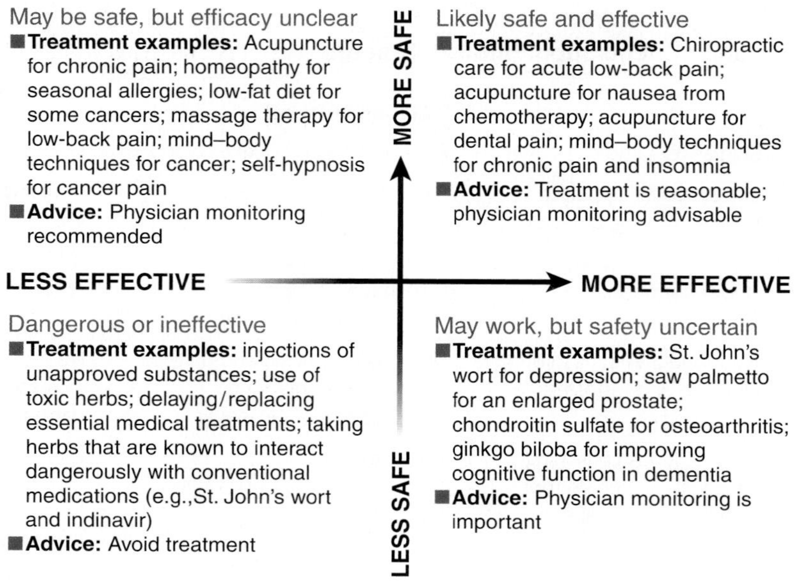

May be safe, but efficacy unclear
- **Treatment examples:** Acupuncture for chronic pain; homeopathy for seasonal allergies; low-fat diet for some cancers; massage therapy for low-back pain; mind–body techniques for cancer; self-hypnosis for cancer pain
- **Advice:** Physician monitoring recommended

Likely safe and effective
- **Treatment examples:** Chiropractic care for acute low-back pain; acupuncture for nausea from chemotherapy; acupuncture for dental pain; mind–body techniques for chronic pain and insomnia
- **Advice:** Treatment is reasonable; physician monitoring advisable

MORE SAFE

LESS EFFECTIVE ⟶ **MORE EFFECTIVE**

Dangerous or ineffective
- **Treatment examples:** injections of unapproved substances; use of toxic herbs; delaying/replacing essential medical treatments; taking herbs that are known to interact dangerously with conventional medications (e.g.,St. John's wort and indinavir)
- **Advice:** Avoid treatment

May work, but safety uncertain
- **Treatment examples:** St. John's wort for depression; saw palmetto for an enlarged prostate; chondroitin sulfate for osteoarthritis; ginkgo biloba for improving cognitive function in dementia
- **Advice:** Physician monitoring is important

LESS SAFE

Figure 23.3

Assessing the Risks and Benefits of CAM Treatments

Medical experts devised this chart to gauge the potential liability of recommending alternative treatments, but it can also help patients choose treatments based on safety and effectiveness by determining how the treatment is categorized.

Source: Figure from M. H. Cohen and D. M. Eisenberg, "Potential Physician Malpractice Liability Associated with Complementary and Integrative Medical Therapies," *Annals of Internal Medicine* 136, no. 8. (2002): 596–603.

of unregulated growth, including an abundance of claims and testimonials about their supposed health-enhancing attributes. With few regulatory controls in place, many get-rich-quick charlatans have jumped into the health food and CAM market. As their profits soar, more and more companies eagerly join them. Unfortunately, this trend means that issues related to consumer safety and protection from fraudulent claims will also grow more urgent and continue to raise serious questions about our current regulatory system. It is important to have as much information as possible to make a smart decision when evaluating CAM options (Figure 23.3).

Strategies to Protect Consumers' Health

The burgeoning popularity of nutraceuticals and functional foods concerns many scientists. According to National Institutes of Health (NIH) nutritional biochemist Dr. Terry Krakower:

NIH does have some concerns about them, and we are looking into them, especially the potential for interaction with other medications. We advise anyone who uses them to talk to their physician. [Functional foods] are so new we don't

know yet if they are good, bad, or indifferent. [Much] of the herb content in these food products is so small that it's probably ineffective, and if it were included in large amounts, it could be harmful. Anyone taking these supplements, whether in pill form or in foods, should do their homework and thoroughly research them rather than rely on health claims made by manufacturers.[55]

By legal definition, herbal supplements and functional foods are neither prescription drugs nor over-the-counter medications. Instead, classified as food supplements, they can be sold without FDA approval. Since they are not regulated by the FDA, these products are not subject to the strict guidelines that govern the research and development of medications. Many are not labeled with the precise amount of chemicals in the product, and the labels provide little guidance on how they should be used. They are not supposed to be accompanied by claims of therapeutic benefit, but they often are. Since they are available without a prescription, this poses risks for unsuspecting consumers, raising issues of consumer safety to new levels.

Even when products are dispensed by CAM practitioners, the situation can be risky. Some homeopaths and herbal-

News from the World of CAM Research

Research is being conducted on complementary and alternative therapies in all areas of health, with investigations into treatments for some conditions making headlines. Recently, experts from Harvard Medical School shared their insights about selected treatments for certain conditions:

CANCER

Although CAM therapies for cancer abound on the Internet and elsewhere, choosing a CAM therapy over conventional treatment is risky business. Promising new research focusing on diet, mind–body techniques, and even shark-cartilage supplements indicates that when CAM is coupled with traditional medicine, treatment may be more bearable and survival rates may improve. Interesting points include:

- "Natural" doesn't always mean "safe." High doses of vitamin E and ginkgo biloba have anticoagulant effects that could cause excessive bleeding during surgery, particularly in those already taking aspirin. Soy contains plant estrogens that have not been ruled out in breast or endometrial cancer.
- Some supplements, such as St. John's wort, seem to counteract the effects of conventional cancer treatment drugs.
- Antioxidants may limit adverse effects of radiation and chemotherapy; however, recent studies suggest they may also sometimes make these treatments less effective.

- Mind–body therapies, acupuncture, massage, and other remedies may help comfort patients going through chemotherapy or radiation treatment by relieving physical symptoms such as pain and insomnia, alleviating nausea, and improving recovery from treatment.

CARDIOVASCULAR DISEASE (CVD)

Diet and exercise provide nearly undisputable benefits for reducing CVD risks. Research on other natural strategies is mixed. Findings include:

- The Harvard Nurses' Health Study and Health Professionals Follow-Up Study found reduced rates of CVD in people whose diets are rich in antioxidants such as vitamin E, vitamin A, and beta-carotene. However, other studies have refuted these results.
- A large study of chelation therapy (a technique used to clear toxic metals from the bloodstream) may provide results within the next five years. Until such time, the jury is out on this one.
- Supplements to watch out for include ginkgo biloba (can cause excessive bleeding) and ephedra (ma huang), which has been banned by the FDA for its serious side effects, including high blood pressure and irregular heartbeat.

ARTHRITIS

Current treatment for arthritis sufferers has been primarily exercise and acetaminophen (Tylenol) plus nonsteroidal anti-inflammatory drugs (NSAIDs) such as aspirin, ibuprofen (Advil), naproxen (Aleve), and celecoxib (Celebrex). Rofecoxib (Vioxx), a widely prescribed choice, was recently

revealed to be linked to an increased risk of heart attack and stroke. People are seeking alternatives, such as:

- *Glucosamine.* Although critics abound, many believe that glucosamine may help those suffering from arthritis pain while reducing the gastrointestinal irritation of NSAIDs. However, newer research also indicates that it can interfere with insulin, causing increases in blood sugar.
- *Chondroitin.* Often used with glucosamine, chondroitin may also elevate blood sugar levels and lead to excessive bleeding, particularly among those already on blood thinners and with other risks.
- *Herbs and supplements.* Although many are touted as arthritis treatments, scientific evidence of pain and symptom relief is lacking.

MEMORY LOSS

While Americans have been buying gingko biloba in search of supposed memory-aiding benefits, most research supports the idea that mental activities, such as playing brain teasers and working on puzzles, are the best remedies for slowed memory.

Sources: Adapted from W. Weiger and D. Eisenberg, "Health For Life: The New Science of Alternative Medicine. Cancer: Easing the Treatment," *Newsweek*, December 2, 2002, p. 49; W. Haskell and David Eisenberg, "Health For Life: The New Science of Alternative Medicine. Cardiac Disease: Ways to Heal your Heart," *Newsweek*, December 2, 2002, p. 52.

---

ists who mix their own tonics may not use standardized measures. Unfortunately, some unskilled and untrained people, who do not fully understand the potential chemical interactions of their preparations, are treating patients.

Consumer groups, members of the scientific community, and government officials are calling for action. Pressure is mounting to establish consistent standards for herbal supplements and functional foods similar to those used in Germany and other countries. Many scientists advocate a more stringent FDA approval process for virtually all supplements sold in the United States.

The German Commission E

The German Commission E has been among the most noteworthy of the international groups attempting to regulate the sale of alternative medicines and supplements. Consisting of an expert panel established in 1970, its mission was to conduct a formal evaluation of the hundreds of herbal remedies that have been part of traditional German medicine for centuries. Commission members carefully analyzed data from clinical trials, observational studies, biological experiments, and chemical analyses. Between 1983 and 1996, they evaluated 383 herbal remedies, approving almost two-thirds of them for use but discounting nearly another third, some of which continue to be sold in the United States.[56]

Essentially, the German Commission E analyzed a growing list of **phytomedicines**, another name for medicinal herbs, many of which are sold over the counter in Europe. Typically, phytomedicines are integrated into conventional medical practice and are prepared in several different ways, usually as tablets or powders.[57] Many are sold in much the same way as over-the-counter remedies in the United States.

Looking to Science for More Answers

Even as CAM treatments gain credibility, this credibility still must be tempered with good science. Although slow in coming, legislators have pushed for better science, increased funding, and an agency designed to garner information useful to consumers. One result is the National Center for Complementary and Alternative Medicine (NCCAM), which has a budget of nearly $70 million with which to fund its own projects. The NCCAM has established research centers at universities and other institutions throughout the United States, where many clinical trials are being conducted[58] (Table 23.4). In addition, numerous studies into alternative treatments such as acupuncture, green tea, fish oil, flaxseed, shark cartilage, and others are taking place across the United States. One of the most promising aspects of this research is the enthusiastic support of professionals who have the training and laboratory expertise to evaluate the efficacy of market-driven claims. To read about test results and new initiatives, go to the NCCAM website (http://nccam.nih.gov).

What do you think?

Why do you think the government has not acted more aggressively to regulate or control herbal and other dietary supplements? ■ *Why are many CAM treatments not covered under typical insurance plans?*

Phytomedicines Another name for medicinal herbs, many of which are sold over the counter in Europe.

Healthy Living in the New Millennium

Clearly, CAM is here to stay. It appears to serve a very real need for consumers. While consumers are making the adjustment to CAM in record numbers, members of the health care delivery system seem slow to act. Although progress has been noted, there is still a long way to go before CAM becomes fully accepted in mainstream medical practice.

Enlisting Support from Insurers and Providers

More and more insurers are hiring alternative practitioners as staff or covering alternative care as a routine benefit, at least to some degree. This is especially true as criticisms of managed care increase and government agencies get involved.

In 1999, over 60 health maintenance groups throughout the United States covered some form of alternative care, nearly three times the number in 1994. The changing nature of health maintenance organizations (HMOs) and health care insurers makes it impossible to determine exactly how many insurance companies cover CAM therapies today. What is known is that the numbers are increasing despite a reimbursement system that is biased in favor of traditional treatments. For example, while the nation's insurers spend over $30 billion a year on bypass and angioplasty for CVD, only 40 companies cover the lifestyle-based program developed by Dr. Dean Ornish—and this despite repeated compelling research which demonstrates that the program is safe, effective, and much cheaper than surgery.[59] In some cases, consumers are offered an optional "extra-cost" rider on their insurance policy, through which they may choose to consult alternative practitioners for a higher premium and co-pay agreement. For many consumers, just knowing they have a choice seems to be worth the extra cost.

Support from professional organizations, such as the AMA, is also increasing, as more physician training programs require or offer electives in alternative treatment modalities. In many cases, medical schools are educating a new generation of medical doctors to be better prepared to advise patients about the pros and cons of alternative treatments and how to follow integrative practices. Studies comparing the efficacy of alternative strategies to that of traditional treatments are becoming more comprehensive. Although alternative medicine is becoming increasingly integrated into today's health care programs and plans, there is still a long way to go. As we learn more, we will be better able to apply both traditional and alternative care.

Self-Care: Protecting Yourself

Any decision you make about your health is important, whether it be what you eat and drink, how you exercise, and other day-to-day decisions. None are more important than

Table 23.4

Selected NCCAM-Funded Centers of Research on Complementary and Alternative Medicine

Name/Website of Center	Institution	Research Specialty
Center for CAM Research in Aging and Women's Health www.rosenthal.hs.columbia.edu	Columbia University	Aging and women's health
Center for Alternative Medicine Research on Arthritis www.compmed.ummc.umaryland.edu	University of Maryland	Arthritis
Center for Frontier Medicine in Biofield Science	University of Arizona	Energy fields
Botanical Center for Age-Related Diseases	Purdue University West Lafayette	Plant-based treatments for CVD, cancer, osteoporosis, cognitive decline
Botanical Dietary Supplements for Women's Health	University of Illinois at Chicago	Herbal supplements and women's health
Center for Dietary Supplements Research: Botanicals	University of California at Los Angeles	Botanicals and cholesterol
Center for Phytomedicine Research	University of Arizona	Botanicals and inflammatory conditions
The Center for Cancer Complementary Medicine www.hopkins-cam.org	Johns Hopkins University	Cancer
Specialized Center of Research in Hyperbaric Oxygen Therapy	University of Pennsylvania	Cancer
CAM Research Center for Cardiovascular Diseases www.med.umich.edu/camrc/index.html	University of Michigan	CVD
Center for Natural Medicine and Prevention www.mum.edu/CNMP	Maharishi University of Management	CVD in older African Americans
Consortial Center for Chiropractic Research www.palmer.edu	Palmer College	Chiropractic
Oregon Center for CAM Research in Craniofacial Disorders	Kaiser Foundation Hospitals	Craniofacial disorders
Oregon Center for CAM Research in Neurological Disorders	Oregon Health Sciences University	Neurological disorders
Center for CAM Research in Neurodegenerative Diseases www.emory.edu/WHSC/MED/NEUROLOGY/CAM/index.html	Emory University	Neurodegenerative diseases
Pediatric Center for Complementary and Alternative Medicine	University of Arizona	Pediatrics
Exploratory Program Grant for Frontier Medicine	University of Connecticut	Touch

Source: National Center for Complementary and Alternative Medicine, "NCCAM's Research Centers Program," 2004, http://nccam.nih.gov/training/centers

the decisions you make about health care treatments and whether or not you use traditional medicines or opt for some of the complementary and alternative medicine treatments discussed in this chapter.

To help you further in making these decisions, review this list of considerations from NCCAM and elsewhere:[60]

- Take charge of your health by being an informed consumer. Find out what scientific studies have been done on the safety and effectiveness of the CAM treatment in which you are interested. Don't rely on friends or testimonials.
- Remember that decisions about treatment should be made in consultation with a qualified health care provider

and based on the condition and needs of each person. Discuss information on CAM with your health care provider before making any decisions.

- If you use any CAM therapy, inform your primary health care provider. This is for your safety and so your health care provider can develop a comprehensive treatment plan. It is particularly important to talk with your provider if you are thinking about replacing your prescribed treatment with one or more supplements; currently taking a prescription drug; have a chronic medical condition; are planning to have surgery; are pregnant or nursing; or are thinking about giving supplements to children or pets.
- If you use a CAM therapy provided by a practitioner, such as acupuncture, choose the practitioner with care. Check

Selecting a CAM Provider

Selecting a CAM practitioner—indeed, any health care provider—can be difficult. Although these recommendations apply to CAM, you should also consider them when selecting any health care product or service. Before starting a CAM therapy or choosing a practitioner, talk with your primary health care provider(s) and others who are knowledgeable about CAM. If they dismiss the therapy, ask why. Check their explanations with other sources to see if their insights are confirmed.

FINDING A CAM PRACTITIONER

- Ask your doctor or other health professional to recommend or refer you to a CAM therapist.
- Ask people you trust who have used CAM practices if they have any recommendations based on experience.
- Contact a nearby hospital or medical school and ask if they could recommend CAM practitioners in your area. Some may actually have CAM providers on staff.
- If your therapy will be covered by insurance, ask your carrier for a list of approved CAM providers.
- Contact a professional organization for the type of practitioner you are seeking.

Often they have standards of practice and websites or publications that list recommended providers. These resources will also answer common questions that you might have. If there is a regulatory or licensing board for this specialty, check to see that your practitioner has the proper credentials.

INTERVIEWING A CAM PRACTITIONER

- Gather information about your options before making your first visit. Ask basic questions about providers' credentials and experience. Where did they obtain their training? What supporting degrees, licenses, or certifications do they have?
- Make a list of questions to ask at your first visit. You may want to bring a friend or family member who can help you ask questions and note answers.
- Bring medical information with you, including any tests you've had, information about your health history, surgical history, allergies, and any medications you take (including prescription, over-the-counter, and herbal or other supplements).
- Ask if there are diseases/health conditions in which the practitioner specializes and how frequently she treats patients with conditions like yours.
- Ask if there is any scientific research supporting the use of this treatment for your condition.

- Is the provider supportive of conventional as well as CAM treatments? Does he have a good relationship for referrals to (and from) conventional practitioners?
- Were questions answered to your satisfaction?
- How many patients per day does the provider see, and how much time is spent with each one?
- Ask about charges and payment options. What percentage of the payment might you have to pay out of pocket?

After the visit, assess the interaction and how you felt about the practitioner.

UNDERSTANDING THE RECOMMENDED TREATMENT

Questions to ask your CAM practitioner include:

- What benefits can I expect from this therapy?
- What are the risks and side effects associated with this therapy? Do the benefits outweigh the risks?
- Will I need to buy any special equipment or take special supplements?
- Will this therapy interfere with any conventional medicine treatments?
- If there are problems, where would I be referred for further treatment?
- What is the history of success in treating this type of condition for someone of my age and health status?

with your insurer to see if the services will be covered. (See the Skills for Behavior Change box for more information on selecting a CAM provider.)

- Consult only reliable sources—texts, journals, periodicals, and government resources. Start with the websites listed at the end of this and every chapter.
- Remember that *natural* and *safe* are not necessarily synonyms. Many people have become seriously ill from seemingly harmless products. For example, some have suffered serious liver damage from sipping teas brewed with comfrey, an herb used in poultices and ointments to treat sprains and bruises and that should not be taken internally. Pregnant women face special risks from herbs such as echinacea, senna, comfrey, and licorice.

- Realize that no one is closely monitoring the purity of herbal supplements. The FDA has verified industry reports that certain shipments of ginseng were contaminated with high levels of fungicides. Other problems with imported herbs have been noted.
- Recognize that dosage levels in many herbal products are not regulated. German manufacturers produce identical batches of herbal remedies as required by law. Look for reputable manufacturers.
- Always look for the word *standardized* on any herbal product you buy. This indicates that manufacturing is monitored to ensure that the dosage and content are the same in every pill or tablet.

- Tell your doctor if you are taking herbal medications. Several may interact with prescription (and over-the-counter) medications.
- Be cautious about combining herbal medications, just as you should be cautious about combining other drugs. Always remember that just because something is natural, it doesn't mean it is safe.
- Remember that no herbal medicine is likely to work miracles. Monitor your health, and seek help if you notice any unusual side effects from herbal products.

As we enter a new era of medicine, more than ever, you are being called upon to take responsibility for what goes into your body. This means you must educate yourself. CAM can offer new avenues toward better health, but it is up to you to make sure that you are on the right path.

What do you think?

What can you do as a consumer to obtain the greatest benefit from CAM? ■ *How can you protect yourself from possible negative risks?*

TAKING CHARGE

MAKE IT HAPPEN!

Assessment: The Assess Yourself box on page 648 investigates your opinions about complementary and alternative medicine. Now that you have considered your results, you may want to take steps to explore your attitudes further or discuss them with others.

Making a Change: In order to change your behavior, you need to develop a plan. Follow these steps.

1. Evaluate your behavior, and identify patterns and specific things you are doing. What can you change now? What can you change in the near future?
2. Select one pattern of behavior that you want to change.
3. Fill out a Behavior Change Contract. It should include your long-term goal for change, your short-term goals, the rewards you'll give yourself for reaching these goals, potential obstacles along the way, and strategies for overcoming these obstacles. For each goal, list the small steps and specific actions that you will take.
4. Chart your progress in a journal. At the end of a week, consider how successful you were in following your plan. What helped you be successful? What made change more difficult? What will you do differently next week?
5. Revise your plan as needed. Are the short-term goals attainable? Are the rewards satisfying?

One Student's Plan: When Melia answered the question about the type of person most likely to seek CAM treatment, she assumed that no one she knew would use anything but traditional treatment. She was surprised when she started asking her friends and family and it turned out that several of them had tried various CAM therapies. Several had positive experiences: Her uncle Louis had developed back problems after a car accident, and a chiropractor had brought him relief. Also, her friend Tony had had acupuncture for his tennis elbow and reported that it had helped. On the other hand, Melia's mother had taken gingko biloba because she felt she needed help with her memory; however, she didn't tell her regular physician that she was taking it and, when she started taking a blood thinner he prescribed for her, the combination of the two caused dangerous bleeding. She had not experienced any memory enhancement from the gingko and was glad to stop it.

Melia had chronic knee pain, and her doctor had not discovered any causes that could be treated with surgery or other conventional treatments. Now that she had thought more about CAM and had seen how widely used some of the therapies are, Melia decided to investigate the most appropriate ones for knee pain and ask her doctor's opinion about pursuing one of them. Based on her mother's experience, she knew she would need to work together with her physician and any CAM provider to be sure that their treatments were compatible. She made an appointment with her doctor to discuss possible treatments and planned to research all of her options, including side effects and insurance coverage.

Summary

- People throughout the world are choosing complementary and alternative medicine options, and these numbers are growing exponentially. Compared to other countries, the United States has been relatively slow to turn to alternative treatment and medicine.

- The National Center for Complementary and Alternative Medicine groups CAM practices into four major domains: (1) biologically-based practices (including substances found in nature, such as herbs, as vitamin megadoses); (2) energy medicine (use of biofields or energy fields); (3) manipulative and body-based practices (manipulation or movement of one or more body parts); and (4) mind–body medicine a variety of techniques designed to enhance the mind's ability to affect bodily function and symptoms. Another area of study is a variety of whole medical systems, which cut across all domains. Acupuncture and acupressure, two derivatives of energy medicine, are among the more popular forms of traditional Chinese medicine in the United States.

- Herbal remedies, largely derived from traditional Oriental medicine, include ginkgo biloba, St. John's wort, echinacea, and green tea. Other herbal remedies have also received widespread attention as potential miracle drugs without having harmful side effects. Special supplements include muscle enhancers, ginseng, glucosamine, chromium picolinate, SAMe, and antioxidants. A number of functional foods may also serve as healing agents.

- Though many positive effects are associated with CAM, there are also many risks. The drive for profits and the lack of strict government regulation make the CAM market a free-for-all. As a consumer, you must be aware of the risks and check reputable sources to ensure that you are not being lured by false claims and promises.

- Health in the new millennium provides an interesting assortment of choices for health care consumers. By enlisting the support of health professionals and health care services and by making informed decisions, you will reap positive rewards in your quest for health enhancement in the days ahead.

Questions for Discussion and Reflection

1. What are some of the potential benefits and risks of CAM? Why do you think these practices and products are becoming so popular?

2. What are some of the major domains of CAM treatments? Have you tried any of them? Would you feel comfortable trying any new ones? Why or why not?

3. What are the major herbal remedies? Special supplements? What are some of the risks and benefits associated with each?

4. What can you do to ensure that you are receiving accurate information regarding CAM treatments or medicines? Which federal agency oversees CAM in the United States?

5. What is being done in the United States to ensure continued growth of CAM?

Accessing Your Health on the Internet

Visit the following Internet sites to explore further topics and issues related to personal health. To visit an organization's website, go to the Companion Website for *Access to Health, Ninth Edition* at www.aw-bc.com/donatelle, click on the book image, and select "Accessing Your Health on the Internet" from the navigation menu.

1. *Acupuncture.com.* Provides resources for consumers regarding traditional Asian therapies, geared to students and practitioners.

2. *Alternative Medicine Links.* Provides links to a number of the best alternative, complementary, and preventive health news pages.

3. *National Center for Complementary and Alternative Medicine.* A division of the National Institutes of Health dedicated to providing the latest information on complementary and alternative practices.

4. *National Institutes of Health, Office of Dietary Supplements.* An excellent resource for information on dietary supplements.

Further Reading

Blumenthal, M., ed. *Complete German Commission E Monographs: Therapeutic Guide to Herbal Medicines.* Austin, TX: The American Botanical Council, 1998.

Overview of German Commission E findings and relevant information about supplement research for consumers. Provides an interesting perspective on international herbal research, policies, recommendations, and future directions.

Cassileth, B. R. *The Alternative Medicine Handbook: The Complete Reference Guide to Alternative and Complementary Therapies.* New York: W. W. Norton & Co., 1998.

A complete reference for patients and physicians alike on possible alternative treatments.

Pelletier, Ken. *The Best Alternative Medicine: What Works? What Does Not?* New York: Simon & Schuster, 2000.

Excellent overview of commonly used CAM techniques with scientific information for consumers.

Turchaninov, R. and C. A. Cox. *Medical Massage.* Scottsdale, AZ: Stress Less Publishing and Phoenix: Aesculapius Books, 1998.

An in-depth review of therapeutic practices from around the world.

HEALTH RESOURCES

Injury Prevention and Emergency Care

Injury Prevention

Unintentional injuries are one of the major public health problems facing the United States today. On an average day, more than a million people will suffer a nonfatal injury; almost 100,000 people die each year as a result of unintentional injuries. Unintentional injuries are the leading cause of death for Americans under the age of 44. In the United States, unintentional injuries are the fifth leading cause of death, after heart disease, cancer, stroke, and lung disease.

Vehicle Safety

The risk of dying in an automobile crash is related to age. Young drivers (aged 16–24) have the highest death rate, owing to their inexperience and immaturity. Each year about 40,000 Americans die in automobile crashes and another 1.9 million are disabled, 140,000 permanently. Most of these car crashes were avoidable. The best way to prevent crashes is to practice risk management driving and accident-avoidance techniques and to be aware of safety technology when purchasing a car.

Risk Management Driving   Risk management driving techniques, which help reduce chances of being involved in a collision, include the following:

- *Surround your car with a bubble space.* The rear bumper of the car ahead of you should be three seconds away. To measure your safety bubble, choose a roadside landmark such as a signpost or light pole as a reference point. When the car in front of you passes this point, count "one-one-thousand, two-one-thousand." Make sure you are not passing the reference point before you've finished saying "three-one-thousand."
- *Scan the road ahead of you and to both sides.*
- *Drive with your low-beam headlights on.* Being seen is an important safety factor. Driving with your low-beam headlights on, *day and night,* makes you more visible to other drivers.

Other important techniques include anticipating other drivers' actions, driving refreshed, driving sober, obeying all traffic laws, and using safety belts.

Accident-Avoidance Techniques   Sometimes when driving, you need to react instantly to a situation. To avoid a more severe accident, you may need to steer into another, less severe collision. The point of accident avoidance is to save lives. Here are the Automobile Association of America's (AAA) rules for avoidance:

- Generally, veer to the right.
- Steer, don't skid, off the road. (It is easy to roll a vehicle over if you swerve suddenly off the edge of the road.)
- If you have to hit a vehicle, hit one moving in the same direction as your own.
- If you have to hit a stationary object, try to hit a soft one (bushes, small trees) rather than a hard one (boulders, brick walls, giant trees).
- If you have to hit a hard object, hit it with a glancing blow.
- Avoid hitting pedestrians, motorcyclists, and bicyclists at all costs.

Safety Technology   The last line of defense against a collision is the car itself. How a car is equipped can mean the difference between life and death. When purchasing a car, the Insurance Institute for Highway Safety recommends that you look for the following features:

- Does the car have airbags? Remember, airbags do not eliminate the need for everyone to wear safety belts. Airbags inflate only in the case of frontal crashes.
- Does the car have antilock brakes? Antilock brakes rapidly pump the brakes to prevent them from locking up and, hence, prevent the car from skidding.
- Does the car have impact-absorbing crumple zones?
- Are there strengthened passenger compartment side walls?
- Is there a strong roof support? (The center door post on four-door models gives you an extra roof pillar.)

In Case of Mechanical Breakdown

- Try to get off the road as far as possible.
- Turn on your car's emergency flashers, and raise the hood. Set out flares or reflective triangles.

- Stay in the car until a law enforcement officer arrives. If others stop to help, ask them to contact the police, sheriff's office, or the state patrol.
- If you must leave your car, leave a note with the car explaining the problem (as best you can), the time and date, your name, the direction in which you are walking, and what you are wearing. This information will help anyone who needs to look for you.
- Remove all valuables from the car if you must leave it.

Safe Refueling   Gasoline is a flammable substance. Follow these guidelines from the Petroleum Equipment Institute any time you are filling up a car, truck, or motorcycle:

- Turn off the engine while refueling.
- Do not reenter your vehicle during refueling. In the unlikely event of a static-caused fire, leave the nozzle in the tank and back away from the vehicle. Notify the attendant immediately.
- Avoid prolonged breathing of gasoline vapors. Keep gasoline away from your eyes and skin; it can cause irritation. Never use it to wash your hands or as a cleaning solvent.
- If you are dispensing gasoline into a container or storing it, be sure the container is approved for such a use.
- Never siphon gasoline by mouth; it can be harmful or fatal if swallowed.

Pedestrian Safety

Each year approximately 13 percent of all motor vehicle deaths involve pedestrians, and another 82,000 pedestrians are injured each year. The highest death rates involving pedestrians occur among the very young and older populations. Pedestrian injuries occur most frequently after dark, in urban settings, and primarily in intersections where pedestrians may walk or dart into traffic. It is not uncommon for alcohol to play a role in the death or injury of a pedestrian. How can you protect yourself from being injured or becoming a fatality? AAA has the following suggestions for joggers and walkers:

- Carry or wear reflective material at night to help drivers see you.
- Cross only at crosswalks. Keep to the right in crosswalks.
- Before crossing, look both ways. Be sure the way is clear before you cross.
- Cross only on the proper signal.
- Watch for turning cars.
- Never enter the roadway from between parked cars.
- Where there is no sidewalk and it is necessary to walk in a roadway, walk on the left side, facing traffic.
- Don't wear headphones for a radio or CD player. These may interfere with your ability to hear sounds of motor vehicles.

Cycling Safety

Currently over 63 million Americans of all ages ride bicycles for transportation, recreation, and fitness. The Consumer Product Safety Commission reports about 800 deaths per year from cycling accidents. The biggest risk factors are failure to wear a helmet, being male, and riding after dark. Children aged 10 to 14 also are at higher risk for injury. Approximately 87 percent of fatal collisions were due to cyclists' errors, usually failure to yield at intersections. Alcohol also plays a significant role in bicycle deaths and injuries. The following are suggestions cyclists should consider to reduce risk of injury or death.

- Wear a helmet. It should be ANSI or Snell approved. This can reduce head injuries by 85 percent.
- Don't drink and ride.
- Respect traffic.
- Wear light reflective clothing that is easily seen at night and during the day.
- Avoid riding after dark.
- Ride with the flow of traffic.
- Know and use proper hand signals.
- Keep your bicycle in good working condition.
- Use bike paths whenever possible.
- Stop at stop signs and traffic lights.

Water Safety

Drowning is the third most common cause of accidental death in the United States, according to the National Safety Council. About 85 percent of drowning victims are teenage males. Many drowned swimmers are strong swimmers. Alcohol plays a significant role in many drowning cases. Most drownings occur in unorganized or unsupervised facilities, such as ponds or pools with no lifeguards present. Swimmers should take the following precautions:

- Don't drink alcohol before or while swimming.
- Don't enter the water unless you can swim at least 50 feet unassisted.
- Know your limitations; get out of the water as soon as you start to feel even slightly fatigued.
- Never swim alone, even if you are a skilled swimmer. You never know what might happen.
- Never leave a child unattended, even in extremely shallow water or wading pools.
- Before entering the water, check the depth. Most neck and back injuries result from diving into water that is too shallow.
- Never swim in muddy or dirty water that obstructs your view of the bottom.
- Never swim in a river with currents too swift for easy, relaxed swimming.

Emergency Care

In certain situations, it may be necessary to administer first aid. Ideally, first aid procedures should be performed by someone who has received formal training from the American Red Cross or some other reputable institution. If you do not have such training, contact a physician or call your local emergency medical service (EMS) by dialing 911 or your local emergency number. In life-threatening situations, however, you may not have time to call for outside assistance. In cases of serious injury or sudden illness, you may need to begin first aid immediately and continue until help arrives. This section contains basic information and general steps to follow for various emergency situations. Simply reading these directions, however, may not prepare you fully to handle these situations. For this reason, you may want to enroll in a first aid course.

Calling for Emergency Assistance

When calling for emergency assistance, be prepared to give exact details. Be clear and thorough, and do not panic. Never hang up until the dispatcher has informed you that he or she has all the information needed. Be ready to answer the following questions:

1. Where are you and the victim located? This is the most important information the EMS will need.
2. What is your phone number and name?
3. What has happened? Was there an accident, or is the victim ill?
4. How many people need help?
5. What is the nature of the emergency? What is the victim's apparent condition?
6. Are there any life-threatening situations that the EMS should know about (for example, fires, explosions, or fallen electrical lines)?
7. Is the victim wearing a medic-alert tag (a tag indicating a specific medical condition such as diabetes)?

Are You Liable?

According to the laws in most states, you are not required to administer first aid unless you have a special obligation to the victim. For example, parents must provide first aid for their children, and a lifeguard must provide aid to a swimmer.

Before administering first aid, you should obtain the victim's consent. If the victim refuses aid, you must respect that person's rights. However, you should make every reasonable effort to persuade the victim to accept your help. In emergency situations, consent is *implied* if the victim is unconscious. Once you begin to administer first aid, you are required by law to continue. You must remain with the victim until someone of equal or greater competence takes over.

Can you be held liable if you fail to provide adequate care or if the victim is further injured? To help protect people who render first aid, most states have "Good Samaritan" laws. These laws grant immunity (protection from civil liability) if you act in good faith to provide care to the best of your ability, according to your level of training. Because these laws vary from state to state, you should become familiar with the Good Samaritan laws in your state.

When Someone Stops Breathing

If someone has stopped breathing, you should perform mouth-to-mouth resuscitation. This involves the following steps:

1. Check for responsiveness by gently tapping or shaking the victim. Ask loudly, "Are you OK?"
2. Call the local EMS for help (usually 911).
3. Gently roll the victim onto his or her back.
4. Open the airway by tilting the victim's head back, placing your hand nearest the victim's head on the victim's forehead, and applying backward pressure to tilt the head back and lift the chin.
5. Check for breathing (3 to 5 seconds): look, listen, and feel for breathing.
6. Give two slow breaths.
   - Keep the victim's head tilted back.
   - Pinch the victim's nose shut.
   - Seal your lips tightly around the victim's mouth.
   - Give two slow breaths, each lasting 1 1/2 to 2 seconds.
7. Check for pulse at side of neck; feel for pulse for 5 to 10 seconds.
8. Begin rescue breathing.
   - Keep the victim's head tilted back.
   - Pinch the victim's nose shut.
   - Give one breath every 5 to 6 seconds.
   - Look, listen, and feel for breathing between breaths.
9. Recheck pulse every minute.
   - Keep the victim's head tilted back.
   - Feel for pulse for 5 to 10 seconds.
   - If the victim has a pulse but is not breathing, continue rescue breathing. If there is no pulse, begin CPR.

There are some variations when performing this procedure on infants and children. For children aged one to eight, at step 8, give one slow breath every 4 seconds. For infants, you should not pinch the nose. Instead, seal your lips tightly around the infant's nose and mouth. Also for infants, at step 8, you should give one slow breath every 3 seconds.

In cases in which the victim has no pulse, cardiopulmonary resuscitation (CPR) should be performed. This technique involves a combination of artificial respiration and chest compressions. You should not perform CPR unless you have received training in it. You cannot learn CPR simply by reading directions; and, without training, you could cause further injury to the victim. The American Red Cross offers courses in mouth-to-mouth resuscitation and CPR as well as general first aid. If you have taken a CPR course in the past, you should be aware that certain changes have been made in the procedure. Consider taking a refresher course.

When Someone Is Choking

Choking occurs when an object obstructs the trachea (windpipe), thus preventing normal breathing. Failure to expel the object and restore breathing can lead to death within 6 minutes. The universal signal of distress related to choking is the clasping of the throat with one or both hands. Other signs of choking include not being able to talk and/or noisy and difficult breathing. If a victim can cough or speak, do not interfere. The most effective method for assisting choking victims is the Heimlich maneuver, which involves the application of pressure to the victim's abdominal area to expel the foreign object. The Heimlich maneuver involves the following steps:

If the Victim Is Standing or Seated

1. Recognize that the victim is choking.
2. Wrap your arms around the victim's waist, making a fist with one hand.
3. Place the thumb side of the fist on the middle of the victim's abdomen, just above the navel and well below the tip of the sternum.
4. Cover your fist with your other hand.
5. Press fist into victim's abdomen, with up to five quick upward thrusts.
6. After every five abdominal thrusts, check the victim and your technique.
7. If the victim becomes unconscious, gently lower him or her to the ground.
8. Try to clear the airway by using your finger to sweep the object from the victim's mouth or throat.
9. Give two rescue breaths. If the passage is still blocked and air will not go in, proceed with the Heimlich maneuver.

If the Victim Is Lying Down

1. Facing the person, kneel with your legs astride the victim's hips. Place the heel of one hand against the abdomen, slightly above the navel and well below the tip of the sternum. Put the other hand on top of the first hand.
2. Press inward and upward using both hands with up to five quick abdominal thrusts.
3. Repeat the following steps in this sequence until the airway becomes clear or the EMS arrives:
   a. Finger sweep.
   b. Give two rescue breaths.
   c. Do up to five abdominal thrusts.

Alcohol Poisoning

Alcohol overdose is considered a medical emergency when an irregular heartbeat or coma occur. The two immediate causes of death in such cases are cardiac arrhythmia and respiratory depression. If a person is seriously uncoordinated and has possibly also taken a depressant, the risk of respiratory failure is serious enough that a physician should be contacted. When dealing with someone who is drunk, remember these points:

1. Stay calm. Assess the situation.
2. Keep the person still and comfortable.
3. Stay with the person if she or he is vomiting. When helping him or her to lie down, turn the head to the side to prevent it from falling back. This helps to keep the person from choking on vomit.
4. Monitor the person's breathing.
5. Keep your distance. Before approaching or touching the person, explain what you intend to do.
6. Speak in a clear, firm, reassuring manner.

When Someone Is Bleeding

External Bleeding   Control of external bleeding is an important part of emergency care. Survival is threatened by the loss of one quart of blood or more. There are three major procedures for the control of external bleeding.

1. *Direct pressure.* The best method is to apply firm pressure by covering the wound with a sterile dressing, bandage, or clean cloth. Wearing disposable latex gloves or an equally protective barrier, apply pressure for 5 to 10 minutes to stop bleeding.
2. *Elevation.* Elevate the wounded section of the body to slow the bleeding. For example, a wounded arm or leg should be raised above the level of the victim's heart.
3. *Pressure points.* Pressure points are sites where an artery that is close to the body's surface lies directly over a bone. Pressing the artery against the bone can limit the flow of blood to the injury. This technique should be used only as a last resort when direct pressure and elevation have failed to stop bleeding.

Knowing where to apply pressure to stop bleeding is critical (see Figure H.1 on the next page). For serious wounds, seek medical attention immediately.

Internal Bleeding   Although internal bleeding may not be immediately obvious, you should be aware of the following signs and symptoms:

1. Symptoms of shock (discussed on page H-6)
2. Coughing up or vomiting blood
3. Bruises or contusions of the skin
4. Bruises on chest or fractured ribs
5. Black, tarlike stools
6. Abdominal discomfort or pain (rigidity or spasms)

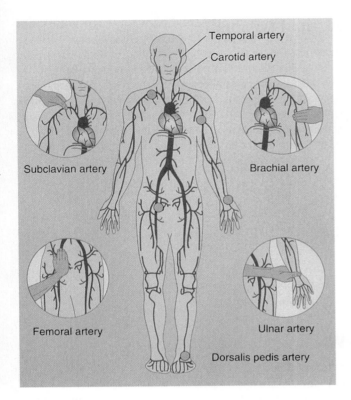

Figure H.1
Pressure Points
Pressure can be applied to these points to stop bleeding. However, unless absolutely necessary, avoid applying pressure to the carotid arteries, which supply blood to the brain. Never apply pressure to both carotid arteries at the same time.

In some cases, a person who has suffered an injury (such as a blow to the head, chest, or abdomen) that does not cause external bleeding may experience internal bleeding. If you suspect that someone is suffering from internal bleeding, follow these steps:

1. Have the person lie on his or her back on a flat surface with knees bent.
2. Treat for shock. Keep the victim warm. Cover the person with a blanket, if possible.
3. Expect vomiting. If vomiting occurs, keep the victim on his or her side for drainage, to prevent inhalation of vomit, and to prevent expulsion of vomit from the stomach.
4. Do *not* give the victim any medications or fluids.
5. Send someone to call for emergency medical help immediately.

Nosebleeds To control a nosebleed, follow these steps:

1. Have the victim sit down and lean slightly forward to prevent blood from running into the throat. If you do not suspect a fracture, pinch the person's nose firmly closed using the thumb and forefinger. Keep the nose pinched for at least 5 minutes.
2. While the nose is pinched, apply a cold compress to the surrounding area.
3. If pinching does not work, gently pack the nostril with gauze or a clean strip of cloth. Do not use absorbent cotton, which will stick. Be sure that the ends of the gauze or cloth hang out so that it can be easily removed later. Once the nose is packed with gauze, pinch it closed again for another 5 minutes.
4. If the bleeding persists, seek medical attention.

Treatment for Burns

Minor Burns   For minor burns caused by fire or scalding water, apply running cold water or cold compresses for 20 to 30 minutes. Never put butter, grease, salt water, aloe vera, or topical burn ointments or sprays on burned skin. If the burned area is dirty, gently wash it with soap and water, and blot it dry with a sterile dressing.

Major Burns   For major burn injuries, call for help immediately. Wrap the victim in a clean, dry sheet. Do not clean the burns or try to remove any clothing attached to burned skin. Remove jewelry near the burned skin immediately, if possible. Keep the victim lying down and calm.

Chemical Burns   Remove clothing surrounding the burn. Wash skin that has been burned by chemicals by flushing with water for at least 20 minutes. Seek medical assistance as soon as possible.

Shock

Shock is a condition in which the cardiovascular system fails to provide sufficient blood circulation to all parts of the body. Victims of shock display the following symptoms:

- Dilated pupils
- Cool, moist skin
- Weak, rapid pulse
- Vomiting
- Delayed or unrelated responses to questions

All injuries result in some degree of shock. Therefore, treatment for shock should be given after every major injury. The following are basic steps for treating shock:

1. Have the victim lie flat with his or her feet elevated approximately 8 to 12 inches. (In the case of chest injuries, difficulty breathing, or severe pain, the victim's head should be slightly elevated if there is no sign of spinal injury.)
2. Keep the victim warm. If possible, wrap him or her in blankets or other material. Keep the victim calm and reassured.
3. Seek medical help.

Electrical Shock

Do not touch a victim of electrical shock until the power source has been turned off. Approach the scene carefully, avoiding any live wires or electrical power lines. Pay attention to the following:

1. If the victim is holding onto the live electrical wire, do not remove it unless the power has been shut off at the plug, circuit breaker, or fuse box.
2. Check the victim's breathing and pulse. Electrical current can paralyze the nerves and muscles that control breathing and heartbeat. If necessary, give mouth-to-mouth resuscitation. If there is no pulse, CPR might be necessary. (Remember that only trained people should perform CPR.)
3. Keep the victim warm and treat for shock. Once the person is breathing and stable, seek medical help or send someone else for help.

Poisoning

Of the 1 million cases of poisoning reported in the United States each year, about 75 percent occur in children under age five, and the majority are caused by household products. Most cases of poisoning involving adults are attempted suicides or attempted murders.

You should keep emergency telephone numbers for the poison control center and the local EMS close at hand. Many people keep these numbers on labels on their telephones. Check the front of your telephone book for these numbers. The National Safety Council recommends that you be prepared to give the following information when calling for help:

- What was ingested? Have the container of the product and the remaining contents ready so you can describe it. You should also bring the container to the emergency room with you.
- When was the substance taken?
- How much was taken?
- Has vomiting occurred? If the person has vomited, save a sample to take to the hospital.
- Are there any other symptoms?
- How long will it take to get to the nearest emergency room?

When caring for a person who has ingested a poison, keep these basic principles in mind:

1. Maintain an open airway. Make sure the person is breathing.
2. Call the local poison control center. Follow their advice for neutralizing the poison.
3. If the poison control center or another medical authority advises you to induce vomiting, then do so.
4. If a corrosive or caustic (that is, acid or alkali) substance was swallowed, immediately dilute it by having the victim drink at least one or two 8-ounce glasses of cold water or milk.

5. Place the victim on his or her left side. This position will delay advancement of the poison into the small intestine, where absorption into the victim's circulatory system is faster.

Injuries of Joints, Muscles, and Bones

Sprains   Sprains result when ligaments and other tissues around a joint are stretched or torn. The following steps should be taken to treat sprains:

1. Elevate the injured joint to a comfortable position.
2. Apply an ice pack or cold compress to reduce pain and swelling.
3. Wrap the joint firmly with a roller bandage.
4. Check the fingers or toes periodically to ensure that blood circulation has not been obstructed. If the bandage is too tight, loosen it.
5. Keep the injured area elevated, and continue ice treatment for 24 hours.
6. Apply heat to the injury after 48 hours if there is no further swelling.
7. If pain and swelling continue or if a fracture is suspected, seek medical attention.

Fractures   Any deformity of an injured body part usually indicates a fracture. A fracture is any break in a bone, including chips, cracks, splinters, and complete breaks. Minor fractures (such as hairline cracks) might be difficult to detect and might be confused with sprains. If there is doubt, treat the injury as a fracture until X rays have been taken.

Do not move the victim if a fracture of the neck or back is suspected because this could result in a spinal cord injury. If the victim must be moved, splints should be applied to immobilize the fracture in order to prevent further damage and to decrease pain. Following are some basic steps for treating fractures and applying splints to broken limbs:

1. If the person is bleeding, apply direct pressure above the site of the wound.
2. If a broken bone is exposed, do not try to move it back into the wound. This can cause contamination and further injury.
3. Do not try to straighten out a broken limb. Splint the limb as it lies.
4. The following materials are needed for splinting:
   - *Splint:* wooden board, pillow, or rolled up magazines and newspapers.
   - *Padding:* towels, blankets, socks, or cloth.
   - *Ties:* cloth, rope, or tape.

5. Place splints and padding above and below the joint. Never put padding directly over the break. Padding should protect bony areas and the soft tissue of the limb.
6. Tie splints and padding into place.

7. Check the tightness of the splints periodically. Pay attention to the skin color, temperature, and pulse below the fracture to make sure the blood flow is adequate.
8. Elevate the fracture and apply ice packs to prevent swelling and reduce pain.

Head Injuries

A head injury can result from an auto accident, a fall, an assault, or a blow from a blunt object. All head injuries can potentially lead to brain damage, which may result in a cessation of breathing and pulse.

For Minor Head Injuries

1. For a minor bump on the head resulting in a bruise without bleeding, apply ice to decrease the swelling.
2. If there is bleeding, apply even, moderate pressure. Because there is always the danger that the skull may be fractured, excessive pressure should not be used.
3. Observe the victim for a change in consciousness. Observe the size of pupils, including whether both pupils are dilated to the same degree, and note signs of inability to think clearly. Check for any signs of numbness or paralysis. Allow the victim to sleep, but wake him or her periodically to check for awareness.

For Severe Head Injuries

1. If the victim is unconscious, check the airway for breathing. If necessary, perform mouth-to-mouth resuscitation.
2. If the victim is breathing, check the pulse. If it is less than 55 or more than 125 beats per minute, the victim may be in danger.
3. Check for bleeding. If fluid is flowing from the ears or nose, do not stop it.
4. Do not remove any objects embedded in the victim's skull.
5. Cover the victim with blankets to maintain body temperature, but guard against overheating.
6. Seek medical help as soon as possible.

Temperature-Related Emergencies

Frostbite Frostbite is damage to body tissues caused by intense cold. Frostbite generally occurs at temperatures below 32°F. The body parts most likely to suffer frostbite are the toes, ears, fingers, nose, and cheeks. When skin is exposed to the cold, ice crystals form beneath the skin. Avoid rubbing frostbitten tissue because the ice crystals can scrape and break blood vessels. To treat frostbite, follow these steps:

1. Bring the victim to a health facility as soon as possible.
2. Cover and protect the frostbitten area. If possible, apply a steady source of external warmth, such as a warm compress. The victim should avoid walking if the feet are frostbitten.

3. If the victim cannot be transported, you must rewarm the body part by immersing it in warm water (100°F to 105°F). Continue to rewarm until the frostbitten area is warm to the touch when removed from the bath. Do not allow the body part to touch the sides or bottom of the water container. After rewarming, dry gently and wrap the body part in bandages to protect from refreezing.

Hypothermia Hypothermia is a condition of generalized cooling of the body, resulting from exposure to cold temperatures or immersion in cold water. It can occur at any temperature below 65°F and can be made more severe by wind chill and moisture. The following are key symptoms of hypothermia:

- Shivering
- Vague, slow, slurred speech
- Poor judgment
- A cool abdomen
- Lethargy, or extreme exhaustion
- Slowed breathing and heartbeat
- Numbness and loss of feeling in extremities

After contacting the EMS, you should take the following steps to provide first aid to a victim of hypothermia:

1. Get the victim out of the cold.
2. Keep the victim in a flat position. Do not raise the legs.
3. Squeeze as much water as possible from wet clothing, and layer dry clothing over wet clothing. Removal of clothing may jostle victim and lead to other problems.
4. Give the victim warm drinks only if he or she is able to swallow. Do not give the victim alcohol or caffeinated beverages, and do not allow the victim to smoke.
5. Do not allow the victim to exercise.

Heatstroke Heatstroke, the most serious heat-related disorder, results from the failure of the brain's heat-regulating mechanism (the hypothalamus) to cool the body. The following are signs and symptoms of heatstroke:

- Rapid pulse
- Hot, dry, flushed skin (absence of sweating)
- Disorientation leading to unconsciousness
- High body temperature

As soon as these symptoms are noticed, the body temperature should be reduced as quickly as possible. The victim should be immersed in a cool bath, lake, or stream. If there is no water nearby, loosen clothing and use a fan to help lower the victim's body temperature.

Heat Exhaustion Heat exhaustion results from excessive loss of salt and water. The onset is gradual, with the following symptoms:

- Fatigue and weakness
- Anxiety

- Nausea
- Profuse sweating
- Clammy skin
- Normal body temperature

To treat heat exhaustion, move the victim to a cool place. Have the victim lie down flat, with feet elevated 8 to 12 inches. Replace lost fluids slowly and steadily. Sponge or fan victim.

Heat Cramps   Heat cramps result from excessive sweating, resulting in an excessive loss of salt and water. Although heat cramps are the least serious heat-related emergency, they are the most painful. The symptoms include muscle cramps, usually starting in the arms and legs. To relieve symptoms, the victim should drink electrolyte-rich beverages or a light saltwater solution or eat salty foods.

First Aid Supplies

Every home, car, or boat should be supplied with a basic first aid kit. In order to respond effectively to emergences, you must have the basic equipment. This kit should be stored in a convenient place, but it should be kept out of the reach of children. Following is a list of supplies that should be included:

- Bandages, including triangular bandages (36 inches by 6 inches), butterfly bandages, a roller bandage, rolled white gauze bandages (2- and 3-inch widths), adhesive bandages
- Sterile gauze pads and absorbent pads
- Adhesive tape (2- and 3-inch widths)
- Cotton-tip applicators
- Scissors
- Thermometer
- Antibiotic ointment
- Aspirin
- Calamine lotion
- Antiseptic cream or petroleum jelly
- Safety pins
- Tweezers
- Latex gloves
- Flashlight
- Paper cups
- Blanket

You cannot be prepared for every medical emergency. Yet these essential tools and a knowledge of basic first aid will help you cope with many emergency situations.

Nutritive Value of Selected Foods and Fast Foods

This section presents nutritional information about a wide array of foods, including many fast foods. Values are given for calories, protein, carbohydrates, fiber, fat, saturated fat, and cholesterol for common foods and serving sizes. Use the EvaluEat code with the EvaluEat nutritional software to assess your diet and make improvements. (This is only a sampling of the most common foods. The EvaluEat database contains an extensive list of foods, and the values for 20 vitamins, minerals, and other food components.)

EvaluEat Code	Food Name	Amt	Wt (g)	Ener (kcal)	Prot (g)	Carb (g)	Fiber (g)	Fat (g)	Sat (g)	Chol (g)
Grains										
18001	Bagel, Plain/Onion/Poppy/Sesame, enriched	1 bagel (4" dia)	89	244.75	9.345	47.526	2.047	1.424	0.196	0
18005	Bagel, cinnamon-raisin	1 bagel (4" dia)	89	243.86	8.722	49.128	2.047	0.597	0.244	0
18003	Bagel, egg	1 large bagel (4-1/2" dia)	131	364.18	13.886	69.43	3.013	0.841	0.552	31.44
18013	Biscuit, Plain or Buttermilk, baked, reduced fat refrig dough,	1 biscuit (2-1/4" dia)	21	62.79	1.638	11.634	0.399	1.092	0.272	0
18641	Bread, Hamburger Rolls/Wonder	1 serving	43	117.39	3.47	21.861	1.118	1.785	0.436	
18035	Bread, Mixed Grain/7-Grain/Whole Grain	1 slice, large	32	80	3.2	14.848	2.048	1.216	0.258	0
18039	Bread, Oatmeal	1 slice (6-1/2" dia)	27	72.63	2.268	13.095	1.08	1.188	0.19	0
18041	Bread, Pita, White, enriched	1 pita, large (6-1/2" dia)	60	165	5.46	33.42	1.32	0.72	0.1	0
18042	Bread, Pita, Whole Wheat	1 pita, large (6-1/2" dia)	64	170.24	6.272	35.2	4.736	1.664	0.262	0
18044	Bread, Rye - Pumpernickel	1 slice, regular	26	65	2.262	12.35	1.69	0.806	0.114	0
18047	Bread, Raisin, enriched	1 slice	26	71.24	2.054	13.598	1.118	1.144	0.281	0
18064	Bread, Wheat (includes wheat berry)	1 slice	25	65	2.275	11.8	1.075	1.025	0.223	0
18055	Bread, Wheat, reduced kcal	1 slice	23	45.54	2.093	10.028	2.76	0.529	0.079	0
18069	Bread, White, commercially prep, crumbs/cubes/slices	1 slice	25	66.5	1.91	12.653	0.6	0.822	0.179	0
18057	Bread, White, reduced kcal	1 slice	23	47.61	2.001	10.189	2.231	0.575	0.126	0
43100	Breakfast bars, oats, sugar, raisins, coconut (include granola bar)	1 cup	186	863.04	18.228	124.062	5.766	32.736	23.603	0
8053	Cereal, 100% Bran (wheat bran & barley)	.333 cup (1 NLEA serving)	29	83.23	3.683	22.678	8.294	0.609	0.087	0
8037	Cereal, Granola (oats & wheat germ) homemade	1 cup	122	597.8	18.141	64.599	10.492	29.719	5.535	0
8284	Cereal, Low Fat Granola with Raisins/Kellogg	.667 cup (1 NLEA serving)	55	201.3	4.4	44	2.75	2.75	0.825	0

EvaluEat Code	Food Name	Amt	Wt (g)	Ener (kcal)	Prot (g)	Carb (g)	Fiber (g)	Fat (g)	Sat (g)	Chol (g)
8180	Cereal, Oats, Regular/Quick/Instant, ckd w/salt	1 cup	234	145.08	6.084	25.272	3.978	2.34	0.421	0
8060	Cereal, Raisin Bran/Kellogg	1 cup (1 NLEA serving)	61	194.59	5.185	46.543	7.259	1.525	0.336	0
8157	Cereal, Wheat, Puffed, fortified	1 cup	12	43.68	1.764	9.552	0.528	0.144	0.024	0
8147	Cereal, Wheat, Shredded, large biscuit	2 biscuits (1 NLEA serving)	46	156.4	5.235	36.138	5.336	1.104	0.207	0
8089	Cereal, Wheaties/Gen Mills	1 cup (1 NLEA serving)	30	106.5	3	24.3	3	0.96	0.18	0
18214	Cracker, Cheese	1 cup, bite size	62	311.86	6.262	36.084	1.488	15.686	5.81	8.06
18620	Cracker, Original Premium Saltine Crackers/Nabisco	1 serving	14	58.8	1.526	9.954	0.364	1.428	0.259	0
18621	Cracker, Ritz/Nabisco	1 serving	16	78.72	1.152	10.272	0.304	3.664	0.627	0
18235	Cracker, Whole Wheat	10 Triscuit Bits	10	44.3	0.88	6.86	1.05	1.72	0.339	0
18457	Crackers, Saltines, fat-free, low-sodium	6 saltines	30	117.9	3.15	24.69	0.81	0.48	0.073	0
18258	English Muffin, Plain/Sourdough, enriched	1 muffin	57	133.95	4.389	26.22	1.539	1.026	0.148	0
20006	Grain, Barley, Pearled, ckd	1 cup	157	193.11	3.548	44.305	5.966	0.691	0.146	0
20013	Grain, Bulgar, ckd	1 cup	182	151.06	5.606	33.816	8.19	0.437	0.076	0
20029	Grain, Couscous, ckd	1 cup, cooked	157	175.84	5.95	36.455	2.198	0.251	0.046	0
20038	Grain, Oats	1 cup	156	606.84	26.348	103.381	16.536	10.764	1.899	0
20037	Grain, Rice, Brown, Long grain, ckd	1 cup	195	216.45	5.031	44.772	3.51	1.755	0.351	0
20345	Grain, Rice, White, Long grain, enriched, ckd w/salt	1 cup	158	205.4	4.25	44.509	0.632	0.442	0.122	0
22005	Macaroni and Cheese Dinner, Kraft Original Flavor, unprepared	1 NLEA Serving (makes about 1 cup prepared)	70	259	11.34	47.53	1.47	2.59	1.26	9.8
20100	Macaroni, enriched, cooked	1 cup elbow shaped	140	197.4	6.678	39.676	1.82	0.938	0.133	0
18274	Muffin, Blueberry, commercially prep	1 medium	113	313.01	6.215	54.24	2.938	7.345	1.579	33.9
18279	Muffin, Corn, commercially prep	1 medium	113	344.65	6.667	57.517	3.842	9.492	1.53	29.38
18283	Muffin, Oatbran	1 medium	113	305.1	7.91	54.579	5.198	8.362	1.228	0
20113	Noodles, Chinese, Chow Mein	1 cup	45	237.15	3.771	25.893	1.755	13.842	1.973	0
20110	Noodles, Egg, enriched, ckd w/salt	1 cup	160	212.8	7.6	39.744	1.76	2.352	0.496	52.8
18293	Pancakes, Plain, homemade	1 pancake (4" dia)	38	86.26	2.432	10.754		3.686	0.806	22.42
20121	Pasta, Spaghetti, enriched, ckd w/o salt	1 cup	140	197.4	6.678	39.676	2.38	0.938	0.133	0
20125	Pasta, Spaghetti, Whole Wheat, ckd	1 cup	140	173.6	7.462	37.156	6.3	0.756	0.139	0
43572	Popcorn, microwave, low fat and sodium	1 cup	148	634.92	18.648	108.617	21.016	14.06	2.094	0
18349	Roll, French	1 roll	38	105.26	3.268	19.076	1.216	1.634	0.366	0
18350	Roll, Hamburger/HotDog, Plain	1 roll	43	119.97	4.085	21.264	0.903	1.862	0.47	0
18348	Roll, Hamburger/HotDog, Whole Wheat	1 medium (2-1/2" dia)	36	95.76	3.132	18.396	2.7	1.692	0.301	0
18353	Roll, Hard/Kaiser	1 roll (3-1/2" dia)	57	167.01	5.643	30.039	1.311	2.451	0.345	0
12166	Seeds, Sesame, Tahini made w/roasted & toasted kernels	1 tbsp	15	89.25	2.55	3.179	1.395	8.064	1.129	0

EvaluEat Code	Food Name	Amt	Wt (g)	Ener (kcal)	Prot (g)	Carb (g)	Fiber (g)	Fat (g)	Sat (g)	Chol (g)
12037	Seeds, Sunflower Kernels, dry roast w/o salt	1 oz	28.35	164.997	5.48	6.824	3.147	14.118	1.48	0
19015	Snack, Granola Bar, Hard, Plain	1 bar (1 oz)	28	131.88	2.828	18.032	1.484	5.544	0.664	0
19020	Snack, Granola Bar, Soft, Plain	1 bar (1 oz)	28	124.04	2.072	18.844	1.288	4.816	2.027	0.28
19034	Snack, Popcorn, air-popped	1 cup	8	30.56	0.96	6.232	1.208	0.336	0.046	0
19051	Snack, Rice Cake, brown rice, Plain	2 cakes	18	69.66	1.476	14.67	0.756	0.504	0.103	0
22901	Tortellini, pasta with cheese filling	1 cup	236	724.52	31.86	110.92	4.484	17.063	8.496	99.12
18449	Tortilla, Corn, w/o salt, ready to cook	1 tortilla, medium (approx 6" dia)	26	57.72	1.482	12.116	1.352	0.65	0.087	0
18364	Tortilla, Flour, ready-to-cook	1 tortilla medium (approx 6" dia)	46	149.5	4.002	25.576	1.518	3.266	0.803	0
18360	Tortilla, Taco Shell, baked	1 large (6-1/2" dia)	21	98.28	1.512	13.104	1.575	4.746	0.681	0
18367	Waffle, Plain, homemade	1 waffle, round (7" dia)	75	218.25	5.925	24.675		10.575	2.149	51.75
18365	Waffle, Plain/Buttermilk, frozen, ready-to-heat	1 waffle square	39	97.89	2.301	15.054	0.858	3.042	0.505	12.48

Protein Sources

EvaluEat Code	Food Name	Amt	Wt (g)	Ener (kcal)	Prot (g)	Carb (g)	Fiber (g)	Fat (g)	Sat (g)	Chol (g)
43212	Bacon bits, meatless	1 cup	186	885.36	59.52	53.196	18.972	25.199	7.542	0
16104	Bacon, vegetarian, meatless	1 strip	5	15.5	0.534	0.316	0.13	1.476	0.231	0
16006	Beans, Baked, Plain or Vegetarian, canned	1 cup	254	236.22	12.167	52.121	12.7	1.143	0.295	0
16015	Beans, Black, mature seeds, boiled w/o salt	1 cup	172	227.04	15.239	40.781	14.964	0.929	0.239	0
16029	Beans, Kidney, mature seeds, canned	1 cup	256	207.36	13.312	38.093	8.96	0.794	0.115	0
16033	Beans, Kidney, Red, mature seeds, boiled w/o salt	1 cup	177	224.79	15.346	40.356	13.098	0.885	0.127	0
16070	Beans, Lentils, mature seeds, boiled w/o salt	1 cup	198	229.68	17.86	39.857	15.642	0.752	0.105	0
16038	Beans, Navy, mature seeds, boiled w/o salt	1 cup	182	258.44	15.834	47.884	11.648	1.037	0.269	0
16039	Beans, Navy, mature seeds, canned	1 cup	262	296.06	19.729	53.579	13.362	1.127	0.293	0
16110	Beans, Soy, mature seeds, roasted w/salt	1 cup	172	810.12	60.578	57.706	30.444	43.688	6.319	0
16162	Beans, Soy, Tofu, Mori-Nu, silken, firm	1 slice	84	52.08	5.796	2.016	0.084	2.268	0.341	0
16050	Beans, White, mature seeds, boiled w/o salt	1 cup	179	248.81	17.417	44.911	11.277	0.626	0.163	0
16051	Beans, White, mature seeds, canned	1 cup	262	306.54	19.021	57.483	12.576	0.76	0.194	0
16137	Beans, Hummus, Garbanzo or Chick Pea Spread, homemade	1 tbsp	15	26.55	0.729	3.018	0.6	0.312	0.168	0
22529	Beef Pot Pie, frozen	1 package yields	198	449.46	13.266	44.154	2.178	24.354	8.514	37.62
13012	Beef, All Cuts, All Grades, lean (1/4" trim) cooked	3 oz	85	183.6	25.143	0	0	8.424	3.222	73.1
13004	Beef, All Cuts, All Grades, lean & fat (1/4" trim) cooked	3 oz	85	259.25	22.049	0	0	18.309	7.259	74.8
13306	Beef, Ground, lean, broiled, well done	3 oz	85	238	23.97	0	0	14.994	5.891	85.85
13313	Beef, Ground, regular, broiled, well done	3 oz	85	248.2	23.12	0	0	16.541	6.503	85.85
13238	Beef, Tenderloin, All Grades, lean & fat (1/4" trim) broiled	3 oz	85	247.35	21.471	0	0	17.221	6.758	73.1

EvaluEat Code	Food Name	Amt	Wt (g)	Ener (kcal)	Prot (g)	Carb (g)	Fiber (g)	Fat (g)	Sat (g)	Chol (g)
13192	Beef, Tip Round, All Grades, lean & fat (1/4" trim) roasted	3 oz	85	198.9	22.874	0	0	11.254	4.267	69.7
13427	Beef, Top Round, All Grades, lean & fat (1/40 trim) braised	3 oz	85	210.8	28.756	0	0	9.716	3.672	76.5
13278	Beef, Top Sirloin, All Grades, lean & fat (1/40 trim) broiled	3 oz	85	219.3	23.639	0	0	13.099	5.219	76.5
7933	Chicken breast, oven-roasted, fat-free, sliced	1 serving 2 slices	42	33.18	7.052	0.911	0	0.164	0.055	15.12
22527	Chicken Pie, frozen/Stouffers	1 package yields	283	571.66	23.206	36.507	3.113	37.073	10.726	76.41
5007	Chicken, Broiler or Fryer, meat & skin, batter fried chicken	Yield from 1 lb ready-to-cook	280	809.2	63.112	26.376	0.84	48.58	12.908	243.6
5009	Chicken, Broiler or Fryer, meat & skin, roasted	1 cup, chopped or diced	140	334.6	38.22	0	0	19.04	5.306	123.2
5012	Chicken, Broiler or Fryer, meat only, no skin, fried	1 cup, chopped or diced	140	306.6	42.798	2.366	0.14	12.768	3.444	131.6
5013	Chicken, Broiler or Fryer, meat only, no skin, roasted	1 cup, chopped or diced	140	266	40.502	0	0	10.374	2.856	124.6
43128	Chicken, meatless	1 cup	186	416.64	43.97	6.77	6.696	13.528	3.385	0
22904	Chili con carne w/beans, canned entree	1 serving	222	255.3	20.18	24.487	8.214	8.147	2.109	24.42
22720	Chili, Vegetarian Chili w/beans, canned entree/Hormel	1 cup	247	205.01	11.93	38.013	9.88	0.692	0.124	0
5140	Duck, Domestic, Meat & Skin, roasted	1 cup, chopped or diced	140	471.8	26.586	0	0	5.11	13.538	117.6
1143	Egg Substitute, liquid	1 cup	251	210.84	30.12	1.606	0	8.308	1.654	2.51
1128	Egg, Whole, fried	1 large	46	92.5	6.27	0.405	0		1.975	210.2
1129	Egg, Whole, hard-cooked	1 large	50	77.5	6.29	0.56	0	5.305	1.633	212
1131	Egg, Whole, poached	1 large	50	73.5	6.265	0.38	0	0.679	1.543	211
1132	Egg, Whole, scrambled	1 large	61	101.26	6.765	1.342	0	7.448	2.244	214.72
15187	Fish, Bass, Freshwater, cooked w/dry heat	3 oz	85	124.1	20.553	0	0	1.156	0.851	73.95
15188	Fish, Bass, Striped, cooked w/dry heat	3 oz	85	105.4	19.32	0	0	0.854	0.553	87.55
15008	Fish, Carp, raw	3 oz	85	107.95	15.156	0	0	1.216	0.921	56.1
15011	Fish, Catfish, Channel, breaded & fried	3 oz	85	194.65	15.377	6.834	0.595	2.826	2.795	68.85
15012	Fish, Caviar, black/red, granular	1 tbsp	16	40.32	3.936	0.64	0	1.185	0.65	94.08
15016	Fish, Cod, Atlantic, baked/broiled (dry heat)	3 oz	85	89.25	19.406	0	0	0.248	0.143	46.75
15192	Fish, Cod, Pacific, cooked w/dry heat	3 oz	85	89.25	19.508	0	0	0.266	0.088	39.95
15034	Fish, Haddock, baked or broiled (dry heat)	3 oz	85	95.2	20.604	0	0	0.263	0.142	62.9
15035	Fish, Haddock, smoked	3 oz	85	98.6	21.445	0	0	0.273	0.147	65.45
15037	Fish, Halibut, Atlantic & Pacific, baked or broiled dry heat)	3 oz	85	119	22.687	0	0	0.799	0.354	34.85
15196	Fish, Halibut, Greenland, cooked w/dry heat	3 oz	85	203.15	15.657	0	0	1.49	2.637	50.15
15040	Fish, Herring, Atlantic, baked or broiled (dry heat)	3 oz	85	172.55	19.576	0	0	2.325	2.223	65.45
15087	Fish, Salmon, Sockeye w/bone, canned, drained	3 oz	85	130.05	17.399	0	0	6.214	1.397	37.4
15086	Fish, Salmon, Sockeye, baked or broiled (dry heat)	3 oz	85	183.6	23.214	0	0	9.325	1.629	73.95
15102	Fish, Snapper, baked or broiled (dry heat)	3 oz	85	108.8	22.355	0	0	1.462	0.31	39.95

EvaluEat Code	Food Name	Amt	Wt (g)	Ener (kcal)	Prot (g)	Carb (g)	Fiber (g)	Fat (g)	Sat (g)	Chol (g)
15176	Fish, Squid, fried	3 oz	85	148.75	15.249	6.622	0	6.358	1.596	221
15111	Fish, Swordfish, baked or broiled (dry heat)	3 oz	85	131.75	21.582	0	0	4.369	1.195	42.5
15128	Fish, Tuna Salad	1 cup	205	383.35	32.882	19.29	0	18.983	3.165	26.65
15126	Fish, White Tuna, canned in H₂0, drained	3 oz	85	108.8	20.077	0	0	2.525	0.673	35.7
15124	Fish, White Tuna, canned in oil, drained	3 oz	85	158.1	22.551	0	0	6.868	1.088	26.35
7945	Frankfurter, beef, heated	1 serving	52	169.52	6.001	1.96	0	15.319	5.947	29.12
17002	Lamb, Domestic, Choice, Composite, lean & fat (1/4" trim) ckd	3 oz	85	249.9	20.842	0	0	17.799	7.506	82.45
7043	Lunch Meat, Beef, thin slices	1 oz	28.35	50.18	7.969	1.619	0	1.089	0.468	11.624
7007	Lunch Meat, Bologna (Beef)	1 slice	28	87.08	2.876	1.114	0	7.893	3.118	15.68
7079	Lunch Meat, Turkey Breast Meat	1 slice	28	26.88	2.044	3.822	0.56	0.378	0.118	3.36
16097	Peanut Butter, chunky w/salt	2 tbsp	32	188.48	8.022	6.749	2.112	15.904	3.066	0
16098	Peanut Butter, smooth w/salt	2 tbsp	32	191.68	7.99	5.894	1.888	16.73	3.209	0
16090	Peanuts, All Types, dry roasted w/salt	1 oz	28.35	165.848	6.713	6.098	2.268	14.079	1.954	0
16363	Peas, Cowpea, Common (blackeyed, crowder, southern) mature seed, boiled w/salt	1 cup	171	198.36	13.218	35.5	11.115	0.906	0.236	0
22903	Pizza, Pepperoni, frozen	1 serving	146	400.04	16.191	36.208	2.336	21.112	7.066	33.58
22902	Pizza, Sausage & pepperoni, frozen	1 serving	146	385.44	15.768	36.179	2.336	19.695	6.336	30.66
10193	Pork Back Rib, Fresh, lean & fat, roasted	1 piece, cooked (yield from 1 lb raw meat)	219	810.3	53.129	0	0	64.78	24.068	258.42
10124	Pork Bacon, Cured, broiled, pan-fried, or roasted	1 slice, cooked	8	43.28	2.963	0.114	0	3.342	1.099	8.8
10188	Pork Composite (leg, loin/shoulder/sparerib) Fresh, lean & fat, ckd	3 oz	85	232.05	23.434	0	0	14.603	5.287	77.35
10220	Pork, Ground, Fresh, ckd	3 oz	85	252.45	21.837	0	0	17.655	6.562	79.9
7019	Sausage, Chorizo (Pork & Beef)	1 link (4" long)	60	273	14.46	1.116	0	22.962	8.628	52.8
7023	Sausage, Frankfurter (weiner) (Beef & Pork)	1 frankfurter (5" long x 3/4" dia, 10 per lb)	45	137.25	5.188	0.774	1.08	12.438	4.846	22.5
7919	Sausage, Turkey, breakfast links, mild	1 serving	56	131.6	8.635	0.874	0	10.13	4.002	33.6
16107	Sausage, Vegetarian, Meatless	1 link	25	64.25	4.633	2.46	0.7	4.54	0.732	0
15159	Shellfish, Clams, boiled/steamed (moist heat)	20 small	190	281.2	48.545	9.747	0	3.705	0.357	127.3
15158	Shellfish, Clams, breaded & fried	3 oz	85	171.7	12.104	8.781		9.477	2.281	51.85
15137	Shellfish, Crab, Alaskan King, boiled/steamed	1 leg	134	129.98	25.929	0	0	2.064	0.178	71.02
15138	Shellfish, Crab, Alaskan King, imitation surimi	3 oz	85	86.7	10.217	8.687	0	1.113	0.221	17
15148	Shellfish, Lobster, Northern, boiled/steamed (moist heat)	3 oz	85	83.3	17.425	1.088	0	0.502	0.091	61.2
15168	Shellfish, Oyster, Eastern, breaded & fried	6 medium	88	173.36	7.718	10.226		11.07	2.813	71.28
15245	Shellfish, Oyster, Eastern, Farmed, raw	6 medium	84	49.56	4.385	4.645	0	1.302	0.372	21

EvaluEat Code	Food Name	Amt	Wt (g)	Ener (kcal)	Prot (g)	Carb (g)	Fiber (g)	Fat (g)	Sat (g)	Chol (g)
15171	Shellfish, Oyster, Pacific, raw	1 medium	50	40.5	4.725	2.475	0	1.15	0.255	25
15151	Shellfish, Shrimp, boiled/ steamed (moist heat)	4 large	22	21.78	4.6	0	0	0.238	0.064	42.9
15150	Shellfish, Shrimp, breaded & fried	4 large	30	72.6	6.417	3.441	0.12	3.684	0.626	53.1
43133	Soyburger	1 cup	186	332.94	33.313	24.924	8.556	11.104	1.337	0
22905	Stew, Beef Stew, canned entree	1 serving	232	218.08	11.461	15.706	3.48	12.482	5.15	37.12
42130	Turkey bacon, cooked	1 ounce	28.34	108.259	8.389	0.879	0	7.907	2.351	27.773
22528	Turkey Pot Pie, frozen	1 serving	397	698.72	25.805	70.269	4.367	34.936	11.434	63.52
5220	Turkey, Fryer/Roaster, Breast, no skin, roasted	1 unit (yield from 1 lb ready-to-cook turkey)	87	117.45	26.152	0	0	0.644	0.209	72.21
5208	Turkey, Fryer/Roaster, Dark Meat w/skin, roasted	1 unit (yield from 1 lb ready-to-cook turkey)	106	192.92	29.351	0	0	7.484	2.247	124.02
5206	Turkey, Fryer/Roaster, Light Meat w/skin, roasted	1 unit (yield from 1 lb ready-to-cook turkey)	123	201.72	35.387	0	0	5.633	1.538	116.85
5306	Turkey, Ground, cooked	1 patty (4 oz, raw)	82	192.7	22.435	0	0	10.783	2.78	83.64
7900	Turkey, pork, and beef sausage, low fat, smoked	1 frankfurter	56	56.56	4.48	6.44	0.336	1.4	0.476	11.76
17089	Veal, Composite, lean & fat, cooked	3 oz	85	196.35	25.585	0	0	9.682	3.638	96.9
43134	Vegetarian fillets	1 cup	186	539.4	42.78	16.74	11.346	33.48	5.299	0
43137	Vegetarian meatloaf or patties	1 cup	186	366.42	39.06	14.88	8.556	16.74	2.65	0
43136	Vegetarian stew	1 cup	186	228.78	31.62	13.02	2.046	5.58	0.883	0

Dairy

EvaluEat Code	Food Name	Amt	Wt (g)	Ener (kcal)	Prot (g)	Carb (g)	Fiber (g)	Fat (g)	Sat (g)	Chol (g)
43276	Cheese spread, cream cheese base	1 cup	186	548.7	13.206	6.51	0	53.196	33.517	167.4
1009	Cheese, Cheddar	1 cup, shredded	113	455.39	28.137	1.446	0	37.448	23.834	118.65
1012	Cheese, Cottage, Creamed, large or small curd	4 oz	113	116.39	14.114	3.028	0	5.096	3.224	16.95
1015	Cheese, Cottage, Lowfat, 2% fat	4 oz	113	101.7	15.526	4.102	0	2.181	1.38	9.04
1014	Cheese, Cottage, Nonfat, Uncreamed, Dry, large or small curd	4 oz	113	96.05	19.515	2.091	0	0.475	0.308	7.91
1017	Cheese, Cream	1 tbsp	14.5	50.605	1.095	0.386	0	5.056	3.185	15.95
1186	Cheese, Cream, fat free	1 ounce	28.34	27.206	4.084	1.644	0	0.385	0.255	2.267
1190	Cheese, Kraft Free Singles American Nonfat Pasteurized Process Cheese Product	1 slice	21	31.08	4.767	2.457	0.042	0.21	0.147	3.36
1004	Cheese, Blue	1 oz	28.35	100.076	6.067	0.663	0	0.227	5.293	21.263
1006	Cheese, Brie	1 cubic inch	17	56.78	3.528	0.076	0	0.14	2.96	17
1168	Cheese, Cheddar or Colby, low fat	1 cup, shredded	113	195.49	27.516	2.158	0	0.251	4.906	23.73
1019	Cheese, Feta	1 oz	28.35	74.844	4.029	1.16	0	0.168	4.237	25.232
1035	Cheese, Provolone	1 oz	28.35	99.509	7.252	0.607	0	0.218	4.842	19.562
1040	Cheese, Swiss	1 oz	28.35	107.73	7.635	1.525	0	0.276	5.04	26.082
1028	Cheese, Mozzarella, Part Skim Milk	1 oz	28.35	72.009	6.878	0.785	0	4.513	2.867	18.144
1026	Cheese, Mozzarella, Whole Milk	1 oz	28.35	85.05	6.285	0.621	0	6.336	3.729	22.397
1032	Cheese, Parmesan, grated	1 tbsp	5	21.55	1.923	0.203	0	1.431	0.865	4.4
42205	Cheese, pasteurized process, cheddar or american, fat-free	1 cup	186	275.28	41.85	24.924	0	1.488	0.937	20.46

EvaluEat Code	Food Name	Amt	Wt (g)	Ener (kcal)	Prot (g)	Carb (g)	Fiber (g)	Fat (g)	Sat (g)	Chol (g)
1035	Cheese, Provolone	1 oz	28.35	99.509	7.252	0.607	0	7.547	4.842	19.562
1037	Cheese, Ricotta, Part Skim Milk	1 cup	246	339.48	28.019	12.644	0	19.459	12.12	76.26
1049	Cream, Half and Half	1 tbsp	15	19.5	0.444	0.645	0	1.725	1.074	5.55
1053	Cream, Heavy Whipping	1 cup, whipped	120	414	2.46	3.348	0	1.649	27.638	164.4
1074	Cream, Sour, Imitation, cultured	1 oz	28.35	58.968	0.68	1.88	0	5.534	5.044	0
42185	Frozen yogurts, chocolate, nonfat milk, with low calorie sweetener	1 cup	186	199.02	8.184	36.642	3.72	1.488	0.939	7.44
42187	Frozen yogurts, flavors other than chocolate	1 cup	186	236.22	5.58	40.176	0	6.696	4.326	24.18
1088	Milk, Buttermilk, Lowfat, Cultured	1 cup	245	98	8.109	11.736	0	2.156	1.343	9.8
1082	Milk, Lowfat, 1% fat w/added vitamin A	1 cup	244	102.48	8.223	12.176	0	2.367	1.545	12.2
1104	Milk, Lowfat, 1% fat, Chocolate	1 cup	250	157.5	8.1	26.1	1.25	2.5	1.54	7.5
1085	Milk, Nonfat/Fat Free, Skim w/added Vit A	1 cup	245	83.3	8.257	12.152	0	0.196	0.287	4.9
16120	Milk, Soy, fluid	1 cup	245	120.05	9.188	11.368	3.185	5.096	0.524	0
1077	Milk, Whole, 3.25% fat	1 cup	244	146.4	7.857	11.029	0	7.93	4.551	24.4
1102	Milk, Whole, Chocolate	1 cup	250	207.5	7.925	25.85	2	8.475	5.26	30
1180	Sour cream, fat free	1 ounce	28.34	20.972	0.879	4.421	0	0	0	2.551
1179	Sour cream, light	1 ounce	28.34	38.542	0.992	2.012	0	3.004	1.87	9.919
19393	Yogurt, Frozen, Chocolate, soft serve	.5 cup (4 fl oz)	72	115.2	2.88	17.928	1.584	4.32	2.614	3.6
43261	Yogurt, fruit variety, nonfat	1 cup	186	174.84	8.184	35.34	0	0.372	0.221	3.72
1121	Yogurt, Lowfat w/fruit, 10 g protein/8 oz	1 cup (8 fl oz)	245	249.9	10.707	46.673	0	2.646	1.708	9.8
1117	Yogurt, Lowfat, Plain, 12 g protein/8 oz	1 cup (8 fl oz)	245	154.35	12.863	17.248	0	3.797	2.45	14.7
1116	Yogurt, Whole Milk, Plain, 8 g protein/8 oz	1 cup (8 fl oz)	245	149.45	8.502	11.417	0	7.963	5.135	31.85

Fruits

EvaluEat Code	Food Name	Amt	Wt (g)	Ener (kcal)	Prot (g)	Carb (g)	Fiber (g)	Fat (g)	Sat (g)	Chol (g)
9103	Fruit Salad (peach, apricot & pineapple, pear, cherry) canned in juice	1 cup	249	124.5	1.27	32.494	2.49	0.075	0.01	0
9003	Fruit, Apple w/skin, raw	1 large (3-1/4" dia) (approx 2 per lb)	212	110.24	0.551	29.277	5.088	0.36	0.059	0
9402	Fruit, Applesauce, canned, sweetened w/added Vit C	1 cup	255	193.8	0.459	50.771	3.06	0.459	0.076	0
9401	Fruit, Applesauce, canned, unsweetened w/added Vit C	1 cup	244	104.92	0.415	27.548	2.928	0.122	0.02	0
9024	Fruit, Apricot w/skin, canned in juice	1 cup, halves	244	117.12	1.537	30.11	3.904	0.098	0.007	0
9023	Fruit, Apricot, peeled, canned in H₂O	1 cup, whole, without pits	227	49.94	1.566	12.44	2.497	0.068	0.005	0
9021	Fruit, Apricot, raw	1 apricot	35	16.8	0.49	3.892	0.7	0.136	0.009	0
9038	Fruit, Avocado, California, peeled, raw	1 fruit without skin and seeds	173	288.91	3.391	14.947	11.764	26.659	3.678	0
9040	Fruit, Banana, peeled, raw, mashed/sliced	1 medium (7" to 7-7/8" long)	118	105.02	1.286	26.951	3.068	0.389	0.132	0
9050	Fruit, Blueberries, raw	1 cup	145	82.65	1.073	21.01	3.48	0.479	0.041	0
9070	Fruit, Cherries, Sweet, raw	1 cup, with pits, yields	117	73.71	1.24	18.732	2.457	0.234	0.044	0
9078	Fruit, Cranberries, raw	1 cup, chopped	110	50.6	0.429	13.42	5.06	0.143	0.012	0

EvaluEat Code	Food Name	Amt	Wt (g)	Ener (kcal)	Prot (g)	Carb (g)	Fiber (g)	Fat (g)	Sat (g)	Chol (g)
9087	Fruit, Dates, Domestic, Natural, dried	1 cup, pitted, chopped	178	501.96	4.361	133.553	14.24	0.694	0.057	0
9092	Fruit, Figs, canned in heavy syrup	1 cup	259	227.92	0.984	59.311	5.698	0.259	0.052	0
9089	Fruit, Figs, raw	1 large (2-1/2" dia)	64	47.36	0.48	12.275	1.856	0.192	0.038	0
9111	Fruit, Grapefruit, Red, White or Pink, peeled, raw	.5 medium (approx 4" dia)	128	40.96	0.806	10.342	1.408	0.128	0.018	0
9131	Fruit, Grapes, American type (slip skin) raw	1 cup	92	61.64	0.58	15.778	0.828	0.322	0.105	0
9148	Fruit, Kiwifruit (Chinese Gooseberry) peeled, raw	1 fruit without skin, medium	76	46.36	0.866	11.142	2.28	0.395	0.022	0
9176	Fruit, Mango, peeled, raw	1 cup, sliced	165	107.25	0.841	28.05	2.97	0.446	0.109	0
9184	Fruit, Melon, Honeydew, peeled, wedges, raw	1 wedge (1/8 of 6" to 7" dia melon)	160	57.6	0.864	14.544	1.28	0.224	0.061	0
9188	Fruit, Mixed (prune, apricot & pear) dried	1 package (11 oz)	293	711.99	7.208	187.696	22.854	1.436	0.117	0
9191	Fruit, Nectarine, raw	1 fruit (2-1/2" dia)	136	59.84	1.442	14.348	2.312	0.435	0.034	0
9193	Fruit, Olives, Ripe, pitted, canned	1 tbsp	8.4	9.66	0.071	0.526	0.269	0.897	0.119	0
9200	Fruit, Orange, All Varieties, peeled, raw	1 fruit (2-5/8" dia)	131	61.57	1.231	15.392	3.144	0.157	0.02	0
9241	Fruit, Peach, canned in heavy syrup	1 cup	262	193.88	1.179	52.243	3.406	0.262	0.026	0
9236	Fruit, Peach, peeled, raw	1 medium (2-1/2" dia) (approx 4 per lb)	98	38.22	0.892	9.349	1.47	0.245	0.019	0
9257	Fruit, Pear, canned in heavy syrup	1 cup	266	196.84	0.532	50.992	4.256	0.346	0.019	0
9252	Fruit, Pear, raw	1 pear, medium (approx 2-1/2 per lb)	166	96.28	0.631	25.664	5.146	0.199	0.01	0
9270	Fruit, Pineapple, canned in heavy syrup	1 cup, crushed, sliced, or chunks	254	198.12	0.889	51.308	2.032	0.279	0.023	0
9268	Fruit, Pineapple, canned in juice	1 cup, crushed, sliced, or chunks	249	149.4	1.046	39.093	1.992	0.199	0.015	0
9279	Fruit, Plum, raw	1 fruit (2-1/8" dia)	66	30.36	0.462	7.537	0.924	0.185	0.011	0
9291	Fruit, Prunes, dried	1 prune	8.4	20.16	0.183	5.366	0.596	0.032	0.007	0
9298	Fruit, Raisins, seedless	1 cup (not packed)	145	433.55	4.451	114.811	5.365	0.667	0.084	0
9302	Fruit, Raspberries, raw	1 cup	123	63.96	1.476	14.686	7.995	0.799	0.023	0
9306	Fruit, Raspberries, Red, frozen, sweetened	1 cup, unthawed	250	257.5	1.75	65.4	11	0.4	0.012	0
9319	Fruit, Strawberries, frozen, whole, sweetened	1 cup, thawed	255	198.9	1.326	53.55	4.845	0.357	0.018	0
9316	Fruit, Strawberries, halves/slices, raw	1 cup, halves	152	48.64	1.018	11.674	3.04	0.456	0.023	0
9326	Fruit, Watermelon, balls, raw	1 cup, balls	154	46.2	0.939	11.627	0.616	0.231	0.025	0

Vegetables

11358	Potatoes, red, flesh and skin, baked	1 potato, large (3" to 4-1/4" dia)	299	266.11	6.877	58.574	5.382	0.449	0.078	0
11356	Potatoes, Russet, flesh and skin, baked	1 potato, large	299	290.03	7.864	64.106	6.877	0.389		0
11702	Vege, Artichokes (Globe or French) boiled w/salt, drained	1 artichoke, medium	120	60	4.176	13.416	6.48	0.192	0.044	0
11705	Vege, Asparagus, boiled w/salt, drained	4 spears (1/2" base)	60	13.2	1.44	2.466	1.2	0.132	0.043	0
11712	Vege, Bamboo Shoots, boiled w/salt, drained	1 cup (1/2" slices)	120	14.4	1.836	2.304	1.2	0.264	0.061	0
11028	Vege, Bamboo Shoots, canned, drained	1 cup (1/8" slices)	131	24.89	2.253	4.218	1.834	0.524	0.121	0

EvaluEat Code	Food Name	Amt	Wt (g)	Ener (kcal)	Prot (g)	Carb (g)	Fiber (g)	Fat (g)	Sat (g)	Chol (g)
11626	Vege, Bean Sprouts, Mung, mature seeds, sprouted, canned, drained	1 cup	125	15	1.75	2.675	1	0.075	0.02	0
11723	Vege, Beans, Snap, Green, boiled w/salt, drained	1 cup	125	43.75	2.362	9.863	4	0.35	0.08	0
11056	Vege, Beans, Snap, Green, canned, drained	1 cup	135	27	1.553	6.075	2.565	0.135	0.03	0
11084	Vege, Beets, canned, drained	1 cup, diced	157	48.67	1.429	11.32	2.669	0.22	0.036	0
11609	Vege, Beets, pickled, canned, solids & liquid	1 cup slices	227	147.55	1.816	36.956	5.902	0.182	0.03	0
11741	Vege, Broccoli Stalks, raw	1 stalk	114	31.92	3.397	5.974		0.399	0.062	0
11742	Vege, Broccoli, boiled w/salt, chopped, drained	.5 cup, chopped	78	21.84	2.324	3.947	2.574	0.273	0.042	0
11745	Vege, Brussels Sprouts, boiled w/salt, drained	.5 cup	78	31.98	1.989	6.763	2.028	0.398	0.082	0
11109	Vege, Cabbage Heads, raw	1 cup, chopped	89	21.36	1.282	4.966	2.047	0.107	0.014	0
11751	Vege, Cabbage, boiled w/salt, drained	.5 cup, shredded	75	16.5	0.765	3.345	1.425	0.322	0.04	0
11960	Vege, Carrots, Baby, raw	1 medium	10	3.5	0.064	0.824	0.18	0.013	0.002	0
11757	Vege, Carrots, boiled w/salt, drained	.5 cup slices	78	27.3	0.593	6.412	2.34	0.14	0.023	0
11135	Vege, Cauliflower head, raw	1 cup	100	25	1.98	5.3	2.5	0.1	0.032	0
11761	Vege, Cauliflower, boiled w/salt, drained	.5 cup (1" pieces)	62	14.26	1.141	2.548	1.674	0.279	0.043	0
11764	Vege, Celery, boiled w/salt, drained	1 cup, diced	150	27	1.245	6.015	2.4	0.24	0.06	0
11143	Vege, Celery, raw	1 cup, diced	120	16.8	0.828	3.564	1.92	0.204	0.052	0
11765	Vege, Chard, Swiss, boiled w/salt, drained	1 cup, chopped	175	35	3.29	7.227	3.675	0.14		0
11768	Vege, Collards, boiled w/salt, drained	1 cup, chopped	190	49.4	4.009	9.329	5.32	0.684	0.089	0
11908	Vege, Corn, White, Sweet, canned, vacuum/regular pack	.5 cup	105	82.95	2.53	20.412	2.1	0.525	0.081	0
11900	Vege, Corn, White, Sweet, ears, raw	1 ear, large	143	122.98	4.605	27.199	3.861	1.687	0.26	0
11176	Vege, Corn, Yellow, Sweet, canned, vacuum/regular pack	.5 cup	105	82.95	2.53	20.412	2.1	0.525	0.081	0
11205	Vege, Cucumber, raw	.5 cup slices	52	7.8	0.338	1.888	0.26	0.057	0.018	0
11783	Vege, Eggplant (Brinjal) boiled w/salt, drained	1 cup (1" cubes)	99	34.65	0.822	8.643	2.475	0.228	0.044	0
11264	Vege, Fungi, Mushrooms, canned, caps/slices, drained	1 can	132	33	2.468	6.719	3.168	0.383	0.05	0
11260	Vege, Fungi, Mushrooms, slices, raw	1 medium	18	3.96	0.56	0.583	0.216	0.061	0.008	0
11790	Vege, Kale, boiled w/salt, drained	1 cup, chopped	130	36.4	2.47	7.319	2.6	0.52	0.068	0
11233	Vege, Kale, raw	1 cup, chopped	67	33.5	2.211	6.707	1.34	0.469	0.061	0
11250	Vege, Lettuce, Butterhead (Boston/Bibb) leaves, raw	1 leaf, medium	7.5	0.975	0.101	0.167	0.083	0.016	0.002	0
11251	Vege, Lettuce, Cos/Romaine, raw	1 inner leaf	10	1.7	0.123	0.329	0.21	0.03	0.004	0
11252	Vege, Lettuce, Iceberg, head, raw	1 head, medium	539	53.9	4.366	11.265	5.39	0.593	0.075	0
11253	Vege, Lettuce, Looseleaf, raw	1 leaf	10	1.5	0.136	0.279	0.13	0.015	0.002	0
11803	Vege, Okra, boiled w/salt, drained	.5 cup slices	80	17.6	1.496	3.608	2	0.168	0.036	0

EvaluEat Code	Food Name	Amt	Wt (g)	Ener (kcal)	Prot (g)	Carb (g)	Fiber (g)	Fat (g)	Sat (g)	Chol (g)
11808	Vege, Parsnip, boiled w/salt, drained	.5 cup slices	78	63.18	1.03	15.233	3.12	0.234	0.039	0
11298	Vege, Parsnip, peeled, raw	1 cup slices	133	99.75	1.596	23.927	6.517	0.399	0.067	0
11300	Vege, Peas w/edible pod-Snow/Sugar, raw	1 cup, chopped	98	41.16	2.744	7.399	2.548	0.196	0.038	0
11811	Vege, Peas, Green, boiled w/salt, drained	1 cup	160	134.4	8.576	25.024	8.8	0.352	0.062	0
11308	Vege, Peas, Green, canned, regular pack, drained	1 cup	170	117.3	7.514	21.386	6.97	0.595	0.105	0
11304	Vege, Peas, Green, raw	1 cup	145	117.45	7.859	20.967	7.395	0.58	0.103	0
11979	Vege, Pepper, Jalapeno, raw	1 cup, sliced	90	27	1.215	5.319	2.52	0.558	0.056	0
11333	Vege, Pepper, Sweet, Green, chopped/sliced, raw	1 medium	119	23.8	1.023	5.522	2.023	0.202	0.069	0
11821	Vege, Pepper, Sweet, Red, raw	1 medium	119	30.94	1.178	7.176	2.38	0.357	0.07	0
11383	Vege, Potato Mashed, granules w/milk, prep w/water & margarine	1 cup	210	243.6	4.599	33.768	2.73	10.059	2.541	4.2
11373	Vege, Potato, Au Gratin, homemade w/butter	1 cup	245	323.4	12.397	27.612	4.41	18.596	11.596	56.35
11833	Vege, Potato, boiled w/o skin & w/salt	1 medium	167	143.62	2.856	33.417	3.34	0.167	0.043	0
11838	Vege, Potato, French Fries, frozen, oven heated, w/salt	10 strips	50	100	1.585	15.595	1.6	3.78	0.631	0
11846	Vege, Pumpkin, canned w/salt	1 cup	245	83.3	2.695	19.796	7.105	0.686	0.358	0
11429	Vege, Radish, slices, raw	1 large (1" to 1-1/4" dia)	9	1.44	0.061	0.306	0.144	0.009	0.003	0
11439	Vege, Sauerkraut, canned, solids & liquid	1 cup	142	26.98	1.292	6.078	3.55	0.199	0.05	0
11854	Vege, Spinach, boiled w/salt, drained	1 cup	180	41.4	5.346	6.75	4.32	0.468	0.076	0
11461	Vege, Spinach, canned, drained	1 cup	214	49.22	6.013	7.276	5.136	1.07	0.173	0
11457	Vege, Spinach, raw	1 cup	30	6.9	0.858	1.089	0.66	0.117	0.019	0
11857	Vege, Squash, Summer, All Varieties, boiled w/salt, drained	1 cup slices	180	36	1.638	7.758	2.52	0.558	0.115	0
11863	Vege, Squash, Winter, All Varieties, baked w/salt	1 cup, cubes	205	79.95	1.824	17.938	5.74	1.291	0.266	0
11861	Vege, Squash, Zucchini w/skin, boiled w/salt, drained	.5 cup slices	90	14.4	0.576	3.537	1.26	0.045	0.009	0
11875	Vege, Sweet Potato, baked in skin w/salt	1 medium (2" dia, 5" long, raw)	114	102.6	2.291	23.609	3.762	0.171	0.039	0
11531	Vege, Tomato, Red, canned, whole	1 cup	240	40.8	1.92	9.384	2.16	0.312	0.043	0
11529	Vege, Tomato, Red, ripe, whole, raw	1 cup, chopped or sliced	180	32.4	1.584	7.056	2.16	0.36	0.081	0
11590	Vege, Waterchestnut, Chinese, canned, solids & liquid	.5 cup slices	70	35	0.616	8.61	1.75	0.042	0.011	0
11591	Vege, Watercress, raw	1 cup, chopped	34	3.74	0.782	0.439	0.17	0.034	0.009	0
11897	Vege, Yam, boiled or baked w/salt	1 cup, cubes	136	157.76	2.026	37.509	5.304	0.19	0.039	0
11578	Vegetable Juice Cocktail, canned	1 cup	242	45.98	1.525	11.011	1.936	0.218	0.031	0
11159	Vegetable Salad, Coleslaw, homemade	.5 cup	60	41.4	0.774	7.446	0.9	1.566	0.231	4.8
11894	Vegetables, Mixed, frozen, boiled w/salt, drained	.5 cup	91	53.69	2.603	11.912	4.004	0.137	0.028	0

EvaluEat Code	Food Name	Amt	Wt (g)	Ener (kcal)	Prot (g)	Carb (g)	Fiber (g)	Fat (g)	Sat (g)	Chol (g)
Fast Food										
Breakfast Items										
21023	Fast Food, French Toast w/butter	2 slices	135	356.4	10.341	36.045		18.765	7.749	116.1
21025	Fast Food, Pancakes w/butter & syrup	2 cakes	232	519.68	8.259	90.898		13.99	5.851	58
21026	Fast Food, Potatoes, Hash Brown	.5 cup	72	151.2	1.944	16.15		9.216	4.324	9.36
21002	Fast Food, Sandwich, Biscuit w/egg	1 biscuit	136	372.64	11.601	31.906	0.816	22.073	4.729	244.8
21003	Fast Food, Sandwich, Biscuit w/egg & bacon	1 biscuit	150	457.5	16.995	28.59	0.75	31.095	7.95	352.5
21004	Fast Food, Sandwich, Biscuit w/egg & ham	1 biscuit	192	441.6	20.429	30.317	0.768	27.034	5.914	299.52
21005	Fast Food, Sandwich, Biscuit w/egg & sausage	1 biscuit	180	581.4	19.152	41.148	0.9	38.7	14.976	302.4
21007	Fast Food, Sandwich, Biscuit w/egg, cheese & bacon	1 biscuit	144	476.64	16.258	33.422		31.392	11.398	260.64
21011	Fast Food, Sandwich, Croissant w/egg & cheese	1 croissant	127	368.3	12.789	24.308		24.701	14.065	215.9
21012	Fast Food, Sandwich, Croissant w/egg, cheese bacon	1 croissant	129	412.8	16.228	23.646		28.354	15.432	215.43
21013	Fast Food, Sandwich, Croissant w/egg, cheese & ham	1 croissant	152	474.24	18.924	24.198		33.577	17.475	212.8
Chicken										
21035	Fast Food, Chicken, breaded, fried, dark meat (drumstick or thigh)	2 pieces	148	430.68	30.074	15.703		26.699	7.049	165.76
21036	Fast Food, Chicken, breaded, fried, light meat (breast or wing)	2 pieces	163	493.89	35.713	19.576		29.519	7.844	148.33
21102	Fast Food, Sandwich, Chicken Filet, plain	1 sandwich	182	515.06	24.115	38.693		29.448	8.527	60.06
Burgers										
21092	Fast Food, Sandwich, Cheeseburger (2 patty) plain	1 sandwich	155	457.25	27.667	22.056		28.474	12.997	110.05
21098	Fast Food, Sandwich, Cheeseburger, large, one meat patty w/condiments & veges	1 sandwich	219	562.83	28.185	38.391		32.938	15.039	87.6
21109	Fast Food, Sandwich, Hamburger, one patty w/condiments & veges	1 sandwich	110	279.4	12.914	27.291		13.475	4.131	26.4
21107	Fast Food, Sandwich, Hamburger, plain	1 sandwich	90	274.5	12.321	30.51		11.817	4.141	35.1
Mexican										
21061	Fast Food, Burrito w/beans & cheese	2 pieces	186	377.58	15.066	54.963		11.699	6.849	27.9
21066	Fast Food, Burrito w/beef	2 pieces	220	523.6	26.598	58.52		20.812	10.459	63.8
21078	Fast Food, Nachos w/cheese	1 portion (6–8 nachos)	113	345.78	9.097	36.33		18.95	7.78	18.08
21080	Fast Food, Nachos w/cheese, beans, ground beef & peppers	1 portion (6–8 nachos)	255	568.65	19.788	55.819		30.702	12.487	20.4
21082	Fast Food, Taco	1 large	263	568.08	31.77	41.107		31.613	17.484	86.79

EvaluEat Code	Food Name	Amt	Wt (g)	Ener (kcal)	Prot (g)	Carb (g)	Fiber (g)	Fat (g)	Sat (g)	Chol (g)
Sides/Beverages/Other										
21118	Fast Food, Hot Dog, plain	1 sandwich	98	242.06	10.388	18.032		14.543	5.109	44.1
21033	Fast Food, Ice Cream Sundae, hot fudge	1 sundae	158	284.4	5.641	47.669	0	8.627	5.023	20.54
14346	Fast Food, Milk Beverage, Chocolate Shake/ McDonald's	1 medium shake (16 fl oz)	333	422.91	11.322	68.265	6.327	12.321	7.702	43.29
14347	Fast Food, Shake, Vanilla/ McDonald's	1 medium shake (16 fl oz)	333	369.63	11.655	59.607	0.333	9.99	6.187	36.63
21130	Fast Food, Onion Rings, breaded, fried	1 portion (8–9 onion rings)	83	275.56	3.702	31.324		15.513	6.953	14.11
21049	Fast Food, Pizza w/cheese	1 slice	63	140.49	7.68	20.5		3.213	1.54	9.45
21050	Fast Food, Pizza w/cheese, meat & veges	1 slice	79	184.07	13.011	21.291		5.364	1.535	20.54
21051	Fast Food, Pizza w/ pepperoni	1 slice	71	181.05	10.125	19.866		6.958	2.236	14.2
21138	Fast Food, Potato, French fried w/vegetable oil	1 large	169	577.98	7.267	67.279	5.915	31.147	6.507	0
21105	Fast Food, Sandwich, Fish w/tartar sauce	1 sandwich	158	431.34	16.938	41.017		22.768	5.235	55.3
Beverages										
14006	Beverage, Alcoholic, Beer, Light	1 can or bottle (12 fl oz)	354	99.12	0.708	4.602	0	0	0	0
14003	Beverage, Alcoholic, Beer, Regular	1 can	356	117.48	1.068	5.732	0.356	0.214	0	0
14010	Beverage, Alcoholic, Daiquiri, prep from recipe	1 cocktail (2 fl oz)	60	111.6	0.036	4.164	0.06	0.036	0.004	0
14049	Beverage, Alcoholic, Distilled Spirits, Gin, Vodka, Rum, Whiskey	1 jigger 1.5 fl oz	42	110.46	0	0	0	0	0	0
14084	Beverage, Alcoholic, Wine (all table)	1 glass 3.5 fl oz	103	79.31	0.206	3.296	0	0	0	0
14209	Beverage, Coffee, Brewed	1 cup (8 fl oz)	237	9.48	0.332	0	0	1.801	0	0
14201	Beverage, Coffee, brewed, prepared with tap water, decaffeinated	1 cup (8 fl oz)	237	9.48	0.332	0	0	1.801	0	0
14400	Beverage, Cola w/caffeine	1 can 12 fl oz	370	155.4	0.185	39.775	0	0	0	0
14177	Beverage Mix, Chocolate Flavor, dry mix, prep w/milk	1 cup (8 fl oz)	266	226.1	8.592	31.681	1.064	0.495	4.948	23.94
14318	Beverage Mix, Chocolate Malted Milk Powder, no added nutrients, prep w/milk	1 cup (8 fl oz)	265	225.25	8.931	29.68	1.325	0.551	4.99	26.5
14351	Beverage Mix, Strawberry Flavor, dry, prep w/milk	1 cup (8 fl oz)	266	234.08	7.98	32.718	0	0.303	5.081	31.92
14182	Beverage, Chocolate Syrup w/o added nutrients, prep w/milk	1 cup (8 fl oz)	282	253.8	8.657	36.04	0.846	0.485	4.74	25.38
14390	Beverage, Cocoa Mix w/aspartame, dry, low kcal, prep w/H$_2$O	1 packet dry mix with 6 fl oz water	192	55.68	2.419	10.445	0.96	0.013	0	0
14418	Beverage, Coffee Mix w/sugar (Cappuccino) dry, prep w/H$_2$O	6 fl oz H$_2$O & 2 rounded tsp mix	192	61.44	0.384	10.752	0	0.038	1.83	0
14419	Beverage, Coffee Mix w/sugar (French) dry, prep w/H$_2$O	6 fl oz H$_2$O & 2 rounded tsp mix	189	56.7	0.567	6.615	0	0.062	2.947	0
14420	Beverage, Coffee Mix w/sugar (Mocha) dry, prep w/H$_2$O	6 fl oz & 2 round tsp mix	188	50.76	0.564	8.46	0.188	0.034	1.609	0

EvaluEat Code	Food Name	Amt	Wt (g)	Ener (kcal)	Prot (g)	Carb (g)	Fiber (g)	Fat (g)	Sat (g)	Chol (g)
14232	Beverage, Coffee Mix, Kraft Intl Sugar Free Fat Free Low Calorie French Vanilla	1 NLEA Serving	7	25.41	0.217	5.32	0.343		0.056	0
14136	Beverage, Soft Drink, Ginger Ale	1 can or bottle (16 fl oz)	488	165.92	0	42.798	0	0	0	0
14145	Beverage, Soft Drink, Lemon-Lime	1 can or bottle (16 fl oz)	491	196.4	0	51.064	0	0	0	0
14153	Beverage, Soft Drink, Pepper type	1 can or bottle (16 fl oz)	491	201.31	0	51.064	0	0.491	0.344	0
14355	Beverage, Tea, Brewed	1 cup (8 fl oz)	237	2.37	0	0.711	0	0	0.005	0
14352	Beverage, Tea, brewed, prepared with tap water, decaffeinated	1 cup (8 fl oz)	237	2.37	0	0.711	0	0	0.005	0
14381	Beverage, Tea, Herbal (not chamomile) Brewed	1 cup (8 fl oz)	237	2.37	0	0.474	0	0	0.005	0
14553	Beverage, Wine, non-alcoholic	1 fl oz	29	1.74	0.145	0.319	0	0	0	0
9206	Fruit Juice, Orange, fresh	1 cup	248	111.6	1.736	25.792	0.496	0.099	0.06	0
9215	Fruit Juice, Orange, frozen concentrate, unsweetened, prep	1 cup	249	112.05	1.693	26.842	0.498	0.03	0.017	0
9016	Fruit Juice, Apple, canned or bottled, unsweetened w/o added Vit C	1 cup	248	116.56	0.149	28.966	0.248	0.082	0.002	0
9018	Fruit Juice, Apple, frozen concentrate, unsweetened w/o added Vit C, prep	1 cup	239	112.33	0.335	27.581	0.239	0.074	0.047	0
11886	Vegetable Juice, Tomato, canned w/o salt	1 cup	243	41.31	1.847	10.303	0.972	0.058	0.019	0

Fats/Sweets/Other

EvaluEat Code	Food Name	Amt	Wt (g)	Ener (kcal)	Prot (g)	Carb (g)	Fiber (g)	Fat (g)	Sat (g)	Chol (g)
16112	Bean Sauce, Fermented Soy Product, Miso	1 cup	275	566.5	32.478	76.89	14.85	9.427	2.414	0
16113	Bean Sauce, Fermented Soy Product, Natto	1 cup	175	371	31.01	25.13	9.45	10.868	2.784	0
16114	Bean Sauce, Fermented Soy Product, Tempeh	1 cup	166	320.38	30.776	15.587		6.353	3.685	0
16424	Bean Sauce, Soy & Wheat (Shoyu) low sodium	1 tbsp	18	9.54	0.931	1.532	0.144	0.006	0.002	0
16124	Bean Sauce, Soy (Tamari)	1 tsp	6	3.6	0.631	0.334	0.048	0.003	0.001	0
1001	Butter, Regular (with salt)	1 tbsp	14.2	101.814	0.121	0.009	0	11.518	5.799	30.53
1002	Butter, Whipped (with salt)	1 tbsp	9.4	67.398	0.08	0.006	0	7.624	4.746	20.586
18096	Cake, Chocolate w/chocolate icing, commercially prep	1 piece (1/8 of 18 oz cake)	64	234.88	2.624	34.944	1.792	10.496	3.053	26.88
18101	Cake, Chocolate, homemade, w/o icing	1 piece (1/12 of 9" dia)	95	340.1	5.035	50.73	1.52	14.345	5.158	55.1
18140	Cake, Yellow w/chocolate icing, commercially prep	1 piece (1/8 of 18 oz cake)	64	242.56	2.432	35.456	1.152	11.136	2.98	35.2
43031	Candies, chocolate covered, caramel with nuts	1 cup	186	874.2	17.67	112.846	7.998	39.06	8.662	0
43046	Candies, nougat	1 cup	186	740.28	6.194	171.845	6.138	3.106	3.101	0
19081	Candy, Chocolate, sweet	1 bar (1.45 oz)	41	207.05	1.599	24.436	2.255	14.022	8.233	0
19120	Candy, Milk Chocolate	1 bar 1.55 oz	44	235.4	3.366	26.136	1.496	13.05	6.271	10.12
19126	Candy, Peanuts, milk chocolate coated	10 pieces	40	207.6	5.24	19.76	1.88	13.4	5.84	3.6
19127	Candy, Raisins, milk chocolate coated	10 pieces	10	39	0.41	6.83	0.42	1.48	0.88	0.3
19434	Cheese puffs and twists, corn based, low fat	1 oz	28.35	122.472	2.41	20.511	3.033	3.43	0.595	0.284
14197	Cocoa Mix, Rich Chocolate Hot Cocoa Mix/Carnation	1 serving	28	112	1.296	24.237	0.672	1.109	0.291	1.68

EvaluEat Code	Food Name	Amt	Wt (g)	Ener (kcal)	Prot (g)	Carb (g)	Fiber (g)	Fat (g)	Sat (g)	Chol (g)
1105	Cocoa, Hot, homemade w/whole milk	1 cup	250	192.5	8.8	26.575	2.5	5.825	3.577	20
2046	Condiment, Mustard, prepared, yellow	1 tsp or 1 packet	5	3.3	0.198	0.389	0.16	0.155	0.008	0
11945	Condiment, Vege, Pickle Relish, Sweet	1 tbsp	15	19.5	0.056	5.258	0.165	0.071	0.008	0
11935	Condiment, Vege, Tomato Catsup	1 tbsp	15	14.25	0.271	3.582	0.195	0.089	0.012	0
18154	Cookie, Brownies, homemade	1 brownie (2" square)	24	111.84	1.488	12.048		6.984	1.757	17.52
18378	Cookie, Chocolate Chip, homemade w/butter	1 cookie, medium (2-1/4" dia)	16	78.08	0.912	9.312		4.544	2.251	11.2
18170	Cookie, Fig Bar	1 individual package (2 oz package containing 2 3" bars)	57	198.36	2.109	40.413	2.622	4.161	0.64	0
18184	Cookie, Oatmeal, homemade w/raisins	1 cookie (2-5/8" dia)	15	65.25	0.975	10.26		2.43	0.485	4.95
1054	Cream, Whipped Cream Topping, Pressurized	1 tbsp	3	7.71	0.096	0.375	0	0.667	0.415	2.28
18242	Croutons, Plain	.5 oz	14.2	57.794	1.69	10.437	0.724	0.937	0.214	0
4002	Fat, Animal, Lard, Pork	1 tbsp	12.8	115.456	0	0	0	12.8	5.018	12.16
18269	French Toast, homemade w/reduced fat (2%) milk	1 slice	65	148.85	5.005	16.25		7.02	1.77	75.4
19270	Ice Cream, Chocolate	.5 cup (4 fl oz)	66	142.56	2.508	18.612	0.792	7.26	4.488	22.44
19271	Ice Cream, Strawberry	.5 cup (4 fl oz)	66	126.72	2.112	18.216	0.594	5.544	3.425	19.14
19095	Ice Cream, Vanilla	1 tsp	4.7	33.793	0.042	0.042	0	3.783	0.705	0
4067	Margarine, Hard, Corn, Soybean-Hydrogenated & Cottonseed-Hydrogenated w/salt	1 tsp	4.7	33.793	0.042	0.042	0	3.783	0.705	0
4611	Margarine, regular, tub, composite, 80% fat, with salt	1 tbsp	12.8	91.648	0.102	0.077	0	10.291	1.66	0
4053	Oil, Vegetable/Salad/ Cooking, Olive	1 tbsp	13.5	119.34	0	0	0	13.5	1.816	0
4510	Oil, Vegetable/Salad/ Cooking, Safflower, linoleic >70%	1 tbsp	13.6	120.224	0	0	0	13.6	0.844	0
18239	Pastry, Croissant, Butter	1 croissant, mini	28	113.68	2.296	12.824	0.728	5.88	3.265	18.76
18245	Pastry, Danish, Cheese	1 pastry	71	265.54	5.68	26.412	0.71	15.549	4.824	11.36
11942	Pickles, cucumber, fresh, (bread and butter pickles)	1 slice	7	5.39	0.063	1.253	0.105	0.014	0.004	0
18301	Pie, Apple, enriched, commercially prep	1 piece (1/8 of 9" dia)	125	296.25	2.375	42.5	2	13.75	4.746	0
18305	Pie, Blueberry, commercially prep	1 piece (1/8 of 9" dia)	125	290	2.25	43.625	1.25	12.5	2.099	0
18308	Pie, Cherry, commercially prep	1 piece (1/8 of 9" dia)	125	325	2.5	49.75	1	13.75	3.203	0
18320	Pie, Lemon Meringue, commercially prep	1 piece (1/6 of 8" pie)	113	302.84	1.695	53.336	1.356	9.831	1.996	50.85
18324	Pie, Pecan, commercially prep	1 piece (1/6 of 8" pie)	113	452	4.52	64.636	3.955	20.905	4.006	36.16
18326	Pie, Pumpkin, commercially prep	1 piece (1/6 of 80 pie)	109	228.9	4.251	29.757	2.943	10.355	1.946	21.8
19823	Potato chips, without salt, reduced fat	1 cup	146	711.02	10.366	98.988	8.906	30.368	6.074	0
19183	Pudding, Chocolate, RTE	1 can (5 oz)	142	197.38	3.834	32.66	1.42	5.68	1.008	4.26
19193	Pudding, Rice, ready-to-eat	1 can (5 oz)	142	231.46	2.84	31.24	0.142	10.65	1.661	1.42
19218	Pudding, Tapioca, ready-to-eat	1 can (5 oz)	142	168.98	2.84	27.548	0.142	5.254	0.852	1.42

EvaluEat Code	Food Name	Amt	Wt (g)	Ener (kcal)	Prot (g)	Carb (g)	Fiber (g)	Fat (g)	Sat (g)	Chol (g)
19201	Pudding, Vanilla, ready-to-eat	4 oz	113	145.77	2.599	24.747	0	4.068	0.644	7.91
4017	Salad Dressing, 1000 Island, regular, w/salt	1 tbsp	16	59.2	0.174	2.342	0.128	5.61	0.815	4.16
4635	Salad dressing, 1000 Island dressing, fat-free	1 tbsp	14.6	19.272	0.08	4.273	0.482	0.212	0.029	0.73
4636	Salad dressing, Italian dressing, fat-free	1 tbsp	14.6	6.862	0.142	1.278	0.088	0.127	0.043	0.292
4114	Salad Dressing, Italian, regular w/salt	1 tbsp	14.7	42.777	0.056	1.533	0	4.17	0.658	0
4641	Salad dressing, mayonnaise, light	1 tbsp	14.6	47.304	0.128	1.197	0	4.831	0.761	5.11
4026	Salad Dressing, Mayonnaise, regular, Safflower/Soybean Oil, w/salt	1 tbsp	13.8	98.946	0.152	0.373	0	10.957	1.187	8.142
4012	Salad dressing, Miracle Whip Light Dressing/Kraft	1 tbsp	16	36.96	0.096	2.304	0.016	2.976	0.464	4.16
4638	Salad dressing, ranch dressing, fat-free	1 tbsp	14.6	17.374	0.036	3.87	0.015	0.28	0.075	1.022
4640	Salad dressing, ranch dressing, reduced fat	1 tbsp	14.6	32.85	0.15	2.365	0.131	2.526	0.194	3.066
4135	Salad Dressing, Vinegar & Oil, homemade	1 tbsp	16	71.84	0	0.4	0	8.016	1.456	0
6930	Sauce, cheese, ready-to-eat	.25 cup	63	109.62	4.227	4.303	0.315	8.373	3.786	18.27
6555	Sauce, hollandaise, with butterfat, dehydrated, prepared with water	1 cup (8 fl oz)	244	224.48	4.441	12.956	0.732	18.593	10.931	48.8
6931	Sauce, Pasta, Spaghetti/Marinara	1 cup	250	142.5	3.55	20.55	4	5.15	0.737	0
6164	Sauce, Salsa	1 cup	259	72.52	3.289	16.162	4.144	0.622	0.078	0
6112	Sauce, Teriyaki	1 tbsp	18	15.12	1.067	2.871	0.018	0	0	0
19097	Sherbet, Orange	.5 cup (4 fl oz)	74	106.56	0.814	22.496	2.442	1.48	0.858	0
4031	Shortening, Vegetable Fat, Soy-hydrogenated & Cottonseed-hydrogenated	1 tbsp	12.8	113.152	0	0	0	12.8	3.2	0
19002	Snack, Beef Jerky	1 piece, large	20	82	6.64	2.2	0.36	5.12	2.17	9.6
19003	Snack, Corn Chips, Plain	1 oz	28.35	152.807	1.871	16.131	1.389	9.469	1.29	0
19422	Snack, Potato Chips, light	1 oz	28.35	133.529	2.013	18.966	1.673	5.897	1.179	0
19411	Snack, Potato Chips, Plain, salted	1 oz	28.35	151.956	1.985	14.997	1.276	9.809	3.107	0
19047	Snack, Pretzel, Hard, Plain, salted	10 twists	60	228.6	5.46	47.52	1.92	2.1	0.45	0
19056	Snack, Tortilla Chips, Plain	1 oz	28.35	142.034	1.985	17.832	1.843	7.428	1.423	0
6008	Soup, Beef Broth or Bouillon, canned	1 cup	240	16.8	2.736	0.096	0	0.528	0.264	0
6070	Soup, Beef, chunky, canned	1 cup	240	170.4	11.736	19.56	1.44	5.136	2.544	14.4
6413	Soup, Chicken Broth, canned, made w/H$_2$O	1 cup	240	38.4	4.848	0.912	0	1.368	0.384	0
6018	Soup, Chicken Noodle, chunky, canned	1 cup	240	175.2	12.72	17.04	3.84	6	1.392	19.2
6468	Soup, Vegetarian Vegetable, canned, made w/H$_2$O	1 cup	241	72.3	2.097	11.978	0.482	1.928	0.289	0
6583	Soup, ramen noodle, any flavor, dehydrated, dry	1 container, individual	64	289.92	5.952	41.92	1.536	1.667	4.883	0
19173	Sweet, Gelatin, dry, prep w/H$_2$O	.5 cup	135	83.7	1.647	19.156	0	0	0	0
19296	Sweet, Honey, strained/extracted	1 tbsp	21	63.84	0.063	17.304	0.042	0	0	0
19283	Sweet, Ice Popsicle	1 bar (1.75 fl oz)	52	37.44	0	9.828	0	0	0	0

EvaluEat Code	Food Name	Amt	Wt (g)	Ener (kcal)	Prot (g)	Carb (g)	Fiber (g)	Fat (g)	Sat (g)	Chol (g)
19297	Sweet, Jams & Preserves	1 tbsp	20	55.6	0.074	13.772	0.22	0.014	0.002	0
19334	Sweet, Sugar, brown	1 tsp packed	4.6	17.342	0	4.477	0	0	0	0
19335	Sweet, Sugar, granulated, white	1 tsp	4.2	16.254	0	4.199	0	0	0	0
19129	Sweet, Syrup, pancake	1 tbsp	20	46.8	0	12.294	0.14	0	0	0
1073	Whipped Dessert Topping, Nondairy, semi solid, frozen	1 tbsp	4	12.72	0.05	0.922	0	1.012	0.871	0
42135	Whipped topping, frozen, low fat	1 ounce	28.34	62.348	0.85	6.688	0	3.713	3.195	0.567
2047	Salt, Table (Sodium Chloride)	1 tsp	6	0	0	0	0	0	0	0

Behavior Change Contract

Complete the Assess Yourself questionnaire, and read the Skills for Behavior Change box describing the stages of change. After reviewing your results and considering the various factors that influence your decisions, choose a health behavior that you would like to change, starting this quarter or semester (see other side for a sample filled-in contract). Sign the contract at the bottom to affirm your commitment to making a healthy change, and ask a friend to witness it.

My behavior change will be:

_____

My long-term goal for this behavior change is:

_____

These are three obstacles to change (things that I am currently doing or situations that contribute to this behavior or make it harder to change):

1. _____

2. _____

3. _____

The strategies I will use to overcome these obstacles are:

1. _____

2. _____

3. _____

Resources I will use to help me change this behavior include:

a friend/partner/relative: _____

a school-based resource: _____

a community-based resource: _____

a book or reputable website: _____

In order to make my goal more attainable, I have devised these short-term goals:

short-term goal	target date	reward
short-term goal	target date	reward
short-term goal	target date	reward

When I make the long-term behavior change described above, my reward will be:

_____ target date: _____

I intend to make the behavior change described above. I will use the strategies and rewards to achieve the goals that will contribute to a healthy behavior change.

Signed: _____   Witness: _____

Sample Behavior Change Contract

Complete the Assess Yourself questionnaire, and read the Skills for Behavior Change box describing the stages of change. After reviewing your results and considering the various factors that influence your decisions, choose a health behavior that you would like to change, starting this quarter or semester. Sign the contract at the bottom to affirm your commitment to making a healthy change, and ask a friend to witness it.

My behavior change will be:

To snack less on junk food and more on healthy foods

My long-term goal for this behavior change is:

Eat junk food snacks no more than once a week

These are three obstacles to change (things that I am currently doing or situations that contribute to this behavior or make it harder to change):

1. The grocery store is closed by the time I come home from school

2. I get hungry between classes, and the vending machines only carry candy bars

3. It's easier to order pizza or other snacks than to make a snack at home

The strategies I will use to overcome these obstacles are:

1. I'll leave early for school once a week so I can stock up on healthy snacks in the morning

2. I'll bring a piece of fruit or other healthy snack to eat between classes

3. I'll learn some easy recipes for snacks to make at home

Resources I will use to help me change this behavior include:

a friend/partner/relative: my roommates: I'll ask them to buy healthier snacks instead of chips when they do the shopping

a school-based resource: the dining hall: I'll ask the manager to provide healthy foods we can take to eat between classes

a community-based resource: the library: I'll check out some cookbooks to find easy snack ideas

a book or reputable website: the USDA nutrient database at www.nal.usda.gov/fnic: I'll use this site to make sure the foods I select are healthy choices

In order to make my goal more attainable, I have devised these short-term goals:

short-term goal	target date	reward
Eat a healthy snack 3 times per week	September 15	new CD
Learn to make a healthy snack	October 15	concert ticket
Eat a healthy snack 5 times per week	November 15	new shoes

When I make the long-term behavior change described above, my reward will be:

Ski lift tickets for winter break   target date: December 15

I intend to make the behavior change described above. I will use the strategies and rewards to achieve the goals that will contribute to a healthy behavior change.

Signed: Elizabeth King   Witness: Susan Bauer

GLOSSARY

Abortion The medical means of terminating a pregnancy.

Abstinence Refraining from an addictive behavior.

Accessory glands The seminal vesicles, prostate gland, and bulbourethral (Cowper's) glands.

Accountability Accepting responsibility for personal decisions, choices, and actions.

Acid deposition The acidification process that occurs when pollutants are deposited in precipitation, directly on the land, or by clouds.

Acquired immunodeficiency syndrome (AIDS) Extremely virulent sexually transmitted disease that renders the immune system inoperative.

Active euthanasia "Mercy killing," in which a person or organization knowingly acts to hasten the death of a terminally ill person.

Activities of daily living (ADLs) Performance of tasks of everyday living, such as bathing and walking up the stairs.

Acupressure Application of pressure to selected body points to balance energy.

Acupuncture The insertion of long, thin needles to affect the energy flow within the body.

Acute bronchitis A form of bronchitis most often caused by viruses.

Adaptive response Form of adjustment in which the body attempts to restore homeostasis.

Adaptive thermogenesis Theoretical mechanism by which the brain regulates metabolic activity according to caloric intake.

Addiction Continued involvement with a substance or activity despite ongoing negative consequences.

Addictive exercisers People who exercise compulsively to try to meet needs of nurturance, intimacy, self-esteem, and self-competency.

Adequate Intake (AI) Best estimates of nutritional needs.

Adjustment The attempt to cope with a given situation.

Adrenocorticotropic hormone (ACTH) A pituitary hormone that stimulates the adrenal glands to secrete cortisol.

Aerobic capacity The current functional status of a person's cardiovascular system; measured as VO_{2max}.

Aerobic exercise Any type of exercise that increases heart rate.

Afterbirth The expelled placenta.

Ageism Discrimination based on age.

Aggravated rape Rape that involves multiple attackers, strangers, weapons, or a physical beating.

Aggressive communicators People who use hostile, loud, and blaming communication styles.

Aging The patterns of life changes that occur in members of all species as they grow older.

Alcohol abuse Use of alcohol that interferes with work, school, or personal relationships or that entails violations of the law.

Alcoholic hepatitis Condition resulting from prolonged use of alcohol in which the liver is inflamed. It can result in death.

Alcoholics Anonymous (AA) An organization whose goal is to help alcoholics stop drinking; includes auxiliary branches such as Al-Anon and Alateen.

Alcoholism (alcohol dependency) Condition when personal and health problems related to alcohol use are severe and stopping alcohol use results in withdrawal symptoms.

Allergy Hypersensitive reaction to a specific antigen or allergen in the environment in which the body produces excessive antibodies to that antigen or allergen.

Allopathic medicine Traditional, Western medical practice; in theory, based on scientifically validated methods and procedures.

Alternative insemination Fertilization accomplished by depositing a partner's or a donor's semen into a woman's vagina via a thin tube; almost always done in a doctor's office.

Alternative medicine Treatment used in place of conventional medicine.

Alveoli Tiny air sacs of the lungs where gas exchange occurs (oxygen enters the body and carbon dioxide is removed).

Alzheimer's disease (AD) A chronic condition involving changes in nerve fibers of the brain that results in mental deterioration.

Amino acids The building blocks of protein.

Amniocentesis A medical test in which a small amount of fluid is drawn from the amniotic sac to test for Down's syndrome and other genetic diseases.

Amniotic sac The protective pouch surrounding the baby.

Amphetamines A large and varied group of synthetic agents that stimulate the central nervous system.

Amyl nitrite A drug that dilates blood vessels and is properly used to relieve chest pain.

Anabolic steroids Artificial forms of the hormone testosterone that promote muscle growth and strength.

Analgesics Pain relievers.

Anal intercourse The insertion of the penis into the anus.

Androgyny Combination of traditional masculine and feminine traits in a single person.

Anemia Iron-deficiency disease that results from the body's inability to produce hemoglobin.

Aneurysm A weakened blood vessel that may bulge under pressure and, in severe cases, burst.

Angina pectoris Chest pain occurring as a result of reduced oxygen flow to the heart.

Angiography A technique for examining blockages in heart arteries. A catheter is inserted into the arteries, a dye is injected, and an X ray is taken to find the blocked areas. Also called cardiac catheterization.

Angioplasty A technique in which a catheter with a balloon at the tip is inserted into a clogged artery; the balloon is inflated to flatten fatty deposits against artery walls, allowing blood to flow more freely.

Anorexia nervosa Eating disorder characterized by excessive preoccupation with food, self-starvation, and/or extreme exercising to achieve weight losses.

Antagonism A type of interaction in which two or more drugs work at the same receptor site.

Antibiotics Prescription drugs designed to fight bacterial infection.

Antibodies Substances produced by the body that are individually matched to specific antigens.

Antidepressants Prescription drugs used to treat clinically diagnosed depression.

Antigen Substance capable of triggering an immune response.

Antioxidants Substances believed to protect active people from oxidative stress and resultant tissue damage at the cellular level.

Anxiety disorders Disorders characterized by persistent feelings of threat and anxiousness in coping with everyday problems.

Appetite The desire to eat; normally accompanies hunger but is more psychological than physiological.

Arrhythmia An irregularity in heartbeat.

Arteries Vessels that carry blood away from the heart to other regions of the body.

Arterioles Branches of the arteries.

Arteriosclerosis A general term for thickening and hardening of the arteries.

Arthritis Painful inflammatory disease of the joints.

Asbestos A substance that separates into stringy fibers and lodges in the lungs, where it can cause various diseases.

Assertive communicators People who use direct, honest communication that maintains and defends their rights in a positive manner.

Asthma A chronic respiratory disease characterized by attacks of wheezing, shortness of breath, and coughing spasms.

Asymptomatic Without symptoms, or symptom-free.

Atherosclerosis Condition characterized by deposits of fatty substances, cholesterol, cellular waste products, calcium, and fibrin in the inner lining of an artery.

Atria The two upper chambers of the heart, which receive blood.

Attitude Relatively stable set of beliefs, feelings, and behavioral tendencies in relation to something or someone.

Autoerotic behaviors Sexual self-stimulation.

Autoinoculation Transmission of a pathogen from one part of the body to another.

Autonomic nervous system (ANS) The portion of the central nervous system that regulates bodily functions that a person does not normally consciously control.

Autonomy The ability to care for oneself emotionally, socially, and physically.

Ayurveda (Ayurvedic medicine) A method of treatment derived largely from ancient India, in which practitioners diagnose by observation and touch, and then assign a largely dietary treatment laced with herbal medicines.

Background distressors Environmental stressors of which people are often unaware.

Bacteria Single-celled organisms that may cause disease.

Barrier methods Contraceptive methods that block the meeting of egg and sperm by means of a physical barrier (such as condom, diaphragm, or cervical cap), a chemical barrier (such as spermicide), or both.

Basal metabolic rate (BMR) The energy expenditure of the body under resting conditions at normal room temperature.

Belief Appraisal of the relationship between some object, action, or idea and some attribute of that object, action, or idea.

Benign Harmless; refers to a noncancerous tumor.

Bereavement The loss or deprivation experienced by a survivor when a loved one dies.

Bidis Hand-rolled flavored cigarettes.

Binge drinking Drinking for the express purpose of becoming intoxicated; five drinks in a single sitting for men and four drinks in a sitting for women.

Binge eating disorder (BED) Eating disorder characterized by recurrent binge eating, without excessive measures to prevent weight gain.

Bioelectrical impedence analysis (BIA) A technique of body fat assessment in which electrical currents are passed though fat and lean tissue.

Biofeedback A technique involving using a machine to self-monitor physical responses to stress.

Biologically-based practices Treatments using substances found in nature, such as herbs, special diets, or vitamin megadoses.

Biopsy Microscopic examination of tissue to determine if a cancer is present.

Biopsychosocial model of addiction Theory of the relationship between an addict's biological (genetic) nature and psychological and environmental influences.

Bipolar disorder Form of depression characterized by alternating mania and depression.

Bisexual Experiencing attraction to and preference for sexual activity with people of both sexes.

Black tar heroin A dark brown, sticky form of heroin.

Blood alcohol concentration (BAC) The ratio of alcohol to total blood volume; the factor used to measure the physiological and behavioral effects of alcohol.

Body mass index (BMI) A technique of weight assessment based on the relationship of weight to height.

Body temperature method A birth control method in which a woman monitors her body temperature for the rise that signals ovulation in order to abstain from intercourse around this time.

Botulism A resistant foodborne organism that is extremely virulent.

Brain death   The irreversible cessation of all functions of the entire brainstem.

Bronchitis   An inflammation of the lining of the bronchial tubes.

Bulbourethral (Cowper's) glands   Glands that secrete a fluid that lubricates the urethra and neutralizes any acid remaining in the urethra after urination.

Bulimia nervosa   Eating disorder characterized by binge eating followed by inappropriate measures to prevent weight gain.

Burnout   Physical and mental exhaustion caused by excessive stress.

Caffeine   A stimulant found in coffee, tea, chocolate, and some soft drinks.

Caffeinism   Caffeine intoxication brought on by excessive use; symptoms include chronic insomnia, irritability, anxiety, muscle twitches, and headaches.

Calendar method   A birth control method in which a woman's menstrual cycle is mapped on a calendar to determine presumed fertile times in order to abstain from penis-vagina contact during those times.

Calorie   A unit of measure that indicates the amount of energy obtained from a particular food.

Cancer   A large group of diseases characterized by the uncontrolled growth and spread of abnormal cells.

Candidiasis (yeast infection, moniliasis)   Yeastlike fungal disease often transmitted sexually.

Capillaries   Minute blood vessels that branch out from the arterioles; their thin walls allow for the exchange of oxygen, carbon dioxide, nutrients, and waste products among body cells.

Capitation   Prepayment of a fixed monthly amount for each patient without regard to the type or number of services provided.

Carbohydrates   Basic nutrients that supply the body with glucose, the energy form most commonly used to sustain normal activity.

Carbon monoxide   A gas found in cigarette smoke that binds at oxygen receptor sites in the blood and motor vehicle emissions.

Carcinogens   Cancer-causing agents.

Cardiorespiratory fitness   The ability of the heart, lungs, and blood vessels to supply oxygen to skeletal muscles during sustained physical activity.

Cardiovascular disease (CVD)   Disease of the heart and blood vessels.

Cardiovascular system   A complex system consisting of the heart and blood vessels that transports nutrients, oxygen, hormones, metabolic wastes, and enzymes throughout the body and regulates temperature, the water levels of cells, and the acidity levels of body components.

Carotenoids   Fat-soluble compounds with antioxidant properties.

Carpal tunnel syndrome   A common occupational injury in which the median nerve in the wrist becomes irritated, causing numbness, tingling, and pain in the fingers and hands.

Cataracts   Clouding of the lens that interrupts the focusing of light on the retina, resulting in blurred vision or eventual blindness.

Celibacy   State of not being involved in a sexual relationship.

Cellulose   Fiber; a major form of complex carbohydrates.

Cerebral cortex   The region of the brain that interprets the nature of an event.

Cerebrospinal fluid   Fluid within and surrounding the brain and spinal cord tissues.

Certified Health Education Specialists (CHES)   Academically trained health educators who have passed a national competency examination for prevention and intervention programming.

Cervical cap   A small cup made of latex that is designed to fit snugly over the entire cervix.

Cervical mucus method   A birth control method that relies upon observation of changes in cervical mucus to determine when the woman is fertile so the couple can abstain from intercourse during those times.

Cervix   Lower end of the uterus that opens into the vagina.

Cesarean section (C-section)   A surgical procedure in which a baby is removed through an incision made in the mother's abdominal and uterine walls.

Chancre   Sore often found at the site of syphilis infection.

Chemotherapy   The use of drugs to kill cancerous cells.

Chewing tobacco   A stringy type of tobacco that is placed in the mouth and then sucked or chewed.

Child abuse   The systematic harming of a child by a caregiver, typically a parent.

Chiropractic medicine   Manipulation of the spine to allow proper energy flow.

Chlamydia   Bacterially caused STI of the urogenital tract.

Chlorofluorocarbons (CFCs)   Chemicals that contribute to the depletion of the ozone layer.

Cholesterol   A form of fat circulating in the blood that can accumulate on the inner walls of arteries.

Chronic bronchitis   A serious respiratory disorder in which the bronchial tubes become so inflamed and swollen that respiratory function is impaired.

Chronic fatigue syndrome (CFS)   A condition of unknown cause characterized by extreme fatigue that is not caused by other illness.

Chronic mood disorder   Experience of persistent sadness, despair, and hopelessness.

Chronic obstructive pulmonary diseases (COPDs)   A collection of chronic lung diseases including asthma, emphysema, and chronic bronchitis.

Cirrhosis   The last stage of liver disease associated with chronic heavy use of alcohol during which liver cells die and damage becomes permanent.

Clitoris   A pea-sized nodule of tissue located at the top of the labia minora.

Cocaine   A powerful stimulant drug made from the leaves of the South American coca shrub.

Codeine   A drug derived from morphine; used in cough syrups and certain painkillers.

Codependence   A self-defeating relationship pattern in which a person is "addicted to the addict."

Cognitive stress system   The psychological system that recognizes stressors and processes emotional responses to stress.

Cohabitation   Living together without being married.

Collateral circulation   Adaptation of the heart to partial damage accomplished by rerouting needed blood through unused or underused blood vessels while the damaged heart muscle heals.

Commercial preparations Commonly used chemical substances including cosmetics, household cleaning products, and industrial by-products.

Common-law marriage Cohabitation lasting a designated period of time (usually seven years) that is considered legally binding in some states.

Communication The transmission of information and meaning from one individual to another.

Comorbidity The presence of a number of diseases at the same time.

Complementary and alternative medicine (CAM) Forms of treatment distinct from traditional allopathic medicine that until recently were neither taught widely in U.S. medical schools nor generally available in U.S. hospitals.

Complementary medicine Treatment used in conjunction with conventional medicine.

Complete (high-quality) proteins Proteins that contain all of the nine essential amino acids.

Complex carbohydrates A major type of carbohydrate, which provides sustained energy.

Compulsion Obsessive preoccupation with a behavior and an overwhelming need to perform it.

Compulsive gambler A person addicted to gambling.

Computed tomography (CT) Use of X-ray for a cross section of the body, which can reveal intraabdominal fat.

Computerized axial tomography (CAT scan) A machine that uses radiation to view internal organs not normally visible in X rays.

Concentric muscle action Force produced while the muscle is shortening.

Conception The fertilization of an ovum by a sperm.

Conflict An emotional state that arises when the behavior of one person interferes with the behavior of another.

Conflict resolution A concerted effort by all parties to resolve points in contention in a constructive manner.

Congeners Forms of alcohol that are metabolized more slowly than ethanol and produce toxic by-products.

Congenital heart disease Heart disease that is present at birth.

Congestive heart failure (CHF) An abnormal cardiovascular condition that reflects impaired cardiac pumping and blood flow; pooling blood leads to congestion in body tissues.

Conjunctivitis Serious inflammation of the eye caused by any number of pathogens or irritants; can be caused by STIs such as chlamydia.

Contraception (birth control) Methods of preventing conception.

Coronary bypass surgery A surgical technique whereby a blood vessel is implanted to bypass a clogged coronary artery.

Coronary thrombosis A blood clot occurring in the coronary artery.

Cortisol Hormone released by the adrenal glands that makes stored nutrients more readily available to meet energy demands.

Counselor A person with a variety of academic and experiential training who deals with the treatment of emotional problems.

Crack A distillate of powdered cocaine that comes in small, hard "chips" or "rocks"; not the same as rock cocaine.

Cross-tolerance The development of a tolerance to one drug that reduces the effects of another, similar drug.

Cunnilingus Oral stimulation of a female's genitals.

Daily Reference Values (DRVs) Recommended amounts for micronutrients such as total fat, saturated fat, and cholesterol.

Daily Values (DVs) The RDIs and DRVs together make up the Daily Values seen on food and supplement labels.

Death The permanent ending of all vital functions.

Dehydration Loss of fluids from body tissues.

Delirium tremens (DTs) A state of confusion brought on by withdrawal from alcohol. Symptoms include hallucinations, anxiety, and trembling.

Dementias Progressive brain impairments that interfere with memory and normal intellectual functioning.

Dengue A disease transmitted by mosquitoes; causes flulike symptoms.

Dengue hemorrhagic fever A more serious form of dengue.

Denial Inability to perceive or accurately interpret the effects of the addictive behavior.

Dentist Specialist who diagnoses and treats diseases of the teeth, gums, and oral cavity.

Depo-Provera An injectable method of birth control that lasts for three months.

Designer drug or **club drug** A synthetic analog (a drug that produces similar effects) of an existing illicit drug.

Detoxification The early abstinence period during which an addict adjusts physically and cognitively to being free from the influences of the addiction.

Diabetes mellitus A disease in which the pancreas fails to produce enough insulin or the body fails to use insulin effectively.

Diagnosis-related groups (DRGs) Diagnostic categories established by the federal government to determine in advance how much hospitals will be reimbursed for the care of a particular Medicare patient.

Diaphragm A latex, cup-shaped device designed to cover the cervix and block access to the uterus; should always be used with spermicide.

Diastolic pressure The lower number in the fraction that measures blood pressure, indicating pressure on the walls of the arteries during the relaxation phase of heart activity.

Dietary Reference Intake (DRI) A new, combined listing of over 26 essential vitamins and minerals developed by Canadian and U.S. researchers.

Digestive process The process by which foods are broken down and either absorbed or excreted by the body.

Dilation and curettage (D&C) An abortion technique in which the cervix is dilated and the uterine walls scraped clean.

Dilation and evacuation (D&E) An abortion technique that combines vacuum aspiration with dilation and curettage; fetal tissue is both sucked and scraped out of the uterus.

Dioxins Highly toxic chlorinated hydrocarbons contained in herbicides and produced during certain industrial processes.

Dipping Placing a small amount of chewing tobacco between the lower lip and front teeth for rapid nicotine absorption.

Disaccharide A combination of two monosaccharides.

Discrimination Actions that deny equal treatment or opportunities to a group, often based on prejudice.

Disease prevention Actions or behaviors designed to keep people from getting sick.

Disenfranchised grief Grief concerning a loss that cannot be openly acknowledged, publicly mourned, or socially supported.

Distillation The process whereby mash is subjected to high temperatures to release alcohol vapors, which are then condensed and mixed with water to make the final product.

Distress Stress that can have a negative effect on health.

Diuretics Drugs that increase the excretion of urine from the body.

Diverticulosis A condition in which bulges form in the walls of the intestine; results in irritation and infection of the intestine.

Documenting Giving specific examples of issues being discussed.

Domestic violence The use of force to control and maintain power over another person in the home environment, including both actual and the threat of harm.

Down syndrome A condition characterized by mental retardation and a variety of physical abnormalities.

Downshifting Conscious attempt to simplify life in an effort to reduce the stresses and strains of modern living.

Drug abuse The excessive use of a drug.

Drug misuse The use of a drug for a purpose for which it was not intended.

Dual energy X-ray absorptiometry (DEXA) Technique using low-dose X rays that read bone and soft tissue mass at the same time.

Ductus (vas) deferens A tube that transports sperm toward the penis.

Dying The process of decline in body functions, resulting in the death of an organism.

Dysfunctional family A family in which the interaction between family members inhibits rather than enhances psychological growth.

Dysmenorrhea Condition that causes pain or discomfort in the lower abdomen just before or after menstruation.

Dyspareunia Pain experienced by women during intercourse.

Dyspnea Shortness of breath, usually associated with disease of the heart or lungs.

Eccentric muscle action Force produced while the muscle is lengthening.

Eclampsia Untreated preeclampsia can develop into this potentially fatal complication that involves maternal strokes and seizures.

Ecological or **Public Health Model** A model in which diseases and other negative health events are viewed as a result of an individual's interaction with his/her social and physical environment.

Ecstasy A club drug that creates feelings of openness and warmth but also raises heart rate and blood pressure.

Ectopic pregnancy Implantation of a fertilized egg outside the uterus, usually in a uterine tube; a medical emergency that can end in death from hemorrhage for the mother.

Editing The process of censoring comments that would be intentionally hurtful or irrelevant to the conversation.

Ejaculation The propulsion of semen from the penis.

Electrocardiogram (ECG) A record of the electrical activity of the heart; may be measured during a stress test.

ELISA Blood test that detects presence of antibodies to the HIV virus.

Embolus A blood clot that becomes dislodged from a blood vessel wall and moves through the circulatory system.

Embryo The fertilized egg from conception until the end of two months' development.

Embryo adoption programs A procedure whereby an infertile couple is able to purchase frozen embryos donated by another couple.

Embryo freezing The freezing of an embryo for later implantation.

Embryo transfer Artificial insemination of a donor with the male partner's sperm; after a time, the embryo is transferred from the donor to the female partner's body.

Emergency contraceptive pills (ECPs) Drugs taken within three days after intercourse to prevent fertilization or implantation.

Emergency minipills Contraceptive pills containing only progestin that can be taken up to three days after unprotected intercourse.

Emotional health The feeling part of psychosocial health, includes your emotional reactions to life.

Emotions Intensified feelings or complex patterns of feelings we constantly experience.

Emphysema A chronic lung disease in which the tiny air sacs in the lungs are destroyed, making breathing difficult.

Enablers People who knowingly or unknowingly protect addicts from the natural consequences of their behavior.

Endemic Describing a disease that is always present to some degree.

Endometriosis A disorder in which uterine lining tissue establishes itself outside the uterus; the leading cause of infertility in the United States.

Endometrium Soft, spongy matter that makes up the uterine lining.

Endorphins Opiate-like hormones that are manufactured in the human body and contribute to natural feelings of well-being.

Energy medicine Therapies using energy fields, such as magnetic fields or biofields.

Environmental tobacco smoke (ETS) Smoke from tobacco products, including secondhand and mainstream smoke.

Enzymes Organic substances that facilitate chemical reactions, some of which cause bodily changes and destruction of microorganisms.

Epidemic Disease outbreak that affects many people in a community or region at the same time.

Epidermis The outermost layer of the skin.

Epididymis A comma-shaped structure atop the testis where sperm mature.

Epilepsy A neurological disorder caused by abnormal electrical brain activity; can be accompanied by altered consciousness or convulsions.

Epinephrine Also called adrenaline, a hormone that stimulates body systems in response to stress.

Episiotomy A straight incision in the mother's perineum in the area between the vulva and the anus.

Erectile dysfunction (impotence) Difficulty in achieving or maintaining a penile erection sufficient for intercourse.

Ergogenic aids Special dietary supplements taken to increase strength, energy, and the ability to work.

Ergogenic drug Substance that enhances athletic performance.

Erogenous zones   Areas of the body of both males and females that, when touched, lead to sexual arousal.

Esophagus   Tube that transports food from the mouth to the stomach.

Essential amino acids   Nine of the basic nitrogen-containing building blocks of protein that must be obtained from foods to ensure health.

Essential hypertension   Hypertension that cannot be attributed to any known cause.

Estrogens   Hormones secreted by ovaries; control the menstrual cycle.

Ethnoviolence   Violence directed randomly at persons affiliated with a particular, usually ethnic, group.

Ethyl alcohol (ethanol)   An addictive drug produced by fermentation and found in many beverages.

Eustress   Stress that presents opportunities for personal growth.

Exercise   Planned, structured, and repetitive bodily movement done to improve or maintain one or more components of physical fitness.

Exercise metabolic rate (EMR)   The energy expenditure that occurs during exercise.

External female genitals   The mons pubis, labia majora and minora, clitoris, urethral and vaginal openings, and the vestibule of the vagina and its glands.

External male genitals   The penis and scrotum.

Faith   Belief that helps each person realize a unique purpose in life.

Family of origin   People present in the household during a child's first years of life-usually parents and siblings.

Fats   Basic nutrients composed of carbon and hydrogen atoms; needed for the proper functioning of cells, insulation of body organs against shock, maintenance of body temperature, and healthy skin and hair.

Fellatio   Oral stimulation of a male's genitals.

Female condom   A single-use polyurethane sheath for internal use by women.

Female orgasmic disorder   The inability to achieve orgasm.

Fermentation   The process whereby yeast organisms break down plant sugars to yield ethanol.

Fertility   A person's ability to reproduce.

Fertility awareness methods (FAMs)   Several types of birth control that require alteration of sexual behavior rather than chemical or physical intervention into the reproductive process.

Fertility drugs   Hormones that stimulate ovulation in women who are not ovulating; often responsible for multiple births.

Fetal alcohol effects (FAE)   A syndrome describing children with a history of prenatal alcohol exposure but without all the physical or behavioral symptoms of FAS. Among its symptoms are low birthweight, irritability, and possible permanent mental impairment.

Fetal alcohol syndrome (FAS)   A disorder that may affect the fetus when the mother consumes alcohol during pregnancy. Among its effects are mental retardation, small head, tremors, and abnormalities of the face, limbs, heart, and brain.

Fetus   The name given the developing baby from the third month of pregnancy until birth.

Fiber   The indigestible portion of plant foods that helps move foods through the digestive system and softens stools by absorbing water.

Fibrillation   A sporadic, quivering pattern of heartbeat resulting in extreme inefficiency in moving blood through the cardiovascular system.

Fibrocystic breast condition   A common, noncancerous condition in which a woman's breasts contain fibrous or fluid-filled cysts.

Fibromyalgia   A chronic, rheumatoid-like disorder that can be highly painful and difficult to diagnose.

Fight-or-flight response   Physiological arousal response in which the body prepares to combat a real or perceived threat.

Flexibility   The measure of the range of motion, or the amount of movement possible, at a particular joint.

Folate   A type of vitamin B that is believed to decrease levels of homocysteine, an amino acid that has been linked to vascular diseases.

Follicle-stimulating hormone (FSH)   Hormone that signals the ovaries to prepare to release eggs and to begin producing estrogens.

Food allergies   Overreaction by the body to normally harmless proteins, which are perceived as allergens. In response, the body produces antibodies, triggering allergic symptoms.

Food intolerance   Adverse effects resulting when people who lack the digestive chemicals needed to break down certain substances eat those substances.

Food irradiation   Treating foods with gamma radiation from radioactive cobalt, cesium, or some other source of X rays to kill microorganisms.

Formaldehyde   A colorless, strong-smelling gas released through outgassing; causes respiratory and other health problems.

For-profit (proprietary) hospitals   Hospitals that provide a return on earnings to the investors who own them.

Fourth trimester   The first six weeks of an infant's life outside the womb.

Freebase   The most powerful distillate of cocaine.

Functional foods   Foods believed to be beneficial and/or to prevent disease.

Fungi   A group of plants that lack chlorophyll and do not produce flowers or seeds; several microscopic varieties are pathogenic.

Gallbladder disease   A disease caused by repeated irritation of the gallbladder, which leads to the formation of gallstones.

Gamete intrafallopian transfer (GIFT)   Procedure in which an egg harvested from the female partner's ovary is placed with the male partner's sperm in her uterine tube, where it is fertilized and then migrates to the uterus for implantation.

Gay   Sexual orientation involving primary attraction to people of the same sex; usually but not always applies to men attracted to men.

Gender   The psychological condition of being feminine or masculine as defined by the society in which one lives.

Gender identity   Personal sense or awareness of being masculine or feminine, a male or a female.

Genderlect   The "dialect," or individual speech pattern and conversational style, of each gender.

Gender roles   Expression of maleness or femaleness in everyday life.

Gender-role stereotypes   Generalizations concerning how males and females should express themselves and the characteristics each possesses.

General adaptation syndrome (GAS) The pattern followed in the physiological response to stress, consisting of the alarm, resistance, and exhaustion phases.

Generalized anxiety disorder (GAD) A constant sense of worry that may cause restlessness, difficulty in concentrating, tension, and other symptoms.

Generic drugs Drugs marketed by chemical name rather than brand name.

Genital herpes STI caused by the herpes simplex virus.

Genital warts Warts that appear in the genital area or the anus; caused by the human papilloma viruses (HPVs).

Gerontology The study of individual and collective aging processes.

Glaucoma Elevation of pressure within the eyeball, leading to hardening of the eyeball, impaired vision, and possible blindness.

Glycogen The polysaccharide form in which glucose is stored in the liver and, to a lesser extent, in muscles.

Gonadotropin-releasing hormone (GnRH) Hormone that signals the pituitary gland to release gonadotropins.

Gonads The reproductive organs in a male (testes) or female (ovaries).

Gonorrhea Second most common STI in the United States; if untreated, may cause sterility.

Graded exercise test A test of aerobic capacity administered by a physician, exercise physiologist, or other trained person; two common forms are the treadmill running test and the stationary bike test.

GRAE list A list of drugs generally recognized as effective, which work for their intended purpose when used properly.

GRAS list A list of drugs generally recognized as safe, which seldom cause side effects when used properly.

Greenhouse gases Gases that contribute to global warming by trapping heat near the Earth's surface.

Grief The state of mental distress that occurs in reaction to significant loss, including one's own impending death, the death of a loved one, or a quasi-death experience.

Grief work The process of accepting the reality of a person's death and coping with memories of the deceased.

Group practice A group of physicians who combine resources, sharing offices, equipment, and staff costs, to render care to patients.

Habit A repeated behavior in which the repetition may be unconscious.

Hallucinogens Substances capable of creating auditory or visual distortions and heightened states.

Hangover The physiological reaction to excessive drinking, including symptoms such as headache, upset stomach, anxiety, depression, diarrhea, and thirst.

Hashish The sticky resin of the Cannabis plant, which is high in THC.

Hay fever A chronic respiratory disorder that is most prevalent when ragweed and flowers bloom.

Hazardous waste Solid waste that, due to its toxic properties, poses a hazard to humans or to the environment.

Health The ever-changing process of achieving individual potential in the physical, social, emotional, mental, sprectual, and environmental dimensions.

Health Belief Model (HBM) Model for explaining how beliefs may influence behaviors.

Health disparities Differences in the incidence, prevalence, mortality, and burden of diseases and other health conditions among specific population groups.

Health promotion Combined educational, organizational, policy, financial, and environmental supports to help people reduce negative health behaviors and promote positive change.

Heart attack A blockage of normal blood supply to an area in the heart.

Heat cramps Muscle cramps that occur during or following exercise in warm or hot weather.

Heat exhaustion A heat stress illness caused by significant dehydration resulting from exercise in warm or hot conditions; frequent precursor to heat stroke.

Heat stroke A deadly heat stress illness resulting from dehydration and overexertion in warm or hot conditions; can cause body core temperature to rise from normal to 105°F to 110°F in just a few minutes.

Hemochromatosis Iron toxicity due to excess consumption.

Hepatitis A virally caused disease in which the liver becomes inflamed, producing symptoms such as fever, headache, and possibly jaundice.

Herbal preparations Substances of plant origin that are believed to have medicinal properties.

Heroin An illegally manufactured derivative of morphine, usually injected into the bloodstream.

Heterosexual Experiencing primary attraction to and preference for sexual activity with people of the other sex.

High-density lipoproteins (HDLs) Compounds that facilitate the transport of cholesterol in the blood to the liver for metabolism and elimination from the body.

Histamines Chemical substances that dilate blood vessels, increase mucous secretions, and produce other symptoms of allergies.

Holographic will A will written in the testator's own handwriting and unwitnessed.

Homeopathic medicine Unconventional Western system of medicine based on the principle that "like cures like."

Homeostasis A balanced physical state in which all the body's systems function smoothly.

Homicide Death that results from intent to injure or kill.

Homophobia Irrational hatred or fear of homosexuals or homosexuality.

Homosexual Experiencing primary attraction to and preference for sexual activity with people of the same sex.

Hope Belief that allows us to look confidently and courageously to the future.

Hormone replacement therapies (HRTs) Therapies that replace estrogen in postmenopausal women.

Hospice A concept of care for terminally ill patients designed to maximize quality of life.

Hostility The cognitive, affective, and behavioral tendencies toward anger and cynicism.

Human chorionic gonadotropin (HCG) Hormone detectable in blood or urine samples of a mother within the first few weeks of pregnancy.

Human immunodeficiency virus (HIV) The slow-acting virus that causes AIDS.

Human papilloma viruses (HPVs) A small group of viruses that cause genital warts.

Hunger An inborn physiological response to nutritional needs.

Hydrocarbons Chemical compounds that contain carbon and hydrogen.

Hydrodensitometry weighing (underwater weighing) Method of determining body fat by measuring the amount of water displaced when a person is completely submerged.

Hymen Thin tissue covering the vaginal opening in some women.

Hyperglycemia Elevated blood sugar levels.

Hyperlipidemia Elevated levels of lipids in the blood.

Hyperplasia A condition characterized by an excessive number of cells.

Hypertension Sustained elevated blood pressure.

Hypertrophy The ability of cells to swell.

Hypervitaminosis A toxic condition caused by overuse of vitamin supplements.

Hypnosis A process that allows people to become unusually responsive to suggestion.

Hypothalamus A section of the brain that controls the sympathetic nervous system and directs the stress response.

Hypothermia Potentially fatal condition caused by abnormally low body core temperature.

Hysterectomy Surgical removal of the uterus.

Ice A potent, inexpensive methamphetamine that has long-lasting effects.

Idiopathic Of unknown cause.

Illicit (illegal) drugs Drugs whose use, possession, cultivation, manufacture, and/or sale are against the law because they are generally recognized as harmful.

Imagined rehearsal Practicing, through mental imagery, to become better able to perform an event in actuality.

"I" messages Messages in which a person takes responsibility for communicating his or her own feelings, thoughts, and beliefs by using statements that begin with "I," not "you."

Immunocompetence The ability of the immune system to respond to assaults.

Immunological competence Ability of the immune system to defend the body from pathogens.

Immunotherapy A process that stimulates the body's own immune system to combat cancer cells.

In vitro fertilization Fertilization of an egg in a nutrient medium and subsequent transfer back to the mother's body.

Incidence The number of new cases.

Incomplete proteins Proteins that are lacking in one or more of the essential amino acids.

Incubation period The time between exposure to a disease and the appearance of the symptoms.

Induction abortion A type of abortion in which chemicals are injected into the uterus through the uterine wall; labor begins, and the woman delivers a dead fetus.

Infertility Difficulties in conceiving.

Influenza A common viral disease of the respiratory tract.

Inhalants Products that are sniffed or inhaled in order to produce highs.

Inhalation The introduction of drugs through the nostrils.

Inhibited sexual desire (ISD) Lack of sexual appetite or simply a lack of interest and pleasure in sexual activity.

Inhibition A type of interaction in which the effects of one drug are eliminated or reduced by the presence of another drug at the receptor site.

Injection The introduction of drugs into the body via a hypodermic needle.

Insomnia Difficulty in falling asleep or staying asleep.

Insulin A hormone produced by the pancreas; required by the body for the metabolism of carbohydrates.

Intact dilation and extraction (D&X) A late-term abortion procedure in which the body of the fetus is extracted up to the head and then the contents of the cranium are aspirated.

Intentional injuries Injuries committed on purpose with intent to harm.

Interconnectedness A web of connections, including our relationship to ourselves, to others, and to a larger meaning or purpose in life.

Interferon A protein substance produced by the body that aids the immune system by protecting healthy cells.

Internal female genitals The vagina, uterus, uterine (fallopian) tubes, and ovaries.

Internal male genitals The testes, epididymides, vasa deferentia, ejaculatory ducts, urethra, and accessory glands.

Internet addiction Compulsive use of computer activities such as fantasy games, online shopping, and chat rooms.

Intersexuality Not exhibiting exclusively female or male primary and secondary sex characteristics.

Interspecies transmission Transmission of disease from humans to animals or from animals to humans.

Intervention A planned process of confronting an addict; carried out by significant others.

Intestate Not having made a will.

Intimate relationships Relationships with family members, friends, and romantic partners, characterized by closeness and understanding.

Intolerance A type of interaction in which two or more drugs produce extremely uncomfortable symptoms.

Intracytoplasmic sperm injection (ICSI) Fertilization accomplished by injecting a sperm cell directly into an egg.

Intramuscular injection The introduction of drugs into muscles.

Intrauterine device (IUD) A T-shaped device that is implanted in the uterus to prevent pregnancy.

Intravenous injection The introduction of drugs directly into a vein.

Inunction The introduction of drugs through the skin.

Ionizing radiation Radiation produced by photons having high enough energy to ionize atoms

Irritable bowel syndrome (IBS) Nausea, pain, gas, or diarrhea caused by certain foods or stress.

Ischemia Reduced oxygen supply to a body organ or part.

Isometric muscle action Force produced without any resulting joint movement.

Jealousy   An aversive reaction evoked by a real or imagined relationship involving a person's partner and a third person.

Ketosis   A condition in which the body adapts to prolonged fasting or carbohydrate deprivation by converting body fat to ketones, which can be used as fuel for some brain activity.

Labia majora   "Outer lips," or folds of tissue covering the female sexual organs.

Labia minora   "Inner lips," or folds of tissue just inside the labia majora.

Lactose intolerance   The inability to produce lactase, an enzyme needed to convert milk sugar into glucose.

Laxatives   Medications used to soften stool and relieve constipation.

Leach   To dissolve and filter through soil.

Leachate   A liquid consisting of soluble chemicals that come from garbage and industrial waste that seeps into the water supply from landfills and dumps.

Lead   A metal found in the exhaust of motor vehicles powered by fuel containing lead and in emissions from lead smelters and processing plants.

Learned behavioral tolerance   The ability of heavy drinkers to modify behavior so that they appear to be sober even when they have high BAC levels.

Learned helplessness   Pattern of responding to situations by giving up because of repeated failure in the past.

Learned optimism   Teaching oneself to think optimistically.

Lesbian   Sexual orientation involving primary attraction of women to other women.

Leukoplakia   A condition characterized by leathery white patches inside the mouth; produced by contact with irritants in tobacco juice.

Leveling   The communication of a clear, simple, and honest message.

Loss of control   Inability to predict reliably whether a particular instance of involvement with the addictive object or behavior will be healthy or damaging.

Love   Acceptance, affirmation, and respect for the self and others.

Low sperm count   A sperm count below 60 million sperm per milliliter of semen; the leading cause of infertility in men.

Low-density lipoproteins (LDLs)   Compounds that facilitate the transport of cholesterol in the blood to the body's cells.

Luteinizing hormone (LH)   Hormone that signals the ovaries to release an egg and to begin producing progesterone.

Lysergic acid diethylamide (LSD)   Psychedelic drug causing sensory disruptions; also called acid.

Macrominerals   Minerals that the body needs in fairly large amounts.

Macular degeneration   Disease that breaks down the macula, the light-sensitive part of the retina responsible for sharp, direct vision.

Magnetic resonance imaging (MRI)   A device that uses magnetic fields, radio waves, and computers to generate an image of internal tissues of the body for diagnostic purposes without the use of radiation.

Mainstream smoke   Smoke that is drawn through tobacco while inhaling.

Major depressive disorder   Severe depression that entails chronic mood disorder, physical effects such as sleep disturbance and exhaustion, and mental effects such as the inability to concentrate.

Male condom   A single-use sheath of thin latex or other material designed to fit over an erect penis and to catch semen upon ejaculation.

Malignant   Very dangerous or harmful; refers to a cancerous tumor.

Malignant melanoma   A virulent cancer of the melanocytes (pigment-producing cells) of the skin.

Managed care   Cost-control procedures used by health insurers to coordinate treatment.

Manipulative and body-based practices   Treatments involving manipulation or movement of one or more body parts.

Marijuana   Chopped leaves and flowers of the Cannabis indica or Cannabis sativa plants (hemp); a psychoactive stimulant that intensifies reactions to environmental stimuli.

Masturbation   Self-stimulation of genitals.

Measles   A viral disease that produces symptoms including an itchy rash and a high fever.

Medicaid   Federal-state health insurance program for the poor.

Medical Model   A model in which health status was focused primarily on the induvidual and a biological or diseased organ perspecive.

Medicare   Federal health insurance program for the elderly and the permanently disabled.

Meditation   A relaxation technique that involves deep breathing and concentration.

Meltdown   An accident that results when the temperature in the core of a nuclear reactor increases enough to melt the nuclear fuel and the containment vessel housing it.

Menarche   The first menstrual period.

Menopausal hormone therapy   Use of synthetic or animal estrogens and progesterone to compensate for decreases in estrogens in a woman's body.

Menopause   The permanent cessation of menstruation, generally between the ages of 40 and 60.

Mental health   The thinking part of psychosocial health; includes your values, attitudes, and beliefs.

Mental illnesses   Disorders that disrupt thinking, feeling, moods, and behaviors, and impair daily functioning.

Mescaline   A hallucinogenic drug derived from the peyote cactus.

Metabolic syndrome   A group of three or more characteristics, including waist circumference and blood pressure, that can cause metabolic problems that raise CVD risk.

Metastasis   Process by which cancer spreads from one area to different areas of the body.

Methadone maintenance   A treatment for people addicted to opiates that substitutes methadone, a synthetic narcotic, for the opiate of addiction.

Methamphetamine   A powerfully addictive drug that strongly activates certain areas of the brain and affects the central nervous system.

Middle-old   People aged 75 to 84.

Midwives   Experienced practitioners who assist with pregnancy and delivery.

Mifepristone   A steroid hormone that induces abortion by blocking the action of progesterone.

Migraine   A condition characterized by localized headaches that possibly result from alternating dilation and constriction of blood vessels.

Mind-body medicine   Techniques designed to enhance the mind's ability to affect bodily function and symptoms.

Mindfulness   Awareness and acceptance of the reality of the present moment.

Minerals   Inorganic, indestructible elements that aid physiological processes.

Miscarriage   Loss of the fetus before it is viable; also called spontaneous abortion.

Modeling   Learning specific behaviors by watching others perform them.

Monogamy   Exclusive sexual involvement with one partner.

Mononucleosis   A viral disease that causes pervasive fatigue and other long-lasting symptoms.

Monosaccharide   A simple sugar that contains only one molecule of a simple sugar.

Mons pubis   Fatty tissue covering the pubic bone in females; in physically mature women, the mons is covered with coarse hair.

Morbidity   The relative incidence of disease.

Morphine   A derivative of opium; sometimes used by medical practitioners to relieve pain.

Mortality   The proportion of deaths to population.

Mourning   The culturally prescribed behavior patterns for the expression of grief.

Multifactorial disease   Disease caused by interactions of several factors.

Multiple sclerosis (MS)   A degenerative neurological disease in which myelin, an insulator of nerves, breaks down.

Municipal solid waste   Solid wastes such as durable goods, nondurable goods, containers and packaging, food wastes, yard wastes, and miscellaneous wastes from residential, commercial, institutional, and industrial sources.

Muscle dysmorphia   Sometimes referred to as "big-arexia," a pathological preoccupation with being larger and more muscular, which can lead to exercise addiction.

Muscular endurance   A muscle's ability to exert force repeatedly without fatiguing.

Muscular strength   The amount of force that a muscle is capable of exerting.

Mutant cells   Cells that differ in form, quality, or function from normal cells.

Myocardial infarction (MI)   Heart attack.

Narcotic   Drugs that induce sleep and relieve pain; primarily the opiates.

Naturopathic medicine   System of medicine that attempts to restore natural processes of the body and promote healing through natural means.

Near-infrared interactance (NIR)   Fiber optic measurement of tissue composition.

Negative consequences   Physical damage, legal trouble, financial problems, academic failure, family dissolution, and other severe problems associated with addiction.

Neoplasm   A new growth of tissue that serves no physiological function and results from uncontrolled, abnormal cellular development.

Neurotransmitters   Biochemical messengers that exert influence at specific receptor sites on nerve cells.

Nicotine   The primary stimulant chemical in tobacco products.

Nicotine poisoning   Symptoms often experienced by beginning smokers, including dizziness, diarrhea, lightheadedness, rapid and erratic pulse, clammy skin, nausea, and vomiting.

Nicotine withdrawal   Symptoms, including nausea, headaches, and irritability, suffered by addicted smokers who cease using tobacco.

Nitrogen dioxide   An amber-colored gas found in smog; can cause eye and respiratory irritations.

Nitrous oxide   The chemical name for "laughing gas," a substance properly used for surgical or dental anesthesia.

Nonassertive communicators   Individuals who tend to be shy and inhibited in their communication with others.

Nonpoint source pollutants   Pollutants that run off or seep into waterways from broad areas of land.

Nonprofit (voluntary) hospitals   Hospitals run by religious or other humanitarian groups that reinvest their earnings in the hospital to improve health care.

Nonsurgical embryo transfer   In vitro fertilization of a donor egg by the male partner's (or donor's) sperm and subsequent transfer to the female partner's or another woman's uterus.

Nonverbal communication   All unwritten and unspoken messages, both intentional and unintentional.

Nuclear family   Parents (usually married, but not necessarily) and their offspring.

Nurse   Health practitioner who provides many services for patients and who may work in a variety of settings.

Nurturing through avoidance   Repeatedly seeking the illusion of relief to avoid unpleasant feelings or situations, a maladaptive way of taking care of emotional needs.

Nutraceuticals   Term often used interchangeably with functional foods; refers to the combined nutritional and pharmaceutical benefit derived through use of foods or food supplements.

Nutrients   The constituents of food that sustain us physiologically: proteins, carbohydrates, fats, vitamins, minerals, and water.

Nutrition   The science that investigates the relationship between physiological function and the essential elements of foods eaten.

NuvaRing   A soft, flexible ring inserted into the vagina that releases hormones, preventing pregnancy.

Obesity   A weight disorder generally defined as an accumulation of fat beyond that considered normal for a person based on age, sex, and body type.

Obesogenic   Society in which several factors make people more prone to obesity.

Obsession   Excessive preoccupation with an addictive object or behavior.

Old-old   People aged 85 and over.

Oncogenes   Suspected cancer-causing genes present on chromosomes.

Oncologists   Physicians who specialize in the treatment of malignancies.

One repetition maximum (1 RM)   The amount of weight/resistance that can be lifted or moved once, but not twice; a common measure of strength.

Open relationship   A relationship in which partners agree that sexual involvement can occur outside the relationship.

Ophthalmologist   Physician who specializes in the medical and surgical care of the eyes, including prescriptions for glasses.

Opium   The parent drug of the opiates; made from the seedpod resin of the opium poppy.

Optometrist   Eye specialist whose practice is limited to prescribing and fitting lenses.

Oral contraceptives   Pills taken daily for three weeks of the menstrual cycle that prevent ovulation by regulating hormones.

Oral ingestion   Intake of drugs through the mouth.

Oral surgeon   Dentist who performs surgical procedures to correct problems of the mouth, jaw, and face.

Organically grown   Foods that are grown without use of pesticides or chemicals.

Ortho Evra   A patch that releases hormones similar to those in oral contraceptives; each patch is worn for one week.

Orthodontist   Dentist who specializes in the alignment of teeth.

Osteoarthritis (OA)   A progressive deterioration of bones and joints that has been associated with the "wear and tear" theory of aging.

Osteopath   General practitioner who receives training similar to a medical doctor's but with an emphasis on the skeletal and muscular systems, often using spinal manipulation as part of treatment.

Osteoporosis   A degenerative bone disorder characterized by increasingly porous bones.

Outpatient (ambulatory) care   Treatment that does not involve an overnight stay in a hospital.

Ovarian follicles (egg sacs)   Areas within the ovary in which individual eggs develop.

Ovaries   Almond-size organs that house developing eggs and produce hormones.

Overload   A condition in which a person feels overly pressured by demands.

Over-the-counter (OTC) drugs   Medications that can be purchased without a physician's prescription.

Overuse injuries   Injuries that result from the cumulative effects of day-after-day stresses placed on tendons, muscles, and joints.

Overweight   Increased body weight in relation to height.

Ovulation   The point of the menstrual cycle at which a mature egg ruptures through the ovarian wall.

Ozone   A gas formed when nitrogen dioxide interacts with hydrogen chloride.

Pairings   Paired associations (such as coffee and a cigarette) that trigger cravings.

Pandemic   Global epidemic of a disease.

Panic attack   Severe anxiety reaction in which a particular situation, often for unknown reasons, causes terror.

Pap test   A procedure in which cells taken from the cervical region are examined for abnormal cellular activity.

Parasitic worms   The largest of the pathogens, most of which are more a nuisance than a threat.

Parasympathetic nervous system   Branch of the autonomic nervous system responsible for slowing systems stimulated by the stress response.

Parkinson's disease   A chronic, progressive neurological condition that causes tremors and other symptoms.

Particulates   Nongaseous air pollutants.

Passive euthanasia   The intentional withholding of treatment that would prolong life.

Passive immunity   Antibodies formed in another person or animal, and then given to someone with a weakened immune system.

Pathogen   A disease-causing agent.

Pelvic inflammatory disease (PID)   An infection that scars the uterine tubes and consequently blocks sperm migration, causing infertility.

Penis   Male sexual organ that releases sperm into the vagina.

Peptic ulcer   Damage to the stomach or intestinal lining, usually caused by digestive juices.

Perception   The process of filtering and interpreting information gathered through the senses.

Perineum   Tissue that forms the "floor" of the pelvic region; it covers a kite-shaped region including the external genitalia and anus.

Periodontal diseases   Diseases of the tissue around the teeth.

Personal control   Belief that one's own internal resources can control a situation.

Pesticides   Chemicals that kill pests.

Peyote   A cactus with small "buttons" that, when ingested, produce hallucinogenic effects.

Phencyclidine (PCP)   A drug, commonly called "angel dust," that causes hallucinations, delusions, and delirium.

Phobia   A deep and persistent fear of a specific object, activity, or situation that results in a compelling desire to avoid the source of the fear.

Photochemical smog   The brownish yellow haze resulting from the combination of hydrocarbons and nitrogen oxides.

Physical activity   Any bodily movement that is produced by the contraction of skeletal muscles and that substantially increases energy expenditure.

Physical fitness   The ability to perform moderate-to-vigorous levels of physical activity on a regular basis without excessive fatigue.

Physician assistant   A midlevel practitioner trained to handle most standard cases of care.

Phytomedicines   Another name for medicinal herbs, many of which are sold over the counter in Europe.

Pica   Iron-deficiency disease characterized by craving for certain foods and substances.

Pilates   Exercise programs that combine stretching with movement against resistance, aided by devices such as tension springs and heavy bands.

Pituitary gland   The endocrine gland located deep within the brain; controls reproductive functions.

Placebo effect   An apparent cure or improved state of health brought about by a substance or product that has no medicinal value.

Placenta   The network of blood vessels, connected to the umbilical cord, that carries nutrients to the developing infant and carries wastes away.

Plaque   Cholesterol buildup on the inner walls of arteries, causing a narrowing of the channel through which blood flows; a major cause of atherosclerosis.

Plateau That point in a weight loss program at which the dieter finds it difficult to lose more weight.

Platelet adhesiveness Stickiness of red blood cells associated with blood clots.

Pneumonia Bacterially caused disease of the lungs.

Point source pollutants Pollutants that enter waterways at a specific point.

Polychlorinated biphenyls (PCBs) Toxic chemicals that were once used as insulating materials in high-voltage electrical equipment.

Polydrug use The use of multiple medications or illicit drugs simultaneously.

Polysaccharide A complex carbohydrate formed by the combination of long chains of saccharides.

Portion The amount of a given food that you choose to eat at a particular time.

Positive reinforcement Presenting something positive following a behavior that is being reinforced.

Positron emission tomography (PET scan) Method for measuring heart activity by injecting a patient with a radioactive tracer that is scanned electronically to produce a three-dimensional image of the heart and arteries.

Postpartum depression The experience of energy depletion, anxiety, mood swings, and depression that women may feel during the postpartum period.

Post-traumatic stress disorder An acute stress disorder caused by experiencing an extremely traumatic event, such as rape or combat.

Power The ability to make and implement decisions.

Preconception care Medical care received prior to becoming pregnant that helps a woman assess and address potential maternal health.

Preeclampsia A complication in pregnancy characterized by high blood pressure, protein in the urine, and edema.

Prejudice A negative evaluation of an entire group of people that is typically based on unfavorable and often wrong ideas about the group.

Premature ejaculation Ejaculation that occurs prior to or almost immediately following penile penetration of the vagina.

Premenstrual dysphoric disorder (PMDD) Collective name for a group of negative symptoms similar to but more severe than PMS, including severe mood disturbances.

Premenstrual syndrome (PMS) Comprises the mood changes and physical symptoms that occur in some women during one or two weeks prior to menstruation.

Prescription drugs Medications that can be obtained only with the written prescription of a licensed physician.

Prevalence The number of existing cases.

Primary aggression Goal-directed, hostile self-assertion that is destructive in character.

Primary care practitioner A medical practitioner who treats routine ailments, advises on preventive care, gives general medical advice, and makes appropriate referrals when necessary.

Primary prevention Actions designed to stop problems before they start.

Prions A recently identified pathogen that infects humans and animals; a self-replicating protein-based agent that systematically destroys brain cells.

Process addictions Behaviors such as money addictions, work addiction, exercise addiction, and sex addictions that are known to be addictive because they are mood-altering.

Progesterone Hormone secreted by the ovaries; helps keep the endometrium developing in order to nourish a fertilized egg; also helps maintain pregnancy.

Proof A measure of the percentage of alcohol in a beverage.

Proprioceptive neuromuscular facilitation (PNF) stretching Techniques that involve the skillful use of alternating muscle contractions and static stretching in the same muscle.

Prostaglandin inhibitors Drugs that inhibit the production and release of prostaglandins associated with arthritis or menstrual pain.

Prostate gland Gland that secretes nutrients and neutralizing fluids into the semen.

Prostate-specific antigen (PSA) An antigen found in prostate cancer patients.

Proteins The essential constituents of nearly all body cells; necessary for the development and repair of bone, muscle, skin, and blood; the key elements of antibodies, enzymes, and hormones.

Protooncogenes Genes that can become oncogenes under certain conditions.

Protozoa Microscopic single-celled organisms.

Psilocybin The active chemical found in psilocybe mushrooms; it produces hallucinations.

Psychedelics Drugs that distort the processing of sensory information in the brain.

Psychiatric nurse specialist A registered nurse specializing in psychiatric practice.

Psychiatrist A licensed physician who specializes in treating mental and emotional disorders.

Psychoactive drugs Drugs that have the potential to alter mood or behavior.

Psychoanalyst A psychiatrist or psychologist with special training in psychoanalysis.

Psychoeducation The teaching of crucial psychological skills, giving people knowledge so they can help themselves.

Psychological hardiness A personality trait characterized by control, commitment, and challenge.

Psychological stress Stress caused by being in an environment perceived to be beyond one's control and endangering one's well-being.

Psychologist A person with a PhD degree and training in psychology.

Psychoneuroimmunology (PNI) Science of the interaction between the mind and the immune system.

Psychosocial health The mental, emotional, social, and spiritual dimensions of health.

Puberty The period of sexual maturation.

Pubic lice (crabs) Parasites that can inhabit various body areas, especially the genitals.

Qi Element of traditional Oriental medicine that refers to the vital energy force that courses through the body. When qi is in balance, health is restored.

Quasi-death experience A loss or experience that resembles death, in that it involves separation, termination, significant loss, a change of personal identity, and grief.

Rabies   A viral disease of the central nervous system; often transmitted through animal bites.

Radiation absorbed doses (rads)   Units that measure exposure to radioactivity.

Radiotherapy   The use of radiation to kill cancerous cells.

Radon   A naturally occurring radioactive gas resulting from the decay of certain radioactive elements.

Rape   Sexual penetration without the victim's consent.

Rational suicide   The decision to kill oneself rather than endure constant pain and slow decay.

Raynaud's syndrome   A disease in which exposure to cold temperatures produces exaggerated constriction of the small arteries in the extremities, causing fingers and toes to go numb, turn white, and then turn deep purple.

Reactive aggression   Emotional reaction brought about by frustrating life experiences.

Rebound effects   Severe withdrawal effects experienced by users of stimulants, including depression, nausea, and violent behavior.

Receptor sites   Specialized cells to which drugs can attach themselves.

Recommended Dietary Allowances (RDAs)   The average daily intakes of energy and nutrients considered adequate to meet the needs of most healthy people in the United States under usual conditions.

Recreational drugs   Drugs that contain chemicals that help people relax or socialize; most, but not all, drugs in this category are legal.

Reference Daily Intakes (RDIs)   Recommended amounts of 19 vitamins and minerals, also known as micronutrients.

Referred pain   Pain that is present at one point, although the source of pain is elsewhere.

Relapse   The tendency to return to the addictive behavior after a period of abstinence.

Relative risk   A measure of the strength of the relationship between risk factors and the condition being studied, such as a particular cancer.

Repetitive stress injury (RSI)   An injury to nerves, soft tissue, or joints due to the physical stress of repeated motions.

Resistance exercise program   A regular program of exercises designed to improve muscular strength and endurance in the major muscle groups.

Respite care   The care provided by substitute caregivers to relieve the principal caregiver from his or her continuous responsibility.

Resting metabolic rate (RMR)   The energy expenditure of the body under BMR conditions plus other daily sedentary activities.

Reticular formation   An area in the brain stem that is responsible for relaying messages to other areas in the brain.

Rh factor   A blood protein related to the production of antibodies. If an Rh-negative mother is pregnant with an Rh-positive fetus, the mother will manufacture antibodies that can kill the fetus, causing miscarriage.

Rheumatic heart disease   A heart disease caused by untreated streptococcal infection of the throat.

Rheumatoid arthritis   A serious inflammatory joint disease.

RICE   Acronym for the standard first-aid treatment for virtually all traumatic and overuse injuries: rest, ice, compression, and elevation.

Rickettsia   A small form of bacteria that live inside other living cells.

Risk behaviors   Behaviors that increase susceptibility to negative health outcomes.

Rosacea   Skin disorder that causes facial redness, puffiness, and other symptoms.

Route of administration   The manner in which a drug is taken into the body.

Rubella (German measles)   A milder form of measles that causes a rash and mild fever in children and may cause damage to a fetus or a newborn baby.

Saliva   Fluid secreted by the salivary glands; enzymes in the fluid aid in the breakdown of certain foods for digestion.

Sarcopenia   Age-related loss of muscle mass.

Satiety   The feeling of fullness or satisfaction at the end of a meal.

Saturated fats   Fats that are unable to hold any more hydrogen in their chemical structure; derived mostly from animal sources; solid at room temperature.

Schizophrenia   A mental illness with biological origins that is characterized by irrational behavior, severe alterations of the senses (hallucinations), and often an inability to function in society.

Scleroderma   A disease in which fibrous growth of connective tissue underlying the skin and body organs hardens and makes movement difficult.

Scrotum   Sac of tissue that encloses the testes.

Seasonal affective disorder (SAD)   A type of depression that occurs in the winter months, when sunlight levels are low.

Secondary hypertension   Hypertension caused by specific factors, such as kidney disease, obesity, or tumors of the adrenal glands.

Secondary prevention (intervention)   Intervention early in the development of a health problem.

Secondary sex characteristics   Characteristics associated with gender but not directly related to reproduction, such as vocal pitch, degree of body hair, and location of fat deposits.

Secondhand smoke (sidestream smoke)   The cigarette, pipe, or cigar smoke breathed by nonsmokers.

Sedatives   Central nervous system depressants that induce sleep and relieve anxiety.

Self-disclosure   The process of revealing one's inner thoughts, feelings, and beliefs to another person.

Self-efficacy   Belief in one's own ability to perform a task successfully.

Self-esteem   Sense of self-respect or self-confidence.

Self-nurturance   Developing individual potential through a balanced and realistic appreciation of self-worth and ability.

Semen   Fluid containing sperm and nutrient fluids that increase sperm viability and neutralize vaginal acid.

Seminal vesicles   Storage areas for sperm where nutrient fluids are added to them.

Senility   A term associated with judgment and orientation problems and the loss of memory occurring in a small percentage of the elderly.

Serial monogamy   A series of monogamous sexual relationships.

Serving   The amount of a given food recommended by materials such as the Food Guide Pyramid.

Setpoint theory A theory of obesity causation that suggests that fat storage is determined by a thermostatic mechanism in the body that acts to maintain a specific amount of body fat.

Sexual abuse of children Sexual interaction between a child and an adult or older child; includes, but is not limited to, sexually suggestive conversations, inappropriate kissing, touching, petting, and oral, anal, or vaginal intercourse.

Sexual addiction Compulsive involvement in sexual activity.

Sexual assault Any act in which one person is sexually intimate with another person without that person's consent.

Sexual aversion disorder Type of desire dysfunction characterized by sexual phobias and anxiety about sexual contact.

Sexual dysfunction Problems associated with achieving sexual satisfaction.

Sexual fantasies Sexually arousing thoughts and dreams.

Sexual harassment Any form of unwanted sexual attention.

Sexual identity Recognition of oneself as a sexual being; a composite of biological sex characteristics, gender identity, gender roles, and sexual orientation.

Sexual orientation A person's enduring emotional, romantic, sexual, or affectionate attraction to other persons.

Sexual performance anxiety A condition of sexual difficulties caused by anticipating some sort of problem with the sex act.

Sexually transmitted infections (STIs) A variety of infections that can be acquired through sexual contact.

Shaping Using a series of small steps to gradually achieve a particular goal.

Sick building syndrome (SBS) Problem that exists when 80 percent of a building's occupants report maladies that tend to lessen or vanish when they leave the building.

Sickle-cell anemia Genetic disease commonly found among African Americans; results in organ damage and premature death.

Simple rape Rape by one person known to the victim that does not involve a physical beating or use of a weapon.

Simple sugar A major type of carbohydrate, which provides short-term energy.

Sinoatrial node (SA node) Cluster of electric-generating cells that serve as a form of natural pace-maker for the heart.

Situational inducement Attempt to influence a behavior through situations and occasions that are structured to exert control over that behavior.

Skinfold caliper technique A method of determining body fat whereby folds of skin and fat at various points on the body are grasped between thumb and forefinger and measured with calipers.

Sleep apnea Disorder in which a person has numerous episodes of breathing stoppage during a normal night's sleep.

Slow-acting viruses Viruses having long incubation periods and causing slowly progressive symptoms.

Small intestine Muscular, coiled digestive organ; consists of the duodenum, jejunum, and ileum.

Snuff A powdered form of tobacco that is sniffed and absorbed through the mucous membranes in the nose or placed inside the cheek and sucked.

Social bonds Degree and nature of interpersonal contacts.

Social death A seemingly irreversible situation in which a person is not treated like an active member of society.

Social health Aspect of psychosocial health that includes interactions with others, ability to use social supports, and ability to adapt to various situations.

Social learning theory Theory that people learn behaviors by watching role models-parents, caregivers, and significant others.

Social phobia A phobia characterized by fear and avoidance of social situations.

Social physique anxiety (SPA) A desire to look good that has a destructive effect on a person's ability to function effectively socially.

Social support Network of people and services with whom you share ties and get support.

Social worker A person with an MSW degree and clinical training.

Socialization Process by which a society communicates behavioral expectations to its individual members.

Solo practitioner Physician who renders care to patients independently of other practitioners.

Spermatogenesis The development of sperm.

Spermicides Substances designed to kill sperm.

Spirituality A belief in a unifying force that gives meaning to life and transcends the purely physical or personal dimensions of existence.

Spontaneous remission The disappearance of symptoms without any apparent cause or treatment.

Staphylococci Round, gram-positive bacteria, usually found in clusters.

Static stretching Techniques that gradually lengthen a muscle to an elongated position (to the point of discomfort) and hold that position for 10 to 30 seconds.

Sterilization Permanent fertility control achieved through surgical procedures.

Stillbirth The birth of a dead baby.

Stomach Large muscular organ that temporarily stores, mixes, and digests foods.

Strain The wear and tear sustained by the body and mind in adjusting to or resisting a stressor.

Streptococcus A round bacterium, usually found in chain formation.

Stress Mental and physical responses to change.

Stress inoculation Newer stress management technique in which a person consciously tries to prepare ahead of time for potential stressors.

Stressor A physical, social, or psychological event or condition that requires our bodies to make an adjustment.

Stroke A condition occurring when the brain is damaged by disrupted blood supply.

Subcutaneous injection The introduction of drugs into the layer of fat directly beneath the skin.

Subjective well-being (SWB) That uplifting feeling of inner peace and wonder that we call happiness.

Sudden cardiac death Death that occurs as a result of sudden, abrupt loss of heart function.

Sudden infant death syndrome (SIDS) The sudden death of an infant under one year of age for no apparent reason.

Sulfur dioxide A yellowish brown gaseous by-product of the burning of fossil fuels.

Superfund Fund established under the Comprehensive Environmental Response Compensation and Liability Act to be used for cleaning up toxic waste dumps.

Suppositories Mixtures of drugs and a waxy medium designed to melt at body temperature that are inserted into the anus or vagina.

Sympathetic nervous system Branch of the autonomic nervous system responsible for stress arousal.

Sympathomimetics Drugs found in appetite suppressants that affect the sympathetic nervous system.

Synergism An interaction of two or more drugs that produces more profound effects than would be expected if the drugs were taken separately.

Synesthesia A (usually) drug-created effect in which sensory messages are incorrectly assigned-for example, the user hears a taste or smells a sound.

Syphilis One of the most widespread STIs; characterized by distinct phases and potentially serious results.

Systemic lupus erythematosus (SLE, or lupus) A disease in which the immune system attacks the body, producing antibodies that destroy or injure organs such as the kidneys, brain, and heart.

Systolic pressure The upper number in the fraction that measures blood pressure, indicating pressure on the walls of the arteries when the heart contracts.

Tai chi An ancient Chinese form of exercise widely practiced in the West today that promotes balance, coordination, stretching, and meditation.

Tar A thick, brownish substance condensed from particulate matter in smoked tobacco.

Target heart rate Calculated as a percentage of maximum heart rate (220 minus age); heart rate (pulse) is taken during aerobic exercise to check if exercise intensity is at the desired level (e.g., 60 percent of maximum heart rate).

Temperature inversion A weather condition occurring when a layer of cool air is trapped under a layer of warmer air.

Teratogenic Causing birth defects; may refer to drugs, environmental chemicals, X rays, or diseases.

Terrorism The use of unlawful force or violence against persons or property to intimidate or coerce a government, the civilian population, or any segment thereof, in furtherance of political or social objectives.

Tertiary prevention Treatment and/or rehabilitation efforts.

Testator A person who leaves a will or testament at death.

Testes Two organs, located in the scrotum, that manufacture sperm and produce hormones.

Testosterone The male sex hormone manufactured in the testes.

Tetrahydrocannabinol (THC) The chemical name for the active ingredient in marijuana.

Thanatology The study of death and dying.

Theory of Reasoned Action Model for explaining the importance of our intentions in determining behaviors.

Thrombolysis Injection of an agent to dissolve clots and restore some blood flow, thereby reducing the amount of tissue that dies from ischemia.

Thrombus Blood clot attached to the wall of a blood vessel.

Tinctures Herbal extracts usually combined with grain alcohol to prevent spoilage.

Tolerable Upper Intake Level (UL) The highest amount of a nutrient that an individual can safely consume every day without risking adverse health effects.

Tolerance Phenomenon in which progressively larger doses of a drug or more intense involvement in a behavior is needed to produce the desired effects.

Total body electrical conductivity (TOBEC) Technique using an electromagnetic force field to assess relative body fat.

Toxic shock syndrome (TSS) A potentially life-threatening disease that occurs when specific bacterial toxins are allowed to multiply unchecked in wounds or through improper use of tampons or diaphragms.

Toxins Poisonous substances produced by certain microorganisms that cause various diseases.

Toxoplasmosis A disease caused by an organism found in cat feces that, when contracted by a pregnant woman, may result in stillbirth or an infant with mental retardation or birth defects.

Trace minerals Minerals that the body needs in only very small amounts.

Traditional Chinese medicine (TCM) Comprehensive system of diagnosis and treatment in which dietary change, touch, massage, medicinal teas, and other herbal medicines are used extensively.

Tranquilizers Central nervous system depressants that relax the body and calm anxiety.

***Trans* fatty acids (*trans* fats)** Fatty acids that are produced when polyunsaturated oils are hydrogenated to make them more solid.

Transgendered Refusing to follow the sexual and gender scripts prescribed based on biology and resisting the division of gender into two distinct categories.

Transient ischemic attacks (TIAs) Brief interruptions of the blood supply to the brain that cause only temporary impairment; often an indicator of impending major stroke.

Transition The process during which the cervix becomes nearly fully dilated and the head of the fetus begins to move into the birth canal.

Transsexuality Condition in which a person is psychologically of one sex but physically of the other.

Traumatic injuries Injuries that are accidental in nature, which occur suddenly and violently (including fractured bones, ruptured tendons, and sprained ligaments).

Trichomoniasis Protozoan infection characterized by foamy, yellowish discharge and unpleasant odor.

Triglycerides The most common form of fat in the body; excess calories are converted into triglycerides and stored as body fat.

Trimester A three-month segment of pregnancy; used to describe specific developmental changes that occur in the embryo or fetus.

Trust The degree of confidence felt in a relationship.

Tubal ligation Sterilization of the female that involves the cutting and tying off or cauterizing of the uterine tubes.

Tuberculosis (TB) A disease caused by bacterial infiltration of the respiratory system.

Tumor A neoplasmic mass that grows more rapidly than surrounding tissue.

U.S. Recommended Daily Allowances (USRDA) Dietary guidelines developed by the Food and Drug Administration (FDA) and the United States Department of Agriculture.

Ulcerative colitis An inflammatory disorder that affects the mucous membranes of the large intestine, producing bloody diarrhea.

Unintentional injuries Injuries committed without intent to harm.

Unsaturated fats Fats that do have room for more hydrogen in their chemical structure; derived mostly from plants; liquid at room temperature.

Urethral opening The opening through which urine is expelled.

Urinary incontinence The inability to control urination.

Uterine (fallopian) tubes Tubes that extend from near the ovaries to the uterus.

Uterus (womb) Hollow, pear-shaped muscular organ whose function is to contain the developing fetus.

Vaccination Inoculation with killed or weakened pathogens or similar, less dangerous antigens in order to prevent or lessen the effects of some disease.

Vacuum aspiration The use of gentle suction to remove fetal tissue from the uterus.

Vagina The passage in females leading from the vulva into the uterus.

Vaginal intercourse The insertion of the penis into the vagina.

Vaginismus A state in which the vaginal muscles contract so forcefully that penetration cannot be accomplished.

Vaginitis Set of symptoms characterized by vaginal itching, swelling, and burning.

Validating Letting your partner know that although you may not agree with his or her point of view, you still respect the fact that he or she thinks or feels that way.

Variant sexual behavior A sexual behavior that is not engaged in by most people.

Vasectomy Sterilization of the male that involves the cutting and tying off of both ductus deferentia.

Vasocongestion The engorgement of the genital organs with blood.

Vegetarian A term with a variety of meanings: vegans avoid all foods of animal origin; lacto-vegetarians avoid flesh foods but eat dairy products; ovo-vegetarians avoid flesh foods but eat eggs; lacto-ovo-vegetarians avoid flesh foods but eat both dairy products and eggs; pesco-vegetarians avoid meat but eat fish, dairy products, and eggs; semivegetarians eat chicken, fish, dairy products, and eggs.

Veins Vessels that carry blood back to the heart from other regions of the body.

Ventricles The two lower chambers of the heart, which pump blood through the blood vessels.

Venules Branches of the veins.

Very low calorie diets (VLCDs) Diets with a daily caloric value of 400 to 700 calories.

Violence A set of behaviors that produce injuries, as well as the outcomes of these behaviors (the injuries themselves).

Virulent Strong enough to overcome host resistance and cause disease.

Viruses Minute parasitic microbes that live inside another cell.

Vitamins Essential organic compounds that promote growth and reproduction and help maintain life and health.

Vulva The female's external genitalia.

Waist circumference measurement Assessment of healthy weight by measurement of the circumference of the waist.

Waist-to-hip ratio Ratio that indicates increased risks due to an unhealthy weight distribution.

Wake or viewing Displaying of the deceased to formalize last respects and increase social support of the bereaved.

Wellness The achievement of the highest level of health possible in each of several dimensions.

Western blot A test more accurate than the ELISA to confirm presence of HIV antibodies.

Whole medical systems Complete systems of theory and practice that involve several CAM domains.

Withdrawal A method of contraception that involves withdrawing the penis from the vagina before ejaculation. Also called coitus interruptus. This term is also used to describe a series of temporary physical and biopsychosocial symptoms that occur when the addict abruptly abstains from an addictive chemical or behavior.

Women's Health Initiative (WHI) National study of postmenopausal women conducted in conjunction with the NIH mandate for equal research priorities for women's health issues.

Work addiction The compulsive use of work and the work persona to fulfill needs for intimacy, power, and success.

Xanthines The chemical family of stimulants to which caffeine belongs.

Yoga A variety of Indian traditions geared toward self-discipline and the realization of unity; includes forms of exercise widely practiced in the West today that promote balance, coordination, flexibility, and meditation.

Young-old People aged 65 to 74.

Yo-yo diets Cycles in which people repeatedly gain weight, and then starve themselves to lose weight. This lowers their BMR, which makes regaining weight even more likely.

CHAPTER 1

1. Writing Group for the Womens' Health Initiative Investigators, "Risks and Benefits of Estrogen Plus Progestin in Health of Postmenopausal Women: Principal Results from the Women's Health Initiative Randomized Controlled Trial," *Journal of the American Medical Association* 288, no. 3 (July 17, 2002): 321–323; J. A. Simon et al., "Postmenopausal Hormone Therapy and Risk of Stroke," *Circulation* 103 (2001): 638–642; American College of Obstetricians and Gynecologists, "Questions and Answers on Hormone Therapy," 2002, www.acog.org/from_home/publication /press_releases/nr08-30-02.cfm; A. L. Hersh, M. L. Stefanick, and R. S. Stafford, "National Use of Postmenopausal Hormone Therapy: Answers and Responses to Recent Evidence," *Journal of the American Medical Association* 291 (2004): 47–53; Womens' Health Initiative Steering Committee, "Effects of Conjugated Equine Estrogen in Postmenopausal Women with Hysterectomy: Women's Health Initiative Randomized Controlled Trial," *Journal of the American Medical Association* 291 (2004),1701–1712; S. B. Hulley and D. Grady, "The WHI Estrogen-Alone Trial: Do Things Look Any Better?" *Journal of the American Medical Association* 291, no. 14 (April 14, 2004): 1769–1771.
2. World Health Organization, "Constitution of the World Health Organization," *Chronicles of the World Health Organization* (Geneva, Switzerland, 1947).
3. R. Dubos, *So Human an Animal* (New York: Scribners, 1968), 15.
4. Department of Health and Human Services, *Healthy People 2000: National Health Promotion and Disease Prevention Objectives for the Year 2000* (Washington, DC: Government Printing Office, 1990).
5. National Center for Health Statistics, "About Healthy People 2010," 2002, www.health.gov/healthypeople/About/hpfact.htm
6. Centers for Disease Control and Prevention (CDC), *Best Practices for Comprehensive Tobacco Control Programs—August 1999* (Atlanta: U.S. Department of Health and Human Services, CDC, National Center for Chronic Disease Prevention and Health Promotion, Office on Smoking and Health, August 1999), reprinted, with corrections; and Institute of Medicine, *The Future of Public Health in the 21st Century* (Washington, DC: National Academies Press, 2003).
7. R. Donatelle and S. Prows, *The Use of Financial Incentives and Social Support to Motivate Smoking Cessation Among High-Risk Pregnant Smokers,* technical report submitted to R. W. Johnson, Smoke-Free Families Office, Birmingham, AL.
8. G. E. Hardy, Jr. "The Burden of Chronic Disease: The Future Is Prevention." *Preventing Chronic Disease* [serial online], April 2004, www.cdc.gov/pcd/issues/2004/apr/04_0006.htm
9. Adapted from "Ten Great Public Health Achievements—United States, 1900–1999," *Morbidity and Mortality Weekly Report* 48, no. 12 (April 1999): 241–243, www.cdc.gov/epo/mmwr /preview/mmwhtml/00056796.htm
10. L. Strohl, "A Special Health Report: A Look at the Future of Medicine," *USA Weekend,* (October 1–3, 1999): 6–9.
11. Institute of Medicine, *Who Will Keep the Public Healthy: Educating Public Health Professionals for the 21st Century* (Washington, DC: National Academies Press, 2003).
12. Ibid.
13. Institute of Medicine, Board on International Health, *America's Vital Interest in Global Health: Protecting Our People, Enhancing Our Economy, and Advancing Our International Interests,* 2002, www.stills.nap.edu/readingroom/books/avi/index.html
14. Ibid.
15. L. Miller, "Medical Schools Put Women in Curricula," *The Wall Street Journal* (May 24, 1994): B1, B7.
16. E. Austin, "Women in Focus," *Shape* (September 1994): 46–47.
17. C. Tavris, *The Mismeasure of Woman* (New York: Touchstone, 1992), 99.
18. Ibid.
19. National Heart, Blood, and Lung Institute, "Facts about the Women's Health Initiative," www.nhlbi.nih.gov
20. M. DiMatteo, *The Psychology of Health, Illness, and Medical Care: An Individual Perspective* (Pacific Grove, CA: Brooks/Cole, 1994), 101–103.
21. Ibid.
22. Ibid.
23. E. P. Sarafino, *Health Psychology* (New York: Wiley, 1990), 189–191.
24. G. D. Bishop, *Health Psychology* (Boston: Allyn & Bacon, 1994), 84–86.
25. K. Glanz, F. Lewis, and B. Rimer, *Health Behavior and Health Education* (San Francisco: Jossey Bass, 2003), Chapters 8 and 9.
26. Ibid.
27. R. Donatelle, et al., "Randomized Controlled Trial Using Social Support and Financial Incentives for High-Risk Pregnant Smokers: Significant Other Supporter (SOS) Program," *Tobacco Control* 9 Suppl. III (2000): iii, 67–69; S. Higgins et al., "Participation of Significant Others in Outpatient Behavioral Treatment Predicts Greater Cocaine Abstinence," *American Journal of Drug and Alcohol Abuse* (1994): 2047.
28. A. Ellis and M. Benard, *Clinical Application of Rational Emotive Therapy* (New York: Plenum, 1985).
29. P. Watson and R. Tharp, *Self-Directed Behavior: Self-Modification for Personal Adjustment* (Pacific Grove, CA: Brooks/Cole, 1993), 13.

CHAPTER 2

1. S. Benton et al., "Changes in Counseling Center Client Problems across 13 years," *Professional Psychology: Research and Practice* 34, no. 1 (2003): 66–72.
2. S. Hyman and G. Fischbach, "Mental Health: A Report of the Surgeon General," 2002, www.surgeongeneral.gov/library /mentalhealth/home.html
3. R. Lazarus, *Emotion and Adaptation* (New York: Oxford Press, 1994).
4. C. Ritter, "Social Supports, Social Networks, and Health Behaviors," in *Health Behavior: Emerging Perspectives*, ed. D. Gochman

(New York: Plenum, 1988); S. Kashubeck and S. Christensen, "Parental Alcohol Use, Family Relationships Quality, Self-Esteem, and Depression in College Students," *Journal of College Health* 36 (1995): 431–445; and L. K. George, *The Health-Promoting Effects of Social Bonds* (Durham, NC: Center for the Study of Aging and Human Development, Duke University, 2003).

5. S. R. Hawks et al., "Review of Spiritual Health: Definition, Role, and Intervention Strategies in Health Promotion," *American Journal of Health Promotion* 9, no. 5 (1995): 371–378.

6. A. Scandurra, "Everyday Spirituality: A Core Unit in Health Education and Lifetime Wellness," *Journal of Health Education* 30, no. 2 (1999): 104–109.

7. Ibid., 106.

8. L. Chapman, "Developing a Useful Perspective on Spiritual Health: Love, Joy, Peace and Fulfillment," *American Journal of Health Promotion* 2 (1987): 121–127.

9. Ibid., 122.

10. Ibid., 124.

11. R. Sloan, E. Bagiella, and T. Powell, "Religion, Spirituality, and Medicine," *The Lancet*, 353 (1999): 664–672.

12. D. Elkins, *Beyond Religion—A Personal Program for Building a Spiritual Life Outside the Walls of Traditional Religion* (Wheaton, IL: Quest Books, 1998).

13. Ibid.

14. D. Elkins, "Spirituality: It's What's Missing in Mental Health," *Psychology Today,* 32, no. 5 (1999): 48.

15. M. Seligman and D. M. Isaacowitz, "Learned Helplessness," in *Encyclopedia of Stress,* ed. F. J. McGuigan. (Boston: Allyn & Bacon, 1999).

16. J. R. Grant (ed.), *Journal of Humanistic Psychology* (special issue on positive psychology), 4, no. 1 (2001): 1–153.

17. S. Proffitt, "Pursuing Happiness with a Positive Outlook, Not a Pill," *Los Angeles Times*, January 24, 1999, www.apa.org /releases/pursuing.html; APA HelpCenter: Mind/Body Connection, "Learned Optimism Yields Health Benefits," http://helping .apa.org; American Psychological Association, "Century of Research Confirms Impact of Psychosocial Factors on Health— Question Is How to Apply that Knowledge to Healthcare Systems," January 19, 2004, www.apa.org/releases/ mind.html

18. M. Seligman, *Learned Optimism: How to Change Your Mind and Your Life* (New York: Free Press, 1998).

19. J. H. Martin, "Motivation Processes and Performance: The Role of Global and Facet Personality," PhD diss., University of North Carolina at Chapel Hill, 2002.

20. American Sleep Apnea Association, "What Is Sleep Apnea?" 2004, www.sleepapnea.org

21. National Institutes of Health, "National Center on Sleep Disorders Research," 2004, www.nhlbi.nih.gov/about/ncsdr/index.htm

22. Ibid.

23. D. G. Myers and E. Diener, "Who Is Happy?" *Psychological Science* 6 (1995): 10–19.

24. Ibid.

25. Ibid.

26. B. L. Fredrickson, "Cultivating Positive Emotions to Optimize Health and Well-Being," *Prevention & Treatment* 3, Article 0001a, March 7, 2000.

27. P. Doskoch, "Happily Ever Laughter," *Psychology Today* 29, no. 4 (1996): 33–35.

28. Frederickson, "Cultivating Positive Emotions."

29. B. Siegel, *Love, Medicine, and Miracles* (New York: Perennial, 1990).

30. Fredrickson, "Cultivating Positive Emotions."

31. Grady, "Think Right, Stay Well," *American Health* 11 (1992): 50–54.

32. L. Temoshock, *The Type C Connection* (New York: Random House, 1995).

33. L. Cool, "Is Mental Illness Catching?" *American Health for Women* 16 (1997).

34. MayoClinic.com, "Mental Health Definitions," 2003, www .mayoclinic.com

35. World Health Organization, "GBD 2001 Estimates by Region," www.who.int/en; Burden of Disease Unit, *The Global Burden of Disease: A Comprehensive Assessment of Mortality and Disability from Diseases, Injuries, and Risk Factors in 1990 and Projected to 2020* (Cambridge, MA: Harvard University Press, 1996).

36. MayoClinic.com, "Lifting the Curtain on Mental Illness: Growing Awareness of a Common Problem," 2001, www.mayoclinic.com

37. L. A. Lefton, *Psychology,* 8th ed., (Boston: Allyn & Bacon, 2002).

38. M. Sullivan, "Widespread Effects of Depression," NIH *Word on Health* newsletter, April 2003, www.nih.gov/news/WordonHealth /apr2003/depression.htm

39. R. Hirshchfeld et al., "The National Depressive and Manic Depression Association Consensus Statement on the Undertreatment of Depression," *Journal of the American Medical Association* 277 no. 4 (1997): 333–340.

40. Lefton, *Psychology.*

41. Lefton, *Psychology,* 543.

42. Adapted by permission of the author from K. R. Gertz, "Mood Probe: Pinpointing the Crucial Differences between Emotional Lows and the Gridlock of Depression," *Self*, November 1990.

43. National Institute for Mental Health, 2004, www.nimh.nih.gov

44. D. R. Rubinow, P .J. Schmidt, and C. A. Roca, "Estrogen-Serotonin Interactions: Implications for Affective Regulation," *Biological Psychiatry* 44, no. 9 (1998): 839–850; P. J. Schmidt et al., "Differential Behavioral Effects of Gonadal Steroids in Women with and in Those without Premenstrual Syndrome," *New England Journal of Medicine* 338 (1998): 209–216.

45. R. G. Gladstone and L. Koenig, "Sex Differences in Depression Across the High School to College Transition," *Journal of Youth and Adolescence* 23 (1994): 643–669.

46. S. Scott, "Biology and Mental Health: Why Do Women Suffer More Depression and Anxiety?" *Maclean's*, 12, 1998.

47. National Institute of Mental Health, "Real Men, Real Depression," 2003, www.menanddepression.nimh.nih.gov

48. Ibid.

49. A. K. Ferketick et al., "Depression as an Antecedent to Heart Disease Among Women and Men in the NHANES I Study National Health and Nutrition Examination Survey," *Archives of Internal Medicine* 60, no. 9 (2002): 1261–1268.

50. I. Levav et al., "Vulnerability of Jews to Affective Disorders," *American Journal of Psychiatry* 154 (1997): 941–947.

51. S. Wood and E. Wood, *The World of Psychology,* 4th ed. (Boston: Allyn & Bacon, 2001).

52. S. Banks and R. Kerns, "Explaining High Rates of Depression in Chronic Pain: A Diathesis-Stress Framework," *Psychological Bulletin* 119 (1996); (NIH Publication No. 00-4779), "Depression: What Every Woman Should Know," National Institute of Mental Health, 2000, www.nimh.nih.gov/publicat/depwomenknows .cfm#ptdep4

53. L. Rabasca, "Psychotherapy May Be as Useful as Drugs in Treating Depression, Study Suggests," *The APA Monitor Online* 30, no. 8 (1999), www.apa.org/monitor

54. U.S. Food and Drug Administration (FDA), "FDA Issues Public Health Advisory on Cautions for Use of Antidepressants in Adults and Children" (FDA Talk Paper, T04-08), March 22, 2004, www.fda.gov/bbs/topics/ANSWERS/2004/ANS01283.html; U.S. FDA, Center for Drug Evaluation and Research, "Antidepressant Use in Children, Adolescents, and Young Adults," March 22, 2004, www.fda.gov/cder/drug/antidepressants/default.htm

55. MayoClinic.com, "Medical and Health Information for a Healthier Life," 2003, www.mayoclinic.com

56. MayoClinic.com, "Bipolar Disorder," 2003, www.mayoclinic.com

57. National Institute of Mental Health, "Anxiety Disorders" (NIH Publication No. 02-3879), 2002, www.nimh.nih.gov/publicat /anxiety.cfm

58. Anxiety Disorders Association of America, "Statistics and Facts about Anxiety Disorders," www.adaa.org/mediaroom/index.cfm

59. P. Zimbardo, A. Weber, and R. Johnson, *Psychology* (Boston: Allyn & Bacon, 2000), 505.

60. MayoClinic.com, "Panic Attacks," 2002, www.mayoclinic.com

61. Ibid.

62. G. Wilson, et al., *Abnormal Psychology*, (Boston: Allyn & Bacon, 1996).

63. Ibid., 147.

64. National Institute of Mental Health, "Women Hold Up Half the Sky: Women and Mental Health Research," 2001, www.nimh.nih.gov/publicat/womensoms.cfm; R. Saltus, "The PMS Debate," *Boston Globe Magazine* (July 25, 1999).

65. National Institute of Mental Health, "Depression" (NIMH Publication No. 00-3561), 2000, www.nimh.nih.gov/publicat/depression.cfm

66. K. Kendler and C. Gardner, "Boundaries of Major Depression: An Evaluation of DSM-IV Criteria," *American Journal of Psychiatry* 155 (1998): 172–176.

67. Ibid.

CHAPTER 3

1. S. Shellenbarger, "Learning How to Work with the Good Stress, Live without the Bad," *The Wall Street Journal* (July 25, 2001): B1.

2. H. Selye, *Stress Without Distress* (New York: Lippincott, 1974), 28–29.

3. D. Kenny, F. J. McGuigan, and J. Sheppard (Eds). *Stress and Health Research and Clinical Applications* (New York: Gordon and Breach Pub., 2000).

4. H. Anismam and Z. Merali, "Cytokines, Stress and Depressive Illness." *Brain, Behavior, and Immunity* 16, no. 5 (2002): 513–524.

5. M. D. Jeremko, "Stress Inoculation Training: A Generic Approach for the Prevention of Stress-Related Disorders," *The Personnel and Guidance Journal* 62 (1984): 544–550; H. S. Friedman and S. Booth-Kewley, "The Disease-Prone Personality: A Meta-Analytic View of the Construct," *American Psychologist* 42 (1987): 539–555.

6. G. E. Vaillant, *Adaptation to Life* (Boston: Little, Brown, 1977).

7. S. A. Lyness, "Predictions of Differences Between Type A and B Individuals in Heart Rate and Blood Pressure Reactivity," *Psychological Bulletin* 114 (1993): 266–295; J. C. Barefoot and M. Schroll, "Symptoms of Depression, Acute Myocardial Infarction, and Total Mortality in a Community Sample, 1976–1980," *Circulation* 93 (1996); and G. R. Schiraldi, G. T. Spalding, and C. Holford, "Expanding Health Educators' Roles to Meet Critical Needs in Stress Management and Mental Health," *Journal of Health Education* (1998): 70.

8. J. Chi and R. Kloner, "Stress and Myocardial Infarction," *Heart* 89, no. 5 (May 2003): 555–556.

9. F. Jones and J. Bright, *Stress: Myth, Theory, and Research* (New York: Prentice Hall, 2001).

10. R. Glaser et al., "Updates Linking Evidence and Experience: Stress-Induced Immunomodulation," *Journal of the American Medical Association* 281, no. 24 (1999): 2268–2270.

11. B. Rabin, *Stress, Immune Function, and Health: The Connection* (New York: Wiley-Liss, 1999).

12. J. Kiecolt-Glaser et al., "Chronic Stress and Age-Related Increases in the Proinflammatory Cytokine IL-6," *Proceedings of the National Academy of Sciences, USA* 100 (2003): 9090–9095.

13. D. Padgett et al., "Social Stress and the Reactivation of Latent Herpes Simplex Virus-Type 1," *Proceedings of the National Academy of Sciences, USA* 9 (1998): 7231–7235.

14. J. Kiecolt-Glaser et al., "Chronic Stress Alters the Immune Response to Influenza Virus Vaccines in Older Adults," *Proceedings of the National Academy of Sciences, USA* 93 (1996): 3043–3047.

15. R. Glaser et al., "The Influence of Psychological Stress on the Immune Response to Vaccines," *Annals of the New York Academy of Sciences* 840 (1998): 649–655.

16. A. Smith, "Breakfast, Stress, and Catching Colds," *Journal of Family Health Care* 13, no. 1 (2003): 2.

17. S. Cohen et al., "Types of Stressors That Increase Susceptibility to the Common Cold in Adults," *Health Psychology* 17 (1998): 214–223.

18. S. Cohen et al., "Social Ties and Susceptibility to the Common Cold," *Journal of the American Medical Association* 277 (1997): 1940–1944.

19. R. Kessler, "The Effects of Stressful Life Events on Depression," *Annual Reviews of Psychology* 48 (1997): 191–214.

20. American Diabetes Association, "Stress," 2004, www.diabetes.org/type-1-diabetes/stress.jsp

21. Schiraldi et al., "Exploring Health Educators' Roles," 69.

22. T. Holmes and R. Rahe, "The Social Readjustment Rating Scale," *Journal of Psychosocial Research* (1967): 213–217.

23. Ibid., 214.

24. R. Lazarus, "The Trivialization of Distress," in *Preventing Health Risk Behaviors and Promoting Coping with Illness,* ed. J. Rosen and L. Solomon (Hanover, NH: University Press of New England, 1985), 279–298.

25. L. Lefton, *Psychology,* 8th ed. (Boston: Allyn and Bacon, 2002).

26. M. Kenny and K. Rice, "Attachment to Parents and Adjustment in College Students: Current Status, Applications, and Future Considerations," *Counseling-Psychologist* 23 (1995): 433–456.

27. K. Nadal, "Ethnic Minority Students' Stressors: Their Impact on Campus Climate Perceptions and Academic Achievement," R. E. McNair Fellowship paper, http://members.tripod.com/~knall/minoritystress.html

28. Ibid.

29. R. C. Kessler, et al., "Social Support, Depressed Mood, and Adjustment to Stress: A Genetic Epidemiological Investigation," *Journal of Personality and Social Psychology* 62 (1992): 257–272.

30. M. Friedman and R. H. Rosenman, *Type A Behavior and Your Heart* (New York: Knopf, 1974).

31. R. Ragland and R. Brand, "Distrust, Rage May Be Toxic Cores That Put Type A Person at Risk," *Journal of American Medical Association* 261 (1989): 813, 814; J. C. Barefoot, W. G.Dahlstrom, and R. B. Williams, "Hostility, CHD Incidence, and Total Mortality: A 25 Year Follow-up Study of 255 Physicians," *Psychosomatic Medicine* 51 (1983): 46–57; J. C. Barefoot et al., "Hostility Patterns and Health Implications: Correlates of Cook-Medley Hostility Scale Scores in a National Survey," *Health Psychology* 10 (1991): 18–24.

32. P. L. Rice, *Stress and Health* (Belmont, CA: Wadsworth Publishing, 1998), 378.

33. Ibid.

34. American College Health Association, *National College Health Assessment: Reference Group Executive Summary* (Baltimore MD: ACHA, 2001).

35. L. Reisberg, "Student Stress Is Rising, Especially Among Women," *Chronicle of Higher Education* 46 (2000): A49–A50.

36. P. Jackson and M. Finney, "Negative Life Events and Psychological Distress among Young Adults," *Social Psychology Quarterly* (2003) (forthcoming) www.homepages.Indiana.edu/101201/text/stress.html

37. L. Towbes and L. Cohen, "Chronic Stress in the Lives of College Students: Scale Development and Prospective Prediction of Distress," *Journal of Youth and Adolescence* 25 (1996): 206–217.

38. C. Crandell, J. Preisler, and J. Ausspring, "Measuring Life Event Stress in the Lives of College Students: The Undergraduate Stress Questionnaire (USQ)," *Journal of Behavioral Medicine* 15 (1992): 627–642.

39. National Mental Health Association, "Finding Hope and Help: College Student and Depression Pilot Initiatives," 2004, www.nmha.org/camh/college/index.cfm

40. R. Niaura et al., "Hostility, Metabolic Syndrome, and Incident Coronary Heart Disease, " *Health Psychology* 21, no. 6 (2002): 588–593.
41. P. Holmes, "Managing Anger: Understanding the Dynamics of Violence, Abuse and Control," SIUC Mental Health Web Site, 2004, www.siu.edu/offices/counsel/anger.htm
42. Ibid.
43. C. Tavris, *Anger: The Misunderstood Emotion* (New York, Touchstone, 1989).

CHAPTER 4
1. D. Zucchio, "Todays's Violent Crime Is an Old Story with a New Twist," *San Jose Mercury News* (November 21, 1994).
2. Bureau of Justice Statistics, "Key Crime and Justice Facts at a Glance," February 2004, www.ojp.usdoj.gov/bjs
3. Bureau of Justice Statistics, "Expenditures and Employment Report: 1997," 1998, www.ojp.usdoj.gov/bjs
4. Bureau of Justice Statistics, "Key Crime and Justice Facts," 2004.
5. CDC Youth Risk Behavioral Surveillance U.S., vol. 53/SS-2, page 3, 2003, www.cdc.gov/mmwr/PDF
6. World Health Organization, Seventh World Conference on Injury Prevention and Safety Promotion, Vienna, Austria, June 6–9 2004, www.who.int/mediacentre/releases/2004/pr40/en/print.html
7. Centers for Disease Control and Prevention, National Center for Injury Control and Prevention, "Costs of Intimate Partner Violence Against Women in the U.S.," 2003, www.cdc.gov/ncipc/pub-res/ipv_cost/IPVBook-Final-Feb18.pdf
8. U.S. Center for Health Statistics, "Health, United States, 2001" (Atlanta: Centers for Disease Control and Prevention, 2001).
9. M. Leeds, Violence Prevention Conference (2002), Oregon State University, Corvallis, OR.
10. Ibid.
11. L. Lamberg, "Prediction of Violence Both Art and Science," *Journal of the American Medical Association* 275 (1996): 1713.
12. Leeds, Violence Prevention Conference.
13. Ibid.
14. Ibid.
15. F. Rivera et al., "Alcohol and Illicit Drugs and the Risk of Violent Death in the Home," *Journal of the American Medical Association* 278 (1997): 569–572.
16. "Substance Abuse: A Significant Characteristic in Domestic Violence Assailants," *Brown University Digest of Addiction Theory and Application* 16: 1–3.
17. M. Swartz et al., "Violence and Severe Mental Illness: The Effects of Substance Abuse and Non-Adherence to Medication," *American Journal of Psychiatry* 155 (1998): 226.
18. Rivera et al., "Alcohol and Illicit Drugs," 571.
19. Federal Bureau of Investigation, "Uniform Crime Reports, January–December 2003," 2004, www.fbi.gov/ucr/ucr.htm
20. U.S. Center for Health Statistics, "Table 32: Leading Causes of Death and Numbers of Deaths by Age," *Health United States, 2003* (Atlanta: Centers for Disease Control and Prevention, 2004)
21. U.S. Center for Health Statistics, *Health, United States, 2003*.
22. Ibid., 44.
23. Ibid., 46.
24. R. Lacyo, "Still Under the Gun?" *Time* (July 6, 1998): 32–56.
25. Federal Bureau of Investigation, "Hate Crime Statistics Report, 2002," 2003, www.fbi.gov/ucr/hatecrime2002.pdf
26. R. Fenske and L. Gordon, "Reducing Racial and Ethnic Hate Crimes on Campus: The Need for Community," in *Violence on Campus: Defining the Problems, Strategies for Action,* ed. A. Hoffman et al. (Gaithersburg, MD: Aspen, 1998).
27. Ibid.
28. Ibid.
29. C. Renninson and M. Rand, "National Crime Victimization Survey, 2002," U.S. Department of Justice, Bureau of Crime Statistics, 2003, www.ojp.usdoj.gov/bjs

30. Ibid.
31. Ibid.
32. National Center for Domestic Violence and Abuse. Fact Sheet (2000).
33. J. Barley et al., "Risk Factors for Violent Death in the Home," *Archives of Internal Medicine* 157 (1997): 786.
34. D. Brookkoff et al., "Characteristics of Participants in Domestic Violence: Assessment at the Scene of Domestic Violence," *Journal of the American Medical Association* 277 (1997): 1369.
35. "Injury and Domestic Violence Prevention," *Nurse Practitioner* 22 (1997): 122.
36. F. Trevino, S. Walker, and G. Ramirez, "Violent Crime in American Society," in *Violence on Campus: Defining the Problems, Strategies for Action,* ed. A. Hoffman et al. (Gaithersburg, MD: Aspen, 1998); and the Federal Bureau of Investigation, *Uniform Crime Report* (Washington, DC: U.S. Department of Justice, 1997).
37. Renninson and Rand, "National Crime Victimization Survey, 2002."
38. A. Joerger and L. McClellan, "Why Men Batter: Why Women Stay," *Community Safety Quarterly* 5 (1992): 22–23.
39. N. West, "Crimes Against Women," *Community Safety Quarterly* 5 (1992): 3.
40. M. A. Straus and R. Gelles, eds., *Physical Violence in American Families: Risk Factors and Adaptions to Violence in 8,145 Families* (New Brunswick, NJ: Transaction, 1993): 101–201.
41. H. Pan, P. Neidig, and K. O'Leary, "Physical Aggression in Early Marriage: Pre-relationship and Relationship Effects," *Journal of Consulting and Clinical Psychology* 62 (1994): 975–981.
42. G. T. Wilson et al., *Abnormal Psychology* (Boston: Allyn & Bacon, 1996).
43. Ibid.
44. Ibid.
45. E. Newberger, "Child Sexual Abuse," in *Violence in America: A Public Health Approach,* ed. M. Rosenberg and M. Fenley (New York: Oxford University Press, 1991), 85.
46. American Academy of Pediatrics, "Child Abuse and Neglect," 2004, www.aap.org/healthtopics/childabuse.cfm
47. M. Whittaker, "The Continuum of Violence Against Women: Psychological and Physical Consequences," *Journal of American College Health* 40 (1992): 155.
48. D. Finkelhor, "Child Sexual Abuse," in *Violence in America: A Public Health Approach,* ed. M. Rosenberg and M. Fenley (New York: Oxford University Press, 1991), 25.
49. N. West, "Children: The Invisible Victims of Domestic Violence," *Community Safety Quarterly* 5 (1992): 20.
50. Whittaker, "The Continuum of Violence," 152.
51. American Academy of Pediatrics, Medical Library "Child Abuse and Neglect."
52. K. Hunnicutt, "Women and Violence on Campus," in *Violence on Campus: Defining the Problems, Strategies for Action,* ed. A. Hoffman et al. (Gaithersburg, MD: Aspen, 1998), 150.
53. Ibid., 149.
54. National Women's Health Information Center, "Sexual Assault," 2004, www.4woman.gov/fag/sexualassault.htm
55. A. Berkowitz, "College Men as Perpetrators of Acquaintance Rape and Sexual Assault: A Review of Recent Literature," *Journal of American College Health* 40 (1992): 175.
56. National Women's Health Information Center, "Sexual Assault."
57. Rennison and Rand, "National Crime Victimization Survey, 2002."
58. National Women's Health Information Center, "Sexual Assault."
59. A. Hoffman, J. Schuh, and R. Fenske, *Violence on Campus* (Gaithersburg, MD: Aspen, 1998), 149–168.
60. D. Benson, C. Charlton, and F. Goohart, "Acquaintance Rape on Campus: A Literature Review," *Journal of American College Health* (1992): 157.

61. Wilson et al., *Abnormal Psychology.*
62. R. K. Bergen, *Violence Against Women Online Resources,* University of Minnesota, 2002, www.vaw.umn.edu/Vawnet/mrape.htm
63. Ibid.
64. Benson et al., "Acquaintance Rape on Campus," 158.
65. M. W. Leidig, "The Continuum of Violence Against Women: Psychological and Physical Consequences," *Journal of American College Health* 40 (1992): 151. Reprinted with permission of the Helen Dwight Reid Education Foundation. Published by Heldref Publications, 1319 Eighteenth Street NW, Washington, DC 20036-1802. Copyright © 1992.
66. Berkowitz, "College Men as Perpetrators," 177.
67. Ibid., 175.
68. Whittaker, "The Continuum of Violence," 153–154.
69. Berkowitz, "College Men as Perpetrators," 718.
70. Ibid., 175.
71. Ibid., 176.
72. Bureau of Justice Statistics, "College Students Victimized Less by Violent Crime than Non-Students According to New Justice Department Study," (press release), December 7, 2003, www.ojp.usdoj.gov/bjs/pub/press/vvcs00pr.htm
73. Hoffman et al., *Violence on Campus,* 1–40.
74. Ibid., 175.
75. Ibid., 183.
76. J. Baier, M. Rosenzweig, and E. Shipple, "Patterns of Sexual Behavior, Coercion, and Victimization of University Students," *Journal of College Student Development* 32 (1991): 178.
77. M. Koss, "Rape: Scope, Impact, Interventions, and Public Policy Responses," *American Psychologist* 48 (1993): 1062–1069.
78. Hoffman et al., *Violence on Campus,* 242.
79. E. Dersinger, C. Cychosz, and L. Jaeger, "Strategies for Dealing with Campus Violence," in *Violence on Campus: Defining the Problems, Strategies for Action,* ed. A. Hoffman et al. (Gaithersburg, MD: Aspen, 1998).
80. American Association of University Professors, *Hostile Hallways, The AAUW Survey on Sexual Harrassment in America's Schools,* 1996; Hunnicutt, "Woman and Violence on Campus," 160.
81. Ibid., 161.
82. Ibid., 162.
83. A. Matthews, "Campus Crime 101," *Eugene Register Guard,* March 1993, 4B.
84. Dersinger et al., "Strategies for Dealing with Campus Violence," 248.
85. B. Moyers, "What Can We Do About Violence?" Public Broadcasting Service, January 1995.
86. Bureau of Labor Statistics, "Injuries, Illnesses, and Fatalities," 2004, www.bls.gov
87. Bureau of Labor Statistics, "National Census of Fatal Occupational Injuries, 1999," 2000, www.bls.gov

CHAPTER 5

1. MayoClinic.com, "Nurture Relationships: A Healthy Investment," Mayo Foundation for Medical Education and Research (MFMER), 2002, www.mayohealth.org/home
2. S. L. Michaud and R. M. Warner, "Gender Differences in Self-Reported Response in Troubles Talk," *Sex Roles: A Journal of Research* 37 (1997): 527–541; and D. J. Canary and M. J. Cody, *Interpersonal Communication* (New York: St. Martin's, 1994), 33.
3. C. Snapp and M. Leary, "Hurt Feelings Among New Acquaintances: Moderating Effects of Interpersonal Familiarity," *Journal of Social and Personal Relationships* 18, no. 3 (June 2001): 1344–1350.
4. D. V. L. Loyer-Carlson, *Pathways to Marriage with RELATE Online Relationship Inventory: Premarital and Early Marital Relationships* (Boston: Allyn & Bacon/Longman, 2003).
5. K. Galvin and P. Cooper, *Making Connections* (Los Angeles: Roxbury Press, 2000), 4.
6. Ibid., 6.
7. R. Adler and G. Rodman, "Perceiving the Self," in *Making Connections,* ed. K. Galvin and P. Cooper (Los Angeles: Roxbury Press, 2000), 23.
8. J. Caputo, H. C. Hazel, and C. McMahon, *Interpersonal Communication* (Boston: Allyn & Bacon, 1994), 224.
9. Ibid., 100.
10. Larry A. Nadig, "Effective Listening," 2004, www.drnadig.com/listening.htm
11. Ibid.
12. Ibid.
13. M. E. Guffy, *Business Communication: Process and Products* (Belmont, CA: Wadsworth, 1994), 38.
14. Ibid., 38.
15. L. A. Nadig, "How to Express Difficult Feelings," 2004, www.drnadig.com/feelings.htm
16. M. Beard, *Interpersonal Relationships* (Dubuque, IA: Kendall/Hunt, 1989); N. Coupland, H. Giles, and W. Wieman, *Miscommunication and Problematic Talk* (London: Sage, 1991).
17. L. A. Nadig. "Relationship Conflict: Healthy or Unhealthy," 2004, www.drnadig.com.conflict.htm
18. H. Lerner, *The Dance of Intimacy* (New York: Perennial, 1990).
19. S. Brehm et al., *Intimate Relationships,* 3rd ed. (New York: McGraw-Hill, 2002), 6–7.
20. L. Lefton and L. Brannon, *Psychology,* 8th ed. (Boston: Allyn & Bacon, 2003), 474.
21. Ibid., 475.
22. J. Holmes, "Healthy Relationships: Their Influence on Physical Health," BC Council for Families, 2004, www.bccf.bc.ca/learn/health_relations.htm
23. J. Turner and L. Rubinson, *Contemporary Human Sexuality* (Englewood Cliffs, NJ: Prentice Hall, 1993), 457.
24. D. McAdams, *Intimacy: The Need to Be Close* (New York: Doubleday, 1989), 87–91.
25. Turner and Rubinson, *Contemporary Human Sexuality,* 457.
26. G. Levinger, "Can We Picture Love?" in *The Psychology of Love,* ed. R. J. Sternberg and M. Barnes (New Haven: Yale University Press, 1988), 139–159.
27. E. Hatfield, "Passionate and Compassionate Love" in *The Psychology of Love,* ed. R. J. Sternberg and M. Barnes (New Haven: Yale University Press, 1988), 191–217.
28. R. A. Baron and D. Byrne, *Social Psychology,* 10th ed. (Boston: Allyn & Bacon, 2004), 310–312.
29. E. Hatfield and G. W. Walster, *A New Look at Love* (Reading, MA: Addison Wesley, 1981).
30. H. Fisher, *Why We Love: The Nature and Chemistry of Romantic Love* (New York: Henry Holt, 2004).
31. A. Toufexis and P. Gray, "What Is Love? The Right Chemistry," *Time* (1993): 47–52.
32. Ibid.
33. Ibid.
34. C. McLoughlin, "Science of Love—Cupid's Chemistry," 2003, www.thenakedscientist.com/HTML/Columnists/clairemccloughlincolumn1.htm
35. Ibid.
36. "I Get a Kick Out of You," *The Economist,* February 12, 2004.
37. D. Tannen, *You Just Don't Understand: Women and Men in Conversation* (New York: William Morrow, 1990).
38. Michaud and Warner, "Gender Differences," 528; K. Pasley, J. Kerpelman, and D. Guilbert, "Gender Conflict; Identity Disruption and Marital Instability. Expanding Gottman's Model," *Journal of Social and Personal Relationships* 18, no. 1 (2001): 1107–1114; L. C. Gallo and T. W. Smith, "Attachment Style in Marriage: Adjustments and Responses to Interaction," *Journal of Social and Personal Relationships* 18, no. 2 (2001): 263–289; and J. Manusov and J. Harvey, eds., *Attribution, Communication Behavior, and Close Relationships* (New York: Cambridge University Press, 2001).

39. C. Gilligan, *In a Different Voice: Psychological Theory and Women's Development* (Cambridge, MA: Harvard University Press, 1982).
40. Ibid.
41. Ibid.
42. C. Morris and A. Maisto, *Psychology: An Introduction,* 12th ed. (Upper Saddle River, NJ: Prentice Hall, 2005).
43. Ibid.
44. M. Brenton, *Sex Talk* (New York: Stein and Day, 1972); J. Gottman, C. Notarius, and H. Markman, *A Couple's Guide to Communication* (Champaign, IL: Research Press, 1976).
45. M. McGill, *The McGill Report on Male Intimacy* (New York: Holt, Rinehart and Winston, 1985), 87–88.
46. M. Klausner and B. Hasselbring, *Aching for Love: The Sexual Drama of the Adult Child* (New York: Harper and Row, 1990).
47. Brehm, *Intimate Relationships.*
48. B. Strong, C. DeVault, and B. Sayad, *Human Sexuality* (Mountain View, CA: Mayfield Publishing, 1999), 219.
49. U.S. Census Bureau, "U.S. Adults Postponing Marriage, Census Bureau Reports," 2001, www.census.gov/Press-Release/www/releases/archives/population/000436.html
50. A. Greeff and H. L. Malherbe, "Intimacy and Marital Satisfaction in Spouses," *Journal of Sex and Marital Therapy* 27, no. 93 (May–June 2001) Special Issue: 247–257; "Is Your Love Life Making You Sick?" *Ebony* 56, no. 9 (July 2001): 38–41; L. Waite and M. Gallagher, *The Case for Marriage: Why Married People Are Healthier, Happier, and Better off Financially* (New York: Doubleday, 2000).
51. M. Young et al., "Sexual Satisfaction Among Married Women," *American Journal of Health Studies* 16, no. 2 (2000): 73–78.
52. R. Alsop, "As Same-Sex Households Grow More Mainstream, Businesses Take Note," *The Wall Street Journal* (August 8, 2001): B1, B4.
53. Ibid.
54. U.S. Census Bureau, "Marital Status of People 15 Years and Older, March 2002," June 2003, www.census.gov/population/www.socdemo/hh-fam.html; and Centers for Disease Control and Prevention, "Advance Data, First Marriage Dissolution, Divorce, and Remarriage: United States," 2001, www.cdc.gov/nchs/data/ad/ad323.pdf
55. Alsop, "As Same-Sex Households Grow."
56. National Center for Health Statistics, *National Vital Statistics Report* 49, no. 6 (August 2001).
57. U.S. Department of Labor Statistics, "Consumer Expenditure Survey," 2004, www.bls.gov/eex/csxover.htm
58. National Center for Health Statistics, "Births, Marriages, Divorces, and Deaths Provisional Data for 2003," *National Vital Statistics Report* 52, no. 22 (2004): 1120.
59. H. Markham, "Love Lessons: 6 New Moves to Improve your Relationship," *Psychology Today* (March/April 1997): 42–49.

CHAPTER 6
1. The National College Health Assessment (Baltimore, MD: American College Health Association [ACHA], 2000).
2. S. Shaw and J. Lee, "Learning Gender in a Diverse Society," *Women's Voices, Feminist Visions: Classic and Contemporary Readings* (Mountain View, CA: Mayfield Publishing, 2001).
3. American Psychological Association, "Lesbian, Gay, and Bisexual Concerns Policy Statements," 2004, www.apa.org/pi/lgbc/policy/statements.html
4. G. M. Herek, J. Roy Gillis, and J. C. Cogan, "Psychological Sequelae of Hate-Crime Victimization Among Lesbian, Gay and Bisexual Adults," *Journal of Consulting and Clinical Psychology* 67, no. 6 (1999): 945–951.
5. A. H. Slyper, "Childhood Obesity, Adipose Tissue Distribution, and the Pediatric Practitioner," *Pediatrics* 102 (1998): 4.
6. J. Endicott et al., "Is Premenstrual Dysphoric Disorder a Distinct Clinical Entity?" *Journal of Women's Health and Gender-Based Medicine* 8 (1999): 663–679; and F. R. Jelovesk, "Premenstrual Syndrome (PMS) vs. Premenstrual Dysphoric Disorder (PMDD)," Women's Diagnostic Cyber, 2000, (www.wdxcyber.com/nmood06.htm
7. Writing Group for the Women's Health Initiative Investigators, "Risk and Benefits of Estrogen Plus Progestin in Healthy Postmenopausal Women: Principal Results from the Women's Health Initiative Randomized Controlled Trial," *Journal of the American Medical Association* 288, no. 3 (2002): 321–333.
8. W. H. Masters and V. Johnson, *Human Sexual Response* (Boston: Little, Brown, 1966).
9. G. F. Kelly, "Sexual Individuality and Sexual Values," in *Sexuality Today: The Human Perspective,* updated 7th ed. (Dubuque, IA: McGraw-Hill, 2004).
10. Ibid.
11. R. T. Michael et al., *Sex in America: A Definitive Survey* (Boston: Little, Brown, 1994).
12. Ibid.
13. J. G. Beck, "Hypoactive Sexual Desire Disorder: An Overview," *Journal of Consulting and Clinical Psychology* 36, no. 6 (1995): 919–927.
14. National Kidney and Urological Diseases Information Clearinghouse, "Erectile Dysfunction," 2004, http://kidney.niddk.nih.gov/kudiseases/pubs/impotence/index.htm
15. B. Handy, "The Potency Pill," *Time* (May 4, 1998): 50–57.
16. Arnot Ogden Medical Center, "Frequently Asked Questions," 1998, www.aomc.org/HOD2/general/ViagraFAQ.html
17. S. A. Lyman, C. Hughes-McLain, and G. Thompson, "'Date-Rape Drugs': A Growing Concern," *Journal of Health Education* 29, no. 5 (1998): 271–274.

CHAPTER 7
1. World Health Organization, "Nonoxynol-9 Ineffective in Preventing HIV Infection," June 28, 2002, www.who.int/mediacentre/notes/release55/en
2. R. A. Hatcher et al., *Contraceptive Technology,* 17th revised ed. (New York: Ardent Media, 1998), 457.
3. R. A. Hatcher et al., *Contraceptive Technology,* 18th revised ed. (New York: Ardent Media, 2004).
4. National Center for Health Statistics, "Fertility, Family Planning, and Women's Health," 23 (1997): 7.
5. "FDA Approves Emergency Contraceptive Kit," College Health Report 1 (1998): 8.
6. Boston Women's Health Collective, *Our Bodies Ourselves for the New Century: A Book by Women and for Women* (New York: Simon and Schuster, 1998).
7. NARAL Pro-Choice America Foundation, "Who Decides? A State-by-State Report on the Status of Women's Reproductive Rights," 2004, www.naral.org
8. Allan Guttmacher Institute, "Facts in Brief: Induced Abortion," 2000, www.agi-usa.org
9. J. Gans Epner, H. Jonas, and D. Seckinger, "Late Term Abortion," *Journal of the American Medical Association* 280 (1998): 726.
10. D. A. Grimes and R. J. Cook, "Mifepristone (RU-486)—An Abortifacient to Prevent Abortion?," *The New England Journal of Medicine* 327, no. 15 (1992): 1041–1044.
11. N. F. Russo and A. J. Dabul, "The Relationship of Abortion to Well-Being: Do Race and Religion Make a Difference?," *Professional Psychology: Research and Practice* 28, no. 1 (2000): 23–31.
12. K. Schmidt, "The Dark Legacy of Fatherhood," *U.S. News and World Report* (December 14, 1992): 94–95.
13. Center for Nutrition Policy and Promotion, "Expenditure on Children by Families, 2003 Annual Report," 2004, www.usda.gov/cnpp/Crc/crc2003.pdf
14. Parenthood.com, "Containing the Costs of Childcare," 2004, www.parenthood.com

15. U.S. Department of Health and Human Services, "The Health Consequences of Smoking: What It Means to You," in *The 2004 Surgeon General's Report* (Washington, DC: Government Printing Office, 2004).

16. H. Klonoff-Cohen et al., "The Effects of Passive Smoking and Tobacco Exposure Through Breast Milk on Sudden Infant Death Syndrome," *Journal of the American Medical Association* 273 (1995): 795–798.

17. Centers for Disease Control and Prevention, "Cigarette Smoking Among Pregnant Women," *Women and Smoking: A Report of the Surgeon General,* 2001, www.cdc.gov/tobacco

18. American College of Obstetricians and Gynecologists, "Nutrition During Pregnancy," *Patient Education Pamphlet* (AP0001), March 1996.

19. National Down Syndrome Society, 2004, www.ndss.org

20. Eleena de Lisser, "Breast-Feeding Boosts Adult IQ, Research Suggests," *The Wall Street Journal* (May 8, 2002): D2.

21. M. Avery et al., "Factors Associated with Very Early Weaning Among Primiparas Intending to Breastfeed," *Maternal and Child Health Journal* 2 (1998): 167–179.

22. Centers for Disease Control and Prevention, "U.S Birth Rate Reaches Record Low," 2003, www.cdc.gov/nchs/releases /03news/lowbirth.htm

23. Centers for Disease Control and Prevention, "Pelvic Inflammatory Disease," 2002, www.cdc.gov.

24. Ibid.

25. K. Powell, "Fertility Treatments: Seeds of Doubt," *Nature* 422 (2003): 656–658.

CHAPTER 8

1. L. Crawford, Acting Commissioner of the FDA, "Remarks," Harvard Medical School 6th Postgraduate Nutrition Symposium, Cambridge, MA, March 10, 2004, www.fda.gov/oc/speeches /2004/harv0310.html

2. American Dietetic Association, "Nutrition and You Survey," 2002, www.eatright.org/pr/2002/052002a.html

3. American Institute of Cancer Research, "Food, Nutrition and the Prevention of Cancer: A Global Perspective," (Washington, DC: author, 1997).

4. Centers for Disease Control, "Health, United States, 2002. Overview of Obesity in the United States," www.cdc.gov

5. F. S. Sizer and E. N. Whitney, *Nutrition: Concepts and Controversies,* 9th ed. (Belmont, CA: Wadsworth, 2003), 590.

6. Ibid., 322.

7. Ibid., 10–11, 323.

8. National Center for Health Statistics, *Prevalence of Overweight and Obesity Among Adults: United States,* 1999, www.cdc.gov /nchs/products/pubs/pubd/hestats/obese/obse99/htm

9. U.S. Department of Health and Human Services, "Surgeon General's Call to Action to Prevent and Decrease Overweight and Obesity," July 7, 2004, www.surgeongeneral.gov/topics/obesity

10. Worldwatch Institute, "State of the World. Trends and Facts: Watching What We Eat," 2004, www.worldwatch.org/features /consumption/sow/trendsfacts/2004/06/02/

11. Ibid.

12. G. Block, "Foods Contributing to Energy Intake in the U.S.: Data from NHANES III and NHANES 1999–2000," *Journal of Food Composition and Analysis* 17, nos. 3–4 (2004): 439–447.

13. J. D. Wright et al., "Trends in Intake of Energy and Macronutrients—United States 1971–2000," *Morbidity and Mortality Weekly Report* (February 6, 2004).

14. D. Ludwig, "Obesity: A New Dietary Treatment for a Major Public Health Threat," paper presented at the Linus Pauling Institute International Conference on Diet and Optimum Health (Portland, OR: May 2001).

15. U.S. Department of Agriculture, "Questions and Answers About the Food Guide Pyramid," 2003, www.usda.gov/news/releases /2003/09/qa0308.htm

16. B. Black, "Healthgate: Just How Much Food IS on That Plate? Understanding Portion Control," 2004, http://community .healthgate.com/getcontent.asp?siteid = contentupdate&docid = /healthy

17. American Dietetic Association, "American Dietetic Association Survey Shows Americans Can Use Some Help in Sizing Up Their Meals," May 20, 2002, www.eatright.org/pr/2002 /052002b.html

18. Sizer and Whitney, *Nutrition,* 38.

19. Ibid.

20. Ibid.

21. "Proteins," *Harvard Women's Health Watch,* 5 (1998): 4.

22. Ibid., 4.

23. J. W. White and M. Wolraich, "Effect of Sugar on Behavior or Cognition in Children: A Meta-Analysis," *Journal of the American Medical Association* 274 (1995): 1617–1621.

24. "Is Sugar Really Addictive?" *Tufts University Health and Nutrition Letter: Special Report* 20, no. 8 (2002): 1–4.

25. "Do Potato Chips Cause Cancer? Don't Panic Yet, Say Experts," *Environmental Nutrition* 25, no. 6 (June 2002): 3.

26. Center for Science in the Public Interest, "New Tests Confirm Acrylamide in American Foods—Snack Chips and French Fries Show Highest Levels of Known Carcinogens," www.cspinet.org /new/200206251.html

27. M. Pereira et al., "Dietary Fiber and Risk of Coronary Heart Disease: A Pooled Analysis of Cohort Studies," *Archives of Internal Medicine* 164, no. 4 (2004): 370–376.

28. Ibid.

29. Ibid., 170.

30. C. Fuchs et al., "Dietary Fiber and the Risk of Colorectal Cancer and Adenoma in Women," *New England Journal of Medicine* 340 (1999): 169–176.

31. M. Pereira et al., "Dietary Fiber and Risk."

32. American Dietetic Association, "Position Statement: Diabetic Care," *Journal of the American Dietetic Association,* 1 (22 suppl.) (1999): 542.

33. R. Mensink and M. Katan, "Effect of Dietary Trans-Fatty Acids on High-Density and Low-Density Lipoprotein and Cholesterol Levels in Healthy Subject," *New England Journal of Medicine* 323, no. 7: 339–343.

34. G. Ruoff, "Reducing Fat Intake with Fat Substitutes," *American Family Physician* 43 (1991): 1235–1242.

35. World Cancer Research Fund and the American Institute for Cancer Research, *Food, Nutrition, and the Prevention of Cancer: A Global Perspective* (1997).

36. W. Willet and A. Ascherio, "Health Effects of Trans-Fatty Acids," *American Journal of Clinical Nutrition* 66 (1997): 1006S–1010S.

37. E. Whitney and S. Rolfes, *Understanding Nutrition,* 8th ed. (Belmont, CA: Wadsworth, 1999), 3–4.

38. American Heart Association, Nutrition Advisory Committee, News Release on *trans* fatty acids, May 13, 1994.

39. Willet and Ascherio, "Health Effects of Trans Fatty Acids."

40. Whitney and Rolfes, *Understanding Nutrition,* 144.

41. E. M. Ward, "Balancing Essential Dietary Fats: When More Might Be Better," *Environmental Nutrition* 24, no. 12 (2002): 1–6.

42. Ibid.

43. "MUFAs and PUFAs," *Food and Fitness Advisor* 9, (September 2002).

44. "The CLA Paradox," *American Institute for Cancer Research Newsletter* 78 (Winter 2003): 8–9.

45. "MUFAs and PUFAs," *Food and Fitness Advisor* (September 2002).

46. Institute of Medicine, "Dietary Reference Intake for Water, Potassium, Sodium, Chloride, and Sulfate," March 4, 2004, www.nap.edu

47. J. Midgley et al., "Effects of Reduced Dietary Sodium on Blood Pressure: A Meta-Analysis of Randomized Controlled Trials," *Journal of the American Medical Association* 275 (1996): 1590–1598.

48. Whitney and Rolfes, *Understanding Nutrition,* 412.

49. A. C. Looker et al., "Prevalence of Iron Deficiency in the United States," *Journal of the American Medical Association* 277 (1997): 973–976; "Recommendations to Prevent and Control Iron Deficiency in the United States," *Morbidity and Mortality Weekly Report* 47 (1998 supplement).

50. G. T. Sempos, A. C. Looker, and R. E. Gillum, "Iron and Heart Disease: The Epidemiological Data," *Nutrition Reviews* 54 (1996): 73–84.

51. Whitney and Rolfes, *Understanding Nutrition,* 412.

52. "Food as Medicine," *Harvard Women's Health Watch* 5 (1998): 4–5.

53. Sizer and Whitney, *Nutrition,* 257.

54. Ibid., 260.

55. M. Manore and J. Thompson, *Sport Nutrition for Health and Performance* (Champaign, IL: Human Kinetics Publishing, 2000), 283.

56. E. Giovanucci et al., "Intake of Carotenoids and Retinol in Relation to Risk of Prostate Cancer," *Journal of the National Cancer Institute* 87 (1995): 1767.

57. H. Gerster, "The Potential Role of Lycopene for Human Health," *Journal of American College Nutrition* 16 (1997): 109–126; T. H. Rissonanen et al. "Low Serum Lycopene Concentration Is Associated with an Excess Incidence of Acute Coronary Events and Stroke," *British Journal of Nutrition* 85 (2001): 749–754.

58. "Kale, Collards and Spinach Beat Carrots for Protecting Aging Eyes," *Environmental Nutrition* 24, 4 (2001).

59. Ibid.

60. J. Carper, "Eat Smart," *USA Weekend* (May 3–5, 2002): p. 6.

61. J. Smythies, *Every Person's Guide to Antioxidants* (Newark, NJ: Rutgers University Press, 1998).

62. B. Frie, Linus Pauling Institute Seminar Series (Portland, OR: 2000).

63. R. Malinow, "Homocysteine, Folic Acid and CVD." Paper presented at the Linus Pauling Institute International Conference on Diet and Optimum Health (Portland, OR: May 2001).

64. Ibid.

65. N. T. Crane, V. S. Hubbard, and C. J. Lewis, "National Nutrition Objectives and Dietary Guidelines for Americans," *Nutrition Today* 33 (1998): 186–188.

66. Ibid.

67. L. K. Mahan and S. Escott-Stump, *Krause's Food, Nutrition, and Diet Therapy* (Philadelphia: Saunders, 2000), 343–345.

68. S. Loft, "Diet, Oxidative DNA Damage and Cancer" and L. Kolonel, "Overview of Diet and Cancer Epidemiology." Papers presented at the Linus Pauling Institute International Conference on Diet and Optimum Health (Portland, OR: May 2001).

69. K. M. Fairfield and R. H. Fletcher, "Vitamins for Chronic Disease Prevention in Adults: Scientific Review," *Journal of the American Medical Association* 287, no. 23 (2001): 3116–3126.

70. D. Bender, "Daily Doses of Multivitamin Tablets," editorial in the *British Medical Journal* 325, no. 174 (July 27): 173–174.

71. Centers for Disease Control and Prevention, Center for Infectious Diseases, "Food Borne Illnesses," 2002, www.cdc.gov; American Medical Association, "Diagnosis and Management of Foodborne Illness: A Primer for Physicians and Other Health Care Professionals," 2004, www.ama-assn.org/ama/org

72. Ibid.

73. Ibid.

74. Ibid.

75. Ibid.

76. L. Hughes, "Don't Let Unexpected Visitors 'Spoil' Summer Meals," *Environmental Nutrition* 25, no. 6 (June 2002): 2.

77. P. Morris, Y. Motarjemi, and F. Kaferstein, "Emerging Food-Borne Diseases," *World Health* 50 (1997): 16–22; Centers for Disease Control and Prevention "Food Borne Illnesses."

78. "Special Report: Irradiation Plants Geared to 'Zap' Meat and Poultry—Is it Safe?" *Tufts University Health and Nutrition Letter* 18, no. 1 (2000): 4–7.

79. Ibid., 5.

80. National Institute of Allergy and Infectious Diseases, "Fact Sheet: Food Allergy and Intolerances," August 2002, www.niaid.gov/factsheets/food.htm

81. Ibid.

CHAPTER 9

1. Centers for Disease Control and Prevention, *Behavioral Risk Factor Surveillance System,* 2003, www.cdc.gov/brfss

2. Ibid.

3. National Center for Health Statistics, "National Health and Nutrition Examination Survey IV—Part I," 2004, www.cdc.gov/nchs/nhanes.htm

4. A. H. Mokdad et al., "Actual Causes of Death in the United States—2000," *Journal of the American Medical Association* 291 (2004): 1238–1245.

5. C. Rodrigues, K. Walker-Thurmond and M. Thun, "Overweight, Obesity, and Cancer Rise," *New England Journal of Medicine* 348 (2003): 1625–1638; S. Konchicah et al., "Obesity and the Rise of Heart Failure," *New England Journal of Medicine* 347 (2002): 305–313.

6. J. P. Boyle et al., *Diabetes Care* 24, no. 11 (2001): 1936–1940.

7. E. A. Finkelstein, I. C. Fiebelkorn, and G. Wang, "National Medical Spending Attributable to Overweight and Obesity: How Much, and Who's Paying?" *Health Affairs,* 2003, http://content.healthaffairs.org/cgi/content/full/hlthaff.w3.219v1/DC1

8. E. A. Finkelstein, I. C. Fiebelkorn, and G. Wang, "State-Level Estimates of Annual Medical Expenditures Attributable to Obesity," *Obesity Research* 12 (2004): 18–24.

9. G. Cowley, "Generation XXL," *Newsweek* (July 3, 2000): 40–46.

10. A. Peeters et al., "Adult Obesity and the Burden of Disability Throughout Life," *Obesity Research* 12 (2004): 1145–1151.

11. National Center for Chronic Disease Prevention and Health Promotion, "Nutrition: Defining Overweight and Obesity," September 2002, www.cdc.gov/nccdphp/dnpa/obesity/defining.htm

12. Weight-Control Information Network, "Statistics Related to Overweight and Obesity," 2003, www.niddk.nih.gov/health/nutrit/pubs/statobes.htm

13. National Center for Chronic Disease Prevention and Health Promotion, "Nutrition."

14. National Center for Health Statistics, "Prevalence of Overweight and Obesity," 2004, www.cdc.gov/nchs/products/pubs/pubd/estats/obese/obse99.htm

15. Ibid.

16. Ibid.

17. Ibid.

18. D. Eberwine, "Globesity: The Crisis of Growing Proportions," *Perspectives in Health* 7, no. 3 (2003): 9.

19. Dietary Guidelines Research Committee, "Dietary Guidelines for Americans," 2000, www.ars.usda.gov/dgac/2kdiet.pdf

20. National Center for Chronic Disease Prevention and Health Promotion, "Nutrition."

21. S. Cummings, K. Goodrick, and J. Foreyt, "Position of the American Dietetic Association: Weight Management," *Journal of the American Dietetic Association* 102 (2002): 1145–1155.

22. J. G. Meisler and S. St. Jeor, "Summary and Recommendations from the American Health Foundation's Expert Panel on Healthy Weight," *American Journal of Clinical Nutrition* 63 (1996): 474S–477S.

23. U.S. Department of Health and Human Services, "The Surgeon General's Call to Action to Prevent and Decrease Overweight and Obesity," 2001, www.surgeongeneral.gov/topics/obesity

24. Weight-Control Information Network, "Statistics Related to Overweight and Obesity."

25. U.S. Department of Health and Human Services, "Surgeon General's Call to Action."

26. S. A. French, M. Story, and R. W. Jeffrey, "Environmental Influences on Eating and Physical Activity," *Annual Review Public Health* 22 (2001): 309–335.

27. L. Young and M. Nestle, "Expanding Portion Sizes in the U.S. Marketplace: Implications for Nutrition Counseling," *Journal of the American Dietetic Association* 103 (2003): 231–234.

28. J. D. Wright et al., "Trends in Intake of Energy and Macronutrients—United States 1971–2000," *Morbidity and Mortality Weekly Report,* February 6, 2004.

29. M. W. Gillman et al., "Risk of Overweight Among Adolescents Who were Breastfed as Infants," *Journal of the American Medical Association* 285 (2001): 2461–2467; M. L. Hediger et al., "Association between Infant Breastfeeding and Overweight in Young Children," *Journal of the American Medical Association* 285 (2001): 2453–2460.

30. National Center for Health Statistics, "Prevalence of Overweight and Obesity."

31. C. J. Crespo et al., "Television Watching, Energy Intake, and Obesity in U.S. Children: Results from the Third National Health and Nutrition Examination Survey," *Archives of Pediatric and Adolescent Medicine* 155 (2001): 360–365; W. H. Dietz, "The Obesity Epidemic in Young Children: Reduce Television Viewing and Promote Playing," *British Medical Journal* 322 (2001): 313–324.

32. M. Dowda et al., "Environmental Influences, Physical Activity, and Weight Status in 8–12 Year Olds," *Archives of Pediatric and Adolescent Medicine* 155 (2001): 711–717.

33. Ibid, 715.

34. E. Snyder et al. "The Human Obesity Gene Map: 2003 Update," *Obesity Research* 12 (2003): 369–439.

35. Mayo Clinic "Special Report: Weight Control," *Women's HealthSource* (1987): 3.

36. R. J. Loos and C. Bouchard, "Obesity—Is It a Genetic Disorder?" *Journal of Internal Medicine* 254, no. 5 (2003): 401–425.

37. Ibid.

38. Ibid.

39. Ibid.

40. L. K. Mahan and S. Escott-Stump, *Krause's Food, Nutrition, and Diet Therapy* (Philadelphia: Saunders, 2004).

41. R. J. Loos, and C. Bouchard, "Obesity—Is It a Genetic Disorder?"

42. Ibid.

43. "Genes and Appetite," *Harvard Women's Health Watch* (January 1996); L. Tartaglia et al., "Identification and Expression Cloning of a Leptin Receptor," *Cell* 83 (1995): 1263–1271.

44. M. Saad et al., "Genes for Hunger Hormones Play Role in Obesity," *Journal of Clinical Endocrinology and Metabolism* 87 (2002): 3997–4000, 4005–4008.

45. D. E. Cummings et al., "Plasma Ghrelin Levels After Diet-Induced Weight Loss or Gastric Bypass Surgery," *New England Journal of Medicine* 346, no. 21 (2002): 1623–1630.

46. M. Turton, D. O'Shea, I. Gunn et al., "A Role of Glucagon-Like Peptide 1 in the Central Regulation of Feeding," *Nature* 379 (1996): 69–72.

47. American Diabetes Association, "Press Release: Gut Hormone Shown to Affect Obesity and Diabetes," June 16, 2003, www.diabetes.org/for-media/scientific-sessions/06-13-03.jsp

48. Mayo Clinic, "Special Report: Weight Control," 4.

49. L. K. Mahan and S. Escott-Stump, *Krause's Food, Nutrition, and Diet Therapy.*

50. G. B. Forbes, "Childhood and Adolescent Obesity: Causes and Consequences, Prevention and Management," *New England Journal of Medicine* 349 (2003): 619.

51. S. Lichman et al., "Discrepancy between Self-Reported and Actual Caloric Intake and Exercise in Obese Subjects," *New England Journal of Medicine* 327 (1992): 1894–1897.

52. Y. Rolland et al., "Muscle Strength in Obese Elderly Women: Effect of Physical Activity in a Cross-Sectional Study," *American Journal of Clinical Nutrition* 79 (2004): 552–557; K. Hallsten et al., "Insulin- and Exercise-Stimulated Skeletal Muscle Blood Flow and Glucose Uptake in Obese Men," *Obesity Research* 11 (2003): 257–265.

53. K. Brownell, "Comments on the Latest Study on Yo-Yo Diets by Steven Blair of the Institute for Aerobics Research" (paper originally presented in 1993, newer report in paper presented at Oregon State University by Steven Blair, Fall, 1998).

54. National Center for Health Statistics, "Prevalence of Sedentary Leisure-Time Behavior Among Adults in the United States," December 2000, www.cdc.gov/nchs/products/pubs/pubd/hestats/3and4/sedentary.htm

55. Ibid.

56. Ibid.

57. "Special Report: Weight Control," 4.

58. I. Rashad and M. Grossman, "Economics of Obesity," *The Public Interest* 156 (2004), www.thepublicinterest.com/previous/article3.html

59. Mayo Clinic, "Special Report: Weight Control," 4.

60. N. Diehl, C. Johnson, and R. Rogers, "Social Physique Anxiety and Disordered Eating: What's the Connection?" *Addictive Behaviors* 23 (1998): 1–16.

61. *USA Today Weekend* (July 14–16, 2000): 6.

62. R. L. Atkinson, "Use of Drugs in the Treatment of Obesity," *Annual Review of Nutrition* 17 (1997): 383–403, as reported in E. Whitney and S. R. Rolfes, *Understanding Nutrition,* 9th ed. (Belmont, CA: Wadsworth, 2002), 278.

63. "Fen-Phen Legal Resources," 2002, www.fen-phen-legal-resources.com

64. Food and Drug Administration, "FDA Approves Orlistat for Obesity," 1999, www.fda.gov/bbs/topics/ANSWERS/ANS00951.html

65. U.S. Food and Drug Administration Center for Drug Evaluation and Research, "Phenylpropanolamine (PPA) Information Page," 2004, www.fda.gov/cder/drug/infopage/ppa

66. E. Whitney and S. R. Rolfes, *Understanding Nutrition,* 279.

67. L. Busetto et al., "Short-Term Effects of Weight Loss on the Cardiovascular Risk Factors in Morbidly Obese Patients," *Obesity Research* 12 (2004): 1256–1263.

68. M. Schwartz et al., "Weight Bias Among Health Professionals Specializing in Obesity," *Obesity Research* 11 (2003): 1033–1039; J. Latner and A. Stunkard, "Getting Worse: The Stigmatization of Obese Children," *Obesity Research* 11 (2003): 452–456.

69. "Eating Disorders," *Harvard Mental Health Letter* 14 (1997): 4.

70. Substance Abuse and Mental Health Services Administration, "SAMHSA's Mental Health Information Center: Eating Disorders," 2004, www.mentalhealth.samhsa.org/publications/allpubs/KEN98-0047

CHAPTER 10

1. Centers for Disease Control and Prevention, "Physical Activity and Health: A Report of the Surgeon General," 1996, www.cdc.gov/nccdphp/sgr/mm.htm; National Center for Chronic Disease Prevention and Health Promotion, "The Surgeon General's Call to Action to Prevent and Decrease Overweight and Obesity," 2002, www.cdc.gov

2. Centers for Disease Control and Prevention, "Physical Activity and Health: The Link between Physical Activity and Morbidity and Mortality," 1996, www.cdc.gov/nccdphp/sgr/mm.htm

3. National Institutes of Mental Health, "Statistics," 2004, www.nimh.nih.gov/healthinformation/statisticsmenu.cfm

4. C. A. Macera et al., "Prevalence of Physical Activity, Including Lifestyle Activities Among Adults—U.S. 2000-2001," *Morbidity and Mortality Weekly Report* 52, no. 32 (2003): 764-769.

5. Centers for Disease Control, "Physical Activity and Health."

6. Ibid.

7. National Center for Chronic Disease Prevention and Health Promotion, "Nutrition and Physical Activity Recommendations," 2004, www.cdc.gov/nccdphp/dnpa/physical/recommendations/index.htm.

8. Ibid.

9. C. B. Corbin and R. Lindsey, *Concepts in Physical Education with Laboratories,* 8th ed. (Dubuque, IA: Times Mirror, 1994).

10. Centers for Disease Control, "Physical Activity and Health."

11. J. C. Bolen et al., "State-specific Prevalence of Selected Health Behaviors by Race and Ethnicity," *Behavioral Risk Factor Surveillance System 1997* 49, ssu 2 (2000): 1-60.

12. C. J. Newscaffer, R. C. Brownson, and L. J. Dusenberry, "Cardiovascular Disease" in *Chronic Disease Epidemiology and Control,* eds. R. C. Brownson, P. L. Remington, and J. R. Davis (Washington, DC: American Public Health Association, 1998).

13. K. J. Stewart, "Exercise Guidance in Hypertension," *The Physician and Sportsmedicine,* 28(10) (Oct 2000).

14. G. A. Colditz, et al. "Physical Activity and Risk of Breast Cancer in Premenopausal Women," *British Journal of Cancer* 89, no. 5 (2003): 847-851.

15. American Cancer Society, "Colon Cancer and Exercise," July 20, 1999, www.cancer.org

16. T. J. Key et al., "Diet, Nutrition, and the Prevention of Cancer," *Public Health Nutrition,* (February 7, 2004) (1A): 187-200.

17. National Osteoporosis Foundation, "Fast Facts," 2004, www.nof.org

18. Osteoporosis and Related Bone Disease National Resource Center, "Fast Facts on Osteoporosis," 2001, www.osteo.org/osteofastfact.html

19. C. M. Snow, J. M. Shaw, and C. C. Matkin, "Physical Activity and Risk for Osteoporosis," in *Osteoporosis,* eds. R. Marcus, D. Feldman, and J. Kelsey (San Diego: Academic Press, 1996), 511-528.

20. C. Snow and T. Hayes, "Bone Health" (guest lecture, Modern Maladies class, Oregon State University, Corvallis, OR, 2001).

21. W. McArdle, F. Katch, and V. Katch, *Exercise Physiology,* 5th ed. (Philadelphia: Lippincott, Williams and Wilkins, 2001), 60-65.

22. J. M. Jakacic et al., "Appropriate Intervention Strategies for Weight Loss and Prevention of Weight Regain for Adults," *Medicine and Science in Sports and Exercise* 33, no. 12 (2001): 2145-2156.

23. R. Ross, J. A. Freeman, and I. Janssen, "Exercise Alone Is an Effective Strategy for Reducing Obesity and Related Comorbidities," *Exercise and Sport Sciences Reviews* 28, no. 4, (2000): 165-170.

24. American Diabetes Association, "Diabetes Risk Test," 2004, www.diabetes.org/risk-test.jsp

25. S. P. Helmrich, D. R. Ragland, and R. S. Paffenbarger, Jr., "Prevention of Non-Insulin-Dependent Diabetes Mellitus with Physical Activity," *Medicine and Science in Sports and Exercise* 26 (1994): 824-830.

26. J. Shaw, "The Deadliest Sin," *Harvard Magazine* (March/April 2004).

27. Centers for Disease Control, "*Physical Activity and Health.*"

28. P. Palatini et al., "Exercise Capacity and Mortality," *New England Journal of Medicine,* 374, no. 4 (2002): 288.

29. E. Quinn, "Exercise and Immunity," *Sports Medicine,* 2004, http://sportsmedicine.about.com/cs/exercisephysiology/a/aa100303a.htm

30. D. C. Neiman, "Is Infection Risk Linked to Exercise Workload?" *Medicine and Science in Sports and Exercise* 32, no. 7 Suppl (2000): S406-S411.

31. E. R. Eichner, "Infection, Immunity, and Exercise: What to Tell Patients?" *The Physician and Sportsmedicine* 21 (January 1993): 125-135.

32. D. C. Neiman, and B. K. Pederson, "Exercise and Immune Function: Recent Developments," *Sports Medicine* 27, no. 2 (1999): 73-80.

33. R. Gates, "Fitness Is Changing the World: For Women," *IDEA Today* (July–August 1992): 58.

34. E. T. Howley and D. B. Franks, *Health Fitness Instructor's Handbook,* 2nd ed. (Champaign, IL: Human Kinetics Books, 1992).

35. Centers for Disease Control and Prevention, "Measuring Physical Activity Intensity," 2004, www.cdc.gov/nccdphp/dnpa/physical/measuring/index.htm

36. American Council on Exercise, "Calorie Burners: Activities That Turn up the Heat," 2004, www.acefitness.org/fitfacts

37. American College of Sports Medicine, "ACSM Position Stand on the Recommended Quantity and Quality of Exercise for Developing and Maintaining Cardiorespiratory and Muscular Fitness, and Flexibility in Adults," *Medicine and Science in Sports and Exercise* 30 (1998): 975-991.

38. Ibid.

39. M. Cyphers, "Flexibility," in *Personal Trainer Manual,* 2nd ed. (San Diego: American Council on Exercise, 1996), 291-308.

40. T. D. Fahey, *Basic Weight Training for Men and Women,* 5th ed. (San Francisco: McGraw-Hill, 2004).

41. Ibid.

42. M. S. Feigenbaum and M. L. Pollock, "Prescription of Resistance Training for Health and Disease," *Medicine and Science in Sports and Exercise* 31 (1999): 38-45.

43. American College of Sports Medicine, "ACSM Position Stand."

44. C. L. Wells, *Women, Sport, and Performance: A Physiological Perspective,* 2nd ed. (Champaign, IL: Human Kinetics, 1991).

45. W. C. Whiting and R. F. Zernicke, *Biomechanics of Musculoskeletal Injury* (Champaign, IL: Human Kinetics, 1998).

46. D. M. Brody, *Clinical Symposia: Running Injuries: Prevention and Management* 39 (1987).

47. J. C. Erie, "Eye Injuries: Prevention, Evaluation, and Treatment," *The Physician and Sportsmedicine* 19 (November 1991): 108-122.

48. Bicycle Helmet Safety Institute, "A Compendium of Statistics," 2004, www.bhsi.org/stats.htm

49. S. M. Simons, "Foot Injuries of the Recreational Athlete," *The Physician and Sportsmedicine* 27 (January 1999): 57-70.

50. C. J. Couture and K. A. Karlson, "Tibial Stress Injuries: Decisive Diagnosis and Treatment of 'Shin Splints,'" *The Physician and Sportsmedicine* 30, no. 6 (2002):

51. G. I. Drosos and J. L. Pozo, "The Causes and Mechanisms of Meniscal Injuries in the Sporting and Non-sporting Environment in a Selected Population," *Knee* 11, no. 2 (2004): 143-149.

52. American Academy of Orthopaedic Surgeons (AAOS), *Athletic Training and Sports Medicine,* 3rd ed., (Park Ridge, IL: AAOS, 2000).

53. N. M. Lugo-Amador, T. Rothenhaus, and P. Mover, "Heat Related Illness," *Emergency Medical Clinics of North America* 22, no. 2 (2004): 315-327.

54. J. J. Mistovich, B. Q. Hafen, and K. J. Karren, *Prehospital Emergency Care,* 6th ed. (Upper Saddle River, NJ: Prentice Hall, 2000).

55. International Fitness Association, *Aerobics and Fitness Institute Certification Coursebook,* 2004, http://ifafitness.com/book1

56. D. J. Casa et al., "National Athletic Trainers' Association Position Statement: Fluid Replacement for Athletes," *Journal of Athletic Training* 35, no. 2, (2000): 212-224.

57. American College of Sports Medicine, "Position Stand—Exercise and Fluid Replacement," *Medicine and Science in Sports and Exercise* 28 (January 1996): i-vii.

58. D. J. Casa et al., "NATA Position Statement: Fluid Replacement for Athletes," *Journal of Athletic Training* 35, no. 2 (2000): 212–224.

59. R. Sallis and C. M. Chassay, "Recognizing and Treating Common Cold-induced Injury in Outdoor Sports," *Medicine and Science in Sports and Exercise* 31, no. 10 (1999): 1367–1373.

60. American College of Sports Medicine, "Position Stand—Heat and Cold Illnesses During Distance Running," *Medicine and Science in Sports and Exercise* 28 (December 1996): i–x.

61. N. Clark, "Muscle Cramps: Do They Cramp Your Style?" *Newsletter of the American College of Sports Medicine* (Summer 2001): 7.

62. Ibid.

63. Ibid.

64. Ibid.

CHAPTER 11

1. H. F. Doweiko, *Concepts of Chemical Dependency* (Belmont, CA: Wadsworth, 2001), 11.

2. R. Goldberg, *Drugs Across the Spectrum* (Pacific Grove, CA: Brooks/Cole, 2002), 17.

3. K. Blum and J. E. Payne, *Alcohol and the Addictive Brain* (New York: The Free Press, 1991), 186.

4. National Institute on Alcohol Abuse and Alcoholism, "Alcohol Alert 18: Genetic Influences," October 2000, www.niaaa.nih .gov/publications.aa18.htm

5. J. Kinney, *Loosening the Grip* (Boston: McGraw-Hill, 2003), 103.

6. G. Hansen and P. Venturelli, *Drugs and Society,* 7th ed. (Sudbury, MA: Jones & Bartlett, 2002), 49.

7. Ibid., 4.

8. Ibid.

9. L. Kurtz, *Self Help and Support Groups: A Handbook for Practitioners* (Thousand Oaks, CA: Sage, 1997), 12.

10. J. R. Wilson and J. A. Wilson, *Addictionary* (New York: Simon & Schuster, 1992), 166.

11. C. Nakken, *The Addictive Personality* (Center City, MN: Hazelden, 1996), 24.

12. National Council on Problem Gambling, "Fact Sheets," September 1, 2004, www.ncpgambling.org

13. J. W. Welte et al., "Gambling Participation and Pathology in the United States," *Addictive Behaviors* 29, no. 5 (2004): 983–989.

14. D. Engwall et al., "Gambling and Other Risk Behaviors on University Campuses," *Journal of American College Health* 56, no. 6 (2004): 245–255.

15. Performance Resource Press, "Health Sentry Newsletter" 15, no. 1 (2002), www.prponline.net

16. B. Yoder, *The Resource Recovery Book* (New York: Simon & Schuster, 1992), 259.

17. R. Olivardia, H. Pope, and J. Hudson, "Muscle Dysmorphia in Male Weightlifters: A Case-Control Study," *American Journal of Psychiatry* 157 (2000): 1291–1296.

18. M. Maine, *Body Wars: Making Peace with Women's Bodies* (Carlsbad, CA: Gurze, 2000), 282.

19. K. Young et al., "Cyber-Disorders: The Mental Health Concern for the New Millennium," paper presented at 107th APA convention, August 20, 1999, www.netaddiction.com/articles /cyberdisorders.htm

20. K. Young, "Net Compulsions: The Latest Trends in the Area of Internet Addiction," 1999, www.netaddiction.com/net _compulsions.htm

21. Ibid.

22. Nakken, *The Addictive Personality,* 16.

23. Wilson and Wilson, *Addictionary,* 167.

24. National Institute on Alcohol Abuse and Alcoholism, Alcohol Alert Number 36, *Patient-Treatment Matching,* April 1997.

CHAPTER 12

1. L. D. Johnson, P. M. O'Malley, and J. G. Bachman, *The Monitoring the Future Study,* 1975–2002, vol. 2 (Rockville, MD: NIDA, 2003).

2. A. Cohen, "Battle of the Binge," *Time* (September 8, 1997).

3. H. Wechsler et al., "Trends in College Binge Drinking During a Period of Increased Prevention Efforts: Findings from Four Harvard School of Public Health College Study Surveys: 1993–2001," *Journal of American College Health* 50, no. 5 (2002): 207.

4. Johnson, O'Malley, and Bachman, *Monitoring the Future Study.*

5. Wechsler et al., "Trends in College Binge Drinking."

6. H. Wechsler et al., "College Binge Drinking in the 1990s: A Continuing Problem," *Journal of American College Health* 28 (2000): 202.

7. J. Knight et al., "Alcohol Abuse and Dependence among U.S. College Students," *Journal of Studies on Alcohol* 63, no. 3 (2002): 263–270.

8. T. M. Nephew et al., "Surveillance Report #62: Apparent per Capita Alcohol Consumption: National, State, and Regional Trends, 1977–2000," 2003, www.niaaa.nih.gov/publications /surveillance62/CONS00.htm

9. National Institutes of Health, "Alcohol: A Women's Health Issue," 2003, www.niaaa.nih.gov/publications/brochurewomen /women.htm

10. C. Ikonomidou et al., "Ethanol-Induced Apoptotic Neurodegeneration and the Fetal Alcohol Syndrome," *Science* 287 (2000): 1056–1060.

11. National Organization on Fetal Alcohol Syndrome, www.nofas.org

12. National Highway Traffic Safety Administration, "Traffic Safety Facts, 2002—Alcohol," 2003, www.nhtsa.dot.gov

13. H. Wechsler et al., "Changes in Binge Drinking and Related Problems among American College Students Between 1993 and 1997," *Journal of American College Health* 47, no. 2 (1998): 57–68.

14. National Highway Traffic Safety Administration, "Traffic Safety Facts, 1996—Alcohol," Washington, DC: National Center for Statistics and Analysis, 1997.

15. National Highway Traffic Safety Administration, "Crash Stats: Alcohol-Related Fatalities by State, 2003," 2004, www .nhtsa.dot.gov

16. National Highway Traffic and Safety Administration, "Traffic Safety Facts, 2002—Alcohol," www.nhtsa.dot.gov

17. Ibid.

18. Insurance Institute for Highway Safety. "Fatality Facts: Alcohol 2003," www.iihs.org

19. Ibid.

20. Substance Abuse and Mental Health Services Administration, *Results from the 2003 National Survey on Drug Use and Health: National Findings* (Office of Applied Studies, NHSDA Series H-24, DHHS Publication No. SMA 04-3963), (Rockville, MD, 2004).

21. F. K. Goodwin and E. M. Gause, "Alcohol, Drug Abuse, and Mental Health Administration," *Prevention Pipeline* 3 (1990): 19.

22. M. A. Shockit, "New Findings on Genetics of Alcoholism," *Journal of American Medical Association* 281, no. 20 (1999): 1875–1976.

23. W. S. Slutske et al., "The Heritability of Alcoholism Symptoms: Indicators of Environmental Influence in Alcohol Dependent Individuals—Revisited," *Alcoholism and Experimental Research* 23, no. 5 (1999): 759.

24. "Adult Children of Alcoholics," *Alcohol Issues and Solutions* 6, no. 2 (2000): 6.

25. B. F. Grant, "Estimates of U.S. Children Exposed to Alcohol Abuse and Dependence in the Family," *American Journal of Public Health* 90, no. 1 (2000).

26. U.S. Department of Health and Human Services, *Tenth Special Report to the U.S. Congress on Alcohol and Health* (2000): 273.

27. F. Blow et al., "Use and Misuse of Alcohol Among Older Women," *Alcohol Research and Health* 26, no. 4 (2002): 308.

28. National Institute on Drug Abuse, "Info Facts: Treatment Methods for Women," August 30, 2004, www.nida.nih.gov/Infofax/treatwomen.html

CHAPTER 13

1. W. Max, "The Financial Impact of Smoking on Health-Related Costs: A Review of the Literature," *American Journal of Health Promotion* 15 (2001): 321–331.

2. Centers for Disease Control and Prevention, "Annual Smoking-Attributable Mortality, Years of Potential Life Lost, and Economic Costs—United States," *Morbidity and Mortality Report*, 51, no. 14 (2002): 300–303.

3. Centers for Disease Control and Prevention, "Trends in Cigarette Smoking Among High School Students—United States, 1991–2001," *Morbidity and Mortality Weekly* 51, no. 19 (2002): 409–412.

4. Centers for Disease Control and Prevention, "Annual Smoking-Attributable Mortality."

5. N. Rigotti, J. Lee, and H. Wechsler, "U.S. College Students' Use of Tobacco Products," *Journal of the American Medical Association* 284 (2000): 699–705.

6. S. A. Everett et al., "Smoking Initiation and Smoking Patterns Among U.S. College Students," *Journal of American College Health* 48 (1999): 55.

7. American Cancer Society, "The Facts About Secondhand Smoke," 2004, www.cancer.org

8. American Lung Association, "Trends in Cigarette Smoking," March 1999, www.lungusa.org

9. S. Hansen, "Bidis," University of Iowa's Student Health Service/Health Iowa, 2003, www.uiowa.edu/~shs

10. American Cancer Society, *Cancer Facts and Figures 2004* (Atlanta: American Cancer Society, 2004), 17.

11. National Institute on Drug Abuse Research Report Series, "Nicotine Addiction." (USDHHS Publication No. 01-4342) (Bethesda, MD, 2001).

12. National Institute on Drug Abuse, "Evidence Builds that Genes Influence Cigarette Smoking." NIDA Notes. (NIDA Publication No. 00–3478) (Bethesda, MD: USDHHS, 2000).

13. American Cancer Society, *Cancer Facts and Figures 2004*, 38.

14. Ibid.

15. Ibid.

16. World Health Organization Collaborative Study of Cardiovascular Disease and Steroid Hormone Contraception, "Acute Myocardial Infarction and Combined Oral Contraceptives: Results of an International Multicentre Case-Control Study," *Lancet* (April 26, 1997): 1202–1209.

17. American Cancer Society, *Cancer Facts and Figures, 2004.*

18. American Academy of Periodontology, "Tobacco Use and Periodontal Disease," 2004, www.perio.org

19. National Cancer Institute, "Health Effects of Exposure to Environmental Tobacco Smoke," Smoking and Tobacco Control Monograph No. 10, (February 2004).

20. Centers for Disease Control and Prevention, "Second National Report on Human Exposure to Environmental Chemicals: Tobacco Smoke." (USDHHS Publication No. 03-0022) (Bethesda, MD: U.S. Department of Health and Human Services, 2003).

21. P. Hilts, "Wide Peril is Seen in Passive Smoking," *New York Times* (May 9, 1990): A25.

22. American Lung Association, "Secondhand Smoke," 2004, http://ala.org

23. D. Mannino, "Children Exposed to ETS Miss More School," *Tobacco Control* (May 1996): 13–18.

24. M. Fogarty, "Public Health and Smoking Cessation," *The Scientist*, 17, no. 6 (2003), 23; Tobacco Control Research Center, Tobacco Litigation Documents, "Multistate Settlement with Tobacco Industry," 2004, www.library.ucsf.edu/tobacco/litigation

25. American Cancer Society, *Cancer Facts and Figures 2004*, 25.

26. Ibid.

27. Your Nutrition and Food Safety Resource, "Questions and Answers about Caffeine and Health," January 2003, http://ific.org

28. Ibid.

CHAPTER 14

1. Substance Abuse and Mental Health Services Administration, "Substance Abuse; A National Health Challenge," October 4, 2001, www.samhsa.gov/oas/oas.html

2. Ibid.

3. Substance Abuse and Mental Health Services Administration, *Results from the 2003 National Survey on Drug Use and Health: National Findings,* (NSDUH Series H-25, DHHS Publication No. SMA 04-3964) (Rockville, MD: Office of Applied Studies, 2004).

4. Ibid.

5. National Institute on Drug Abuse, "National Survey Results on Drug Use, 1975–2002: College Students and Adults," *Monitoring the Future,* (2003), 227.

6. Ibid.

7. M. Fisherman and C. Johanson, "Cocaine," in *Pharmacological Aspects of Drug Dependence: Towards an Integrated Neurobehavior Approach (Handbook of Experimental Pharmacology),* ed. C. Schuster and M. Kuhar (Hamburg: Springer Verlag, 1996): 159–195.

8. Ibid.

9. Substance Abuse and Mental Health Services Administration, *Results from 2003 Survey.*

10. H. C. Ashton, "Pharmacology and Effects of Cannabis: A Brief Review," *British Journal of Psychiatry* 178 (2001): 101–106.

11. American Academy of Ophthalmology, Medical Library, "The Use of Marijuana in the Treatment of Glaucoma," 2003, www.medem.com

12. R. Mathias, "Marijuana Impairs Driving-Related Skills and Workplace Performance," *NIDA Notes 11,* no. 1 (January/February 1996): 6.

13. Office of National Drug Control Policy, "Fact Sheet Heroin," 2002, www.whitehousedrugpolicy.gov/publications/factsht/heroin/index.html

14. National Institute on Drug Abuse, "National Survey Results on Drug Use: 1975–2003," *Monitoring the Future* (2004).

15. National Institute on Drug Abuse, "National Survey Results on Drug Use: 1975–2002."

16. National Institute on Drug Abuse, "NIDA Launches Initiative to Combat Club Drugs," *NIDA Notes* 14, no. 2 (2000).

17. National Institute on Drug Abuse, "Anabolic Steroid Abuse," *NIDA Research Report Series* (2000).

18. Office of National Drug Control Strategy, "2002 National Drug Control Strategy" 2002, www.whitehousedrugpolicy.gov

19. Ibid.

20. National Institute on Drug Abuse, "Worker Drug Use and Workplace Policies and Programs: Results from the 1994 and 1997 National Household Survey on Drug Abuse," (1999).

21. Ibid.

CHAPTER 15

1. World Health Organization, *The World Health Report,* 2004, www.who.int/whr/2004/en

2. American Heart Association, *Heart Disease and Stroke Statistics* (Dallas: American Heart Association, 2004), 3.

3. Ibid., 3.

4. Ibid.

5. Ibid., 2.

6. Ibid., 3.

7. American Heart Association, *Heart Facts 2004: African Americans* (Dallas: American Heart Association, 2004).

8. American Heart Association, *Heart Facts 2004: Latino/Hispanic Americans* (Dallas: American Heart Association, 2004).

9. American Heart Association, *Heart Disease and Stroke Statistics* (Dallas: American Heart Association, 2004).

10. Ibid.

11. Ibid.

12. Ibid.

13. Ibid.

14. Ibid., 4.

15. Ibid.

16. Ibid.

17. Ibid.

18. R. Ross, "Atherosclerosis—An Inflammatory Disease," *New England Journal of Medicine* 340 (1999): 115–126.

19. American Heart Association, *Heart Disease and Stroke Facts,* (Dallas: American Heart Association, 2004), 3.

20. C. Napoli et al., "Fatty Streak Formation Occurs in Human Fetal Aortas and Is Greatly Enhanced by Maternal Hypercholesterolemia: Intimal Accumulation of Low-Density Lipoprotein and its Oxidative Precede Monocyte Recruitment into Early Atherosclerotic Lesions," *Journal of Clinical Investigation* 100 (1997): 2680–2690.

21. World Health Organization, *The World Health Report,* 2004; American Heart Association, *Heart Disease and Stroke Facts.*

22. Ross, "Atherosclerosis—An Inflammatory Disease."

23. J. C. Kaski et al., "Inflammation Markers and Rapidly Advancing Coronary Disease," *Circulation* (September 24, 2004).

24. A. Forman, "The Threat of Insulin Resistance to Your Heart," *Environmental Nutrition* 23, no. 8 (2000): 4–6.

25. American Heart Association, *Heart Disease and Stroke Statistics.*

26. Ibid.

27. Ibid., 12.

28. Ibid., 23.

29. Ibid, 61.

30. Ibid., 53.

31. Ibid., 58.

32. Ibid., 13.

33. Ibid.

34. Ibid., 14.

35. Ibid.

36. Ibid, 27.

37. Ibid.

38. "Women Benefit More From Quitting Smoking than Men," *NIH News,* June 2, 2003, www.nhlbi.nih.gov/news/press

39. National Heart, Lung, and Blood Institute, "Third Report of the National Cholesterol Education Program (NCEP) Expert Panel on Detection, Evaluation, and Treatment of High Blood Cholesterol in Adults (Adult Treatment Panel III)," 2001, www.nhlbi.nih.gov/guidelines/cholesterol/index.htm

40. Ibid.

41. S. M. Marovina et al., "NHLBI Workshop on Lipoprotein(a) and CVD: Recent Advances and Future Directions," 2004, www.nhlbi.nih.gov; A. Ariyo, C. Thach, and R. Tracy, "Lp(a) Lipoprotein, Vascular Disease, and Mortality in the Elderly," *New England Journal of Medicine* 349, no. 22 (2003): 2108–2115.

42. National Heart, Lung, and Blood Institute, NCEP.

43. Ibid.

44. Ibid.

45. Center for Science in the Public Interest, *Nutrition Action Health Letter* 22 (1995): 4.

46. American Heart Association, *Heart Disease and Stroke Facts;* United States Department of Health and Human Services, "Surgeon General's Report on Physical Activity and Health," 1996, www.cdc.gov/nccdphp/sgr/summary.htm

47. L. E. Fields et al, "The Burden of Adult Hypertension in the United States 1999 to 2000: A Rising Tide," *Hypertension* 44 (2004): 1–7.

48. American Heart Association, *Heart Disease and Stroke Statistics.*

49. National Heart, Lung, and Blood Institute, "Understanding High Blood Pressure," 2002, www.nhlbi.nih.gov/hbp/hbp/intro.htm

50. Ross, "Atherosclerosis—An Inflammatory Disease."

51. L. L. Yan et al., "Psychosocial Factors and Risk of Hypertension," *Journal of the American Medical Association* 290, no. 16 (2003): 2138–2148.

52. R. Eliot, "Changing Behavior: A New Comprehensive and Quantitative Approach" (keynote address, Annual Meeting of the American College of Cardiology on Stress and the Heart, Jackson Hole, WY, July 3, 1987).

53. A. G. Boston et al., "Elevated Plasma Lipoprotein(a) and Coronary Heart Disease in Men Aged 55 Years and Younger: A Prospective Study," *Journal of the American Medical Association* 276 (1996): 555–558.

54. Ibid., 555.

55. Ibid., 556.

56. National Heart, Lung, and Blood Institute, "Heart Memo: The Cardiovascular Health of Women" (Bethesda, MD: NHLBI, 1995), 5.

57. Ibid., 5.

58. American Heart Association, *Heart Disease and Stroke Facts.*

59. J. E. Willard, R. A. Lange, and D. L. Hillis, "The Use of Aspirin in Ischemic Heart Disease," *New England Journal of Medicine* 327 (1992): 175–179.

60. Agency for Healthcare Policy and Research, "Cardiac Rehabilitation: Exercise, Training, Education, Counseling, and Behavioral Interventions" (Publication #96-0672) (Rockville, MD: Author, 1996).

CHAPTER 16

1. American Cancer Society, *Cancer Facts and Figures 2004* (Atlanta: American Cancer Society, 2004).

2. American Cancer Society, *Cancer Facts and Figures 2003* (Atlanta: American Cancer Society, 2003).

3. American Cancer Society, *Cancer Facts and Figures 2004.*

4. American Cancer Society, *Cancer Facts and Figures 2003.*

5. American Cancer Society, *Cancer Facts and Figures 2004.*

6. B. D. Smedley, A. Y. Stith, and A. R. Nelson, eds., *Unequal Treatment: Confronting Racial and Ethnic Disparities in Health Care* (Washington, DC: National Academies Press, 2003).

7. H. P. Freeman, "Commentary on the Meaning of Race in Science and Society," *Cancer Epidemiology Biomarkers and Prevention* 12, no. 3 (2003): 232S–236S.

8. American Cancer Society, *Cancer Facts and Figures 2004,* 24.

9. Ibid, 22–30.

10. Ibid., 3.

11. J. Peto, "Cancer Epidemiology in the Last Century and Next Decade," *Nature* 411 (2001): 390–395.

12. American Cancer Society, *Cancer Facts and Figures 2004.*

13. American Cancer Society, *Cancer Facts and Figures 2003.*

14. Ibid.

15. Ibid.

16. American Cancer Society, *Cancer Facts and Figures 2004.*

17. M. Osborne, P. Boyle, and M. Lipkin, "Cancer Prevention," *The Lancet* 349 (1997): 1–8 (special oncology supplement).

18. International Agency for Research on Cancer (IARC), *Hormonal Contraception and Post-Menopausal Hormonal Therapy* (IARC Monographs on the Evaluation of Carcinogenic Risks to Humans, 72) (Lyon, France: IARC, 1999).

19. Peto, "Cancer Epidemiology in the Last Century."

20. American Cancer Society, *Cancer Facts and Figures 2003.*

21. Osborne, Boyle, and Lipkin, "Cancer Prevention."

22. Peto, "Cancer Epidemiology in the Last Century."

23. American Cancer Society, *Cancer Facts and Figures 2004.*

24. Ibid.

25. Ibid.

26. Ibid.

27. Ibid.
28. Ibid.
29. Ibid.
30. Ibid.
31. Ibid.
32. Ibid.
33. Ibid.
34. Peto, "Cancer Epidemiology in the Last Century."
35. A. Bergstrom et al., "Overweight as an Avoidable Cause of Cancer in Europe," *International Journal of Cancer* 91 (2001): 421–430.
36. Ibid
37. Ibid
38. Ibid.
39. P. A. Janne and R. J. Mayer, "Chemoprevention of Colorectal Cancer," *New England Journal of Medicine* 342 (2000): 1960–1968; Writing Group—WHI, "Risks and Benefits of Estrogen Plus Progesterone on the Health of Postmenopausal Women," *Journal of the American Medical Association,* 288, no. 3 (July 17, 2002).
40. American Cancer Society, *Cancer Facts and Figures 2004.*
41. L. Seeff et al., "Screening for Colorectal Cancer in the U.S.," *Journal of Family Practice* 51 (2002): 761–766.
42. American Cancer Society, *Cancer Facts and Figures 2004.*
43. Ibid.
44. Ibid.
45. Ibid.
46. Ibid.
47. Ibid.
48. Ibid.
49. University of Wisconsin Health Service, "Sunburn: Prevention /Treatment" (2002) www.uhs.wisc.edu/ex/selfcare/resource /sunburn.php
50. American Cancer Society, *Cancer Facts and Figures 2004.*
51. University of Wisconsin Health Service, "Sunburn: Prevention/ Treatment."
52. American Cancer Society, *Cancer Facts and Figures 2004.*
53. University of Wisconsin Health Service, "Sunburn: Prevention/Treatment."
54. Ibid.
55. American Cancer Society, *Cancer Facts and Figures 2004.*
56. Ibid.
57. Ibid.
58. Ibid.
59. National Cancer Institute, "Ovarian Cancer and You," 2004, www.cancer.gov/cancerinfo/pdq/screening/ovarian/patient
60. American Cancer Society, *Cancer Facts and Figures 2004.*
61. Ibid.
62. A. Harvey et al., "Dietary Fat Intake and Risk of Epithelial Ovarian Cancer," *Journal of the National Cancer Institute* 86 (1994): 21.
63. G. C. Zografos, M. Panou, and N. Panou, "Common Risk Factors of Breast and Ovarian Cancer: Recent Review," *International Journal of Gynecological Cancer* 14, no. 5 (2004): 721–740; C. T. Berkelman, "Risk Factors and Risk Reduction of Breast and Ovarian Cancer," *Current Opinion in Obstetrics and Gynecology* 15, no. 1 (2003): 63–68.
64. American Cancer Society, *Cancer Facts and Figures 2004.*
65. Ibid.
66. Ibid.
67. National Cancer Institute, "Endometrial Cancer Overview," 2004, www.nci.gov
68. American Cancer Society, *Cancer Facts and Figures 2004.*
69. Ibid.
70. Ibid.
71. Ibid.
72. Ibid.
73. Ibid.

CHAPTER 17

1. K. Nelson, C. Williams, and N. Graham, *Infectious Disease Epidemiology: Theory and Practice* (Gaithersburg, MD: Aspen, 2001), 17–39.
2. University of Michigan Health System,"TSS," 2003, www.med .umich.edu/1libr/aha/aha_toxic_crs.htm
3. Centers for Disease Control and Prevention, "Group B Streptococcal Infections," 2000, www.cdc.gov/ncidod/diseases/bacter /strep_b.htm
4. Childbirth Solutions, "Group B Streptoccocal Disease (GBS) Frequently Asked Questions," 2004, www.childbirthsolutions.com /articles/pregnancy/groupb/index.php
5. National Institute of Allergy and Infectious Diseases, "Pneumoccocal Pneumonia Fact Sheet," 2001, www.niaid.nih.gov /factsheets/pneumonia.htm
6. *British Medical Journal,* "Editorial: New Outbreak of Legionnaire's Disease in the United Kingdom," *British Medical Journal* 325 (2002): 347–348.
7. National Center for HIV, STD, and TB Prevention, "Surveillance Report: Reported Tuberculosis in the United States, 2003," 2004, www.cdc.gov/nchstp/tb/surv/surv2003/default.htm
8. Ibid.
9. Centers for Disease Control and Prevention, "Trends in Tuberculosis—United States, 1998–2003," *Morbidity and Mortality Weekly Report* 53 (2004): 209–214. (http://jama.ama-assn.org/ cgi/reprint/291/15/1827.pdf)
10. National Institute of Allergy and Infectious Diseases, "Tuberculosis Fact Sheet," 2002, www.niaid.nih.gov/factsheets/tb.htm
11. World Health Organization, "Coordinates 2002: Charting Progress against AIDS, TB, and Malaria," 2002, www.synergyaids .com/documents/3854_unaids_coordinates2002.pdf
12. Ibid.
13. Global Tuberculosis Program, "Tuberculosis Fact Sheet No. 104," wwwwho.int/inffs/en/fact104.html
14. Centers for Disease Control and Prevention, "Rocky Mountain Spotted Fever Epidemiology," 2000, www.cdc.gov/ncidod /dvrd/rmsf/epidemiology.htm
15. A. Evans and R. Kaslow, *Viral Infections in Humans: Epidemiology and Control,* 4th ed. (New York: Plenum, 1997), 6–11.
16. Benton County Health Department, "Flu Info," 2004, www.co .benton.or.us/health/health_alerts/flu_info.htm
17. National Center for Infectious Diseases, "Disease Burden from Hepatitis A, B, and C in the United States," 2002, www.cdc.gov .ncidod/diseases/hepatitis/resource/dz_burden02.htm
18. National Digestive Diseases Information Clearinghouse, "Promote Prevention: Hepatitis—Education and Information for Patients and Professionals," 2000, www.niddk.nih.gov/health .digest/digest.htm
19. National Center for Infectious Diseases, "Viral Hepatitis B Fact Sheet," 2004, www.cdc.gov/ncidod/diseases/hepatitis/b/fact.htm
20. National Digestive Diseases Information Clearinghouse, "Promote Prevention."
21. Ibid.
22. National Center for Infectious Diseases, "Viral Hepatitis B Fact Sheet."
23. National Digestive Diseases Information Clearinghouse, "Promote Prevention."
24. Ibid.
25. National Center for Infectious Diseases, "Viral Hepatitis C Fact Sheet," 2004, www.cdc.gov/ncidod/diseases/hepatitis/c /fact.htm
26. National Immunization Program, "Viral Hepatitis Vaccines," 2004, www.cdc.gov/nip/vaccine/hep/default.htm
27. Seattle Biomedical Research Institute, "Global Connections, Infectious Diseases Hinder Environment," 2003, www.sbri.org .news/GC%20summer03.pdf
28. Nelson, Williams, and Graham, *Infectious Disease Epidemiology,* 17–39.

29. National Center for Infectious Diseases, "BSE and CJD Information and Resources," 2003, www.cdc.gov/ncidod/diseases/cjdcjd.htm
30. Ibid.
31. Nelson, Williams, and Graham, *Infectious Disease Epidemiology,* 315–318.
32. Ibid.
33. Centers for Disease Control and Prevention, "Diseases—Ebola Hemorrhagic Fever," 2004, www.cdc.gov/ncidod/dvrd/spb/mnpages/dispages/ebola.htm
34. Ibid.
35. Nelson, Williams, and Graham, *Infectious Disease Epidemiology,* 325.
36. R. Fenner, *The History of Smallpox and Its Spread Around the World* (Geneva, Switzerland: World Health Organization, 1988).
37. T. J. Torok, R. V. Tauxe, and R. P. Wise, "A Large Community Outbreak of Salmonellosis Carried by Intentional Contamination of Restaurant Salad Bars," *Journal of the American Medical Association* 279 (1997): 389–395.
38. New York State Department of Health, "Streptococcal Infections," 2004, www.health.state.ny.us/nysdoh/communicable_diseases/en/gas.htm
39. National Center for HIV, STD, and TB Prevention, "STD Surveillance 2002," 2004, www.cdc.gov/std/stats/toc2002.htm
40. Ibid.
41. National Institute of Allergy and Infectious Diseases, "Profile Fiscal Year 2003. Sexually Transmitted Infections," 2004, www.niaid.nih.gov/facts/profile_fy2003/PDF/SSAR_SEXUALLY.pdf
42. Centers for Disease Control and Prevention, "STDs Today," 2004, www.cdcnpin.org/scripts/std/std.asp
43. National Centers for Chronic Disease Prevention and Health Promotion, "Healthy Youth, Sexual Behaviors," 2004, www.cdc.gov/HealthyYouth/sexualbehaviors/index.htm
44. Centers for Disease Control and Prevention, "STDs Today."
45. Ibid.
46. National Centers for Chronic Disease Prevention and Health Promotion, "Healthy Youth, Sexual Behaviors."
47. National Center for HIV, STD, and TB Prevention, "Chlamydia Fact Sheet," 2004, www.cdc.gov/std/Chlamydia/STDFact-Chlamydia.htm
48. National Center for HIV, STD, and TB Prevention, "PID Fact Sheet," 2004, www.cdc.gov/std/PID/STDFact-PID.htm
49. Ibid.
50. National Center for HIV, STD, and TB Prevention, "Gonorrhea Fact Sheet," 2004, www.cdc.gov/std/Gonorrhea/STDFact-Gonorrhea.htm
51. Ibid.
52. A. Evans and P. Brachman, *Bacterial Infections of Humans: Epidemiology and Control,* 3rd ed. (New York: Plenum, 1998).
53. National Center for HIV, STD, and TB Prevention, "Genital Herpes Fact Sheet," 2004, www.cdc.gov/std/herpes/STDFact-Herpes.htm
54. Ibid.
55. Ibid.
56. National Institute of Allergy and Infectious Diseases, "HIV/AIDS Statistics," 2004, www.niaid.nih.gov/factsheets/aidsstat.htm
57. Ibid.
58. Ibid.
59. National Institute of Allergy and Infectious Disease, "HIV Infection in Women—Fact Sheet," 2002, www.niaid.nih.gov/factsheets/womenhiv.htm
60. National Institute of Allergy and Infectious Diseases, "HIV/AIDS Statistics."
61. National Institute of Allergy and Infectious Diseases, "HIV Infection in Women," 2004. www.niaid.nih.gov/factsheets/womenhiv.htm
62. National Institute of Allergy and Infectious Diseases, "HIV Infection in Infants and Children," 2004, www.niaih.nih.gov/factsheets/hivchildren.htm
63. National Center for HIV, STD, and TB Prevention, "HIV and Its Transmission," 2003, www.cdc.gov/hiv/pubs/facts/transmission.htm
64. National Institute of Allergy and Infectious Diseases, "HIV Infection in Infants and Children."
65. F. Cox, *The AIDS Booklet,* 6th ed. (Boston: McGraw-Hill Higher Education, 2000), 27–30.
66. R. Conviser, "Changing Care Costs for HIV/AIDS," 2002, http://hab.hrsa.gov/reports/changingcost/sld001.htm
67. National Institute of Allergy and Infectious Diseases, "Developing a Safe and Effective AIDS Vaccine," 2003, www.niaid.nih.gov/daids/vaccine/optimisim.htm

CHAPTER 18
1. National Heart, Lung, and Blood Institute, "Chronic Obstructive Pulmonary Disease Facts," (NIH Publication No. 03-5229), 2003, http://nhlbi.nih.gov/health/public/lung/other/copd_fact.pdf
2. Ibid.
3. Asthma and Allergy Foundation of America, 2004, www.aafa.org
4. National Center for Health Statistics, "Allergies and Hay Fever," 2004, www.cdc.gov/nchs/fastats/allergies.htm
5. MayoClinic.com, "Asthma Signs and Symptoms," 2004, www.mayoclinic.com/invoke.cfm?id = DS00021
6. Asthma and Allergy Foundation, 2004.
7. Ibid.; Patient Health International, "Asthma Facts and Figures," 2004, www.patienthealthinternational.com/article/501252.aspx
8. R. Brownson, P. Remington, and J. Davis, eds., *Chronic Disease Epidemiology and Control* (Washington, DC: American Public Health Association, 1998), 389.
9. MayoClinic.com, "Bronchitis," 2003, www.mayclinic.com/invoke.cfm?id = DS00031
10. National Sleep Foundation, "Sleep Apnea," 2002, www.sleepfoundation.org/publications/sleepap.cfm; American Sleep Apnea Association, "Information about Sleep Apnea," 2004, www.sleepapnea.org/geninfo.html
11. Ibid.
12. National Headache Foundation, 2004, www.headaches.org
13. Ibid.
14. Ibid.
15. Ibid.
16. MayoClinic.com, "Migraine," 2004, www.mayoclinic.com/invoke.cfm?id = DS00120
17. J. Adler and A. Rogers, "The New War Against Migraines," *Newsweek,* January 11, 1999, 46–55.
18. J. Allen, "Oh, My Aching Head," *Life,* 1994, 66–76.
19. Ibid., 72.
20. J. Adler and A. Rogers, "The New War Against Migraines."
21. MayoClinic.com, "Cluster Headache," 2003, www.mayoclinic.com/invoke.cfm?id = DS00487
22. National Headache Foundation, 2004.
23. MayoClinic.com, "Epilepsy," 2003, www.mayoclinic.com/invoke.cfm?id = DS00342
24. Ibid.
25. National Parkinson Foundation, "Parkinson Primer," 2004, www.parkinson.org
26. Ibid.
27. R. Schapiro, "What Is Multiple Sclerosis?" International MS Support Foundation, 2001, www.msnews.org/
28. J. Gerberding, "Diabetes: Disabling, Deadly, and on the Rise. At A Glance 2004," 2004, www.cdc.gov/nccdphp/aag/aag_ddt.htm; Centers for Disease Control and Prevention, "Diabetes Surveillance System," 2004, www.cdc.gov/diabetes/statistics
29. Ibid.
30. Ibid.

31. Ibid.
32. Ibid.
33. Ibid.
34. J. Koplan, "Diabetes Is a Growing Public Health Concern," 2002, www.cdc.gov/diabetes/pubs/glance.htm
35. Ibid.
36. J. Adler and C. Kalb, "An American Epidemic: Diabetes," *Newsweek* (September 4, 2000): 40–48; Centers for Disease Control and Prevention, "Diabetes Surveillance System."
37. Centers for Disease Control and Prevention, "Diabetes Surveillance System."
38. P. Lustman and A. Keegan, "Depression," *Diabetes Forecast* 51 (1998): 56–64.
39. J. Gerberding, "Diabetes: Disabling, Deadly, and on the Rise."
40. R. Brownson, P. Remington, and J. Davis, eds., *Chronic Disease Epidemiology and Control,* 424.
41. Arthritis Foundation, "Disease Center," 2002, www.arthritis.org /conditions/DiseaseCenter/oa.asp
42. Arthritis Foundation, "Osteoarthritis," 2004, www.arthritis .org/conditions/DiseaseCenter/oa.asp
43. Ibid.
44. Ibid.
45. Ibid.
46. R. Brownson, P. Remington, and J. Davis, eds., *Chronic Disease Epidemiology and Control.*
47. "Is the Prevalence of Back Pain Rising?" *The Back Letter* 17, no. 11 (2002).
48. N. Hadler and T. Carey, "Low Back Pain: An Intermittent Predicament in Life," *Annals of the Rheumatic Diseases* 57 (1998): 1–3.
49. K. Nelson, C. Williams, and N. Graham, *Infectious Disease Epidemiology* (Gaithersburg, MD: 2001), 348–349.

CHAPTER 19

1. J. Kavenaugh, *Adult Development and Aging* (Pacific Grove, CA: Brooks/Cole/ITP, 1996), 45.
2. C. Garnett, "Keys to Successful Aging," *The NIH Word on Health,* June 2002, www.nih.gov/news/WordonHealth/jun2002 /successfulaging.htm
3. National Institute on Aging, "Life Extension: Science Fact or Science Fiction?," *Age Page,* September 2002, www.niapublications .org/engagepages/lifeext.asp
4. Illinois Department on Aging, "Facts on Aging," June 1, 2002, www.state.il.us/aging/1news_pubs/onage53.htm
5. W. Madar, "Life Stories as Well as Theory Needed to Understand Aging," *Center for the Humanities Newsletter* (Corvallis, OR: Consortium of Humanities Centers and Institutes, Oregon State University, Spring 2000), 8.
6. U.S. Department of Health and Human Services, Administration on Aging, *A Profile of Older Americans: 2003.* Projections of the population by age are taken from the January 2004 Census Internet Release. Historical data are from "65 + in the United States," Current Population Reports, Special Studies, P23-190. Data for 2000 are from the 2000 census. www.aoa.gov/prof /Statistics/profile/2003/4_pf.asp
7. "Press Briefing by the World Health Organization," Second World Assembly on Aging, Madrid, Spain, April 8–12, 2002, www.un.org/ageing/coverage/pr/briefingwho.htm
8. U.S. Department of Health and Human Services, Administration on Aging, "A Profile of Older Americans 2003: Future Growth," March 8, 2004, www.aoa.gov/prof/Statistics/profile /2003/4.asp
9. U.S. Department of Health and Human Services, Administration on Aging, "A Profile of Older Americans 2003: The Older Population," www.aoa.gov/prof/Statistics/profile/2003/3.asp
10. U.S. Department of Health and Human Services, Administration on Aging, "A Profile of Older Americans 2003: Health and Health Care," March 8, 2004, www.aoa.gov/prof/Statistics /profile/2003/14.asp
11. Alliance for Health Reform, "Sourcebook," 2002, www.allhealth .org/sourcebook/2002
12. National Institutes of Health, Osteoporosis and Related Bone Diseases—National Resource Center, "Osteoporosis Overview," revised January 2003, www.osteo.org/newfile.asp?doc = osteo&doctitle = Osteoporosis + Overview&doctype = HTML + Fact + Sheet
13. National Kidney and Urologic Diseases Information Clearinghouse, "Kidney and Urologic Disease Statistics for the United States" (NIH Publication No. 04-3895), February 2004, www .kidney.niddk.nih.gov/kudiseases/pubs/kustats/index.htm#up
14. Ibid.
15. National Eye Institute, News and Events, NEI Press Release, "Vision Loss from Eye Diseases Will Increase as Americans Age," April 12, 2004, www.nei.nih.gov/news/pressreleases /041204.asp
16. National Eye Institute, "Cataract: What You Should Know," August 2004, www.nei.nih.gov/health/cataract/cataract_facts .asp#1
17. National Eye Institute, "Vision Loss from Eye Diseases."
18. National Eye Institute, "Glaucoma: What You Should Know," revised August 2004, www.nei.nih.gov/health/glaucoma/ glaucoma_facts.asp#13
19. National Eye Institute, "Vision Loss from Eye Diseases."
20. Philadelphia Corporation for Aging, *Health Matters,* no. 14, August 2004, www.pcaphl.org/healthmatters/agingsexuality.pdf
21. National Council on Aging, "Half of Older Americans Report They Are Sexually Active, 4 in 10 Want More Sex, Says New Survey," September 28, 1998, http://ncoa.org/mews/archives .sexsurvey.htm
22. Alzheimer's Association, "Fact Sheet," April 5, 2004, www.alz .org/Resources/FactSheets/FSAlzheimerStats.pdf
23. Ibid.
24. Alzheimer's Association, "Data Suggest Benefits to Shedding the Spare Tire," 2004, www.alz.org/Perspective/shedding.asp
25. Alzheimer's Association, "Fact Sheet: Cholinesterase Inhibitors," 2002, www.alz.org/ResourceCenter/ByTopic/cholinesterase.htm
26. Alzheimer's Association, "Standard Prescriptions for Alzheimer's," 2004, www.alz.org/AboutAD/Treatment/Standard.asp

CHAPTER 20

1. *Oxford English Dictionary* (Oxford, UK: Oxford University Press, 1969), 72, 334, 735.
2. President's Commission for the Study of Ethical Problems in Medicine and Biomedical and Behavioral Research, *Deciding to Forgo Life-Sustaining Treatment* (New York: Concern for Dying, 1983), 9.
3. Ad Hoc Committee of the Harvard Medical School to Examine the Definition of Brain Death, "A Definition of Irreversible Coma," *Journal of the American Medical Association* 205 (1968): 377.
4. L. R. Aiken, *Dying, Death, and Bereavement,* 3rd ed. (Boston: Allyn & Bacon, 1994), 4.
5. *Civilization,* 6, no. 6 (2000): 30, 33–34.
6. E. Kübler-Ross, *On Death and Dying* (New York: Macmillan, 1969), 113.
7. C. Corr, C. Nabe, and D. Corr, *Death and Dying: Life and Living,* 4th ed. (Belmont, CA: Wadsworth, 2003).
8. R. J. Kastenbaum, *Death, Society, and Human Experience,* 8th ed. (Boston: Allyn & Bacon, 2003).
9. Ibid.
10. K. J. Doka (ed.), *Disenfranchised Grief: Recognizing Hidden Sorrow* (Lexington, MA: Lexington Books, 1989).
11. J. W. Worden, *Grief Counseling and Grief Therapy: A Handbook for the Mental Health Practitioner,* 3rd ed. (New York: Springer, 2001).

12. Public Health Advisory Board. *Health and the American Child: A Focus on Mortality Among Children, 2001 Update,* 2001, http://phpab.org/HealthandtheAmericanChild/ReportPortal1.htm

13. J. W. Worden, *Children and Grief: When a Parent Dies* (New York: Guilford Press, 1996).

14. The term *quasi-death experience* was coined by J. B. Kamerman, *Death in the Midst of Life* (Englewood Cliffs, NJ: Prentice Hall, 1988), 71.

15. C. M. Parkes, *Bereavement* (New York: International Universities Press, 1972), 6.

16. National Cancer Institute, "Advance Directives, Cancer Facts 8.12," 2000, http://cis.nci.nih.gov/fact/8_12.htm

17. Public Agenda, "Right-to-Die," 2004, www.publicagenda.org

18. Oregon Department of Human Services, "Oregon's Death with Dignity Act," 2004, www.dhs.state.or.us/publichealth/chs/pas/pas.cfm

CHAPTER 21

1. G. Moore, *Living with the Earth,* 2nd ed. (Boca Raton, FL: Lewis Publisher/CRC Press, 2002), 519–542.

2. Ibid.

3. A. Yassi et al., *Basic Environmental Health* (New York: Oxford University Press, 2001), 14.

4. R. Caplan, *Our Earth, Ourselves* (New York: Bantam, 1990), 247.

5. G. Moore, *Living with the Earth,* 60.

6. A. Nadakavukaren, *Our Global Environment* (Long Grove, IL: Waveland Press, 2000), 45–80.

7. Population Reference Bureau, "2004 World Population Data Sheet," 2004, www.prb.org

8. L. R. Brown, M. Renner, and C. Flavin, *Vital Signs 1998: The Environmental Trends That Are Shaping Our Future* (New York: W. W. Norton & Co., 1998).

9. Ibid.

10. G. Moore, *Living with the Earth,* 62.

11. A. Nadakavukaren, *Our Global Environment,* 76.

12. Ibid.

13. Population Reference Bureau, "2004 World Population Data Sheet."

14. National Cancer Institute, "Tobacco and Smoking Control Monographs: Monograph 10: Health Effects of Exposure to Environmental Tobacco Smoke: The Report of California's EPA," 2003, http://cancercontrol.cancer.gov/tcrb/monographs/10; National Center for Environmental Health, "Second National Report on Human Exposure to Environmental Chemicals," 2003, www.cdc.gov/exposurereport/2nd

15. R. Sargent, R. Shepard, and S. Glantz, "Reduced Incidence of Admissions for Myocardial Infarction Associated with Public Smoking Ban: Before and After Study," *British Medical Journal* 328 (2004): 977–980.

16. J. Medlin, "Sweet Candy, Bitter Poison," 2004, http://ehp.niehs.nih.gov/docs/2004/112-14/forum.html#swee

17. Environment Agency, "Acid Rain," 2004, www.environment-agency.gov.uk/yourenv/eff/pollution/acid_rain

18. L. Brown, "A New Era Unfolds," in *State of the World, 1993,* ed. L. Brown (New York: W. W. Norton Co., 1993), 107.

19. Environmental Protection Agency (EPA), "2003 Status Report Shows U.S. Air Cleanest Ever Since 1970," September 2004, www.epa.gov/newsroom

20. EPA, "The Inside Story: A Guide to Indoor Air Quality" (EPA Document #402-K-93-007), January 2002, http://epa.gov/iaq/pubs/insidest.html.

21. Ibid.

22. Ibid.

23. National Cancer Institute, "Radon and Cancer: Questions and Answers," 2004, http://cis.nci.nih.gov/fact3_52.htm

24. EPA, "The Inside Story."

25. EPA, "Air-Indoor Air Quality," 2004, www.epa.gov/iaq

26. N. Carpenter, " 'Sick' Buildings Can Be Root of Work-Related Maladies," *Boston Business Journal* 20 (2000): 36–37.

27. U.S. EPA, *Questions and Answers on Ozone Depletion* (Washington, DC: Stratospheric Protection Division, 1998).

28. EPA, "Global Warming-Climate," 2002, http://yosemite.epa.gov/oar/globalwarming.nsf/content/climate.html

29. Ibid.

30. J. Abramovitz, *Taking a Stand: Cultivating a New Relationship with the World's Forests* (Washington, DC: Worldwatch Institute, 1998).

31. American Water Works Association, "Drop by Drop: A Guide to Starting a Water Conservation Program," 2002, www.awwa.org/community

32. U.S. Geological Survey, "New Reports on Our Nation's Water Quality," 2004, http://water.usgs.gov/pubs/fs/2004/3045

33. World Health Organization, "Meeting the Millennium Development Goals Drinking Water and Sanitation Target—A Mid-term Assessment of Progress," 2004, www.who.int/water_sanitation_health/monitoring/jmp2004

34. P. Hamilton, T. Miller, and D. Meyers, "Water Quality in the Nations Streams and Aquifers—Overview of Selected Findings," U.S. Geological Survey Circular 1265, 20: 2004.

35. U.S. Environmental Protection Agency, *Water on Tap: A Consumer's Guide to the Nation's Drinking Water* (Washington, DC: Safe Drinking Water Information System, 1997).

36. Ibid.

37. Ibid.

38. G. Moore, *Living with the Earth,* 203.

39. G. Moore, *Living with the Earth,* 203.

40. G. Moore, *Living with the Earth,* 248.

41. Global Programme of Action for the Protection of the Marine Environment from Land-Based Activities, "Inputs of POPs in Coastal and Marine Environment," 2001, http://pops.gpa.unep.org/031marin.htm

42. A. Hoyer, "Organochlorine Exposure and Risk of Breast Cancer," *Lancet* 352 (1998): 1816–1831.

43. Environment News Service, "Europe Secures Victory over Aircraft Noise," 2001, http://ens-news.com/ans/oct2001/2001-10-08-05.asp

44. Ibid.

45. EPA, "Superfund National Accomplishments Summary Fiscal Year 2004," 2004, www.epa.gov/superfund/action/process/numbers04.htm

46. Ibid.

47. Ibid.

48. National Institute of Environmental Health Sciences, "EMF Questions and Answers June 2002: Results of EMF Research," 2002, www.niehs.nih.gov/emfrapid/booklet/results.htm

CHAPTER 22

1. L. C. Baker and L. S. Baker, "Excess Cost of Emergency Department Visits for Nonurgent Care," *Health Affairs* (Winter 1994): 162–180.

2. A. B. Bernstein et al., "Introduction," *Health Care in America: Trends in Utilization.* Hyattsville, Maryland: National Center for Health Statistics, 2003, www.cdc.gov/nchs/data/misc/healthcare.pdf

3. American Academy of Orthopaedic Surgeons, "Advisory Statement: The Importance of Good Communication in the Physician-Patient Relationship," September 4, 2003, www.aaos.org/wordhtml/papers/advistmt/1017.htm

4. C. Huggins, "Poll Shows Most Americans Trust Their Doctors," *Medline Plus Health Information,* 2002, www.nlm.nih.gov/medlineplus/news/fullstory_10844.html

5. National Center for Health Statistics, "New Study Shows Critical Role for Primary Care Specialists. National Ambulatory Medical Care Survey: 2002 Summary," August 26, 2004, www.cdc.gov /nchs/pressroom/04facts/primarycare.htm

6. Ibid.

7. J. Rowley et al., "Insomnia," June 17, 2004, www.emedicine .com/neuro/topic418.htm

8. U.S. Food and Drug Administration, "Phenylpropanolamine (PPA) Information Page," 2002, www.fda.gov/cder/drug /infopage/ppa/default.htm

9. Institute for Global Ethics, "Malpractice Fears Are Hurting Nation's Health Care, Group Warns," *Ethics Newsline* 5, no. 16 (April 22, 2002), www.globalethics.org/newsline/members/issue .tmpl?articleid = 04210222410961

10. "Patient Rights: Informed Consent," *Consumer Health,* www.emedicinehealth.com/articles/12033-3.asp

11. D. E. Mittman, "Explaining Rxs with a PA or an NP Signature," *Clinician Reviews,* February 2003, www.findarticles.com/p /articles/mi_m0BUY/is_2_13/ai_98312977

12. J. Silverman, "Consumer Report Spotlights Patient 'Dumping,'" *OB/GYN News,* September 1, 2001, www.findarticles.com/p /articles/mi_m0CYD/is_17_36/ai_78542014

13. National Center for Health Statistics, "Hospital Stays Grow Shorter; Heart Disease Leading Cause of Hospitalization," April 24, 2001, www.cdc.gov/nchs/pressroom/01news/99hospit.htm

14. Centers for Disease Control, "Indicators for Chronic Disease Surveillance," *Morbidity and Mortality Weekly Report, Recommendations and Reports,* 53, no. RR11 (September 10, 2004): 1–6, www.cdc.gov/mmwr/preview/mmwrhtml/rr5311a1.htm

15. National Center for Chronic Disease Prevention and Health Promotion, "Chronic Disease Overview," 2002, www.cdc.gov /nccdphp/overview.htm

16. Centers for Medicare and Medicaid Services, "National Health Care Expenditures Projections: 2002–2012," February 11, 2003, www.cms.hhs.gov/statistics/nhe/projections-2002 /highlights.asp

17. L. Kohn, J. Corrigan, and M. Donaldson, eds., *To Err Is Human: Building a Safer Health System* (Washington, D.C.: The National Academies Press, 2000).

18. J. A. Rhoades and J. W. Cohen, *The Uninsured in America, 1996–2003: Estimates for the U.S. Population under Age 65* (Statistical Brief #45 Rockville, MD: July 2004), Agency for Healthcare Research and Quality, www.meps.ahrq.gov/papers/st45 /stat45.htm

19. P. Lee and C. Estes, *The Nation's Health*, 7th ed. (Sudbury, MA: Jones and Bartlett, 2003).

20. Centers for Medicare & Medicaid Services, "Medicare Celebrates 35 Years of Keeping Americans Healthy," *HHS News,* July 12, 2000, www.cms.hhs.gov/media/press/release.asp?Counter = 219

21. "Medicaid May Restrict Emergency Care," January 17, 2003, www.cbsnews.com/stories/2003/01/17/national/main536916 .shtml

22. M. McFarlane and M. Sinnott, "Managed Care: Nursing's Friend or Foe?" *Nursing Spectrum,* Education/CE Self-Study Module, 2003, http://nsweb.nursingspectrum.com/ce/ce169.htm

23. *Medical Group Practice Digest: Managed Care Digest Series 1998* (Kansas City: Hoechst Marion Roussel, Inc., 1998).

24. McFarlane and Sinnott, "Managed Care."

25. *Medical Group Practice Digest;* McFarlane and Sinnott, "Managed Care."

26. Ibid.

27. V. Kemper, "National Health Insurance Recommended," *The Miami Herald,* January 15, 2004, www.miami.com/mld /miamiherald/news/nation/7714716.htm?1c

28. Ibid.; S. Woolhandler and D. Himmelstein, "Paying for National Health Insurance and Not Getting It," *Health Affairs* 21, no. 4 (2002): 90.

CHAPTER 23

1. National Center for Complementary and Alternative Medicine, "NCCAM-Funded Research for FY 2003," 2004, http://nccam .nih.gov/research/extramural/awards/2003/index.htm

2. Ibid.

3. D. M. Eisenberg, R. Davis, and S. Ettner, "Trends in Alternative Medicine Use in the United States, 1990–97: Results of a Follow-up National Study," *Journal of the American Medical Association* 280 (1998): 1569–1579.

4. National Center for Complementary and Alternative Medicine, "What Is Complementary and Alternative Medicine (CAM)?" 2004, http://nccam.nih.gov/health/whatiscam

5. Ibid.

6. Ibid.

7. D. M. Eisenberg et al., "Unconventional Medicine in the United States," *New England Journal of Medicine* 328 (1993): 246–252.

8. Eisenberg et al., "Unconventional Medicine," 247; Eisenberg et al., "Trends in Alternative Medicine Use," 1570.

9. P. Barnes et al., "CDC Advance Data Report #343: Complementary and Alternative Medicine among Adults: United States, 2002," 2004, http://nccam.nih.gov/news/camsurvey.htm

10. Ibid.

11. Ibid.

12. Barnes et al., "CDC Advance Data Report"; "Terms and Concepts in Alternative Medicine," 2004, www.worddig.com /definitions/terms_and_concepts_in_alternative_medicine

13. National Center for Complementary and Alternative Medicine, "What Is CAM?"

14. "Presentations," Second International Scientific Conference on Complementary, Alternative and Integrative Medicine Research, Boston, MA, April 12–14, 2002; N. Rasmussen and J. Morgall, "The Use of Alternative Treatments in the Danish Adult Population," *Complementary Medicine Research* 4 (1990): 16–22; A. MacLennan, D. Wilson, and A. Taylor, "Prevalence and Cost of Alternative Medicine in Australia," *The Lancet* 347 (1996): 569–573; P. Fisher and A. Ward, "Complementary Medicine in Europe," *British Medical Journal* 309 (1994): 107–111; W. Miller, "Use of Alternative Health Care Practitioners by Canadians, *Canadian Journal of Public Health* 88 (1997): 154–158.

15. Barnes et al., "CDC Advance Data Report."

16. University of Washington School of Medicine, "Chiropractic Medicine," 2004, www.fammed.washington.edu/predoctoral /CAM/images/chiro.pdf; D. C. Cherkin et al., "A Review of the Evidence of the Effectiveness, Safety, and Cost of Acupuncture, Massage Therapy, and Spinal Manipulation for Back Pain," *Annals of Internal Medicine* 138, no. 11 (2003): 898–906.

17. National Center for Complementary and Alternative Medicine, "What Is CAM?"

18. Ibid.

19. Ibid.

20. Ibid.

21. Ibid.

22. J. Greenwald, "Herbal Healing," *Time* (November 23, 1998): 63–65.

23. A. Weil, *Spontaneous Healing* (New York: Fawcett Columbine, 1995).

24. B. Seaward, *Managing Stress,* 4th ed. (Sudbury, MA: Jones and Bartlett, 2004).

25. Ibid., 51.

26. Food and Drug Administration, Center for Food Safety and Applied Nutrition, "Consumer Advisory," 2002, (www.cfsan.fda .gov/~dms/ds-ltr29.html).

27. Ibid.

28. J. Kleignene and P. Knipschild, "Ginkgo Biloba," *Lancet* 340 (1992): 1136–1139.

29. P. L. LeBars et al., "A Placebo-Controlled, Double Blind, Randomized Trial of an Extract of Ginkgo Biloba for Dementia," *Journal of the American Medical Association* 278 (1997): 1327–1332.

30. National Center for Complementary and Alternative Medicine, "What is CAM?"

31. Ibid.

32. "St. John's Wort," Nature's Life Brochure, 1998.

33. H. Schultz, "St. John's Wort for Depression," *British Medical Journal* 7052 (1996): 313–319.

34. H. Schultz et al., "Effects of Hypericum Extract on the Sleep EEG in Older Volunteers," *American Journal of Geriatric Psychiatry,* Supplement 1 (1994): 65–68; K. Linde et al., "St. John's Wort for Depression: A Overview and Meta-analysis of Randomized Clinical Trials," *British Medical Journal* 313 (1996): 253–258.

35. R. J. Davidson et al., "Effect of SJW in Major Depressive Disorder: A Randomized, Controlled Trial," *Journal of the American Medical Association* 287 (2002): 1807–1814.

36. D. Rejali, A. Sivakumar, and N. Balaji, "Gingko Biloba Does Not Benefit Patients with Tinnitus: A Randomized Placebo-controlled Double-blind Trial and Meta-analysis of Randomized Trials," *Clinical Otolaryngology* 29, no. 3 (2004): 226–231; S. M. Yu, R. M. Ghandour, and Z. J. Haung, "Herbal Supplement Use among U.S. Women, 2000," *Journal of the American Medical Women's Association* 59, no. 1 (2004): 17–24; U. S. Sierpina, B. Wollschlaeger, and M. Blumenthal, "Ginkgo Biloba," *American Family Physician* 68, no. 5 (2003): 923–926.

37. "Stacking Up the Benefits of Three Popular Herbs," *Johns Hopkins Medical Letter: Health After 50* 15, no. 6 (2003): 3, 7.

38. Schultz et al., "Effects of Hypericum Extract," 66.

39. A. Cieza, P. Maier, and E. Poppel, "Effects of Gingko on Mental Functioning in Healthy Volunteers," *Archives of Medical Research* 34, no. 5 (2003): 373–381.

40. National Center for Complementary and Alternative Medicine, "What Is CAM?"

41. H. Martin, "St. John's Wort vs. Tricyclic Antidepressants," *American Journal of Naturopathic Medicine* 2 (1995): 42.

42. S. M. Yu, R. M. Ghandour, and Z. J. Haung, "Herbal Supplement Use among U.S. Women, 2000"; B. Barrett, "Efficacy and Safety of Echinacea in Treating Upper Respiratory Tract Infections in Children: A Randomized, Controlled Trial," *Journal of Pediatrics* 145, no. 1 (2004): 135–136; "Does an Echinacea Preparation Prevent Colds? The Debate Continues," *Child Health Alert,* April 22, 2004: 1–2; S. Shaber, "Echinacea for the Common Cold," *Annals of Internal Medicine* 139, no. 7 (2003): 600.

43. A. Sparreboom et al., "Herbal Remedies in the United States: Potential Adverse Interactions with Anti-cancer Agents," *Journal of Clinical Oncology* 22, no. 12 (2004): 2489–2503.

44. J. O. Ciocon, D. G. Ciocon, and D. J. Galioto, "Dietary Supplements in Primary Care: Botanicals Can Affect Surgical Outcomes and Follow-up," *Geriatrics* 59, no. 9 (2004): 20–24.

45. S. Momiyama, "Green Tea as Protection from Heart Attack," *American Journal of Cardiology* (2002), 909: 1150–1153.

46. U.S. Food and Drug Administration, "Sales of Supplements Containing Ephedrine Alkaloids (Ephedra) Prohibited," 2004, www.fda.gov/oc/initiatives/ephedra/february2004

47. D. Ahrendt, "Ergogenic Aids: Counseling the Athlete," *American Family Physician* (2002), 63: 913–922, www.aafp.org/afp/2001/0301/913.htm

48. E. Ernst, "The Risk-benefit Profiles of Commonly Used Herbal Therapies: Ginkgo, St. John's Wort, Ginseng, Echinacea, Saw Palmetto and Kava," *Annals of Internal Medicine* 136, no. 1 (2002), 42–53.

49. Ibid., 45.

50. B. A. Biggee and T. McAlindon, "Glucosamine for Osteoarthritis: Part I, Review of the Clinical Evidence," *Medicine and Health Rhode Island* 87, no. 6 (2004): 176–179; B. A. Biggee and T. McAlindon, "Glucosamine for Osteoarthritis: Part II, Biologic and Metabolic Controversies," *Medicine and Health Rhode Island* 87, no. 6 (2004): 180–181.

51. Ahrendt, "Ergogenic Aids," 915.

52. Agency for Healthcare Research and Quality, "S-Adenosyl-L-Methionine for Treatment of Depression, Osteoarthritis, and Liver Disease," *Evidence Report/Technology Assessment: Number 64"* (August 2002), www.ahrq.gov/clinic/epcsums/samesum.htm

53. Ibid.

54. Ibid.

55. S. Dixon, "Food for Thought: Prebiotic and Probiotics: What Are They and Why Should You Eat Them?" University of Michigan Comprehensive Cancer Center (January 15, 2003). (www.cancer.med.umich.edu/newspro09spr02.htm)

56. D. Wilson, "Health Food Masquerade," *Corvallis Gazette Times,* August 11, 1999, C-4.

57. American Botanical Council. "Commission E." January, 2003. (www.herbab/ram.org/default.asp?c = comm_e_catalog)

58. Ibid.

59. National Center for Complementary and Alternative Medicine, "CAM Centers of Research; Overview of the Specialty Centers," 2004, http://nccam.nih.gov/nccam/research/centers.html

60. "Health for Life: Inside the Science of Alternative Medicine," *Newsweek* (December 2, 2002).

61. National Center for Complementary and Alternative Medicine, "Are You Considering Using Complementary and Alternative Medicine (CAM)?" 2002, http://nccam.nih.gov/health/decisions/index.htm

Page references which end with *fig* indicates an illustrated figure; with *t* indicates a table; with *p* indicates a photograph.

botulism, 110, 483
Bradley method, 212
brain
  benefits of exercise to, 307
  damage due to methamphetamines, 397
  effects of drug Ecstasy on, 414p
  images of normal and individual with schizophrenia, 62p
brain death, 570
BRCA 1 gene, 462, 463
BRCA 2 gene, 462, 463
breast cancer, 458, 461–465fig
breast-feeding, 212p–213
breathalyzer, 356
BRFSS (Behavioral Risk Factor Surveillance System), 8, 304
British Medical Journal, 260, 657
bronchitis, 527–528
Browning, R., 550
BSE (bovine spongiform encephalopthy), 496
BSE (breast self-examination), 462, 463fig–464
bulbourethral (Cowper's glands), 172
bulimia nervosa, 269, 297–298t
burnout stress, 80
burns and residential safety, 123
burns, treatment for, H-7
Burros, M., 221

C

CAD (coronary artery disease), 430
caffeine
  addiction to, 391–392
  content in various products, 391t
  described, 391
  health consequences of long-term use, 392
caffeinism, 392
CAH (congenital adrenal hyperplasia), 163
calcium, 243, 564
calendar birth control method, 197–198fig
calisthenics (body weight resistance), 316–317
caloric intake trends, 224fig–225
calories
  ACSM recommended daily intake of, 306
  defining, 224
  weight management and understanding, 291
CAM (complementary and alternative medicine)
  acupressure, 654
  acupuncture, 645, 654
  assessing risks and benefits of, 662fig
  Ayurveda (or Ayurvedic medicine), 651
  biologically-based practices, 655–660
  chiropractic medicine, 652–653
  defining, 646, 648–649
  emergence in the U.S., 650
  energy medicine, 650, 653–654
  evaluating, 648
  evaluating resources on the Internet, 647
  German Commission E on, 664
  healthy living through, 664

historical perspective of, 649–650
homeopathy and naturopathy, 651–652
major domains of, 650
manipulation therapies, 652–653
mind-body medicine, 650, 654–655
new research on, 663
popular types of, 652t
protecting consumers/regulating claims of, 660, 662–664
selecting provider of, 666
self-care using, 664–667
TCM (traditional Chinese medicine), 651
used in U.S., 646fig
who seeks treatment using, 649
who, what, and why uses of, 650–651
campus ethnoviolence, 107
Campus Sexual Assault Victim's Bill of Rights (Ramstad Act) [1992], 119
cancer causes
  biological factors, 458
  cellular change/mutation theories, 454–455
  chemicals in foods, 459
  lifestyle risks, 455–458
  medical factors, 460
  social and psychological factors, 459
  viral factors, 460
cancer pathway, 476
cancers
  alcohol and, 359, 474
  assessing your personal risk for, 456–457
  causes of, 454–460
  defining, 453–454
  detecting, 473–475t
  disparities in rates of, 452–453
  fiber as protection, 238–239, 474
  new hope in treatments of, 475–476
  new research findings on, 474
  physical fitness and reduced risk of, 305
  recommendations for early detection in asymptomatic people, 464t
  research on CAM treatment for, 663
  survival rates at stage of diagnosis, 477t
  talking with your doctor about, 476–477
  tobacco and, 382–383fig
  types of, 460–473
  vaccine for cervical, 451
cancer's seven warning signals, 475t
cancer survivors, 477–478
cancer types
  breast, 458, 461–465fig
  cervical and endometrial (uterine), 472–473
  classifications of, 460
  colon and rectal, 465t–466
  leading sites of new cases/deaths, 461fig
  leukemia, 460, 473

lung, 382–383fig, 460–461
ovarian, 471–472
pancreatic, 473
prostate, 466–468
skin, 468p–470, 472
testicular, 470–471
"cancer virus," 460
candidiasis (moniliasis), 509
capillaries, 429
capitation, 639
carbohydrate loading, 237
carbohydrates
  athletic performance and, 237
  carcinogens and, 237
  defining, 235–236
  diets low in, 221; 286–287
  myth of sugar and hyperactivity, 237
  trends in intake of, 224fig
carbon monoxide, 378, 595–596
carcinogens, 237, 455
carcinomas, 460
cardiac rehabilitation, 446
cardiorespiratory fitness
  aerobic fitness programs for, 309–311
  benefits of, 305
  evaluating your, 309
  improving, 308–309
cardiovascular disease (CVD)
  advances made against, 445
  angioplasty versus bypass surgery for, 444–445
  aspirin for, 444, 445
  cardiac rehabilitation, 446
  cardiorespiratory fitness and reduced risk of, 305
  death due to, 425fig, 430fig
  diabetes and, 437–438, 445, 537
  epidemiological overview of, 424fig–426
  fiber as protection against, 239
  gender bias in research on, 441
  high blood sugar and risk of, 423
  hostility as a risk factor for, 89
  HRT controversy and, 170–171, 440, 442–443
  new techniques of diagnosing, 441–443
  personal advocacy and heart-smart behaviors, 446–447
  reducing your risk for, 435–439
  research on CAM treatment for, 663
  role of homocysteine in, 431
  stress and, 76–77
  sudden cardiac deaths due to, 424
  thrombolysis, 445–446
  tobacco and, 384
  trends in death from, 425fig
  Type A/Type B personalities and, 76, 438, 439
  understanding your risk for, 427–428
  women and, 440–441
  See also CHD (coronary heart disease)
cardiovascular system
  alcohol effects on, 358
  described, 428
  the heart, 428–430

Carey, B., 69
carotenoids, 252
carpal tunnel syndrome, 545
cataracts, 558
category A diseases, 110–111
category B diseases, 111
category C diseases, 111
CAT scan (computerized axial tomography), 473–474
CDC (Centers for Disease Control and prevention)
  Best Practices for Comprehensive Tobacco Control Programs, 11
  BRFSS survey conducted by, 8, 304
  consumer alerts provided by, 7
  on C-sections, 213
  Division of Violence Prevention of, 100
  on greatest public health achievements of 20th century, 18–19
  physical fitness recommendations by, 304
  programs on dealing with terrorism by, 109
  on smoking as leading cause of mortality in U.S., 5
celibacy, 174, 176
cell phones health hazard, 612
cellular theory of aging, 555–556
cellulose, 236
cerebral cortex, 71
cerebral palsy, 543t
cerebrospinal fluid, 356
certified nurse-wives, 204
cervical cancer, 458, 472–473
cervical cancer vaccine, 451
cervical cap, 191–192
cervical mucus method, 196
cervix, 167fig
CFCs (chlorofluorocarbons), 602
CFS (chronic fatigue syndrome), 543–544
change agents
  family as, 27
  your social bonds as, 27–28p
  See also behavior change
changing self-talk
  blocking/thought stopping, 32
  Meichenbaum's self-instructional methods, 31
  rational-emotive therapy, 29–30
CHD (coronary heart disease), 424, 431–433
chemical agents (bioterrorism), 111
chemical contaminants, 604–605
chemotherapy, 475
Chernobyl accident (1980s), 458, 613
CHESs (Certified Health Education Specialists), 17
chewing tobacco, 380
CHF (congestive heart failure), 433
chickenpox (HVZV), 491
child abuse, 113
childbirth
  alternatives for, 212
  choosing location for, 210
  labor and delivery process, 210–211fig
  medical/nonmedical approaches to, 211–212
  See also pregnancy

emergency minipills, 196

emerging/resurgent diseases, 496–502

EMFs (electromagnetic fields), 610–611

emotional attachment, 141

emotional availability, 141

emotional health, 10, 43–44

emotional response management, 88

emotions

anger, 89–90, 102–103, 104

defining, 44

hostility, 88–89

love, 143*fig*–144

physical health and positive, 54

stress management by dealing with negative, 95

See also feelings

emphysema, 384, 526–527

EMR (exercise metabolic rate), 291

enablers, 342

enabling factors, 24*fig*–25

endemic, 488

endometrial (uterine) cancer, 472–473

endometriosis, 215, 532–533

endometrium, 167*fig*

endorphins, 411

energy medicine, 650, 653–654

environmental factors

biopsychosocial model of addiction on, 336–337

cancer risk and, 458–459

stress and, 82

environmental health

air pollution, 594–603

cell phones and risks to health, 612

defining, 10

land pollution, 608*p*–610

noise pollution, 608

overpopulation, 592–594

taking action to improve, 607

water pollution, 603–606

environmental molds, 601

environmental racism, 611

enzymes, 492–493

EPA (U.S. environmental Protection Agency), 378, 591, 595, 600, 609

ephedra (ma huang), 658

epidemics, 482

epidermis, 485

epididymis, 172

epilepsy, 530–531

epinephrine, 72

episiotomy, 211

Epstein-Barr virus, 460, 488, 544

EQ (eating quotient) assessment, 226–228

erectile dysfunction (impotence), 17

ergogenic aids, 659

ergogenic drugs, 417

Ericsson method, 210

Erikson, E., 556

erogenous zones, 176

erotic touching, 176

Escherichia coli (E. coli), 261

esophagus, 232

essential amino acids, 233

essential hypertension, 438

estrogens, 168, 440–441, 460

ethical dilemmas and gender differences, 145

ethnicity. *See* racial/ethnic differences

ethnoviolence, 107

ethyl alcohol (ethanol), 353

ETS (environmental tobacco smoke), 385–386

eustress, defining, 70

evaluating personal risk, 30–31

Every Person's Guide to Antioxidants (Smythies), 252

exercise

addictive and obsessive, 308, 332*p*, 339–340

aerobic, 308

avoiding dehydration during, 323*p*

benefits to brain and body, 307

body composition and, 318

in cold weather, 326

cramps during, 326

creating your own program for, 327

CVD risk reduced by, 437

defining, 304

determining frequency, intensity, and duration of, 310–311*fig*

eating disorders combined with excessive, 308

EIA (exercise-induced asthma), 526

enhancing psychosocial health through, 51

fighting technostress with, 81

flexibility and stretching, 312–315*fig*, 563

healthy aging and, 563

heat stress and, 322–323

improving muscular strength/endurance, 315–318

overcoming obstacles to, 324–325

pregnancy and, 204–205*p*

recommendations for, 304

resistance training, 316–318, 563

starting routine of, 312

stress management using, 91

study on pets/owners and, 303

weight management through, 290, 291

See also physical fitness

exercise addiction, 308, 332*p*, 339–340

exercise equipment

injury prevention and, 319

picking your workout, 327*t*

tips for buying, 320–321

external female genitals, 165–166*fig*

external locus of control, 84

external male genitals, 171

eyesight, 558–559

F

FAE (fetal alcohol effects), 359

fallopian (uterine) tubes, 167*fig*

fall-proofing home, 123

faltering relationships

building better relationships, 156–157

getting help for, 155–156

key factors predicting success or, 156*t*

reasons for, 153–155

families

addiction intervention by, 343

adopting children, 217

as alcohol abuse/alcoholism factor, 361, 363

changing types of, 153*fig*

decision to have children or not, 153

dysfunctional, 48, 148, 364–365

how addiction affects, 342

impact of alcoholism on the, 364–365

intimate relationships of, 141

nuclear, 141

role in alcoholism recovery, 366

See also parents; relationships

family history. *See* genetics

family of origin, 141

FAMs (fertility awareness methods), 196

FAS (fetal alcohol syndrome), 204, 359

fast foods, 258–259, H-10

fatal workplace injuries, 124–125

fats

CVD risk and saturated, 436

defining, 240–241

new research findings on, 242–243

reducing dietary, 241–242

saturated and unsaturated, 241

trans, 242

trends in intake of, 224*fig*

FDA (U.S. Food and Drug Administration), 169, 185, 196, 222, 296, 389, 523, 561, 612, 617, 624

feelings, 146

See also emotions

Feldenkrais therapy, 654

fellatio, 176

female athlete triad disorder, 308, 332*p*, 339–340

female condom, 187*t*, 190, 191*p*

female orgasmic disorder, 179

female sexual anatomy/physiology, 165–171

female sterilization, 194

FermCap, 188

fermentation, 353

fertility

defining, 186

managing, 186–202

planning a pregnancy, 202–203

See also infertility

fertility awareness methods, 196–198*fig*

fertility cycle, 197*fig*

fertility drugs, 215

fertility management

abstinence and outercourse, 196

barrier methods of, 186, 188, 190–192

contraceptives research, 188

costs of, 195*t*

emergency contraceptive pills, 196

fertility awareness methods, 196–198*fig*

hormonal methods of, 192–194

IUDs (intrauterine devices), 195

surgical methods of, 194

withdrawal, 195–196

fertilization, 206*fig*

fetoscopy, 209

fetus

defining, 208

development of the, 207*p*

exposed to cocaine, 405

hysterotomy or surgical removal of, 200

miscarriage of, 213–214

fever immune response, 494

fiber, 237–240, 474

fibrillation, 433

fibrocystic breast condition, 532

fight-or-flight response, 70, 73*p*, 79

final arrangements

funerals, 584–585

hospice care, 582–583

organ donation, 585–586*p*

wills, 585

See also death/deaths

first aid (seizures), 531

first aid supplies, H-9

first trimester, 207–208

fitness-related injuries

causes of, 318

overtraining and, 318

prevention of, 318–319

fixed resistance, 317

flaxseed, 240

flexibility

defining, 312

stretching exercises to improve, 312–315*fig*

flexibility (emotional), 559–560

flu, 489*fig*

FOBT (fecal occult blood tests), 466

folate, 252, 254

food additives, 263

food allergies, 263–264

foodborne illnesses, 260–261, 262*t*

Food Guide Pyramid, 225*fig*, 228–229*fig*, 230, 231

Food Guide Pyramid (vegetarian), 257*fig*–258

food intolerance, 264

food irradiation, 262–263*fig*

food labels, 255*p*–256*fig*

Food and Nutrition Board report (1945), 233

foods

cancer risk due to chemicals in, 459

common interactions between medication and, 249*t*–250*t*, 629*t*

cultural and social meanings attached to, 223

digestive process and, 231–232

eating nutrient-dense, 231

examining medicinal value of, 248, 254

fast foods, 258–259

Food Guide Pyramid, 225*fig*, 228–229*fig*, 230, 231

functional, 223

as healing agents, 660

nutritive value of, H-10

organically grown, 264*fig*

vegetarian Food Guide Pyramid, 257*fig*–258

whole grains, 238

See also healthy eating; nutrition

food safety

avoiding risks in the home, 261–262

food additives, 263

food allergy or intolerance, 263–264

intravenous injection, 399
intruders (preventing), 123–124
intuition development, 95
inunction, 400
in vitro fertilization, 216
ionizing radiation, 610
IR (ionizing radiation), 458–459
iron, 243
iron-deficiency anemia, 248
ischemia, 433
ISD (inhibited sexual desire), 177
ISH (isolated systolic hypertension), 438
isometric muscle action, 316, 317*fig*
IUDs (intrauterine devices), 195

J

Jacoby, S., 116
James, W., 47
Janofsky, M., 591
JCAHO (Joint Commission on Accreditation of Healthcare Organizations), 622
jealousy, 148–149
JE (Japanese encephalitis), 501
Jeremko, M. D., 73
Johnson, V., 174
joints (older adults), 556
Journal of the American Medical Association, 77, 260, 549, 657
Jung, C., 47
Just the Facts program (Oregon State University), 350–351

K

Kaposi's sarcoma, 516*p*
Kegel exercises, 558
keptin, 283
ketamine, 180
ketosis, 293
Kevorkian, J., 582
Kile, D., 426*p*
killer T cells, 77
kissing, 176
Klinefelter's syndrome, 163
Kobasa, S., 83
Krakower, T., 662
Kübler-Ross, E., 573
Kübler-Ross's stages of dying, 573*fig*–574
Kushner, R., 303

L

labia majora, 166*fig*
labia minora, 166*fig*
labor
    medical/nonmedical approaches to managing, 211–212
    process of delivery and, 210–211*fig*
lactose intolerance, 538
Lamaze method, 212
Lance Armstrong Foundation, 471
landfills, 604
land pollution
    hazardous waste, 609–610*t*
    solid waste, 608–609
Latinos. *See* racial/ethnic differences
laughter, 52–54, 88
laxatives, 626
lay midwives, 204
Lazarus, R., 44
LBP (low back pain), 542–543

LDLs (low-density lipoproteins), 241, 242, 286, 436*t*
leach, 598–599
leachate, 604
lead pollution, 597, 606
The Leapfrog Group, 635
learned behavioral tolerance, 354
learned helplessness, 49
learned optimism, 49
Lea's Shield, 188
Leavitt, M. O., 591
Leboyer method, 212
leg cramps, 326
Legionnaire's disease, 485
Lerner, H. G., 139
lesbian, 165
lesbian partnerships, 150
leukemias, 460, 473
leukoplakia, 380
leveling communication technique, 146
Levenkron, S., 61
Levitra, 178
LH (luteinizing hormone), 168
Liebman, B., 221
life-and-death decision making
    directive to physicians, 580*fig*
    physical-assisted suicide (PAS), 581
    rational suicide, 579, 581–582
    right to die, 578–579
life span
    physical fitness and longer, 306
    relationship between maturity and, 49
lifestyle
    cancer risks due to, 455–458, 459*t*
    CVD risk and, 437
    obesity and, 288
lifetime risk, 455
lipoprotein profile, 305
liposuction, 295
Liptak, A., 569
listening
    benefits of active, 135
    learning to really listen, 134
    stress management by, 95
    three basic modes of, 133–135
listening modes
    active or reflective, 135
    competitive or combative, 134
    passive or attentive, 135
listeriosis, 500–501
liver disease, alcohol and, 358
"LiveStrong" wristbands, 471
living will, 579
locus of control
    external vs. internal, 84
    jealousy and fear of losing, 149
    psychological hardiness and, 83
loneliness, 156
loss of control, 334
love, 143*fig*–144
lovers (common bonds of), 142*fig*
low back pain (LBP), 542–543
low-carb diets, 221, 286–287
low sperm count, 215
LSD (lysergic acid diethylamide), 412–413
Lunelle, 193–194
lung cancer, 382–383*fig*, 460–461
lungs (older adults), 558

lupus, 541
lutein, 252
lymphomas, 460

M

McGwire, M., 417
macrominerals, 243
macular degeneration, 252, 559
mad cow disease, 496
Madden, J., 58
MADD (Mothers Against Drunk Driving), 360
mainstream smoke, 385
major depressive disorder, 54–55
malaria, 501
male condom, 186, 187*t*, 188, 190*fig*
male sexual anatomy/physiology, 171–172
male sterilization, 194
malignant melanoma, 468–469
malignant tumor, 545
Malkin, E., 3
malpractice, 636, 637
mammograms, 463
managed care, 639–640
manipulation therapies, 652–653
manipulative and body-based practices, 650
manual stimulation, 176
marijuana, 407–410
marijuana medical use debate, 409
marital rape, 116
marriage
    as committed relationship, 149–150
    common-law, 150
    decision to have children or not, 153
    single status versus, 151
    See also divorce
Maslow, A., 47
massage therapy, 93
Master, W. H., 174
masturbation, 176
maturity-life span relationship, 49
Mayer, J., 92
May, R., 47
Mead, M., 592
measles, 491
Medicaid, 638–639
medical abortions, 201
medical model, defining, 6
medical practices, 632
Medicare
    administrative expenses of, 635
    described, 638–639
    health care costs and concerns about, 554
    increasing out-of-pocket costs of, 553
medications
    Alzheimer's disease (AD), 561
    for angina pectoris condition, 433
    antibiotic resistance, 498–499
    antidepressants, 57*t*–58, 623*t*
    arthritis pill Vioxx, 617
    aspirin for CVD, 444, 445
    cancer treatments, 475–476
    for CHF (congestive heart failure), 433
    common interactions between foods and, 249*t*–250*t*, 629*t*
    generic drug, 623

older adults and use of prescription, 562
OTC (over-the-counter) drugs, 399, 562
prescription, 399, 622–623
women and, 629–630
    See also drugs
meditation, 93
Meichenbaum's self-instructional methods, 31
meltdown, 613
Memantine, 561
memory changes, 59
memory loss treatments, 59, 663
men
    bereavement experience of, 577
    blood alcohol concentration in, 357*t*
    depression in, 56
    as domestic violence victims, 112
    gender-role stereotypes of, 163
    infertility in, 215–216
    male sexual anatomy/physiology, 171–172
    nutritional needs of, 254
    percentage who are overweight/obese, 282
    prevalence of sexual problems in, 178*fig*
    See also gender differences; women
menarche, 168
Men Are from Mars, Women Are from Venus, 147
menopausal hormone therapy, 170–171
menopause, 170–171
menstrual cycle
    calendar birth control method using, 197–198*fig*
    menopause and ending of, 170–171
    phases of, 168*fig*
    problems during, 169–170
    puberty and onset of, 167–169
mental action (stress reduction), 90–91
mental changes (older adults), 559–560
mental health
    defining, 41–43
    physical fitness and improved, 307
    stress and, 79
mental illnesses
    anxiety disorders, 58–60
    defining, 54
    depression disorders, 54–58
    SAD (seasonal affective disorder), 60
    schizophrenia, 60–62
Merck Laboratories, 451
mercury pollution, 591
mescaline, 413–414
metabolic syndrome, 431
metastasis, 454
methadone maintenance, 412
methamphetamine, 406–407*p*
MicroSort method, 210
middle-old category, 552
midwives, 204
mifepristone (RU-486), 185, 201
migraine headaches, 529–530

mind-body connection and, 51–52

spirituality as key to, 46, 47

wellness continuum, 9*fig*

Wellness Institute (Northwestern Memorial Hospital), 303

Western blot, 516

West Nile virus, 500–501

Weuve, J., 549

When You Say Yes But Mean No (Perlow), 53

Whittaker, M., 113

WHI (Women's Health Initiative), 21

whole grains, 238

whole medical systems, 650

WHO (World Health Organization)

on acrylamide as carcinogen, 237

on health care gap, 3

health as defined by, 8

on prevalence of anxiety disorders, 58

on tuberculosis health threat, 486

UNICEF report (2004), 604

wills

holographic, 585

living, 579

Winning the Fight Between You and Your Desk (Mayer), 92

withdrawal

addiction, 332, 334

caffeine, 392

contraception method using, 195–196

nicotine, 387

women

addiction treatment for, 345

AIDS (acquired immunodeficiency syndrome) and, 513

alcoholism and, 365–366

bereavement experience of, 577

in blood alcohol concentration, 357*t*

breast cancer as leading cause of death in, 458, 461–465*fig*

cardiovascular disease (CVD) and, 440–441

debate over hormone patch for, 161

as domestic violence victims, 110–112

drug abuse and, 405

female sexual anatomy/physiology, 165–171

gender-role stereotypes of, 163

heart attack symptoms in, 441, 444

infertility in, 215–216

marriage success and ethnicity/age of, 154*fig*

medications and, 629–630

nutritional needs of, 254

obesity impact on, 288–289

percentage who are overweight/obese, 282

PMS (premenstrual syndrome) and, 55–56, 62

prevalence of sexual problems in, 178*fig*

rape assault against, 114–116

reproductive years of, 205–207

smoking and, 385

See also gender differences; men; pregnancy

Worden's model of grieving tasks, 576

Worden, W., 576

work addiction, 338–339, 338–339*fig*

workout machines, 319, 320–321, 327*t*

workplace drug use, 418–419

workplace safety, 124–125

World Bank, 3

World Trade Center attack (2001), 101, 106, 108*p*

X, Y, Z

xanthines, 391

X rays (pregnancy and), 204

yoga, 53, 90, 313–314*p*

You Just Don't Understand (Tannen), 144

"you" messages, 136, 137

young-old category, 552

yo-yo diets, 288

YRAS (Youth Risk Assessment Survey) [1991], 374

Zyban, 389

CREDITS

Chapter Opening Art

Chapter 1, **p. 2**: Getty Images Inc.; Chapter 2, **p. 38**: Photodisc/Getty Images; Chapter 3, **p. 68**: Photodisc/Getty Images; Chapter 4, **p. 98**: Mary-Arthur Johnson/Taxi/Getty Images; Chapter 5, **p. 128**: Stockbyte; Chapter 6, **p. 160**: Getty Images/Digital Vision; Chapter 7, **p. 184**: Michelangelo Gratton/Digital Vision Ltd.; Chapter 8, **p. 220**: Peter Cade/Image Bank/Getty Images; Chapter 9, **p. 268**: Getty Images Inc./Comstock Images; Chapter 10, **p. 302**: Photodisc/Getty Images; Chapter 11, **p. 330**: Eric Bean/ Image Bank/Getty Images; Chapter 12, **p. 348**: Ryan McVay/Photodisc/Getty Images; Chapter 13, **p. 372**: Picture Arts Coporation; Chapter 14, **p. 396**: Stockbyte; Chapter 15, **p. 422**: Getty Images/Digital Vision; Chapter 16, **p. 450**: David Becker/ Stone/Getty Images; Chapter 17, **p. 480**: Arthur Tilley/Taxi/Getty Images; Chapter 18, **p. 522**: Mel Curtis/Photodisc/Getty Images; Chapter 19, **p. 548**: Jim Naughten/Taxi/Getty Images; Chapter 20, **p. 568**: Keith Brofsky/Photodisc/Getty Images; Chapter 21, **p. 590**: Getty Images Inc./Comstock Images; Chapter 22, **p. 616**: Stockbyte; Chapter 23, **p. 644**: Mel Yates/Photodisc/Getty Images

Photo Credits

Chapter 1, **p. 6**: Digital Stock/CORBIS; **p. 10**: Scott Barbour/ALLSPORT/ Getty Images; **p. 28**: Roy Morsch/CORBIS; Chapter 2, **p. 46**: Kent Meireis/The Image Works; **p. 56**: Penny Tweedie/Stone; **p. 59**: Najlah Feanny/Corbis; **p. 62**: Monte S. Buschbaum, M.D; Chapter 3, **p. 73**: Marc Romanelli/Getty Images; **p. 83**: Leland Bobbe/Getty Images; **p. 84**: Robin Sachs/PhotoEdit; **p. 92**: Chuck Savage/CORBIS; Chapter 4, **p. 107**: Zed Nelson-IPG/Matrix; **p. 108**: Rudi Von Briel/ PhotoEdit; **p. 112**: Bill Aron/PhotoEdit; **p. 124**: James Lauritz/Getty Images; Chapter 5, **p. 133**: Charles Gupton/CORBIS; **p. 136**: Jose Luis Pelaez, Inc./CORBIS; **p. 149**: AP Photo/The Holland Sentinel, Dan Irving; **p. 151**: Ellen Senisi/The Image Works; Chapter 6, **p. 164**: Michael Pole/CORBIS; **p. 165**: SAM MIRCOVICH/Reuters/Landov; **p. 177**: Color Day Production/ Getty Images Inc- Image Bank; **p. 180**: Bill Stanton/ Rainbow; Chapter 7, **p. 191**: Dorling Kindersley; **p. 193**: Joel Gordon Photography; **p. 160**: Michael Newman/PhotoEdit; **p. 207a**: Claude Edelman/Photo Researchers; **p. 207b**: Petit Format-Nestle/Photo Researchers; **p. 207c**: Petit Format-Nestle/Photo Researchers; **p. 212**: Getty Images/Photodisc Blue; Chapter 8, **p. 222**: Reg Charity/ CORBIS; **p. 255**: Stone/Getty Images; Chapter 9, **p. 271**: Guang Niu/CORBIS; **p. 278 (left)**: C Squared Studios/Getty Images; **p. 278 (right)**: James Noble/CORBIS; **p. 279**: David Young-Wolff/PhotoEdit; **p. 281**: Ariel Skelley/CORBIS; **p. 300 (left)**: David Young-Wolff/PhotoEdit; **p. 300 (right)**: Esbin-Anderson, The Image Works; Chapter 10, **p. 310 (left)**: David Young-Wolff/ PhotoEdit; **p. 310 (right)**: Esbin-Anderson/The Image Works; **p. 306**: David Stoecklein/CORBIS; **p. 314**: Image Source/SuperStock; **p. 322**: David Sacks/Getty Images; **p. 323**: Bob Daemmrich/The Image Works; Chapter 11, **p. 332**: Bonnie Kamin/ PhotoEdit; **p. 337**: Mary Kate Denny/PhotoEdit; **p. 339**: Peter Cade/Stone; **p. 343**: Rick Bostick/ Index Stock Imagery, Inc.; Chapter 12, **p. 350**: Chuck Savage/CORBIS; **p. 361**: Yva Momatiuk & John Eastcott/Stock Boston; **p. 362**: Jon Feingersh/CORBIS; Chapter 13, **p. 375**: Jon Riley/Getty Images; **p. 378**: David Young-Wolff/PhotoEdit; **p. 380**: Courtesy of Romano & Associates Inc./Oral Health America; **p. 387**: Doug Martin/Photo Researchers, Inc.; Chapter 14, **p. 407**: SPL/Photo Researchers, Inc.; **p. 408**: Tom & Dee Ann McCarthy/ CORBIS; **p. 414**: Courtesy of NIDA; **p. 418**: Luc Beziat/Getty Images; Chapter 15, **p. 426**: Mike Fiala/CORBIS; **p. 434**: Michal Heron/CORBIS; **p. 441**: Keith Brofsky/Getty Images; **p. 440**: Thinkstock/Getty Images; Chapter 16, **p. 455**: Jonathan A. Meyers/Photo Researchers, Inc.; **p. 462**: Charles Gupton/Stock Boston; **p. 468 (left)**: James Stevenson/ SPL/Photo Researchers, Inc.; **p. 468 (middle and right)**: Dr. P. Marazzi/ SPL/Photo Researchers, Inc.; **p. 471**: AFP Photo/ Joel Saget/Getty Images, Inc.-Agence France Presse; **p. 476**: Bill Greenblatt/ Newsamakers/Liaison Agency; Chapter 17, **p. 491**: Mark Hanauer/ CORBIS; **p. 496**: Richard Hutchings/PhotoEdit; **p. 507**: SPL/Photo Researchers, Inc; **p. 508**: Dr. P. Marazzi/SPL/Photo Researchers, Inc; **p. 510**: Steven J. Nussenblatt/Custom Medical Stock Photo; **p. 514**: Dan McCoy/Rainbow; **p. 516**: A Ramy/Stock Boston; Chapter 18, **p. 526**: John Millar/Stone; **p. 530**: Elena Dorfman/Offshoot Stock; **p. 534**: Donna Day/Getty Images; **p. 540**: Bonnie Kamin; **p. 544**: ; Chapter 19, **p. 522 (left)**: Fred Prouser/CORBIS; **p. 522 (middle)**: AP/Wide World Photos; **p. 522 (right)**: Nancy Kaszerman/ZUMA/Corbis; **p. 558**: Dan Bosler/Stone; **p. 560**: Yva Momatiuk & John Eastcott/Stock Boston; **p. 564**: John Henley/CORBIS; Chapter 20, **p. 571**: Arvind Garg/Photo Researchers; **p. 578**: Mark Reinstein/The Image Works; **p. 579**: Mark Richards/PhotoEdit; **p. 586**: Ben Edwards/Stone; Chapter 21, **p. 592**: AP/Wide World Photos; **p. 599**: Will and Demi McIntyre/Photo Researchers; **p. 606**: Seth Resnick/Stock Boston; **p. 608**: Bonnie Kamin/ Photo Edit; Chapter 22, **p. 618**: Jim Sulley/Image Works; **p. 631**: Superstock; **p. 633**: Paul Conklin/PhotoEdit; **p. 634**: Fotopic/Index Stock Imagery, Inc.; Chapter 23, **p. 653**: The Stock Connection/Novastock; **p. 654**: Willie Hill, Jr./The Image Works; **p. 656**: Michael Newman/ PhotoEdit